9/25/02

4442

$1 ~~3̶7̶0̶~~

$1 130⁰⁰

9¹⁰   Tax

8⁰⁰   S&H

$ 147¹⁰

D1716932

Acute Renal Failure

A COMPANION TO

Brenner & Rector's **THE KIDNEY**

Acute Renal Failure

A COMPANION TO

Brenner & Rector's THE KIDNEY

Bruce A. Molitoris, MD
Professor of Medicine
Director, Nephrology
Indiana University School of Medicine
Indianapolis, Indiana

William F. Finn, MD
Professor of Medicine
University of North Carolina at Chapel Hill
Chapel Hill, North Carolina

W.B. SAUNDERS COMPANY
A Harcourt Health Sciences Company
Philadelphia London New York St. Louis Sydney Toronto

W.B. SAUNDERS COMPANY
A Harcourt Health Sciences Company

The Curtis Center
Independence Square West
Philadelphia, Pennsylvania 19106

Library of Congress Cataloging-in-Publication Data

Acute renal failure: a companion to Brenner and Rector's The kidney / [edited by]
Bruce A. Molitoris, William F. Finn.—1st ed.

p.   cm.

ISBN 0–7216–9174–9

1. Acute renal failure.   I. Molitoris, Bruce A. II. Finn, William F.
   (Francis).   III. Brenner and Rector's The kidney.
   [DNLM: 1. Kidney Failure, Acute. WJ 342 A18945 2001]

RC918.R4 A336 2001 616.6′14—dc21

00–063525

Editor-in-Chief: Richard Zorab
Acquisitions Editor: Richard Zorab
Developmental Editor: Jennifer Shreiner
Project Manager: Marian Bellus
Production Manager: Natalie Ware
Illustration Specialist: Rita Martello
Book Designer: Jonel Sofian

ACUTE RENAL FAILURE: A Companion to Brenner & Rector's
The Kidney

ISBN 0–7216–9174–9

Printed in the United States of America.

Last digit is the print number: 9   8   7   6   5   4   3   2   1

Contributors

Emaad M. Abdel-Rahman, MD, MSc, PhD
Assistant Professor of Internal Medicine and Nephrology, University of Virginia, Charlottesville, Virginia
Acute Renal Failure in Burns

Mahendra Agraharkar, MD, FACP
Assistant Professor of Medicine, University of Texas Medical Branch; Director of Chronic Home Dialysis, Director of Acute Dialysis, Nephrology Staff, University of Texas Medical Branch Galveston, Texas
Acute Renal Failure Associated With Cancer

Robert J. Anderson, MD
Professor of Medicine, Head, Division of General Internal Medicine, University of Colorado Health Sciences Center, Denver, Colorado
Clinical and Laboratory Diagnosis of Acute Renal Failure

Simon J. Atkinson, PhD
Associate Professor of Medicine, Biochemistry, and Molecular Biology, Indiana University School of Medicine, Indianapolis, Indiana
Cytoskeletal Alterations as a Basis of Cellular Injury in Acute Renal Failure

Robert L. Bacallao, MD
Associate Professor of Medicine, Indiana University School of Medicine, Indianapolis, Indiana
Tight Junction and Adherens Junction Dysfunction During Ischemic Injury

Peter H. Bach, PhD
Khaya Lami House, Surrey, United Kingdom
Acute Renal Failure Associated With Occupational and Environmental Settings

Priya Visweswaran Balakrishnan, MD
Clinical Fellow in Nephrology, Department of Internal Medicine, Division of Renal Diseases and Hypertension, University of Texas, Houston, Medical School, Houston, Texas
Osmotic Nephropathy

Radhakrishna Baliga, MD
Professor, Department of Pediatrics, University of Mississippi Medical Center, Jackson, Mississippi
Oxidant Mechanisms in Acute Renal Failure

Rinaldo Bellomo, MD
Professor of Medicine; Director of Research, Department of Anesthesia and Intensive Care, Austin E Repatriation Medical Center, Heidelberg-Victoria, Australia
Dialysis: Continuous Versus Intermittent Renal Replacement Therapy in the Treatment of Acute Renal Failure

Ori S. Better, MD
Professor of Medicine, Faculty of Medicine, Crush Syndrome Center, Technion-Israel Institute of Technology, Haifa, Israel
Post-Traumatic Acute Renal Failure With Emphasis on the Muscle Crush Syndrome

Joseph V. Bonventre, MD, PhD
Robert H. Ebert Professor of Molecular Medicine, Harvard Medical School; Director, Harvard-Massachusetts Institute of Technology, Division of Health Sciences and Technology, Boston, Massachusetts
Growth Factors, Signaling, and Renal Injury and Repair

Emmanuel A. Burdmann, MD, PhD
Associate Professor of Nephrology, Division of Nephrology, São José Rio Preto School of Medicine-FAMERP São José Rio Preto, São Paulo, Brazil
Metabolic and Electrolyte Disturbances: Secondary Manifestations; Acute Renal Failure as a Result of Infectious Diseases

Andrew I. Choi, MD
Staff Radiologist, Department of Radiology, Durham Regional Hospital, Durham, North Carolina
Imaging Techniques in Acute Renal Failure

Richard L. Clark, MD
Professor of Radiology and Director of Genitourinary Radiology, The University of North Carolina of Chapel Hill, North Carolina Department of Radiology, The University of North Carolina Hospitals, Chapel Hill, North Carolina
Imaging Techniques in Acute Renal Failure

John D. Conger, MD
Professor, Department of Medicine, University of Colorado Health Sciences Center, Denver, Colorado
Vascular Alterations in Acute Renal Failure: Roles in Initiation and Maintenance

Eric P. Cohen, MD
Associate Professor of Medicine, Medical College of Wisconsin; Staff Physician, Froedtert Hospital, Milwaukee, Wisconsin
Acute Renal Failure After Bone Marrow Transplantation

Taigen Cui, MD
Assistant Professor, Medical School of Peking University; Attending Physician, Institute of Nephrology, First Hospital, Peking University, Beijing, People's Republic of China
Biological Nephrotoxins

Carlos T. da Silva, Jr., MD, MPH
Assistant Professor of Medicine, Boston University Medical School; Staff Physician, Renal Section, Boston Medical Center, Boston, Massachusetts
Acute Renal Failure as a Result of Malignancy

Marc E. De Broe, MD, PhD
Professor of Medicine, University of Antwerp; Nephrologist and Head, Department of Nephrology, University Hospital Antwerp, Antwerp, Belgium
Inflammatory Cells in Renal Damage and Regeneration

Kathleen E. De Greef, MD
University of Antwerp; University Hospital Antwerp, Antwerp, Belgium
Inflammmatory Cells in Renal Damage and Regeneration

An S. De Vriese, MD, PhD
Physician, Renal Unit, University Hospital Ghent, Ghent, Belgium
Renal Failure in Disasters

John J. Dillon, MD
Assistant Professor, The University of Chicago, Chicago, Illinois
Nephrotoxicity From Antibacterial, Antifungal, and Antiviral Drugs

Wilfred Druml, MD
Professor of Medicine, Vienna Medicinal School, University of Vienna; Director, Acute Dialysis Unit; Vienna General Hospital, Vienna, Austria
Nutritional Support in Patients With Acute Renal Failure

Thomas D. Du Bose, Jr., MD
Peter T. Bohan Professor of Internal Medicine, University of Kansas School of Medicine, Kansas City, Kansas
Osmotic Nephropathy

Garabed Eknoyan, MD
Professor of Medicine, Baylor College of Medicine, Houston, Texas
Acute Renal Failure and Nonsteroidal Anti-Inflammatory Drugs

Murray Epstein, MD, FACP
Professor of Medicine, University of Miami School of Medicine; Attending Physician, University of Miami-Jackson Medical Center and Miami Veterans Administration Medical Center, Miami, Florida
Acute Renal Failure in Liver Disease

Christiane M. Erley, MD
Associate Professor, University of Tübingen; Intensive Care Unit, Medizinische Universitäts-Klinik und Poliklinik, Tübingen, Germany
Acute Renal Failure Associated With Radiocontrast Agents

Steven W. Falen, MD, PhD
Assistant Professor, Department of Radiology, University of North Carolina at Chapel Hill, Chapel Hill, North Carolina
Imaging Techniques in Acute Renal Failure

William F. Finn, MD
Professor of Medicine, University of North Carolina at Chapel Hill, Chapel Hill, North Carolina
Recovery From Acute Renal Failure

Juan Fort, MD
Autonomous University of Barcelona; Staff Physician, Nephrology Department, Vall d'Hebron Hospital, Barcelona, Spain
Acute Renal Failure With Cardiovascular Disease

Shobha Gopalakrishnan, PhD
Research Associate, Indiana University School of Medicine, Indianapolis, Indiana
Tight Junction and Adherens Junction Dysfunction During Ischemic Injury

Susan C. Guba, MD
Division of Nephrology, University of Texas Medical Branch, Galveston, Texas; Texas Cancer Associates, Dallas, Texas
Acute Renal Failure Associated With Cancer Chemotherapy

Susan Hou, MD
Professor of Medicine, Loyola University, Stritch School of Medicine; Loyola University Medical Center, Maywood, Illinois
Acute Renal Failure in Pregnancy

Takaharu Ichimura, PhD
Instructor, Harvard Medical School; Assistant in Biology, Massachusetts General Hospital, Boston, Massachusetts
Growth Factors, Signaling, and Renal Injury and Repair

Sharan Kanakiriya, MD
Fellow in Nephrology, Mayo Clinic, Rochester, Minnesota
Heme Oxygenase and Acute Renal Injury

Dieter Kleinknecht, MD
Honorary Maître de Conférences Libre, University of Paris, France; Formerly Honorary Head, Department of Nephrology and Intensive Care, Centre Hospitalier, Montrevil-Sous-Bois, France
Multiple Organ System Failure

James P. Knochel, MD
Professor, Department of Internal Medicine, University of Texas Southwestern Medical Center; Chairman, Department of Internal Medicine, Presbyterian Hospital of Dallas, Dallas, Texas
Nontraumatic Rhabdomyolysis

Norbert H. Lameire, MD, PhD
Renal Division, University Hospital, Ghent, Belgium
Renal Failure in Disasters

Jerrold S. Levine, MD
Assistant Professor of Medicine, University of Chicago Medical School; Visiting Physician, University of Chicago Hospital, Chicago, Illinois
Terminal Pathways to Cell Death

Fernando Liaño, MD, PhD
Associate Professor of Medicine, Department of Medicine, Facultad de Medicina, Universidad de Alcalá; Nephrologist, Department of Nephrology, Hospital Ramón y Cajal, Madrid, Spain
Predictive Factors and Scoring

Wilfred Lieberthal, MD
Professor of Medicine, Visiting Physician, Boston University Medical Center, Boston, Massachusetts
Terminal Pathways to Cell Death

Colm C. Magee, MRCPI
Instructor in Medicine, Harvard Medical School; Staff Physician, Brigham and Women's Hospital, Boston, Massachusetts
Acute Renal Failure in Solid-Organ Transplantation

James A. Marrs, PhD
Assistant Professor of Medicine, Physiology, and Biophysics, Indiana University School of Medicine, Indianapolis, Indiana
Tight Junction and Adherens Junction Dysfunction During Ischemic Injury

Philip R. Mayeux, PhD
Associate Professor, Department of Pharmacology and Toxicology, University of Arkansas for Medical Sciences, Little Rock, Arkansas
Oxidant Mechanisms in Acute Renal Failure

Ravindra Mehta, MD, PhD
University of California, San Francisco, Medical Center, San Francisco, California
Renal Failure in Disasters

Douglas E. Mesler, MD, MPH
Assistant Professor, Boston University School of Medicine; Clinical Director, Renal Section, Boston Medical Center, Boston, Massachusetts
Acute Renal Failure as a Result of Malignancy

Bruce A. Molitoris, MD
Professor of Medicine, Director, Nephrology, Department of Medicine, Indiana University School of Medicine, Indianapolis, Indiana
Cytoskeletal Alterations as a Basis of Cellular Injury in Acute Renal Failure

A. Vishnu Moorthy, MD
Associate Professor, Department of Medicine and Pathology, University of Wisconsin; William S. Middleton Memorial Veterans Hospital, Madison, Wisconsin
Acute Renal Failure in Burns

Patrick H. Nachman, MD
Assistant Professor of Medicine, Division of Nephrology and Hypertension, University of North Carolina at Chapel Hill, Chapel Hill, North Carolina
Acute Renal Failure in Vasculitis

Karl A. Nath, MBChB
Professor of Medicine, Staff Consultant, Mayo Medical School, Mayo Clinic, Rochester, Minnesota
Heme Oxygenase and Acute Renal Injury; Hemoglobinuria

Julio Pascual, MD, PhD
Servicio de Nefrología, Hospital Ramón y Cajal, Madrid, Spain
Predictive Factors and Scoring

Hamid Rabb, MD
Associate Professor of Medicine, University of Minnesota Medical School; Director, MMRF Endowed Kidney Laboratory, Nephrologist, Hennepin County Medical Center, Minneapolis, Minnesota
Inflammatory Response and Its Consequences in Acute Renal Failure

Lorraine C. Racusen, MD
Associate Professor of Pathology, The Johns Hopkins University School of Medicine; Director, Renal Biopsy Service, The Johns Hopkins Hospital and Johns Hopkins Bayview Hospital, Baltimore, Maryland
The Morphologic Basis of Acute Renal Failure

Claudio Ronco, MD
Professor of Medicine, Università Degli Studi, Padova, Italy; Associate in Clinical Nephrology, Department of Nephrology, St. Bortolo Hospital, Vicenza, Italy
Dialysis: Continuous Versus Intermittent Renal Replacement Therapy in the Treatment of Acute Renal Failure

Irit Rubinstein, PhD
Senior Investigator, Faculty of Medicine, Department of Physiology and Biophysics and Crush Syndrome Center, Technion-Israel Institute of Technology, Haifa, Israel
Post-traumatic Acute Renal Failure With Emphasis on the Muscle Crush Syndrome

Robert L. Safirstein, MD
Professor, Department of Medicine, University of Arkansas for Medical Sciences; Chief, Medical Services, Central Arkansas Veterans Healthcare System, Little Rock, Arkansas
Acute Renal Failure Associated With Cancer

Dipti Shah, MD
Attending Physician, St. John's Hospital, Santa Monica, California
Acute Renal Failure in Pregnancy

Sudhir V. Shah, MD
Professor of Medicine, Director, Division of Nephrology, University of Arkansas for Medical Science; Chief, Renal Medicine Section, Central Arkansas Veterans Healthcare System, Little Rock, Arkansas
Oxidant Mechanism in Acute Renal Failure

Norman J. Siegel, MD
Professor of Pediatrics and Medicine, Department of Pediatrics, Yale University School of Medicine; Physician-in-Chief, Yale-New Haven Children's Hospital, New Haven, Connecticut
Heat Shock Proteins: Role in Prevention and Recovery From Acute Renal Failure

Robert Star, MD
Chief, Renal Diagnostics & Therapeutics, NIDDK, National Institutes of Health, Bethesda, Maryland
Inflammatory Response and Its Consequences in Acute Renal Failure

John H. Turney, MD, FRCP
Senior Clinical Lecturer, University of Leeds; Consultant Renal Physician, Leeds General Infirmary, Leeds, United Kingdom
Acute Renal Failure Associated With Recreational Drug Use

Norishi Ueda, MD
Director, Department of Pediatrics, Tokoname City Hospital, Tokoname, Aichi, Japan
Oxidant Mechanisms in Acute Renal Failure

Raymond Vanholder, MD, PhD
Renal Division, University Hospital, Ghent, Belgium
Renal Failure in Disasters

Scott K. Van Why, MD
Associate Professor, Department of Pediatrics, Yale University School of Medicine, New Haven, Connecticut
Heat Shock Proteins: A Role in Prevention and Recovery From Acute Renal Failure

Joseph J. Walshe, MB, PhD
Consultant Nephrologist, Beaumont Hospital, Dublin, Ireland
Acute Renal Failure in Solid-Organ Transplantation

Hai Yan Wang, MD
Professor, Medical School of Peking University; Institute of Nephrology, First Hospital, Peking University, Beijing, People's Republic of China
Biological Nephrotoxins

Mei Wang, MD
Department of Nephrology, The First Teaching Hospital, Beijing Medical University, Beijing, People's Republic of China
Biological Nephrotoxins

Michelle Whittier, MD
Clinical Fellow in Nephrology, Division of Nephrology and Hypertension, University of North Carolina at Chapel Hill, Chapel Hill, North Carolina
Biological Nephrotoxins

Dirk K. Ysebaert, MD, PhD
Assistant Professor in Surgery, University of Antwerp; Staff Surgeon, University Hospital Antwerp, Antwerp, Belgium
Inflammatory Cells in Renal Damage and Regeneration

Luis Yu, MD, PhD
Associate Professor of Nephrology, University of São Paulo School of Medicine; Chief of Acute Renal Failure Group, Hospital das Clinicas da Faculdade de Medicina da Universidade de São Paulo, São Paulo, Brazil
Metabolic and Electrolyte Disturbances: Secondary Manifestations; Acute Renal Failure as a Result of Infectious Diseases

Preface

Acute Renal Failure (ARF) represents a significant and persistent problem with serious implications for those so afflicted. Indeed, it has come to be the most common reason for seeking nephrology consultation in hospitalized patients. Consider that patients with ARF may account for 5% of hospital admissions and occupy 50% of beds in intensive care units. The spectrum of factors leading to the development of ARF is broad and varies considerably among various populations. To mention a few: snake-bites in India, leptospirosis in Brazil, ethylene glycol poisoning in Haiti, crushing injuries in Turkey and other earthquake-prone regions of the World, trauma in civilian and military settings, and exposure to an increasing number of therapeutic agents that themselves cause ARF. In the United States, ARF is primarily a hospital-acquired disease process with up to 50% of the cases relating directly to ischemic injury, 35% to exposure to nephrotoxin injury, and the remaining 15% to obstructive uropathy, interstitial disease processes, and acute glomerular nephritis.

The true incidence of ARF is difficult to determine in large part because of the diversity in causes and predisposing conditions and also to some extent because of uncertainty in the definition of ARF. One might argue that a transient, self-limited rise in the serum creatinine concentration (S_{Cr})—as may occur following exposure to radiocontrast agents—is of little importance. However, even here the data are clear that hospitalization is prolonged and mortality rates are increased. The use of predefined increases in the S_{Cr} must take into consideration that an increase in the S_{Cr} of 0.5 mg/dL has a different implication when a baseline value is 1.0 mg/dL as opposed to 3.0 mg/dL. The former represents a much greater reduction in the creatinine clearance (C_{Cr}) than does the latter. This distinction is important when group comparisons are made without consideration of baseline values. Nevertheless, if a small change in the C_{Cr} is the difference in the need for renal replacement therapy, the definition of what constitutes a significant change in the C_{Cr} takes on a new meaning.

Despite these semantic issues, it is agreed by all that ARF carries with it a substantial degree of morbidity and an unacceptably high mortality rate. While it may be argued that the illnesses that precede the ARF and the other co-morbid conditions are more responsible for the eventual outcome, this explanation falls short. Not only are outcome variables specifically affected by the presence of ARF but also recent data indicate that ARF *per se* is a major risk factor for the development of nonrenal complications. Thus, the increased patient morbidity and mortality associated with ARF is due to the interaction of a number of factors—not the least of which is the ARF itself.

The clinical course of ARF remains highly variable without adequate markers to assist the physician in determining the severity of the renal injury or the prognosis for recovery. It is surprising that little has been added to our understanding of the microscopic appearance of renal tissue during the period after the initial diagnosis. With the exception of studies performed following renal transplantation, scant information exists about sequential changes in structure as the kidney attempts to recover. This helps to explain the relative lack of other biological markers of injury and/or repair and the complete absence of specific therapeutic tools. Indeed, many patients with ARF, once stabilized, are discharged to outpatient dialysis facilities in the hope that they will eventually recover renal function. Many do not.

This is not to say that little progress has been made, for the material contained in this volume will dispel that notion if it exists. Indeed, extensive investigation has been undertaken in the laboratory in order to more completely understand the pathophysiology of ischemic and nephrotoxic ARF. This has resulted in a wealth of important information leading directly to the development of a number of therapeutic maneuvers that are now known to prevent or treat ARF in animal models. Translation of these data for the prevention of clinical ARF and the promotion of recovery has resulted in important additions to the care of our patients. This is especially true in the understanding of the importance of maximizing the patient's volume status prior to the administration of any nephrotoxin. The most obvious manifestation of the success in preventing ARF and treating its complications comes from the spectacular results achieved in Turkey following the 1999 earthquakes. Yet, our ability to treat patients with ARF and alter the clinical course has not fully benefited from the fundamental insights gained in the laboratory. Several large clinical trials utilizing different therapeutic approaches have shown little or no differences in outcomes. The reasons for the unsatisfactory results may not relate to the individual agents used or the hypothesis on which the therapy was based. Rather, the problems may be more related to the innate heterogeneity of the clinical population studied, the lack of appropriate sample size, the lack of early treatment, and our persistence in using one agent to treat a multi-factorial disease process. Thus, there is and will continue to be a need for well-designed, comprehensive clinical studies in order to translate the success of the laboratory to the treatment of the patient with ARF.

In this companion textbook to *The Kidney* by Dr. Barry M. Brenner, we have extended the concepts presented in the parent textbook by presenting new and exciting information on the pathophysiology of ARF and then complementing this with individual chapters addressing the clinical aspects of the different forms of ARF. In these chapters, the authors have specifically approached the clinical nature of the disease process, the differential diagnosis, and the therapeutic options for prevention and treatment. It is our intention to provide an integrative approach to patient care based on clinical as well as basic science knowledge. Our strategy was to have each chapter be self-contained and provide the reader with a thorough review of the topic and a complete list of key references. Diagnostic and treatment algorithms have been included where appropriate.

We thank the contributing editors for their extremely important and scholarly input; we also thank Richard Zorab, Editor-in-Chief, Medicine, and Jennifer Shreiner, Associate Developmental Editor, and the production staff at W.B. Saunders for their excellent guidance and attention to detail. Finally, we thank Dr. Barry M. Brenner for commissioning this text, as we hope this allows us to maintain this as a textbook in progress with periodic updates as the rapid basic science and clinical advances in the field of ARF continue to unfold.

Contents

NOTICE

Medicine is an ever-changing field. Standard safety precautions must be followed, but as new research and clinical experience broaden our knowledge, changes in treatment and drug therapy may become necessary or appropriate. Readers are advised to check the product information currently provided by the manufacturer of each drug to be administered to verify the recommended dose, the method and duration of administration, and the contraindications. It is the responsibility of the treating physician, relying on experience and knowledge of the patient, to determine dosages and the best treatment for each individual patient. Neither the publisher nor the editor assumes any liability for any injury and or damage to persons or property arising from this publication.

THE PUBLISHER

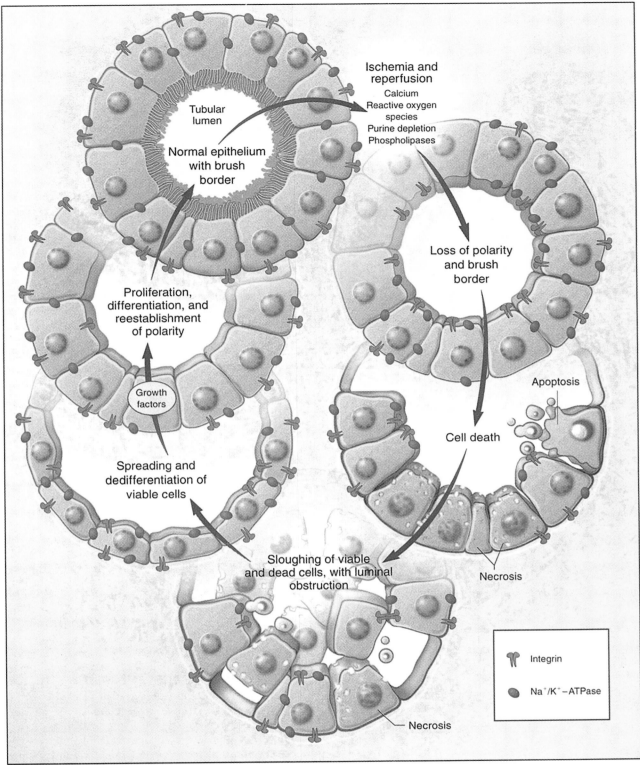

FIGURE 7–1 ■ Tubular-cell injury and repair in ischemic acute renal failure. After ischemia and reperfusion, morphologic changes occur in the proximal tubules, including loss of the brush border, loss of polarity, and redistribution of integrins and Na⁺/K⁺-ATPase to the apical surface. Calcium, reactive oxygen species, purine depletion, and phospholipases probably have a role in these changes in morphology and polarity as well as in the subsequent cell death that occurs as a result of necrosis and apoptosis. There is a sloughing of viable and nonviable cells into the tubular lumen resulting in the formation of casts and luminal obstruction and contributing to the reduction in the glomerular filtration rate. The severely damaged kidney can completely restore its structure and function. Spreading and dedifferentiation of viable cells occur during recovery from ischemic acute renal failure, which duplicates aspects of normal renal development. A variety of growth factors probably contribute to the restoration of a normal tubular epithelium. (From Thadhani R, Pascual M, Bonventre JV: Acute renal failure. N Engl J Med 1996; 334: 1448–1460; with permission.)

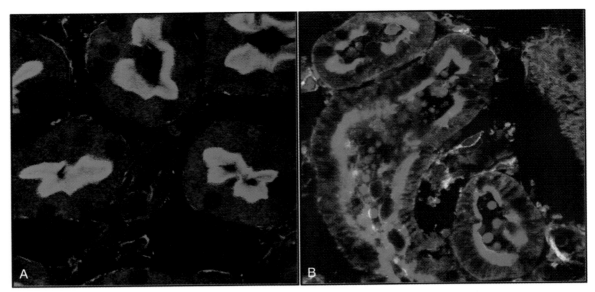

FIGURE 8–2 ■ Effect of ischemia on PTC F-actin and ADF localization (*A–D*). Renal PTC under physiologic conditions (*A* and *C*) and following 25 minutes of ischemia (*B* and *D*) were stained for F-actin with fluorescein isothiocyanate (FITC)-phalloidin and actin depolymerizing factor (ADF) using a Texas-Red secondary (*A* and *B*). Ischemia resulted in marked disruption of apical microvillar F-actin and redistribution of ADF to the apical domain and into the lumen in membrane sealed vesicles. Low power electron micrographs show marked apical damage following mild to moderate ischemic injury with loss of individual microvillar structure, internalization of microvillar membrane and formation of membrane-bound vesicles in the lumen. (From Schwartz N, Hosford M, Sandoral RM, et al: Ischemia activates actin depolymerizing factor: role in proximal tubule microvillar actin alterations. Am J Physiol 1999; 276:F544–F551; with permission.)

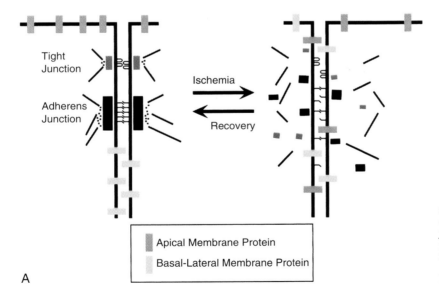

A

FIGURE 9–1 ■ *A,* Ischemia affects epithelial phenotype by disrupting actin cytoskeleton, junctional complexes and cell polarity. Epithelial cell recovery from ischemic injury requires that these features be re-established.

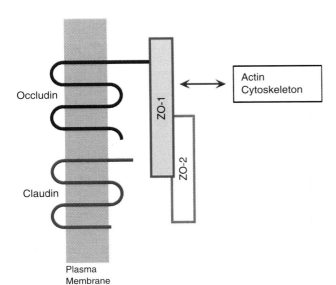

FIGURE 9–2 ▪ Tight junction proteins form a multi-protein complex that controls paracellular permeability. Occludin and claudin are integral membrane proteins. Both are four-pass transmembrane integral membrane proteins. There are numerous members of the claudin family that may create cell-type specific permeability pores. Occludin cytoplasmic domain sequences bind ZO-1 directly. ZO-1 and ZO-2 form a complex with one another, and each of these proteins contain domains that could interact with other tight junction proteins. ZO-1 also binds actin filaments.

FIGURE 9–3 ▪ Adherens junctions are organized by cadherin cell adhesion molecules. Dimers are probably required for cadherin cell adhesion activity. The extracellular cadherin repeat sequences require calcium binding for proper conformation. The extracellular domain repeats are also responsible for determining homophilic binding activity. Cadherins are single-pass transmembrane integral membrane proteins with a highly conserved cytoplasmic domain that interacts with numerous membrane cytoskeletal proteins and signal transduction molecules. Both β- and γ-catenin bind cadherin cytoplasmic domain sequences, and both these proteins bind α-catenin. α-Catenin is an actin binding protein that also interacts with other adherens junction components, including vinculin, α-actinin, and IQGAP.

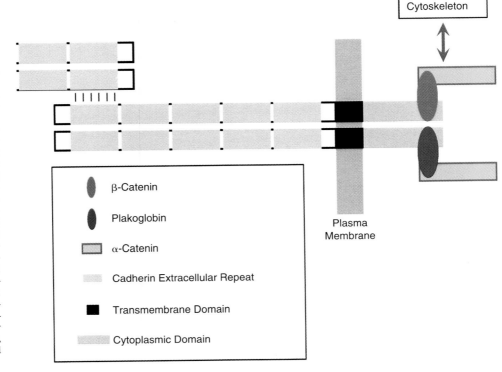

15 Minutes   2 Hours   6 Hours

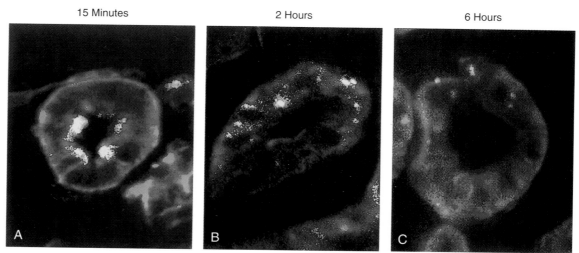

FIGURE 10–3 ■ After 45 minutes of ischemia and reflow of 15 minutes *(A)*, 2 hours *(B)*, and 6 hours *(C)*, rat kidneys were perfusion-fixed in situ. Proximal tubules were examined by fluorescence microscopy after treatment with separately labelled antibodies to HSP-72 (in *orange*) and Na/K ATPase (in *green*). Co-localization appears in *yellow*. At 15 minutes of reflow HSP-72 co-localizes with Na$^+$, K$^+$-ATPase in the apical domain of proximal tubules. At two hours of reflow, the two proteins have redistributed and co-localize in an aggregated pattern. By 6 hours of reflow HSP-72 remains in an aggregated pattern in the cytoplasm, but Na$^+$, K$^+$-ATPase has returned to the basolateral domain; minimal co-localization is present.

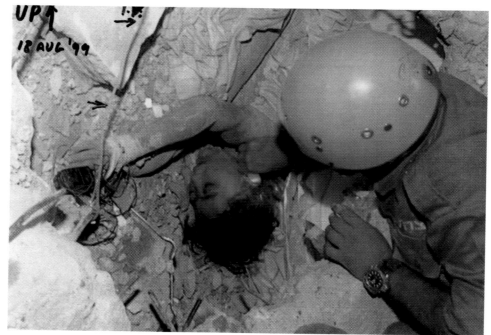

FIGURE 16–2 ■ Rescue of a Turkish girl who was buried during the major earthquake in Turkey on August 17, 1999. Note the intravenous line *(arrow)* for early volume replacement for hours prior to complete extrication of the casualty. Such an infusion may contribute to the prevention of myoglobinuric ARF in casualties suffering from the crush syndrome.[13] (Courtesy of the spokesman of the Israeli Defense Forces (IDF) to whom we are indebted.)

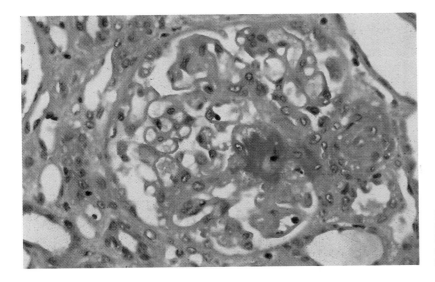

FIGURE 23–1 ▪ Fibrin thrombus extending from the afferent arteriole to the glomerular capillary in a pregnant patient with hemolytic uremic syndrome. (Photograph courtesy of Melvin Schwartz MD)

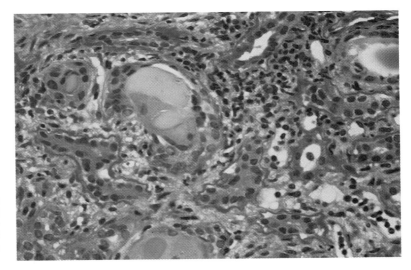

FIGURE 24–4 ▪ Intraluminal cast formation in myeloma kidney. Note reactive inflammation and giant cell formation in surrounding tubule. (Periodic acid–Schiff × 350). (Courtesy of Helmut Rennke, MD of Brigham and Women's Hospital, Boston, MA.)

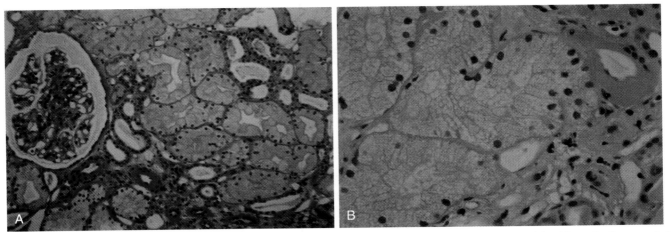

FIGURE 31–1 ▪ Percutaneous biopsy of the kidney. Light microscopy. *A,* Periodic acid–Schiff-stained section with markedly expanded proximal convoluted tubules, which in some examples have obliterated lumina. Note pale cytoplasm and flattened brush border (×200) *B,* Hematoxylin-eosin–stained section of proximal tubules, which display uniform distribution of vacuoles in cytoplasm (×400).

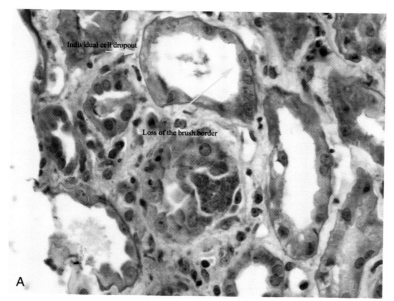

Individual cell dropout

Loss of the brush border

A

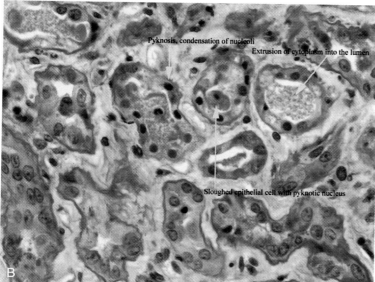

Pyknosis, condensation of nucleoli

Extrusion of cytoplasm into the lumen

Sloughed epithelial cell with pyknotic nucleus

B

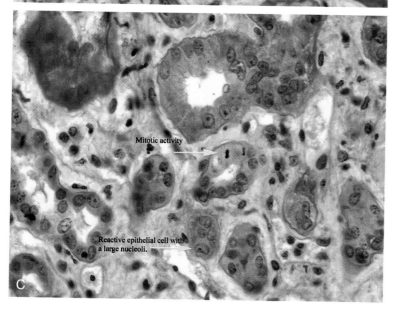

Mitotic activity

Reactive epithelial cell with a large nucleoli.

C

FIGURE 35–3 ■ Light micrographs of a percuta-neous renal biopsy specimen obtained during the early recovery phase from ischemic injury following renal transplantation. *A*, Individual cell dropout can be seen along with the absence of the brush border membrane. *B*, Tubular lumina contain sloughed epi-thelial cells with pyknotic nucleus and extruded cyto-plasm. *C*, Mitotic activity is apparent. Also seen is a reactive epithelial cell with large nucleoli (Courtesy of Dr. David Thomas).

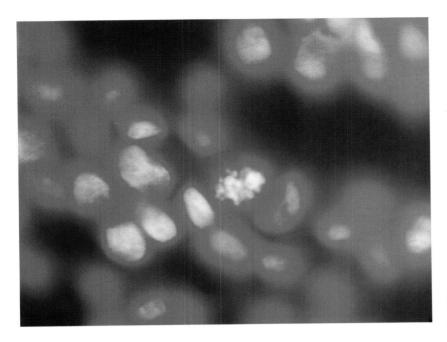

FIGURE 35–12 ■ LLC-PK₁ cells in culture incubated with Angiotensin II demonstrating apoptotic changes.

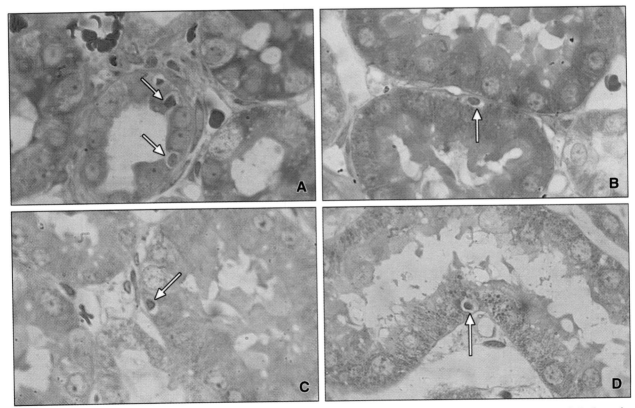

FIGURE 35–13 ■ Histologic evidence of the apoptosis of postischemic kidney from rats on a low-salt diet. *A* and *B*, 1 week after unilateral renal ischemia, *C* and *D*, 2 weeks after unilateral renal ischemia. *Arrows* indicate apoptotic bodies (H&E).

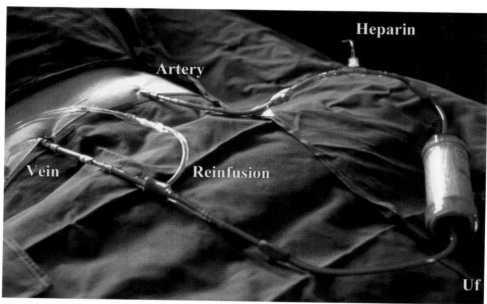

FIGURE 39–1 ■ The extracorporeal circuit in continuous arteriovenous hemofiltration. No pumps are used.

Section I
THE PATHOPHYSIOLOGY OF ACUTE RENAL FAILURE

CHAPTER **1**

The Morphologic Basis of Acute Renal Failure

Lorraine C. Racusen

INTRODUCTION

An understanding of the structural and ultrastructural changes that occur in the kidney in acute renal failure (ARF) is critical in defining the pathophysiology of renal dysfunction in this common clinical syndrome. Moreover, optimal and innovative treatment can be defined only in the context of an understanding of patterns of tissue injury. Morphologic changes underlie and reflect the functional changes that occur in the kidney in renal failure states. This chapter sets the stage for the remainder of the text to follow, providing a framework for consideration of the pathophysiology, clinical spectrum, and management of ARF. The focus of this chapter is on the pathologic findings in the most common form of ARF, so-called acute tubular injury. In the first section of this chapter, the emphasis is on clinical ARF in humans, with particular attention to changes in tubular cells with sublethal injury, lethal injury, and changes of apoptotic cell death. In the second part of the chapter, morphologic findings in various experimental models are discussed, with particular emphasis on those that seem most relevant to clinical ARF. In addition, acute tubular injury in the native kidney is compared with injury in the renal allograft.

MORPHOLOGIC OBSERVATIONS IN ACUTE TUBULAR INJURY IN HUMANS

Before the advent of the renal biopsy, morphologists investigating acute renal injury had to rely largely on observations of human kidney tissue obtained at autopsy to define pathology. In general, postmortem tissue shows substantial artifact. In the kidney, the tubules in particular suffer autolytic changes with artifactual separation of cells from basement membrane and loss of cellular integrity. It is not surprising, therefore, that only the most severe forms of tubular injury could be confidently recognized in this setting.

With the advent of renal biopsy, renal tissue could be obtained during life and fixed rapidly in newer buffered fixatives, preserving cellular detail and enabling more accurate definition of tubular cell structure. In this newer era, a range of morphologic changes have been defined in the kidney with injury, varying with the time at which kidney tissue is examined following injury. The extent and severity of the morphologic changes depend on the nature of the injurious agent and the duration of the injury process. Variable patterns of morphologic change within the kidney result from the complex structure of the kidney, with its heterogeneous nephron segments and substantial regional differences in blood flow and oxygenation.

The most common causes of ARF are disease processes that affect the tubulointerstitium. It is true, of course, that severe glomerular and vascular disease can also produce ARF, in large part by reducing renal blood flow and glomerular filtration rate. Even in these settings, almost invariably there are alterations in the tubulointerstitium, often related to ischemia. Indeed some clinical studies suggest that it is the severity of the tubulointerstitial damage that ultimately determines prognosis, regardless of the primary disease process.[1]

Acute Tubular Cell Injury

We now recognize that the process of renal tubular injury and repair is very complex, encompassing more than simply cell death followed by proliferation. Histologic assessment of renal tissue in clinical ARF had led many early investigators to conclude that in many cases tubular cell injury was not as severe as the level of renal dysfunction would lead one to expect. However, tubular injury at that time was defined primarily as tubular cell necrosis, and less severe changes were not recognized, largely because of suboptimal tissue preparations. Indeed some investigators had concluded that there was no correlation between morphologic evidence of tubular injury and severity of renal failure.[2] While renal dysfunction due to acute tubular cell injury is still often referred to clinically as "acute tubular necrosis," the changes found on pathologic examination are generally more subtle. Indeed, as we shall see, "acute tubular injury" is a more suitable term for this most common form of ARF. The results of microdissection studies[3] and the recognition of these more subtle morphologic manifestations of nonlethal cell injury have led to the recognition that there is quite a good correlation between histologic findings and function.[4] These various morphologic changes and the insights they provide regarding the mechanisms of injury and repair in the renal tubule are reviewed here.

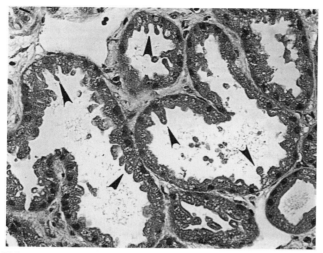

FIGURE 1–1 ■ Injured tubules with loss of cellular brush border and formation of blebs from apical cytoplasm *(arrows)* (PAS ×400).

Morphologic changes in acute tubular injury can be divided into three phases. First, cells may undergo reversible injury, with changes in ultrastructure and molecular interactions in the cell surface and cell cytoskeleton and altered intracellular ion concentrations and gradients. Some cells may then go on, more or less rapidly, to some form of cell death. The cells remaining in the injured epithelium then progress to a third phase of repair and regeneration. While proliferation is an important component of the repair process, alterations in cell shape and cell motility are probably equally important in the earliest phase of recovery and repair. Careful observation of the morphology of renal injury has provided major clues to the important cellular events involved in this dynamic process, and these clues are also reviewed in this section.

One of the earliest morphologic changes following tubular cell injury is the simplification of apical and basal cell surfaces. An increase in cytosolic calcium apparently underlies many of these changes, either directly or via activation of calcium-dependent proteolytic enzymes[5] (see later). The complex structure of the apical brush border of tubular cells is held in place by cytoskeletal elements, including actin and actin bundling proteins. With injury, the microvilli of the brush border begin to shorten and disappear, or detach from the apical cell surface. Brush border may be sloughed from the cell surface, and some may be internalized, appearing within vacuoles in the cells.[6] This loss of brush border is best seen in periodic acid–Schiff (PAS)–stained sections, since PAS stains the glycocalyx of intact brush border bright pink. Fragments of brush border may be seen in tubular lumina. The enzymes of the brush border such as gamma-glutamyl transpeptidase (GGTP) and alkaline phosphatase, detectable in voided urine, serve as markers of brush border loss. Indeed, biochemical assays for brush border enzymes have been used to detect tubular injury in clinical studies of nephrotoxicity.[7] Membrane-bound blebs form very early from the apical

surface as well, and detach into the tubular lumen (Fig. 1–1).

Loss of the apical brush border in the proximal tubule is best documented by electron microscopy; the true extent of loss of apical cell surface area is best appreciated with this technique. This loss of microvillar surface area in turn leads to loss of enzymes and loss of transport sites for apical uptake and transcellular absorption. In addition, by electron microscopy, loss of the complex interdigitating infoldings on the basolateral surface of the cells can be seen.[8] This, too, results in loss of transport surface area and of the Na^+,K^+-ATPase that is localized to this membrane and that drives many transapical and transepithelial transport processes.

Tubular cell loss is a frequent feature on histologic examination in clinical acute tubular injury. Cell detachment, in turn, probably results from cytoskeletal changes and consequent altered cell-cell and cell-matrix attachments.[9] Areas of denuded tubular basement membrane may be seen in the tubular epithelium where cells have been lost (Fig. 1–2). This feature may be difficult to quantify, since adjacent cells spread to cover these denuded areas. As a consequence of cell loss and reactive changes in surviving cells, the tubular epithelium appears flattened and paucicellular (see Fig. 1–2). Morphometric assessment with quantitation of cell numbers per unit of tubular cross-sectional area may be needed to fully appreciate the extent of this phenomenon.

Sloughed tubular epithelial cells are often seen in the lumen of tubules, either at the site of injury or downstream, having been swept along by filtrate within the tubule (Fig. 1–3A). These exfoliated cells may appear in aggregates (Fig. 1–3B), with the potential for impacting in the lumen of the nephron, especially in the outer medulla where the luminal diameter is narrowed. While some of these cells are overtly necrotic, many appear morphologically intact (see Fig.

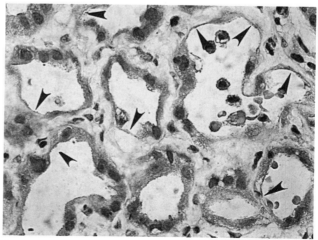

FIGURE 1–2 ■ Renal tubules showing focal exfoliated cells and numerous sites where cells have detached *(arrows)*, leaving denuded basement membrane covered by, at most, a very attenuated layer of cytoplasm caused by spreading of surviving cells. Some surviving cells have large hyperchromatic nuclei (H&E ×630).

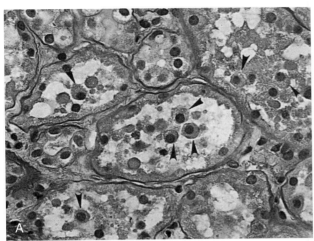

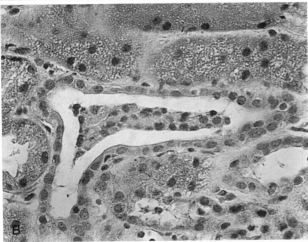

FIGURE 1–3 ■ *A*, Numerous intact tubular cells *(arrows)*, many with nuclei, in the lumen of cortical tubules (PAS ×630). *B*, Aggregation of exfoliated cells in the lumen of a tubule in a kidney with ischemic injury. Most of the aggregated cells are morphologically intact (H&E ×500).

1–3*A*). In addition, it has been shown quite definitively that at least some of these exfoliated tubular cells are viable. In a study of patients with acute renal injury, tubular epithelial cells were retrieved from the urine and shown to exclude the vital dye trypan blue. Moreover, when placed in culture medium, some of the retrieved cells grew in in vitro culture.[10, 11]

Cell exfoliation is one consequence of loosening or loss of cell-cell and cell-matrix attachment. However, it is likely that in some cases, such cells may remain in situ, still within the epithelium but with altered adhesion to adjacent cells and not functioning to maintain transepithelial electrochemical gradients, at least until normal attachments are restored as the epithelium recovers. In addition, loosening of cell-matrix attachments may trigger apoptosis in some of these cells[12] (see later).

While changes in the proximal nephron may predominate in some animal models of tubular cell injury, clinical biopsies often show prominent injury in the distal nephron segments in the cortex and outer medulla. In a large early series of autopsy cases of ARF,

Lucke and coworkers[13] were struck by this phenomenon, which led to the concept of "lower nephron nephrosis." It should be noted, however, that more subtle changes in proximal nephrons may not have been appreciable in autopsy material because of autolytic changes. Injury to the medullary thick ascending limb and to the distal nephron is commonly seen, and it is not infrequent in clinical renal biopsies to see injured distal tubules while proximal tubules remain relatively intact. In experimental models, the medullary thick ascending limb in the outer medulla has been shown to be sensitive to hypoxic and some forms of toxic injury, and especially injury produced by toxins such as radiocontrast agents and cyclosporine, which can reduce renal perfusion.[14, 15] However, morphologic changes in these tubular segments may be missed in clinical cases of ARF, since the outer medulla may not be sampled on renal biopsy, and these changes may be under-appreciated. There is an ongoing debate regarding the nephron segment or segments most severely injured in ARF induced by an ischemic or toxic insult.[16] Because clinical tubular injury often occurs in a very complex setting, with several potential injurious factors occurring simultaneously, and because "dose" of drug or severity of ischemia may result in different patterns of injury, it is likely that "pure" patterns of injury cannot be defined for many cases of clinical acute renal injury.

Impaction of exfoliated cells or cell debris forms casts (see Fig. 1–3*B*) that may obstruct the nephron. These casts often contain Tamm-Horsfall protein as a component. With reduction in glomerular filtration rate (GFR) in injury states, cast formation may be potentiated by relative stasis of tubular fluid flow. Oliver and coworkers[3] definitively demonstrated how finite areas of injury or obstruction in the nephron may be, in microdissection studies in an animal model; obstruction of a relatively short segment is potentially enough to cause shut-down of the affected nephron. Since actual sites of obstruction may be short, they may not be captured on biopsy. What is often seen, however, is dilatation of portions of the tubular system proximal to the site of obstruction. However, this phase only persists as long as glomerular filtration or the integrity of the epithelial lining of the tubule is maintained. Defects developing in the wall of the tubule as cells are injured and exfoliate or decline in GFR allow the tubule to decompress, and the dilatation will disappear. Persistent reabsorption of tubular fluid in relatively uninjured portions of the nephron also serves to decompress obstructed nephrons.

Swelling, edema, and vacuolization of cell cytosol are histologic signs of tubular cell injury often seen on clinical renal biopsy (Fig. 1–4). These cell changes reflect derangements in fluid homeostasis as critical cellular ion gradients are dissipated.[17] These overt changes, of course, antecede more subtle fluid accumulations appreciable largely at the ultrastructural level.

Cell death does occur, of course, with clinical renal injury. Typically, however, cell death detectable on renal biopsy is usually focal and almost never as severe

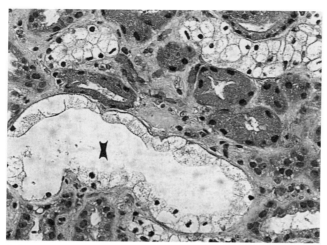

FIGURE 1–4 ■ Severe hydropic swelling and vacuolization of one large dilated tubule and several smaller tubules. Cells in affected tubules have a pale "watery" appearance. The latter show complete obstruction of the tubular lumen caused by cell swelling (H&E ×400).

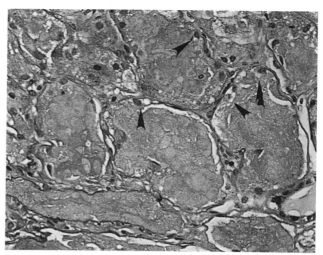

FIGURE 1–5 ■ Injured tubules with necrotic cells and granular cell debris filling the lumens. A few residual intact tubular cells can be identified (arrows) (PAS ×440).

as that seen in the most commonly used in vivo models of injury (see later). Cell death occurs in two forms, coagulative necrosis and apoptosis. The latter is more subtle than the former, but both may be evanescent and difficult to detect or quantify in all but the most extreme forms of clinical renal injury.

Coagulative necrosis represents the extreme of a spectrum of morphologic changes occurring in injured tubular cells. Cells with coagulative necrosis have recognizable changes in both the cell nucleus and the cell cytoplasm. The nucleus of the cell may shrink and become dense, an appearance referred to as pyknotic. Nuclear membranes break down, and nuclear chromatin begins to break up (karyorrhexis) and disappear (karyolysis). Associated with these nuclear changes, the cell cytoplasm becomes brightly eosinophilic as cell proteins "coagulate." If there is complete disruption of the cell membrane, the cell may disintegrate. These necrotic cells may be seen in situ within the epithelium or in tubular lumina (Fig. 1–5). These morphologic changes, in turn, reflect a complex injury cascade that includes ATP depletion, alterations in metabolic function, altered permeabilities and ion distributions, dysfunction of critical enzymes, and resultant degradation of structural molecules within the cells. The exact point along the cascade at which the cell loses the potential for recovery is impossible to detect morphologically. What can be appreciated is the morphologic end-stage, the overtly necrotic cell.

In contrast, apoptosis is a form of cell death characterized by nuclear and cytoplasmic condensation with shrinkage of the cells (Fig. 1–6) and cell fragmentation into membrane-bound "apoptotic bodies" that may contain nuclear fragments. These changes are the result of endonuclease activation, resulting in a distinctive pattern of DNA fragmentation; these enzymes cause a relatively specific "laddering" pattern of nuclear chromatin fragments on electrophoresis.[18] The apoptotic cells and remnants are usually phagocytosed

by neighboring cells and macrophages or are shed into the urine (see Fig. 1–6), so that the phenomenon may be difficult to quantify in vivo. End-labeling techniques using radioactive label that links to cleavage sites has been used to stain cells with DNA fragmentation and enhance recognition of apoptosis. However, the extent of labeling using this technique may be misleading. A complicating factor is the observation that ladder-like DNA fragmentation has been described with coagulative necrosis as well as with apoptosis.[19] It seems clear that endonuclease activation and apoptosis are separable processes. Experimental studies (see later) provide evidence that these two types of cell death are not mutually exclusive and may be coincident. Apoptosis can also be seen in renal tubule and tubular cell culture. This phenomenon is discussed in detail in Chapter 8 on cell death. Morphologic, biochemical, and molecular methods can be used to define apoptosis.[20] It remains a matter of controversy whether morphologic or molecular criteria are best for identifying

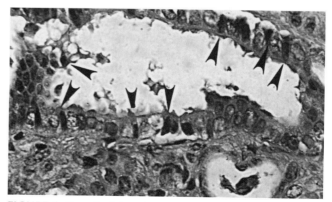

FIGURE 1–6 ■ An injured renal tubule showing numerous apoptotic cells in the wall and others that have become detached and are in the lumen (arrowheads). These cells can be recognized by their condensed compacted appearance and the dark staining of their nuclei and cytoplasm (H&E ×630).

apoptotic cell death. Apoptotic cells may be seen in ischemic tubular injury in both native and transplant human kidneys.[8, 21] It has been suggested that it may be more common in the renal allograft[21] (see later).

Ultimately, the adequacy of repair and regeneration following injury to the tubular epithelium determines the speed and completeness of return of function in the injured nephrons. Early phases of repair are characterized by reactive changes in surviving cells, changes that precede cell proliferation. Flattening and spreading of the remaining cells can be seen on histologic examination in clinical renal biopsy specimens that are examined following injury (see Fig. 1–2). Sponsel and coworkers[22] and Kartha and Toback[23] have studied the cellular response to renal epithelial wounding in vitro. After wounding of renal tubular cell monolayers, the repair process is seen to begin almost immediately. Cells migrate into the wound and fill the defect within 24 to 48 hours, even without cell proliferation. Spreading and realigning of the response axis of tubular cells occurs in this process, correlating to the flattening and spreading of cells seen in situ in injured tubules. Alterations in cell cytoskeleton and attachment molecules have also been documented in this process.

Cell regeneration in the proliferative phase following cell death or cell loss is also a challenge to quantify. Mitoses can, of course, be detected in clinical renal biopsies by light microscopy. Immunostaining for nuclear factors such as proliferating cell nuclear antigen (PCNA) and Ki67 helps to highlight and enable quantitation of the proliferation response in tubular cells on biopsy (Fig. 1–7). Using antibodies to PCNA in human "acute tubular necrosis," Nadasdy and coworkers[24] have found an increased proliferative index in both transplant and native kidneys; the proliferative index was lower with cyclosporine treatment. Both proximal and distal tubules showed positive staining, though positive cells in distal tubules were predominant in native kidney "ATN." Both "regenerating" and normal tubules showed increased staining. Cells

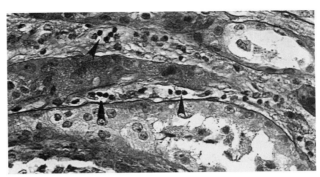

FIGURE 1–8 ▪ Marginating inflammatory cells *(arrowheads)* in peritubular capillaries in a kidney with ischemic injury. Note exfoliated cells in one tubule (PAS ×400).

labeled with PCNA have reached late G_I or early S phase in the cell cycle, an indication that the cells may indeed be in the early phase of proliferation. However, PCNA is also expressed during DNA repair,[25] so that it must be noted that some of the labeled cells may be undergoing repair rather than mitosis. Regenerating cells have hyperchromatic nuclei and a high nucleus-to-cytoplasm ratio.

Interstitium

Interstitial edema is often a prominent feature in ARF. Accumulation of interstitial fluid is in part due to altered capillary permeability. In addition, edema also correlates with tubular dilatation,[26] suggesting that the presence of increased intratubular pressure and interstitial edema may be related, perhaps via "backleak" through the wall of the distended or injured tubules.

Although inflammatory cells are usually not a prominent feature in ischemic and tubulotoxic injury, there may be a generally mild inflammatory infiltrate, often localized in peritubular capillaries (Fig. 1–8). Special stains for leukocytes may reveal larger numbers of inflammatory cells than are readily apparent by routine histology. Indeed, ill-defined methods for identifying leukocytes have led to controversy regarding the role of leukocytes in this setting.[27] These inflammatory cells may be responding to tubular cell injury. However, some experimental studies suggest that inflammatory cells may also have some role in initiation or maintenance of renal dysfunction and tissue injury. Leukocyte-depleted animals[28, 29] or animals treated with anti-ICAM antibody or deficient in ICAM-1[30, 31] have milder ischemia-induced renal injury, suggesting a significant role for leukocytes and leukocyte adhesion in the pathogenesis of tubular injury or renal dysfunction. Intracapillary leukocytes are considered later.

Vessels

The most striking vascular changes in ischemic ARF are those in peritubular capillaries, especially in the

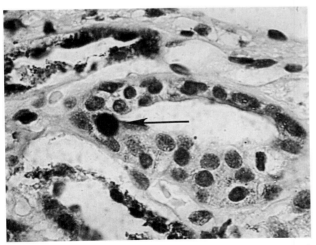

FIGURE 1–7 ▪ Immunostain for Ki67, a transcription factor, staining the nucleus *(arrow)* of an injured tubular cell in an ischemic kidney (immunoperoxidase ×1000).

outer medulla. Vascular congestion, detectable grossly as hyperemia often localized to the corticomedullary junction, has been described with reduced renal perfusion in humans. Peritubular capillaries may also be compressed in ARF. Klingebiel and coworkers[32] compared morphometric findings from semithin silver sections of kidney from control subjects with those from individuals in the oliguric or polyuric phase of ARF due to a variety of causes, including obstruction, drug toxicity, burns, and sepsis. They found a decrease in the apparent number of peritubular and intertubular capillaries, with distention of detectable capillaries. These changes were significantly different from the morphologic findings in controls and were seen throughout the cortex. The authors suggested that distended tubules, found with increased frequency in both renal failure groups, may compress some vessels, resulting in dilatation in the remaining vessels.

The finding of inflammatory cells in the capillaries of the medullary vasa recta is a fairly constant morphologic feature in ischemic ARF[26] (see Fig. 1–8). Solez and coworkers[33] showed that intravascular leukocyte accumulation occurred in the setting of reduced medullary plasma flow. Kelly and coworkers[31] have postulated that aggregation of leukocytes, as well as platelets and red blood cells, may contribute to obstruction of peritubular capillaries. The mechanisms potentially contributing to aggregation and obstruction include enhanced leukocyte-endothelium interactions with injury, mediated by ICAM and other adhesion molecules, and concentration of these cellular elements because of enhanced permeability and resultant fluid loss from the local intravascular space. With a fall in renal perfusion pressures, sluggish intracapillary flow rates would enhance this process.

In contrast, the arteries and arterioles in common forms of renal injury due to ischemia or tubulotoxins show only subtle morphologic changes. Vacuolization of smooth muscle cells may be observed (Fig. 1–9), especially if there has been severe or relatively prolonged vasoconstriction, as is seen in hypotension and ischemia. Spasm of the arteries may be detectable as reduction of luminal diameter. Some nephrotoxins, such as cyclosporine and amphotericin, also have primary vascular effects and can produce morphologic changes in vessels, including endothelial activation and a prominent vacuolization of smooth muscle cells in the vessel wall (see later).

Glomeruli

The most prominent glomerular change in ischemic injury with hypoperfusion is a collapse of the glomerular tuft. On stains such as PAS and silver stains, which highlight the glomerular basement membrane, wrinkling and collapse of glomerular capillaries may be seen. By electron microscopy, this change is nicely documented. In addition, some investigators have described changes in endothelial or epithelial cells. Solez and coworkers[34] described a reduction in fenestrae in the endothelium on freeze-fracture electron micros-

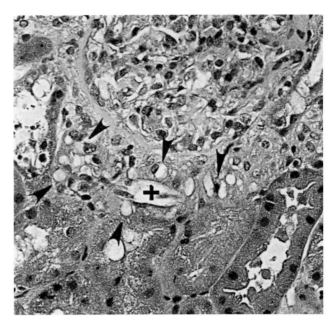

FIGURE 1–9 ■ A cross marks the lumen of an arteriole with severe vacuolization of smooth muscle cells; *arrowheads* mark a few of the vacuoles (H&E ×44).

copy in ischemic human kidneys. This finding, however, has not been universally confirmed.

Visceral epithelial cell changes have also been described. Solez and coworkers[34] have described thickening and coarsening of foot processes in glomerular renal epithelial cells in the early phase of ischemic injury induced by pedicle clamping in rabbits, and in the postperfusion biopsy in renal allografts that had early clinical ischemic injury. These investigators suggested that this change could lead to abnormally high filtration of protein, which in turn could contribute to intratubular cast formation. Barnes and coworkers[35] described a similar phenomenon in the glomeruli of rat kidney with ischemia. However, other investigators have not found these changes in other models. Parietal epithelial cells may become more cuboidal, reflecting reactive and regenerative changes in the epithelial cells of the proximal tubule, with which they are in direct continuity (Fig. 1–10). Finally, the juxtaglomerular apparatus may be enlarged in ARF. Bohle and coworkers[36] have documented this change in renal biopsies obtained in the oligoanuric phase, but not in the nonoliguric phase, of ARF.

MORPHOLOGIC OBSERVATIONS IN ACUTE TUBULAR INJURY IN EXPERIMENTAL MODELS

While the morphology of the kidney is typically assessed at a single time point in clinical biopsies, the cellular changes reflecting injury and adaptation are very dynamic. It requires repeated observations at defined intervals to develop a complete picture of relevant cellular responses to injury. This is most optimally

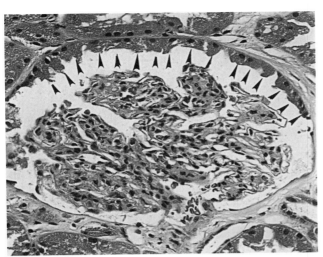

FIGURE 1–10 ▪ A glomerulus with striking reactive changes of some of the parietal epithelial cells lining Bowman's capsule *(arrowheads)*. Note the similarity of these cells to the adjacent tubular cells. Cells lining Bowman's capsule closer to the hilum have a more typical flattened appearance (H&E ×325).

achieved in experimental models. Unfortunately, however, most of the widely used in vivo models are not particularly good models of clinical renal injury.[37] While ischemic injury is generally induced in animals by renal artery or pedicle clamping, clinical ischemic injury is generally the result of hypoperfusion, rather than vascular obstruction. Similarly, toxic injury in human kidneys results from concentrations of drug or toxin lower than those used to model toxic injury experimentally. Moreover, while many cases of clinical ARF are multifactorial, only a few investigators have modeled concomitant renal insults. However, the models do represent a first approximation of clinical injury and have led to some central morphologic observations reflecting the range and complexity of cell changes that occur, so that a totally nihilistic view of their usefulness should be avoided. In addition, some valuable studies in in vitro models have considerably advanced our understanding of cellular behavior with injury. Indeed, kinetic observations can be made in vitro that would be impossible to make in vivo.

Histology and immunohistology have proved very valuable in elucidating the mechanisms of injury in these models. An early morphologic change defined in animal models of ischemic and toxic injury is loss of integrity of the actin cytoskeleton in tubular cells demonstrable by staining with rhodamine phalloidin. This alteration occurs within minutes of injury. Actin redistributes from the apical pole of tubular cells into the cytoplasm and also detaches from basolateral surface proteins, including Na$^+$, K$^+$-ATPase and integrins.[38–41] Using electron microscopy techniques, Molitoris and coworkers[42] and Canfield and coworkers[43] have defined very early alterations in the integrity of tubular epithelial tight junctions with experimental ischemic injury. Loss of tight junctions and of normal cytoskeletal attachments to membrane proteins results in redistribution of Na$^+$, K$^+$-ATPase to the apical sur-

face of the cells, a change occurring largely in proximal tubular cells. This change is demonstrable by immunohistochemistry and biochemical studies of the two membrane domains in vivo and in vitro.[44, 45] Alterations in tight junctions occur early[41] and involve disruption of cytoskeletal attachments.

Studies of renal tubular cells in vitro have demonstrated altered cell attachment as a manifestation of sublethal cell injury, analogous to changes seen in clinical tubular cell injury in humans. Cultured cells exposed to hypoxia or oxidant injury showed retraction and rounding,[41, 46] eventual disruption of actin filaments, and altered distribution of epithelial adhesion molecules.[41] Redistribution of β$_1$ integrin, an attachment molecule critical in cell-to-cell and cell-matrix attachments in these cells, has also been shown by immunohistochemistry in in vivo models of ischemia.[47] Impaired adhesion of mouse proximal tubular cells has also been documented with ATP depletion, an effect that was fully reversible with recovery[48]; associated with these changes, there is disruption of actin filaments and loss of surface adhesion sites. Expression of osteopontin, a secreted glycosylated phosphoprotein containing a GRGDS motif that can mediate cell attachment, increases with ischemic injury in vivo[49] and following oxidant injury to renal epithelial cells in vitro.[50]

In a rat model of ischemic renal injury produced by 40 minutes of ischemia and 1 hour of reperfusion, microtubules have been shown to be disrupted in the S3 segment, with variable loss in thick ascending limbs as well. On staining with anti-tubulin antibody, injured cells showed reduced intensity of staining and fragmentation of tubulin.[51] This change results from the reperfusion phase, because no change was seen without reperfusion. Alteration in microtubules may also contribute to loss of cell polarity and to disruption of intracellular transport.

In these models, intermediate filaments have also been shown to be altered with tubular cell injury. While the role of these cytoskeletal elements in cell physiology and pathophysiology is not well defined, alterations in these filaments reflect altered differentiation in these cells and are likely to have functional consequences. Vimentin is the best studied of these molecules in renal injury. Normally not found in epithelial cells, vimentin has been shown to be expressed by tubular epithelium following injury.[52, 53] Vimentin has been demonstrated by immunohistochemistry in experimental ischemic injury in the S3 segment 2 to 5 days after injury, following a wave of mitogenesis.[53] This protein is also expressed in injured tubular segments following toxic injury.[52]

Brush border loss and apical blebbing analogous to that in the human have been documented in animal models with less severe injury. Using electron microscopy, Venkatachalam and coworkers[6] have shown in a rat model of ischemic injury (25 to 60 minutes of pedicle clamping) that sloughed microvillar fragments and blebs can swell and impact in the proximal straight segment. Impaction of cells and cell fragments may also occur in the distal nephron, where cellular casts or casts containing cells may be seen apparently obstructing tubules. Some investigators have proposed that redistribution of cell adhesion molecules around the cell surface may enhance aggregation and impaction of cells in the nephron (see earlier).[41]

The pattern of tubular cell swelling has been studied in an experimental model of renal ischemia in the rat. Investigators measured diameters of the lumen and the entire tubular cross-section in different nephron segments.[54] They found that the pattern varied, depending on the nephron segment. Proximal tubular segments appear to accumulate fluid and expand basolaterally, compressing interstitium and peritubular capillaries; this swelling appears to contribute to stasis and vascular congestion in the cortex and outer stripe of the outer medulla. In contrast, cells of the thick ascending limb swell into and reduce the volume of the tubular lumen, which could contribute to nephron obstruction.

Striking vascular congestion may be seen in the outer medulla in ischemic models of ARF. Mason and coworkers[55] found that by lowering hematocrit or raising perfusion pressure this congestion was reduced, and there was improved GFR and tubular reabsorption, normalized renal blood flow and renal vascular resistance, and reduced epithelial damage. Inhibition of thrombus formation was not effective, suggesting red cell aggregation but not thrombosis as the critical pathogenic factor. Using laser-Doppler flowmetry, others have shown marked reduction of blood flow in outer medulla and moderate reduction in cortex with ischemic injury (60-minute pedicle clamp) in the rat,[56] with extensive trapping of red blood cells in outer medulla. In these studies, reduced outer medullary blood and erythrocyte trapping were normalized by hemodilution. Administration of indomethacin plus radiocontrast medium to salt-depleted uninephrectomized rats is also associated with increased residual red cell mass in the outer medulla, which correlated with medullary thick ascending limb (MTAL) necrosis.[14] Tubular cell injury and swelling in the outer stripe may lead to vascular stasis as well.[23, 57, 58] As noted previously, leukocyte adhesion and intracapillary aggregation have been proposed as contributing to capillary obstruction and stasis.[31]

Mitotic activity has been shown to increase in both experimental ischemic and toxic renal injury.[59-61] Of course, while occasional mitoses may be seen at the time of sampling, proliferation is an ongoing and evanescent process, and quantitation of mitotic figures surely underestimates proliferative activity. In experimental models of toxic and ischemic renal injury, immunostaining for antibodies to PCNA and Ki67 has demonstrated large numbers of labeled cells in tubules of renal cortex and outer medulla.[54, 62, 63]

Shimuza and Yamanaka[64] have described focal apoptotic cells in early experimental ischemic acute tubular injury but found the most marked increase in apoptosis following the proliferative response to injury, suggesting that apoptosis occurs as the epithelium remodels. Using a more clinically relevant model of transient occlusion and reperfusion, Schumer and cowork-

ers[20] found that apoptosis occurred in the reperfusion phase after a short duration of ischemia (15 minutes), with a peak at 24 and 48 hours of reperfusion. With 30 and 45 minutes of ischemia, both apoptosis and coagulative necrosis were seen. At 1 hour of ischemia or more, extensive coagulative cell necrosis was detected. Rapid DNA fragmentation is also seen within 15 minutes of hypoxia in the MTAL in the isolated perfused rat kidney, as well as in vivo in radiocontrast-induced ARF.[65] In recent studies, a second wave of cell death by apoptosis, found morphologically and by identification of clusterin, was detected in distal tubules and collecting ducts in experimental aminoglycoside nephrotoxicity in the rat,[66] perhaps resulting from reduction of blood flow due to the edema caused by the drug-induced proximal tubule injury. There is clearly an elaborate choreography here, with a balance between necrosis and apoptosis in ARF, which is being actively explored experimentally.[67, 68]

ACUTE TUBULAR INJURY IN THE TRANSPLANT KIDNEY

Acute tubular injury is a common cause of renal failure in the renal allograft. The differential diagnosis includes ischemia, acute rejection, drug toxicity, and infection. Even these processes, however, also ultimately affect renal function by producing changes in the tubulointerstitium.[69] The interstitial inflammation in acute rejection is often targeted toward the tubular epithelium, with inflammation in the epithelium and tubular cell injury as prominent features (Fig. 1–11). Cyclosporine/tacrolimus can produce vasospasm and isometric vacuolization in tubular cells (see later) and prolong ischemic tubular cell injury. Infection of tubular cells can likewise lead to cell injury.

Ischemic injury is, of course, a common cause of dysfunction in the renal allograft. While there are many similarities between allograft and native kidney

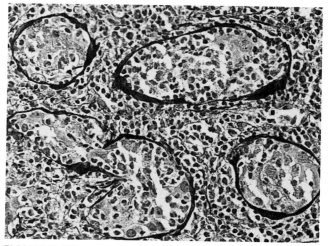

FIGURE 1–11 ■ Renal tubules in a kidney with severe tubulointerstitial rejection. Injured tubular cells can be seen in inflamed tubular epithelium (silver ×400).

ischemic tubular injury, there are some interesting differences as well; these observations have been reviewed.[21] Inflammatory infiltrates may be more prominent, not surprising in view of the fact that allografted kidneys often contain subclinical infiltrates. Deposits of calcium oxalate are more frequently seen in injured tubules and tubular cells (Fig. 1–12). These crystalline deposits reflect the often elevated circulating oxalate levels in these patients. Diminished GFR, diminished intratubular flow rates, and ischemic epithelial cell damage undoubtedly all contribute to the deposition of quite extensive oxalate deposits. It has been shown that if these deposits are extensive, recovery of renal function may be delayed or prevented.[70]

Frank coagulative necrosis of cells is more frequently seen in the allograft kidney. To some extent, this may be due to more frequent biopsy sampling of these kidneys—biopsy examination of native kidneys with ischemic injury is not often carried out, especially in the early phases. However, there are other possible explanations for these findings, including the cold as well as warm ischemia that allograft kidneys undergo and the potential synergy with toxic effects of immunosuppressive agents. As in the native kidney, inflammatory adhesion molecules play a role in reperfusion injury in the grafted kidney.[71] Ischemic injury in the transplant kidney may have a significant impact on acute renal function. In a rat model, acute ischemic injury to a solitary kidney with impairment of function after injury was associated with widespread tubulointerstitial disease, with tubular atrophy, cystic tubules, dilatation, reduction of tubular cell volume, and atubular glomeruli.[72] Inflammatory processes triggered by ischemic injury may lead to progressive renal damage denoted in the allograft as chronic allograft nephropathy.[73]

Apoptosis may also be more common in the allograft kidney,[21] perhaps reflecting ongoing often subclinical injury and repair. Interestingly, the number of apoptotic tubular epithelial cells in donor kidney biopsies taken at the time of implantation predicts early renal allograft function.[74] In this experiment a significantly higher percentage of apoptotic cells were found in the distal tubule than in the proximal tubule. Another apparent risk factor for apoptosis of tubular cells in the allograft is cyclosporin A, which has been shown to induce apoptosis in renal tubular epithelial cells in vitro.[75, 76] As with ischemic injury, there is a balance between apoptosis and necrosis, depending on the dose of the drug.[76] Of note, mycophenolate mofetil appears to decrease the apoptotic rate in renal transplant kidneys[77] without affecting proliferation.

Although not as extensively investigated as acute injury in the native kidney, acute injury in the allograft results in alterations in matrix factors that may provide clues to the differential diagnosis and to potential mechanisms of late allograft damage.[78, 79] The appearance of monocyte/macrophages as transitional cells in the response to acute injury appears to signal initiation of a process leading to diminished graft function.

Cyclosporine-FK506 treatment, especially with high doses, can produce an "isometric" vacuolization of tubular cells, with many equal-sized vacuoles (Fig. 1–13). While not specific, this change is suggestive of drug toxicity. This finding, while common in the allograft, may also be seen in native kidney of nonrenal

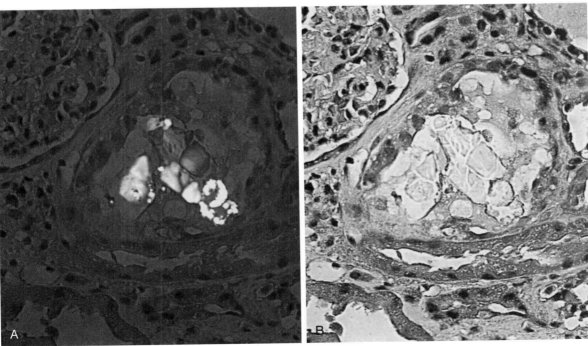

FIGURE 1–12 ■ Oxalate crystals in an injured tubule in biopsy tissue from a renal allograft. Polarized light *(A)* and light microscopy *(B)* showing characteristic appearance of oxalate (H&E ×400).

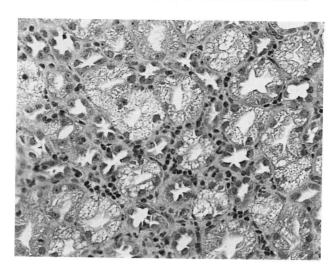

FIGURE 1–13 ■ Many small equal-sized (isometric) vacuoles in tubular cells in a renal allograft biopsy from a patient with toxic levels of tacrolimus (H&E ×400).

allograft patients treated with these drugs. With cyclosporine-FK506 toxicity, vascular changes may be seen as well, primarily in arterioles. Individual muscle cells may become necrotic and be replaced by nodular hyaline deposits, characteristically around the periphery of the vessels; extensive hyalinization of arterioles may result with prolonged exposure.

SUMMARY

Histopathologic studies of both native and allograft kidney continue to be useful in investigations of renal injury. Figure 1–14 shows a summary schema of tubular cell morphologic changes with injury. Morphologic changes may be appreciated as important observations

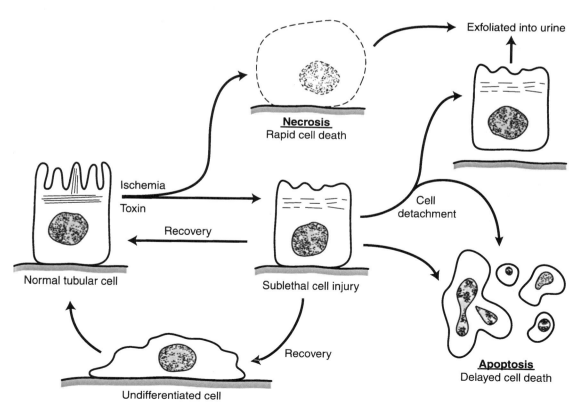

FIGURE 1–14 ■ Schema of tubular cell morphologic changes with injury.

in their own right and are seminal in introducing and guiding new avenues of investigation. Morphologic studies, broadly defined as including light and electron microscopy, immunohistology and immunoelectron microscopy, and molecular histology, are and will remain a critical component of ARF investigations.

REFERENCES

1. Bohle A, Mackensen-Haen S, von Gise H: Significance of tubulointerstitial changes in the renal cortex for the excretory function and concentration ability of the kidney: a morphometric contribution. Am J Nephrol 1987; 7:421.
2. Finckh ES, Jeremy D, Whyte HM: Structural renal damage and its relation to clinical features in acute oliguric renal failure. Q J Med 1962; 31:429.
3. Oliver J, MacDowell M, Tracy A: The pathogenesis of acute renal failure associated with traumatic and toxic injury: renal ischemia, nephrotoxic damage, and the ischemuric episode. J Clin Invest 1951; 30:1305–1440.
4. Solez K, Finckh ES: Is There a Correlation Between Morphologic and Functional Changes in Human Acute Renal Failure? Data of Finckh, Jeremy, and Whyte Re-examined Twenty Years Later. In: Solez K, Whelton A, eds: *Acute Renal Failure: Correlations between Morphology and Function.* New York: Marcel Dekker Inc; 1984.
5. Edelstein CL, Schrier RW: The Role of Calcium in Cell Injury. In: Goligorsky M, Stein JH, eds. *Acute Renal Failure.* New York: Churchill-Livingstone; 1995:3–216.
6. Venkatachalam MA, Jones DB, Rennke HG, et al: Mechanism of proximal tubule brush border loss and regeneration following mild ischemia. Lab Invest 1981; 45:355.
7. Wedeen PR, Udasin I, Fiedler N, et al: Urinary biomarkers as indicator of renal disease. Ren Fail 1999; 21:241–249.
8. Olsen TS, Olsen HS, Hansen HE: Tubular ultrastructure in acute renal failure in man: epithelial necrosis and regeneration. Virchows Arch 1985; 406:75–89.
9. Racusen LC: Alterations in tubular epithelial cell adhesion and mechanisms of acute renal failure. Lab Invest 1992; 67:158–165.
10. Racusen LC, Fivush BA, Li Y-L, et al: Dissociation of tubular cell detachment and tubular cell death in clinical and experimental "acute tubular necrosis." Lab Invest 1991; 64:546–556.
11. Racusen LC: Epithelial cell shedding in acute renal injury. Clin Exp Pharmacol Physiol 1998; 5:273–275.
12. Ruoslahti E, Reed JC: Anchorage dependence, integrins, and apoptosis. Cell 1994; 77:477.
13. Lucke B: Lower nephron nephrosis. Mil Surg 1946; 99:371.
14. Brezis M, Rosen S: Hypoxia of the renal medulla—its implications for disease. N Engl J Med 1995; 32:647–655.
15. Rosen S, Brezis M, Stillman I: The pathology of nephrotoxic injury: a reappraisal. Miner Electrolyte Metab 1994; 20:174–180.
16. Lieberthal W, Nigam SK:. Acute renal failure. I. Relative importance of proximal vs distal tubular injury. Am J Physiol 1998; 275:F623–F631.
17. Lefurgey A, Spencer AJ, Jacobs WR, et al: Elemental microanalysis of organelles in proximal tubules. I. Alterations in transport and metabolism. J Am Soc Nephrol 1991; 1:1305–1320.
18. Wyllie AH: Glucocorticoid-induced thymocyte apoptosis is associated with endogenous endonuclease activation. Nature 1980; 284:555.
19. Iwata M, Myerson D, Torok-Storb B, Zager RA: An evaluation of DNA laddering in response to oxygen deprivation and oxidant injury. J Am Soc Nephrol 1994; 5:1307–1313.
20. Schumer M, Colombel MC, Sawczuk IS, et al: Morphological, biochemical and molecular evidence of apoptosis during the reperfusion phase following brief periods of renal ischemia. Am J Pathol 1992; 140:831.
21. Olsen TS, Burdick JF, Keown PA, et al: Primary acute renal failure ("acute tubular necrosis") in the transplanted kidney: morphology and pathogenesis. Medicine 1989; 68:173.
22. Sponsel HT, Breckon R, Hammond W, et al: Mechanisms of recovery from mechanical injury of renal tubular epithelial cells. Am J Physiol 1994; 267:F257.
23. Kartha S, Toback FG: Migration of Kidney Epithelial Cells During Recovery From Acute Renal Failure. In: Goligorsky M, Stein JH, eds: *Acute Renal Failure.* New York: Churchill-Livingstone; 1995:287–319.
24. Nadasdy T, Laszik Z, Blick KE, et al: Lectin and immunohistochemical studies in human acute tubular necrosis. Human Pathol 1995; 26:230–239.
25. Nichols AF, Sancar A: Purification of PCNA as a nuclear excision repair protein. Nucleic Acid Res 1992; 20:2441–2445.
26. Solez K, Morel-Maroger L, Sraer J-D: The morphology of "acute tubular necrosis" in man: analysis of 57 biopsies and a comparison with the glycerol model. Medicine 1979;58:362–376.
27. Ghielli M, Verstrepen W, Nouwen E, DeBroe ME: Regeneration processes in the kidney after acute injury: role of infiltrating cells. Exp Nephrol 1998; 6:502–507.
28. Hellberg POA, Kallskog OK: Neutrophil-mediated post-ischemic tubular leakage in the rat kidney. Kidney Int 1988; 36:555.
29. Klausner JM, Paterson FS, Goldman G, et al: Postischemic renal injury is mediated by neutrophils and leukotrienes. Am J Physiol 1989; 256:F794.
30. Kelly KJ, Williams LWW, Colvin RB, Bonventre JV: Antibody to intracellular adhesion molecule-l protects the kidney against ischemic injury. Proc Natl Acad Sci USA 1994; 91:812.
31. Kelly KJ, Williams WW Jr, Colvin RB, et al: Intercellular adhesion molecule-1–deficient mice are protected against ischemic renal injury. J Clin Invest 1996; 97:1056–1063.
32. Klingebiel TH, von Gise H, Bohle A: Morphometric studies on acute renal failure in humans during the oligoanuric and polyuric phases. Clin Nephrol 1983; 20:1–10.
33. Solez K, Kramer EC, Fox JA, Heptinstall RH: Medullary plasma flow and intravascular leukocyte accumulation in acute renal failure. Kidney Int 1974; 6:24–37.
34. Solez K, Racusen LC, Whelton A: Glomerular epithelial cell changes in early postischemic acute renal failure in rabbits and man. Am J Pathol 1981; 103:163–173.
35. Barnes JL, Osgood RW, Reineck HJ, Stein JH: Glomerular alterations in an ischemic model of acute renal failure. Lab Invest 1981; 45:378–386.
36. Bohle A, Christensen J, Kokot F, et al: Acute renal failure in man: New aspects concerning pathogenesis. Am J Nephrol 1990; 10:374.
37. Zager R: Partial aortic ligation: a hypoperfusion model of ischemic acute renal failure and a comparison with renal artery occlusion. J Lab Clin Med 1987; 110:396–405.
38. Kellerman PS, Clark RAF, Hoilien CA, et al: Role of microfilaments in the maintenance of proximal tubule structural and functional integrity. Am J Physiol 1990; 259:F279.
39. Kellerman PS, Bogusky RT: Microfilament disruption occurs very early in ischemic proximal tubule injury. Kidney Int 1992; 42:896.
40. Molitoris BA, Geerdes AE, McIntosh JR: Dissociation and redistribution of Na$^+$, K$^+$-ATPase from its surface membrane actin cytoskeleton complex during cellular ATP depletion. J Clin Invest 1991; 88:462.
41. Gailit J, Coldflesh D, Rabiner I, et al: Redistribution and dysfunction of integrins in cultured renal epithelial cell exposed to oxidative stress. Am J Physiol 1993; 264:F149.
42. Molitoris BA, Falk SA, Dahl RH: Ischemia-induced loss of epithelial polarity: role of the tight junction. J Clin Invest 1989; 84:1334.
43. Canfield PE, Geerdes AE, Molitoris BA: Effect of reversible ATP depletion on tight junction integrity. Am J Physiol 1991; 261:F1038.
44. Molitoris BA, Dahl R, Geerdes AE: Cytoskeleton disruption and apical redistribution of proximal tubule Na$^+$, K$^+$-ATPase during ischemia. Am J Physiol 1992; 263:F488.
45. Paller MS: Lateral mobility of Na,K-ATPase and membrane lipids in renal cells. Importance of cytoskeletal integrity. J Membr Biol 1994; 142:127–135.
46. Racusen LC: Alterations in human proximal tubule attachment in response to hypoxia—role of microfilaments. J Lab Clin Med 1994; 123:357–364.
47. Zak A, Bonventre JV, Brown D, Matlin KS: Polarity, integrin and extracellular matrix dynamics in the postischemic rat kidney. Am J Physiol 1998; 275:C711–C731.

48. Kroshian VM, Sheridan AM, Lieberthal W: Functional and cytoskeletal changes induced by sublethal injury in proximal tubular epithelial cells. Am J Physiol 1994; 266:F21.

49. Kleinman JG, Worcester EM, Beshensky AM, et al: Upregulation of osteopontin expression by ischemia in rat kidney. Ann NY Acad Sci 1995; 760:321–323.

50. Hwang SM, Wilson PD, Larkin JD, Denhardt DT: Age and development-related changes in osteopontin and nitric oxide synthase mRNA levels in human kidney proximal tubule epithelial cells: contrasting responses to hypoxia and reoxygentation. J Cell Physiol 1994; 160:61–68.

51. Abbate M, Bonventre JV, Brown D: The microtubule network of renal epithelial cells is disrupted by ischemia and reperfusion. Am J Physiol 1994; 267:F971–F978.

52. Wallin A, Zhang G, Jones TW, et al: Mechanisms of the nephrogenic repair response: studies on proliferation and vimentin expression after 35S–1,2-dichlorovinyl-l-cysteine nephrotoxicity in vivo and in cultured proximal tubule epithelial cells. Lab Invest 1992; 66:474–484.

53. Witzgall R, Brown D, Schwarz C, Bonventre JV: Localization of proliferating nuclear antigen, vimentin, c-Fos and clusterin in the postischemic kidney. J Clin Invest 1994; 93:2175–2188.

54. Mason J, Joeris B, Welsch J, Kriez W: Vascular congestion in ischemic renal failure: the role of cell swelling. Miner Electrolyte Metab 1989; 15:114–124.

55. Mason J, Welsch J, Torhorst J: The contribution of vascular obstruction to the functional defect that follows renal ischemia. Kidney Int 1987; 31:65–71.

56. Hellberg POA, Kallskog O, Wolgast M: Red cell trapping and postischemic renal blood flow: differences between the cortex, outer and inner medulla. Kidney Int 1991; 40:625.

57. Yamamoto K, Wilson DR, Baumal R: Outer medullary circulatory defect in ischemic acute renal failure. Am J Pathol 1984; 116:253–261.

58. Hellberg POA, Kallskog O, Wolgast M: Nephron function in the early phase of ischemic renal failure: significance of erythrocyte trapping. Kidney Int 1990; 38:432–439.

59. Humes HD, Cieslinski DA, Coimbra TM, et al: Epidermal growth factor enhances renal tubular cell regeneration and repair and accelerates the recovery of renal function in postischemic acute renal failure. J Clin Invest 1989; 84:1757–1761.

60. Coimbra TM Cielsinski DA, Humes HD: Epidermal growth factor accelerates renal repair in mercuric chloride nephrotoxicity. Am J Physiol 1990; 259:F438–F443.

61. Norman J, Tsau Y-K, Bacay A, Fine LG: Epidermal growth factor accelerates functional recovery from ischaemic acute tubular necrosis in the rat: role of the epidermal growth factor receptor. Clin Sci 1990; 78:445–450.

62. Nouwen EJ, Verstepen WA, Byssens N, et al: Hyperplasia, hypertrophy and phenotypic alterations in the distal nephron after acute proximal tubular injury in the rat. Lab Invest 1994; 70:479.

63. Zager RA, Fuerstenberg SM, Baehr PH, et al: An evaluation of antioxidant effects on recovery from postischemic acute renal failure. J Am Soc Nephrol 1994; 4:1588–1597.

64. Shimuza A, Yamanaka N: Apoptosis and cell desquamation in repair process of ischemic tubular necrosis. Virchows Arch B Cell Pathol Incl Mol Pathol 1993; 64:171.

65. Beeri R, Symon Z, Brezis M, et al: Rapid DNA fragmentation from hypoxia along the thick ascending limb of rat kidneys. Kidney Int 1995; 47:1806–1810.

66. Nouwen EJ, Verstrepen WA, Buyssens N, et al: Hyperplasia, hypertrophy, and phenotypic alterations in the distal nephron after acute proximal tubular injury in the rat. Lab Invest 1994; 70:479–493.

67. Lieberthal W, Koh JS, Levine JS: Necrosis and apoptosis in acute renal failure. Semin Nephrol 1998; 18:505–518.

68. Lieberthal W, Menza SA, Levine JS: Graded ATP depletion can cause necrosis or apoptosis of cultured mouse proximal tubular cells. Am J Physiol 1998; 274:F315–F327.

69. Racusen LC, Solez K, Colvin R, et al: The Banff 97 Working Classification of renal allograft pathology. Kidney Int 1999; 55:713–723.

70. Sanders HM, Moura LAR, Pestana JOM, et al: Intragraft calcium oxalate deposits are associated with post-transplant acute tubular necrosis and decreased allograft survival. J Am Soc Nephrol 1997; 8:720A.

71. Dragun D, Tullius SG, Park JK, et al: I-CAM-1 antisense oligodesoxynucleotides prevent reperfusion injury and enhance immediate graft function in renal transplantation. Kidney Int 1998; 54:590–602.

72. Pagtalunan ME, Olson JL, Tilney NL, Meyer TW: Late consequences of acute ischemic injury to a solitary kidney. J Am Soc Nephrol 1999; 10:366–373.

73. Halloran PF: Renal Injury and Preservation in Transplantation. In: Racusen L, Solez K, Burdick JF, eds. Kidney Transplant Rejection. 3rd ed. New York: Marcel Dekker Inc, 1998:149–176.

74. Oberbauer R, Rohrmoser M, Regele H, et al: Apoptosis of tubular epithelial cells in donor kidney biopsies predicts early renal allograft function. J Am Soc Nephrol 1999; 10:2006–2013.

75. Ortiz A, Lorz C, Catalan M, et al: Cyclosporine A induces apoptosis in murine tubular epithelial cells: role of caspases. Kidney Int Suppl 1998; 68:S25–S29.

76. Healey E, Dempsey M, Lally C, Ryan MP: Apoptosis and necrosis: mechanisms of cell death induced by cyclosporine A in a renal proximal tubular cell line. Kidney Int 1998; 54:1955–1966.

77. Pardo-Mindian FJ, Errasti P, Panizo A, et al: Decrease of apoptotic rate in patients with renal transplantation treated with mycophenolate mofetil. Nephron 1999; 82:232–237.

78. Abrass CK, Berfield AK, Stehman-Breen C, et al: Unique changes in interstitial extracellular matrix composition are associated with rejection and cyclosporine toxicity in human renal allograft biopsies. Am J Kidney Dis 1999; 33:11–20.

79. Croker BP, Clapp WL, Abdel RF, et al: Macrophages and chronic renal allograft nephropathy. Kidney Int Suppl 1996; 57:S42–S49.

CHAPTER 2

Vascular Alterations in Acute Renal Failure: Roles in Initiation and Maintenance

John D. Conger

INTRODUCTION

Despite the emphasis placed on renal tubular cell injury, no one would deny the pathophysiologic importance of the vasculature in acute renal failure (ARF). In particular, this is true of ischemic forms of this disorder. On the other hand, the precise roles played by the vasculature in the initiation, evolution, and established phases of ARF are neither well understood nor widely appreciated. Over the past several years, new information has accumulated regarding not only the vascular events connected with the onset of ischemic injury but also the intrarenal structural and functional alterations of resistance vessels that follow ischemia and contribute to the course of the established phase and the duration of ARF.

This chapter focuses on the sequence of changes in the renal arterial vessels that accompany an ischemic insult. The initial vascular responses to significant reductions in renal perfusion are examined. Next, ischemic injury to the blood vessels themselves is described along with associated functional aberrations. The potential consequences of these functional abnormalities are considered in terms of their effects on the course of ARF. Finally, clinical correlations of these postischemic renovascular abnormalities are explored as they relate to the overall management of patients with ARF. An obvious deficiency in this presentation is the paucity of direct human data. Nearly all of the information regarding the renal vasculature in ARF is based on studies in animal models. Where available, corresponding human findings are reported. The reader is reminded that while the animal data reported are quite consistent, much of the discussion relating these finding to human ischemic ARF is, at best, reasonable speculation.

Prior to beginning a presentation of the vascular events in renal ischemia and the subsequent pathophysiologic aberrations, it is important to review salient features of normal vascular function that make the kidney unique. These very features predispose the kidney to ischemia. In addition, it is worthwhile to review the fundamentals of mammalian microvascular tone and reactivity, since these vessels are the most important, both functionally and structurally, in postischemic injury. The focus obviously is on the kidney; however, identifying organ-specific differences aids in understanding the special sensitivity of the renal vasculature.

UNIQUE FEATURES OF THE RENAL CIRCULATION

Renal resistance vessels begin with the interlobular arteries, which give rise to lateral afferent arteriolar branches, and terminate in afferent arterioles (AAs) in the superficial cortex. Near the vascular pole of the glomeruli, the smooth muscle cells (SMCs) of AAs are modified to renin granule–containing epithelioid cells that contain rudimentary myofibrils. Upon entering the glomerular capsule, AAs promptly divide into primary glomerular capillaries that give rise to the anastomosing capillary network. The hydraulic permeability coefficient for glomerular capillaries is approximately 300 times that of skeletal muscle capillaries and 50 times that of mesenteric capillaries. Within the glomerulus, the capillaries converge to form the efferent arteriole (EA).[1] The intraglomerular portion of the EA is surrounded by mesangial cells. Upon exit from the glomerulus, the EA is encircled by a relatively sparse (compared with the AA) single layer of SMCs. In the middle and outer cortex, EAs divide into a capillary network that surrounds the proximal and distal tubules largely from the same nephron. A similar capillary network arises from EAs in the juxtamedullary cortex. However, juxtamedullary EAs also give rise to the vasa rectae capillaries, which form hairpin loops that course into and out of the renal medulla. Venous outflow from the cortex follows the pattern of the arterial system and can be clearly identified beginning at the interlobular vessel level.

While the combined weight of two adult human kidneys is only 300 g, they receive approximately one fifth of the cardiac output. Glomerular filtration, which is dependent on the high blood flow, is the principal functional process carried out by the kidneys. The process of glomerular filtration is controlled by a combination of physical forces. The vascular pressure profile through the kidney, based primarily on measurements in the rat,[2] is shown in Figure 2–1. The glomerular capillary hydraulic pressure of approximately 45 to 50 mm Hg is maintained by variations in the preglomerular and postglomerular arteriolar resistances. At the afferent end of the glomerular capillary network, the intracapillary colloid osmotic pressure is approximately 20 mm Hg. The hydraulic conductivity coefficient of glomerular capillaries measured directly in the Munich Wistar rat kidney is 2520 nL/min per mm Hg per cm.[2, 3] The filtration process increases the plasma protein concentration and colloid osmotic pressure of the plasma remaining in the efferent end of the glomerular capillary network to approximately 35 mm Hg. When the proximal tubular hydraulic pressure of approximately 10 mm Hg is added to the colloid osmotic pressure, the net efferent driving pressure for ultrafiltration is reduced to near 0. Thus, under basal physiologic conditions, near filtration

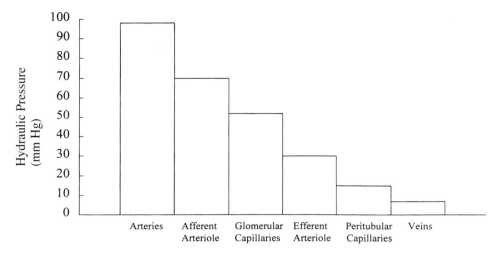

FIGURE 2–1 ■ The pressure profile along the renal vasculature, based on direct micropuncture measurements in rat kidneys.

equilibrium exists at the efferent end of the glomerular capillary network.

Glomerular filtration rate (GFR) remains relatively constant despite variations in renal perfusion pressure. This is the result of autoregulation of renal blood flow (RBF). Over a wide range of renal perfusion pressures (estimated to be 80–160 mm Hg in humans), RBF remains the same. Two mechanisms are primarily responsible for the autoregulatory phenomenon: myogenic adjustments in periglomerular arteriolar tone[4] and tubuloglomerular feedback.[5]

Several factors can increase or decrease basal RBF. Table 2–1 gives a number of endogenous humoral factors and their influence on RBF and GFR. Some of these agents have differential effects on afferent and efferent arteriolar resistances and the glomerular ultrafiltration coefficient and, therefore, can have unique effects on RBF and glomerular filtration that could not be predicted from their generally recognized systemic vascular effects.

TABLE 2–1. Effects of Vasoactive Agents on Renal Blood Flow and Glomerular Filtration

	RBF	GFR
Catecholamines		
Norepinephrine	↓	→ or ↓
Dopamine	↑	↑
Peptides		
Antidiuretic hormone	→	→
Parathyroid hormone	↑ or →	→ or ↓
Atrial natriuretic peptide	→	→ or ↑
Angiotensin II	↓	→ or ↓
Bradykinin	↑	→
Glucagon	↑	↑
Endothelin	↓	↓
Arachidonate Metabolites		
Prostaglandins E_2, I_2	↑	→
Thromboxane A_2	↓	↓
Leukotrienes C_4, D_4	↓	↓
Other		
Adenosine	↓ then ↑	↓
Histamine	↑	→
Platelet-activating factor	↓	↓
Acetylcholine	↑	→

VASCULAR TONE AND REACTIVITY

Basal Vascular Tone

Under resting conditions, the level of tone within the small arteries and arterioles of the systemic and pulmonary vasculature is the major factor in resistance to blood flow within the general circulation. In turn, this basal tone maintains appropriate arterial pressures at physiologic levels of cardiac output. Systemic vessels have relatively high basal tone (compared to the lungs), a function of vessel structure and smooth muscle tension that affords the presumed advantage of maintaining high systemic pressure that offsets the effects of gravity in upright animals and, perhaps, provides dilator reserve for increased perfusion demands during exercise.

Resting tone reflects basal properties intrinsic to the smooth muscle and the modulating influence of several well-defined extrinsic factors. These include metabolic demand, neural and humoral influences, locally generated paracrine modulators, and physical forces (stretch and shear). The influence of these modulators varies greatly among organs. In heart, skeletal muscle, and brain, metabolic demand is a preeminent regulator, while in lung and kidney the blood flows are high compared with energy requirements and are largely unrelated to them. The arterial vessels of the heart and brain are relatively resistant to neurohumoral constriction, whereas those of the kidney are highly responsive.

Resistance vessels isolated in vitro have very little basal tone compared with those in vivo—a difference that is independent of neurohumoral effects and is thus termed *myogenic* (intrinsic to the vessel). Myogenic tone is characterized by an increase in response to stretch (increased intraluminal pressure) and weaker relaxation in response to shear forces (flow). The myogenic response that increases smooth muscle tone in response to stretch is mediated largely by specialized, distinct stretch-operated Ca^{2+} channels.[6-13] These channels, located on the surface of SMCs, respond to stretch by augmenting entry of extracellular calcium and increasing contraction.

The other major mechanism that intrinsically regulates blood vessels in the in vivo circulation is the transduction of flow-related stimuli. Flow produces shear. Shear stress is most readily detected by endothelial cells, which are largely responsible for sensing and mediating responses to altered flow. Vasomotor responses to flow are predominantly of a dilatory nature, although weak constrictor responses are observed in some beds.[14–18] The dominant dilator response has the potentially useful purpose of normalizing shear forces at the surface of the vessel wall when flow is increased. To varying degrees, the shear stress response is found in arterial vessels of all sizes both in vivo and in vitro. Flow-induced dilation can overcome and inhibit stretch-related vasoconstriction,[14, 15, 19] an observation with particular relevance to the renal vasculature in ischemic ARF.

Most studies show that the shear effect is largely, but not entirely, dependent on the endothelium. It is attenuated or lost after endothelial denudation. Translation of the endothelial shear response into smooth muscle relaxation implicates a diffusible messenger. Much evidence assigns a major role to endothelial-derived nitric oxide (NO),[20] but endothelial cyclooxygenase products have also been implicated.[21] The role of NO in the normal circulation is indicated by responses to its inhibition by administration of arginine analogs that block its production and produce increases in basal resistance in essentially all vascular beds. This finding would indicate that basal NO activity is an important determinant of resting vascular tone. Indeed, these effects on resting physiologic vascular tone are substantially greater than those produced by inhibiting other endogenous constrictors or dilators, including the alpha adrenergic nervous system, angiotensin II (AII), endothelins, and prostaglandins, and suggest a dominant role for NO in the regulation of the resting circulation. Some of these effects may be constitutive and unrelated to flow. For example, observations in isolated arterial preparations with physiologic pressure but no flow have shown vasoconstrictor responses to NO inhibitors.[22]

Adjustment of vascular tone and blood flow to meet local metabolic demands is, as mentioned, a prominent feature of high oxygen demand organs such as the exercising muscle, heart, and brain, but it is much less evident under physiologic conditions in high basal blood flow beds such as the kidney. This metabolic demand response is locally regulated, but it is not likely to be intrinsic to the vessel itself. Numerous studies suggest that signals responsible for vasodilation in response to increased energy consumption originate in organ parenchyma and are mediated by vascular actions of several factors with synergistic effects that include decreased oxygen and increased carbon dioxide tensions, decreased pH, increased extracellular K^+, and release of adenosine.[23–25] The adenosine triphosphate (ATP)-sensitive K^+ channel seems to play an important role because blockage of this channel with sulfonylurea compounds greatly attenuates the dilator response to metabolic demand as in reactive hyperemia.[26]

The numerous extrinsic modulators of vascular tone include humoral and neural factors such as adrenergic and cholinergic mediators, prostanoids, and angiotensin. Studies with inhibitors suggest that their influence may be greater in stimulated or stress states than under resting circumstances.

In summary, basal vascular tone is essential for perfusion of complex and distinct vascular beds. Vascular resistance is dictated, in large part, by intrinsic factors that set resting tone and is modulated by factors linked to the requirements of individual organs, eg, in the heart it is energy consumption, whereas in the kidney it is blood pressure and flow and glomerular filtration.

Vascular Reactivity

Responses to extrinsic stimuli are commonly used to assess changes in vascular function. This entails measured responses to vasomotor, neural, or humoral stimuli, as well as to imposed physical forces (stretch and shear). Some of these factors, such as catecholamines, AII, and atrial natriuretic peptides (ANPs), circulate and act globally. Other factors, such as thromboxane A_2 (TXA$_2$), PGH$_2$, endothelin-1 (ET-1), adenosine, platelet-activating factor (PAF), neuropeptide Y, kinins, histamine, serotonin, NO, and PGI$_2$ have predominantly local paracrine or autocrine effects (Table 2–2). Their actions vary among individual organs, based on differences in receptor density and affinity, postreceptor signaling events, and interactions with other vasoactive factors. For example, the kidney has greater vasoconstrictor sensitivity to ET-1 than other organs,[27] and adenosine, which is a potent vasodilator in coronary circulation, has both dilator and constrictor effects in the renal arterial bed.[28]

A particularly important dimension of vasoreactivity is the tendency for vascular tone to respond in a fash-

TABLE 2–2. Endogenous Agents That Modify Vascular Tone and Mediate Vasoactivity

CIRCULATING FACTORS	
Constrictors	**Dilators**
Norepinephrine	Natriuretic peptides
Angiotensin II	Acetylcholine
Endothelin-1	

LOCAL FACTORS	
Constrictors	**Dilators**
Thromboxane A_2	Nitric oxide
Prostaglandin H_2	Kinins
Leukotrienes	Dopamine
Endothelin-1	Histamine
Platelet activating factor*	Serotonin
Neuropeptide Y	Prostaglandins I_2, $E_{1,2}$
Adenosine*	Adenosine*
	Platelet activating factor*
	Acetylcholine

*An agonist may be a constrictor or a dilator, based on local concentration and site of action.

ion that keeps organ blood flow constant. Renal, coronary, and cerebral circulation demonstrate autoregulatory capacity. In part, autoregulation reflects the action of the myogenic response, wherein changes in intraluminal pressure act directly on stretch-operated channels of vascular smooth muscle to alter calcium influx and contraction. There are also length-dependent changes in contractile protein function and endothelial modulation of SMC tone.[29] Other factors may also participate. In the kidney, for instance, characteristics of tubular fluid flow in the distal nephron modulate arteriolar tone and autoregulation of glomerular filtration to maintain fluid and electrolyte balance. In the coronary circulation and, to a lesser extent, in the cerebral circulation, metabolic demand is a major factor in autoregulation.

In summary, vascular reactivity is the responsiveness of the blood vessels to extrinsic neural, humoral, and local stimuli and to changes in the physical forces that modify vascular tone. The integrity of these responses is critical to maintenance of organ function and viability in the setting of cardiocirculatory changes and hypovolemia. Loss of normal responsiveness is an important indicator of vascular injury.

INITIATION OF ISCHEMIC RENAL INJURY

Most explanations of ischemic injury to the kidney begin with a description of the consequences of an ischemic event. It is assumed that a finite period of reduction in RBF occurs as an antecedent to a series of damaging biological reactions about which there is an ever-expanding scientific appreciation. While this is an appropriate approach to the discussion of renal tubular cell injury, it is not the correct starting point for describing the vascular component of ischemia pathophysiology. It must be kept in mind that the initial process of ischemia begins as a vascular event.

As pointed out in the preceding review of normal renovascular physiology, the kidneys have a remarkably high blood flow per unit of tissue weight and a relatively low oxygen extracting fraction. Intuitively, it would be assumed that these features would make the kidneys relatively resistant to ischemic injury. However, it is well established that the kidney is one of the organs most susceptible to ischemia that is related to changes in systemic hemodynamics. This apparent paradox is explained, at least in part, by the special functional anatomy of the kidney circulation. Phylogenetically speaking, the renal arterial system is adapted primarily for the preservation of glomerular filtration. As illustrated in Figure 2–2, pre- and postglomerular arteriolar resistances change reciprocally to maintain the relative constancy of both glomerular plasma flow and hydraulic pressure when there are substantial alterations in systemic arterial pressure. While this autoregulatory mechanism protects the clearance function of the kidney, which ensures systemic nitrogen balance and nonvolatile waste elimination, it has the potential to negatively affect postglomerular and peritubular capillary blood flow when

systemic arterial pressure is reduced to a level that is at or below the lower limit of autoregulation for some finite interval. Under these conditions baseline peritubular capillary pressure is reduced well below its already low normal level of 10 to 12 mm Hg. (Normal postglomerular capillary pressure is about half that in a skeletal muscle capillary bed.) Maximal efferent arteriolar constriction in the presence of decreased systemic blood pressure drops peritubular capillary pressure and flow to near zero. Ischemic injury can result, therefore, with seemingly minor declines in systemic hemodynamics.

It is of interest that documented episodes of surgical hypotension lasting no more than 15 minutes can be causally associated with ischemic ARF, while other patients have undergone more than an hour of similar intraoperative hypotension and had no evidence of renal impairment. Thus, while the organization and function of the renal microcirculation itself predisposes the kidney to ischemic ARF, there are less well defined factors that determine the actual magnitude of organ hypoperfusion and tubular cell susceptibility to ischemia. Broadly stated, factors that appear to enhance the likelihood of ARF occurring when renal blood perfusion is reduced include those that increase both pre- and postglomerular vascular resistance and those that increase the metabolic work and energy demand of renal tubular cells. The former include volume depletion, heart failure, increased sympathetic tone, chronic renal failure, renal artery stenosis, nonsteroidal anti-inflammatory drugs, anesthesia, cyclosporine, and physiologic vasoconstrictors, including norepinephrine, AII, and endothelin.[30] Theoretically, any condition that increases metabolic demand or interferes with energy utilization may increase renal tubular cell sensitivity to ischemia. A clearly documented example is hyperthermia. Zager and coworkers[31, 32] have shown that an increased body temperature is a critical variable in the severity of ischemic injury in a renal artery cross-clamp model in rats.

Several studies have been carried out that demonstrate that inhibition of vasodilators amplifies, while antagonists of vasoconstrictors attenuate, the severity of ischemic kidney insults in animal models.[33] Unfortunately, it is difficult to interpret the results of these studies in terms of their specificity. When these inhibitors or antagonists are given prior to ischemia, it is uncertain whether the effect is simply a resetting of basal renal hemodynamics. Moreover, the postinsult residual plasma level of the pharmacologic test agent may nonspecifically increase RBF, rather than directly attenuate causal factors in ischemic injury. This, in turn, may influence the post-insult GFR. The observation that pretreatment with a broad array of different vasoconstrictor antagonists, including PGH_2,[34] TXA_2,[35] AII,[36–37] endothelin[38, 39] sympathetic agonists,[40, 41] and PAF,[42, 43] achieves similar levels of protection supports the likelihood that the effect is nonspecific. It is probably reasonable to conclude that any pharmacologic vasoactive agent that alters pre- and postglomerular arteriolar balance of tone alters either the magnitude or the effects of a standard ischemic insult. It is diffi-

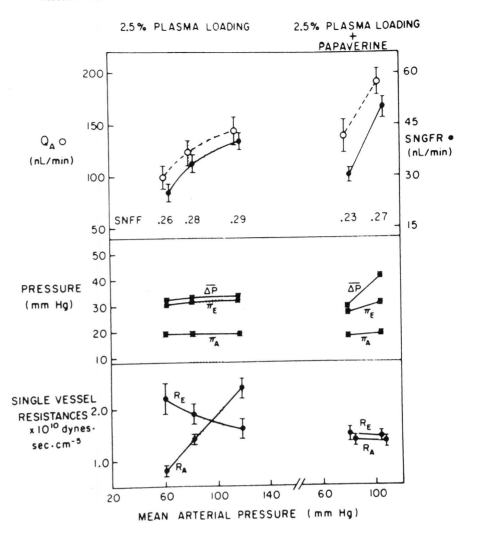

FIGURE 2–2 ■ Effects of graded reductions in renal perfusion pressure on glomerular plasma flow (GPF) and single nephron glomerular filtration rate (SNGFR): glomerular capillary (P_{GC}) and proximal tubular (P_T) hydraulic, efferent (II_{AA}), and efferent arteriolar (II_{EA}) oncotic pressures; and afferent (R_A) and efferent arteriolar (R_E) resistances. (From Robertson CR, Deen WM, Troy JL, et al: Dynamics of glomerular ultrafiltration in the rat. III. Hemodynamics and autoregulation. Am J Physiol 1972; 223:1193; with permission.)

cult to conclude that the activity of any endogenous constrictor agonist or the absence of any physiologic vasodilator is a unique mediator of the initial phase of renal ischemia. Regardless of the uncertainty as to specific cofactors, it is clear that there are conditions and, perhaps, specific substances that increase the likelihood of tissue injury following a transient reduction in RBF. The better understood these modifying factors are, the better the opportunity to identify patients at high risk for ischemic ARF and develop useful preventive treatments.

PATHOPHYSIOLOGY OF THE EVOLUTION OF ISCHEMIC ACUTE RENAL FAILURE

Historically, the mechanism underlying the abrupt decline in kidney function in ARF has been variously identified, depending on human and animal pathologic observations and functional studies carried out mostly in dogs and rodents. Basically, all proposed mechanisms can be reduced to three: tubular obstruction, persistent reduction in glomerular hemodynamics, and tubular fluid backleak. Each of these has been

championed in different eras, depending on the model and the techniques of study available at the time. The reader is referred to classic articles by Oliver and coworkers,[44] Biber and coworkers,[45] Bank and coworkers,[46] Oken and coworkers,[47] and Tanner and coworkers.[48] In a sequential micropuncture study performed on rats with norepinephrine-induced ischemic ARF for a period of 7 days in the author's laboratory (Fig. 2–3), a random examination of tubular pressures and single-nephron GFRs (SNGFR) measured at the existing tubular pressures was carried out.[49] At 24 hours after ischemia induction, tubular pressures varied widely in different nephrons, from distinctly below normal to markedly above normal. Single-nephron GFRs were uniformly reduced to less than one fourth of normal so long as existing tubular pressures were maintained during tubular fluid collections. The SNGFR closely paralleled the percentage decline in whole-kidney GFR. Re-examination of these same parameters at 48 hours showed the same wide spectrum of tubular pressures with uniformly reduced SNGFR. At 72 hours there was a trend toward normalization of tubular pressures, and by 7 days the mean tubular pressure was nearly normal with the variance only

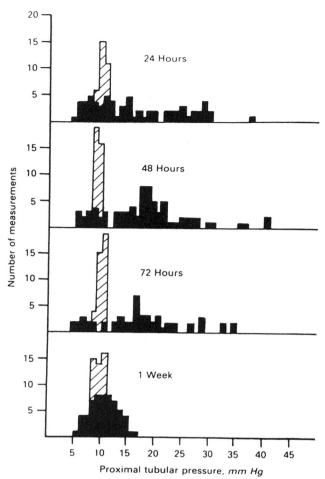

FIGURE 2–3 ■ Proximal tubular pressures in NE-ARF *(solid bars)* and sham-infused ARF control rats *(hatched bars)*. (From Conger JD, Robinette JB, Kelleher SP: Nephron heterogeneity in ischemic acute renal failure. Kidney Int 1984; 26:425; with permission.)

slightly greater than that in control animals. Of interest, when the tubules with elevated pressures were decompressed to normal pressures during tubular fluid collections, SNGFR measurements were increased to the range of normal values. Taken together, these data suggest strongly that there are at least two pathogenetic mechanisms operating simultaneously in ischemic ARF: tubular obstruction and persistent reduction in glomerular blood flow. Some nephrons are primarily obstructed, with the potential for normal function if the obstruction is eliminated, and others have negligible glomerular blood flow independent of any tubular obstruction. The variable pressure measurements indicate that there are gradations and combinations of these pathogenetic factors operating throughout the majority of the nephron population. This nephron heterogeneity may frustrate the notion of a simple pathogenetic process. However, it appears to be a biological reality. Direct data in the norepinephrine ARF (NE-ARF) model would not support an important role for tubular fluid backleak.[49] Other data collected later in the course of ischemic ARF from both rodents and humans do suggest that backleak may play at least a partial pathogenetic role.[46, 50]

The best investigative efforts to define the pathophysiology of ischemic ARF in humans have been carried out by Myers,[51] whose principal work has been in renal transplant recipients with initial renal dysfunction. In a study reported in 1995 using both direct measurements and indirect estimates of GFR determinants, he and his coworkers attempted to identify the mechanisms of reduced renal function.[52] Results in that study showed that renal plasma flow and the calculated net hydraulic driving force for primary glomerular filtration (ΔP) were low. The glomerular ultrafiltration coefficient was normal, and there was no evidence of obstruction as measured by morphometry of biopsy tissue. They concluded that the likely principal mechanism of renal failure was afferent arteriolar constriction. Subsequently, using para-aminohippurate extraction, phase-contrast cine magnetic resonance imaging, and intraoperative Doppler flowmeter determinations,[53, 54] they found, as did others,[55–57] only small depressions in RBF despite profound reductions in GFR. In other studies, the results supported a role for tubular fluid backleak and possible increased sodium delivery from the proximal tubule to activate the tubuloglomerular feedback system and reflex afferent arteriolar constriction.[58, 59] It is obviously difficult to draw simple conclusions from these data regarding pathogenetic mechanisms for ischemic ARF. Myers recognizes the apparent contradictions in some of the data obtained in this human "model" of ischemic ARF. Nonetheless, it is his belief that the reduced ΔP is important, and he would lean toward a reduction in glomerular hydraulics over tubular obstruction as a mechanism. There is uncertainty regarding the quantitative role of tubular fluid backleak. As yet, no other investigators have carried out similar levels of direct measurement and analysis in other forms of human ischemic ARF.

The purpose of reviewing this information is to put the role of the vascular abnormalities in perspective when discussing the evolutionary and established phases of ischemic ARF. As an ongoing pathogenetic mechanism, glomerular hypoperfusion (as a vascular factor) may account for up to 50 percent of the acute renal dysfunction but probably not more than that. The partial recovery in RBF without a parallel increase in whole kidney GFR and the overall lack of success in improving renal function with vasodilator agents support the contention that renal dysfunction in established ARF is more complex than glomerular hypoperfusion. Thus, in the larger picture, vascular abnormalities following ischemia are of great interest and of considerable importance. However, they are only a part of the pathophysiology of ischemic ARF.

ISCHEMIC INJURY TO THE RENAL VASCULATURE

In both human and animal models of ischemic ARF, there has been little focus on injury to the vasculature itself. There are several reasons for this: the impressive preservation of glomerular morphology in the presence of substantial tubular injury, the relative paucity of fresh biopsy material in human ischemic ARF, the limited number of arteriolar vessels that can be visualized in comparison to tubules, the frequent requirement for special staining to highlight vascular necrosis and fibrosis, and the generally greater interest in tubular pathology. Nonetheless, when specifically sought out, substantial and similar morphologic changes in renal arterial vessels have been shown in both the renal artery clamp and norepinephrine models of ischemic ARF in rats.[60]

Vascular Pathology in Models of Ischemic ARF

Figure 2–4 shows sequential representative cross sections of interlobular and afferent arteriolar vessels from NE-ARF rats immediately after and up to 7 days post ischemic insult. The pathologic profile is similar

and, in fact, more frequent in the renal artery clamp (RAC) model.[61, 62] The earliest changes of vacuoles in the muscular layers appear within 4 to 6 hours of ischemic insult. By 24 hours, there is evidence of focal necrosis in the smooth muscle. By 48 hours, there is the appearance of immature fibroblasts surrounding the vessels in addition to continued evidence of patchy smooth muscle necrosis. Over the ensuing 5 days there is diminishing evidence of necrosis, but the circumferential perivascular fibrosis becomes increasingly dense. By 4 weeks after insult there is some remaining fibrosis surrounding the microvasculature but substantially less than that at 7 days.[60] Evidence of pathologic changes can be detected in roughly one half of small arterial vessels from renal artery clamp and approximately one third of those from norepinephrine models of ARF.

Interestingly, there has been no evidence of consistent abnormalities of the endothelium in the postischemic renal vasculature at any point in the previously mentioned chronologic sequence.[60] There were no

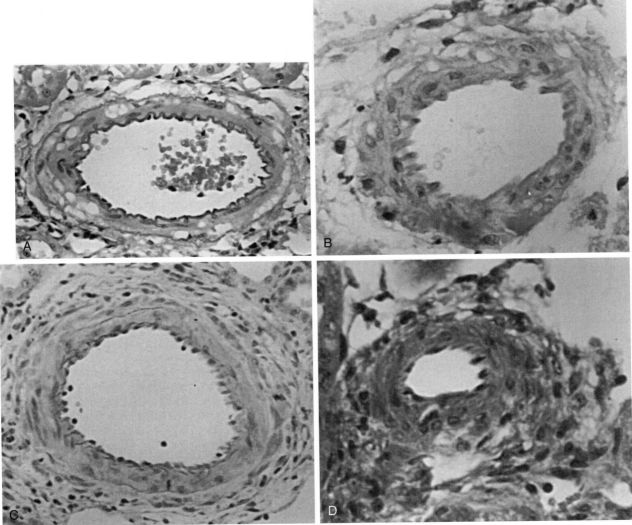

FIGURE 2–4 ■ Sequential changes in interlobular arteries in ischemic NE-ARF in rats. *A,* At 6 hours post ischemic insult, there are vacuoles in the smooth muscle layer. *B,* At 24 hours, there is patchy necrosis in the vessel wall. *C,* At 96 hours, there is an abundance of immature fibroblasts surrounding the smooth muscle cells. *D,* At 1 week, the perivascular fibrosis persists and is well organized. (*A–D,* ×500).

findings of neutrophil adhesion or endothelial denudation. This does not negate, nor does it give support to, a role for decreased activity of endothelium-derived relaxing factor or oxidant injury in these animal models of ischemic ARF. As can be seen from the injury mechanisms to be described, the weight of data suggests that the endothelium plays a critical role even though the morphologic correlation is elusive in our studies.

Although it often may be difficult to differentiate the separate effects of ischemia and reperfusion in severe insults, the role of reperfusion is strongly evident following episodes of brief ischemia in which the injury induced by reperfusion is dominant. This appears to be true particularly of such organs as heart, lung, brain, skeletal muscle, and intestine. The data regarding the kidney and kidney vasculature are more controversial. Nonetheless, it is important to review the process of reperfusion injury for the purpose of understanding its potential relevance. As illustrated in Figure 2–5, an important feature of early ischemia is the depletion of high-energy chemical stores, such as ATP, with accumulation of purine degradation products and the conversion of the enzyme xanthine dehydrogenase to an oxidase. Subsequent reperfusion and resupply of oxygen (the oxygen paradox) permit xanthine oxidase to act on its purine substrate, with the resulting generation of oxidants. This process probably occurs in organ parenchymal cells and in the endothelium.

In some organs, microvascular endothelium is the major locus of xanthine oxidase. Even though it is difficult to document in the kidney, the other important event in early reperfusion is the inflow of neutrophils, which are sequestered in the small vessels of the postischemic organ—an effect attributed to expression of adhesion molecules on both the endothelium and the neutrophils. Adherence, activation, and migration of neutrophils is generally considered a critical contributor to reperfusion injury, mediated by further release of oxidants and accompanied by proteases and elastases and activation of phospholipases.[63, 64]

Following ischemia-reperfusion and, to a lesser extent, ischemia alone, the endothelium produces pro-inflammatory substances, including ET-1,PAF, leukotriene B_4 (LTB_4) and oxygen metabolites while down-regulating production of "stabilizing" substances, including adenosine, NO, and PGI_2.[64] There is early increased expression of leukocyte components (CD11/CD18, LAM-1, L-selectin) and endothelial components (ICAM-1, ELAM-1, P-selectin) of the adhesion molecule system, resulting in leukocyte (primarily polymorphonuclear neutrophil [PMN]) adherence and the subsequent release of additional pro-inflammatory mediators from both endothelial cells and PMN (tumor necrosis factor alpha [TNF_α], interleukin-1 [IL-1], proteinases, O_2 metabolites, PAF, and other cytokines).[65, 66]

The endothelial cells undergo morphologic changes as a consequence of ischemia and ischemia-reperfusion. In the cerebral vasculature, for example, ultrastructural abnormalities have ranged from thick finger-like projections, dark osmophilic cytoplasm, clustering of ribosomal structures, and dilation of tight junctions to frank necrosis and endothelial blebbing, depending on the severity of the ischemia.[66] In the coronary arteries, total ischemia and reperfusion result in partial detachment and blebbing of the endothelial cells and both thickening and thinning of the basal lamina.[67] When one compares the cerebral and coronary vessels with the renal vasculature, there are differences in postischemic endothelial cell morphologic changes based on the author's own pathology studies, as alluded to previously.[60, 68] In both the RAC- and the NE-ARF models in rats, the renal endothelium shows negligible definitive changes by either light or electron microscopy.

The basal lamina of the arterial resistance vasculature, consisting predominantly of collagen type IV, laminin, entactin, heparan sulfate, and fibronectin,[69] provides the attachment ligands for endothelial cell integrins and a supplemental barrier to diffusion of endothelial-generated and circulating cytotoxic substances into the vessel wall. While there is evidence indicating that the permeability of postglomerular capillaries and vasa rectae following renal ischemia is increased,[70] there are no studies examining disruption of endothelial cell-to-cell attachment or of the basal lamina in the resistance arterial vasculature. Ischemia-reperfusion–related injury of tubular basement membrane matrix has been reported by Walker and coworkers.[71] The marked reduction of the laminin component was consistent with enzymatic degradation. Recently, this same group identified a metalloproteinase from tubular epithelial cells that caused laminin degradation.[72] While not exclusively related to ischemia, several studies have demonstrated glomerular basement membrane lysis by proteinases (elastase, cathepsin G, B, and L, and serine proteinases) produced by inflammatory

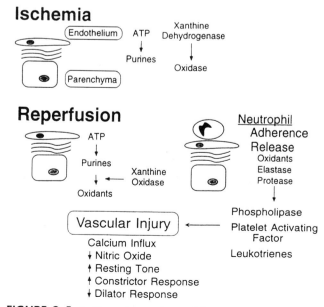

FIGURE 2–5 ■ The primary sites and known common events in ischemia-reperfusion injury to the arterial vasculature. (From Conger JD, Weil JV: Abnormal vascular function following ischemia-reperfusion injury. J Invest Med 1995; 43:434; with permission.)

leukocytes.[71, 73] The matrix proteins degraded were identical to those found in normal arterial vascular basal lamina. Thus, while the evidence is indirect, there are studies that support the possibility that post-ischemia disruption of the basal lamina occurs. This disruption, due primarily to matrix component degradation by proteinases from leukocytes or endothelial cells, could both promote diapedesis and cytokine entry into the vessel wall and contribute to the detachment of endothelial cells by modifying expression of integrin receptors.

Loss of an effective endothelium and basal lamina protective barrier exposes vessel wall cells to a variety of pro-inflammatory agents that can produce cytotoxicity. In addition, there is a second consequence, ie, loss of the paracrine "cross talk" function between the intima and the vessel wall cells. As a general function, the normal endothelium has a modulating role regarding vessel wall cell function and structural expression. Local production of PGI$_2$, NO, cyclic nucleotides, and proteoglycans (heparan sulfate) is critical to the maintenance of normal SMC and fibroblast growth in the arterial vessel walls.[74] As illustrated in Figure 2–6, the vessel walls of the resistance renal vasculature at 48 hours show rare areas of patchy necrosis, intracellular and intercellular fluid accumulation, and early perivas-

cular fibroblast infiltration, all potential consequences of endothelial and leukocyte cytokine effects, as well as loss of normal endothelial modulating influence on smooth muscle cells.

Potentially important changes also are evident in the recovery stage when "fibroblast-like" cells appear in the outer smooth muscle layer and adventitia. Several indicators suggest that, following ischemia-reperfusion, SMCs may shift from their usual adult "contractile" nonproliferative phenotype to a more primitive "synthetic" and proliferative phenotype, which may alter SMC function.[75, 76] These ultrastructural changes could have important implications for resting and stimulated behavior of postischemic vascular beds, but the responsible mechanisms are not yet clear.

VASCULAR DYSFUNCTION IN ISCHEMIC ACUTE RENAL FAILURE

Before discussing the functional aberrations of the renal vasculature, it is well to keep in mind two important points alluded to earlier. First, the detailed observations are derived principally from animal models of renal ischemia and ischemia-reperfusion injury. While there are human data that support the animal findings, they are indirect. Thus, there are uncertainties about the level of identity that can be assumed among species. The second point is that the vascular injury and dysfunction are partial. Not all microvessels undergo the same changes—qualitatively or quantitatively. Thus, the "net" functional disturbances for the whole kidney are generally less than that predicted from descriptions of the most severe pathophysiologic aberrations.

Postischemic abnormalities of the kidney vasculature are of three fundamental types: an increase in basal arterial tone, disordered reactivity to normal mechanical and neurohumoral stimuli, and increased permeability of the peritubular capillary system. These same basic abnormalities of postischemic vascular function are observed in the heart, the brain, and the lung,[77] as well as in the kidney.

Increase in Basal Vascular Tone

Demonstrations of altered basal vascular tone following an ischemic insult are both model and time dependent. Regarding the RAC model in rodents, brief clamp time (less than 1 hr), bilateral rather than unilateral clamping, and prior nephrectomy all tend to attenuate the postischemia reduction in RBF to the extent that increased vascular tone is not considered a factor in the reduction in GFR. On the other hand, reduced RBF following ischemia is increasingly profound and pathophysiologically relevant if renal artery occlusion is longer, more complete, or unilateral in a two-kidney model.[30] In the NE-ARF model in rats, blood flow returns slowly to about 65 percent of normal by 48 hours after 90 minutes of intrarenal norepinephrine infusion and to 85 to 90 percent of normal

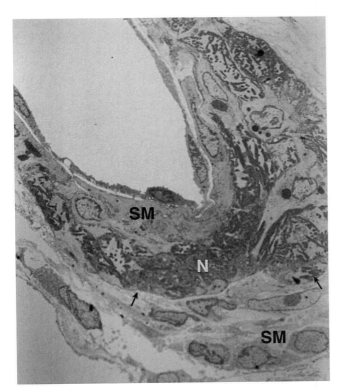

FIGURE 2–6 ■ Necrotic smooth muscle cells (N) in interlobular artery of a NE-ARF kidney at 48 hours. These cells are characterized by loss of nuclei and by aggregates of dense fibrillar material (*arrows*) in a loose cytoplasmic matrix devoid of organelles. A few viable smooth muscle cells (SM) remain. Endothelial cells appear normal. Note the presence of immature fibroblasts in the adventitia. (×2000). (From Conger JD, Robinette JB, Hammond WS: Differences in vascular reactivity in models of ischemic acute renal failure. Kidney Int 1991; 39:1095; with permission.)

by 1 week.[78, 79] As pointed out earlier, in nearly all human studies, using a variety of techniques, there is agreement that there is a 20 to 40 percent reduction in RBF following an ischemic insult sufficient to produce ARF.[53–57] Thus, the bulk of evidence indicates that there is a small to moderate increase in overall tone in the renal microvasculature. Micropuncture measurements of glomerular and periglomerular hemodynamics from the author's laboratory and others, using the RAC- and NE-ARF models, support a uniform decrease in the net glomerular driving pressure for filtration.[49, 80] As pointed out previously, this may be partially the result of an elevated tubular pressure (P_T) and, in part, attributable to a reduced glomerular capillary hydraulic pressure (P_{GC}).

Since it is not possible to examine the basis for a reduced P_{GC} in an in vivo experimental model, the author's laboratory adapted a technique from Edwards[81] that allowed us to isolate individual AAs and EAs from normal and ARF rat kidneys and perfuse them in vitro at physiologic pressure where lumen diameters and SMC cytosolic calcium ($[Ca^{2+}]_i$) could be measured.[82–84] The majority of experiments have been carried out at 48 hours after NE-ARF induction, because this was a time of consistent residual RBF reduction. Mean lumen diameters of both AAs and EAs from NE-ARF kidneys were significantly less than those from sham-ARF kidneys at identical lumen pressures of 80 mm Hg for AAs and 30 mm Hg for EAs, respectively (Fig. 2–7). SMC $[Ca^{2+}]_i$ was higher in AAs and EAs from NE-ARF kidneys,[85] consistent with a higher level of active tone. The addition of antagonists to local physiologic constrictor agonists, including those to AII, TXA_2, PGH_2, and ET-1 did not change the lumen diameter in AAs or EAs, suggesting that at least these agonists were not responsible for the postischemic increase in vascular tone and SMC $[Ca^{2+}]_i$. The potential role of agonists, including catecholamines, adenosine, and PAF, obviously needs to be determined. Another possibility, based on hypoxia studies in pulmonary artery SMCs,[86] is that there is a postischemic Ca^{2+} leak secondary to cell membrane depolarization or injury. The observation that SMC $[Ca^{2+}]_i$ falls rapidly when NE-ARF arterioles are placed in low Ca^{2+} media is consistent with this possibility.[85]

One of the more interesting findings both in vivo and in vitro in the NE-ARF model at 48 hours is

that endothelial nitric oxide synthase (NOS) activity is normal to increased, not decreased, in the renal vasculature.[87] While there is a reduced response to endothelium-dependent dilators such as acetylcholine and bradykinin, the vasoconstrictor response to inhibition of NOS by N(G)-nitro-L-arginine-methyl ester (L-NAME) is increased. By histochemistry, the intensity of staining for vascular constitutive NOS is comparable to, or greater than that of, control vessels, as shown in Figure 2–8. These vessels do show minimal dilator responses to cAMP-dependent PGI_2 but not to the NO donor sodium nitroprusside.[87] Collectively, these findings suggest that NOS activity in this preparation is operating at high intensity with maximal stimulation of dilator pathway guanylate cyclase such that NO agonists and donors have a reduced effect. It could be that this apparent increase in NOS activity acts as a protective counter-regulatory modulator of the response to an underlying vasoconstrictor stimulus produced by ischemia. The stimulus and mechanism of this vasoconstriction are unknown, as noted previously.

Disordered Vasoreactivity

The most significant features of postischemic abnormal reactivity in models of ischemic ARF are loss of RBF autoregulation, hypersensitivity to constrictor agonists, and increased peritubular capillary permeability. The first two defects have the potential for aggravating ischemia in the established phase of the disease.

A now well-described form of abnormal vascular reactivity in models of established ischemic ARF is loss of RBF autoregulation. A number of investigators,[61, 88, 89] including the author's group,[60, 90–92] have found an attenuated autoregulatory response from 2 to 7 days after ARF induction in the RAC model in rats. In the NE-ARF model in rats there was an actual paradoxical vasoconstriction with renal perfusion pressure (RPP) reduction in the autoregulatory range,[60, 92, 93] as shown in Figure 2–9. In the latter model RBF fell by 75 to 80 percent when mean RPP was lowered only from 120 to 90 mm Hg, the lower limit of RBF autoregulation in normal rats.[92] In subsequent studies, it was shown that transient reduction in mean RPP to only 90 mm Hg for 4 hours in rats 1 week after NE-ARF induction resulted in worsening azotemia and recurrent focal

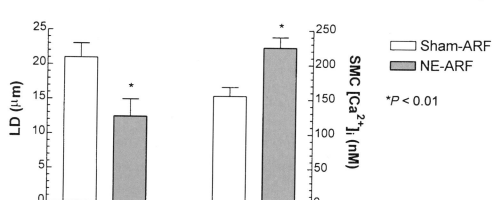

FIGURE 2–7 ▪ In NE-ARF AAs, the mean lumen diameter (LD) is smaller and the mean smooth muscle cell cytosolic calcium (SMC $[Ca^{2+}]_i$) is larger than that in sham-ARF AAs at 48 hours. The results are similar in EAs.

□ Sham-ARF
▨ NE-ARF

*$P < 0.01$

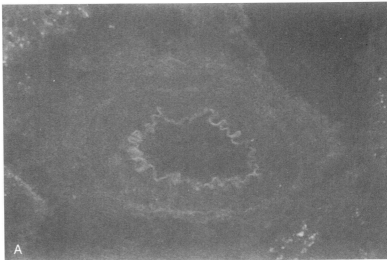

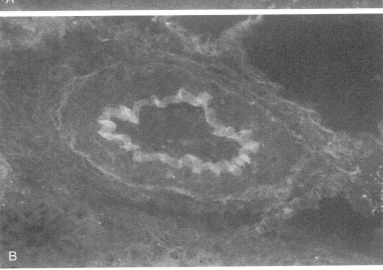

Figure 2–8 ■ Immunofluorescence demonstration of representative sections of distal interlobular arteries incubated with mouse anti-NOS monoclonal antibody. *A,* Anti-NOS in sham-ARF kidney. *B,* anti-NOS in NE-ARF kidney. The intensity of anti-NOS immunofluorescence was at least similar, if not greater, in the endothelium of NE-ARF compared with sham-ARF kidneys. (From Conger JD, Robinette JB, Villar A: Increased nitric oxide synthase activity despite lack of response to endothelium-dependent vasodilators in postischemic acute renal failure. J Clin Invest 1995; 96:636; with permission.)

ischemic injury that prolonged recovery from ARF[91, 93], as shown in group II rats in Figure 2–10. Group III rats with NE-ARF were not subjected to RPP reduction. Group I rats underwent sham-ARF induction, had normal RBF autoregulation, and no measurable effects of 4-hour RPP reduction.

The paradoxical vasoconstriction to a reduction in RPP in the autoregulatory range in NE-ARF kidneys is unexplained. However, there is an interesting correlation observed in the isolated arterioles from these kidneys as illustrated in Figure 2–11. In AAs and EAs from normal kidneys there is an increase in SMC $[Ca^{2+}]_i$ as lumen pressure is increased from 0 to 80 mm Hg in the former and 0 to 30 mm Hg in the latter.[85] This finding is consistent with the development of physiologic myogenic tone. Contrariwise, there are opposite responses in AAs and EAs from 48-hour postischemic kidneys. SMC $[Ca^{2+}]_i$ is elevated at 0 mm Hg lumen pressure and falls as pressure in increased. There is no explanation for this response. However, it is consistent with the paradoxical response to changes in RPP observed in the intact NE-ARF kidney and suggests that the defect is intrinsic to the postischemic microvasculature.

Hypersensitivity to Neurohumoral Agents

The second feature of hypersensitivity in the postischemic vasculature, amplified response to renal nerve stimulation and physiologic constrictor agonists, has been found only in the NE-ARF kidney and not the RAC-ARF kidney. In response to similar frequencies of renal nerve stimulation, there was a significantly greater fall in RBF at 1 week in NE-ARF kidneys.[92] The enhanced sensitivity to renal nerve stimulation could be attenuated by AII and TXA₂ inhibition, which correlated with a reduction in increased norepinephrine release during nerve stimulation in the NE-ARF kidneys.[79]

Infusion of AII and ET-1 produces a significantly greater constrictor response in 48-hour NE-ARF kidneys than in control kidneys.[94] Similar hypersensitivity to AII and ET-1 is found in AAs and EAs isolated from these same kidneys.[22, 85, 94] Interpretation of these data is complicated, since the basal lumen diameters are less in the vessels from the NE-ARF kidneys, indicating a higher basal tone. Smooth muscle cell $[Ca^{2+}]_i$ in these arterioles was increased slightly, but significantly, in the basal state. In response to the median effective

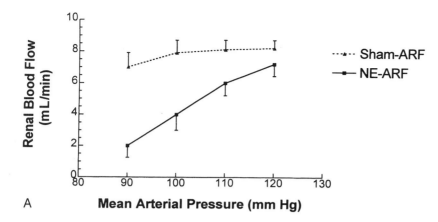

A

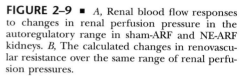

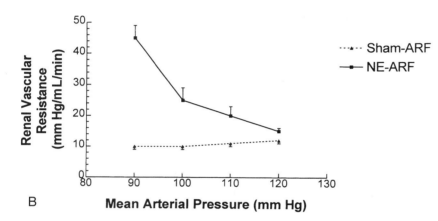

B

FIGURE 2–9 ■ *A,* Renal blood flow responses to changes in renal perfusion pressure in the autoregulatory range in sham-ARF and NE-ARF kidneys. *B,* The calculated changes in renovascular resistance over the same range of renal perfusion pressures.

concentration (EC_{50}) of AII, there was a striking spike-profile increase in SMC $[Ca^{2+}]_i$, suggestive of sarcoplasmic reticulum (SR) mobilization, coupled with near-total constriction.[10] The SMC $[Ca^{2+}]_i$ spikes in AA and EA were reproduced by addition of ryanodine, an SR Ca^{2+} releasing agent. These SMC $[Ca^{2+}]_i$ response patterns were markedly different from those in sham-ARF control arterioles as shown in Figure 2–11. Based on these data from AAs and EAs of 48-hour ARF kidneys, it is attractive to hypothesize that ischemic injury to the vasculature itself results in increased SMC membrane leak of Ca^{2+} which, in turn, is buffered by intracellular organelles, including SR. Agonists that operate, at least in part, through SR Ca^{2+} mobilization, such as AII and ET-1, appear to cause a superphysiologic Ca^{2+} release to the constrictor agonists and an exaggerated constrictor response.

While these studies shed some light, they do not define clear mechanisms underlying the postischemic hypersensitivity of the renal vasculature. The experiments in isolated arterioles do indicate, however, that the basic defects are intrinsic to the vessels and are not the result of systemic or organ parenchymal secondary humoral effects. It also is of interest that postischemic vascular hypersensitivity is found in several vital organs, based on evidence from a variety of models.[77] Thus, it is unlikely that the abnormal vascular reactivity de-

scribed in this section for the kidney is peculiar to the NE-ARF model.

Increased Capillary Permeability

Vascular congestion with RBCs, particularly in the outer medulla following ischemia, has been widely reported in both animals and humans. The dense packing of the erythrocytes and the scarcity of blood plasma around them have been interpreted as a pathologic condition of increased capillary permeability since the study by Mason et al[95] using salicylate and heparin appeared to exclude the possibility of a thrombotic origin. Studies by Hellberg and coworkers[96] and Ojteg and associates,[97] using molecular tracing, confirm that there is increased peritubular capillary permeability following ischemia.

The functional importance of RBC trapping, particularly in the outer medulla, is unclear. Most studies have shown that blood flow in the outer medulla is reduced following ischemia.[95, 98–100] However, blood flow in the inner medulla is increased or unchanged.[96, 101] Reduction in cortical blood could not be correlated with RBC trapping. Mason et al[95] have found that maneuvers that reduce medullary hyperemia, such as increasing postischemia blood pressure

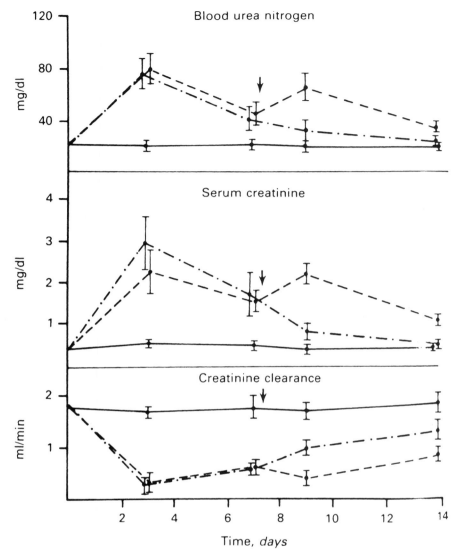

FIGURE 2–10 ■ Effect of hemorrhagic reduction in blood pressure (BP) to 90 mm Hg on blood urea nitrogen (BUN), S_{cr}, and C_{cr} in NE-ARF. Hemorrhagic reduction of BP on day 7 is indicated by the arrow. Hemorrhagic reduction in BP had no effect on renal function in group I (—) sham-infused rats, but in group II (- - -) NE-ARF rats it induced a recurrent rise in BUN and S_{cr} and decrement C_{cr}. Group III (-•-) NE-ARF rats that did not have BP reduction had no recurrent loss of renal function. (Reprinted with permission from Kelleher SP, Robinette JB, Miller F, Conger JD: Effect of hemorrhagic reduction in blood pressure on recovery from acute renal failure. Kidney Int 31:725–730, 1987.)

or using pre-ischemia hemodilution, preserved renal function. On the other hand, Hellberg and coworkers,[102] Bayati and coworkers,[103] and Nygren and coworkers[104] could find little correlation between RBC trapping in the outer medulla and whole kidney RBF and GFR. However, this latter group of investigators has raised questions about the possible long-term effects of secondary hypoxia on the metabolically active outer medulla.

CLINICAL CORRELATES OF VASCULAR FACTORS IN ISCHEMIC ACUTE RENAL FAILURE

It is self-evident that prevention is the key issue when considering the clinical implications of the initiation phase of ischemic ARF. As noted earlier, the likelihood of developing ischemic kidney failure is enhanced not only by the anatomy of the renal vasculature itself but also by a variety of associated risk

factors, including volume depletion, pre-existing renal failure, heart failure, vasoconstrictor hormones or drugs, and elevated body temperature. Awareness of these added risk factors when there is the potential for systemic hypotension or renal hypoperfusion probably could do more to reduce morbidity and mortality than any therapy currently available for established ARF.

There is very little evidence to indicate that any form of treatment is efficacious in reducing the likelihood that renal hypoperfusion will evolve into ischemic ARF. Mannitol or calcium entry blockers may be of value in transplant recipients to prevent primary renal dysfunction.[105] Otherwise, there is neither circumstance nor treatment in which a pharmacologic regimen has been shown to be superior to saline or other modes of volume replacement.[105, 106]

Regarding factors in the early established phase of ischemic ARF, it is difficult to come to any firm conclusions about the clinical importance of increased basal vascular tone. Both the animal data and the human data cited earlier indicate that reduced RBF may play

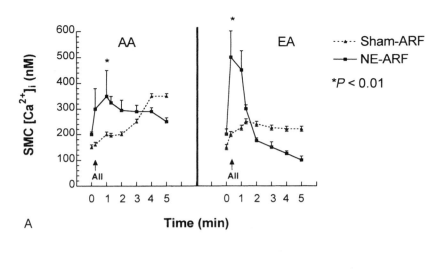

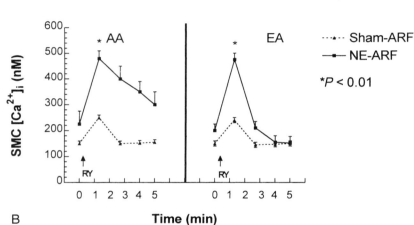

FIGURE 2–11 ■ A, SMC [Ca²⁺]ᵢ responses to bath addition of EC₅₀ AII in isolated perfused AAs and EAs from sham-ARF and NE-ARF rat kidneys. Note that both AAs and EAs from postischemic NE-ARF kidneys have exaggerated spike responses consistent with augmented calcium release from SR.[110] B, Comparatively greater increases in SMC [Ca²⁺]ᵢ are observed in AAs and EAs from NE-ARF than in those from sham-ARF kidneys in response to identical concentrations of ryanodine, an SR calcium-releasing agent.

a partial pathogenetic role in impaired glomerular filtration, but it is not the sole factor. Prior experience with the use of vasodilator agents to improve glomerular perfusion has been of limited benefit in the clinical arena.[106] There may be instances in ischemic ARF in which increased vascular tone plays a major role in the ongoing pathophysiology and vasodilator agents might be of benefit, but it is not possible with current diagnostic capabilities to determine which episodes of ARF may be of this type. Another factor that deserves attention is the mechanism of increased vascular tone in postischemic ARF. From the studies in the author's laboratories on postischemic isolated renal arterioles, it appears that the spontaneous constrictor potency is dramatic when unmasked by NOS inhibition.[22, 85, 94] Until this constrictor mechanism is better understood, common vasodilators that operate through cAMP, cGMP, or calcium entry blockade may not have the targeted capacity to relax these arterioles, as suggested by a recent study examining the lack of effectiveness of atrial natriuretic peptide.[107]

Probably of more relevance are the clinical implications of the altered vascular reactivity in established ischemic ARF. There is a risk of either reducing residual renal function or inducing further renal ischemic injury. For example, the beneficial effect of the systemic administration of pharmacologic agents with vasoconstrictor activity must be weighed against possible deleterious effects on the hypersensitive renal vasculature that may prolong kidney dysfunction. Another consequence of the abnormal vascular reactivity, related to the loss of autoregulation, is the risk of recurrent renal ischemic injury prolonging the course of ARF. Studies by Kelleher and coworkers[91] and Conger and coworkers[93] have shown deleterious effects on kidneys caused by small reductions in RPP in NE-ARF rats. As pointed out earlier, rats with NE-ARF at 1 week that had relatively small reductions in mean arterial pressure had worsening azotemia and prolongation of the course of ARF. Morphology showed fresh ischemic lesions in the kidneys after these modest arterial pressure reductions. The fresh ischemic lesions observed in the NE-ARF model with transient arterial pressure reduction and recurrent azotemia were reminiscent of those described by Solez and coworkers[108] in patients with ARF of longer than three weeks' duration. Taken together, these studies suggest that the postischemic ARF kidney, because of the loss of autoregulation and paradoxical vasoconstriction in response to reduction in arterial pressure, is at risk for recurrent ischemia, as might occur with intermittent hemodialysis, volume depletion, or systemic vasodilators. Measurements by Mann and coworkers[109] suggest that intermittent hemodialysis, when associated with hypotension, may significantly reduce residual renal function in ARF patients. Additional studies are required to determine whether more careful monitoring and support of systemic hemodynamics during dialysis have a positive effect on decreasing the duration of ARF. Unfortunately, studies to date have not been able to address adequately whether continuous-mode dialysis might give better outcomes in these patients.

REFERENCES

1. Kriz W, Kaissling B: Structural Organization of the Mammalian Kidney. In Seldin DW, Giebisch G, eds: *The Kidney: Physiology and Pathophysiology.* New York: Raven Press; 1991:25.
2. Brenner BM, Humes HD: Mechanics of glomerular ultrafiltration. N Engl J Med 1977; 297:197.
3. Farquhar MG: The primary glomerular filtration barrier—basement membrane or epithelial slits? Kidney Int 1975; 8:197.
4. Robertson CR, Deen WM, Troy JL, et al: Dynamics of glomerular ultrafiltration in the rat. III. Hemodynamics and autoregulation. Am J Physiol 1972; 223:1191.
5. Schnermann J: Vascular Tone as a Determinant of Tubuloglomerular Feedback Responsiveness. In: Fernstrom EK, ed: Symposium on the Juxtaglomerular Apparatus. Amsterdam: Elsevier; 1988:393.
6. Hwa JJ, Bevan JA: A nimodipine-resistant Ca^{2+}-resistant Ca^{2+} pathway is involved in myogenic tone in a resistant artery. Am J Physiol 1986; 251:H182.
7. Cabanac M: Keeping a cool head. News Physiol Sciences 1986; 1:41.
8. Laher I, Bevan JA: Stretch of vascular smooth muscle activates tone and $^{45}Ca^{2+}$ influx. Hypertension 1989; 7:S17.
9. Laher I, van Breemen C, Bevan JA: Stretch-dependent calcium uptake associated with myogenic tone in rabbit facial vein. Circ Res 1988; 63:669.
10. Jackson PA, Duling BR: Myogenic response to wall mechanics of arterioles. Am J Physiol 1989; 257:H1147.
11. McCalden TA, Nath RG: Cerebrovascular autoregulation is resistant to calcium channel blockage with nimodipine. Experienta 1989; 45:305.
12. Harris RJ, Banston NM, Symon L, et al: The effects of a calcium antagonist, nimodipine, upon physiologic responses of the cerebral vasculature: its possible influence upon focal cerebral ischaemia. Stroke 1982; 13:759.
13. Pearce WJ, Bevan JA: Diltiazem and autoregulation of canine cerebral blood flow. J Pharmacol Exp Ther 1987; 242:812.
14. Garcia-Roldan JL, Bevan JA: Flow-induced constriction and dilation of cerebral resistance arteries. Circ Res 1990; 66:1445.
15. Bevan JA, Joyce EH: Flow-induced resistance artery tone: a balance between constrictor and dilator mechanisms. Am J Physiol 1990; 258:H663.
16. Bevan JA, Laher I: Pressure- and flow-dependent vascular tone. FASEB J 1991; 5:2267.
17. Joyce EH, Bevan JA: Unique sensitivity of flow-induced changes in tone to extracellular sodium concentrations. FASEB J 1991; 5:A1751.
18. Koller A, Kaley G: Endothelium regulates skeletal muscle microcirculation by a blood flow velocity sensing mechanism. Am J Physiol 1988; 258:H916.
19. Vallance P, Collier J, Moncada S: Effects of endothelium-derived nitric oxide on peripheral arteriolar tone in man. Lancet 1989; 2:997.
20. Tolins JP, Palmer RMJ, Moncada S, et al: Role of endothelium-derived relaxing factor in regulation of renal hemodynamic responses. Am J Physiol 1990; 258:H655.
21. Pohl V, Holtz J, Busse R, et al: Crucial role of the endothelium

22. in the vasodilator response to increased flow in vivo. Hypertension 1986; 8:37.
23. Conger JD, Falk SA: Abnormal vasoreactivity of isolated arteriole from rats with ischemic acute renal failure (ARF). J Am Soc Nephrol 1993; 4:733A.
24. Olsson RA, Bugni WJ: Coronary Circulation. In: Fozzard HA, Haber E, et al, eds: *The Heart and Cardiovascular System.* New York: Raven Press; 1986:987.
25. Kanatsku H, Lamping KG, Eastham CL, et al: Comparison of the effects of increased myocardial oxygen consumption and adenosine on the coronary microvascular resistance. Circ Res 1989; 65:1296.
26. Madden JA: The effect of carbon dioxide on cerebral arteries. Pharmacol Ther 1993; 59:229.
27. Vanelli G, Hussain SNA: Effects of potassium channel blockers on basal vascular tone and reactive hyperemia of canine diaphragm. Am J Physiol 1994; 226:H43.
28. Goetz KL, Wang BC, Madwed JB, et al: Cardiovascular, renal, and endocrine responses to intravenous endothelin in conscious dogs. Am J Physiol 1988; 255:R1064.
29. Spielman WS, Arend LJ: Adenosine receptors and signaling in the kidney. Hypertension 1991; 17:117.
30. Meininger GA, Davis MJ: Cellular mechanisms involved in the vascular myogenic response. Am J Physiol 1992; 263:H647.
31. Yaqoob MM, Alkunaizi AM, Edelstein CL, et al: Acute Renal Failure: Pathogenesis, Diagnosis and Management. In: Schrier RW,ed: *Renal and Electrolyte Disorders.* Philadelphia: Lippincott-Raven; 1997:449.
32. Zager RA, Altschuld R: Body temperature: an important determinant of severity of ischemic injury. Am J Physiol 1986; 251:F87.
33. Zager RA, Gmur DJ, Bredk CR, et al: Degree and time sequence of hypothermic protection against experimental ischemic acute renal failure. Circ Res 1989; 65:1263.
34. Conger JD: The Role of Vasodilatory Substances in Acute Renal Failure. In: Goligorsky MS, Stein JH, eds: *Acute Renal Strategies.* New York: Livingstone; 1995:355.
35. Conger JD, Kim GE, Robinette JB: Effects of angiotensin II, endothelin A, and thromboxane A_2 receptor antagonists on cyclosporin A renal vasoconstriction. Am J Physiol 1994; 267:F443.
36. Kramer HJ, Mohaupt MG, Backer A, et al: Effects of thromboxane A_2 receptor blockade on oliguric ischemic acute renal failure in conscious rats. J Am Soc Nephrol 1993; 4:50.
37. Ishikawa I, Hollenberg NK: Pharmacologic interruption of the renin-angiotensin system in myohemoglobinuric acute renal failure. Kidney Int 1976; 10:S183.
38. Bauereiss K, Hofbauer KG, Konrads A, et al: Effect of saralasin and serum in myohemoglobinuric acute renal failure in rats. Clin Sci Mol Med 1978; 54:555.
39. Chan L, Chittinandana A, Shapiro JI, et al: Effect of an endothelin-receptor antagonist on ischemic acute renal failure. Am J Physiol 1994; 266:F135.
40. Gellai M, Jugus M, Fletcher T, et al: Reversal of postischemic acute renal failure with a selective endothelin A receptor antagonist in the rat. J Clin Invest 1994; 93:900.
41. Iaina A, Solomon S, Eliahou HE: Reduction in severity of acute renal failure in rats by beta-adrenergic blockade. Lancet 1975; 2:158.
42. Solez K, Ideura R, Silva CB, et al: Clonidine after renal ischemia to lessen acute renal failure and microvascular damage. Kidney Int 1980; 18:309.
43. Kelly KJ, Tolkoff-Rubin RH, Williams WW Jr, et al: An oral platelet-activating factor antagonist, Ro-24-4736, protects the rat kidney from ischemic injury. Am J Physiol 1996; 271(5):F1061.
44. Lopez-Novoa JM: Potential role of platelet activating factor in acute renal failure. Kidney Int 1999; 55:1672.
45. Oliver J, MacDowell M, Tracy A: Pathogenesis of acute renal failure associate with traumatic and toxic injury: renal ischemia, nephrotoxic damage and the ischemic episode. J Clin Invest 1951; 30:1305.
46. Biber TUL, Mylle M, Baines AD, et el: A study by micropuncture and microdissection of acute renal damage in rats. Am J Med 1968; 44:664.

46. Bank N, Mutz BF, Aynedjian HS: Role of "leakage" of tubular fluid in anuria due to mercury poisoning. J Clin Invest 1967; 46:695.
47. Oken DE, Arce ML, Wilson DR: Glycerol-induced hemoglobinuric acute renal failure in the rat: I. Micropuncture study of the development of oliguria. J Clin Invest 1966; 45:724.
48. Tanner GA, Sloan KL, Sophasan S: Effects of renal artery occlusion on kidney function in the rat. Kidney Int 1973; 4:377.
49. Conger JD, Robinette JB, Kelleher SP: Nephron heterogeneity in ischemic acute renal failure. Kidney Int 1984; 26:422.
50. Kwon O, Nelson WJ, Sibley R, et al: Backleak, tight junctions and cell-cell adhesion in postischemic injury to the renal allograft. J Clin Invest 1998; 101:2054.
51. Myers BD: Pathogenetic processes in human acute renal failure. Semin Dialysis 1996; 9:144.
52. Alejandro V, Scandling JD, Siblet RK, et al: Mechanisms of filtration failure during postischemic injury of the human kidney: a study of the reperfused renal allograft. J Clin Invest 1995; 95:820.
53. Myers BD, Sommers G, Li K, et al: Determination of blood flow to the transplanted kidney. Transplantation 1994; 10:1445.
54. Corrigan G, Ramaswamy D, Kwon O, et al: PAH extraction and estimation of plasma flow in human postischemic acute renal failure. Am J Physiol 1999; 277:F312–F318.
55. Reubi FC, Gurtler R, Gossweiler N: A dye dilution method of measuring renal blood flow in man with special reference to the anuric subject. Proc Soc Exp Biol Med 1962; 111:760.
56. Hollenberg NK, Birtch A, Rashid A, et al: Relationships between intrarenal perfusion and function: serial hemodynamic studies in the transplanted human kidney. Medicine 1972; 51:95.
57. Hollenberg NK, Epstein M, Rosen SM, et al: Acute oliguric renal failure in man: evidence for preferential renal cortical ischemia. Medicine 1968; 47:455.
58. Alejandro VSJ, Nelson WJ, Huie P, et al: Postischemic injury, delayed function and Na⁺/K⁺-ATPase distribution in the transplanted kidney. Kidney Int 1995; 48:1308.
59. Kwon O, Corrigan G, Myers BD, et al: Sodium reabsorption and distribution of Na⁺/K⁺-ATPase during postischemic injury to the renal allograft. Kidney Int 1999; 55:963.
60. Conger JD, Robinette JB, Hammond WS: Differences in vascular reactivity in models of ischemic acute renal failure. Kidney Int 1991; 39:1087.
61. Matthys E, Patton M, Osgood R, et al: Alterations in vascular function and morphology in ischemic ARF. Kidney Int 1983; 23:717.
62. Terry BE, Jones DB, Mueller CB: Experimental ischemic renal arterial necrosis with resolution. Am J Pathol 1970; 58:69.
63. Lefer AM. Physiologic and pathophysiologic role of cyclo-oxygenase metabolites of arachidonic acid in circulating disease states. Cardiovasc Clin 1987; 18:85.
64. Lefer AM, Lefer DJ: Pharmacology of the endothelium in ischemia-reperfusion and circulatory shock. Annu Rev Pharmacol Toxicol 1993; 33:71.
65. Pober JS, Contran RS: Cytokinases and endothelial cell biology. Physiol Rev 1990; 70:427.
66. Pomfy M, Huska J: The state of the microcirculatory bed after total ischaemia of the brain. Funct Dev Morphol 1992; 2:253.
67. VanBenthuysen KM, McMurty IF, Horwitz LD: Reperfusion after acute coronary occlusion in dogs impairs endothelium-dependent relaxation to acetylcholine and augments contractile reactivity in vitro. J Clin Invest 1987; 76:265.
68. Conger JD, Hammond WS: Renal vasculature and ischemic injury. Renal Failure 1992; 14:307.
69. Defilippi P, Van Hinsbergh V, Bertolotto A, et al: Differential distribution and modulation of expression of alpha 1/beta 1 integrin on human endothelial cells. J Cell Biol 1991; 114:855.
70. Ojteg G, Nygren K, Wolgast M: Permeability of renal capillaries. II. Transport of neutral and charged protein molecular probes. Acta Physiol Scand 1986; 129:287.
71. Walker PD, Kaushal GP, Shah SV: Presence of a distinct extracellular matrix–degrading metalloproteinase activity in renal tubules. J Am Soc Nephrol 1994; 5:55–61.
72. Walker PD, Kaushal GP, Shah SV: Presence of a distinct extra-

73. cellular matrix-degrading metalloproteinase activity in renal tubules. J Am Soc Nephrol 1994; 5:55–61.
73. Humes HD, Nakamura T, Cieslinski DA, et al: Role of proteoglycans and cytoskeleton in the effects of TGF-β1 on renal proximal tubule cells. Kidney Int 1993; 43:575.
74. De Mey JGR, Schifferes PM: Effects of the endothelium on growth responses in arteries. J Cardiovasc Pharmacol 1993; 21:S22.
75. Glukhova MA, Kabakov AE, Frid MG, et al: Modulation of human aorta smooth muscle cell phenotype: a study of muscle-specific variants of vinculin, caldesmon, and actin expression. Proc Natl Acad Sci USA 1988; 85:9542.
76. Newcomb PM, Herman IM: Pericyte growth and contractile phenotype: modulation by endothelial-synthesized matrix and comparison with aortic smooth muscle. J Cell Physiol 1993; 155:385.
77. Conger JD, Weil JV: Abnormal vascular function following ischemia-reperfusion injury. J Invest Med 1995; 43:431.
78. Conger JD, Robinette JB: Effects of acetylcholine on postischemic acute renal failure. Kidney Int 1981; 19:399.
79. Robinette JB, Conger JD: The roles of angiotensin II and thromboxanes in the hypersensitivity to renal nerve stimulation in acute renal failure. J Clin Invest 1990; 86:1532.
80. Finn WF, Arendshorst WJ, Gottschalk CW: Pathogenesis of oliguria in acute renal failure. Circ Res 1975; 36:675.
81. Edwards RM: Segmental effects of norepinephrine and angiotensin II on isolated renal microvessels. Am J Physiol 1983; 244(13):F526.
82. Yuan BH, Conger JD: Effects of angiotensin II and norepinephrine on isolated rat afferent and efferent arterioles. Am J Physiol 1990; 258:F741.
83. Lanese DM, Yaun BH, Conger JD: The effects of AP III on the isolated afferent and efferent arterioles of the rat kidney. Am J Physiol 1991; 261:F1102.
84. Conger JD< Falk SA, Robinette JB: Angiotensin II–induced changes in smooth muscle calcium in isolated renal arterioles. J Am Soc Nephrol 1993; 3:1792.
85. Conger JD, Falk SA, Robinette JB: Cytosolic smooth muscle calcium [Ca²⁺]ᵢ kinetics in the 48-hr postischemic renal vasculature. J Am Soc Nephrol 1994; 5:895A.
86. Salvaterra CG, Goldman WF: Acute hypoxia increases cytosolic calcium in cultured pulmonary arterial myocytes. Am J Physiol 1993; 264:L323.
87. Conger JD, Shultz P, Raij L, et al: Increased NOS activity despite lack of response to endothelium-dependent vasodilators in postischemic acute renal failure in rats. J Clin Invest 1995; 96:631.
88. Adams PL, Admas PF, Bell PD, et al: Impaired renal blood flow autoregulation in ischemic acute renal failure. Kidney Int 1980; 18:68.
89. Williams RH, Thomas CE, Navar LG, et al: Hemodynamic and single nephron function during maintenance phase of ischemic acute renal failure in the dog. Kidney Int 1981; 19:503.
90. Conger JD: The role of blood flow autoregulation in pathophysiology in acute renal failure. Circ Shock 1983; 11:235.
91. Kelleher SP, Robinette JB, Miller F, et al: Effect of hemorrhagic reduction in blood pressure on recovery from acute renal failure. Kidney Int 1987; 31:725.
92. Kelleher SP, Robinette JB, Conger JD: Sympathetic nervous system in the loss of autoregulation in acute renal failure. Am J Physiol 1984; 15:F379.
93. Conger JD, Schultz MF, Miller F, et al: Responses to hemorrhagic arterial pressure reduction in different ischemic renal failure models. Kidney Int 1994;46:318.
94. Conger JD: Unpublished observations.
95. Mason J, Welsch J, Torhorst J: The contribution of vascular obstruction to the functional defect that follows renal ischemia. Kidney Int 1987; 31:65.
96. Hellberg POA, Kallskog O, Wolgast M: Red cell trapping and postischemic renal blood flow: differences between the cortex, outer and inner medulla. Kidney Int 1991; 40:625.
97. Ojteg G, Nygren K, Wolgast M: Permeability of renal capillaries. I. Preparation of neutral and charged protein probes. Acta Physiol Scand 1986; 129:277.
98. Karlberg L, Ojteg G, Norlen BJ, et al: Impaired medullary

circulation in post ischemic renal failure. Acta Physiol Scand 1981; 118:11.

99. Vetterlein F, Prthho A, Schmidt G: Distribution of capillary blood flow in the renal kidney during postischemic renal failure. Am J Physiol 1986; 251:H510.

100. Karlberg L, Norlen BJ, Ojteg G, et al: Impaired medullary circulation in postischemic acute renal failure. Acta Physiol Scand 1983; 118:11.

101. Hellberg O, Bayati A, Kallskog O, et al: Red cell trapping after ischemia and long-term kidney damage: influence of hematocrit. Kidney Int 1990; 37:1240.

102. Hellberg O, Nygren A, Hansell P, et al: Postischemic administration of hyperosmolar mannitol enhances erythrocyte trapping in outer medullary vasculature in the rat kidney. Renal Physiol 1990; 13:328.

103. Bayati A, Hellberg O, Odlind B, et al: Prevention of acute renal failure with superoxide dismutase and sucrose. Acta Physiol Scand 1981; 130:367.

104. Nygren A, Hansell P, Hellberg I, et al: Red Cell Congestion in Renal Microvasculature Induced by Low Osmolar Contrast Media and Mannitol. In: Contrast Media and Regional Blood Flow. 1981:1.

105. Conger JD: Interventions in clinical acute renal failure—what are the data? Am J Kidney Dis 1995; 26:565.

106. Conger JD: Drug therapy in acute renal failure. In Lazarus JM, Brenner BM,eds: Acute Renal Failure. New York: Churchill-Livingstone; 1993:527.

107. Vinot O, Bialek J, Canaan-kuhl S, et al: Endogenous ANP in postischemic acute renal allograft failure. Am J Physiol 1995; 269:F125.

108. Solez L, Morel-Maroger L, Sraer J: The morphology of acute tubular necrosis in man: Analysis of 57 renal biopsies and comparison with glycerol model. Medicine 1979; 58:362.

109. Manns M, Sigler MH, Teehan BP: Intradialytic renal haemodynamics—potential consequences for the management of the patient with acute renal failure. Nephrol Dial Transplant 1997; 12:870.

110. Conger J, Falk S: KCl and angiotensin responses in isolated rat renal arterioles: effects of diltiazem and low-calcium medium. Am J Physiol 1993; 264:F134.

CHAPTER **3**

Terminal Pathways to Cell Death

Jerrold S. Levine ▪ Wilfred Lieberthal

INTRODUCTION

Acute tubular necrosis (ATN) is the term conventionally used in clinical practice to identify the form of acute renal failure (ARF) that results from acute ischemic or toxic injury to the kidney. While this term is accurate in identifying renal tubular cells as the major target of injury in this disease, the term is misleading in that it suggests that necrosis is the predominant manifestation of tubular cell injury.[1] In response to injury, the renal tubular cell can suffer a number of fates other than necrosis.[2] The evidence demonstrating a role for sublethal, reversible injury to tubular cells in the pathophysiology of ATN is now substantial (see Chapter 8). In addition, once lethally injured, tubular cell death can occur by two distinct mechanisms, apoptosis or necrosis. There is increasing evidence that apoptosis of renal tubular cells plays an important role in the tubular cell loss associated with ARF.[3]

Overview of the Morphologic Differences Between Necrosis and Apoptosis

Necrosis and apoptosis have their own characteristic and distinct morphologic features (Table 3–1). In the early stages of necrosis, cells become swollen because of an accumulation of sodium and water within the cytosol. Next, the mitochondria develop marked morphologic abnormalities, becoming enlarged with loss of the normal folding of the mitochondrial cristae. Eventually, the plasma membrane loses functional and structural integrity. In the final stages of necrosis, plasma membrane injury becomes so severe that there is leakage of cytosolic contents from the cell. The resulting injury and inflammation to surrounding tissues is a characteristic feature of necrosis[2, 3] (see Table 3–1).

In contrast to necrosis, cells undergoing apoptosis become smaller as the result of a reduction in cytosolic volume and condensation of nuclear chromatin[4–6] (see Table 3–1). In parallel with the decrease in cell volume, apoptotic cells lose cell-cell and cell-matrix adhesion early on and round up into a spherical shape. Simultaneously, they begin a process of plasma membrane blebbing.[7] On time-lapse video microscopy, the cell membrane appears to bubble, with small blebs protruding and then retracting from the cell surface.[7] This process eventually leads to fragmentation of the cell into apoptotic bodies, which are membrane-enclosed vesicles containing nuclear fragments of condensed chromatin and cytosolic organelles such as mitochondria.[2, 3, 5] Apoptotic bodies, like intact apoptotic cells, are rapidly ingested by phagocytes.[2, 3] It should be stressed that throughout this process the organelles within apoptotic bodies retain a virtually normal mor-

TABLE 3–1. Morphologic Differences Between Apoptosis and Necrosis

MORPHOLOGIC FEATURE	APOPTOSIS	NECROSIS
Cell size	Decreased	Increased ("oncosis")
Plasma membrane integrity	Relatively normal (trypan blue–impermeable)	Absent (trypan blue–permeable)
Plasma membrane "blebbing"	Characteristic	Absent
Mitochondria	Normal appearance	Swollen, distorted cristae
Cell-cell adhesion	Lost early	Remains relatively intact
Cell-matrix adhesion	Lost early	Lost late
Exfoliation	Early (as single cells)	Late (as sheets of cells)
Chromatin condensation and nuclear fragmentation	Characteristic	Absent
Nuclear morphology (Hoechst staining)	Homogeneous intense fluorescence, absence of nucleoli	Relatively normal
Nuclear morphology (electron microscopy)	Collapse of chromatin into one or more electron-dense masses	Disintegration of chromatin without electron-dense masses
Release of cytosolic contents	Absent	Characteristic
Pattern of cell death in tissue	Individual scattered cells dying asynchronously	Groups of contiguous cells dying together
Tissue inflammation	Absent	Characteristic
Apoptotic bodies*	Characteristic	Absent
Phagocytosis of dying cells	Characteristic	Absent

*Plasma membrane shedding of apoptotic bodies leads to the disintegration of the cell into multiple plasma membrane-bound "apoptotic bodies" that contain fragments of condensed chromatin, cytosol, and subcellular organelles.

30

phology and that the integrity of the plasma membrane of apoptotic cells and bodies is preserved. As a result, cells dying by apoptosis do not release their cytosolic contents into the extracellular space and do not cause surrounding tissue injury or inflammation (see Table 3–1).

Both the absence of surrounding injury and the rapid clearance of apoptotic cells by phagocytosis account for the difficulty in identifying apoptotic cells in tissue samples. For these reasons, the quantification of apoptosis in tissues may require examination of several thousand cells. Even if a fraction of a percent of the cells in a section of tissue are identified as apoptotic, the overall cellular loss caused by apoptosis occurring over a few hours or days may still be substantial.[8, 9] The inconspicuous nature of apoptosis in tissue sections probably accounts for the fact that its importance in ischemic and toxic injury was not recognized until relatively recently.[8, 9]

Mitochondrial Dysfunction: The "Common Denominator" of Both Apoptosis and Necrosis

Apoptosis and necrosis differ from each other not only in their morphology but also in the biochemical pathways that lead to each form of cell death. Nevertheless, it is crucial to appreciate that apoptosis and necrosis do have one thing in common: both forms of cell death are initiated by changes in mitochondrial function.[10, 11]

Necrosis is usually the result of overwhelming cellular injury that causes severe mitochondrial dysfunction and impaired oxidative phosphorylation. The resultant severe depletion of cellular adenosine 5'-triphosphate (ATP) stores leads to the general metabolic "collapse" of the cell. Thus, necrosis, sometimes referred to as "accidental" death, is the combined result of a multitude of injurious biochemical events that are the consequences of ATP depletion (Fig. 3–1). By contrast, apoptosis, or "cell suicide," is an ATP-requiring process that proceeds in an orderly, genetically determined manner. Mitochondria play two roles in apoptosis. First, they provide the ATP necessary to fuel the energy-dependent biochemical events mediating apoptosis.[10] Second, mitochondria release a number of specific molecules into the cytosol that activate the biochemical pathways leading to apoptosis.[10, 11]

In this chapter, the distinct biochemical pathways that mediate necrosis and apoptosis are described, as well as how the morphologic features of each form of cell death are determined by these pathways. The fundamental role of mitochondria in initiating both forms of cell death is also discussed. Finally, the evidence indicating that both necrosis and apoptosis represent important mechanisms of renal tubular cell loss following ischemic or toxic injury to the kidney is presented, and the speculation regarding the potential clinical significance of these two forms of cell death in ARF is also presented.

CELL BIOLOGY OF NECROSIS

Cellular necrosis results from the combined deleterious effects of a number of biochemical pathways that are simultaneously precipitated by extremely severe injury to the cell. In contrast, although apoptosis is often precipitated by the same injurious stimuli as is necrosis, apoptosis is ultimately mediated by an organized, genetically predetermined final common pathway. Thus, necrosis and apoptosis differ fundamentally from each other not only morphologically but also biochemically.[2, 3] The multiple biochemical pathways that are activated by severe cell injury and lead to cell necrosis include all of the following: severe depletion of cell energy stores; an increase in cytosolic free calcium; the generation of reactive oxygen species (ROS); and the activation of multiple enzymes, including phospholipases, proteases, and endonucleases (see Fig. 3–1).

Adenosine 5'-Triphosphate (ATP) Depletion

When necrosis is caused by a severe deficiency of oxygen (due to ischemia, hypoxia, or anoxia), a fall in the level of cell adenosine 5'-triphosphate (ATP) stores is the proximate event leading to cell necrosis. When cells are subjected to cytotoxic injury, such as oxidant stress, the initial damage may not be ATP depletion, but rather injury to cellular components such as cell membranes and proteins. However, these cytotoxic events rapidly lead to mitochondrial injury, so that depletion of cell ATP stores ultimately occurs as a secondary event. Therefore, whether as the result of oxygen deprivation or cytotoxic injury, profound depletion of energy stores is a fundamental pathophysiologic event leading to necrosis[1, 12] (see Fig. 3–1).

Oxygen deprivation results in the rapid degradation of available ATP to adenosine 5'-diphosphate (ADP) and adenosine 5'-monophosphate (AMP). Restoration of oxygen before AMP is further metabolized allows rapid resynthesis of ATP. However, if ischemia is prolonged, AMP is further metabolized to nucleosides (adenosine and inosine) and hypoxanthine. These purine metabolites are then able to diffuse passively from the cell. As a result, metabolites that serve as a reservoir for the rapid resynthesis of ATP during reperfusion become depleted.[1, 13] Under such circumstances of prolonged ischemia, restitution of cell ATP requires de novo synthesis of ATP from nonpurine precursors. As this process itself requires a substantial amount of energy, de novo synthesis probably does not play much of a role in the recovery of ATP after ischemia. Prolonged ischemia also ultimately results in an irreversible loss of mitochondrial function, further impairing rapid regeneration of ATP following reperfusion. Thus, the rate of recovery of cell ATP following reperfusion and, consequently, the ability of the cell to survive ischemia are dependent upon the duration of the ischemic period.[12, 13] The beneficial effect of maintaining stores of adenosine and adenosine nucleotides within cells subjected to ischemia has been shown

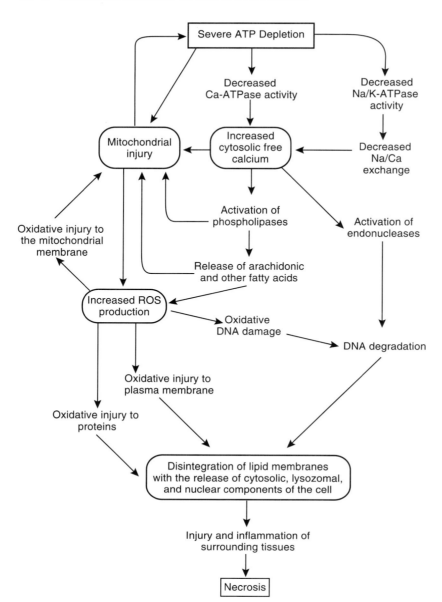

FIGURE 3–1 ■ Biochemical pathways leading to necrosis. Severe depletion of cell ATP stores results in a number of diverse and uncoordinated biochemical events that act in an additive fashion to cause necrosis (see text for details).

by studies in which inhibitors of nucleotide metabolism such as 5'-nucleotidase (which catalyzes the dephosphorylation of AMP to adenosine)[14] and adenosine deaminase (which catalyzes the metabolism of adenosine to inosine)[15] were both able to ameliorate ischemic injury.

The three most important factors that determine the sensitivity of individual renal tubular cells to ischemic renal injury are the cell's energy requirements, its glycolytic capacity, and the severity of the hypoxia to which the cell is exposed.[16, 17] ATP can be generated via both glycolysis and oxidative phosphorylation. Cells that have a high glycolytic capacity are generally less sensitive to oxygen deprivation than are cells that depend predominantly or exclusively on mitochondrial respiration. It is therefore not surprising that the proximal tubule, which depends largely on mitochondrial respiration for its energy supply,[18] is generally more susceptible to ATP depletion and ischemic renal injury

than are more distal nephrons.[17] Another important factor that determines the severity of cell injury is the degree of hypoxia to which cells are subjected following ischemia. Oxygen tensions vary widely within different regions of the kidney following ischemia, with the medulla becoming far more hypoxic than the cortex.[16] This probably explains the observation that the medullary straight portion of the proximal tubule (pars recta), which has more glycolytic capacity than the cortical segments of the proximal tubule, is more sensitive than cortical segments to ischemic injury in vivo but more resistant than cortical segments to injury when isolated tubular segments are subjected to hypoxia in vitro.[17] Another determinant of ischemic injury is the amount of energy that tubular cells require for transport activity.[19] While the inner medulla becomes far more hypoxic than the outer medulla after ischemia-reperfusion, the tubular segments within the inner medulla suffer little injury in response to renal ischemia, probably because of their low energy requirements for transport in this region. Thus, the more prominent injury to the pars recta in experimental models of ARF is likely due to the combined effects of persistent hypoperfusion, medullary hypoxia, and the high energy requirements of this tubular segment.[17, 20]

Cell Swelling

In the presence of adequate energy stores, the Na^+,K^+-ATPase actively extrudes sodium from the cell. Loss of intracellular chloride, to which cells are highly permeable, is also indirectly the result of Na^+, K^+-ATPase activity; the active pumping of sodium from the cell causes a negative intracellular potential, which leads to passive movement of chloride from the cytosol. The resultant accumulation of sodium, chloride, and water within the cell is initially offset by diffusion of potassium out of the cell. However, continued accumulation of sodium, chloride, and water within the cytosol leads to cell swelling, or "oncosis." Oncosis is an early and typical morphologic feature of necrosis and one of the many morphologic features that distinguishes necrosis from apoptosis, in which a reduction in cytosolic volume and cell size occurs[1, 12] (see Table 3–1).

Increased Intracellular Free Calcium

Substantial evidence now suggests that an increase in the concentration of cytosolic free ionized calcium ($[Ca]_i$) plays an important role in necrosis.[21] When renal tubular cells are exposed to hypoxia, $[Ca]_i$ increases from its normal value of $\sim$100 nM to >500 nM within 5 minutes.[12, 22, 23] With more prolonged oxygen deprivation, $[Ca]_i$ can increase further into the low micromolar range.[12] The increase in $[Ca]_i$ associated with ATP depletion precedes lethal cell injury and is reversible if oxygen supply is restored before necrosis occurs.[12, 22, 23]

Like the accumulation of intracellular sodium, the increase in $[Ca]_i$ that occurs in response to hypoxia is the result of depletion of energy stores. $[Ca]_i$ requires tight regulation because the concentration of calcium in extracellular fluid exceeds the intracellular concentration by approximately 10,000-fold. This steep gradient is maintained by a number of mechanisms. A calcium ATPase, localized in the plasma membrane, pumps calcium from the cytosol into the extracellular space. A second calcium ATPase, present in the membrane of the endoplasmic reticulum (ER), pumps calcium from the cytosol into the ER.[12] In addition to these two calcium ATPases, a sodium/calcium exchanger, present in the basolateral membrane of tubular cells, provides another important route for extrusion of calcium. While sodium/calcium exchange is a passive process, it depends indirectly on an adequate supply of energy, because Na^+,K^+-ATPase is required for pumping sodium from the cell and maintaining the sodium gradient needed by the sodium/calcium exchanger. Thus, depletion of cell energy stores impairs all three available transport mechanisms responsible for maintenance of a normal $[Ca]_i$ level.[12]

The evidence that increased $[Ca]_i$ contributes to cell injury comes from multiple sources. Hypoxic injury to renal tubular cells can be reduced by removal of extracellular calcium.[21] Chelation of intracellular calcium, which attenuates the rise in $[Ca]_i$ associated with hypoxia, also ameliorates injury.[23] Finally, calcium channel blockers ameliorate injury in experimental ischemic injury both in vivo[24] and in vitro.[12] Importantly, the administration of calcium channel blockers has been shown to ameliorate ischemic renal failure in humans. These agents reduce the incidence of ARF immediately following cadaveric kidney transplant if they are given to both the recipient and the donor.[25] However, the mechanism or mechanisms by which calcium channel blockers protect against ARF remains unclear and may not solely relate to a reduction of $[Ca]_i$. In addition to improving renal blood flow, calcium channel blockers may also have effects on cell function independent of their effect on $[Ca]_i$.[12] Nonetheless, when evaluated in aggregate, the evidence that an increase in $[Ca]_i$ is an important event in the evolution of renal cell necrosis remains convincing.

There are several potential mechanisms by which an increase in $[Ca]_i$ may contribute to cell injury. Calcium activates a number of enzymes, including phospholipases, proteases, and endonucleases,[21] all of which probably contribute to cell necrosis (see Fig. 3–1). Increased $[Ca]_i$ can also directly injure mitochondria. When the $[Ca]_i$ level exceeds 400 nM, the calcium uptake capacity of the ER becomes saturated. A $[Ca]_i$ level >400 nM is buffered by mitochondria via a calcium uniporter present in the inner mitochondrial membrane.[12] Mitochondrial overload of calcium results in uncoupling of oxidative phosphorylation, which has two adverse effects. The first effect is impaired production of ATP, thereby exacerbating the primary depletion in cell ATP stores and setting up a vicious cycle[12] (see Fig. 3–1). The second effect of uncoupling oxidative phosphorylation is the release of superoxide. Mitochondria are but one of many sources of superoxide during and following injury and thus contribute to oxidant injury of the cell[26] (see Fig. 3–1).

Phospholipase Activation

Phospholipases are enzymes that hydrolyze phospholipids and can be divided into two distinct classes. Acyl hydrolases release fatty acids from the phospholipid backbone. Phospholipase A_1 (PLA_1) acts at the sn-1-acyl ester bond, PLA_2 at the sn-2 position, and PLB at both the sn-1 and the sn-2 positions. The second class of phospholipases includes phosphodiesterases, among which are PLC (which cleaves the glycerolphosphate bond) and PLD (which removes the alcohol head group from phospholipids).[27] The activation of multiple phospholipases is a characteristic feature of ischemic cell injury.[27]

The observed increase in cell diacylglycerol and phosphatidic acid associated with ATP depletion is indirect evidence of activation of PLC and PLD.[28] Elevations in the levels of all classes of free fatty acids[28] are consistent with a generalized disruption of lipid metabolism. The equimolar release of lysophospholipid together with fatty acids[28] suggests that PLA_2 accounts for most of the free fatty acids released in association with ATP depletion.[12, 28] Deficiency of ATP may further exacerbate the accumulation of fatty acids and other lipid metabolites within the cytosol, because both reacylation of fatty acids into phospholipid and de novo synthesis of phospholipids are energy-dependent processes.[12]

Several isoforms of PLA_2, both calcium-dependent[29] and calcium-independent,[30] have been demonstrated in cytosolic, mitochondrial, and microsomal fractions of rat kidneys. Ischemia-reperfusion results in activation of both classes of PLA_2.[30, 31] PLA_2 activation is an important mediator of ischemic injury to brain, heart, intestine, and kidney.[12, 32, 33] Activation of PLA_2 and other phospholipases contributes to cell injury and necrosis in a number of ways. Plasma membrane degradation by phospholipases leads to the early loss of plasma membrane integrity and increased permeability that is characteristic of necrosis (see Fig. 3–1). In addition, the release of arachidonic acid, the predominant fatty acid released by PLA_2, can independently exacerbate cell injury in a number of ways. Arachidonic acid directly compromises oxidative phosphorylation, thereby worsening cellular depletion of ATP stores.[34] Arachidonic acid also impairs Na^+,K^+-ATPase activity.[35] Arachidonic acid is the essential precursor of a number of metabolites, such as thromboxanes, leukotrienes, and platelet-activating factor (PAF), all of which can exacerbate ischemia by their vasoconstrictor and proinflammatory activity.[36, 37] Finally, the enzymatic conversion of arachidonic acid to some of its metabolites leads to the release of superoxide as a byproduct that can then contribute to oxidant injury (see Chapters 4 and 5 by Shah and Nath, respectively).

While activation of PLA_2 appears to play an important role in cell injury, there is also some evidence suggesting a protective role for PLA_2. Zager and colleagues[38, 39] have demonstrated that exposure of isolated proximal tubules to exogenous PLA_2 protects renal tubular cells from hypoxic injury. However, both the mechanism underlying this protective effect of PLA_2 and the relevance of exposing tubular cells to exogenous PLA_2 remain uncertain. Finally, a specific class of phospholipids called plasmalogens that have a vinyl-ether group instead of a fatty acid at the sn-1 position have been shown to protect cells from ischemic injury, possibly by acting as scavengers of oxygen radicals.[40]

Protease Activation

Lysosomal proteases such as cathepsin B and L do not appear to play an important role in necrotic cell death.[41, 42] However, activation of calpain, a nonlysosomal calcium-dependent neutral cysteine protease, does appear to contribute to cell necrosis. Calpain

regulates multiple intracellular events, including membrane channel activity, membrane receptor function, kinase activation (eg, protein kinase C), and interactions between cytoskeletal proteins. Calpain is activated following hypoxic and toxic stress in renal tubular cells, and inhibitors of calpain ameliorate necrosis induced by hypoxia[42, 43] (see Fig. 3–1).

Increased $[Ca]_i$ also activates a calmodulin-dependent protease that alters the enzymatic activity of xanthine dehydrogenase by converting it to xanthine oxidase.[44] Xanthine dehydrogenase and xanthine oxidase both convert hypoxanthine (a metabolite of purine nucleotides) to xanthine. However, xanthine oxidase, unlike xanthine dehydrogenase, generates superoxide that can contribute to oxidant injury following ischemia-reperfusion[1, 44] (see Fig. 3–1).

Dong and coworkers[45] have described the activation of a calcium-dependent serine protease that activates an endonuclease or endonucleases that appear to be partly responsible for the DNA degradation that occurs in necrosis (discussed later).

Caspases, a distinct family of cysteine proteases that play a central role in the execution phase of apoptosis, are discussed in detail later.[6, 8, 46] The role of caspases in necrosis, if any, remains uncertain.

Endonuclease Activation

Extensive and random degradation of nuclear DNA is a typical feature of advanced necrosis and produces a "smear" of low-molecular-weight DNA fragments in electrophoretic gels.[2] By contrast, apoptosis leads to the cleavage of DNA between nucleosomes and results in a "ladder" pattern on gel electrophoresis.

A nucleosomal form of DNA degradation has been described in necrosis of renal tubular cells.[45, 47] Interestingly, the endonuclease activation and nucleosomal DNA cleavage associated with necrosis is not due to caspases (as is the case in apoptosis), but rather to the activation of a calcium-dependent serine protease. The results of Dong and coworkers[45] suggest a novel pathway of endonuclease activation during necrosis that occurs after the loss of plasma membrane integrity but precedes the random DNA fragmentation associated with the terminal stages of necrosis. These studies are important from a practical point of view because they suggest that DNA laddering, long regarded as a specific marker of apoptosis, may not completely discriminate between these two forms of cell death.[45]

Oxidant Injury, Nitric Oxide, and Peroxynitrite

The role of oxidant stress in ischemic and toxic injury to renal tubular cells is discussed in detail in Chapters 4 and 5. Some of the numerous potential sources of superoxide generation following tubular cell injury, including xanthine oxidase, cyclooxygenase activity, and injured mitochondria, have been discussed previously. Superoxide is converted to hydrogen peroxide by superoxide dismutase. Hydrogen peroxide is in turn converted to the highly reactive hydroxyl radical by a reaction that requires catalytic "free" iron.[48] The role of superoxide, hydrogen peroxide, free iron, and the hydroxyl radical in cell injury is discussed in detail in Chapters 4 and 5 by Shah and Nath, respectively.

It is important to recognize recent evidence demonstrating that superoxide, by reacting with nitric oxide (NO), can be the precursor of another reactive species, distinct from the hydroxyl radical, called peroxynitrite. An important difference between peroxynitrite and the hydroxyl radical is that generation of peroxynitrite does not require the presence of catalytic "free" iron.[48] Peroxynitrite, like the hydroxyl radical, can induce oxidant injury to all cellular components. Furthermore, peroxynitrite can contribute to protein dysfunction by nitrosylating tyrosine residues.[41, 48] A number of studies have shown a role for increased production of NO and peroxynitrite in the necrosis of tubular cells exposed to hypoxia and to cytotoxic stimuli.[49, 50] Studies in knockout mice lacking either constitutive nitric oxide synthase (cNOS), inducible NOS (iNOS), or neuronal NOS (nNOS) suggest that activation of iNOS is the major source of NO production by tubular cells during hypoxia[51] (see Fig. 3–1).

CELL BIOLOGY OF APOPTOSIS

Causes of Apoptosis

Apoptosis occurs in response to a wide variety of stimuli. These may conveniently be grouped into five broad categories: embryo apoptosis (programmed cell death), receptor-mediated apoptosis, loss of "survival factors," cytotoxic stimuli, and DNA damage. It should be stressed that all nucleated mammalian cells appear to express constitutively the machinery needed to undergo apoptosis and that once induced, irrespective of the trigger, the morphologic features of apoptosis are remarkably similar, if not universal, for all cell types.

PROGRAMMED CELL DEATH

Apoptosis during embryo development involves two distinct genetically mediated events, one that determines the time of onset of apoptosis and a second that carries out the death program itself. Programmed cell death (PCD) is essential for normal renal development. However, once embryogenesis is complete, PCD plays little if any role in renal disease and is not involved in ARF.[2]

RECEPTOR-MEDIATED APOPTOSIS

Nearly all cells possess membrane receptors whose engagement can induce apoptosis. The best characterized receptor family of this type is the tumor necrosis factor (TNF) receptor superfamily, of which Fas (CD95) is the most prominent member.[52] Engagement of Fas by its ligand (FasL), or the type I TNF receptor (TNF-R1) by TNF-α, leads to apoptosis of the target cell. Receptor-mediated apoptosis is not limited to soluble ligands. Cytotoxic T lymphocytes (CTL) and natural killer (NK) cells also rely on receptor-triggered events to induce apoptosis in their target cells.[53] This occurs via one of two mechanisms. The first is Fas-dependent and entails interaction of FasL on the CTL or NK cell with Fas on the target cell. In the second mechanism, which is independent of Fas, apoptosis is induced via injection of serine proteases called granzymes into target cells by CTL. CTL and NK cells create pores in their target cells, through which to inject granzymes, by the release of perforin. The list of receptors whose engagement induces apoptosis expands each year.[54] Additional examples of physiologic ligands with potential relevance for renal epithelial cells include glucocorticoids, which induce apoptosis of thymocytes, transforming growth factor-β (TGF-β), which induces apoptosis in a number of epithelial cell lines, and angiotensin II, which induces apoptosis of rat cardiomyocytes via the AT2 receptor.[2]

An interesting paradigm for the regulation of cell fate by receptor-mediated events has emerged. Both TNF-α and angiotensin II bind with high affinity to two distinct receptor subtypes, with opposing effects on cell fate. In the case of TNF-α, activation of TNF-R1 induces apoptosis, whereas activation of TNF-R2 protects against apoptosis and stimulates cell proliferation.[52, 54] Similarly for angiotensin II, the AT2 receptor promotes apoptosis, whereas the AT1 receptor signals proliferation.[55] Thus, it is not possible a priori to predict the effect that receptor-mediated stimuli such as TNF-α and angiotensin II will have on a given cell without knowledge of the specific receptor subtypes expressed by that cell. A similar paradigm will probably be found to apply to other factors capable of inducing apoptosis.

APOPTOSIS DUE TO A DEFICIENCY OF "SURVIVAL FACTORS"

Most, if not all, cells undergo apoptosis if grown in the absence of so-called "survival factors."[56] Appreciation of this phenomenon has led to the concept that all cells possess a genetically inbuilt "default pathway" capable of initiating apoptotic death unless specifically inhibited by signals from the extracellular environment.[56] Thus, to maintain viability, a cell must receive a more or less continuous stream of extracellular "survival signals" so as to keep its "default pathway" in a state of constant inactivation. Inhibition of apoptosis by survival factors is therefore said to be under negative regulation, meaning that in the absence of "survival factors," cells automatically undergo apoptosis. This is as opposed to the positive regulation seen with receptor-mediated and cytotoxic inducers of apoptosis, which trigger cell death by their presence. The "default pathway" of apoptosis probably evolved as a "fail-safe" to protect against uncontrolled proliferation and neoplasia.

Competition for survival factors provides an elegant means for ensuring that normal adult tissues maintain a fairly constant size by striking a balance between the number of cells produced by cell division and those eliminated by cell death.[56] Thus, if a given level of a survival factor supports a certain number of cells, any increase in cell number would tend to increase competition and lead to increased cell death, thereby returning cell number to its original value. Similarly, a decrease in cell number would lessen competition and allow proliferation of cells back to the original number.

Three distinct classes of survival signals have been described:

1. Cytokines and soluble growth hormones as survival factors. Most soluble survival factors are either proteins or steroid-based lipids. Specific examples include testosterone, which acts on prostatic epithelial cells; cytokines such as interleukin-2, which act on lymphoblasts; and growth factors for renal epithelial cells, such as epidermal growth factor (EGF), insulin-like growth factor-1 (IGF-1), and hepatocyte growth factor (HGF).[2, 57] Additional classes of survival factors with potential importance for renal epithelial cells are lipid-derived factors such as lysophosphatidic acid, which exists in serum complexed to albumin,[58, 59] and cyclooxygenase-derived prostaglandins and eicosanoids.[60]
2. Cell-matrix adhesion as a survival factor. Many adherent cells, especially epithelial and endothelial cells, undergo apoptosis upon loss of normal cell-matrix interaction.[61, 62] This process has been termed *anoikis* ("homelessness"). However, aside from representing a specific cause of apoptosis, anoikis appears comparable in all aspects to apoptosis induced by any other trigger. Survival signals are transmitted to the cell from the extracellular matrix via integrins and perhaps other adhesion molecules that mediate cell-matrix adhesion interaction.[61, 62] Several studies have shown the importance of cell-matrix adhesion in maintaining the survival of renal epithelial cells in culture.[63, 64] Importantly, not all integrins are equally effective in inhibiting anoikis.[65, 66] For example, in one study, endothelial cells adhering solely through $\alpha_2\beta_1$ integrins underwent apoptosis even in the presence of soluble survival factors.[65] In addition, inhibition of anoikis may depend as much on changes in cell shape that result from cell spreading[66] as on integrin-mediated activation of specific intracellular signaling pathways.[65, 66]
3. Cell-cell interactions as a survival factor. Cell-cell adhesion has also been shown to act as a survival signal for epithelial cells. Inhibition of apoptosis by cell-cell contact may be mediated by members of either the integrin or the cadherin families.[63, 64]

APOPTOSIS INDUCED BY DNA DAMAGE

The tumor suppressor gene p53 mediates apoptosis in cells whose DNA has been damaged by a variety of mechanisms, including γ-radiation, UV irradiation, and chemotherapeutic drugs.[67] This has an obvious evolutionary advantage. When DNA damage cannot be repaired, p53 mediates apoptosis, thereby preventing the proliferation and transmission of mutated cells. DNA damage may contribute to the death of renal epithelial cells seen in association with the administration of chemotherapeutic agents such as cisplatin.[68]

APOPTOSIS INDUCED BY CELL INJURY

Apoptosis appears to represent a generalized response to cellular injury. A wide variety of cytotoxic events that cause necrosis, including ischemia, toxins, infection, and oxidative injury, can also cause apoptosis within the same cell type.[69] In general, the mechanism of cell death is determined by the severity of injury, with extremely severe insults causing metabolic collapse and necrosis, and milder insults of the same sort causing apoptosis.[69] The relationship between severity of injury and the mechanism of cell death has been most clearly delineated using cells in culture. However, a number of studies have shown that a similar relationship also exists in vivo.[69, 70] For example, in both myocardial infarction and stroke, cell death outside the central zone of necrosis occurs by apoptosis,[69, 70] presumably because the degree of ischemia in this surrounding zone is too severe to permit cell repair and recovery but not severe enough to cause extreme depletion of cellular ATP, metabolic collapse, and necrosis.

Cellular Events Associated With Apoptosis

OVERVIEW

The striking characteristic morphologic features of apoptosis were described previously and are summarized in Table 3–1. The entire process of apoptosis may conveniently be divided into two phases[4, 71, 72] (Fig. 3–2). During the first phase, called the commitment phase, an individual cell "decides" whether to undergo apoptosis. This decision is based upon signals both intrinsic and extrinsic to the cell and, as discussed previously, occurs in response to a wide variety of triggers (see Table 3–1). The second, or execution, phase entails the genetically controlled activation of effector mechanisms that lead to the classic morphologic features of apoptosis[5, 71] (see Table 3–1). The execution phase, once initiated, is typically brief, lasting between 15 minutes and 2 hours.[4, 71] While the duration of the execution phase demonstrates remarkable uniformity among cells of a given population, the commitment phase is highly stochastic in nature and can last anywhere from 2 to 48 hours[4, 71] (see Fig. 3–2). Not only is it impossible to predict which cells of a population will die by apoptosis but also it is clear that the cells that die by apoptosis do so after a variable and completely random time interval following the apoptotic stimulus.[4, 71] This randomness is so inherent to apoptosis, that even the two daughter cells of a mitotic cell do not die at the same time.[71] The stochastic nature of apoptosis explains one of the key features of apoptotic cell death, namely, that cells die individually in an asynchronous manner over hours or days after a

FIGURE 3–2 ■ The stochastic nature of apoptosis. When a population of cells (in tissue or culture) is exposed to an apoptotic trigger, the cells destined to die pass through two sequential phases, the "commitment" phase and the "execution" phase. The commitment phase is very variable in duration, lasting from minutes to hours. During the commitment phase, cells appear normal morphologically. Once the cells pass the "point of no return," the excecution phase occurs which, in contrast to the commitment phase, is relatively constant in duration (15 minutes to 1 hour) and is associated with the classic morphologic features of apoptosis (see text and Table 3—1). However, variation in the duration of the commitment phase results in the asynchronous death of cells exposed simultaneously to a single apoptotic stimulus. (Modified from Lieberthal W, Levine J: Mechanisms of apoptosis and its potential role in renal tubular epithelial cell injury. Am J Physiol 1996; 271:F477–F488; with permission.)

single apoptotic trigger[4, 71] (see Fig. 3–2). In sharp contrast, overwhelming injury, severe enough to cause necrosis, typically leads to the near-simultaneous death of cells in large contiguous masses[68, 73] (see Table 3–1).

Morphologic and biochemical events occurring within the commitment and execution phases of apoptosis involve nearly all the cellular compartments, with the most prominent alterations occurring in the nucleus, mitochondria, cytoskeleton, and cell membrane. While the asynchronous nature of apoptosis has made it difficult to determine the precise order of these events, two important generalizations can be made. First, it appears that mitochondrial changes are primary to the execution of apoptosis.[10] Not only is it evident that loss of mitochondrial transmembrane potential precedes all apoptotic changes within both the nucleus[74] and the cell membrane,[75] but also the release of mitochondrial cytochrome *c* into the cytosol seems to be an essential inciting event for setting in motion the multiple proteolytic cascades ultimately responsible for all the characteristic features of apoptosis.[10] Second, once initiated, apoptotic events

within each cellular compartment seem to proceed more or less independently of one another. Thus, for example, cell membrane changes typical of apoptosis occur in enucleated cells.[75] Similarly, isolated nuclei exposed to mitochondrial extracts from apoptotic cells manifest all the usual features of apoptosis, despite the absence of a plasma membrane.[76]

NUCLEAR CHANGES

Endonuclease Activation and DNA Fragmentation. Apoptosis is associated with the activation of a specific endonuclease that causes internucleosomal cleavage of DNA.[46, 76, 77] The resulting pattern of DNA fragmentation is usually referred to as a "ladder." The basis for this so-called "ladder" pattern is best appreciated by reviewing the structural organization of nuclear chromatin (Fig. 3–3). Chromatin, which refers to the complex of double-stranded DNA (dsDNA) and nuclear histones, is organized into repeating units called nucleosomes (see Fig. 3–3). Each nucleosome consists of an octameric core of eight histone proteins (4 pairs

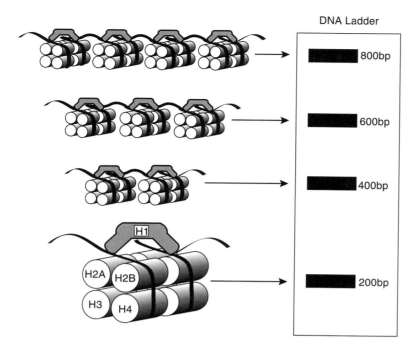

DNA Ladder

800bp

600bp

400bp

200bp

FIGURE 3–3 ■ Nucleosomal structure and its relationship to DNA fragmentation in apoptosis. Each nucleosome consists of an octameric core consisting of four pairs of each of the histone proteins H2A, H2B, H3 and H4. Wrapped around this octamer is a segment of double-stranded DNA approximately 170 base pairs in length whose ends are secured to the octamer by a single H1 histone. The DNA connecting one octamer with the next forms the "linking region" and is the site of cleavage by endonucleases in apoptosis. The length of DNA between the cleavage sites on either side of a single octamer is approximately 200 base pairs. On the left of this figure is shown the intact nucleosomes, and on the right is a schematic portrayal of the DNA ladder observed when nucleosomes from apoptotic cells are disrupted and the unbound fragments of DNA (multiples of 200 base pairs in size) are separated by gel electrophoresis. (Modified from Levine JS, Koh JS: Role of apoptosis in autoimmunity: immunogen, antigen, and accelerant. Semin Nephrol 1999; 19:34–37; with permission.)

of the histones H2A, H2B, H3, and H4) and approximately 170 base pairs of dsDNA, which wind around the outside of this octameric nucleosomal core. The dsDNA is tightly attached to the nucleosomal core via ionic bonds between the negatively charged phosphate groups of dsDNA and the positively charged histones. The two ends of the dsDNA are secured to the octameric core by a single H1 histone. This nucleosomal structure serves two functions: to protect the dsDNA from cleavage by nucleases and to aid in the tight packing of dsDNA. Individual nucleosomes are connected to one another by a 40– to 60–base pair segment of dsDNA called the "linking region." As a result of this arrangement, chromatin has the appearance of nucleosomal beads evenly spaced along a string of linker dsDNA. The specific endonuclease or endonucleases activated during apoptosis cleave DNA at the "linking regions," thereby generating mono- and polynucleosomes.[46, 76, 77] Ex vivo, when nucleosomes are disrupted and their DNA is extracted and separated by gel electrophoresis, a ladder pattern is visible. The rungs of the ladder correspond to DNA fragments increasing in size by multiples of approximately 200 base pairs (consisting of core plus linker DNA) (see Fig. 3–3).

As already discussed, DNA fragmentation also occurs during necrosis, but the resulting pattern is usually different from that seen in apoptosis. The release of lysosomal enzymes and proteases leads to the proteolytic degradation of histones so that the entire length of dsDNA becomes unprotected and accessible to endonuclease cleavage. As a result, dsDNA from necrotic cells is rapidly degraded into short fragments of random length. When DNA from necrotic cells is separated by electrophoresis, a "smear" pattern is the typical result. However, recent evidence suggests that a "ladder" pattern may also occur early during necro-

sis.[45, 78] Therefore, a "ladder" pattern may not be so specific for apoptosis as once believed. Such considerations increase the importance and utility of end-labeling assays (described later) as a more specific means of distinguishing between apoptosis and necrosis.

End-Labeling Assays. Consistent with the fact that apoptosis leads to the activation of a specific endonuclease, the DNA cleavage patterns in apoptotic versus necrotic nuclei are quite different.[79, 80] Apoptotic dsDNA cleavage is characterized by the presence of single nucleotide 3' overhangs. The overhanging 3'-nucleotides terminate in hydroxyl groups, whereas the recessed 5'-nucleotides terminate in phosphate groups. In contrast, the DNA cleavage seen in necrosis typically produces much longer overhangs as well as single strands of DNA. Single nucleotide 3' overhangs either do not occur in necrotic nuclei or are present at far lower concentrations than in apoptotic nuclei. While blunt ends are found in both apoptotic and necrotic nuclei, they occur at a higher frequency in apoptotic nuclei. Unfortunately, the commonly used TUNEL (terminal deoxynucleotidyl transferase-mediated dUTP nick end-labeling) assay, based on the enzyme TdT (terminal deoxynucleotidyl transferase), detects 3' hydroxyl ends of all types (single-stranded DNA as well as blunt, recessed, or overhanging ends of dsDNA) and therefore labels DNA cleavages seen in both necrosis and apoptosis.[79] This nonspecificity of TdT-based assays was demonstrated using tissue samples from a number of organs subjected to known apoptotic and necrotic stimuli.[79] A recently developed assay by Didenko and coworkers,[79, 80] based on the Taq DNA polymerase, is specific for the single nucleotide 3' overhangs found only in apoptotic DNA cleavage. TdT-based assays do retain an important role in apoptosis research. Once the mechanism of cell death has been established by morphologic or other methods, then TdT-based assays are a simple and sensitive means of identifying individual dead or affected cells. However, if the mechanism of cell death is in question, TdT-based assays do not reliably distinguish necrosis from apoptosis, and alternative assays such as that described by Didenko and coworkers[79, 80] must be used.

Condensation and Fragmentation of Nuclear Chromatin. Condensation and fragmentation of nuclear chromatin are highly specific features of apoptosis.[4, 5] While the biochemical events responsible for condensation and fragmentation remain poorly characterized,[81] their presence is extremely useful for morphologic identification of apoptotic cells[2, 57, 58, 59, 68, 73] (see Table 3–1). The two best means for detecting these nuclear events are electron microscopy[2, 57, 58, 73] or fluorescent staining with supravital DNA dyes such as Hoechst dye.[2, 57–59, 68, 73] On electron microscopy, nuclear condensation is characterized by collapse of chromatin toward the nuclear periphery in one of several characteristic electron-dense patterns: a single dense mass, a cluster of smaller dense masses, or a crescent moon plastered against the nuclear envelope. At this stage, the nuclear envelope is usually intact. On fluorescent staining with dyes such as Hoechst, nuclear condensation results in a homogeneous, more intense fluorescence with loss of nucleoli and other nuclear structural detail. Depending upon whether the chromatin condenses into single or multiple dense masses, the nucleus appears as intact or fragmented. It is important to emphasize that the nuclear chromatin of cells dying by necrosis undergoes neither condensation nor fragmentation so that the morphology of necrotic nuclei examined under fluorescent microscopy is indistinguishable from that of viable cells.[2, 57, 58, 68, 73] On electron microscopy, the chromatin of necrotic nuclei is often disintegrated, but condensation into electron-dense masses does not occur.[68, 73]

Loss of the Nuclear Envelope. The eukaryotic nucleus is surrounded by two phospholipid membranes, collectively referred to as the nuclear envelope. The inner nuclear membrane defines the nucleus, whereas the outer membrane is continuous with the endoplasmic reticulum. These two membranes appear to fuse at the nuclear pores, which are holes connecting the nucleus and cytoplasm. The inner aspect of the inner nuclear membrane is lined by a proteinaceous and filamentous layer consisting of three different lamins (lamins A, B, and C). This nuclear lamina serves to anchor regions of chromatin to the nuclear membrane.

During apoptosis, as chromatin condenses against the nuclear envelope, the nuclear pores slide away from and aggregate between areas of condensed chromatin.[81] It appears that both processes, chromatin condensation and movement of nuclear pores, are dependent upon caspase-mediated proteolytic cleavage of the nuclear lamina.[82, 83] In cells expressing mutant uncleavable forms of lamin A or B that were induced to undergo apoptosis, no nuclear condensation was observed.[83] Instead, the nuclear envelope broke down, while the nuclear lamina remained intact.[83] Cell death and DNA fragmentation eventually occurred but were delayed by up to 12 hours.[83] Apoptotic events in other cell compartments, such as membrane blebbing and formation of apoptotic bodies, were unaffected.[83] The dissolution of the nuclear lamina and envelope in normal cells is followed by the packaging and shedding of condensed chromatin in apoptotic bodies.

PLASMA MEMBRANE CHANGES

Loss of Plasma Membrane Asymmetry. Phospholipids are distributed in an asymmetric manner throughout the plasma membrane of viable cells.[84, 85] Anionic phospholipids, such as phosphatidylserine (PS), are localized almost entirely to the inner cytoplasmic leaflet of the cell membrane and are virtually absent from the external leaflet.[84, 85] However, upon induction of apoptosis, PS is redistributed from the inner to the outer face of the cell membrane.[85, 86] This loss of membrane asymmetry is a very early feature of cells undergoing apoptosis, and precedes membrane blebbing and nuclear condensation.[87, 88]

At least two mechanisms appear to contribute in varying degrees to the loss of membrane asymmetry during apoptosis. Under normal circumstances, membrane asymmetry appears to be maintained by a so-called "aminophospholipid translocase."[84, 89] This enzyme translocates PS and, to a lesser degree, phosphatidylethanolamine from the external to the internal leaflet of the cell membrane in an ATP-dependent manner.[84, 88, 89] The limited capacity of this enzyme suggests that its main role is in the preservation, rather than the generation, of lipid asymmetry. Indeed, inhibition of the translocase in normal cells itself does not lead to a significant loss of membrane asymmetry.[84] The main role of this translocase may therefore be to protect the cell membrane from the perturbations in lipid distribution that occur during processes such as endocytosis and exocytosis.[84] Thus, while apoptosis is, in fact, associated with down-regulation of the activity of the aminophospholipid translocase, it seems highly unlikely that inhibition of this translocase alone accounts for redistribution of PS to the external leaflet.[88] Rather, apoptosis also leads to the activation of a nonspecific lipid scramblase that results in bidirectional transmembrane movement of all lipid classes.[88]

The presence of PS on the surface of apoptotic cells forms the basis of a number of useful assays for detecting apoptotic cells. Both annexin V and β2-glycoprotein 1 (β2GP1) are proteins that selectively interact with anionic phospholipids, such as PS. Apoptotic cells may therefore be identified by the binding of fluorescently labeled annexin V or β2GP1 to the apoptotic cell surface.[86] In addition, the loss of membrane asymmetry results in a looser packing of phospholipids that can be detected by the lipophilic dye merocyanine 540.[85]

Membrane Blebbing and Shedding of Apoptotic Bodies. The membrane of cells dying by apoptosis undergoes a dynamic process of blebbing.[71] Blebbing begins during the commitment phase and extends into the execution phase. Eventually, the cell fragments into membrane-enclosed apoptotic bodies containing condensed chromatin or entire organelles.[5, 7] Despite this intense blebbing, the membranes of apoptotic cells and bodies remain impermeable to vital dyes, such as trypan blue and propridium iodide, that readily enter necrotic cells[68, 71] (see Table 3–1). It is unclear at present whether the shedding of apoptotic bodies from the surface of apoptotic cells is a more extended and intense version of membrane blebbing or whether the two represent distinct processes.

The biochemical events regulating these two processes are still obscure, but at least in the case of blebbing, a number of studies clearly implicate the involvement of the actin cytoskeleton.[90–94] Not only has polymerized actin (F-actin) been shown to accumulate at the base of blebs in apoptotic cells[90–94] but also its concentration correlates directly with bleb size.[94] Treatment of apoptotic cells with the actin depolymerizer cytochalasin D markedly decreases blebbing.[90] Similarly, blebbing can be blocked by inhibition of the cytoplasmic G protein Rho, a regulator of the actin cytoskeleton, or by inhibition of myosin light chain kinase, a protein kinase that catalyzes the motor interaction of myosin and actin.[90] In addition, gelsolin, a regulator of actin polymerization, is specifically cleaved by caspases during apoptosis.[91] Expression of this caspase-generated gelsolin fragment in viable cells leads to the rounding up and detachment of the cells in association with membrane blebbing.[91] Moreover, cells from knockout mice lacking gelsolin showed a delayed onset of blebbing after an apoptotic stimulus.[91] Thus, caspase-mediated cleavage of gelsolin may be a key event in the initiation of membrane blebbing. Finally, although the contribution of the actin cytoskeleton seems established, the microtubular network does not seem to be involved in blebbing, because treatment of cells with Taxol (paclitavel) or nocodazole, two agents that stabilize or destabilize microtubules, respectively, had little or no effect on blebbing.[90]

Much less is understood about the biochemistry underlying the formation of apoptotic bodies, although the actin cytoskeleton appears to play a role in this process.[90] Caspase-mediated cleavage of the p21-activated kinase 2 (PAK2), a class of serine-threonine kinases, generates a constitutively active PAK2 fragment that appears to be necessary for the shedding of apoptotic bodies.[7] In cells carrying a dominant negative mutant form of PAK2, the formation of apoptotic bodies was dramatically reduced.[7] The nuclear changes of apoptosis occurred normally in these same cells, and interestingly the surface expression of PS appeared to be increased.[7]

MITOCHONDRIAL CHANGES

Role of the Mitochondrion in Determining the Mode of Cell Death. Evidence is accumulating that implicates a major role for mitochondria in controlling the fate of a cell. In effect, mitochondrial events seem to determine whether a cell lives or dies and, if the cell dies, whether death is carried out by apoptosis or by necrosis.[10, 11] While the role of the mitochondrion as an arbiter of cell fate is well supported, the precise mechanisms by which the mitochondrion senses damage and integrates the disparate signals reaching it from throughout the cell are much less clear.[10, 11] As discussed previously, mitochondrial events are among the earliest in the execution of apoptosis, and events such as release of cytochrome c into the cytosol may in fact represent a "point of no return" in the cell's decision to undergo apoptosis.[10, 11] Moreover, mitochondrial events, such as loss of mitochondrial transmembrane potential, seem to trigger events within other cell compartments, so that interventions that prevent loss of mitochondrial transmembrane potential can also prevent apoptotic nuclear and cell membrane changes.[10, 11]

One of the critical functions performed by the mitochondrion is the production of ATP, the major energy substrate of the cell. Apoptosis is an active, energy-requiring process.[3, 5, 72] For this reason, a key factor in determining whether a cell dies by necrosis or by apoptosis is the capacity of the cell's mitochondria to produce enough ATP to allow the apoptotic pathway to occur. In contrast to the energy requirements needed for apoptosis to occur, necrosis takes place as the result of catastrophic cell injury associated with an inability of the cell to sustain vital ATP-dependent functions. Thus, in renal epithelial cells subjected to graded ATP depletion by means of chemical anoxia, severe ATP depletion ($\leqq15\%$ of control levels) induced necrosis, whereas more moderate degrees of ATP depletion (25% to 75% of control levels) induced apoptosis.[73] Moreover, the mechanism of cell death in two separate cell lines, both exposed to an agonistic anti-Fas antibody, could be converted from apoptosis to necrosis by reducing intracellular ATP levels.[95, 96] A similar conversion from apoptotic to necrotic cell death was shown with two other known inducers of apoptosis, the calcium ionophore A23187 and the broad-spectrum kinase inhibitor staurosporine.[95, 96] Several distinct apoptotic events, including loss of plasma membrane asymmetry, internucleosomal cleavage of DNA, and activation of selective caspases, appear to be dependent on ATP levels.[95, 96]

Taken together, these studies suggest that the ability of a cell to undergo apoptosis, and thereby protect its neighbors from its toxic and inflammatory intracellular contents, is dependent on the cell's possessing sufficient ATP stores to complete the apoptotic pathway and maintain the vital cell functions necessary for warding off necrosis. Mitochondria thus contribute to apoptosis in two important ways—first, as determinants of the availability of cell energy stores and, second (as discussed later), as the source of specific molecules whose release into the cytosol initiates a sequence of proteolytic cascades culminating in nearly all the classic morphologic and biochemical events of apoptosis. It is important to emphasize that despite the essential role of mitochondria in apoptosis the mitochondria of cells undergoing apoptosis appear morphologically normal. In contrast, the mitochondria of necrotic cells are usually swollen and disrupted.

Release of Mitochondrial Proteins. During apoptosis, mitochondria release cytochrome c into the cytosol.[97–99]

Cytochrome c, a relatively small molecule (~15 kDa), is a peripheral membrane protein of the inner mitochondrial membrane that is part of the electron transport chain. Once in the cytoplasm, cytochrome c binds to a protein known as Apaf-1 (apoptosis protease-activating factor 1), an event that requires deoxyadenosine 5'-triphosphate (dATP).[97-99] The interaction of cytochrome c and Apaf-1 induces a conformational change in Apaf-1 that permits the binding of procaspase-9.[97-99] Proteolytic cleavage leads to activation of caspase-9, which then processes and activates caspase-3, beginning the execution phase of apoptosis.[97-99] The complex of cytochrome c, Apaf-1, and procaspase-9 is often referred to as the "apoptosome."

Other mitochondrial proteins important to the execution of apoptosis are also released during apoptosis. Apoptosis-inducing factor (AIF) is a partially characterized 50-kDa protein that apparently activates nuclear endonucleases and procaspase-3.[100] AIF itself may be a caspase, as its activity in vitro is blocked by the caspase inhibitor zVAD-fmk.[100] In addition, the mitochondria of certain cell types contain procaspase-3, which can be released during apoptosis.[101]

While mitochondrial release of cytochrome c is thought to represent a "point of no return" in terms of a cell's commitment to die, the mechanism of death following release of cytochrome c is not necessarily apoptotic. As discussed previously, the mitochondrial function present must be sufficient to generate the ATP needed for both the execution of apoptosis and the maintenance of vital cell functions. This poses something of a dilemma, inasmuch as cytochrome c is a vital enzyme in the electron transport chain. As suggested in a recent review,[11] the form of cell death may depend on the cell type. In cells where cytochrome c and/or caspases are present in excess, enough cytochrome c may remain bound to the inner mitochondrial membrane to permit ongoing ATP production while caspases carry out the execution phase of apoptosis. Conversely, in cells containing a limited amount of cytochrome c or an excess of caspase inhibitors, release of cytochrome c may fail to activate caspases, so that the eventual loss of electron chain transport leads instead to necrosis.

Loss of the Mitochondrial Transmembrane Potential ($\Delta\psi_m$). Mitochondria are surrounded by two membranes. The outer membrane has the unusual feature of being highly porous, permitting the free passage of proteins as large as 10 kDa, and is therefore unable to sustain an electrochemical gradient. The inner membrane, which is much more impermeable, is composed of a number of infoldings called cristae. All of the multiprotein complexes involved in electron chain transport span the inner mitochondrial membrane. Cytochrome c resides in the intermembrane space and is tightly bound to two of the inner-membrane–spanning multiprotein complexes. Electron chain transport generates an unequal distribution of ions (mostly H^+) across the inner mitochondrial membrane that is the basis of $\Delta\psi_m$.

A number of cationic lipophilic dyes that partition across the inner mitochondrial membrane based on charge have been developed to monitor $\Delta\psi_m$.[10, 11] These dyes include rhodamine-123, $DiOC_6$,[10] JC-1, and CMXRos.[10, 11] Use of these dyes has shown that loss of $\Delta\psi_m$ constitutes a very early and irreversible event in apoptosis. Thus, loss of $\Delta\psi_m$ precedes all the nuclear and cell membrane apoptotic changes discussed previously.[74, 75] Moreover, purified cells with a low $\Delta\psi_m$ but no other apoptotic changes proceed to apoptotic death despite removal of the apoptotic stimulus.

Loss of $\Delta\psi_m$ implies the opening of a conductance channel, known as the permeability transition (PT) pore.[10, 11, 102] The complete structure and composition of the PT pore are unknown, but its constituents include proteins found in both the inner and the outer membranes, so presumably they occur at contact points between the inner and the outer mitochondrial membranes.[10, 11] Opening of PT pores leads to dissipation of the H^+ gradient across the inner membrane, loss of $\Delta\psi_m$, and uncoupling of the respiratory chain from oxidative phosphorylation.[10, 11] Several inhibitors of the PT pore, including bongkrekic acid (which blocks the adenine nucleotide transporter [ANT] located in the inner membrane), provide protection against apoptosis in certain systems.[10, 11, 75, 103] Conversely, several activators of the PT pore, including atractyloside (which activates ANT) and protoporphyrin IX, disrupt $\Delta\psi_m$ and induce apoptosis.[10, 11, 75, 103]

Of major clinical importance is the fact that cyclophilin D, a protein found in the mitochondrial matrix and a ligand for the immunosuppressant cyclosporin A, is also a constituent of the PT pore.[102] Cyclophilin D associates with the inner membrane PT pore constituent ANT.[102] A number of studies have shown that cyclosporin A can prevent or retard both loss of $\Delta\psi_m$ and cell death in response to various lethal stimuli.[10, 103, 104] The protective effect of cyclosporin A is seen for apoptotic as well as necrotic stimuli, once again emphasizing the critical role of the mitochondrion in both these forms of cell death.[104] Protection also occurs with the cyclosporin A derivative, N-methyl-Val-cyclosporin A, which retains binding to cyclophilin D but lacks an inhibitory effect on calcineurin and therefore has markedly diminished immunosuppressant activity.[75]

It has been suggested that the PT pore complex, which is regulated by a diverse array of endogenous physiologic effectors, may act as a sensor of cellular stress or damage. In general, opening of the PT pore and loss of $\Delta\psi_m$ occur in response to any major change in energy balance or redox state.[10] In addition, several second messengers, such as ceramide, and increases in cytosolic Ca^{2+} can also facilitate opening of the PT pores.[10] Apoptosome-activated caspases are also able to induce PT pore opening, raising the possibility of self-amplification via positive feedback.[10, 11]

Finally, an as yet unresolved issue is the relationship between opening of the PT pores and the release of cytochrome c into the cytosol.[10, 11] While in most cases release of cytochrome c seems to occur after loss of $\Delta\psi_m$, some studies have suggested that release of cytochrome c and activation of caspase-9 can occur in the absence of any detectable change in $\Delta\psi_m$.[105] It is possible that integrity of the inner and outer membranes is regulated separately and that a distinct protein channel in the outer mitochondrial membrane is responsible for the release of cytochrome *c*.

Phagocytic Clearance of Cells Undergoing Apoptosis

In sharp contrast to necrosis, apoptotic cell death almost always occurs without inflammation or injury to the surrounding tissue (see Table 3–1). This remarkable feature of apoptotic death occurs for two main reasons. First, as previously noted, the cell membrane of cells undergoing apoptosis remains intact until relatively late. Second, apoptotic cells express unique surface markers that permit their rapid recognition and ingestion by phagocytes.[106, 107] Hence, as long as phagocytic clearance of an apoptotic cell occurs before breakdown of its cell membrane, none of the cytosolic contents of the apoptotic cell are released into the extracellular space. In this way, despite the billions of cells that each day die by apoptosis, tissues are protected from an otherwise harmful exposure to the inflammatory contents of dying cells.[106] Indeed, as noted previously, the uptake and digestion of apoptotic cells by phagocytes is so rapid and efficient that apoptotic cells are very rarely observed in histologic sections. This is true even in cases where there is major cell loss by apoptosis, such as the developing thymus, in which as many as 25% of cells may undergo apoptosis within a single day. Conversely, because clearance of apoptotic cells occurs so rapidly, the existence of even very small numbers of apoptotic cells on histologic sections may be indicative of substantial cell death.

Recent data have uncovered an additional important reason for the absence of inflammation in association with apoptotic death. The mechanism described previously—namely, rapid phagocytic clearance preceding breakdown of the apoptotic cell membrane—may be viewed as essentially a passive, or defensive, phenomenon. It appears, however, that phagocytosis of apoptotic cells may also be actively anti-inflammatory. Uptake of apoptotic neutrophils by human monocyte-derived macrophages has been shown to inhibit the endotoxin-induced production of a number of inflammatory mediators, including interleukin-1β (IL-1β), IL-8, TNF-α, thromboxane B_2, and leukotriene C_4.[97, 98] Inhibition of inflammation occurred via the autocrine release of such anti-inflammatory factors as TGF-β, prostaglandin E2, PAF, and IL-10.[108]

Apoptotic clearance may therefore represent an active limiting process by which injured tissues can contain and even act to resolve an inflammatory focus. This is in sharp contrast to necrotic death, where a vicious cycle often ensues in which release of inflammatory intracellular material promotes the recruitment of inflammatory cells and the release of additional inflammatory mediators, leading to yet more necrotic death. Thus, the initial balance between apop-

totic and necrotic death, as determined by the magnitude of the inciting cytotoxic stimulus, may determine which of these opposite tendencies prevails, whether the anti-inflammation of apoptosis or the pro-inflammation of necrosis.

Monocytes and macrophages are the major cell lineages involved in phagocytic uptake of apoptotic cells.[106] Although less efficient than macrophages, other cell types, including fibroblasts, mesangial cells, and epithelial cells, are also capable of ingesting apoptotic cells and bodies.[106, 109] Indeed, in electron micrographs of primary cultures of murine renal epithelial cells, we have observed phagocytosis of apoptotic cells by the remaining viable cells.[3] In accord with the evolutionary importance of clearance of apoptotic cells, phagocytes possess multiple distinct cell surface receptors that act in parallel in order to mediate the recognition and uptake of apoptotic cells. Because the cell membranes of apoptotic cells are intact, recognition of apoptotic cells by phagocytes requires that the apoptotic cell express some unique marker on its cell surface announcing itself as being ready for ingestion. While the exact ligands on the apoptotic cell surface recognized by the phagocyte have yet to be identified, a number of potentially important changes have been shown to occur at the surface membrane of apoptotic cells. These include alterations in glycosylation,[110] surface charge,[110] and phospholipid composition,[85] as well as the specific binding of several circulating plasma proteins.[86, 89] Further details regarding the several incompletely characterized ligand-receptor interactions that mediate phagocytic uptake of apoptotic cells are reviewed in detail elsewhere.[3, 107, 110]

Molecular Biology of Apoptosis

INDUCERS, POSITIVE REGULATORS, AND MEDIATORS OF APOPTOSIS

Caspases. Caspases constitute the major family of proteases involved in the execution phase of apoptosis[6, 8, 9] (Fig. 3–4). They should not be viewed solely as degradative enzymes, but more properly as signaling molecules or enzymes that specifically activate or inactivate key cellular proteins by site-specific cleavage. Like the complement and coagulation systems, caspases are part of a proteolytic system in which inactive precursors (called pro-caspases) are irreversibly cleaved and activated in a tightly regulated, sequential, and most likely self-amplifying cascade, whose ultimate expression is responsible for virtually all the classic features of apoptosis.

To date, 14 caspases have been identified (Table 3–2).[9, 111] The founding member of this family, caspase-1, is also known as IL-1β–converting enzyme (ICE) because of its role in activating pro-IL-1β and was originally identified by virtue of its sequence homology to the gene product CED-3 in the nematode *Caenorhabditis elegans*.[111] Mutant nematodes lacking CED-3 have an almost complete absence of developmental apoptosis.[111] While caspase-1 appears to play a more

FIGURE 3–4 ▪ Schematic representation of the major biochemical events associated with apoptosis. The core machinery of apoptosis consists of two converging pathways, one initiated by ligand-receptor interactions, the other by cell injury. Cell injury leads to the translocation of Bax and other proapoptotic proteins from the cytosol to the mitochondrial membrane, resulting in the release of cytochrome c into the cytosol. Cytochrome c activates apoptosis-activating factor (Apaf) and enables Apaf to activate procaspase-9. The complex of cytochrome c, Apaf, and procaspase-9 is called the apoptosome. Caspase-9 activates caspase-3. Caspase-3, together with other downstream caspases, induces apoptosis by cleaving specific cytosolic and nuclear substrates within the cell. By contrast, apoptosis mediated by ligand-receptor interactions is mediated primarily by the recruitment of procaspase-8 to the cytosolic domain of the receptor (the "death receptor"). This leads to activation of caspase-8, which directly activates caspase-3, leading to apoptosis. In addition, the receptor-mediated pathway is augmented by caspase-8–mediated activation of Bax, release of cytochrome *c*, and activation of caspase-9. A characteristic feature of the apoptotic pathway is that it is opposed at almost every level by a number of different sets of inhibitors (eg, Bcl-2, decoy receptors, and caspase inhibitors) (see text for details).

significant role in cytokine processing than in apoptosis,[112] most of the other caspases, cloned on the basis of similarity to caspase-1, have been shown to be critical to both normal development and the successful execution of apoptosis.[6, 8, 9]

All caspases share a number of structural and functional features, two of which are reflected in the name caspase itself. The "c" refers to the fact that caspases are cysteine proteases, with the catalytic site cysteine contained within a conserved QACXG motif (single letter amino acid code), whereas the "aspase" refers to the absolute predilection of all caspases for cleaving proteins after aspartic acid residues.[6, 8, 9, 111] Caspase activity also depends upon recognition of the 3 amino acids immediately adjacent to the N-terminal side of the aspartic acid.[113] The sequence preferences for these 3 amino acids permit the caspases to be divided into 3 groups (see Table 3–2), which correlate fairly well with the functional division of caspases into apop-

totic initiators, apoptotic effectors, and cytokine processors.[6, 113] Apoptotic "initiators" are defined as the caspases that are the first to be activated by an apoptotic trigger and whose predominant function is to regulate the activity of other caspases. Apoptotic "effectors" are the caspases that mediate the site-specific cleavage of noncaspase cell proteins, leading to the classic morphologic and biochemical features of apoptosis.[6, 8, 9]

All caspases are synthesized as proenzymes with three domains: an N-terminal prodomain, a large subunit domain containing the catalytic cysteine, and a C-terminal small subunit domain.[6, 8, 9] Activation requires cleavage at caspase consensus site or sites in the linker region between the large and the small domains. The N-terminal prodomain, which contains recognition motifs that act to bring together procaspases with upstream activators, is usually also removed by cleavage at a caspase consensus site located between the pro-

TABLE 3–2. Properties of Caspases

CASPASE	PREVIOUS NAMES	OPTIMAL TETRAPEPTIDE*	UPSTREAM ACTIVATOR	SYNTHETIC INHIBITORS	VIRAL/ MAMMALIAN INHIBITORS
Apoptotic initiators					
Caspase-2	ICH-1, NEDD-2	DXXD†	RAIDD	zVAD^c	p35
Caspase-8	FLICE-1, MACH, Mch5	(L/V/D)EXD	FADD	zVAD, DEVD	FLIP, CrmA
Caspase-9	ICE-LAP6, Mch6	(I/V/L)EHD	Apaf-1	—	ARC, CrmA
Caspase-10	FLICE-2, Mch4	Unknown	FADD	DEVD	p35
Apoptotic effectors					
Caspase-3	CPP32, YAMA, apopain	DEXD	NA	DEVD, zVAD	IAP, p35, CrmA
Caspase-6	Mch-2	(V/T/I)EXD	NA	VEID, zVAD	p35, CrmA
Caspase-7	Mch-3, ICE-LAP3, CMH-1	DEXD	NA	DEVD	IAP, CrmA
Cytokine processors					
Caspase-1	ICE	(W/Y/F)EHD	Unknown	zVAD, YVAD, DEVD	p35
Caspase-4	ICE$_{rel\ II}$, ICH-2, TX	(W/L/F)EHD	Unknown	zVAD, YVAD, DEVD	p35
Caspase-5	ICE$_{rel\ III}$, TY, Ich-3	(W/L/F)EHD	Unknown	Unknown	CrmA
Caspase-11 (murine)	—	Unknown	Unknown	Unknown	Unknown
Caspase-12 (murine)	—	Unknown	Unknown	Unknown	Unknown
Caspase-13	—	Unknown	Unknown	Unknown	Unknown
Caspase-14 (murine)	—	Unknown	Unknown	Unknown	Unknown

*Peptides are given in the N-terminal to C-terminal direction. Cleavage occurs after the C-terminal aspartic acid (D) residue.

†Single letter amino acid code: D, aspartic acid; E, glutamic acid; F, phenylalanine; H, histidine; I, isoleucine; L, leucine; T, threonine; V, valine; W, tryptophan; X, almost any amino acid; Y, tyrosine.

Apaf-1, apoptosis protease-activating factor 1; *ARC*, apoptosis repressor with caspase recruitment domain; *CrmA*, cytokine response modifier A; *FADD*, Fas-associated death domain; *FLIP*, FADD-like ICE inhibitory protein; *IAP*, inhibitors of apoptosis proteins; *NA*, not applicable; *RAIDD*, RIP-associated Ich-1/CED-3 homologous protein with a death domain; *RIP*, receptor interacting protein; *zVAD*, benzyloxycarbonyl-Val-Ala-Asp.

Adapted from Wolf BB, Green DR: Suicidal tendencies: apoptotic cell death by caspase family proteases. J Biol Chem 1999; 274:20048–20052; Kidd VJ: Proteolytic activities that mediate apoptosis. Annu Rev Physiol 1998; 60:533–573.

domain and the large subunit. While a role for autoactivation of procaspases has not been definitively ruled out, cleavage of procaspases is thought to occur via transactivation by the same or other caspases or even by noncaspase proteases, such as granzyme B, as found in NK and cytotoxic T cells.[6, 8, 9, 53] Once cleaved, two large and two small subunits assemble into an active tetramer. Each of the two heterodimers contains a catalytic site composed of residues from both the small and the large subunits.

With this schema in mind, it is helpful to re-examine the activation of caspase-9, an apoptotic initiator, after mitochondrial release of cytochrome *c*.[97, 98, 99] Cytoplasmic procaspase-9 is recruited to the cytochrome *c*-Apaf-1 complex through interaction of its prodomain with a conformationally exposed recognition motif on Apaf-1. Subsequent oligomerization of procaspase-9 permits reciprocal transactivation. Activated caspase-9 then commences the apoptotic cascade by activating the apoptotic effector, caspase-3. The activation of procaspase-8, another apoptotic initiator, by Fas follows a similar model and is discussed later.[52, 54]

As opposed to the case with the coagulation and complement cascades, it is not yet possible to provide a complete flow diagram of the precise cascade of reactions by which caspases activate one another. As discussed previously, different triggers of apoptosis lead to the activation of distinct apoptotic initiators. More important, the pattern of cascade activation generated by a given apoptotic trigger may differ among cell types. This difference among cells may depend

upon many factors, including the expression pattern and relative concentrations within the cell of the individual caspases, various cofactors such as Apaf-1, and the growing array of endogenous caspase inhibitors, as well as upon the so far largely unidentified feedback loops and signaling pathways that modulate the activity of individual activation reactions.

Effector caspases cleave an ever increasing and almost bewildering array of targets during the execution phase of apoptosis[6, 8, 9, 111] (Table 3–3). A discussion of all these targets is beyond the realm of this chapter, but selected examples from the various classes of substrates highlight the scope and precision involved in the successful completion of the apoptotic program. The first major class of caspase substrates are regulatory proteins directly involved in the initiation or commitment phase of apoptosis. This class includes proteins such as the procaspases themselves, which are specifically activated by caspase-mediated cleavage, as well as antiapoptotic proteins, such as Bcl-2 and Bcl-xL (discussed later),[114, 115] which are inactivated by cleavage. The combined effect of such activation of proapoptotic proteins and inactivation of antiapoptotic proteins is most likely one of both signal amplification and irrevocable commitment to the execution of apoptosis.

A second class of caspase substrates directly participate in the execution phase of apoptosis[6, 8, 9, 111] (see Tables 3–2 and 3–3). Several members of this class have already been discussed. For example, caspase-mediated cleavage of the kinase PAK2 leads to a constitutively active PAK2 fragment that contributes to the

TABLE 3–3. Targets of Caspases

TARGET	CELL FUNCTION	CONSEQUENCE OF CLEAVAGE
Procaspases	Zymogen proteases	Activation
Bcl-2 family members or associated proteins		
Bcl-2	Antiapoptotic factor	Inactivation, conversion to proapoptotic factor
Bcl-xL	Antiapoptotic factor	Inactivation, conversion to proapoptotic factor
Bid	Latent proapoptotic factor activation	
p28 Bap31	Docking protein for Bcl-2 in ER	Inactivation
DNA endonuclease inhibitors		
ICAD/DFF-45	Inhibitor of apoptosis-specific DNA endonuclease	Inactivation
Structural or cytoskeletal-associated proteins		
β-actin	Cytoskeletal component	? Blebbing, loss of adhesion
β-catenin	Cell-cell junction component	? Disruption of cell-cell adhesion
FAK	Cytoskeleton-associated kinase	? Disruption of cell-matrix adhesion
Fodrin	Cystoskeletal component	Inactivation
Gas2	Cystoskeletal component	Inactivation
Gelsolin	Regulator of actin polymerization	Generation of active fragment with novel properties
Keratin 18	Intermediate filament component	Inactivation
Lamins A, B, C	Nuclear envelope components	Dissolution of nuclear envelope
Signal transduction proteins		
cPLA2	Phospholipid cleavage	Activation
D4-GDI	Regulator of small G proteins	Unknown
MEKK1	Protein kinase	Activation
PAK2	Protein kinase	Activation
PITSLRE kinase	Protein kinase	Activation
PKC-δ	Protein kinase	Activation
PKC-θ	Protein kinase	Activation
PRK2	Protein kinase	Inactivation
Transcription factors or regulators		
IκB-α	Inhibitor of nuclear factor-κB	Inactivation
MDM2	Regulator of p53	Inactivation
Retinoblastoma protein	Cell cycle regulation	Inactivation
Sp1	Transcription factor	Inactivation
SREBP 1, 2	Regulator of sterol responses	Inactivation
DNA/RNA metabolism		
DNA-PKcs	DNA repair	Inactivation
hnRNP C1, C2	pre-mRNA splicing	Inactivation
PARP	DNA repair	Inactivation
RFC140	DNA replication	Inactivation
U1 snRNP	pre-mRNA splicing	Inactivation
Miscellaneous		
DRPLA	Disease-associated protein	?
Huntington protein	Disease-associated protein	?
Presenilins 1, 2	Disease-associated protein	?
Rabaptin-5	Endosomal fusion	Inactivation

cPLA2, cytosolic phospholipase A2; D4-GDI, GDP dissociation inhibitor type 4; DFF-45, DNA fragmentation factor of 45 kDa; DNA-PKcs, catalytic subunit of DNA-dependent protein kinase; DRPLA, dentatorubral pallidoluyian atrophy protein; ER, endoplasmic reticulum; FAK, focal adhesion kinase; hnRNP, heterogeneous nuclear ribonucleoprotein; ICAD, inhibitor of caspase-activated deoxyribonuclease; IκB-α, inhibitor of nuclear factor-κB type α; MDM2, murine double minute gene product 2; MEKK1, mitogen-activated protein kinase/extracellular signal-related kinase kinase 1; PAK2, p21-activated kinase 2; PARP, poly(ADP-ribose) polymerase; PITSLRE kinase, Pro-Iso-Thr-Ser-Leu-Arg-Glu kinase; PKC-δ, protein kinase C-δ; PKC-θ, protein kinase C-θ; PRK2, PKC-related kinase 2; RFC140, replication factor c of 140 kDa; SREBP, sterol-response-element binding protein; U1 snRNP, U1 small nuclear ribonucleoprotein.
Adapted from Cryns V, Yuan J: Proteases to die for. Genes Dev 1998; 12:1551–1570; Tan X, Wang JY: The caspase-RB connection in cell death. Trends Cell Biol 1998; 8:116–120.

packaging and shedding of apoptotic bodies.[7] Cleavage of the actin-regulating protein gelsolin leads to a gelsolin fragment whose unique properties appear to promote membrane blebbing.[91] Caspase-mediated cleavage is also responsible for the activation of the apoptosis-specific endonuclease that generates the "ladder" pattern of DNA fragmentation. This endonuclease, variously called CAD (caspase-activated DNase) or DFF (DNA fragmentation factor), is normally present in cell nuclei as an inactive complex with an inhibitor known as ICAD (inhibitor of CAD).[76, 77] During apoptosis, caspases cleave and inactivate ICAD, so that CAD/DFF may carry out internucleosomal fragmentation of dsDNA.[77]

A third class of caspase substrates are structural proteins of the nucleus and cytoskeleton (see Table 3–3). As previously discussed, cleavage of the nuclear lamins facilitates nuclear condensation.[53–55] Similarly, caspases may promote breakdown of the actin microfilaments and intermediate filaments of the cytoskeleton by specific cleavage of cytoskeletal proteins, such as α-fodrin, β-actin, and keratins.[116] Cleavage of the proteins β-catenin[117] and FAK (focal adhesion kinase)[118] are attractive candidates for explaining the early loss of cell-cell and cell-matrix adhesions, respectively, observed in individual apoptotic cells within a monolayer.

Other classes of caspase substrates cleaved during

apoptosis include the following: homeostatic proteins involved in DNA repair (eg, the catalytic subunit of DNA-dependent protein kinase [DNA-PK$_{cs}$] and poly (ADP-ribose) polymerase [PARP]) or RNA processing (eg, the 70-kDa component of the U1 ribonucleoprotein); classic signal transduction molecules (eg, PKC and cPLA$_2$); transcriptional and cell-cycle regulators (eg, retinoblastoma protein); and miscellaneous proteins with an unclear but potentially intriguing connection to several neurodegenerative diseases (eg, presenilins and huntingtin protein)[6] (see Table 3–3).

As in most proteolytic cascades, the caspase system can be modulated by an assortment of viral, endogenous, and chemical inhibitors[8, 9] (see Fig. 3–4). Four distinct classes of viral inhibitors have been described, two of which have mammalian homologues. Mammalian ARC (apoptosis repressor with caspase recruitment domain) has the same recruitment domain as procaspase-9 but lacks caspase activity.[8, 9] ARC inhibits activation of procaspase-9 by competing with procaspase-9 for binding to the conformationally exposed Apaf-1 recruitment domain in the Apaf-1–cytochrome c complex.[8] Similarly, the inactive caspase homologues, mammalian and viral FLIP (FADD-like ICE inhibitory protein), inhibit the activation of the apoptotic initiator procaspase-8 by competing with procaspase-8 for binding to its cofactor FADD (Fas-associated death domain protein).[9, 119] The IAP proteins (inhibitors of apoptosis proteins) make up a broad family of viral and mammalian proteins that inhibit a number of apoptotic effector caspases through unclear mechanisms.[8, 9, 120, 121] The last two classes of viral inhibitors, for which no mammalian homologues have been described, include the cowpox-virus encoded CrmA (cytokine response modifier A), which inhibits Fas- and TNF-induced apoptosis, and the baculoviral protein p35, which inhibits several effector and cytokine processor caspases.[8, 9, 122]

A number of synthetic cell-permeable peptide inhibitors have been developed based on the caspase recognition sequences of the different classes of caspases (see Table 3–2).[8, 9] These peptide inhibitors are generally small (3 to 4 amino acids in length), water-soluble, and stable (half-lives of up to 4 hours), and they inhibit caspase activation in a dose-dependent manner. The major synthetic inhibitors currently being used include zVAD-fmk (benzyloxycarbonyl-Val-Ala-Asp-fluoromethylketone), YVAD-fmk (acetyl-Tyr-Val-Ala-Asp-fluoromethylketone), DEVD-fmk (acetyl-Asp-Glu-Val-Asp-fluoromethylketone), and VEID-fmk (acetyl-Val-Glu-Ile-Asp-fluoromethylketone).[8, 9]

Fas and Related Cell-Surface Death Receptors. Fas (CD95) is the prototypical member of a family of so-called death receptors that includes the type I TNF-α receptor (TNF-R1), death receptor 3 (DR3), DR4, and DR5.[52, 54] Although the majority of studies on Fas have focused on its role in immune homeostasis, Fas is widely expressed throughout the body, most notably in the thymus, liver, heart, and kidney.[52, 54] Such broad expression is consistent with an emerging major role for Fas in the regulation of apoptosis outside the immune system. In most, but certainly not all, cases engagement of Fas by its ligand FasL (CD95L) induces cell death by apoptosis.[52, 54] In contrast, TNF-α rarely triggers apoptosis through TNF-R1 unless protein synthesis is also inhibited.[52, 54] Signaling through DR3 closely resembles that by TNF-R1, whereas signaling through DR4 and DR5 more closely resembles that by Fas.[52, 54] In this section, discussion is restricted to the signaling pathways, regulatory mechanisms, and molecular biology of Fas and TNF-R1.

Signal transduction via Fas and TNF-R1 requires cross-linking of the receptor molecules, rather than their mere engagement.[52, 54] While FasL is predominantly a cell-surface molecule expressed on lymphocytes and NK cells, FasL can also exist in a soluble form (sFasL) following metalloproteinase-mediated cleavage.[123] Human sFasL is biologically active, whereas murine sFasL is not.[123] Biologic activity may relate to the fact that human, but not murine, sFasL exists as a trimer, enabling oligomerization of cell surface Fas. Like human sFasL, TNF-α exists as a trimer in solution and is processed from a biologically active membrane-bound form by metalloproteinase cleavage.[52, 54] In addition to TNF-α, lymphotoxin-α (TNF-β) also binds to TNF-R1.[52, 54]

The cytoplasmic tails of Fas and TNF-R1 share an approximately 70–amino acid cytoplasmic domain that is responsible for transducing the apoptotic signal and that has been colorfully named a "death domain." Death domains tend to self-aggregate, so that upon trimerization of Fas by FasL or TNF-R1 by TNF-α, the three cytoplasmic death domains interact and cluster.[52, 54] In the case of Fas, this leads to the recruitment of a cytoplasmic protein called FADD (also known as MORT-1), which interacts via its own death domain with the clustered Fas death domains.[52, 54] In addition to its death domain, FADD also possesses a second domain called a "death effector domain" (DED), which serves to recruit the apoptotic initiator procaspase-8.[52, 54, 124] Like death domains, DEDs self-associate, so that recruitment of procaspase-8 by FADD entails interaction between the DED in FADD and the two DEDs present in the N-terminal prodomain of procaspase-8.[124] The resultant oligomerization of procaspase-8 permits reciprocal cleavage and transactivation, thereby initiating the apoptotic cascade.

Trimerization of TNF-R1 by TNF-α also leads to the activation of procaspase-8, but with one large difference. Whereas Fas binds directly to FADD, TNF-R1 recruits FADD indirectly via an intermediary adapter called TRADD (TNF-R1–associated death domain protein).[125] TRADD accomplishes this through its own death domain, which binds both to the aggregated death domains of TNF-R1 and to the death domain of FADD. Once FADD has been recruited, activation of procaspase-8 then proceeds analogously as in the case of Fas.[52, 54] The essential role of FADD in the induction of apoptosis by both Fas and TNF-R1 has been confirmed in knockout mice lacking FADD.[126]

Once activated by either Fas or TNF-R1, caspase-8 may trigger at least two distinct apoptotic cascades.[127] First, caspase-8 may cleave and activate apoptotic effectors, such as caspase-3, -6, and -7. Second, caspase-8 can trigger release of cytochrome *c* from mitochondria, leading to the activation of the apoptotic initiator caspase-9 by the Apaf-1–dependent pathway, discussed previously.[97–99] Release of cytochrome *c* occurs following caspase-8–mediated cleavage and activation of the Bcl-2 family protein Bid, which normally exists as an inactive cytoplasmic precursor.[127] Activated Bid then translocates to mitochondria, where it induces the release of almost 100% of mitochondrial cytochrome *c*. Intriguingly, release of cytochrome *c* seems to occur in the absence of loss of $\Delta\psi_m$, a finding that lends credence to the idea that the opening of mitochondrial PT pores and the release of cytochrome *c* into the cytosol may be separable events.[11, 105, 127]

Importantly, recent studies have shown that engagement of TNF-R1 by TNF-α, as well as Fas by FasL, leads to the simultaneous activation of both death-promoting and life-promoting signaling pathways.[128] This effect is more pronounced for TNF-R1 than for Fas, accounting for the fact that signaling through TNF-R1 rarely induces apoptosis unless protein synthesis is also inhibited.[54] In the case of Fas, life-promoting signals are mediated through a so-called "salvation domain" located at the tail of the cytoplasmic portion of Fas. This "salvation domain" binds a protein tyrosine phosphatase, FAP-1 (Fas-associated phosphatase 1), that confers resistance to FasL. Cells expressing FAP-1 are resistant to Fas-mediated apoptosis, whereas cells lacking FAP-1 are sensitive. The life-promoting pathways activated by TNF-R1 are more elaborate. The adapter protein TRADD, which links TNF-R1 to FADD, recruits two additional proteins, the death domain–containing RIP (receptor-interacting protein) and TRAF-2 (TNFR-associated factor 2).[52, 54] RIP and TRAF-2 contribute to the activation of the nuclear transcription factor kappa B (NF-κB). Inhibition of NF-κB clearly sensitizes cells to TNF-α induced apoptosis.[128] The details of the mechanism by which NF-κB may regulate survival is discussed later in a separate section. TRAF-2 also binds to two endogenous caspase inhibitors, cIAP1 and cIAP2, both members of the IAP family discussed previously.[8, 9, 121]

Just as for caspases, endogenous mechanisms exist for restraining and modulating the activity of both Fas and TNF-R1. Constitutive signaling via spontaneous aggregation of TNF-R1 cytoplasmic death domains is prevented by the protein SODD (silencer of death domains), which binds to the TNF-R1 death domain under resting conditions and is released following engagement of TNF-R1 by TNF-α.[129] Signaling via Fas can be inhibited by a soluble decoy receptor, termed *decoy receptor 3* (DcR3), that binds to and sequesters FasL.[129] Finally, as previously discussed, viral FLIP is an inactive caspase homologue that competes with procaspase-8 for binding to FADD.[9, 119] The issue of whether endogenous cellular FLIP has a similar function is somewhat controversial at present.[9, 119]

p53. The tumor suppressor gene p53 encodes a nuclear transcription factor whose abundance increases dramatically in response to DNA damage or genotoxic stress.[67, 130, 131] p53 is an integral component of an overall DNA damage response system, one of

whose functions is to protect the organism from the acquisition and transmission of potentially neoplastic mutations that might arise in genetically damaged cells.[130] The guiding philosophy of this system seems to be that, as no single cell is indispensable to the organism, it is safer to incapacitate or even eliminate cells whose DNA damage is beyond repair than to risk the development of neoplasia. The DNA damage response involves a number of discrete elements, including a sensor that must continuously monitor the integrity of the genome plus effector limbs that mediate the various possible responses of repair, growth arrest, and apoptosis. p53 has the responsibility of initiating the growth arrest and apoptotic limbs of the DNA damage response.[67, 130] The importance of p53 is evidenced by the fact that mutations of p53 can be found in approximately 50% of all human cancers.[67]

Cellular levels of p53 protein are normally quite low as the result of ubiquitin-mediated proteasomal degradation, signaled through p53's association with the mouse double minute 2 (MDM2) protein.[67, 130, 131] In addition, interaction with MDM2 keeps what p53 is present in an inactive state. DNA damage or genotoxic stress results in a rapid increase in cellular levels of p53 in addition to full activation of p53 as a transcription factor protein.[67, 130, 131] These changes are mediated in part by nuclear kinases that recognize DNA damage in the form of double-strand breaks or repair intermediate protein.[67, 130, 131] DNA damage-activated kinases mediate a rapid increase in functional p53 both by phosphorylating MDM2, leading to its dissociation from p53, and by phosphorylating p53 itself, leading to its full activation. The relevant kinases vary with the DNA-damaging agent, but include DNA-PK, previously discussed as a caspase target, and ATM, whose mutation leads to the disorder ataxia-telangiectasia.[132]

Activated p53 then binds to the promoter elements of a number of genes whose products largely carry out the p53-dependent functions of growth arrest and apoptosis protein.[67, 130, 131, 133] Growth arrest is mediated by several genes that block progression through the cell cycle at a number of so-called "restriction points." Arrest in the pre-DNA synthetic G_1 growth phase is predominantly mediated by the cyclin-dependent kinase inhibitor p21 (also known as WAF1 or CIP1),[134] whereas arrest in the premitotic G_2 growth phase is mediated by both p21 and the protein 14-3-3.[134] Also, p53 induces the production and secretion of IGF-BP3 (insulin-like growth factor binding protein 3), which binds to and inhibits signaling by the mitogen IGF-1.[135] In addition to induction of target genes, p53 also induces growth arrest through transcriptionally independent mechanisms, involving direct interaction with proteins such as the tyrosine kinase c-Abl, which itself mediates growth arrest in response to DNA damage, and several basal transcription factors within RNA polymerase II.[67, 136]

As in the case of growth arrest, p53-dependent apoptosis also occurs through both transcriptionally dependent and independent mechanisms.[67, 130] Key apoptotic genes induced by p53 include the proapoptotic Bcl-2 family member Bax[137] and the GADD45α, β, and γ (growth arrest and DNA damage–induced) proteins, which trigger apoptosis by activating the Jun N-terminal kinase (JNK) pathway.[138] p53-dependent triggering of apoptosis in the absence of transcription may occur through a novel Fas-dependent pathway.[139] Activated p53 increased surface expression of Fas in vascular smooth muscle cells by stimulating transport of Fas from the Golgi complex to the cell membrane.[139] Also, p53 induced transient association of the death domains of Fas and FADD and sensitized cells to Fas-induced apoptosis.[139] It is unclear whether this connection between p53 and Fas generalizes to other cell types. Indeed, p53-dependent regulation of both growth arrest and apoptosis appears to be quite complex, with the specific pathways utilized by p53 being determined by the cell type and stimulus.[67, 130, 131]

In addition to such classic stimuli as ultraviolet light, γ-irradiation, and DNA-damaging chemotherapeutic drugs such as etoposide, mitomycin C, cisplatin, Adriamycin (doxorubicin hydrochloride), and 5-fluorouracil,[67, 130, 131, 139, 140] a variety of insults not classically associated with DNA damage have also been suggested to turn on p53. These include growth factor deprivation in certain neoplastic cell lines, ribonucleotide depletion, heat shock, and expression of certain oncogenes.[67, 130] Moreover, MDM2, which targets p53 for degradation and inhibits p53's transcriptional activity through direct physical interaction, is a caspase target, suggesting that p53 may even be part of the general executionary apparatus during apoptosis.[141]

Another well-characterized inducer of p53 with relevance to renal injury is hypoxia.[142, 143] Oncogenically transformed cells containing wild-type p53 underwent apoptosis in response to hypoxia, whereas cells deficient in p53 as the result of mutation were resistant to the effects of hypoxia.[142] Hypoxia-induced activation of p53 is not limited to neoplastic cells and may occur through the hypoxia-inducible transcription factor HIF-1α (hypoxia-inducible factor 1α), which stabilizes p53 through direct physical interaction.[142, 143]

Finally, it should be mentioned that p53 may be the first of a family of tumor suppressors. Overexpression of either p73α or p73β, two recently cloned structural and functional homologues of p53, has been shown to mediate growth arrest and apoptosis.[144] The physiologic function of p73 is at present uncertain, because, unlike p53, p73 is neither stabilized nor activated by DNA damage.[144]

SURVIVAL PATHWAYS AND ANTAGONISTS OF APOPTOSIS

NF-κB. NF-κB is the general name for a family of nuclear transcription factors that activate transcription of a number of genes involved in the immune and inflammatory responses.[145, 146] It has become evident that activation of NF-κB plays an important role in opposing apoptosis and therefore in determining cell fate in response to a number of apoptotic triggers[128] (see Fig. 3–4). In unstimulated cells, NF-κB resides in the cytoplasm in an inactive form complexed to one of several inhibitory proteins, known collectively as IκB, which prevent NF-κB from entering the nucleus. An extremely wide range of stimuli, many involving some form of cellular stress, activate a specific kinase, NIK (NF-κB–inducing kinase), which phosphorylates IκB and thereby signals its rapid proteasomal degradation. This allows free active NF-κB to translocate to the nucleus, where it binds to specific motifs in the promoter regions of its multiple target genes. NF-κB typically exists as a heterodimer, the most abundant of which is composed of relA (p65) coupled with NF-κB1 (p50).[145, 146]

The antiapoptotic effect of NF-κB was first clearly demonstrated for TNF-α.[128] As previously discussed, TNF-α binds with high affinity to two distinct receptors, TNF-R1 and TNF-R2, with opposing effects on cell fate.[52, 54] The death receptor TNF-R1 induces apoptosis through recruitment and activation of the death domain–containing proteins TRADD and FADD, ultimately leading to the activation of the apoptotic initiator procaspase-8.[52, 54] Signaling through TNF-R2, which lacks a death domain and so does not activate TRADD and FADD, generally promotes survival and proliferation. However, the division in signaling pathways induced by TNF-R1 versus TNF-R2 is not absolute. Signaling through both receptors leads to the activation of the life-promoting NF-κB.[146] In the case of TNF-R2, activation occurs via recruitment of TRAF-2 to the cytoplasmic tail of TNF-R2, followed by TRAF-2–mediated recruitment and activation of NIK.[146] In the case of TNF-R1, activation of NF-κB also occurs via TRAF2 (or possibly RIP), both of which are recruited to TRADD.[125] The strong induction of NF-κB by both TNF-R1 and TNF-R2 accounts for the otherwise puzzling observation that induction of apoptosis by TNF-α generally requires the concomitant addition of a protein synthesis inhibitor, such as cycloheximide.[54]

Recent studies have provided a number of potential mechanisms by which NF-κB protects against apoptosis. These mechanisms include the following: transcriptional induction of various members of the IAP family of apoptosis inhibitors[147] as well as of the antiapoptotic Bcl-2 family member Bfl-A1[148]; induction of a novel inhibitor of apoptosis, named IEX-1L[149]; inhibition of p53 activity through competition for a limiting shared cofactor[150]; and increased expression of TNF receptor-associated proteins, such as TRAF-2.[147] It is probable that the contribution and magnitude of these prosurvival effects of NF-κB depend on the cell type and inducing stimulus. Finally, it is important to note that, because many growth factors are known to activate NF-κB, the role of NF-κB is unlikely to be limited to TNF-α. Indeed, inhibition of NF-κB has been shown to diminish the survival activity of several renal survival factors, including insulin, platelet-derived growth factor (PDGF), and lysophosphatidic acid (LPA).[58, 151, 152]

Phosphatidylinositol 3-Kinase. As previously discussed, most, if not all, mammalian cells undergo apoptosis unless grown in the continuous presence of so-called "survival factors."[56] These survival factors activate specific intracellular signaling pathways that maintain the cell's "default pathway" of apoptosis in a state of constant deactivation.[130] Considerable progress has been made in recent years in determining the identity and mechanism of action of these survival pathways.

One of the key mediators of survival signaling is the combined lipid and protein kinase phosphatidylinositol 3-kinase (PI3K)[153–155] (see Fig. 3–4). PI3K is activated by all three classes of survival factors—cytokines and soluble growth factors[58, 59]; cell-matrix adhesion[156]; and cell-cell adhesion.[63] Like NF-κB, PI3K is the general name for a family of proteins.[153] There are two broad classes of PI3K, which roughly correlate with the major categories of survival factors responsible for their activation. Class I (heterodimer-type) PI3Ks are typically activated by adhesive interactions (cell-matrix and cell-cell) and by soluble survival factors whose receptors have intrinsic tyrosine kinase activity or are directly coupled to tyrosine kinases, such as those for EGF or (IGF-I).[153] Heterodimeric PI3K consists of a 110-kDa catalytic subunit (p110α or p110β) and a regulatory subunit encoded by at least three distinct genes (p85α, p85β, or p55γ).[153] Not only is p85α the most abundantly expressed regulatory subunit, but also, as shown in mice with targeted deletion of the p85α gene, it is the most important biologically.[157] Class II (p110γ-type) PI3Ks are activated by soluble survival factors, such as LPA, that bind to G-protein–coupled receptors (GPCR).[59, 153] They differ from p85/p110 isoforms in two major aspects: they are not associated with a p85 regulatory subunit and they are less sensitive to inhibition by the irreversible PI3K inhibitor wortmannin.[153]

Activation of both classes of PI3K follows a similar theme. Heterodimeric PI3Ks are activated following recruitment of the p85α regulatory subunit to specific phosphotyrosine motifs within the receptor complex.[153] In the case of soluble survival factors, p85α interacts with the cytoplasmic tail of the receptor either directly (eg, EGF) or indirectly via an intermediary protein (eg, IGF-I). Cell-matrix adhesion induces activation of p85α through recruited interaction with the integrin-associated kinase FAK.[156] The recruiting protein in the case of cell-cell interactions is at present unknown. Activation of p110γ (class II) isoforms of PI3K by GPCR also occurs via targeted interaction, in this case directly between catalytic p110γ and the βγ subunit of GPCR.[158]

Once activated, both classes of PI3K have similar substrate specificity. The lipid kinase activity of PI3K catalyzes the transfer of the terminal phosphate of ATP to the D-3 position of membrane-associated phosphatidylinositol (PtdIns), PtdIns-4-monophosphate (PtdIns-4-P), and PtdIns-4,5-P_2 to form PtdIns-3-P, PtdIns-3,4-P_2, and PtdIns-3,4,5-P_3, respectively.[153] PtdIns-3,4,5-P_3 is thought to be the main in vivo product of PI3K.[153] Formation of PtdIns-3,4,5-P_3 then leads to the recruitment and activation of PtdIns-3,4,5-P_3–dependent kinase (PDK1), a recently cloned serine/threonine kinase that contributes to the activation of many of the key downstream mediators of the survival activity of PI3K.[159] Among these mediators are the following: Akt (protein kinase B [PKB]),[159, 160] pp70s6k,[161] and several novel and atypical isoforms of protein kinase C (PKC).[162] In contrast to its lipid kinase activity, the protein kinase activity of PI3K is apparently inhibited by membrane localization.[163] Cytoplasmic PI3K leads to the activation of extracellular signal-related kinases 1 and 2 (ERK1/2) within the mitogen-activated protein kinase (MAPK) pathway, which in many cells is associated with induction of proliferation.[163]

The most important target of PI3K for survival signaling is the serine/threonine kinase Akt/PKB[154, 155] (see Fig. 3–4). In several systems, activation of Akt/PKB has been shown to be both necessary and sufficient for inhibition of the default pathway of apoptosis.[154, 155] Although the mechanism of action of Akt/PKB is likely to be multifactorial and complex, at least one antiapoptotic pathway induced by Akt/PKB has been clearly delineated.[164] Upon activation, Akt/PKB phosphorylates the proapoptotic Bcl-2 family member BAD. Phosphorylated BAD then binds to and is sequestered by the protein 14-3-3τ. This prevents BAD from triggering apoptosis by heterodimerizing with and inactivating mitochondrial prosurvival Bcl-2 family members, such as Bcl-2 and Bcl-xL.[164] Another downstream target of Akt/PKB with potential relevance to cell survival is glycogen synthase kinase-3,[165] which participates in several intracellular signaling pathways, including control of the MAPK-regulated transcription factor AP1 as well as the tumor suppressor product APC (adenomatous polyposis coli).[165]

PI3K also induces the activation of at least two other kinases that contribute to inhibition of the default pathway of apoptosis.[161, 162] pp70s6k, the target of the immunosuppressant rapamycin, plays a critical role in cell cycle progression.[166] Inhibition of pp70s6k with rapamycin blocked up to 50% of the antiapoptotic activity of several known renal tubular survival factors, including EGF and LPA.[59] Rapamycin also enhanced the degree of cell death in response to several known apoptotic stimuli. Several isoforms of PKC with both pro- and antiapoptotic activity are also activated by PI3K via PDK1.[162] The atypical isoform aPKC-ζ apparently protects against apoptosis, whereas the novel isoform nPKC-δ promotes apoptosis.[167]

While most survival signaling seems to proceed through PI3K and Akt/PKB, additional cellular pathways apparently exist that are independent of one or both of these kinases. The best characterized of these pathways involves the adapter protein Shc, which forms part of the multiprotein signaling complex assembled in response to most soluble survival factors and some, but not all, integrin-matrix interactions.[65] Shc is thought to activate the Ras/MAPK pathway and to promote cell cycle progression. However, at least in the case of one soluble survival factor, inhibition of apoptosis was independent of the Ras/MAPK pathway and seemed to depend on induction of the proto-oncogene c-Myc (discussed later).[168] With respect to cell-matrix interactions, inhibition of anoikis occurred only for those integrins that recruited Shc.[21, 22] Adhesion through integrins that did not recruit Shc failed to inhibit anoikis, despite activation of FAK (a known recruiter of PI3K), even in the presence of soluble survival factors.[21, 22] Finally, it should be noted that activation of Akt/PKB can also occur in a PI3K-independent manner in response to cellular stresses, such as heat shock or hyperosmolarity.[168]

PATHWAYS AND FACTORS WITH THE CAPACITY TO EITHER INDUCE OR ANTAGONIZE APOPTOSIS

Bcl-2 Family. Bcl-2 and related proteins are a growing family whose members can be divided into two groups, those with prosurvival activity and those with pro-apoptotic activity[114, 169] (Table 3–4). Family members are defined by the presence of at least one of four conserved protein motifs, known as Bcl-2 homology.[114, 169] Most prosurvival members can inhibit apoptosis induced by an extremely wide range of triggers, including survival factor deprivation,[170] Fas- and TNF-RI receptor activation, cytotoxic stimuli such as hydrogen peroxide or oxidative free radicals,[171] and DNA damage–inducing agents such as chemotherapeutic drugs or γ-irradiation.[172]

Bcl-2 family members bind to one another to form heterodimers.[114, 169] Interaction occurs between members, with both similar and antagonistic effects on apoptosis. In the latter instance, dimerization often

results in a seeming titration of the effect of one of the two interacting family members' homology.[114, 169] Even in the absence of direct interaction, titration of effect by opposing family members may also occur, eg, via competition for downstream targets homology.[114, 169] Such considerations have led to the concept that the balance between survival and apoptosis is determined by the relative concentrations of prosurvival and proapoptotic Bcl-2 family members' homology.[114, 169] An additional layer of complexity arises from the fact that not all family members interact with all others, so that the cellular distribution and promiscuity of interaction of an individual Bcl-2 family member may prove as important as its concentration homology.[114, 169]

Bcl-2, the founding member of this family, is found on the cytoplasmic face of the nuclear envelope, endoplasmic reticulum, and mitochondrial outer membrane homology.[114, 169] While a C-terminal hydrophobic domain is important for membrane anchoring, deletion of this domain does not eliminate the prosurvival activity of Bcl-2. Moreover, while most Bcl-2 family members possess membrane anchoring domains, some, such as Bax, are nonetheless predominantly cytosolic in the absence of an apoptotic stimulus.[169] Given the large number of proteins with which Bcl-2 family members interact,[114] cellular distribution may be determined less by membrane localization domains than by specific targeted protein-protein interactions. As discussed later, the most clearly demonstrated effects of Bcl-2 family members are on mitochondrial regulation of apoptosis, but evidence exists for effects on other cellular organelles, such as the endoplasmic reticulum.[173] Indeed, the subcellular locations where Bcl-2 family members exert their major effects may very well depend on the cell type in question.[174]

In general, Bcl-2 family members influence cell fate during the commitment phase of apoptosis. While a number of potential mechanisms have been proposed, Bcl-2 proteins appear to regulate apoptosis in two major ways. The first involves the direct interaction of Bcl-2 family members with procaspase activating complexes such as that for procaspase-9. It may be recalled that activation of procaspase-9 occurs within a so-called "apoptosome," in which cytoplasmic Apaf-1 binds via separate domains to procaspase-9 and mitochondrially released cytochrome c.[99, 100] Prosurvival Bcl-2 family members, such as Bcl-xL, also bind to Apaf-1 and can prevent or mask the cytochrome c–induced conformational change that leads to the recruitment of procaspase-9.[175, 176] By this means, prosurvival Bcl-2 family members may block initiation of the execution phase of apoptosis, even after mitochondrial permeability transition and release of cytochrome c.[177] Proapoptotic Bcl-2 family members, such as Bik, may counteract the protective effects of Bcl-xL by binding to and sequestering Bcl-xL.[175, 176]

The second mechanism of action of Bcl-2 family members involves maintenance of mitochondrial membrane integrity, and perhaps that of other organelles. Overexpression of Bcl-2 or Bcl-xL has been shown to prevent mitochondrial permeability transition and

TABLE 3–4. Bcl-2 Family of Proteins

Bcl-2 FAMILY MEMBER	MEMBRANE ANCHOR	PORE-FORMING ABILITY
Bcl-2 subfamily (prosurvival)		
Bcl-2	+	+
Bcl-xL	+	+
Bcl-w	+	?*
Mcl-1	+	?
Bfl-A1	−	?
Bax subfamily (proapoptosis)		
Bax	+	+
Bak	+	?
Bok	+	?
BH3 subfamily (proapoptosis)		
Bik	−	Unlikely†
Blk	−	Unlikely
Hrk	−	Unlikely
BNIP3	−	Unlikely
Bim$_L$	−	Unlikely
Bad	−	Unlikely
Bid	−	Unlikely
Viral family members (pro-survival)		
BHRF1	+	?
LMW5-HL	−	?
ORF16	+	?
KS-Bcl-2	+	?
E1B-19 kDa	−	?

*These Bcl-2 family members possess Bcl-2 homology (BH) domains BH1 and BH2 thought to confer pore-forming ability, but have not yet been shown to produce pores in lipid bilayers.
†These Bcl-2 family members lack BH1 and BH2 domains, and are therefore unlikely to form pores.
Adapted from Adams JM, Cory S: The Bcl-2 protein family: arbiters of cell survival. Science 1998; 281:1322–1326; with permission.

release of apoptosis-promoting substances such as cytochrome *c* or AIF, in response to several triggers of apoptosis.[100, 178] Combining these two mechanisms of action, prosurvival Bcl-2 family members may therefore protect cells by acting at two discrete steps along the pathway to activation of the apoptotic initiator caspase-9: first, by inhibiting release of mitochondrial cytochrome *c*, and second, assuming some cytochrome *c* does manage to leak into the cytosol, by inhibiting cytochrome *c*–catalyzed cleavage and activation of procaspase-9. In contrast to the stabilizing effects of prosurvival members, proapoptosis Bcl-2 proteins such as Bax or Bid may directly induce mitochondrial permeability transition or release of cytochrome *c*, or both.[127, 179]

The ability of Bax to promote the opening of mitochondrial pores and loss of mitochondrial transmembrane potential may relate to its three-dimensional structure (see Table 3–4). The structure of several Bcl-2 family members, including Bax and the prosurvival members Bcl-2 and Bcl-xL, resembles the pore-forming domains of bacterial toxins, such as diphtheria toxin.[180] Like the bacterial toxins, these Bcl-2 proteins can insert into synthetic lipid vesicles or planar lipid bilayers and form ion-conducting channels with distinct characteristics[180] (see Table 3–4). While it is unclear how membrane insertion and pore formation by Bcl-2 or Bcl-xL might protect against apoptosis, a plausible argument can be made for induction of apoptosis by Bax through pore formation in mitochondrial membranes.

Finally, there are several notable examples of regulation of the activity of Bcl-2 family members. Such regulation may occur within either the commitment or the execution phase of apoptosis. Within the commitment phase, regulation is exercised primarily via phosphorylation events. As previously discussed, serine phosphorylation of the proapoptotic member BAD by survival factor–induced Akt/PKB leads to its sequestration within the cytosol, thereby preventing access of BAD to mitochondria, where it can heterodimerize with and inactivate prosurvival Bcl-2 family members.[164] Phosphorylation events have also been suggested to regulate the activity, both positively and negatively, of prosurvival family members, such as Bcl-2 and Bcl-xL.[114, 169] Within the execution phase, caspase-mediated cleavage of Bcl-2 proteins can convert them from a latent to an active state. For example, upon FADD-mediated activation by Fas or TNF-R1, caspase-8 cleaves the proapoptotic member Bid, thereby converting it from a latent cytoplasmic form to an active moiety that moves to mitochondria and promotes their nearly complete release of cytochrome *c*.[127] In some cases, caspase-mediated cleavage can even convert proteins from prosurvival to proapoptotic activity. Thus, cleavage of Bcl-2 abrogates its prosurvival activity and converts the protein into a Bax-like proapoptotic factor.[115] These examples highlight the complexity of regulation not only among Bcl-2 family members but also between Bcl-2 family members and other components of the apoptotic machinery.

Cell Cycle Components. An intimate connection exists between movement through the cell cycle and apoptosis. It appears that the pathways for cell proliferation and cell apoptosis are coupled, so that a normal consequence of a cell's undergoing proliferation is activation of the cell's "default pathway" of apoptosis.[181] Thus, unless the default pathway of apoptosis is inhibited by survival signals, proliferating cells automatically die by apoptosis.

This connection between proliferation and apoptosis was first documented for the nuclear transcription factor c-*Myc*. Levels of c-*Myc* correlate directly with the degree of cellular proliferation.[182] This relationship is causal, in that increasing c-*Myc* leads to increased proliferation, whereas down-regulation of c-*Myc* is needed for growth arrest. Intriguingly, as first demonstrated by Evan et al,[183] c-*Myc* can be shown to promote both apoptosis and proliferation. Interestingly, mutational mapping of c-*Myc* shows complete concordance between the domains essential for induction of proliferation and those essential for induction of apoptosis.[130, 184]

Evan and colleagues[130, 183] have proposed the following model to explain the dual roles of c-*Myc* in cell proliferation and apoptosis. They suggest that sensitization to apoptosis is a normal and obligate function of c-*Myc*. The viability of a cell expressing c-*Myc* therefore requires active inhibition of apoptosis by survival factors. Coupling apoptosis and proliferation in this way provides a built-in fail-safe against uncontrolled proliferation. According to this model, neoplastic transformation of a cell would require two separate mutations, one within a proliferative pathway promoting cell cycle entry and the other within the fail-safe pathway inactivating apoptosis.[130]

Linkage of proliferation and apoptosis, although first described in fibroblasts,[183] is not limited to any single cell type.[182] Also, several genes other than c-*Myc* have been shown to intimately link apoptosis to cell-cycle progression. The transcription factor E2F,[185] the cell cycle phosphatase Cdc25a,[186] and the retinoblastoma protein (Rb)[187, 188] all have a dual role in promoting both proliferation and apoptosis in a variety of cell types. Furthermore, linkage of proliferation and apoptosis does not appear to apply exclusively to growth factor–mediated events but extends to nonsoluble survival and proliferative factors, including cell-matrix and, possibly also, cell-cell interactions.[189, 190]

The pathways by which cell cycle–regulating genes such as c-*Myc* sensitize cells to apoptosis are obscure.[130] Although the protein domains responsible for proliferation and apoptosis exactly coincide in all cell cycle–regulating genes examined,[130] the proliferative and apoptotic limbs do eventually diverge. Thus, the prosurvival protein Bcl-2 suppresses only the apoptotic ability of c-*Myc* without affecting its proliferative ability.[191] As recently proposed, these data may be resolved by an alternative model in which cell cycle–regulating genes such as c-*Myc* do not themselves trigger apoptosis, but rather lower the threshold of the cell to any apoptotic trigger that is present.[130] Thus, for example, cells subjected to a cytotoxic trigger might undergo apoptosis at a lower degree of cell damage in the presence of c-*Myc* than in its absence.

Finally, there are a number of proteins collectively known as cyclin-dependent kinase inhibitors (CDKI) that promote exit from the cell cycle.[192] One of these, p21, is induced by p53 and is largely responsible for the growth arrest mediated by p53.[134, 193] In much the same way that genes promoting cell-cycle progression sensitize cells to apoptosis, CDKI may protect against apoptosis by turning off the default pathway of apoptosis that is coupled to cell proliferation. Specific examples of CDKI that have been shown to confer protection against apoptosis in selected models include p21[194] and p27[Kip1].[195]

MISCELLANEOUS FACTORS AND PATHWAYS

Reactive Oxygen Species. The role of oxidant injury in mediating necrotic cell death has been described previously. Reactive oxygen species (ROS) have also been implicated in apoptotic cell death, although their role remains to be defined. Antioxidants and ROS scavengers have been shown to be protective in multiple models of apoptosis.[196] In the case of renal epithelial cells, antioxidants and ROS scavengers have been demonstrated to inhibit apoptosis induced by both survival factor withdrawal and by cytotoxic stimuli, such as cisplatin.[57, 68] In cell death induced by growth factor deprivation, ROS appear to act upstream of caspases,[57] presumably during the commitment, rather than the execution, phase of cell death.

There are at least three general mechanisms by which ROS may theoretically contribute to apoptosis: (1) as effectors of cell death during the execution phase of apoptosis; (2) as cytotoxic stimuli capable of inducing apoptotic or necrotic cell death, depending upon the degree of cellular damage; and (3) as specific signaling intermediates or second messengers capable of triggering apoptosis within the commitment phase of apoptosis. Each of these is discussed in its turn.

While ROS are clearly increased in apoptosis induced by multiple stimuli,[196] a significant role for ROS in the execution phase of apoptosis seems unlikely for the following reasons. First, several models of apoptosis proceeded normally in cells cultured under near-anaerobic conditions ($[O_2]$ <10 parts per million) in which the generation of ROS should, at the very least, be greatly reduced. Dead cells showed all the classic morphologic features of apoptosis. Second, the broad nonspecific nature of the oxidative damage produced by ROS seems inconsistent with the precise highly coordinated protein cleavages and morphologic changes characteristic of apoptosis. ROS may contribute to the ultimate demise of a cell, as their production is bound to increase with continued mitochondrial release of cytochrome c and disruption of the electron transport chain.[10, 11] However, any specific early role for ROS during the execution phase of apoptosis is likely to be minor in comparison with that of caspases.

Both the second and the third mechanisms involving ROS, take place during the commitment phase of apoptosis and represent probable or emerging roles for ROS. The second mechanism is a specific example of an apoptotic trigger within the broader category of cytotoxic stimuli. As previously discussed, a wide variety of cytotoxic stimuli can induce either apoptosis or necrosis in the same cell, depending on the severity of the injury.[68–70, 73] Cytotoxic stimuli known to generate ROS include UV light and γ-irradiation.[196] In addition, in a recent study examining the genes induced by p53 before the visible onset of apoptosis, a surprising number were found to encode proteins that either generate or respond to oxidant stress.[133]

The third mechanism is perhaps the most intriguing. Recent evidence suggests that ROS, including superoxide anion and hydrogen peroxide, can act as second messengers in a variety of signal transduction pathways.[197] The pathways in which ROS participate are quite diverse and affect many signaling molecules with a positive or negative effect on apoptosis, including PI3K, NF-κB, and MAPK family members.[197] In addition, several of the signal transduction pathways initiated by renal epithelial cell survival factors, including EGF[198] and LPA,[199] are at least partially dependent on the production of intracellular ROS, such as hydrogen peroxide. It is presumed that ROS that function as signaling intermediates, rather than oxidative effectors (eg, in phagocytic killing of bacteria), are produced in lower concentrations and in highly restricted regions of the cell.[197]

Several examples serve to illustrate how ROS may act as signaling intermediates within the commitment phase of apoptosis. Oxidative and nitrosative agents may modulate the activity of proteins by modifying cysteine residues that are strategically located at catalytic or allosteric sites. The addition of nitric oxide (NO) to cells, either directly as a gas or indirectly in the form of sodium nitroprusside, led to the redox-triggered activation of Ras, followed by its association with and activation of PI3K.[200] Mutation of a single cysteine residue in Ras abolished its activation by NO but had no effect on activation of Ras through other routes.[200] A similar redox-triggered mechanism might explain the putative role of ROS in activating caspases, which are cysteine-dependent proteases and presumably therefore sensitive to redox changes.[57, 201] Other proteins whose activity can be modulated by the redox state include the nuclear transcription factors NF-κB and AP-1. The recently cloned protein SAG (sensitive to apoptosis gene), which itself is induced by redox changes, protects cells from apoptosis by binding to copper and zinc ions and thereby inhibiting peroxidative reactions.[202] Finally, oxidative stress has been shown to play a role in the regulation of the recently identified kinase ASK-1 (apoptosis signal-regulating kinase 1), a member of the MAPK signaling cascade whose overexpression triggers apoptosis.[203] ASK-1 is held in check by interaction with the protein thioredoxin.[203] Oxidative changes in the redox state of the cell lead to the dissociation of thioredoxin, with resultant ASK-1 activation and apoptosis.[203]

ROLE OF NECROSIS AND APOPTOSIS IN ACUTE RENAL FAILURE IN VIVO

The relative contribution made by necrosis and apoptosis to the renal dysfunction associated with ARF remains uncertain and an important issue for further research. The issue is complicated by the fact that necrosis of renal tubular cells is far more prominent in animal models of ARF than in humans with acute tubular necrosis (ATN).[1] Therefore, caution is necessary when one extrapolates studies of apoptosis in animal models of acute renal injury to humans with ARF. Nevertheless, morphologic studies that demonstrate both necrosis and apoptosis in animals and humans with ARF suggest a role for both forms of cell death. In animals, brief periods of renal ischemia induce apoptosis of renal tubular cells 1 to 2 days later without much evidence of necrosis.[204] Longer periods of renal ischemia in animals induce necrosis as well as apoptosis.[204, 205] Furthermore, while evidence supporting a role for apoptosis in humans with ARF remains sparse, the presence of apoptotic tubular cells has been demonstrated in the kidneys of humans with ATN induced by ischemic and toxic stimuli.[206–208]

Potential Causes of Apoptosis In Acute Renal Failure

While the causes of necrosis in response to renal injury are well defined, the triggers of apoptosis in ARF are less well established. We have already described in detail the many factors that have been identified that can induce apoptosis of cells. We now discuss the potential role of each of these apoptotic triggers in ARF.

ISCHEMIC AND CYTOTOXIC TUBULAR CELL INJURY

The realization that the same causes of cell necrosis can also cause apoptosis represents the most important stimulus to the increasing interest in the role of apoptosis in ARF. It is now clear that the severity of an injurious agent determines the mode of cell death. If injury is severe enough to reduce cell ATP to critically low levels, cells die by necrosis. In response to more modest injury, cells die by apoptosis.[68, 69, 73]

The severity of injury suffered by a tubular cell in response to an ischemic or toxic insult depends upon many factors. Tubular cells in the outer medulla are more sensitive to ischemia than are cells in the cortex because the oxygen tension in the medulla falls to far lower levels than those in the cortex.[16] Susceptibility to injury is also related to the ATP requirements of the cell, which are determined in large part by the energy-requiring solute transport activity of the cell.[16] This explains the resistance of tubular cells of the inner medulla to cell death, despite the profound reduction in oxygen tension in this zone of the kidney after renal ischemia. The mechanism of cell death in response to nephrotoxic agents is related partly to the predominant site of reabsorption of the toxin. For example, both gentamycin and cisplatin are reabsorbed by the proximal tubule, the major site of injury in ARF caused by both agents.[1] The mode of cell death that results probably depends upon the intracellular concentration of the drug in each cell.[68]

Thus, it is probable that the severity of ATP depletion suffered by individual tubular cells following acute renal injury varies greatly, depending on many factors, including the degree of hypoxia, the energy requirements of the cell, and, in the case of cytotoxic injury, the concentration of the toxic factor reached within the tubular cell. Substantial evidence has demonstrated a relationship between the severity of the hypoxia and the mode of cell death in the heart[70] and brain.[209] Both myocardial infarction and stroke result in necrosis of cells most distant from the nearest source of oxygen, while cells at the periphery of the ischemic area die by apoptosis. Although it seems likely that the mode of death in kidneys following acute injury is governed by similar principles, the effect of graded injury on the mechanism of renal tubular cell death has so far been demonstrated only in cultured cells.[68, 73]

SURVIVAL FACTORS AND APOPTOSIS IN ACUTE RENAL FAILURE

The role of growth factors, cell-matrix adhesion, and cell-cell attachment as survival signals and inhibitors of the default pathway of apoptosis has already been discussed in detail in this chapter. A relative or absolute deficiency of soluble growth factors may occur in ARF.[210, 211] A deficiency of growth factors may be responsible for the loss of some tubular cells via the "default" pathway of apoptosis. The well-established therapeutic benefit of growth factors in experimental ARF[212] may be due not only to stimulation of proliferation but also to inhibition of apoptosis.[57, 213] Another potential cause of apoptosis by the default pathway in ARF is loss of normal cell-matrix adhesion. Loss of the normal adhesion between tubular cells and the basement membrane has been shown to occur in response to injury in vitro[214, 215] as well as in humans with ATN.[216, 217] Finally, recent evidence that renal tubular cells that have lost cell-matrix attachment can escape apoptosis and survive as the result of cadherin-mediated cell-cell aggregation provides potentially novel insights into the mechanism of cast formation in ARF.[63]

APOPTOSIS INDUCED BY DNA DAMAGE IN ACUTE RENAL FAILURE

It is likely that apoptosis of renal tubular cells contributes to the tubular dysfunction and ARF associated with cytotoxic agents, such as cisplatin[1, 68] and ifosfamide.[1] Apoptosis induced by these agents is the result, at least in part, of irreparable DNA damage and activation of p53[67] (discussed in detail earlier). Thus, the very mechanism responsible for the efficacy of these agents in treating neoplasms probably contributes to their nephrotoxicity.

RECEPTOR-MEDIATED APOPTOSIS IN ACUTE RENAL FAILURE

Stimulation with endotoxin and cytokines, such as IL-1β and interferon-γ increases the expression of Fas and TNF-α by renal tubular cells in culture.[218] Furthermore, ARF induced by endotoxin in mice in vivo is associated with substantial apoptosis of renal tubular cells.[218] Fas-mediated events may also contribute to apoptosis associated with hypoxic injury to renal tubular cells.[219, 220] Thus, available evidence points toward a role for these receptor-mediated events in ARF associated with sepsis and renal ischemia.

Therapeutic Implications

When cells undergo severe injury, necrotic cell death rapidly ensues and is mediated by a number of disparate biochemical pathways (see Fig. 3–1). It is therefore difficult to prevent severely injured tubular cells from dying by necrosis even when the protective agent is administered before kidneys are subjected to a severe insult. However, our current understanding of the pathways that lead to apoptosis (see Fig. 3–4), which have been described in detail in this chapter, suggests that this form of cell death may be more amenable to reversal by therapeutic intervention.[221] The presence of a commitment phase (see Fig. 3–2), during which the balance of multiple pro- and anti-apoptotic factors determines cell fate (see Fig. 3–4), provides a potential therapeutic "window of opportunity" during which death can potentially be averted. Also, because apoptosis is executed by a caspase-dependent "final common pathway," it provides another potential target for inhibiting this form of cell death (see Fig. 3–4)

INHIBITION OF APOPTOTIC CELL DEATH: BENEFICIAL OR HARMFUL?

It is important to recognize that the effect of interventions that block apoptosis, whether beneficial or harmful, depends on the role of apoptosis in each disease process.[8] For example, in situations in which irreparable DNA damage has occurred (eg, in response to chemotherapeutic agents or irradiation), the apoptotic death of cells is necessary to prevent the development of a malignancy. A defect in this mechanism, caused, for example, by mutations in p53 is an important cause of a variety of cancers.

On the other hand, it is not at all clear that apoptosis induced in response to mild ischemic or toxic injury serves any useful "homeostatic role".[8, 222] In fact, it has become apparent that apoptosis actually contributes to or exacerbates some disease processes, such as neurodegenerative diseases, stroke, and ischemia-reperfusion injury.[8] The complexity of the pathways involved in apoptosis provides a number of potential targets for therapeutic interventions.

POTENTIAL STRATEGIES FOR PREVENTING APOPTOTIC CELL DEATH: ROLE OF CASPASE INHIBITORS

Therapeutic interventions can potentially be directed at a multitude of factors, both pro- and anti-apoptotic, that ultimately determine the fate of the cell exposed to an apoptotic stimulus (see Fig. 3–4). The availability of cell-permeable inhibitors of caspases (see Table 3–2) has resulted in a great deal of interest regarding the efficacy of caspase inhibition in preventing apoptosis and in ameliorating disease processes.[8]

Interestingly, the ability of inhibitors of apoptosis to prevent cell death has resulted in variable effects. In some studies, caspase inhibitors, while effective in blocking many of the biochemical events associated with apoptosis (eg, chromatin condensation and DNA laddering), have been ineffective in preventing cell death.[223] In these situations, caspase inhibitors change the morphologic form of cell death from apoptosis to one more consistent with necrosis.[223] However, many other studies have demonstrated that caspase inhibitors can prevent cell death.[8] This seeming paradox suggests the possibility that the efficacy of caspases in preventing cell death may depend upon both the cell type and the apoptotic trigger. Interestingly, in situations in which caspases have been reported to be ineffective, cell death has been due to DNA damage or oncogene dysregulation.[223] On the other hand, caspase inhibitors have been shown to prevent renal tubular cell death in response to ischemic injury.[8, 224] Available information regarding the hierarchy of caspase activation (see Table 3–3) suggests that it is likely that inhibition of caspases that act as "initiators" of apoptosis or play a signaling role are more likely to be effective in preventing cell death than inhibitors of caspase that act as "executioners."

However, we still have a great deal to learn before we can determine whether the development of therapeutic agents that safely and effectively alter the course of ARF by modulating renal tubular cell apoptosis is feasible. The complex, overlapping, and probably redundant pathways involved in the activation and modulation of the determinants of cell fate need to be further elucidated. Moreover, there may be subtle but important variations in the response among different cell types to the multitude of factors that can trigger apoptosis; if so this adds another layer of complexity to the problem. Nonetheless, despite these reservations and anticipated difficulties, continued intense investigation into the mechanisms mediating apoptosis of renal tubular cells may yield substantial rewards in the treatment of ARF.

REFERENCES

1. Brady HR, Brenner BM, Lieberthal W: Acute Renal Failure. In: Brenner B, ed: *The Kidney.*. Philadelphia: WB Saunders; 1996:1200–1252.
2. Lieberthal W, Levine J: Mechanisms of apoptosis and its potential role in renal tubular epithelial cell injury. Am J Physiol 1996; 271:F477–F488.
3. Lieberthal W, Koh JS, Levine JS: Necrosis and apoptosis in acute renal failure. Semin Nephrol 1998; 18:505–518.
4. Earnshaw W: Nuclear changes in apoptosis. Cur Opin Cell Biol 1995; 7:337–343.
5. Majno G, Joris I: Apoptosis, oncosis, and necrosis: an overview of cell death. Am J Pathol 1995; 146:3–15.

6. Wolf BB, Green DR: Suicidal tendencies: apoptotic cell death by caspase family proteases. J Biol Chem 1999; 274:20048–20052.

7. Rudel T, Bokoch GM: Membrane and morphologic changes in apoptotic cells regulated by caspase-mediated activation of PAK2. Science 1997; 276:1571–1574.

8. Thornberry NA, Lazebnik Y: Caspases: enemies within. Science 1998; 281:1312–1316.

9. Kidd VJ: Proteolytic activities that mediate apoptosis. Annu Rev Physiol 1998; 60:533–573.

10. Kroemer G, Dallaporta B, Resche-Rigon M: The mitochondrial death/life regulator in apoptosis and necrosis. Annu Rev Physiol 1998; 60:619–642.

11. Green DR, Reed JC: Mitochondria and apoptosis. Science 1998; 281:1309–1312.

12. Weinberg JM: The cell biology of ischemic renal injury. Kidney Int 1991; 39:476–500.

13. Lieberthal W: Biology of acute renal failure: therapeutic implications. Kidney Int 1997; 52:1102–1115.

14. Waarde AV, Stromski ME, Thulin G, et al: Protection of the kidney against ischemic injury by inhibition of 5'-nucleotidase. Am J Physiol 1989; 256:F298–F305.

15. Stromski ME, Waarde Av, Avison MJ, et al: Metabolic and functional consequences of inhibiting adenosine deaminase during renal ischemia in rats. J Clin Invest 1988; 82:1694–1699.

16. Epstein F, Agmon Y, Brezis M: Physiology of renal hypoxia. Ann N Y Acad Sci 1994; 718:72–81.

17. Lieberthal W, Nigam SK: Acute renal failure. I. Relative importance of proximal vs. distal tubular injury. Am J Physiol 1998; 275:F623–F631.

18. Bagnasco S, Good D, Balaban R, Burg M: Lactate production in isolated segments of the rat nephron. Am J Physiol 1985; 248:F522–F526.

19. Brezis M, Rosen S, Silva P, et al: Transport activity modifies thick ascending limb damage in the isolated perfused kidney. Kidney Int 1984; 25:65–72.

20. Epstein FH: Oxygen and renal metabolism. Kidney Int 1997; 51:381–385.

21. Edelstein CL, Schrier RW: The role of calcium in cell injury. In: Goligorsky MS, ed: Contemporary Issues in Nephrology. New York: Churchill Livingtone; 1995:1–21.

22. McCoy CE, Selvaggio AM, Alexander EA, Schwartz JH: Adenosine triphosphate depletion induces a rise in cytosolic free calcium in canine renal epithelial cells. J Clin Invest 1988; 82:1326–1332.

23. Kribben A, Wieder ED, Wetzels JF, et al: Evidence for a role of cytosolic free calcium in hypoxia-induced proximal tubular injury. J Clin Invest 1994; 93:1922–1929.

24. Burke TJ, Arnold PE, Gordon JA, et al: Protective effect of intrarenal calcium membrane blockers before or after renal ischemia: functional, morphological, and mitochondrial studies. J Clin Invest 1984; 74:1830–1841.

25. Wagner K, Albrecht S, Neumayer HH: Prevention of postransplant acute tubular necrosis by the calcium antagonist diltiazem. Am J Nephrol 1986; 7:287–291.

26. Caraceni P, Ryu HS, van Thiel DH, Borle AB: Source of oxygen free radicals produced by rat hepatocytes during postanoxic reoxygenation. Biochim Biophys Acta 1995; 1268:249–254.

27. Bonventre JV: The 85-kD cytosolic phospholipase A_2 knockout mouse: a new tool for physiology and cell biology. J Am Soc Nephrol 1999; 10:404–412.

28. Matthys E, Patel Y, Kreisberg J, et al: Lipid alterations induced by renal ischemia: pathogenic factor in membrane damage. Kidney Int 1984; 26:153–161.

29. Gronich J, Bonventre J, Nemenoff R: Identification and characterization of a hormonally regulated form of phospholipase A_2 in rat renal mesangial cells. J Biol Chem 1988; 263:16645–16651.

30. Portilla D, Crew MD, Grant D, et al: cDNA cloning and expression of a novel family of enzymes with calcium-independent phospholipase A_2 and lysophospholipase activities. J Am Soc Nephrol 1998; 9:1178–1186.

31. Nakamura H, Nemenoff R, Gronich J, Bonventre JV: Subcellular characteristics of phospholipase A_2 activity in the rat kidney. J Clin Invest 1991; 87:1810–1818.

32. Bonventre JV, Huang Z, Taheri MR, et al: Reduced fertility and postischemic brain injury in mice deficient in cytosolic phospholipase A_2. Nature 1997; 390:622–625.

33. Takasaki J, Kawauchi Y, Urasaki T, et al: Antibodies against type II phospholipase A_2 prevent renal injury due to ischemia and reperfusion in rats. FEBS Lett 1998; 440:377–381.

34. Zager RA, Conrad DS, Burkhart K: Phospholipase A_2: a potentially important determinant of adenosine triphosphate levels during hypoxic-reoxygenation tubular injury. J Am Soc Nephrol 1996; 7:2327–2339.

35. Schonefeld M, Noble S, Bertorello AM, et al: Hypoxia-induced amphiphiles inhibit renal Na^+, $K(^+)$-ATPase. Kidney Int 1996; 49:1289–1296.

36. López-Novoa JM: Potential role of platelet activating factor in acute renal failure. Kidney Int 1999; 53:1672–1682.

37. Smith SR, Creech EA, Schaffer AV, et al: Effects of thromboxane synthase inhibition with CGS 13080 in human cyclosporine nephrotoxicity. Kidney Int 1992; 41:199–205.

38. Zager RA, Schimpf BA, Gmur DJ, Burke TJ: Phospholipase A_2 activity can protect renal tubules from oxygen deprivation injury. Proc Natl Acad Sci USA 1993; 90:8297–8301.

39. Zager RA, Burkhart KM, Conrad DS, et al: Phospholipase A_2-induced cytoprotection of proximal tubules: potential determinants and specificity for ATP depletion-mediated injury. J Am Soc Nephrol 1996; 7:64–72.

40. Zoeller RA, Lake AC, Nagan N, et al: Plasmalogens as endogenous antioxidants: somatic cell mutants reveal the importance of the vinyl ether. Biochem J 1999; 338:769–776.

41. Edelstein CL, Wieder ED, Yaqoob MM, et al: The role of cysteine proteases in hypoxia-induced rat renal proximal tubular injury. Proc Natl Acad Sci USA 1995; 92:7662–7666.

42. Schnellman RG, Williams SW: Proteases in cell death. Ren Fail 1998; 20:679–686.

43. Edelstein CL, Yaqoob MM, Alkhunaizi AM, et al: Modulation of hypoxia-induced calpain activity in rat renal proximal tubules. Kidney Int 1996; 50:1150–1157.

44. McCord J: Oxygen-derived free radicals in postischemic tissue injury. N Engl J Med 1985; 159–163.

45. Dong Z, Saikumar P, Weinberg JM, Venkatachalam MA: Internucleosomal DNA cleavage triggered by plasma membrane damage during necrotic cell death. Involvement of serine but not cysteine proteases. Am J Pathol 1997; 151:1205–1213.

46. Enari M, Sakahira H, Yokayama H, et al: A caspase-activated endonuclease that degrades DNA during apoptosis, and its inhibitor ICAD. Nature 1998; 391:43–50.

47. Ueda N, Walker P, Hsu S, Shah S: Activation of a 15-kDa endonuclease in hypoxia/reoxygenation injury without morphologic features of apoptosis. Proc Natl Acad Sci USA 1995; 92:7202–7206.

48. Beckman JS, Koppenol WH: Nitric oxide, superoxide and peroxynitrite: the good, the bad, and the ugly. Am J Physiol 1996; C1424–C1437.

49. Yu L, Gengaro PE, Niederberger M, et al: Nitric oxide: a mediator in rat tubular hypoxia/reoxygenation injury. Proc Natl Acad Sci USA 1994; 91:1691–1695.

50. Peresleni T, Noiri E, Bahou WF, Goligorsky MS: Antisense oligodeoxynucleotides to inducible NO synthase rescue epithelial cells from oxidative stress injury. Am J Physiol 1996; 270:F971–F977.

51. Ling H, Gengaro PE, Edelstein CL, et al: Effect of hypoxia on proximal tubules isolated from nitric oxide synthase knockout mice. Kidney Int 1998; 53:1642–1646.

52. Nagata S: Apoptosis by death factor. Cell 1997; 88:355–365.

53. Berke G: The CTL's kiss of death. Cell 1995; 81:9–12.

54. Ashkenazi A, Dixit VM: Death receptors: signaling and modulation. Science 1998; 281:1305–1308.

55. Yamada T, Horiuchi M, Dzau VJ: Angiotensin type 2 receptor mediates programmed cell death. Proc Natl Acad Sci USA 1996; 93:156–160.

56. Raff M: Social controls on cell survival and cell death. Nature 1992; 356:397–400.

57. Lieberthal W, Triaca V, Koh JS: Role of superoxide in apoptosis induced by growth factor withdrawal. Am J Physiol 1998; 44:F691–F702.

58. Levine JS, Koh JS, Triaca V, Lieberthal W: Lysophosphatidic

acid: a novel growth and survival factor for renal proximal tubular cells. Am J Physiol 1997; 273:F575–F585.

59. Koh JS, Lieberthal W, Heydrick S, Levine JS: Lysophosphatidic acid is a major serum noncytokine survival factor for murine macrophages which acts via the phosphatidylinositol 3-kinase signaling pathway. J Clin Invest 1998; 102:716–727.

60. Tsujii M, DuBois RN: Alterations in cellular adhesion and apoptosis in epithelial cells overexpressing prostaglandin endoperoxide synthase 2. Cell 1995; 83:493–501.

61. Meredith J, Schwartz M: Integrins, adhesion and apoptosis. Trends Cell Biol 1997; 7:146–150.

62. Frisch SM, Ruoslahti E: Integrins and anoikis. Curr Opin Cell Biol 1997; 9:701–706.

63. Bergin E, Levine JS, Lieberthal W: Mouse proximal tubular cell-cell adhesion inhibits apoptosis by a cadherin-dependent mechanism. Am J Physiol 2000; 278:F578–F768.

64. Bates RC, Buret A, Van Helden DF: Apoptosis induced by inhibition of intercellular contact. J Cell Biol 1994; 125:403–415.

65. Wary KK, Mainiero F, Isakoff SJ, et al: The adapter protein Shc couples a class of integrins to the control of cell cycle progression. Cell 1996; 87:733–743.

66. Chen CS, Mrksich M, Huang S, et al: Geometric control of cell life and death. Science 1997; 276:1425–1428.

67. Levine A: p53, the cellular gatekeeper for growth and division. Cell 1997; 88:323–331.

68. Lieberthal W, Triaca V, Levine J: Mechanisms of death induced by cisplatin in proximal tubular epithelial cells: apoptosis vs. necrosis. Am J Physiol 1996; 270:F700–708.

69. Thompson C: Apoptosis in the pathogenesis and treatment of disease. Science 1995; 267:1456–1462.

70. Gottlieb RA, Burleson KO, Kloner RA, et al: Reperfusion injury induces apoptosis in rabbit cardiomyocytes. J Clin Invest 1994; 94:1621–1628.

71. Messam CA, Pittman RN: Asynchrony and commitment to die during apoptosis. Exp Cell Res 1998; 238:389–398.

72. Steller H: Mechanisms and genes of cellular suicide. Science 1995; 267:1445–1449.

73. Lieberthal W, Menza SA, Levine JS: Graded ATP depletion can induce apoptosis or necrosis of cultured mouse proximal tubular cells. Am J Phyiol 1998; 274:F315–F327.

74. Zamzami N, Susin SA, Marchetti P, et al: Mitochondrial control of nuclear apoptosis. J Exp Med 1996; 183:1533–1544.

75. Castedo M, Hirsch T, Susin SA, et al: Sequential acquisition of mitochondrial and plasma membrane alterations during early lymphocyte apoptosis. J Immunol 1996; 157:512–521.

76. Liu X, Zou H, Slaughter C, Wang X: DFF, a heterodimeric protein that functions downstream of caspase-3 to trigger DNA fragmentation during apoptosis. Cell 1997; 89:175–184.

77. Sakahira H, Enari M, Nagata S: Cleavage of CAD inhibitor in CAD activation and DNA degradation during apoptosis [see comments]. Nature 1998; 391:96–99.

78. Hagar H, Ueda N, Shah S: Endonuclease activation induced DNA damage and cell death in chemical hypoxic injury to LLC-PK1 cells. Kidney Int 1996; 49:355–361.

79. Didenko VV, Hornsby PJ: Presence of double-strand breaks with single-base 3' overhangs in cells undergoing apoptosis but not necrosis. J Cell Biol 1996; 135:1369–1376.

80. Didenko VV, Turnstead JR, Hornsby PJ: Biotin-labeled hairpin oligonucleotides: probes to detect double-strand breaks in DNA in apoptotic cells. Am J Pathol 1998; 152:897–902.

81. Earnshaw W: Apoptosis: lessons from in vitro systems. Trends Cell Biol 1995; 5:217–220.

82. Lazebnik YA, Takahashi A, Moir RD, et al: Studies of the lamin proteinase reveal multiple parallel biochemical pathways during apoptotic execution. Proc Natl Acad Sci USA 1995; 92:9042–9046.

83. Rao L, Perez D, White E: Lamin proteolysis facilitates nuclear events during apoptosis. J Cell Biol 1996; 135:1441–1455.

84. Comfurius P, Bevers EM, Galli M, Zwaal RF: Regulation of phospholipid asymmetry and induction of antiphospholipid antibodies. Lupus 1995; 4(suppl 1):S19–S22.

85. Fadok VA, Voelker DR, Campbell PA, et al: Exposure of phosphatidylserine on the surface of apoptotic lymphocytes triggers specific recognition and removal by macrophages. J Immunol 1992; 148:2207–2216.

86. Price B, Rauch J, Shia M, et al: Anti-phospholipid autoantibodies bind to apoptotic, but not viable, thymocytes in a β2-glycoprotein 1–dependent manner. J Immunol 1996; 157:2201–2208.

87. Mower DA, Jr, Peckham DW, Illera VA, et al: Decreased membrane phospholipid packing and decreased cell size precede DNA cleavage in mature mouse B cell apoptosis. J Immunol 1994; 152:4832–4842.

88. Verhoven B, Schlegel RA, Williamson P: Mechanisms of phosphatidylserine exposure, a phagocyte recognition signal, on apoptotic T lymphocytes. J Exp Med 1995; 182:1597–1601.

89. Devaux PF: Phospholipid flippases. FEBS Lett 1988; 234:8–12.

90. Mills JC, Stone NL, Erhardt J, Pittman RN: Apoptotic membrane blebbing is regulated by myosin light chain phosphorylation. J Cell Biol 1998; 140:627–635.

91. Kothakota S, Azuma T, Reinhard C, et al: Caspase-3–generated fragment of gelsolin: effector of morphological change in apoptosis. Science 1997; 278:294–298.

92. Laster SM, Mackenzie JM, Jr: Bleb formation and F-actin distribution during mitosis and tumor necrosis factor–induced apoptosis. Microsc Res Tech 1996; 34:272–280.

93. Pitzer F, Dantes A, Fuchs T, et al: Removal of proteasomes from the nucleus and their accumulation in apoptotic blebs during programmed cell death. FEBS Lett 1996; 394:47–50.

94. Cunningham CC: Actin polymerization and intracellular solvent flow in cell surface blebbing. J Cell Biol 1995; 129:1589–1599.

95. Leist M, Single B, Castoldi AF, et al: Intracellular adenosine triphosphate (ATP) concentration: a switch in the decision between apoptosis and necrosis. J Exp Med 1997; 185:1481–1486.

96. Eguchi Y, Shimizu S, Tsujimoto Y: Intracellular ATP levels determine cell death fate by apoptosis or necrosis. Cancer Res 1997; 57:1835–1840.

97. Liu X, Naekyung C, Yang J, et al: Induction of apoptotic program in cell-free extracts: requirement for dATP and cytochrome c. Cell 1996; 86:147–157.

98. Zou H, Henzel WJ, Liu X, et al: Apaf-1, a human protein homologous to C. elegans CED-4, participates in cytochrome c–dependent activation of caspase-3 [see comments]. Cell 1997; 90:405–413.

99. Li P, Nijhawan D, Budihardjo I, et al: Cytochrome c and dATP-dependent formation of Apaf-1/caspase-9 complex initiates an apoptotic protease cascade. Cell 1997; 91:479–489.

100. Susin SA, Zamzami N, Castedo M, et al: Bcl-2 inhibits the mitochondrial release of an apoptogenic protease. J Exp Med 1996; 184:1331–1341.

101. Mancini M, Nicholson DW, Roy S, et al: The caspase-3 precursor has a cytosolic and mitochondrial distribution: implications for apoptotic signaling. J Cell Biol 1998; 140:1485–1495.

102. Zoratti M, Szabo I: The mitochondrial permeability transition. Biochim Biophys Acta 1995; 1241:139–176.

103. Marchetti P, Castedo M, Susin SA, et al: Mitochondrial permeability transition is a central coordinating event of apoptosis. J Exp Med 1996; 184:1155–1160.

104. Pastorino J, Snyder J, Serroni A: Cyclosporin and carnitine prevent the anoxic death of cultured hepatocytes by inhibiting the mitochondrial permeability transition. J Biol Chem 1993; 268:13791–13798.

105. Bossy-Wetzel E, Newmeyer DD, Green DR: Mitochondrial cytochrome c release in apoptosis occurs upstream of DEVD- specific caspase activation and independently of mitochondrial transmembrane depolarization. EMBO J 1998; 17:37–49.

106. Savill J, Fadok V, Henson P, Haslett C: Phagocyte recognition of cells undergoing apoptosis. Immunol Today 1993; 14:131–136.

107. Platt N, da Silva RP, Gordon S: Recognizing death: the phagocytosis of apoptotic cells. Trends Cell Biol 1998; 8:365–372.

108. Fadok VA, Bratton DL, Konowal A, et al: Macrophages that have ingested apoptotic cells in vitro inhibit proinflammatory cytokine production through autocrine/paracrine mechanisms involving TGF-beta, PGE$_2$, and PAF. J Clin Invest 1998; 101:890–898.

109. Hall SE, Savill JS, Henson PM, Haslett C: Apoptotic neutrophils are phagocytosed by fibroblasts with participation of the fibroblast vitronectin receptor and involvement of a mannose/fucose–specific lectin. J Immunol 1994; 153:3218–3227.

110. Duvall E, Wyllie A, Morris R: Macrophage recognition of cells undergoing programmed cell death (apoptosis). Immunology 1985; 56:351–358.

111. Cryns V, Yuan J: Proteases to die for [published erratum appears in Genes Dev 1999, Feb 1;13(3):371]. Genes Dev 1998; 12:1551–1570.

112. Kuida K, Lippke JA, Ku G, et al: Altered cytokine export and apoptosis in mice deficient in interleukin-1 beta converting enzyme. Science 1995; 267:2000–2003.

113. Thornberry NA, Rano TA, Peterson EP, et al: A combinatorial approach defines specificities of members of the caspase family and granzyme B: functional relationships established for key mediators of apoptosis. J Biol Chem 1997; 272:17907–17911.

114. Adams JM, Cory S: The Bcl-2 protein family: arbiters of cell survival. Science 1998; 281:1322–1326.

115. Cheng EH, Kirsch DG, Clem RJ, et al: Conversion of Bcl-2 to a Bax-like death effector by caspases. Science 1997; 278:1966–1968.

116. Mashima T, Naito M, Fujita N, et al: Identification of actin as a substrate of ICE and an ICE-like protease and involvement of an ICE-like protease but not ICE in VP-16–induced U937 apoptosis. Biochem Biophys Res Commun 1995; 217:1185–1192.

117. Brancolini C, Lazarevic D, Rodriguez J, Schneider C: Dismantling cell-cell contacts during apoptosis is coupled to a caspase-dependent proteolytic cleavage of beta-catenin. J Cell Biol 1997; 139:759–771.

118. Wen LP, Fahrni JA, Troie S, et al: Cleavage of focal adhesion kinase by caspases during apoptosis. J Biol Chem 1997, 272:26056–26061.

119. Irmler M, Thome M, Hahne M, et al: Inhibition of death receptor signals by cellular FLIP. Nature 1997, 388:190–195.

120. Rothe M, Pan M-G, Wenzel WJ, Nothing A: The TNFR2-TRAF signaling complex contains two novel proteins related to baculoviral inhibitors of apoptosis. Cell 1995; 274:782–784.

121. Liston P, Roy N, Tamai K, et al: Suppression of apoptosis in mammalian cells by NAIP and a related family of IAP genes. Nature 1996; 379:349–353.

122. Bump N, Hackett M, Hugunin M, et al: Inhibition of ICE family proteases by baculovirus antiapoptotic protein p35. Science 1995; 269:1885–1888.

123. Tanaka M, Suda T, Takahashi T, Nagata S: Expression of the functional soluble form of human fas ligand in activated lymphocytes. EMBO J 1995; 14:1129–1135.

124. Boldin M, Goncharov T, Goltsev Y, Wallach D: Involvement of MACH, a novel MORT1/FADD-interacting protease, in FasAPO-1– and TNF receptor–induced cell death. Cell 1996; 85:803–815.

125. Hsu H, Shu HB, Pan MG, Goeddel DV: TRADD-TRAF2 and TRADD-FADD interactions define two distinct TNF receptor 1 signal transduction pathways. Cell 1996; 84:299–308.

126. Zhang J, Cado D, Chen A, et al: Fas-mediated apoptosis and activation-induced T-cell proliferation are defective in mice lacking FADD/Mort1. Nature 1998; 392:296–300.

127. Luo X, Budihardjo I, Zou H, et al: Bid, a Bcl2 interacting protein, mediates cytochrome c release from mitochondria in response to activation of cell surface death receptors. Cell 1998; 94:481–490.

128. Berg A, Baltimore D: An essential role for NF-κB in preventing TNF-α–induced cell death. Science 1996; 274:782–784.

129. Jiang Y, Woronicz JD, Liu W, Goeddel DV: Prevention of constitutive TNF receptor 1 signaling by silencer of death domains [published erratum appears in Science 1999, Mar 19; 283(5409):1852]. Science 1999; 283:543–546.

130. Evan G, Littlewood T: A matter of life and cell death. Science 1998; 281:1317–1322.

131. Prives C: Signaling to p53: breaking the MDM2-p53 circuit. Cell 1998; 95:5–8.

132. Banin S, Moyal L, Shieh S, et al: Enhanced phosphorylation of p53 by ATM in response to DNA damage. Science 1998; 281:1674–1677.

133. Polyak K, Xia Y, Zweier JL, et al: A model for p53-induced apoptosis. Nature 1997; 389:300–305.

134. Deng C, Zhang P, Harper JW, et al: Mice lacking p21CIP1/WAF1 undergo normal development, but are defective in G1 checkpoint control. Cell 1995; 82:675–684.

135. Buckbinder L, Talbott R, Velasco-Miguel S, et al: Induction of the growth inhibitor IGF-binding protein 3 by p53. Nature 1995; 377:646–649.

136. Kharbanda S, Ren R, Pandey P, et al: Activation of the c-Abl tyrosine kinase in the stress response to DNA damaging agents. Nature 1995; 376:785–788.

137. Miyashita T, Reed JC: Tumor suppressor p53 is a direct transcriptional activator of the human bax gene. Cell 1995; 80:293–299.

138. Takekawa M, Saito H: A family of stress-inducible GADD45-like proteins mediate activation of the stress-responsive MTK1/MEKK4 MAPKKK. Cell 1998; 95:521–530.

139. Lowe S, Schmitt E, Smith S, et al: p53 is required for radiation-induced apoptosis in mouse thymocytes. Nature 1993; 362:847–862.

140. Clarke AR, Purdie CA, Harrison DJ, Nothing N: Thymocyte apoptosis induced by p53-dependent and independent pathways. Nature 1993; 362:849–852.

141. Erhardt P, Tomaselli KJ, Cooper GM: Identification of the MDM2 oncoprotein as a substrate for CPP32-like apoptotic proteases. J Biol Chem 1997; 272:15049–15052.

142. Graeber T, Osmanian C, Jacks T, et al: Hypoxia-mediated selection of cells with diminished apoptotic potential in solid tumours. Nature 1996; 379:88–91.

143. An WG, Kanekal M, Simon MC, et al: Stabilization of wild-type p53 by hypoxia-inducible factor 1 alpha. Nature 1998; 392:405–408.

144. Oren M: Lonely no more: p53 finds its kin in a tumor suppressor haven. Cell 1997; 90:829–832.

145. Siebenlist U, Franzoso G, Brown K: Structure, regulation and function of NF-kappa B. Annu Rev Cell Biol 1994; 10:405–455.

146. Van Antwerp DJ, Martin SJ, Verma IM, Green DR: Inhibition of TNF-induced apoptosis ny NFκB. Trends Cell Biol 1998; 8:107–111.

147. Wang CY, Mayo MW, Korneluk RG, et al: NF-kappaB antiapoptosis: induction of TRAF1 and TRAF2 and c-IAP1 and c-IAP2 to suppress caspase-8 activation. Science 1998; 281:1680–1683.

148. Zong WX, Edelstein LC, Chen C, et al: The prosurvival Bcl-2 homolog Bfl-1/A1 is a direct transcriptional target of NF-kappaB that blocks TNFalpha-induced apoptosis. Genes Dev 1999; 13:382–387.

149. Wu MX, Ao Z, Prasad KVS, et al: IEX-1L, an apoptosis inhibitor involved in NF-κB–mediated cell survival. Science 1998; 281:998–1001.

150. Webster GA, Perkins ND: Transcriptional cross talk between NF-κB and p53. Mol Cell Biol 1999; 19:3485–3495.

151. Besancon F, Atfi A, Gespach C, et al: Evidence for a role of NF-κB in the survival of hematopoietic cells mediated by interleukin 3 and the oncogenic TEL/platelet-derived growth factor receptor beta fusion protein. Proc Natl Acad Sci USA 1998; 95:8081–8086.

152. Bertrand F, Atfi A, Cadoret A, et al: A role for nuclear factor kappaB in the antiapoptotic function of insulin. J Biol Chem 1998; 273:2931–2938.

153. Toker A, Cantley LC: Signalling through the lipid products of phosphoinositide-3-OH kinase. Nature 1997;387:673–676.

154. Franke TF, Kaplan DR, Cantley LC: PI3K: downstream AKTion blocks apoptosis. Cell 1997; 88:435–437.

155. Downward J: Mechanisms and consequences of activation of protein kinase B/Akt. Curr Opin Cell Biol 1998; 10:262–267.

156. King WG, Mattaliano MD, Chan TO, et al: Phosphatidylinositol 3-kinase is required for integrin-stimulated AKT and Raf-1/mitogen-activated protein kinase pathway activation. Mol Cell Biol 1997; 17:4406–4418.

157. Suzuki H, Terauchi Y, Fujiwara M, et al: Xid-like immunodeficiency in mice with disruption of the p85alpha subunit of phosphoinositide 3-kinase. Science 1999; 283:390–392.

158. Stoyanov B, Volinia S, Hanck T, et al: Cloning and characterization of a G protein–activated human phosphoinositide-3 kinase. Science 1995; 269:690–693.

159. Alessi DR, James SR, Downes CP, et al: Characterization of a 3-phosphoinositide-dependent protein kinase which phosphorylates and activates protein kinase B alpha. Curr Biol 1997; 7:261–269.

160. Stokoe D, Stephens LR, Copeland T, et al: Dual role of phosphatidylinositol-3,4,5-trisphosphate in the activation of protein kinase B. Science 1997; 277:567–570.

161. Alessi DR, Kozlowski MT, Weng QP, et al: 3-Phosphoinositide–dependent protein kinase 1 (PDK1) phosphorylates and activates the p70 S6 kinase in vivo and in vitro. Curr Biol 1998; 8:69–81.

162. Le Good JA, Ziegler WH, Parekh DB, et al: Protein kinase C isotypes controlled by phosphoinositide 3-kinase through the protein kinase PDK1. Science 1998; 281:2042–2045.

163. Bondeva T, Pirola L, Bulgarelli-Leva G, et al: Bifurcation of lipid and protein kinase signals of PI3Kgamma to the protein kinases PKB and MAPK. Science 1998; 282:293–296.

164. Dudek H, Datta SR, Franke TF, et al: Regulation of neuronal survival by the serine-threonine protein kinase Akt. Science 1997; 275:661–665.

165. Cross DAE, Alessi DR, Cohen P, et al: Inhibition of glycogen synthase kinase-3 by insulin mediated by protein kinase B. Nature 1995; 378:785–789.

166. Chou M, Blenis J: The 70 kDa S6 kinase: regulation of a kinase with multiple roles in mitogenic signalling. Cur Opin Cell Biol 1995; 806–814.

167. Ghayur T, Hugunin M, Talanian RV, et al: Proteolytic activation of protein kinase C delta by an ICE/CED 3–like protease induces characteristics of apoptosis. J Exp Med 1996; 184:2399–2404.

168. Konishi H, Matsuzaki H, Tanaka M, et al: Activation of RAC-protein kinase by heat shock and hyperosmolarity stress through a pathway independent of phosphatidylinositol 3-kinase. Proc Natl Acad Sci USA 1996; 903:7639–7643.

169. Reed JC: Double identity for proteins of the Bcl-2 family. Nature 1997; 387:773–776.

170. Nunez G, London L, Hockenbery D, et al: Deregulated Bcl-2 gene expression selectively prolongs survival of growth factor–deprived hemopoietic cell lines. J Immunol 1990; 144:3602–3610.

171. Kane D, Sarafian T, Anton R, et al: Bcl-2 inhibition of neural death: decreased generation of reactive oxygen species. Science 1993; 262:1274–1277.

172. Miyashita T, Reed JC: Bcl-2 gene transfer increases relative resistance of S49.1 and WEHI7.2 lymphoid cells to cell death and DNA fragmentation induced by glucocorticoids and multiple chemotherapeutic drugs. Cancer Res 1992; 52:5407–5411.

173. He H, Lam M, McCormick TS, Distelhorst CW: Maintenance of calcium homeostasis in the endoplasmic reticulum by Bcl-2. J Cell Biol 1997; 138:1219–1228.

174. Zhu W, Cowie A, Wasfy GW, et al: Bcl-2 mutants with restricted subcellular location reveal spatially distinct pathways for apoptosis in different cell types. EMBO 1996; 15:4130–4141.

175. Pan G, O'Rourke K, Dixit VM: Caspase-9, Bcl-xL and Apaf-1 form a ternary complex. J Biol Chem 1998; 273:5841–5845.

176. Hu Y, Benedict MA, Wu D, et al: Bcl-xL interacts with Apaf-1 and inhibits Apaf-1–dependent caspase-9 activation. Proc Natl Acad Sci USA 1998; 95:4386–4391.

177. Rosse T, Olivier R, Monney L: Bcl-2 prolongs cell survival after Bax-induced release of cytochrome c. Nature 1998; 391:496–499.

178. Kluck RM, Bossy-Wetzel E, Green DR, Newmeyer DD: The release of cytochrome c from mitochondria: a primary site for Bcl-2 regulation of apoptosis [see comments]. Science 1997; 275:1132–1136.

179. Minn AJ, Velez P, Schendel SL, et al: Bcl-x(L) forms an ion channel in synthetic lipid membranes. Nature 1997; 385:353–357.

180. Antonsson B, Conti F, Ciavatta A, et al: Inhibition of Bax channel-forming activity by Bcl-2. Science 1997; 277:370–372.

181. Cohen J, Duke R: Glucocorticoid activation of a calcium-dependent endonuclease in thymocyte nuclei leads to cell death. J Immunol 1984; 132:38–42.

182. Thompson EB: The many roles of c-Myc in apoptosis. Annu Rev Physiol 1998; 60:575–600.

183. Evan G, Wyllie A, Gilbert C, et al: Induction of apoptosis in fibroblasts by c-myc protein. Cell 1992; 69:119–128.

184. Amati B, Littlewood T, Evan G, Land H: The c-Myc protein induces cell cycle progression and apoptosis through dimerization with Max. EMBO J 1994;12:5083–5087.

185. Qin X-Q, Livingston DM, Kaelin WG, Adams PD: Deregulated transcription factor E2F-1 expression leads to S-phase entry and p53-mediated apoptosis. Proc Natl Acad Sci USA 1994; 91:10918–10922.

186. Galaktionov K, Chen X, Beach D: Cdc25 cell-cycle phosphatase as a target of c-myc. Nature 1996; 382:511–517.

187. Tan X, Wang JY: The caspase-RB connection in cell death. Trends Cell Biol 1998; 8:116–120.

188. Almasan A, Yin Y, Kelly RE, et al: Deficiency of retinoblastoma protein leads to inappropriate S-phase entry, activation of E2F-responsive genes, and apoptosis. Proc Natl Acad Sci USA 1995; 92:5436–5440.

189. Khawaja A, Rodriguez-Viciana P, Wennström S, et al: Matrix adhesion and Ras transformation both activate a phosphoinositide 3-OH kinase and protein kinase B/Akt cellular survival pathway. EMBO J 1997; 16:2783–2793.

190. Day ML, Foster RG, Day KC, et al: Cell anchorage regulates apoptosis through the retinoblastoma tumor suppressor/E2F pathway. J Biol Chem 1997; 272:8125–8128.

191. Fanidi A, Harrington EA, Evan GI: Cooperative interaction between c-myc and bcl-2 proto-oncogenes. Nature 1992; 359:554–556.

192. Kranenburg O, Van der Eb AJ, Zantema A: Cyclin D1 is an esssential mediator of apoptotic neuronal cell death. EMBO J 1996; 15:46–54.

193. Bunz F, Dutriaux A, Lengauer C, et al: Requirement for p53 and p21 to sustain G2 arrest after DNA damage. Science 1998; 282:1497–1501.

194. Poluha W, Poluha DK, Chang B, et al: The cyclin-dependent kinase inhibitior p21WAF1 is required for survival of differentiating neuroblastoma cells. Mol Cell Biol 1996; 16:1335–1341.

195. Hiromura K, Pippin JW, Fero ML, et al: Modulation of apoptosis by the cyclin-dependent kinase inhibitor p27(Kip1). J Clin Invest 1999; 103:597–604.

196. Jacobson M: Reactive oxygen species and programmed cell death. Trends Biol Sci 1996; 21:83–86.

197. Finkel T: Oxygen radicals and signaling. Curr Opin Cell Biol 1998; 10:1248–1253.

198. Bae YS, Kang SW, Seo MS, et al: Epidermal growth factor (EGF)–induced generation of hydrogen peroxide. J Biol Chem 1997; 272:217–222.

199. Chen Q, Olashaw N, Wu J: Participation of reactive oxygen species in the lysophosphatidic acid–stimulated mitogen-activated protein kinase kinase activation pathway. J Biol Chem 1995; 270:28499–29502.

200. Deora AA, Win T, Vanhaesebroeck B, Lander HM: A redox-triggered ras-effector interaction: recruitment of phosphatidylinositol 3'-kinase to Ras by redox stress. J Biol Chem 1998; 273:29923–29928.

201. Hampton MB, Orrenius S: Redox regulation of apoptotic cell death. Biofactors 1998; 8:1–5.

202. Duan H, Wang Y, Aviram M, et al: SAG, a novel zinc RING finger protein that protects cells from apoptosis induced by redox agents. Mol Cell Biol 1999; 19:3145–3155.

203. Saitoh M, Nishitoh H, Fujii M, et al: Mammalian thioredoxin is a direct inhibitor of apoptosis signal- regulating kinase (ASK) 1. EMBO J 1998; 17:2596–2606.

204. Schumer M, Colombel MC, Sawchuk TS, et al: Morphologic, biochemical, and molecular evidence of apoptosis during the reperfusion phase after brief periods of renal ischemia. Am J Pathol 1992; 140:831–838.

205. Shimizu A, Yamanaka N: Apoptosis and cell desquamation in repair process of ischemic tubular necrosis. Virchows Archiv Cell Pathol 1993; 64:171–180.

206. Takase K, Takeyama Y, Nishikawa J, et al: Apoptotic cell death of renal tubules in experimental severe acute pancreatitis. Surgery 1999; 125:411–420.

207. Dharnidharka VR, Nadeau K, Cannon CL, et al: Ciprofloxacin overdose: acute renal failure with prominent apoptotic changes. Am J Kidney Dis 1998; 31:710–712.

208. Jaffe R, Ariel I, Beeri R, et al: Frequent apoptosis in human kidneys after renal hypoperfusion. Exp Nephrol 1997; 5:399–403.

209. Martinou JC, Dubois-Dauphin M, Staple JK, et al: Overexpression of BCL-2 in transgenic mice protects neurons from natu-

rally occurring cell death and experimental ischemia. Neuron 1994; 13:1017–1030.

210. Price PM, Megyesi J, Saggi S, Safirstein RL: Regulation of transcription by the rat EGF gene promoter in normal and ischemic murine kidney cells. Am J Physiol 1995; 268:F664–F670.

211. Safirstein R, Price P, Saggi S, Harris R: Changes in gene expression after temporary renal ischemia. Kidney Int 1990; 37:1515–1521.

212. Hammerman MR, O'Shea M, Miller SB: Role of growth factors in regulation of renal growth. Annu Rev Physiol 1993; 55:305–321.

213. Liu Y, Sun AM, Dworkin LD: Hepatocyte growth factor protects renal epithelial cells from apoptotic cell death. Biochem Biophys Res Commun 1998; 246:821–826.

214. Kroshian VM, Sheridan A, Lieberthal W: Functional and cytoskeletal changes induced by sublethal injury in proximal tubular epithelial cells. Am J Physiol 1994; 266:F21–F30.

215. Lieberthal W, McKenney JB, Kiefer CR, et al: β integrin–mediated adhesion between renal tubular cells following anoxic injury. J Am Soc Nephrol 1997; 8:175–183.

216. Racusen LC, Fivush BA, Li Y-L, et al: Dissociation of tubular cell detachment and tubular cell death in clinical and experimental "acute tubular necrosis." Lab Invest 1991; 64:546–556.

217. Racusen L: Alterations in human proximal tubule attachment in response to hypoxia. J Lab Clin Med 1994; 123:357–364.

218. Ortiz-Arduan A, Danoff TM, Kalluri R, et al: Regulation of Fas and Fas ligand expression in cultured murine renal cells and in the kidney during endotoxemia. Am J Physiol 1996; 271:F1193–F1201.

219. Feldenberg LR, Thevananther S, del Rio M, et al: Partial ATP depletion induces fas- and caspase-mediated apoptosis in MDCK cells. Am J Physiol 1999; 276:F837–F846.

220. Nogae S, Miyazaki M, Kobayashi N, et al: Induction of apoptosis in ischemia-reperfusion model of mouse kidney: possible involvement of Fas. J Am Soc Nephrol 1998; 9:620–631.

221. Deigner HP, Kinscherf R: Modulating apoptosis: current applications and prospects for future drug development. Curr Med Chem 1999; 6:399–414.

222. Honig LS, Rosenberg RN: Apoptosis and neurologic disease. Am J Med 2000; 108:317–330.

223. McCarthy NJ, Whyte MKB, Gilbert CS, Evans GI: Inhibition of Ced-3/ICE-related proteases does not prevent cell death induced by oncogenes, DNA damage, or the Bcl-2 homologue BAK. J Cell Biol 1997; 136:215–227.

224. Kaushal GP, Ueda N, Shah SV: Role of caspases (ICE/CED3 proteases) in DNA damage and cell death in response to a mitochondrial inhibitor, antimycin A. Kidney Int 1997; 52:438–445.

CHAPTER **4**

Oxidant Mechanisms in Acute Renal Failure

Norishi Ueda ▪ Philip R. Mayeux ▪ Radhakrishna Baliga ▪ Sudhir V. Shah

INTRODUCTION

A large body of evidence accumulated over the last decade indicates that partially reduced oxygen metabolites are important mediators of ischemic, toxic, and immune-mediated tissue injury.[1–8] Additionally, in the last few years, a new class of oxidants, nitric oxide–derived reactive nitrogen species, have emerged as important mediators of injury. This chapter summarizes the recent evidence implicating reactive oxygen and nitrogen metabolites in several forms of acute renal failure (ARF).

Reactive Oxygen Species

Oxygen normally accepts four electrons and is converted directly to water. However, partial reduction of oxygen can and does occur in biological systems leading to the generation of partially reduced and potentially toxic reactive oxygen intermediates.[8, 9] Thus, sequential reduction of oxygen along the univalent pathway leads to the generation of superoxide anion, hydrogen peroxide, hydroxyl radical, and water[8, 9] (Fig. 4–1). Superoxide and hydrogen peroxide appear to be the primary species generated. These may then play a role in the generation of additional and more reactive oxidants, including the highly reactive hydroxyl radical (or a related highly oxidizing species) in which iron salts play a catalytic role in a reaction, commonly referred to as the metal-catalyzed Haber-Weiss reaction.[6] Additional reactive oxygen metabolites can be formed as a result of the metabolism of hydrogen peroxide by neutrophil-derived myeloperoxidase (MPO, the enzyme responsible for the green color of pus) to produce highly reactive toxic products, including hy-

pochlorous acid. Myeloperoxidase reacting with hydrogen peroxide forms an enzyme substrate complex that has the capacity to oxidize various halides, producing highly reactive toxic products. Because of the wide distribution of chloride ion in biological systems, the formation of hypochlorous acid (HOCl, the active ingredient in Chlorox Bleach) is probably the most significant product.[7, 10–12] These oxygen metabolites, including the free radical species superoxide and hydroxyl radical, and other metabolites such as hydrogen peroxide and hypohalous acids are often collectively referred to as reactive oxygen metabolites.

The notion that reactive oxygen metabolites may be important in inflammation was initiated by a publication in 1969, in which McCord and Fridovich[13] described an enzyme, superoxide dismutase (SOD), that scavenges superoxide anion. McCord reasoned that because phagocytosing neutrophils, the effector cells of the acute inflammatory response, release large amounts of superoxide extracellularly and because superoxide dismutase, an enzyme that scavenges superoxide, possesses anti-inflammatory activity, superoxide anion and other oxygen metabolites may be important chemical mediators of the inflammatory process.[14] This hypothesis has received considerable support from a large number of studies in which the effect of reactive oxygen metabolites produced either by an enzymatic generating system such as xanthine-xanthine oxidase or by activated leukocytes has been examined in a variety of biological systems as well as in in vivo studies in which scavengers of reactive oxygen metabolites have been shown to be protective.

Reactive Nitrogen Species

Nitric oxide (NO) is an important signaling molecule generated by a five-electron oxidation of the guanidino nitrogen group of the amino acid L-arginine. This reaction is catalyzed by the nitric oxide synthase (NOS) family of enzymes. In 1980, Furchgott and Zawadzki[15] reported that vascular endothelial cells produced a substance that causes underlying smooth muscle cells to relax. The identification of this substance as NO[16, 17] and the understanding of its mechanism of action[18, 19] triggered an explosion of research into this new pathway of signal transduction (Fig. 4–2).

Although it is a free radical gas, NO is relatively benign. Activation of soluble guanylyl cyclase to generate cGMP is the major pathway through which NO regulates vascular tone and ion transport in the kidney. Yet, in an environment of oxidant stress, NO formation can lead to the generation of reactive nitrogen species.

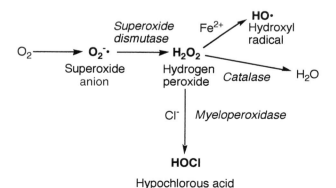

FIGURE 4–1 ▪ Pathways of oxygen-derived reactive species. (From Massry SG, Glassock RS, eds: Textbook of Nephrology. 4th ed. Philadelphia: Lippincott Williams & Wilkins; 1999; with permission.)

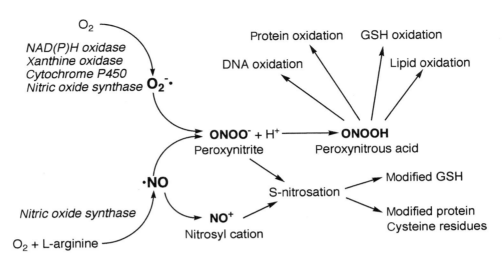

FIGURE 4–2 ▪ Pathways of nitric oxide (NO) signaling and formation of reactive nitrogen species. GSH, reduced glutathione; NADPH, reduced form of nicotinamide adenine dinucleotide phosphate; ONOO⁻, anionic form of peroxynitrite; ONOOH, protonated form of peroxynitrite. (From Massry SG, Glassock RS, eds: Textbook of Nephrology. 4th ed. Philadelphia: Lippincott Williams & Wilkins; 1999; with permission.)

There is growing experimental evidence suggesting that reactive nitrogen species may, in some disease states, be the ultimate reactive oxidant. In the presence of superoxide anion (O_2^-), NO and superoxide react very rapidly to generate peroxynitrite ($ONOO^-$).[20] Neither NO nor superoxide is a strong oxidant toward most types of organic compounds. Peroxynitrite, on the other hand, is a potent oxidant and nitrating species that can attack a broad range of biological targets, including proteins, lipids, and DNA. In the anionic form ($ONOO^-$), it is relatively stable, which allows it to deliver a range of reactivities over a relatively long distance. It is the protonated form (ONOOH) that exhibits hydroxyl radical–like activity and can carry out oxidation reactions involving 1- or 2-electron processes. In addition, peroxynitrite may react with carbon dioxide, yielding nitrosoperoxycarbonate anion ($^-ONOOCO_2$), an even more reactive species. The nitrosation species NO^+ (nitrosyl cation) can also be generated. There is growing interest in the S-nitrosation at sulfur of thiol groups as a pathway for regulating the activity of enzymes and proteins. Glutathione is also a substrate for these reactions and, along with cysteine, is a major intracellular defense against peroxynitrite.[21]

It is becoming increasingly clear from studies in animals that overproduction of NO plays a role in several models of ARF. Generation of NO is critical to normal physiology of the kidney, as discussed previously. However, excessive production of NO may upset the hemodynamic balance within the kidney and affect filtration, absorption, and excretion. Expression of type II NOS, the inducible isoform (iNOS), results in an elevated production of NO. Normally, the kidney is able to compensate for moderate hemodynamic changes. It is under conditions of oxidant stress that elevated levels of NO can become particularly toxic because the generation of peroxynitrite is pathogenic. It is only within the last few years that the importance of peroxynitrite as an oxidant has been realized. Hydroxyl radical scavenging antioxidants, shown to be protective in several models of ARF, also scavenge peroxynitrite. Furthermore, the iron chelator deferoxamine, used to implicate a role for Fenton chemistry–derived reactive oxygen species, is also an effective scavenger of peroxynitrite.[22]

ISCHEMIA-REPERFUSION INJURY

Reactive Oxygen Species

The demonstration that administration of superoxide dismutase provided almost complete protection against ischemia-induced tissue injury to the intestine[23, 24] led to the hypothesis that free radicals play a major role in the progression of ischemia-reperfusion–induced tissue injury. Oxidant stress has been proposed as one of the mechanisms of cellular injury in ischemia-reperfusion injury in brain,[25] heart,[26–28] lung,[29] intestine,[23, 24, 30–33] and kidney.[34–42]

McCord[1] proposed the idea that the primary source of superoxide in reperfused tissues is the enzyme xanthine oxidase. Xanthine oxidase exists in cells predominantly as oxidized nicotinamide adenine dinucleotide (NAD^+)–dependent dehydrogenase.[43] This form of enzyme uses NAD^+ instead of O_2 as the electron acceptor during oxidation of purines and does not produce superoxide or hydrogen peroxide. Ischemia results in more of the radical-producing form of the enzyme.[1] Although there are conflicting results,[44, 45] it has been suggested that the activity of the free radical–producing enzyme xanthine oxidase (type O xanthine oxidase) increases during reperfusion in ischemic kidneys,[36, 46] during hypoxia-reoxygenation in isolated perfused kidney,[39] and in other ischemic organs.[1, 30, 47, 48] Conversion of xanthine dehydrogenase to xanthine oxidase (D to O conversion) occurs by a number of mechanisms, including limited proteolysis and chemical modification, or oxidation of sulfhydryl groups.[49, 50] During ischemia there is also a massive breakdown of the adenine nucleotide pool because of the low energy status of the tissue, and adenosine is converted to inosine and then to hypoxanthine, resulting in its accumulation. Thus, after a period of ischemia, there is an accumulation of xanthine oxidase (preexisting and newly converted) and of its purine substrate, hypoxanthine. After reperfusion, the remaining substrate, molecular oxygen, re-enters the tissues and a burst of superoxide production ensues. The importance of this enzyme in kidney ischemia-reperfusion is still unclear.[44, 45]

Mitochondria are potentially one of the major sources of oxygen free radicals in the various organs under physiologic and pathologic conditions. Mitochondria produce superoxide anions at two sites in the electron transport chain. The first site of superoxide formation is the ubiquinone–to–cytochrome b region on the internal mitochondrial membrane.[51] Ubisemiquinone reduces oxygen to superoxide that dismutates spontaneously or by the action of superoxide dismutase, which is rich in mitochondria, to generate hydrogen peroxide. This auto-oxidation of ubisemiquinone in the coenzyme Q cycle (ubiquinone) is the predominant source of mitochondrial superoxide production.[51] The second site of superoxide formation is on the NADH-dehydrogenase that exists in the inner mitochondrial membrane.[52] The auto-oxidation of the reduced flavin mononucleotide of NADH-dehydrogenase also generates superoxide.[52, 53] During ischemia, the lack of an electron acceptor, molecular oxygen, and an inhibition of electron transfer lead to a high reduction of the components of the mitochondrial respiratory chain. Upon reperfusion, a burst of superoxide production occurs by the increased auto-oxidation of the major intramitochondrial sources of superoxide, ubisemiquinone and NADH-dehydrogenase flavin semiquinone because of steady inhibition of electron transfer.

Microsomal and nuclear membranes also contain the electron transport systems cytochrome P-450 and cytochrome b_5 that generate reactive oxygen metabolites,[54–56] and peroxisomes contain oxidases that generate hydrogen peroxide directly, without superoxide intermediate formation.[57] Although there is little information about the role of suborganelles as a source of reactive oxygen metabolites in the kidney, Campos and coworkers[58] have shown that the renal microsomes have the potential to generate superoxide upon reperfusion after ischemia. Arachidonic acid metabolism via PGH synthase and lipooxygenase has been shown to produce superoxide in the presence of NADH or NADPH.[59] The auto-oxidation of catecholamines[60–62] or heme proteins such as myoglobin[63] generates superoxide and hydrogen peroxide.

Another potentially important source of reactive oxygen metabolites is leukocytes. Indeed, neutrophils have been shown to play an important role in ischemia-reperfusion injury in several organ systems, including the heart,[64] intestines,[65] liver,[48] and kidneys.[66–68] However, the contribution of neutrophils to ischemic ARF is controversial. Thornton and coworkers[69] and Paller[70] have used antineutrophil antiserum to show that neutropenia fails to protect rats from ischemia-reperfusion renal injury. In contrast, Linas and coworkers[66, 68] have shown that infusion of neutrophils into ischemic isolated perfused kidneys enhanced renal injury. In addition, Hellberg and Kallskog[67] have shown that renal ischemia-induced transtubular leakage is reduced in

neutropenic rats compared with non-neutropenic controls. Studies of intracellular adhesion molecules[71] suggest that leukocytes may play an indirect but nonetheless important role in ischemia-reperfusion renal injury.

Several lines of evidence have been presented to indicate a role of reactive oxygen metabolites in the pathogenesis of ischemia-reperfusion injury (Table 4–1).[34–42, 46, 72–79] Various scavengers of reactive oxygen metabolites, such as superoxide dismutase,[34, 38, 80] dimethylthiourea,[34, 38, 81] catalase,[38, 42] reduced glutathione,[74, 75] N-acetylcysteine,[82] or antioxidants such as vitamin E,[83] have been reported to be protective against ischemia-reperfusion injury, although conflicting results were obtained by some investigators.[84–86] In addition, feeding a selenium-deficient diet (which results in a marked reduction in glutathione peroxidase [GSH-Px], an enzyme that metabolizes hydrogen peroxide) and vitamin E, an antioxidant, has been shown to result in a marked susceptibility to ischemia-reperfusion injury.[40] Transgenic mice with increased activity of superoxide dismutase have been shown to be less susceptible to ischemia-reperfusion of the kidney.[76] In contrast, inhibition of catalase resulted in an exacerbation of injury following ischemia-reperfusion.[41] While these observations present evidence of a role of reactive oxygen metabolites in ischemia-reperfusion injury, the exact nature of the oxidant or oxidants responsible for injury is still debated.

Iron, presumably because of its ability to participate in the generation of powerful oxidant species (eg, hydroxyl radical), has been shown to be important in various models of tissue injury.[6] In ischemia-reperfusion injury, there is no significant change in total nonheme or ferritin iron in the kidney, but there is a marked and specific increase in the bleomycin-detectable (capable of catalyzing radical reactions) iron after reperfusion, but not during the ischemic period.[87] Interestingly, despite a drastic reduction in iron content in the kidney, an iron-deficient diet does not prevent a marked increase in bleomycin-detectable iron and

TABLE 4–1. Evidence Suggesting a Role of Reactive Oxygen and Nitrogen Metabolites in Ischemic Acute Renal Failure

- Enhanced generation of reactive oxygen metabolites[37, 38] and xanthine oxidase[36] and increased conversion of xanthine dehydrogenase to oxidase[39, 46] occur in in vitro and in vivo models of injury.
- Lipid peroxidation occurs in in vitro and in vivo models of injury,[34, 35, 38, 72, 73] and this can be prevented by scavengers of reactive oxygen metabolites,[34, 38] xanthine oxidase inhibitors,[35, 37] or iron chelators.[38, 72]
- Scavengers of reactive oxygen metabolites,[34, 38, 42] antioxidants,[74, 75] xanthine oxidase inhibitors,[34, 37, 39] and iron chelators[36, 38, 72] are protective against injury.
- A diet deficient in selenium and vitamin E increases susceptibility to injury.[40]
- Inhibition of catalase exacerbates injury,[41] and transgenic mice with increased superoxide dismutase activity are less susceptible to injury.[76]
- Inhibition of the expression of iNOS in the kidney with antisense DNA greatly reduces injury.[77]
- Appearance of nitrotyrosine-protein adducts indicates the generation of peroxynitrite.[78, 79]

does not protect against ischemia-reperfusion injury. A similar increase in deferoxamine-chelatable iron (ferric iron) in rabbit kidneys exposed to ischemia[88] and in low-molecular-weight iron in isolated rat heart subjected to ischemia-reperfusion[89, 90] has been reported. Iron chelators, such as deferoxamine, that inhibit the generation of hydroxyl radical[91] have also been shown to be protective against ischemia-reperfusion injury in heart[6, 27] gut,[6, 32] and lung[6, 92] and in toxic and immune injury,[93] as well as in ischemic injury to kidney.[36, 38, 72]

Lipid peroxidation as detected by malondialdehyde and ethane has been shown to occur during reoxygenation or reperfusion in a variety of ischemic tissues, including heart,[28] liver,[94] intestine,[31, 33] lung,[29] brain,[25] and kidney.[34, 35, 73, 90]

Lipid peroxidation is an autocatalytic mechanism leading to oxidative destruction of cellular membranes. A number of reactive and toxic aldehyde metabolites can be released. These include malondialdehyde (MDA) and 4-hydroxynonenal (4-HNE).[95] MDA and 4-HNE protein adducts can be detected in the kidney after only 30 minutes of ischemia.[96] Inhibitors of lipid peroxidation, such as lazaroid (21-aminosteroid)[97-99] and bioflavonoids,[100] have been shown to reduce the formation of free radicals, lipid peroxidation, and kidney dysfunction in ischemia-reperfusion injury.

The glutathione redox ratio—oxidized glutathione:reduced glutathione + oxidized glutathione (GSSG:[GSH + GSSG])—has been considered as a parameter for assessing oxidant stress because GSH is oxidized to GSSG through GSH-Px, which can destroy hydrogen peroxide and lipid hydroperoxides, and then can be reduced back to GSH by glutathione reductase.[101] The glutathione redox ratio has been reported to be decreased during ischemia.[99, 101, 102] Ischemia-reperfusion injury to the kidneys also affects the enzymatic antioxidant defense system, resulting in a significant decrease in the levels of SOD, catalase, and GSH-Px in the kidneys.[103-105] The intrinsic cellular properties of the antioxidant enzymes in kidney tubule cells may be an important factor in susceptibility to injury. It was shown that ischemia-reperfusion injury results in proximal tubular damage, but not distal tubular damage, and that the expression of the SOD gene was up-regulated in distal tubular cells, whereas it was down-regulated in proximal tubular cells.[106] This difference in the distribution and regulation of antioxidant enzymes may account for the susceptibility of proximal tubules to ischemia-reperfusion injury.[107]

Reactive Nitrogen Species

Oxidant stress not only may unmask the toxic potential of NO in the kidney but also may be augmented by the generation of NO and reactive nitrogen species. Kidney epithelial and endothelial cells need not be the only source of NO and ROS. Infiltrating inflammatory cells recruited to the site of injury are also capable of generating these species and can extend the kidney's exposure to these oxidants. As discussed previously, there is much speculation as to the source of superox-

ide in the kidney. It must be noted that proximal tubule NOS itself is capable of generating superoxide along with NO.[108] The ratio of generation of superoxide to NO shifts to favor superoxide when the concentration of L-arginine decreases. It is reasonable to speculate that under conditions of reduced blood flow (ischemia or shock) L-arginine concentration in the kidney may fall low enough to favor the generation of superoxide along with NO, and thus peroxynitrite would be generated.

Selective inhibitors of iNOS activity and iNOS expression have been used to investigate the roles of NO and peroxynitrite in several models of ARF. The model most extensively investigated is renal ischemia-reperfusion. The nature of the mediators of renal ischemia-reperfusion injury is still controversial, but reactive nitrogen species appear to play an important role (see Table 4–1). As described previously, treatment with oxygen radical scavengers and antioxidants, such as SOD, dimethylthiourea, allopurinol, and deferoxamine, is protective in some models of ischemia-reperfusion injury but not all, and direct evidence of the generation of hydroxyl radical is absent.[86] The aforementioned inhibitors have another property in common. They all directly scavenge or inhibit the formation of peroxynitrite ($ONOO^-$).[20, 22, 109] When Noiri and coworkers[77] blocked the expression of iNOS in the kidney using antisense oligonucleotides, both functional and morphologic indices of renal failure following ischemia-reperfusion were greatly reduced. Furthermore, selective inhibition of iNOS activity produces a similar protective effect.[78] Support for the generation of peroxynitrite comes from immunohistochemical detection of nitrotyrosine-protein adducts in the kidney following ischemia-reperfusion.[78, 79] The appearance of nitrotyrosine-protein adducts indicates not only the cogeneration of superoxide and NO but also that antioxidant defense mechanisms were not capable of fully suppressing the actions of peroxynitrite.

LIPOPOLYSACCHARIDE-INDUCED RENAL INJURY

Reactive Oxygen Species

Lipopolysaccharide (LPS), a component of the gram-negative bacterial cell wall released during septicemia, is a major cause of septic shock.[110] LPS triggers the synthesis and release of cytokines and NO. A major contributor to the increase in NO production is LPS-stimulated expression of iNOS. This occurs in the vasculature and most organs, including the kidney.[111-113] Although hypotension and reduced renal blood flow can contribute to the renal failure associated with septicemia and septic shock, animal models have shown that LPS can cause renal injury in the absence of significant falls in systemic blood pressure or renal blood flow.[114]

In addition to increasing the synthesis of NO, LPS also causes the synthesis of ROS such as superoxide in the lung,[115, 116] liver,[117] and kidney.[118, 119] Higher doses of LPS (8–10 mg/kg bolus, IV) produce ARF in the

TABLE 4–2. Evidence Suggesting a Role for Reactive Oxygen and Nitrogen Metabolites in Lipopolysaccharide-Induced Renal Injury

- Antioxidants such as SOD and dimethylthiourea are protective against low-dose LPS challenge[118, 119] but not against high-dose challenge.[120]
- LPS induces iNOS expression in the kidney.[112, 113, 121]
- LPS is directly cytotoxic to isolated proximal tubules[122] via a signaling pathway triggered by a rise in intracellular calcium concentration.[123] Cytotoxicity is mediated by NOS-derived oxidant stress.[108, 124]
- Pharmacologic inhibition of iNOS reduces oxidant stress and renal injury.[121]
- Appearance of nitrotyrosine-protein adducts indicates the generation of peroxynitrite.[121]

iNOS, inducible nitric oxide; *LPS,* lipopolysaccharide; *SOD,* superoxide dismutase.

rat that at 24 hours is unaffected by treatment with SOD, catalase, dimethylthiourea, or deferoxamine.[120] However, lower doses (5 mg/kg infused over 1 hour) cause a progressive decline in renal function that can be delayed by administration of SOD or dimethylthiourea.[118] These studies suggest that oxidant stress may play a role in the early development of renal injury (Table 4–2)[108, 112, 113, 118–124] but is not the sole cause of injury leading to renal failure.

The potential for direct toxicity of LPS in renal cells has been examined in vitro. The biologically active component of LPS, lipid A, is toxic to tubular epithelial cell cultures (LLC-PK$_1$ cells) as well as isolated rat proximal tubules.[124, 125] Lipid A triggers a rapid rise in intracellular calcium concentration in the proximal tubule. This response is mediated, at least in part, by the release of intracellular calcium stores. This initiating event leads to oxidant stress, lipid peroxidation, and eventually cell death.[123, 124] Toxicity is prevented by inhibiting calcium release, by the antioxidants butylated hydroxytoluene and N,N'-diphenyl-1-phenylenediamine, SOD, deferoxamine, diethylenetriaminepentaacetic acid, and by increasing intracellular GSH levels.[123, 124] Clearly, oxidant stress plays a role in this in vitro model. Oxidant stress also occurs in vivo. Kidneys from rats treated with LPS (3 mg/kg, IV) show reduced levels of GSH equivalents and evidence of lipid peroxidation at 6 hours after treatment.[121]

Reactive Nitrogen Species

Reactive nitrogen species also appear to play a role in this model of renal injury (see Table 4–2). The role of iNOS-derived reactive nitrogen species on renal injury was evaluated in the rat using the selective iNOS inhibitor L-iminoethyl-lysine (L-NIL). At 6 hours after administration of LPS (2 mg/kg, IV), plasma levels of nitrate and nitrite (markers of NO synthesis) are elevated 100-fold. Expression of iNOS occurs, and oxidant stress becomes evident.[121] There is also immunohistochemical staining for nitrotyrosine-protein adducts throughout the kidney (except for the glomeruli), in-

dicating the formation of peroxynitrite. Treatment with L-NIL inhibits plasma nitrate and nitrite levels by more than 90% and reduces oxidant stress. GSH levels return toward normal, and lipid peroxidation is significantly reduced. LPS administration causes the appearance of 4-hydroxynonenal–protein adducts that are dependent on the activity of iNOS (Fig. 4–3). Inhibiting iNOS also reduces nitrotyrosine-protein adducts, but not completely. This suggests that other isoforms of NOS may be generating NO that is converted to peroxynitrite under conditions of oxidant stress. Reduced glutathione and GSH-Px constitute a major defense system against ONOO$^-$-mediated oxidations.[21, 126] L-NIL significantly reduced oxidant injury and apparent peroxynitrite formation. These data suggest that NO and ONOO$^-$ contribute to the development of oxidant injury. Furthermore, the source of NO may be iNOS. However, other isoforms of NOS are expressed by the kidney, and their activity may increase following LPS administration.[127] The cell types responsible for NO and superoxide generation in the kidney in response to LPS are not known. Interestingly, proximal tubule constitutive NOS and iNOS are both capable of generating superoxide in addition to

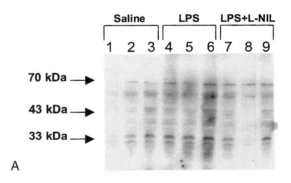

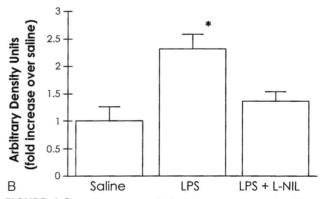

FIGURE 4–3 ■ Generation of 4-hydroxynonenal-protein adducts in kidney following lipopolysaccharide (LPS) administration. *A,* Western blot analysis of 4-hydroxynonenal-protein adducts was performed in whole kidney homogenates 6 hours after LPS (2 mg/kg IV) administration. Shown are lanes 1–3, saline; lanes 4–6, LPS; lanes 7–9, LPS + the inducible nitric oxide synthase (iNOS) inhibitor L-iminoethyl-lysine (L-NIL, 3 mg/kg IP). *B,* Densitometric analysis of the Western blot. Adducts were significantly increased in LPS-treated animals ($P < 0.05$). L-NIL prevented the increase in adduct formation.

NO.[108, 128] Addition of lipid A to isolated rat proximal tubules triggers the generation of superoxide preceded by the synthesis of NO (as measured by the appearance of nitrite). Superoxide generation occurs when the substrate for NO synthesis, L-arginine, becomes depleted. The addition of L-arginine inhibits NOS generation of superoxide.[108]

GENTAMICIN NEPHROTOXICITY

A major complication of the use of aminoglycoside antibiotics, including gentamicin, which are widely used in the treatment of gram-negative infections, is nephrotoxicity, which accounts for 10% to 15% of all cases of ARF.[129] The precise mechanism or mechanisms of gentamicin nephrotoxicity remain unknown. Following is a summary of the current information concerning the role of reactive oxygen and nitrogen species in gentamicin-induced nephrotoxicity (Table 4–3).[130–144]

Reactive Oxygen Species

The ability of gentamicin to alter mitochondrial respiration has been well documented by both in vitro and in vivo studies.[129] Several agents that affect mitochondrial respiration have been shown to enhance the generation of hydrogen peroxide. Based on gentamicin's ability to alter mitochondrial respiration, we pos-

TABLE 4–3. Evidence Suggesting a Role for Reactive Oxygen and Nitrogen Metabolites in Gentamicin-Induced Acute Renal Failure

- Gentamicin enhances the generation of superoxide anion, hydrogen peroxide, and hydroxyl radical by renal cortical mitochondria.[130–132]
- There is enhanced in vivo generation of hydrogen peroxide in renal cortex in the gentamicin-treated rat.[132]
- Gentamicin enhances the release of iron from renal cortical mitochondria.[134]
- Gentamicin-iron complex causes lipid peroxidation in vitro and is a potent catalyst for free radical formation.[135]
- Hydroxyl radical scavengers are protective in gentamicin-induced acute renal failure in rats.[136–138]
- Iron chelators are protective in gentamicin-induced hydroxyl radical formation by renal cortical mitochondria[131] and acute renal failure in the rat.[136]
- Administration of superoxide dismutase provides a marked protection against gentamicin-induced impairment of renal function.[137, 139]
- Iron supplementation enhances gentamicin nephrotoxicity in vivo.[141, 142]
- Pretreatment with zinc prevents gentamicin nephrotoxicity by inducing metallothionein that can scavenge reactive oxygen metabolites.[132]
- Co-administration of the antioxidants vitamin E and vitamin C as well as selenium is protective against gentamicin-induced nephrotoxicity.[138, 140, 143]
- Nonselective inhibition of NOS worsens injury[144]; however, selective iNOS inhibitors have not been evaluated.

NOS, nitric oxide synthase.
Modified from Baliga R, Veda N, Walker PD, Shah SV: Oxidant mechanisms in toxic acute renal failure. Drug Metab Rev 1999; 31:971–998, by courtesy of Marcel Dekker, Inc.

tulated that gentamicin may enhance the generation of reactive oxygen metabolites by renal cortical mitochondria.[130] The hydrogen peroxide generation by mitochondria was enhanced from less than 0.5 nmol/mg per minute in the absence of gentamicin to over 6 nmol/mg per minute in the presence of gentamicin. Recently, gentamicin has also been shown to enhance the generation of superoxide anion and hydroxyl radical in renal cortical mitochondria.[131, 132]

We have also examined whether enhanced in vivo generation of hydrogen peroxide could be demonstrated in rats treated for 5 days with gentamicin.[133] Previous studies by several groups of investigators have established that pure catalase is inactivated by aminotriazole only in the presence of hydrogen peroxide because aminotriazole reacts with the catalase intermediate, compound I, forming an inactive covalent complex with the protein. The profound inhibition of tissue catalase by aminotriazole has been interpreted to indicate the presence of (catalase–hydrogen peroxide) compound I in vivo and has been utilized as a qualitative measure of hydrogen peroxide production. With the use of this method, injection of aminotriazole resulted in much greater inhibition of catalase activity in gentamicin-treated rats, thus providing evidence of enhanced net generation of hydrogen peroxide by renal cortex and in the gentamicin-treated rat.[133]

Despite compelling evidence for the role of iron in various forms of tissue injury, the source of iron available to participate in the generation of hydroxyl radical or other iron-oxygen species remains largely unknown. Most of the iron is bound to heme and nonheme proteins in vivo and does not directly catalyze the generation of hydroxyl radical. Recently, based on the ability of superoxide to release iron from iron-storage protein ferritin (which normally provides a secure means of storing iron in an inert form), ferritin has been suggested as a possible source of iron for the generation of powerful oxidant species. A source of iron not previously considered is iron-rich mitochondria that contain heme as well as nonheme iron. We have found that gentamicin enhances the release of iron from renal cortical mitochondria.[134] Furthermore, gentamicin-induced iron mobilization from mitochondria is mediated by hydrogen peroxide. Thus, mitochondria should be considered as a potential source of iron for the generation of other oxidant species or the initiation of lipid peroxidation in other models of tissue injury. In one study, it was shown that gentamicin-iron complex, but not gentamicin itself, causes lipid peroxidation in vitro and is a potent catalyst of free radical formation.[135]

In vitro and in vivo studies indicate enhanced generation of hydrogen peroxide and release of iron in response to gentamicin. Most, if not all, of the hydrogen peroxide generated by mitochondria is derived from the dismutation of superoxide. Thus, the enhanced generation of hydrogen peroxide by gentamicin suggests that superoxide anion production is also increased. Superoxide and hydrogen peroxide may interact (with trace metals such as iron as the redox agent) to generate highly reactive and unstable oxidizing species, including the hydroxyl radical. Several studies have shown, in fact, that agents that enhance the generation of hydrogen peroxide and superoxide anion by mitochondria also enhance the generation of hydroxyl radical. Indeed, hydroxyl radical scavengers and iron chelators provide a marked protective effect on renal function in gentamicin-induced ARF in the rat[136] (Fig. 4–4), and administration of superoxide dismutase or dimethylthiourea provides protection against impairment of renal function, lipid peroxidation, and tubular damage.[137–139]

It was reported that despite amelioration of gentamicin-induced lipid peroxidation by treatment with an antioxidant, diphenylphenylenediamine, nephrotoxicity still occurred.[145] However, it was also demonstrated that co-administration of the antioxidants vitamin E and selenium is protective against gentamicin-induced nephrotoxicity.[138, 140] In addition, an in vivo study has shown that gentamicin results in a decrease in manganese superoxide dismutase (Mn-SOD), GSH-Px, and catalase activity in the kidney[139, 143] and that co-administration of vitamin E and vitamin C completely abrogates this suppression.[141] It is not clear why the contradictory results were obtained, but one explanation is that they may be due to the difference in the mechanisms of the protective effect of antioxidants. Additional support for a role of iron-catalyzed free radical generation has been provided by demonstrating that gentamicin-induced generation of hydroxyl radicals is reduced by iron chelators in vitro,[131] and iron supplementation enhances gentamicin nephrotoxicity in vivo.[141, 142] Pretreatment of rats with zinc has been shown to prevent gentamicin nephrotoxicity by inducing production of metallothionein, which can scavenge reactive oxygen metabolites.[132] Taken together, it appears that reactive oxygen metabolites are one of the mediators responsible for gentamicin nephrotoxicity.

While most studies have evaluated the ability of gentamicin to cause tubular damage, a study has examined the effect of gentamicin on glomerular cells. In vitro study has shown that gentamicin results in mesangial contraction and an increase in platelet-activating factor, thromboxane B_2, and prostaglandin E2, which are inhibited by an inhibitor of phospholipase A_2.[146] The authors suggest that these glomerular and vascular effects may contribute to the fall in glomerular filtration rate (GFR) observed in gentamicin nephrotoxicity.

Reactive Nitrogen Species

The role reactive nitrogen species may play in gentamicin nephrotoxicity has not been fully examined (see Table 4–3). Glomeruli isolated from gentamicin-treated rats show increased levels of cGMP, suggesting that production of NO is increased.[147] The effect of gentamicin on tubule NO production is not known.

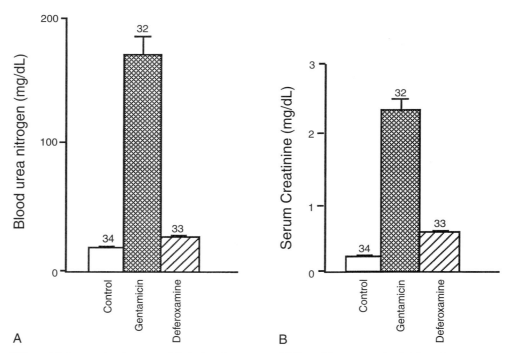

FIGURE 4–4 ■ Effect of deferoxamine in gentamicin-induced acute renal failure. The rats received daily subcutaneous injections of either sterile isotonic saline (1 mL) or gentamicin (100 mg/kg per day) for 8 consecutive days. Twenty-four hours after the last injection, the rats were sacrificed, and plasma was obtained for the measurement of blood urea nitrogen (A) and serum creatinine (B). Deferoxamine (20 mg/rat) was administered just before the first gentamicin injection. At the same time, deferoxamine or 2,3-dihydroxybenzoic acid was administered via an osmotic pump that was implanted subcutaneously. The drugs were reconstituted at a concentration of 175 mg/mL, and the pumps delivered ~20 mg of the iron chelator per rat per day at a continuous rate of 5 μL/h. The number of animals used was collated from several experiments. (From Walker PD, Barri Y, Shah SV: Oxidant mechanisms in gentamicin nephrotoxicity. Ren Fail 1999; 21[3,4]:433–442, by courtesy of Marcel Dekker, Inc.)

Nonselective inhibition of NOS with N^G-nitro-L-arginine methyl ester (L-NAME) worsens gentamicin-induced nephrotoxicity.[144] However, concluding that endogenous NO production is protective in this model is premature because L-NAME raises blood pressure and may affect GFR. Selective inhibitors of iNOS have not yet been examined in this model. There is the potential for NO and its metabolites to participate in mitochondrial injury. Both NO and peroxynitrite inhibit mitochondrial function.[148, 149] Nitric oxide inhibits cytochrome-c oxidase,[150] and peroxynitrite inhibits mitochondrial complexes I, II, and III.[151] Mitochondria are capable of synthesizing NO.[152, 153] Thus, in the presence of superoxide, both NO and peroxynitrite could be affecting mitochondrial function and could augment or even mediate gentamicin-induced mitochondrial dysfunction.

MYOGLOBINURIC ACUTE RENAL FAILURE

During the Battle of Britain, Bywaters and Beall[154] described the first causative association between ARF and skeletal muscle injury with release of muscle cell contents, including myoglobin, into plasma (rhabdomyolysis). Since then, the spectrum of etiologies of rhabdomyolysis, myoglobinuria, and renal failure has been markedly expanded with the recognition of both traumatic and, more recently, nontraumatic causes.[155–157] It is estimated that about one third of patients with rhabdomyolysis develop ARF[155] and that rhabdomyolysis may account for about 10% of all cases of ARF.[156] The most widely used model of myoglobinuric ARF is produced by subcutaneous or intramuscular injection of hypertonic glycerol.[158]

Reactive Oxygen Species

The role of reactive oxygen metabolites in renal failure induced by muscle injury has been examined with the use of the glycerol model (Table 4–4).[159–167] We have demonstrated enhanced generation of hydrogen peroxide in glycerol-induced ARF[159] utilizing the method described for demonstrating enhanced in vivo generation of hydrogen peroxide in response to gentamicin. Zager[168] has provided evidence that mitochondria constitute a critical site of heme-induced free radical formation. When heme-laden proximal tubular segments were exposed to mitochondrial respiratory chain inhibitors, there was a marked alteration in lipid peroxidation: blockade at site 2 or site 3 prevented heme-induced lipid peroxidation, whereas blockade at site 1 increased oxidative damage.

The recognition that hydrogen peroxide is produced in excessive amounts in this model motivated the examination of the potential efficacy of pyruvate, an alpha-ketoacid.[160] A property shared by a wide range of alpha-ketoacids is the ability of these metabolites to scavenge hydrogen peroxide through a nonenzymatic oxidative decarboxylation reaction.[169] The administration of pyruvate following the intramuscular injection

TABLE 4–4. Evidence Suggesting a Role for Reactive Oxygen and Nitrogen Metabolites in Myoglobinuric Acute Renal Failure

- There is enhanced in vivo generation of hydrogen peroxide in renal cortex in rats with glycerol-induced acute renal failure.[159]
- Pyruvate, a scavenger of hydrogen peroxide, is protective in glycerol-induced acute renal failure.[160]
- Hydroxyl radical scavengers and iron chelators are protective in glycerol-induced acute renal failure in the rat.[161]
- Iron chelator is protective in two experimental models of pigment-induced acute renal failure, intramuscular glycerol injection, and intravenous hemoglobin infusion without and with concurrent ischemia in the rat.[162]
- Iron chelator and mannitol can each protect against myohemoglobinuric acute renal failure.[163]
- The protective effect of glutathione and the detrimental effect of either depletion of glomerular-stimulating hormone (GSH) or interference with recycling of oxidized glutathione (GSSG) into GSH indicate an important role of glutathione in glycerol-induced acute renal failure.[164]
- There is increase in both the heme-oxygenase mRNA and the enzyme activity in glycerol-induced acute renal failure.[165] It appears to serve a protective role because inhibiting the enzyme worsens renal failure.
- A lipid peroxidation inhibitor, 21-aminosteroid, prevents heme protein–induced lipid peroxidation and cytotoxicity in in vitro and in vivo models of glycerol-induced acute renal failure.[166, 167]

GSSG, oxidized glutathione; *GSH,* reduced glutathione.
Modified from Baliga R, Veda N, Walker PD, Shah SV: Oxidant mechanisms in toxic acute renal failure. Drug Metabolism Reviews 1999; 31(4):971–998, by courtesy of Marcel Dekker, Inc.

of glycerol resulted in improved renal function, as measured by serum creatinine determinations, and marked reduction in structural injury.[160]

We have also demonstrated the functional and histologic protective effect of hydroxyl radical scavengers and iron chelators in glycerol-induced ARF in the rat.[161] Paller[162] has also demonstrated that deferoxamine treatment was protective in three models of myoglobinuric renal injury, namely, hemoglobin-induced nephrotoxicity, glycerol-induced ARF, and a combined renal ischemia–hemoglobin insult. Similarly, Zager[163] has demonstrated the protective effect of an iron chelator in myohemoglobinuric injury. In addition, studies have shown that a lipid peroxidation inhibitor, 21-aminosteroid, with or without diuretics, prevented heme protein–induced lipid peroxidation and cytotoxicity in renal tubular cells in vitro and in kidneys in vivo in a model of glycerol-induced ARF.[166, 167] Taken together, the histologic and functional protective effect of hydroxyl radical scavengers and the iron chelator and lipid peroxidation inhibitor implicate a role for free radicals in glycerol-induced ARF.

The current dogma is that myoglobin from the muscle serves as an important source of iron in glycerol-induced ARF. This is not surprising because myoglobin released from injured muscles is rich in heme iron. However, numerous experimental studies have demonstrated that myoglobin has an inconsistent and relatively weak nephrotoxic effect. An alternative or additional potential rich source of iron is cytochrome P-450,[170] first described in research on reperfusion injury of the rabbit lung[171] and, more recently, in the kidney.[172]

We measured the bleomycin-detectable iron (iron capable of catalyzing free radical reactions) in the kidneys and examined the role of cytochrome P-450 as a source of catalytic iron in a glycerol-induced model of myoglobinuric ARF.[173] There was a marked and specific increase in the bleomycin-detectable iron content accompanied by a marked decrease in the cytochrome P-450 content in the kidneys of glycerol-treated rats (Fig. 4–5). Two different cytochrome P-450 inhibitors significantly prevented an increase in bleomycin-detectable iron and the loss of cytochrome P-450 content in the kidneys, and provided histologic protection, indicating that cytochrome P-450 may be a significant source of iron in glycerol-induced ARF.

Reduced glutathione, a tripeptide, occurs in high concentrations in virtually all mammalian cells and is the most prevalent intracellular thiol.[174–176] The importance of GSH in protecting cells against oxidant injury has been delineated in numerous in vitro studies where depletion of GSH resulted in markedly enhanced toxicity,[177–180] and elevated nonprotein sulfhy-dryl content provided protection.[177, 181, 182] We have shown that there is a marked depletion of renal GSH early after glycerol injection and a return almost to the baseline level by 24 hours.[164] Rats that received L-buthionine-(S,R)-sulfoximine (BSO) to deplete GSH had significantly higher blood urea nitrogen (BUN) and serum creatinine levels than rats receiving either glycerol alone or glycerol and GSH. Rats that received GSH in addition to glycerol had significantly lower BUN and serum creatinine levels than those receiving glycerol alone or glycerol and BSO. These functional differences between the GSH and the BSO groups were also confirmed histologically. Taken together, these results provide evidence of the role of GSH in glycerol-induced ARF.

Reactive Nitrogen Species

The role of NO or NO-derived reactive nitrogen species has not been examined in myoglobinuric ARF

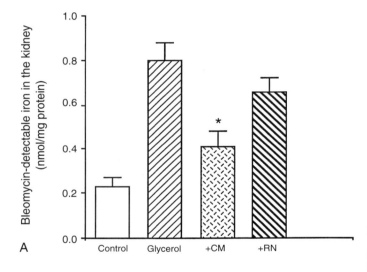

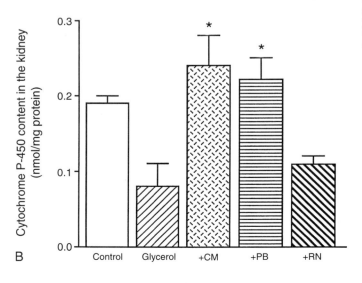

FIGURE 4–5 ■ *A,* Effect of cimetidine (CM) and ranitidine (RN, used as a control) on the bleomycin-detectable iron content in the kidneys of glycerol-treated rats. The assay was performed in five rats from each group. *B,* Effect of cytochrome P-450 inhibitors on cytochrome P-450 content in the kidneys of glycerol-treated rats. Values are means ± SE. N = 5, $P < 0.01$ compared with glycerol treatment alone. *PB,* piperonyl butoxide. (Reprinted with permission from Baliga R, Zhang Z, Baliga M, et al: Evidence for cytochrome P-450 as a source of catalytic iron in myoglobinuric acute renal failure. Kidney Int 1996; 49:362–369, with permission.)

(see Table 4–4). There are, however, compelling reasons for studying NO in this disease. Myoglobin, like hemoglobin, is a potent scavenger of NO. It is conceivable that delivery of myoglobin to the kidney would remove the vasodilatory activity of NO in the renal vasculature. This may in fact be at least part of the mechanism of renal vasoconstriction associated with this disease. It is unknown whether iNOS expression is increased in the kidney. Given the ischemia component of this disease, it is likely that iNOS is induced, because hypoxia[183] or oxidants[184] trigger iNOS gene expression.

There are also interactions between NO and heme oxygenase that may play a role in this model. Nitric oxide can modulate many steps in heme and iron metabolism. The action of heme oxygenase causes release of iron from heme. Thus, for heme oxygenase to defend against oxidant damage there must be a coordinated transfer of iron to a storage form, presumably ferritin, that does not readily permit iron-catalyzed oxidant generation. The interactions of NO with these processes are very complex. Nitric oxide induces heme oxygenase-1 gene expression in mesangial cells[185, 186] but can inhibit expression of ferritin.[187] This could potentially make iron release from heme more available for oxidant generation. However, NO production leads to nitrosylation of heme and prevents the degradation of heme by heme oxygenase.[188] Although this may be thought of as protective (iron is not released by heme oxygenase), nitrosyl-heme formation is reversible. Juckett and coworkers[188] proposed that nitrosyl-heme that escapes heme oxygenase may release free heme later in a lipid environment (cell membrane) that promotes oxidant generation and oxidant damage.

Heme-containing proteins, such as catalase and cytochrome P-450, are also targets for NO.[189] Nitric oxide produces an irreversible inhibition of cytochrome P-450.[190] The inhibitory effect of NO on cytochrome P-450 is particularly intriguing in light of the protective effect that inhibitors of cytochrome P-450 have in this model, as discussed earlier. Clearly, the role of NO and NO-derived species needs to be specifically studied for this cause of ARF.

CYCLOSPORIN A NEPHROTOXICITY

Reactive Oxygen Species

Recent data implicate a role for reactive oxygen and nitrogen metabolites in the pathogenesis of cyclosporine A nephrotoxicity (Table 4–5).[191–207] Enhanced generation of reactive oxygen metabolites has been shown in both in vitro and in vivo models of cyclosporin A nephrotoxicity. For example, several studies demonstrate the generation of hydrogen peroxide by cyclosporin A in mesangial cells[191] and enhanced generation of superoxide anion, hydrogen peroxide, in glomeruli.[192] In addition, an in vivo study showed enhanced generation of reactive free radicals by cyclosporin A in the kidney[195] that can be blocked by antioxidants.[191, 192]

TABLE 4–5. Evidence Suggesting a Role for Reactive Oxygen and Nitrogen Metabolites in Cyclosporin A–Induced Acute Renal Failure

- Cyclosporin A enhances generation of hydrogen peroxide in vitro[191–194] and in vivo.[195–197]
- There is enhanced lipid peroxidation, reduced renal microsomal NADPH cytochrome P-450 and renal glutathione ratio (GSH/GSSG) in kidney cortex, microsomes, or mitochondria in vitro and in vivo.[198–201]
- Superoxide dismutase or catalase can restore a decrease in renal function induced by cyclosporin A,[193] and an inhibitor of xanthine oxidase, oxipurinol, attenuates cyclosporine-induced cytotoxicity in vitro.[202]
- Cyclosporin A reduces the levels of glutathione and antioxidant,[203] and administration of antioxidants such as vitamin E[198, 199, 204, 205] or reduced glutathione[197] results in marked attenuation of the deleterious effects of cyclosporin A.
- Greater lipid peroxidation and renal injury is observed in cyclosporin A–treated rats with antioxidant deficiency.[199]
- Cyclosporine-induced lipid peroxidation is blocked by an inhibitor of cytochrome P-450.[196, 197]
- Initial studies suggest that NO derived from endothelial type III NOS may be beneficial by preserving renal blood flow.[206, 207]

GSH, glomerular-stimulating hormone; *GSSG*, oxidized glutathione; *NADPH*, nicotinamide adenine dinucleotide phosphate, oxidized form.
Modified from Baliga R, Veda N, Walker PD, Shah, SV: Oxidant mechanisms in toxic acute renal failure. Drug Metabolism Reviews 1999; 31(4):971–998, by courtesy of Marcel Dekker, Inc.

There is also evidence suggesting that cytochrome P-450 may play a role in the generation of oxidants[196, 197] by functioning as an iron donor, leading to generation of reactive oxygen metabolites, as well as by regulating arachidonic acid metabolism. Cyclosporin A has been shown to result in increased activity of arachidonic acid omega-hydroxylation that produces omega-hydroxyarachidonic acid, a potent vasoconstrictor, by induction of cytochrome P-450 (CYP4A2) in renal microsomes.[208]

Cyclosporin A also appears to affect antioxidant defense systems in the kidney. Cyclosporin A has been shown to reduce the levels of glutathione and vitamin E.[198–200, 203] This may be due to inhibition of glutathione S-transferase activity, thereby reducing the GSH-mediated detoxification mechanism.[209]

The beneficial effects of scavengers of reactive oxygen metabolites and antioxidants provide additional support for a role of reactive oxygen metabolites in cyclosporin A nephrotoxicity. Cyclosporin A has been shown to result in glomerular contraction that leads to a marked reduction in GFR, and administration of superoxide dismutase or catalase can restore a decrease in renal function.[193] Administration of vitamin E[204] or lazaroids, radical-quenching antioxidants,[205] has been shown to attenuate cyclosporine-induced renal microvascular vasoconstriction and hypoperfusion, resulting in marked preservation of GFR and significant suppression of urinary excretion of vasoactive prostaglandins.[204] Similarly, an inhibitor of xanthine oxidase, oxypurinol, has been shown to attenuate cyclosporine-induced distortion of mitochondria with loss of cristae and cytotoxicity in renal tubular cells.[202] Administration of antioxidants such as vitamin E[198, 199] and GSH[197] has also resulted in marked attenuation of lipid peroxidation and renal toxicity induced by cyclosporin A. Furthermore, administration of cyclosporin A to antioxidant-deficient animals[199] and depletion of glutathione[210] has been reported to result in greater lipid peroxidation and renal injury. These data indicate that reactive oxygen metabolites play a role in the pathogenesis of cyclosporin A nephrotoxicity.

It has been suggested that cyclosporin A induces apoptosis characterized by internucleosomal DNA cleavage due to endonuclease activation, chromatin condensation, and apoptotic bodies in hematopoietic cells.[211, 212] Since oxidants are capable of inducing apoptosis in various types of cells,[213] including renal tubular epithelial cells,[214] it is conceivable that reactive oxygen metabolites may play a role in apoptotic mechanisms of cyclosporin A–induced nephrotoxicity.

Reactive Nitrogen Species

Relatively little is known of the role of NO or its metabolites in the development of cyclosporin A nephrotoxicity. However, the available studies suggest that in this cause of ARF, NO may be beneficial (see Table 4–5). Cyclosporin A nephrotoxicity is characterized by renal vasoconstriction and hypertension that can progress to irreversible structural damage. The vasodilatory action of NO may serve to buffer vasoconstrictor substances, such as endothelin, angiotensin II, and thromboxane. This notion is supported by studies showing that cyclosporin A can cause the induction of endothelial type III NOS in the kidney.[206, 207]

CISPLATIN-INDUCED NEPHROTOXICITY

Reactive Oxygen Species

Cisplatin is a widely used antineoplastic agent, for which nephrotoxicity is a major side effect. Although the underlying mechanism of this nephrotoxicity is still not well known, the role of reactive oxygen metabolites has been implicated (Table 4–6).[215–235] Several in vitro studies have shown that cisplatin enhances the generation of hydrogen peroxide in the S3 segment of mouse proximal tubular cells[212] as well as other reactive oxygen species through inhibition of complex I of the mitochondrial respiratory chain in porcine proximal tubular cells.[216] In addition, with the use of a cell-free system, the formation of reactive metabolites from cis-diammine-(1,1-cyclobutanedicarboxylato)-platinum(II)(carboplatin) that are able to bind to DNA has been shown to be enhanced in the presence of reactive oxygen metabolites as well as hemoglobin.[236] These data indicate that cisplatin not only can enhance the generation of reactive oxygen metabolites but also can convert to more reactive metabolites of platinum in cisplatin nephrotoxicity.

The role of reactive oxygen metabolites in the pathogenesis of cisplatin nephrotoxicity has been supported by the beneficial effect of scavengers of these

TABLE 4–6. Evidence Suggesting a Role for Reactive Oxygen and Nitrogen Metabolites in Cisplatin-Induced Acute Renal Failure

- Cisplatin enhances in vitro generation of hydrogen peroxide in proximal tubular cells.[215, 216]
- In vitro cisplatin increases catalytic iron in LLC-PK$_1$ cells,[217] and iron chelators are protective in vitro[217, 218] and in vivo.[217, 219]
- Scavengers of reactive oxygen metabolites, including catalase[215, 218] and hydroxyl radical scavengers,[217] are protective in vitro and in vivo.[217, 219–221]
- Cisplatin increases renal cytochrome P-450 content,[222] and bleomycin iron[223] and cytochrome P-450 inhibitors prevent increase in bleomycin iron[223] and are protective in vitro and in vivo.[223, 224]
- Cisplatin induces rapid peroxidation in vitro and in vivo.[225]
- Cisplatin induces reduced levels of GSH and thiol in vitro[216] and in vivo[226, 227]; glutathione ester[228, 229] is protective; and inhibition of glutathione[229] and deficiency of selenium[230] accelerate nephrotoxicity in vivo.
- Cisplatin reduces the levels of antioxidants in the cancer patient,[231] and antioxidants[220, 221, 232] are protective in vivo and in vitro.[233]
- Cisplatin induces heme oxygenase[234] and heme protein[222]; however, inhibition of heme oxygenase accelerates cisplatin nephrotoxicity.[234]
- Cisplatin does cause the expression of iNOS in the kidney, and inhibition of NOS activity appears to lessen injury.[235]

GSH, reduced glutathione.

metabolites in this model of renal injury. In vitro studies have shown that catalase, a scavenger of hydrogen peroxide, protects against cisplatin-induced cell death.[215] In vivo studies have also shown the beneficial effect of SOD and dimethylthiourea[219] or N-N'-diphenyl-p-phenylenediamine[220, 221] in cisplatin nephrotoxicity. Although these scavengers of reactive oxygen metabolites have been shown to be beneficial, it was shown that dimethylthiourea protects against tubular damage, but not damage to renal blood flow, whereas SOD can preserve renal blood flow but does not protect against tubular damage induced by cisplatin.[219] Taken together, these data suggest that reactive oxygen metabolites play a role in cisplatin nephrotoxicity; however, different reactive oxygen metabolites may exert different effects in this model of renal injury.

We have examined the catalytic iron content and the effect of iron chelators in an in vitro model of cisplatin-induced cytotoxicity in LLC-PK$_1$ cells and in an in vivo model of cisplatin-induced ARF in the rat.[217] Exposure of LLC-PK$_1$ cells to cisplatin resulted in a significant increase in bleomycin-detectable iron (iron capable of catalyzing free radical reactions) released into the medium. Concurrent incubation of LLC-PK$_1$ cells with iron chelators, including deferoxamine and 1,10-phenanthroline, significantly attenuated cisplatin-induced cytotoxicity, as measured by lactate dehydrogenase release. Bleomycin-detectable iron content was also markedly increased in the kidneys of rats treated with cisplatin, and administration of deferoxamine in rats provided marked functional (as measured by BUN and creatinine levels) and histologic protection against cisplatin-induced ARF. In an additional study, incubation of LLC-PK$_1$ cells with cisplatin caused an increase in hydroxyl radical formation. Hydroxyl radical scavengers significantly reduced cisplatin-induced cytotoxicity and provided significant protection against cisplatin-induced ARF.[217] Taken together, our data strongly support a critical role for iron in mediating tissue injury via hydroxyl radical (or a similar oxidant) in this model of nephrotoxicity.

The source of this iron in cisplatin-induced nephrotoxicity is still not known. We have examined the role of cytochrome P-450 as a source of catalytic iron in cisplatin-induced nephrotoxicity both in vivo and in vitro.[223] In cisplatin-treated rats, there was a marked decrease in the cytochrome P-450 content specifically in the kidney, accompanied by a significant increase in the catalytic iron in the kidney. Co-administration of a cytochrome P-450 inhibitor significantly prevented cisplatin-induced loss of cytochrome P-450 as well as an increase in bleomycin-detectable iron in the kidney, along with both functional (as measured by BUN and plasma creatinine levels) and histologic protection against cisplatin-induced ARF. In an in vitro study, inhibitors of cytochrome P-450 also prevented the increase of catalytic iron from LLC-PK$_1$ cells exposed to cisplatin, accompanied by a marked protection against cisplatin-induced cytotoxicity (Fig. 4–6). Taken together, our data demonstrated that cytochrome P-450, a group of heme proteins, may serve as a significant source of catalytic iron in cisplatin-induced nephrotoxicity.

Heme oxygenase is induced by oxidants and its induction has been shown to be a protective response in renal injury. The study by Agarwal and coworkers[234] has demonstrated that cisplatin induces mRNA and protein of heme oxygenase and that inhibition of heme oxygenase accelerates reduction of renal blood flow, increased renal vascular resistance, and renal dysfunction in cisplatin nephrotoxicity.

Cisplatin results in a reduction of the antioxidant system that detoxifies reactive oxygen metabolites. Cisplatin reduces the levels of antioxidants vitamin C and vitamin E in the cancer patient,[231] and administration of α-tocopherol has been shown to be protective against cisplatin nephrotoxicity.[220, 221] An in vitro study has shown that cisplatin reduces mitochondrial GSH levels by inhibiting GSH reductase in renal tubular cells subjected to cisplatin.[216] In addition, an in vivo study has demonstrated that the concentration of glutathione is increased in the outer medulla after cisplatin treatment, whereas the concentration of protein thiols in the proximal tubules is decreased,[226] which may account for the susceptibility of proximal tubular cells to cisplatin nephrotoxicity. The role of glutathione as a detoxifying system for reactive oxygen metabolites in this model of renal injury has also been supported by the following observations: (1) administration of glutathione ester has been shown to be

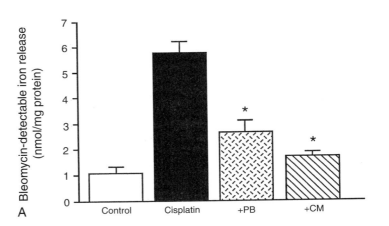

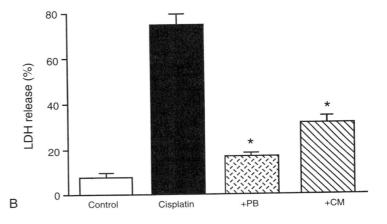

FIGURE 4–6 ▪ Effect of cytochrome P-450 inhibitors on both bleomycin-detectable iron release (*A*) and cytotoxicity (*B*) in cisplatin-treated LLC-PK$_1$ cells. Cells were incubated with a cytotoxic dose of cisplatin (200 μg/mL) for a period of time necessary for substantial cell killing to occur (2.5 h, *Panel A*) or for the induction of consistent cytotoxicity (4 h, *Panel B*) in the presence or absence of cytochrome P-450 inhibitors, cimetidine (CM) (2 mM) and piperonyl butoxide (PB) (1 mM). Values are means ± SE. N = 3–4. *P* < 0.01 compared with cisplatin alone. (Reprinted with permission from Baliga R, Zhang Z, Baliga M, et al: Role of cytochrome P-450 as a source of catalytic iron in cisplatin-induced nephrotoxicity. Kidney Int 1998; 54:1562–1569.)

protective,[228, 229] (2) inhibition of glutathione by BSO[229] and deficiency of selenium[230] have been shown to accelerate cisplatin nephrotoxicity, and (3) administration of selenium was shown to prevent cisplatin nephrotoxicity.[227]

Reactive Nitrogen Species

Cisplatin does cause the expression of iNOS in the kidney,[235] and inhibition of NOS activity does reduce lipid peroxidation and renal injury despite the potential for increased renal vasoconstriction[237] (see Table 4–6). It is also clear that reactive nitrogen metabolites potentiate cisplatin cytotoxicity in cultured fibroblasts.[238] These limited studies indicate the potential importance of reactive nitrogen species in cisplatin nephrotoxicity and suggest that additional studies are warranted.

CONCLUSION

The authors believe that there is compelling evidence implicating reactive oxygen metabolites in gentamicin nephrotoxicity and in myoglobinuric ARF and in cisplatin nephrotoxicity, as well as emerging evidence for their role in cyclosporin A nephrotoxicity. Many questions regarding the mechanisms remain to be elucidated, including the cellular and molecular mechanisms and signal transduction pathways by which reactive oxygen metabolites induce renal injury. Based on recent evidence of important interactions between reactive oxygen metabolites and endonuclease activation, it appears that this would be a fruitful area of investigation. In addition, potential interactions between oxygen metabolites and NO–derived reactive nitrogen species should also be investigated. Ultimately, it is obviously important to learn whether these mechanisms are applicable to ARF in humans. This collective body of evidence suggests an important role for reactive oxygen metabolites in toxic ARF and may provide therapeutic opportunities for preventing or treating ARF in humans. The discovery that reactive nitrogen species can be generated in the kidney and participate in the development of ARF has uncovered a new therapeutic target. Over the past few years, much effort has been directed toward the development of selective iNOS inhibitors to be used in the treatment of a number of human diseases, in particular, septic shock. Nonselective NOS inhibitors that inhibit constitutive isoforms regulating vascular tone in addition to iNOS not only are ineffective but also can increase mortality.[239] Animal studies show that nonselective NOS inhibitors may also worsen ischemia-reperfusion injury presumably by reducing reflow.[77, 78] It may prove difficult to develop truly selective iNOS inhibitors. An alternative approach is to target reactive nitrogen species directly. The iron chelator deferoxamine is one such drug. Its ability to scavenge peroxynitrite may be responsible for many of the beneficial effects observed with deferoxamine treatment, not simply its activity as

an iron chelator. The potential usefulness of reactive nitrogen scavengers may emerge as more of these drugs are developed and tested.

REFERENCES

1. McCord JM: Oxygen-derived free radicals in postischemic tissue injury. N Engl J Med 1985; 312:159–163.
2. Fantone JC, Ward PA: Role of oxygen-derived free radicals and metabolites in leukocyte-dependent inflammatory reactions. Am J Pathol 1982; 107:397–418.
3. Weiss SJ: Oxygen, ischemia, and inflammation. Acta Physiol Scand 1986; 126:9–37.
4. Baud L, Ardaillou R: Reactive oxygen species: production and role in the kidney. Am J Physiol 1986; 251:F765–F776.
5. Freeman BA, Crapo JD: Biology of disease: free radicals and tissue injury. Lab Invest 1982; 47:412–426.
6. Halliwell B, Gutteridge JMC: Role of free radicals and catalytic metal ions in human disease: an overview. Methods Enzymol 1990; 186:1–85.
7. Cross CE, Halliwell B, Borish ET, et al: Oxygen radicals and human disease. Ann Intern Med 1987; 107:526–545.
8. McCord JM, Fridovich I: The biology and pathology of oxygen radicals. Ann Intern Med 1978; 89:122–127.
9. Fridovich I: The biology of oxygen radicals: the superoxide radical is an agent of oxygen toxicity; superoxide dismutases provide an important defense. Science 1978; 201:875–880.
10. Lampert MB, Weiss SJ: The chlorinating potential of the human monocyte. Blood 1983; 62:645–651.
11. Klebanoff SJ: Oxygen metabolism and the toxic properties of phagocytes. Ann Intern Med 1980; 93:480–489.
12. Weiss SJ, LoBuglio AF: Phagocyte-generated oxygen metabolites and cellular injury. Lab Invest 1982; 47:5–18.
13. McCord JM, Fridovich I: Superoxide dismutase: an enzymic function for erythrocuprein (hemocuprein). J Biol Chem 1969; 244:6049–6055.
14. McCord JM: Free radicals and inflammation: protection of synovial fluid by superoxide dismutase. Science 1974; 185:529–531.
15. Furchgott RF, Zawadzki JV: The obligatory role of endothelial cells in the relaxation of arterial smooth muscle by acetylcholine. Nature 1980; 288:373–376.
16. Palmer RMJ, Ferrige AG, Moncada S: Nitric oxide release accounts for the biological activity of endothelium-derived relaxing factor. Nature 1987; 327:524–526.
17. Palmer RMJ, Ashton DS, Moncada S: Vascular endothelial cells synthesize nitric oxide from L-arginine. Nature 1988; 333:664–666.
18. Ignarro LJ, Lippton H, Edwards JC, et al: Mechanism of vascular smooth muscle relaxation by organic nitrates, nitrites, nitroprusside and nitric oxide: evidence for the involvement of S-nitrosothiols as active intermediates. Pharmacol Exp Ther 1981; 218:739–749.
19. Gruetter CA, Gruetter DY, Lyon JE, et al: Relationship between cyclic guanosine 3′:5′-monophosphate formation and relaxation of coronary arterial smooth muscle by glyceryl trinitrate, nitroprusside, nitrite and nitric oxide: effects of methylene blue and methemoglobin. J Pharmacol Exp Ther 1981; 219:181–186.
20. Pryor WA, Squadrito GL: The chemistry of peroxynitrite: a product from the reaction of nitric oxide with superoxide. Am J Physiol 1995; 268:L699–L722.
21. Arteel GE, Briviba K, Sies H: Protection against peroxynitrite. FEBS Lett 1999; 445:226–230.
22. Denicola A, Souza JM, Gatti RM, et al: Desferrioxamine inhibition of the hydroxyl radical-like reactivity of peroxynitrite: role of the hydroxamic groups. Free Radic Biol Med 1995; 19:11–19.
23. Granger DN, Rutili G, McCord JM: Superoxide radicals in feline intestinal ischemia. Gastroenterology 1981; 81:22–29.
24. Parks DA, Bulkley GB, Granger DN: Role of oxygen-derived free radicals in digestive tract diseases. Surgery 1983; 94:415–422.
25. Oliver CN, Starke-Reed PE, Stadtman ER, et al: Oxidative dam-

age to brain proteins, loss of glutamine synthetase activity, and production of free radicals during ischemia-reperfusion–induced injury to gerbil brain. Proc Natl Acad Sci USA 1990; 87:5144–5147.

26. Das DK, Engelman RM, Clement R, et al: Role of xanthine oxidase inhibitor as free radical scavenger: a novel mechanism of action of allopurinol and oxypurinol in myocardial salvage. Biochem Biophys Res Comm 1987; 148:314–319.

27. Williams RE, Zweier JL, Flaherty JT: Treatment with deferoxamine during ischemia improves functional and metabolic recovery and reduces reperfusion-induced oxygen radical generation in rabbit hearts. Circ 1991; 83:1006–1014.

28. Di Pierro D, Tavazzi B, Lazzarino G, et al: Malondialdehyde is a biochemical marker of peroxidative damage in the isolated reperfused rat heart. Mol Cell Biochem 1992; 116:193–196.

29. Fisher AB, Dodia C, Tan Z, et al: Oxygen-dependent lipid peroxidation during lung ischemia. J Clin Invest 1991; 88:674–679.

30. Parks DA, Williams TK, Beckman JS: Conversion of xanthine dehydrogenase to oxidase in ischemic rat intestine: a reevaluation. Am J Physiol 1988; 254:G768–G774.

31. Otamiri T, Tagesson C: Role of phospholipase A_2 and oxygenated free radicals in mucosal damage after small intestinal ischemia and reperfusion. Am J Surg 1989; 157:562–565.

32. Smith JK, Carden DL, Grisham MB, et al: Role of iron in postischemic microvascular injury. Am J Physiol 1989; 256:H1472–H1477.

33. Horton JW, Walker PB: Oxygen radicals, lipid peroxidation, and permeability changes after intestinal ischemia and reperfusion. J Appl Physiol 1993; 74:1515–1520.

34. Paller MS, Hoidal JR, Ferris TF: Oxygen free radicals in ischemic acute renal failure in the rat. J Clin Invest 1984; 74:1156–1164.

35. Paller MS, Hebbel RP: Ethane production as a measure of lipid peroxidation after renal ischemia. Am J Physiol 1986; 251:F839–F843.

36. Ratych RE, Bulkley GB: Free-radical–mediated postischemic reperfusion injury in the kidney. Free Radic Biol Med 1986; 2:311–319.

37. Greene EL, Paller MS: Xanthine oxidase produces O_2 in posthypoxic injury of renal epithelial cells. Am J Physiol 1992; 263:F251–F255.

38. Paller MS, Neumann TV: Reactive oxygen species and rat renal epithelial cells during hypoxia and reoxygenation. Kidney Int 1991; 40:1041–1049.

39. Linas SL, Whittenburg D, Repine JE: Role of xanthine oxidase in ischemia-reperfusion injury. Am J Physiol 1990; 258:F711–F716.

40. Nath KA, Paller MS: Dietary deficiency of antioxidants exacerbates ischemic injury in the rat kidney. Kidney Int 1990; 38:1109–1117.

41. Paller MS: Hydrogen peroxide and ischemic renal injury: effect of catalase inhibition. Free Radic Biol Med 1991; 10:29–34.

42. Kaneko H, Schweizer RT: Venous flushing with vasodilators aids recovery of vasoconstricted and warm ischemic injured pig kidneys. Transplant Proc 1989; 21:1233–1235.

43. Battelli MG, Della Corte E, Stirpe F: Xanthine oxidase type D (dehydrogenase) in the intestine and other organs of the rat. Biochem J 1972; 126:747–749.

44. Joannidis M, Gstraunthaler G, Pfaller W: Xanthine oxidase: evidence against a causative role in renal reperfusion injury. Am J Physiol 1990; 258:F232–F236.

45. Cighetti G, Del Puppo M, Paroni R, et al: Lack of conversion of xanthine dehydrogenase to xanthine oxidase during warm renal ischemia. FEBS Lett 1990; 274:82–84.

46. Sanhueza J, Valdes J, Campos R, et al: Changes in the xanthine dehydrogenase/xanthine oxidase ratio in the rat kidney subjected to ischemia-reperfusion stress: preventive effect of some flavanoids. Res Commun Chem Pathol Pharmacol 1992; 78:211–218.

47. Brass CA, Narciso J, Gollan JL: Enhanced activity of the free radical producing enzyme xanthine oxidase in hypoxic rat liver. Regulation and pathophysiologic significance. J Clin Invest 1991; 87:424–431.

48. Gonzalez-Flecha B, Cutrin JC, Boveris A: Time course and mechanism of oxidative stress and tissue damage in rat liver subjected to in vivo ischemia-reperfusion. J Clin Invest 1993; 91:456–464.

49. Della Corte E, Stirpe F: The regulation of rat liver xanthine oxidase: involvement of thiol groups in the conversion of the enzyme activity from dehydrogenase (type D) into oxidase (type O) and purification of the enzyme. Biochem J 1972; 126:739–745.

50. Waud WR, Rajagoplan KV: The mechanism of conversion of rat liver xanthine dehydrogenase from an NAD^+-dependent form (type D) to an O_2-dependent form (type O). Arch Biochem Biophys 1976; 172:365–379.

51. Turrens JF, Alexandre A, Lehninger AL: Ubisemiquinone is the electron donor for superoxide formation by complex III of heart mitochondria. Arch Biochem Biophys 1985; 237:408–414.

52. Turrens JF, Boveris A: Generation of superoxide anion by the NADH dehydrogenase of bovine heart mitochondria. Biochem J 1980; 191:421–427.

53. Turrens JF, Beconi M, Barilla J: Mitochondrial generation of oxygen radicals during reoxygenation of ischemic tissues. Free Radic Res Commun 1991; 12–13:681–689.

54. Aust SD, Roerig DL, Pederson TC: Evidence for superoxide generation by NADPH-cytochrome c reductase of rat liver microsomes. Biochem Biophys Res Commun 1972; 47:1133–1137.

55. Kuthan H, Ullrich V: Oxidase and oxygenase function of the microsomal cytochrome P450 monooxygenase system. Eur J Biochem 1982; 126:583–588.

56. Rashba-Step J, Cederbaum AI: Generation of reactive oxygen intermediates by human liver microsomes in the presence of NADPH or NADH. Mol Pharmacol 1994; 45:150–157.

57. Masters C, Holmes R: Peroxisomes: new aspects of cell physiology and biochemistry. Physiol Rev 1977; 57:816–882.

58. Campos R, Garrido A, Guerra R, et al: Increased resistance against oxidative stress is observed during a short period of renal reperfusion after a temporal ischemia. Free Radic Res Commun 1990; 10:259–264.

59. Kukreja RC, Kontos HA, Hess ML, et al: PGH synthase and lipoxygenase generate superoxide in the presence of NADH or NADPH. Circ Res 1986; 59:612–619.

60. Misra HP, Fridovich I: The role of superoxide anion in the autoxidation of epinephrine and a simple assay for superoxide dismutase. J Biol Chem 1972; 247:3170–3175.

61. Cohen G: Oxy-radical toxicity in catecholamine neurons. Neurotoxicology 1984; 5:77–82.

62. Bors W, Michel C, Saran M, et al: The involvement of oxygen radicals during the autoxidation of adrenalin. Biochim Biophys Acta 1978; 540:162–172.

63. Grisham MB: Myoglobin-catalyzed hydrogen peroxide–dependent arachidonic acid peroxidation. Free Radic Biol Med 1985; 1:227–232.

64. Lucchesi BR: Complement activation, neutrophils, and oxygen radicals in reperfusion injury. Stroke 1993; 24:I41–I45.

65. Zimmerman BJ, Grisham MB, Granger DN: Role of oxidants in ischemia-reperfusion–induced granulocyte infiltration. Am J Physiol 1990; 258:G185–G190.

66. Linas SL, Shanley PF, Whittenburg D, et al: Neutrophils accentuate ischemia-reperfusion injury in isolated perfused rat kidneys. Am J Physiol 1988; 255:F728–F735.

67. Hellberg PO, Kallskog TO: Neutrophil-mediated postischemic tubular leakage in the rat kidney. Kidney Int 1989; 36:555–561.

68. Linas SL, Whittenburg D, Parsons PE, et al: Mild renal ischemia activates primed neutrophils to cause acute renal failure. Kidney Int 1992; 42:610–616.

69. Thornton MA, Winn R, Alpers CE, et al: An evaluation of the neutrophil as a mediator of in vivo renal ischemic-reperfusion injury. Am J Pathol 1989; 135:509–515.

70. Paller MS: Effect of neutrophil depletion on ischemic renal injury in the rat. J Lab Clin Med 1989; 113:379–386.

71. Kelly KJ, Williams WW Jr, Colvin RB, et al: Antibody to intercellular adhesion molecule 1 protects the kidney against ischemic injury. Proc Natl Acad Sci USA 1994; 91:811–816.

72. Paller MS, Hedlund BE: Role of iron in postischemic renal injury in the rat. Kidney Int 1988; 34:474–480.

73. Kako K, Kato M, Matsuoka T, et al: Depression of membrane-bound Na^+ K^+-ATPase activity induced by free radicals and by ischemia of kidney. Am J Physiol 1988; 254:C330–C337.

74. Paller MS: Renal work, glutathione and susceptibility to free radical–mediated postischemic injury. Kidney Int 1988; 33:843–849.

75. Mandel LJ, Schnellmann RG, Jacobs WR: Intracellular glutathione in the protection from anoxic injury in renal proximal tubules. J Clin Invest 1990; 85:316–324.

76. Shanley PF, White CW, Avraham K, et al: Renal ischemia-reperfusion in transgenic mice with endogenous high levels of superoxide dismutase (SOD). J Am Soc Nephrol 1990; 1:604.

77. Noiri E, Peresleni T, Miller F, et al: In vivo targeting of inducible NO synthase with oligodeoxynucleotides protects rat kidney against ischemia. J Clin Invest 1996; 97:2377–2383.

78. Walker LM, Walker PD, Imam SZ, et al: Evidence for peroxynitrite formation in renal ischemia-reperfusion injury: studies with the inducible nitric oxide synthase inhibitor L-N⁶-(1-iminoethyl) lysine. J Pharmacol Exp Ther 2000; 295:417–422.

79. Chiao H, Kohda Y, McLeroy P, et al: α-Melanocyte-stimulating hormone protects against renal injury after ischemia in mice and rats. J Clin Invest 1997; 99:1165–1172.

80. Bratell S, Haraldsson B, Herlitz H, et al: Protective effects of pretreatment with superoxide dismutase, catalase and oxypurinol on tubular damage caused by transient ischemia. Act Physiol Scand 1990; 139:417–425.

81. Sabbatini M, Sansone G, Uccello F, et al: Functional versus structural changes in the pathophysiology of acute ischemia renal failure in aging rats. Kidney Int 1994; 45:1355–1361.

82. DiMari J, Megyesi J, Udvarhelyi N, et al: N-Acetyl cysteine ameliorates ischemic renal failure. Am J Physiol 1997; 272:F292–F298.

83. Marubayashi S, Dohi K, Sugino K, et al: The protective effect of administered alpha-tocopherol against hepatic damage caused by ischemia-reperfusion or endotoxemia. Ann NY Acad Sci 1989; 570:208–218.

84. Scaduto J, RC, Gattone VH, Grotyohann LW, et al: Effect of an altered glutathione content on renal ischemic injury. Am J Physiol 1988; 255:F911–F921.

85. Zager RA: Hypoperfusion-induced acute renal failure in the rat: an evaluation of oxidant tissue injury. Circ Res 1988; 62:430–435.

86. Zager RA, Gmur DJ, Schimpf BA, et al: Evidence against increased hydroxyl radical production during oxygen deprivation-reoxygenation proximal tubular injury. J Am Soc Nephrol 1992; 2:1627–1633.

87. Baliga R, Ueda N, Shah SV: Increase in bleomycin-detectable iron in ischemia-reperfusion injury to rat kidneys. Biochem J 1993; 291:901–905.

88. Gower J, Healing G, Green C: Measurement by HPLC of desferrioxamine-available iron in rabbit kidneys to assess the effect of ischemia on the distribution of iron within the total pool. Free Radic Res Comm 1989; 5:291–299.

89. Boucher F, Pucheu S, Coudray C, et al: Evidence of cytosolic iron release during post-ischemic reperfusion of isolated rat hearts. FEBS Lett 1992; 302:261–264.

90. Voogd A, Sluiter W, van Eijk HG, et al: Low molecular weight iron and the oxygen paradox in isolated rat hearts. J Clin Invest 1992; 90:2050–2055.

91. Gutteridge JMC, Richmond R, Halliwell B: Inhibition of the iron-catalyzed formation of hydroxyl radicals from superoxide and of lipid peroxidation by desferrioxamine. Biochem J 1979; 184:469–472.

92. Johnson KJ, Ward PA, Kunkel RG, et al: Mediation of IgA–induced lung injury in the rat: role of macrophages and reactive oxygen products. Lab Invest 1986; 54:499–506.

93. Shah SV: Role of reactive oxygen metabolites in experimental glomerular disease. Kidney Int 1989; 35:1093–1106.

94. Foschi D, Castoldi L, Lesma A, et al: Effects of ischemia and reperfusion on liver regeneration in rats. Eur J Surg 1993; 159:393–398.

95. Esterbauer H, Schraur RJ, Zollner H: Chemistry and biochemistry of 4-hydroxynonenal, malonedialdehyde and related aldehydes. Free Radic Biol Med 1991; 11:81–128.

96. Eschwege P, Paradis V, Conti M, et al: In situ detection of lipid peroxidation by-products as markers of renal ischemia injuries in rat kidneys. J Urol 1999; 162:553–557.

97. Paroni R, De Vecchi E, Lubatti L, et al: Influence of the 21-aminosteroid U74389F on ischemia-reperfusion injury in the rat. Eur J Pharmacol 1995; 294:737–742.

98. Garvin PJ, Niehoff ML, Robinson SM, et al: Renoprotective effects of the 21-aminosteroid U74389G in ischemia-reperfusion injury and cold storage preservation. Transplantation 1997; 63:194–201.

99. De Vecchi E, Lubatti L, Beretta C, et al: Protection from renal ischemia-reperfusion injury by the 2-methylaminochroman U83836E. Kidney Int 1998; 54:857–863.

100. Shoskes DA: Effect of bioflavonoids quercetin and curcumin on ischemia renal injury: a new class of renoprotective agents. Transplantation 1998; 66:147–152.

101. McCoy RN, Hill KE, Ayon MA, et al: Oxidant stress following renal ischemia: changes in the glutathione redox ratio. Kidney Int 1988; 33:812–817.

102. Bauer P, Belleville-Nabet F, Watelet F, et al: Selenium, oxygen-derived free radicals, and ischemia-reperfusion injury. An experimental study in the rat. Biol Trace Element Res 1995; 47:157–163.

103. Sela S, Shasha SM, Mashiach E, et al: Effect of oxygen tension on activity of antioxidant enzymes and on renal function of the postischemia reperfused rat kidney. Nephron 1993; 63:199–206.

104. Singh I, Gulati S, Orak JK, et al: Expression of antioxidant enzymes in rat kidney during ischemia-reperfusion injury. Mol Cell Biochem 1993; 125:97–104.

105. Rosenberg ME, Paller MS: Differential gene expression in the recovery from ischemic renal injury. Kidney Int 1991; 39:1156–1161.

106. Kiyama S, Yoshioka T, Burr IM, et al: Strategic locus for the activation of the superoxide dismutase gene in the nephron. Kidney Int 1995; 47:539–546.

107. Gwinner W, Deters-Evers U, Brandes RP, et al: Antioxidant-oxidant balance in the glomerulus and proximal tubule of the rat kidney. J Physiol 1998; 509:559–606.

108. Traylor LA, Mayeux PR: Superoxide generation by renal proximal tubule nitric oxide synthase. Nitric Oxide 1997; 1:432–438.

109. Whiteman M, Halliwell B: Thiourea and dimethylthiourea inhibit peroxynitrite-dependent damage: nonspecificity as hydroxyl radical scavengers. Free Radic Biol Med 1997; 22:1309–1312.

110. Mayeux PR: Pathobiology of lipopolysaccharide. J Toxicol Environ Health 1997; 51:415–435.

111. Forstermann U, Gath I, Schwarz P, et al: Isoforms of nitric oxide synthase: properties, cellular distribution and expressional control. Biochem Pharmacol 1995; 50:1321–1332.

112. Morrissey JJ, McCracken R, Kaneto H, et al: Location of an inducible nitric oxide synthase mRNA in the normal kidney. Kidney Int 1994; 45:998–1005.

113. Mohaupt MG, Elzie JL, Ahn KY, et al: Differential expression and induction of mRNAs encoding two inducible nitric oxide synthases in rat kidney. Kidney Int 1994; 46:653–665.

114. Millar CGM, Theimermann C: Intrarenal hemodynamics and renal dysfunction in endotoxemia: effects of nitric oxide synthase inhibition. Br J Pharmacol 1997; 121:1824–1830.

115. Milligan SA, Hoeffel JM, Goldstein IM, et al: Effect of catalase on endotoxin-induced acute lung injury in unanesthetized sheep. Am Rev Respir Dis 1988; 137:420–428.

116. Demling RH, Lalonde C, Jin LJ, et al: Endotoxemia causes increased lung tissue lipid peroxidation in unanesthetized sheep. J Appl Physiol 1986; 60:2094–2100.

117. Bautista AP, Spitzer J: Superoxide anion generation by in situ perfused rat liver: effect of in vivo endotoxin. Am J Physiol 1990; 259:G907–G912.

118. Zurovsky Y, Gispaan I: Antioxidants attenuate endotoxin-induced acute renal failure in rats. Am J Kidney Dis 1995; 25:51–57.

119. Faas MM, Schuiling GA, Valkhof N, et al: Superoxide-mediated glomerulopathy in the endotoxin-treated pregnant rat. Kidney Blood Press Res 1998; 21:432–437.

120. Walker PD, Shah SV: Reactive oxygen metabolites in endotoxin-induced acute renal failure in rats. Kidney Int 1990; 38:1125–1132.

121. Zhang C, Walker LM, Mayeux PR: Role of nitric oxide in lipopolysaccharide-induced oxidant stress in the rat kidney. Biochem Pharmacol 2000; 59:203–209.

122. Traylor LA, Proksch JW, Beanum VC, et al: Nitric oxide generation by renal proximal tubules: role of nitric oxide in the cytotoxicity of lipid A. J Pharmacol Exp Ther 1996; 279:91–96.

123. Proksch JW, Traylor LA, Mayeux PR: Effects of lipid A on calcium homeostasis in proximal tubules. J Pharmacol Exp Ther 1996; 276:555–560.

124. Traylor LA, Mayeux PR: Nitric oxide generation mediates lipid A–induced oxidant injury in renal proximal tubules. Arch Biochem Biophys 1997; 338:129–135.

125. Mayeux PR, Shah SV: Intracellular calcium mediates the cytotoxicity of lipid A in LLC-PK$_1$ cells. J Pharmacol Exp Ther 1993; 266:47–51.

126. Sies H, Sharov VS, Klotz L-O, et al: Glutathione peroxidase protects against peroxynitrite-mediated oxidations. J Biol Chem 1997; 272:27812–27817.

127. Mayeux PR, Garner HR, Gibson JD, et al: Effect of lipopolysaccharide on nitric oxide synthase activity in rat proximal tubules. Biochem Pharmacol 1995; 49:115–118.

128. Xia Y, Zweier JL: Superoxide and peroxynitrite generation from inducible nitric oxide synthase in macrophages. Proc Natl Acad Sci USA 1997; 94:6954–6958.

129. Walker PD, Barri Y, Shah SV: Oxidant mechanisms in gentamicin nephrotoxicity. Renal Failure 1999; 21(3,4):433–442.

130. Walker PD, Shah SV: Gentamicin-enhanced production of hydrogen peroxide by renal cortical mitochondria. Am J Physiol 1987; 253:C495–C499.

131. Yang CL, Du XH, Han YX: Renal cortical mitochondria are the source of oxygen free radicals enhanced by gentamicin. Ren Fail 1995; 17:21–26.

132. Du XH, Yang CL: Mechanism of gentamicin nephrotoxicity in rats and the protective effect of zinc-induced metallothionein synthesis. Nephrol Dial Transplant 1994; 9:135–140.

133. Guidet BR, Shah SV: In vivo generation of hydrogen peroxide by rat kidney cortex and glomeruli. Am J Physiol 1989; 256:F158–F164.

134. Ueda N, Guidet B, Shah SV: Gentamicin-induced mobilization of iron from renal cortical mitochondria. Am J Physiol 1993; 265:F435–F439.

135. Priuska EM, Schacht J: Formation of free radicals by gentamicin and iron and evidence for an iron-gentamicin complex. Biochem Pharmacol 1995; 50:1749–1752.

136. Walker PD, Shah SV: Evidence suggesting a role for hydroxyl radical in gentamicin-induced acute renal failure in rats. J Clin Invest 1988; 81:334–341.

137. Nakajima T, Hishida A, Kato A: Mechanisms for protective effects of free radical scavengers on gentamicin-mediated nephropathy in rats. Am J Physiol 1994; 266:F425–F431.

138. Zurovsky Y, Haber C: Antioxidants attenuate endotoxin-gentamicin–induced acute renal failure in rats. Scand J Urol Nephrol 1995; 29:147–154.

139. Ali BH: Gentamicin nephrotoxicity in humans and animals: some recent research. Gen Pharmacol 1995; 26:1477–1487.

140. Ademuyiwa O, Ngaha EO, Ubah FO: Vitamin E and selenium in gentamicin nephrotoxicity. Human Exp Toxicol 1990; 9:281–288.

141. Ben Ismail TH, Ali BH, Bashir AA: Influence of iron, deferoxamine and ascorbic acid on gentamicin-induced nephrotoxicity in rats. Gen Pharmacol 1994; 25:1249–1252.

142. Kays SE, Crowell WA, Johnson MA: Iron supplementation increases gentamicin nephrotoxicity in rats. J Nutr 1991; 121:1869–1875.

143. Kavutcu M, Canbolat O, Ozturk S, et al: Reduced enzymatic antioxidant defense mechanism in kidney tissues from gentamicin-treated guinea pigs: effects of vitamins E and C. Nephron 1996; 72:269–274.

144. Rivas-Cabanero L, Rodriguez-Barbero A, Arevalo M, et al: Effect of N(G)-nitro-ʟ-arginine methyl ester on nephrotoxicity induced by gentamicin in rats. Nephron 1995; 71:203–207.

145. Ramsammy LS, Josepovitz C, Ling KY, et al: Effects of diphenylphenylenediamine on gentamicin-induced lipid peroxidation and toxicity in rat renal cortex. J Pharmacol Exp Ther 1986; 238:83–88.

146. Martinez-Salgado C, Rodriguez-Barbero A, Rodriguez-Puyol D, et al: Involvement of phospholipase A$_2$ in gentamicin-induced rat mesangial cell activation. Am J Physiol 1997; 273:F60–F66.

147. Rivas-Cabanero L, Montero A, Lopez-Novoa JM: Increased glomerular nitric oxide synthesis in gentamicin-induced renal failure. Eur J Pharmacol 1994; 270:119–121.

148. Bolanos JP, Peuchen S, Heales SJR, et al: Nitric oxide–mediated inhibition of the mitochondrial respiratory chain in cultured astrocytes. J Neurochem 1994; 63:910–916.

149. Szabo C, Day BJ, Salzman AL: Evaluation of the relative contribution of nitric oxide and peroxynitrite to the suppression of mitochondrial respiration in immunostimulated macrophages using a manganese mesoporphyrin superoxide dismutase mimetic and peroxynitrite scavenger. FEBS Lett 1996; 381:82–86.

150. Brown GC: Nitric oxide regulates mitochondrial respiration and cell functions by inhibiting cytochrome oxidase. FEBS Lett 1995; 369:136–139.

151. Lizasoain I, Moro MA, Knowles RG, et al: Nitric oxide and peroxynitrite exert distinct effects on mitochondrial respiration which are differentially blocked by glutathione or glucose. Biochem J 1996; 314:877–880.

152. Giulivi C, Poderoso JJ, Boveris A: Production of nitric oxide by mitochondria. J Biol Chem 1998; 273:11038–11043.

153. Tatoyan A, Guilivi C: Purification and characterization of a nitric oxide synthase from rat liver mitochondria. J Biol Chem 1998; 273:11044–11048.

154. Bywaters EGL, Beall D: Crush injuries with impairment of renal function. BMJ 1941; 1:427–432.

155. Gabow PA, Kaehny WD, Kelleher SP: The spectrum of rhabdomyolysis. Medicine 1982; 61:141–152.

156. Grossman RA, Hamilton RW, Morse BM, et al: Nontraumatic rhabdomyolysis and acute renal failure. N Engl J Med 1974; 291:807–811.

157. Koffler A, Friedler RM, Massry SG: Acute renal failure due to nontraumatic rhabdomyolysis. Ann Intern Med 1976; 85:23–28.

158. Hostetter TH, Wilkes BM, Brenner BM: Renal Circulatory and Nephron Function in Experimental Acute Renal Failure. In: Brenner BM, Lazarus JM, eds: Acute Renal Failure. Vol. 1. Philadelphia: WB Saunders; 1983:99–115.

159. Guidet B, Shah SV: Enhanced in vivo H$_2$O$_2$ generation by rat kidney in glycerol-induced renal failure. Am J Physiol 1989; 257:F440–F445.

160. Salahudeen AK, Clark EC, Nath KA: Hydrogen peroxide–induced renal injury: a protective role for pyruvate in vitro and in vivo. J Clin Invest 1991; 88:1886–1893.

161. Shah SV, Walker PD: Evidence suggesting a role for hydroxyl radical in glycerol-induced acute renal failure. Am J Physiol 1988; 255:F438–F443.

162. Paller MS: Hemoglobin- and myoglobin-induced acute renal failure in rats: role of iron in nephrotoxicity. Am J Physiol 1988; 255:F539–F544.

163. Zager RA: Combined mannitol and deferoxamine therapy for myohemoglobinuric renal injury and oxidant tubular stress: mechanistic and therapeutic implications. J Clin Invest 1992; 90:711–719.

164. Abul-Ezz SR, Walker PD, Shah SV: Role of glutathione in an animal model of myoglobinuric acute renal failure. Proc Natl Acad Sci USA 1991; 88:9833–9837.

165. Nath KA, Balla G, Vercellotti GM, et al: Induction of heme oxygenase is a rapid, protective response in rhabdomyolysis in the rat. J Clin Invest 1992; 90:267–270.

166. Nath KA, Balla J, Croatt AJ, et al: Heme protein-mediated renal injury: a protective role for 21-aminosteroids in vitro and in vivo. Kidney Int 1995; 47:592–602.

167. Salahudeen AK, Wang C, Bigler SA, et al: Synergistic renal protection by combining alkaline-diuresis with lipid peroxidation inhibitors in rhabdomyolysis: possible interaction between oxidant and non-oxidant mechanisms. Nephrol Dial Transplant 1996; 11:635–642.

168. Zager RA: Mitochondrial free radical production induces lipid peroxidation during myohemoglobinuria. Kidney Int 1996; 49:741–751.

169. Bunton CA: Oxidation of α-diketones and α-keto-acids by hydrogen peroxide. Nature 1949; 163:444.

170. Orrenius S, Ellin A, Jakobsson SV, et al: The cytochrome P-450-containing mono-oxygenase system of rat kidney cortex microsomes. Drug Metab Dispos 1973; 1:350–357.

171. Bysani GK, Kennedy TP, Ky N, et al: Role of cytochrome P-450

in reperfusion injury of the rabbit lung. J Clin Invest 1990; 86:1434–1441.

172. Paller MS, Jacob HS: Cytochrome P-450 mediates tissue-damaging hydroxyl radical formation during reoxygenation of the kidney. Proc Natl Acad Sci USA 1994; 91:7002–7006.

173. Baliga R, Zhang Z, Baliga M, et al: Evidence for cytochrome P-450 as a source of catalytic iron in myoglobinuric acute renal failure. Kidney Int 1996; 49:362–369.

174. Meister A: Selective modification of glutathione metabolism. Science 1983; 220:472–477.

175. Meister A: New developments in glutathione metabolism and their potential application in therapy. Hepatology 1984; 4:739–742.

176. Meister A, Anderson ME, Hwang O: Intracellular cysteine and glutathione delivery systems. J Am Coll Nutr 1986; 5:137–151.

177. Olson CE: Glutathione modulates toxic oxygen metabolite injury of canine chief cell monolayers in primary culture. Am J Physiol 1988; 254:G49–G56.

178. Dethmers JK, Meister A: Glutathione export by human lymphoid cells: depletion of glutathione by inhibition of its synthesis decreases export and increases sensitivity to irradiation. Proc Natl Acad Sci USA 1981; 78:7492–7496.

179. Arrick BA, Nathan CF, Griffith OW, et al: Glutathione depletion sensitizes tumor cells to oxidative cytolysis. J Biol Chem 1982; 257:1231–1237.

180. Andreoli SP, Mallett CP, Bergstein JM: Role of glutathione in protecting endothelial cells against hydrogen peroxide oxidant injury. J Lab Clin Med 1986; 108:190–198.

181. Doroshow JH, Locker GY, Ifrim I, et al: Prevention of doxorubicin cardiac toxicity in the mouse by N-acetylcysteine. J Clin Invest 1981; 68:1053–1064.

182. Lash LH, Hagen TM, Jones DP: Exogenous glutathione protects intestinal epithelial cells from oxidative injury. Proc Natl Acad Sci USA 1986; 83:4641–4645.

183. Melillo G, Musso T, Sica A, et al: A hypoxia-responsive element mediates a novel pathway of activation of the inducible nitric oxide synthase promoter. J Exp Med 1995; 182:1683–1693.

184. Duval DL, Sieg DJ, Billings RE: Regulation of hepatic nitric oxide synthase by reactive oxygen intermediates and glutathione. Arch Biochem Biophys 1995; 316:699–706.

185. Sandau K, Pfeilschifter J, Brune B: Nitrosative and oxidative stress induced heme oxygenase-1 accumulation in rat mesangial cells. Eur J Pharmacol 1998; 342:77–84.

186. Datta PK, Lianos EA: Nitric oxide induces heme oxygenase-1 gene expression in mesangial cells. Kidney Int 1999; 55:1734–1739.

187. Weiss G, Goossen B, Doppler W, et al: Translational regulation via iron-responsive elements by the nitric oxide/NO-synthase pathway. EMBO J 1993; 12:3651–3657.

188. Juckett M, Zheng Y, Yuan H, et al: Heme and the endothelium: effects of nitric oxide on catalytic iron and heme degradation by heme oxygenase. J Biol Chem 1998; 273:23388–23397.

189. Kim Y-M, Bergonia HA, Muller C, et al: Loss and degradation of enzyme-bound heme induced by cellular nitric oxide synthesis. J Biol Chem 1995; 270:5710–5713.

190. Minamiyama Y, Takemura S, Imaoka S, et al: Irreversible inhibition of cytochrome P-450 by nitric oxide. J Pharmacol Exp Ther 1997; 283:1479–1485.

191. Perez de Lema G, Arribas I, Prieto A, et al: Cyclosporin A–induced hydrogen peroxide synthesis by cultured human mesangial cells is blocked by exogenous antioxidants. Life Sci 1998; 62:1745–1753.

192. Parra T, de Arriba G, Arribas I, et al: Cyclosporine A nephrotoxicity: role of thromboxane and reactive oxygen species. J Lab Clin Med 1998; 131:63–70.

193. Wolf A, Clemann N, Frieauff W, et al: Role of reactive oxygen formation in the cyclosporine A–mediated impairment of renal functions. Transplant Proc 1994; 26:2902–2907.

194. Wolf A, Trendelenburg CF, Diez-Fernandez C, et al: Role of glutathione in cyclosporine A in vitro hepatotoxicity. Transplant Proc 1994; 26:2912–2914.

195. Zhong Z, Arteel GE, Connor HD, et al: Cyclosporin A increases hypoxia and free radical production in rat kidneys: prevention by dietary glycine. Am J Physiol 1998; 275:F595–F604.

196. Ahmed SS, Napoli KL, Strobel HW: Oxygen radical formation

during cytochrome P-450–catalyzed cyclosporine metabolism in rat and human liver microsomes at varying hydrogen ion concentrations. Mol Cell Biochem 1995; 151:131–140.

197. Serino F, Grevel J, Napoli KL, et al: Generation of oxygen free radicals during the metabolism of cyclosporine A: a cause-effect relationship with metabolism inhibition. Mol Cell Biochem 1993; 122:101–112.

198. Inselmann G, Blank M, Baumann K: Cyclosporine A–induced lipid peroxidation in microsomes and effect on active and passive glucose transport by brush border membrane vesicles of rat kidney. Res Comm Chem Pathol Pharmacol 1988; 62:207–220.

199. Wang C, Salahudeen AK: Lipid peroxidation accompanies cyclosporine nephrotoxicity: Effects of vitamin E. Kidney Int 1995; 47:927–934.

200. Walker PD, Das C, Shah SV: Cyclosporin A–induced lipid peroxidation in renal cortical mitochondria. Kidney Int 1986; 29:311.

201. Walker RJ, Lazzaro VA, Duggin GG, et al: Evidence that alterations in renal metabolism and lipid peroxidation may contribute to cyclosporine nephrotoxicity. Transplantation 1990; 50:487–492.

202. Yang JJ, Finn WF: Effect of oxypurinol on cyclosporine toxicity in cultured EA, LLC-PK$_1$ and MDCK cells. Ren Fail 1998; 20:85–101.

203. al Khader A, al Sulaiman M, Kishore PN, et al: Quinacrine attenuates cyclosporine-induced nephrotoxicity in rats. Transplantation 1996; 62:427–435.

204. Kanji VK, Wang C, Salahudeen AK: Vitamin E suppresses cyclosporine A–induced increase in the urinary excretion of arachidonic acid metabolites including F2-isoprostanes in the rat model. Transplant Proc 1999; 31:1724–1728.

205. Krysztopik RJ, Bentley FR, Spain DA, et al: Lazaroids prevent acute cyclosporine-induced renal vasoconstriction. Transplantation 1997; 63:1215–1220.

206. Lopez-Ongil S, Saura M, Rodriguez-Puyol D, et al: Regulation of endothelial NO synthase expression by cyclosporin A in bovine aortic endothelial cells. Am J Physiol 1996; 271:H1072–H1078.

207. Bobadilla NA, Gamba G, Tapia E, et al: Role of NO in cyclosporin nephrotoxicity: effects of chronic NO inhibition and NO synthase gene expression. Am J Physiology 1998; 274:F791–F798.

208. Nakamura M, Imaoka S, Miura K, et al: Induction of cytochrome P-450 isozymes in rat renal microsomes by cyclosporin A. Biochem Pharmacol 1994; 48:1743–1746.

209. Hoffman DW, Wiebkin P, Rybak LP: Inhibition of glutathione-related enzymes and cytotoxicity of ethacrynic acid and cyclosporine. Biochem Pharmacol 1995; 49:411–415.

210. Inselmann G, Lawerenz HU, Nellessen U, et al: Enhancement of cyclosporin A–induced hepato- and nephrotoxicity by glutathione depletion. Eur J Clin Invest 1994; 24:355–359.

211. Gottschalk AR, Boise LH, Thompson CB, et al: Identification of immunosuppressant-induced apoptosis in a murine B-cell line and its prevention by Bcl-x but not Bcl-2. Proc Natl Acad Sci USA 1994; 91:7350–7354.

212. Kitagaki K, Niwa S, Hoshiko K, et al: Augmentation of apoptosis in bronchial exuded rat eosinophils by cyclosporin A. Biochem Biophys Res Commun 1996; 222:71–77.

213. Buttke TM, Sandstrom PA: Oxidative stress as a mediator of apoptosis. Immunol Today 1994; 15:7–10.

214. Ueda N, Shah SV: Endonuclease-induced DNA damage and cell death in oxidant injury to renal tubular epithelial cells. J Clin Invest 1992; 90:2593–2597.

215. Tsutsumishita Y, Onda T, Okada K, et al: Involvement of H$_2$O$_2$ production in cisplatin-induced nephrotoxicity. Biochem Biophys Res Commun 1998; 242:310–312.

216. Kruidering M, Van de Water B, de Heer E, et al: Cisplatin-induced nephrotoxicity in porcine proximal tubular cells: mitochondrial dysfunction by inhibition of complexes I to IV of the respiratory chain. J Pharmacol Exp Ther 1997; 280:638–649.

217. Baliga R, Zhang Z, Baliga M, et al: In vitro and in vivo evidence suggesting a role for iron in cisplatin-induced nephrotoxicity. Kidney Int 1998; 53:394–401.

218. Kim YK, Jung JS, Lee SH, et al: Effects of antioxidants and

Oxidant Mechanisms in Acute Renal Failure ■ 77

Ca^{2+} in cisplatin-induced cell injury in rabbit renal cortical slices. Toxicol Appl Pharmacol 1997; 146:261–269.

219. Matsushima H, Yonemura K, Ohishi K, et al: The role of oxygen free radicals in cisplatin-induced acute renal failure in rats. J Lab Clin Med 1998; 131:518–526.

220. Gemba M, Fukuishi N, Nakano S: Effect of N-N'-diphenyl-p-phenylenediamine pretreatment on urinary enzyme excretion in cisplatin nephrotoxicity in rats. Jpn J Pharmacol 1988; 46:90–92.

221. Sugihara K, Gemba M: Modification of cisplatin toxicity by antioxidants. Jpn J Pharmacol 1986; 40:353–355.

222. Jollie DR, Maines MD: Effect of cis-platinum on kidney cytochrome P-450 and heme metabolism: evidence for the regulatory role of the pituitary hormones. Arch Biochem Biophys 1985; 240:51–59.

223. Baliga R, Zhang Z, Baliga M, et al: Role of cytochrome P-450 as a source of catalytic iron in cisplatin-induced nephrotoxicity. Kidney Int 1998; 54:1562–1569.

224. Sleijfer DT, Offerman JJG, Mulder NH, et al: The protective potential of the combination of verapamil and cimetidine on cisplatin-induced nephrotoxicity in man. Cancer 1987; 60:2823–2828.

225. Hannemann J, Baumann K: Cisplatin-induced lipid peroxidation and decrease of gluconeogenesis in rat kidney cortex: different effects of antioxidants and radical scavengers. Toxicology 1988; 51:119–132.

226. Mistry P, Merazga Y, Spargo DJ, et al: The effects of cisplatin on the concentration of protein thiols and glutathione in the rat kidney. Can Chemother Pharmacol 1991; 28:277–282.

227. Sugiyama S, Hayakawa M, Kato T, et al: Adverse effects of antitumor drug, cisplatin, on rat kidney mitochondria: disturbances in glutathione peroxidase activity. Biochem Biophys Res Commun 1989; 159:1121–1127.

228. Babu E, Gopalakrishnan VK, Sriganth NP, et al: Cisplatin-induced nephrotoxicity and the modulating effect of glutathione ester. Mol Cell Biochem 1995; 144:7–11.

229. Anderson ME, Naganuma A, Meister A: Protection against cisplatin toxicity by administration of glutathione ester. FASEB J 1990; 4:3251–3255.

230. Satoh M, Naganuma A, Imura N: Deficiency of selenium intake enhances manifestation of renal toxicity of cis-diamminedichloroplatinum in mice. Toxicol Lett 1987; 38:155–160.

231. Weijl NI, Hopman gD, Wipkink-Bakker A, et al: Cisplatin combination chemotherapy induces a fall in plasma antioxidants of cancer patients. Ann Oncol 1998; 9:1331–1337.

232. Bull JM, Strebel FR, Sunderland BA, et al: o-(beta-Hydroxyethyl)-rutoside–mediated protection of renal injury associated with cis-diamminedichloroplatinum(II)/hyperthermia treatment. Can Res 1988; 48:2239–2244.

233. Gemba M, Fukuishi N: Amelioration by ascorbic acid of cisplatin-induced injury in cultured renal epithelial cells. Contrib Nephrol 1991; 95:138–142.

234. Agarwal A, Balla J, Alam J, et al: Induction of heme oxygenase in toxic renal injury: a protective role in cisplatin nephrotoxicity in the rat. Kidney Int 1995; 48:1298–1307.

235. Srivastava RC, Farookh A, Ahmad N, et al: Evidence for the involvement of nitric oxide in cisplatin-induced toxicity in rats. Biometals 1996; 9:139–142.

236. Tonetti M, Giovine M, Gasparini A, et al: Enhanced formation of reactive species from cis-diammine-(1,1-cyclobutanedicarboxylato)-platinum(II) (carboplatin) in the presence of oxygen free radicals. Biochem Pharmacol 1993; 46:1377–1383.

237. Li Q, Bowner CJ, Yates MS: The protective effect of glycine in cisplatin nephrotoxicity: inhibition with N(G)-nitro-l-arginine methyl ester. J Pharm Pharmacol 1994; 46:346–351.

238. Wink DA, Cook JA, Christodoulou D, et al: Nitric oxide and some nitric oxide donor compounds enhance the cytotoxicity of cisplatin. Nitric Oxide 1997; 1:88–94.

239. Petros A, Lamb G, Leone A, et al: Effects of a nitric oxide synthase inhibitor in humans with septic shock. Cardiovasc Res 1994; 28:34–39.

CHAPTER 5

Heme Oxygenase and Acute Renal Injury

Sharan Kanakiriya ▪ Karl A. Nath

INTRODUCTION

After a lifespan of some 120 days, senescent red blood cells are culled from the circulation and dismantled, and in the course of this degradative pathway, the heme-containing, oxygen-transporting constituent of red blood cells, hemoglobin, undergoes progressive oxidation and denaturation. It was in the course of studies seeking to understand the means for disposing of this heme prosthetic group, released from denatured hemoglobin, that the enzyme heme oxygenase (HO) was discovered.[1] HO facilitates the opening of the heme ring and its conversion to biliverdin; biliverdin is subsequently converted to bilirubin by the cytosolic enzyme biliverdin reductase (Fig. 5–1); the conversion of heme to biliverdin requires oxygen and NADPH and is accompanied by the liberation of iron and the emission of carbon monoxide.[1-4]

For much of the time since this initial discovery, HO was studied largely within the confines of the metabolism and pathophysiology of heme.[1, 2, 3] The prospect that HO may be involved in biological phenomena extending way beyond the parochial concerns of heme metabolism was raised by studies that identified HO as that recondite 32-kDa protein so commonly induced in cells exposed to assorted insults.[5] Recognizing that many of these stimuli were prooxidant in nature, the hypothesis was advanced that increased expression of HO conferred distinct, yet complementary, antioxidant effects in cells so stressed[6] (see later). Evidence in support of this hypothesis and the cytoprotective properties of HO was first derived in a kidney-based model of tissue injury, namely, the glycerol model of acute renal failure (ARF).[7] Subsequently, induction of HO was described in other forms of acute renal injury, including other acute toxic nephropathies,[8, 9] ischemic renal injury,[10] renal inflammation,[11, 12] endotoxin-induced renal injury,[13] and obstruction to the urinary tract[14] (Table 5–1); in several of these models of acute renal injury, induction of HO conferred protective effects.

Three isozymes, each the product of a specific gene, possess HO activity[15–19]: HO-1, HO-2, and HO-3. HO-1 is the inducible isozyme that largely accounts for increased HO activity observed in stressed organs and tissues; HO-1 is arguably one of the most readily inducible genes, responding to an array of stimuli that includes diverse types of oxidative stress, heavy metals, ischemia, irradiation, cytokines, lypopolysaccharide, hypoxia, hyperoxia, nitric oxide, hemodynamic stress, the diabetic milieu, aging, and hyperthermia. HO-2 is the constitutive isozyme and is inducible by corticosteroids; HO-3 resembles HO-2 in some aspects.

Focusing on the involvement of HO-1, this chapter reviews the induction and functional significance of HO in acute renal injury. In instances in which studies in tissues other than the kidney provide added and relevant insights regarding the induction of HO-1 in acutely injured tissue, such studies are also discussed.

CELLULAR METABOLISM OF HEME

The first step in the series of reactions that culminates in the synthesis of heme (iron protoporphyrin IX) involves the synthesis of δ-aminolevulinic acid from glycine and succinyl CoA; the final step in the synthesis of heme involves the insertion of iron in the protoporphyrin ring by the mitochondrial enzyme, ferrochelatase[2, 3, 20] (Fig. 5–2). Heme, so synthesized, has one of two fates: heme is employed as a prosthetic group in diverse proteins—hemoglobin, myoglobin, mitochondrial and microsomal cytochromes, nitric oxide synthase, prostaglandin synthetase, guanylate cyclase, catalase, peroxidases, NADPH oxidase—involved in myriad ways in the sustenance of cellular vitality. Alternatively, heme can undergo degradation by the enzyme HO, with the attendant release of iron, the generation of bile pigments, and the production of carbon monoxide. HO activity is linked to the synthesis of the major iron-storage protein in cells, namely, ferritin,[21, 22] and to a recently described iron-exporting protein.[23] Thus,

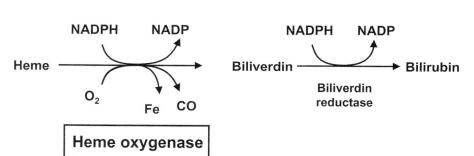

FIGURE 5–1 ▪ The degradation of heme by the enzyme heme oxygenase. (Modified from Nath KA, Agarwal A, Vogt B: Functional consequences of induction of heme oxygenase. In: Goligorsky MS, ed: Contemporary Issues in Nephrology: Acute Renal Failure: Emerging Concepts and Therapeutic Strategies. New York: Churchill Livingstone; 1995: 97; with permission.)

TABLE 5–1. Types of Acute Renal Injury in Which HO-1 Is Induced

Heme protein-induced nephropathy
Assorted toxic nephropathies
Acute ischemia
Acute glomerulonephritides
Acute allograft rejection
Sepsis-related renal insufficiency
Acute obstruction to the urinary tract

iron released from the heme ring, under the facilitatory effect of HO, can be safely stored in the cell or exported to the extracellular compartment, thereby minimizing the risk of iron-mediated oxidative injury.

TOXICITY OF HEME

The heme-degrading action of HO guards against the buildup of cellular levels of heme. Such a function of HO is a critical homeostatic one, because heme, when present in relatively large amounts, can damage cells and their organelles.[4, 6, 7, 24–26] Heme impairs the lipid bilayer in cell membranes, in part, through the peroxidation of membrane lipid; heme can destabilize the attached cytoskeleton and membrane-associated proteins, thereby compromising the structural, transport-related, and other functions of such proteins. The hydrophobic nature of heme allows it to permeate the plasma membrane and to be readily distributed throughout the intracellular compartment via the in-

tracellular canalicular delivery system.[25] In addition to the lipid bilayer and the cytoskeleton, heme could impair the activity of a number of cytosolic enzymes and mitochondrial enzymes; in contrast, heme may activate proteolytic and lysosomal enzymes. DNA is another target that can be oxidatively denatured by heme in vitro. Even relatively small amounts of heme can be potentially injurious if oxidants are concomitantly present. As an example, amounts of heme that are not toxic to cells, when accompanied by nonlytic concentrations of hydrogen peroxide, exert marked cytotoxicity.[26]

That large amounts of heme can be nephrotoxic is supported by substantial literature in disease models[27, 28] and by clinical observations in humans.[29] Heme, the endproduct of porphyrin synthesis, exerts feedback inhibition on porphyrin synthesis by inhibiting the enzyme ALA synthetase.[2, 3] This capacity of heme to suppress porphyrin synthesis is exploited as a stratagem in inducing remissions in acute intermittent porphyria, the latter disease characterized by abnormally increased rates of synthesis of porphyrins.[29] However, when large amounts of heme in the form of hematin are administered to patients with this condition, acute oliguric tubular necrosis develops with markedly pigmented urine, concentrations of blood urea nitrogen approaching 100 mg/dL, and plasma creatinine concentrations exceeding 10 mg/dL, respectively.[29]

The study of the toxicity of heme proteins and heme is facilitated by the glycerol model of ARF[7, 27, 28]: the intramuscular injection of hypertonic glycerol induces myolysis and hemolysis, thereby subjecting the kidney to large amounts of the heme proteins, myoglobin and hemoglobin. Renal damage in this model arises as a consequence of the interdigitation of three main pathways of injury: renal vasoconstriction, direct cytotoxicity, and nephron cast formation.[27, 28] In each of these pathways, heme proteins are pathogenically involved. Heme proteins scavenge nitric oxide, the endogenous vasodilator,[30] while heme proteins, by virtue of their capacity to promote oxidative stress, stimulate the production of such potent vasoconstrictors as 8-isoprostanes.[31, 32] Heme proteins provide large amounts of heme that serve as one source for oxidative stress,[31, 33] the latter contributing to renal injury in this model, as indicated by a substantial body of literature.[28, 31, 33] Additionally, oxidative stress can be sustained by the redox cycling between ferric and ferryl states of iron in the heme prosthetic group of heme proteins.[32] Finally, heme proteins promote the formation of obstructing casts in nephrons.[28]

The cellular basis for renal injury in the glycerol model involves, at least in part, oxidative injury to such organelles as the plasma membrane, nuclear DNA, and the mitochondrion.[28, 31–34] The mitochondrion may be particularly prone to heme-mediated toxicity: the lipid-enriched mitochondrial membranes are readily permeated by heme, a lipophilic substance, while the normal endogenous generation of peroxides by mitochondria may render otherwise innocuous amounts of heme quite toxic to mitochondria.[33] In the glycerol model, the mitochondrial content of heme is increased 10-

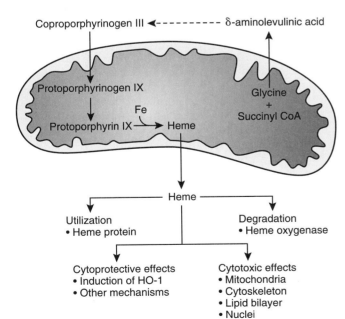

FIGURE 5–2 ■ Overview of synthetic pathways for heme, the fate of heme so synthesized, and the cytotoxic and cytoprotective effects of heme. (Modified from Stocker R: Induction of heme oxygenase as a defense against oxidative stress. Free Rad Res Comms 1990; 9:101, and Abraham NG, Drummond GS, Lutton JD, et al: The biological significance and physiological role of heme oxygenase. Cell Physiol Biochem 1996; 6:129; with permission.)

fold three hours after the administration of glycerol and is accompanied by oxidative stress as indicated by increased lipid peroxidation.[33] Even at this early time point, alterations in mitochondrial function are observed and are characterized by diminished state 3 respiration and uncoupled respirations, when respiration is sustained by either glutamate/malate or succinate/rotenone; mitochondrial respiration is further depressed by 24 hours. These abnormalities in mitochondrial function are accompanied by ultrastructural evidence of mitochondrial injury.[33] Increased amounts of heme present in mitochondria may contribute to such mitochondrial dysfunction as indicated by studies in which mitochondria, harvested from rats with disease-free kidneys, are exposed to heme concentrations that reproduce the levels observed in the myohemoglobinuric model. Such exposure to heme significantly altered oxygen consumption: mitochondria initially displayed increased respiration that gave way to a persistent decline in oxygen consumption until oxygen was no longer consumed; the early stimulation and the subsequent decline in the utilization of oxygen by mitochondria, induced by heme, occurred through iron-dependent and iron-independent processes, respectively; higher concentrations of heme hastened the decline in mitochondrial respiration.[33] Heme is also a potent stimulus for cellular generation of hydrogen peroxide,[31] and such generation of oxidants may contribute to the injurious effects of heme on the plasma membrane, cytoskeleton, mitochondria, and DNA.[28, 31, 33, 34]

The toxic effects of heme in mitochondria and other organelles when heme is present in relatively large amounts contrast with the cytoprotective effects of heme when present in lower amounts; indeed, the exposure of cells in culture to heme in generally smaller quantities, and under certain conditions, can mitigate the severity of necrosis and apoptosis provoked by a number of stimuli (see later). Heme thus represents a study in contrasts: as a prosthetic group, heme indispensably contributes to the functionality of the specific heme proteins, and yet when freed from its protein moiety heme, in copious amounts, may be decidedly toxic; heme, present in lower amounts, and in the appropriate setting, can exert potent protective effects, the latter channeled through the induction of HO-1, and possibly other cellular actions (see Fig. 5–2).

INDUCTION OF HO-1 AS A PROTECTIVE RESPONSE IN ACUTE HEME PROTEIN-MEDIATED RENAL INJURY

The identification of HO-1 as the 32-kDa protein ubiquitously expressed in cells exposed to various stressors led to the thesis that such induction of HO-1 exerted an antioxidant response that enables cells to resist the injurious effect of these stressors.[5, 6] Because many of these stressors that induce HO-1 are prooxidant, it was suggested that the induction of HO-1 in these circumstances provided a protective antioxidant response.[6] Such benefits of induced HO-1 would arise from two complementary actions: on the one hand, HO activity removes heme, a prooxidant that would appear in increasing amounts because of scission of destabilized intracellular heme proteins in oxidant-stressed cells; concomitantly, increased HO activity would generate bilirubin, a metabolite recognized for its potent antioxidant effects.[35–37] In essence, this thesis posited that HO activity would replace a prooxidant (heme) with an antioxidant (bilirubin).

To test the hypothesis that induction of HO-1 occurs in settings in which tissues such as the kidney are exposed to oxidant stress and to examine the functional significance of such induction of HO-1, studies were undertaken in the glycerol model of acute heme protein-induced nephrotoxicity.[7] In view of the presence of oxidant stress in general and the presence of large amounts of heme in the kidney in particular, it was reasoned that the kidney would draw upon HO-1 so as to degrade heme and mitigate the oxidative stress imposed in this state.[7]

In these studies, expression of HO-1 mRNA was observed as early as three hours after the administration of glycerol; intense up-regulation of this gene was observed at six hours.[7] Such expression of HO-1 mRNA was accompanied by a robust increase in enzyme activity as measured either by the generation of bilirubin in microsomal fractions of the kidney or the production of carbon monoxide by cortical slices. That the induction of HO-1 was not a nonspecific antioxidant response was demonstrated by the absence of up-regulation in other antioxidant enzymes, such as catalase and glutathione peroxidase. The functional contribution of the induction of HO-1 was examined in two approaches.[7] The first utilized the competitive inhibitor of HO, tin protoporphyrin. The administration of tin protoporphyrin significantly worsened renal insufficiency in the glycerol model such that on five sequential days the serum creatinine was significantly higher in rats so treated compared with rats similarly treated with glycerol but in which vehicle was administered.[7] However, tin protoporphyrin did not affect serum creatinine in rats with intact, disease-free kidneys. Thus, the inhibition of HO with a competitive inhibitor worsens the course of acute renal insufficiency, thereby indicating that the induction of HO-1 was protective in this disease model.[7]

In a complementary approach, it has been reasoned that if HO-1 subserved a protective role in this disease model, then the prior induction of HO-1 in the kidney would reduce renal injury that ensued after the administration of glycerol.[7] To induce HO-1, small, nontoxic doses of hemoglobin were administered some 18 hours prior to the administration of hypertonic glycerol. Rats so treated, as compared to vehicle-treated rats, were markedly protected against renal insufficiency induced by hypertonic glycerol. In this protocol, a dose of glycerol (10 mL/kg body weight) was used, which was associated with fulminant ARF and 100% mortality in vehicle-pretreated rats. In contrast, rats pretreated with hemoglobin exhibited mild and reversible renal insufficiency and markedly improved survival (14% mortality) following the administration of glycerol.[7]

This potent protective effect of induced HO-1 in the glycerol model is observed even when HO-1 is induced by stimuli that are intrinsically injurious.[12, 13] For example, the prior administration of endotoxin protects against glycerol-induced ARF.[13] Such protection conferred by endotoxin is associated with induction of HO-1, and is lost when HO is concomitantly inhibited.[13] Similarly, the administration of nephrotoxic serum nephritis is a potent inducer of HO-1 in renal tubules and confers a protective effect that is lost when such HO activity is inhibited with tin protoporphyrin.[12] Such examples demonstrate the acquisition of resistance to ARF originating from induced HO-1.[12, 13]

The availability of genetically engineered mice in which there is homozygous deletion of HO-1 provided another approach by which to assess injury induced by heme proteins and heme in general, and the role of HO-1, in particular, in protecting against such renal injury.[38, 39] In this model, the administration of hypertonic glycerol was associated with mild acute reversible renal insufficiency in the wild-type mouse (HO-1 +/+) without any mortality.[39] In contrast, HO-1 −/− mice subjected to the same dose of glycerol, exhibited acute fulminant renal insufficiency and extensive tubular necrosis.[39] Notably, the cumulative mortality from renal failure and other organ dysfunction in HO-1 −/− mice subjected to the glycerol model was 100% compared with 0% in similarly treated HO-1 +/+ mice. In these studies, the absence of expression of HO-1 mRNA or HO-1 protein in HO-1 −/− mice was confirmed in the basal state and following the administration of glycerol; in contrast, HO-1 +/+ mice subjected to the glycerol model exhibited striking expression of HO-1 mRNA and protein, the latter localized, by immunoperoxidase studies, to the proximal and distal tubules in the kidney.[39] In response to glycerol-induced ARF, HO-1 −/− mice demonstrated a pronounced inability to degrade heme as reflected by an eightfold greater increment in heme content in the kidney compared with HO-1 +/+ mice; exacerbation of acute renal insufficiency and markedly increased mortality in the HO-1 deficiency state was thus associated with a rapid accumulation of heme in the kidney.[39]

In the glycerol model, heme proteins represent the major, but not the only, renal insult. To determine whether HO-1 −/− mice were uniquely sensitive to a specific heme protein, the renal effect of single heme protein, hemoglobin, was examined in HO-1 +/+ and HO-1 −/− mice.[39] Such administration of hemoglobin to HO-1 −/− mice led to ARF with marked and rapid rise in serum creatinine and extensive tubular necrosis and cast formation; HO-1 +/+ mice administered a similar dose of mouse hemoglobin demonstrated no rise in serum creatinine and essentially normal kidney structure.[39] Thus, in addition to exquisite sensitivity to heme protein-induced ARF, as imposed by the glycerol model, the HO-1 deficiency state renders the kidney uniquely sensitive to a specific

heme protein.[39] Studies in vitro support the importance of HO-1 in protecting cells against the toxic effects of heme and hemoglobin. For example, transfection of the human HO-1 gene into rabbit coronary microvessel endothelial cells confers remarkable resistance to cell injury induced by heme and hemoglobin.[40]

Induced HO-1 exerts protective actions, in part, by restraining the rise in renal heme content that would otherwise occur. Other possible mechanisms for the protective effects of HO-1 include the fostering of the synthesis of ferritin, the generation of bilirubin, and the production of carbon monoxide.[16–18] Ferritin is the dominant endogenous intracellular storage site for iron, with one molecule of ferritin binding 4500 atoms of iron.[22] The exposure of fibroblasts or endothelial cells to heme induces HO-1 and stimulates the synthesis of ferritin, the latter occurring as a consequence of the release of iron from the heme ring[21, 22]; such increments in cytosolic iron act at a post-transcriptional level to increase the synthesis of ferritin.[21, 22] That increased ferritin synthesis correlated with the protective effects of HO-1 is demonstrated in the glycerol model, where increased ferritin content is associated with the induction of HO-1[7]: maneuvers such as the prior induction of HO-1 by hemoglobin (which is protective) are associated with increased ferritin synthesis, whereas the inhibition of HO activity (which exacerbates injury in this model) is associated with diminished ferritin content.[7] Thus, the induction of ferritin may be one of the mechanisms through which the expression of HO-1 protects against heme protein-induced toxicity. Direct evidence for such protective effects was provided in a model of cytotoxicity in which cells were loaded with heme and then exposed to hydrogen peroxide.[22] In such circumstances, the prior loading of these cells with ferritin protected against injury induced by heme and hydrogen peroxide. Such protection arose from the chelation of intracellular iron and the capacity of the ferritin H-chain to exhibit ferroxidase activity, the latter serving to interrupt the redox cycling of iron.[22]

Heme proteins not only may induce ARF but also, if repetitively administered, can elicit inflammatory responses in the kidney.[41, 42] Such repetitive insults interrupt the reparative processes that facilitate recovery from acute tubular necrosis; repetitive insults expose and amplify inflammatory processes that are instigated by any acute ischemic or nephrotoxic insult. A triphasic response evolves in the kidney subjected to repetitive exposure to heme proteins: initially, sensitivity is manifested in the kidney as a result of the first insult; resistance is then acquired to second and subsequent insults; finally, a third component is provided by a progressive inflammatory response.[41, 42] The role of HO-1 in these phases has been explored in HO-1 −/− mice. When HO-1 −/− and HO-1 +/+ mice are repetitively injected at weekly intervals with hemoglobin, HO-1 −/− mice demonstrate heightened initial sensitivity, as reflected by a marked rise in serum creatinine, following the first and second injections of hemoglobin; thereafter, HO-1 −/− mice as well as the HO-1 +/+ mice acquire resistance to renal injury, at least as measured by serum creatinine levels.[42] However, the inflammatory responses that ensue following such repetitive exposure to hemoglobin is markedly amplified in the HO-1 −/− mice compared with such responses in the HO-1 +/+ mice: HO-1 −/− mice exhibit marked tubulointerstitial injury and cellular infiltration, accompanied by up-regulation of the transcription factor NF-κB, and chemokines such as MCP-1.[42] Thus, inflammatory responses that are instigated by such acute renal insults as heme proteins can be governed by HO-1: in the absence of expression of HO-1, cellular infiltration and the underlying driving processes, such as proinflammatory chemokines and transcription factors, are markedly enhanced.[42] That HO-1 may down-regulate inflammatory responses is especially relevant to ARF since it is now increasingly appreciated that inflammatory processes significantly contribute to the pathogenesis of ischemic and nephrotoxic acute tubular necrosis.

CISPLATIN NEPHROPATHY

Cisplatin nephropathy is another model of toxic nephropathy wherein there is persuasive evidence attesting to the involvement of oxidative stress in the pathogenesis of renal injury.[27] After initial studies in the glycerol-model of ARF,[7] subsequent studies were undertaken in cisplatin-induced renal injury to determine whether acute toxic renal injury, imposed by insults other than heme proteins, would also recruit HO-1 as a protective response.[8] The administration of cisplatin elicited a time-dependent induction of HO-1 mRNA accompanied by increased expression of HO-1 protein and enzyme activity. Inhibition of HO worsened the course of renal injury as evidenced by a higher serum creatinine from the third day onward after the administration of cisplatin; this exacerbation of renal function induced by inhibition of HO was accompanied by worsened structural injury, the latter reflected by a greater volume density of necrotic tubules and tubular casts.[8] Moreover, renal hemodynamic studies demonstrated that such inhibition of HO activity led to greater reductions in renal blood flow as a consequence of increased renal vascular resistances; these findings point to a vasodilatory effect of induced HO-1 in this model.[8] Interestingly, in this disease model, heme content was increased in whole kidney homogenates as well as various cellular fractions, thereby raising the possibility that the inhibition of HO worsened tissue injury, at least in part, through the further elevation in renal heme content.[8] Such elevations in heme, incurred by inhibiting HO, may also be linked to these hemodynamic alterations. Heme, for example, may bind nitric oxide, thereby removing an endogenous vasodilator. Additionally, the inhibition of HO may deprive the kidney of carbon monoxide, the latter serving to offset the hemodynamic actions of vasoconstrictive agonists (see later). An additional mechanism accounting for the protective effects of induced HO-1 in cisplatin nephropathy may relate to increased ferritin content observed in the kidney in this model.[8]

That the induction of HO is a protective response in cisplatin nephropathy is supported by studies undertaken in HO-1 −/− mice.[43] HO-1 −/− mice, when compared with similarly treated HO-1 +/+ mice, exhibit greater deterioration in renal function and more severe histologic injury and apoptosis in the kidneys when subjected to cisplatin nephropathy.[43] In complementary studies conducted in vitro, induction of HO-1 by hemin in human renal tubular epithelial cells rendered these cells resistant to cisplatin-induced apoptosis and necrosis; such protective effects of hemin were attenuated when HO activity was inhibited.[43] Additionally, overexpression of HO-1 by transfection of these cells with human HO-1 also reduced cisplatin-induced cell injury, the latter assessed morphologically and by the LDH release assay; moreover, in these studies overexpression of HO-1 protected mitochondria in cisplatin-exposed cells, mitochondria representing organelles that are prone to the damaging effect of cisplatin.[43]

The mechanism by which HO-1 protects against apoptosis in cisplatin-induced cell injury and other models of apoptosis is very much one of conjecture. It is possible that increased expression of HO-1 may block a key signal in the mediation of the apoptotic cascade, namely, cytochrome c–dependent activation of caspases.[44] Cytochrome c is a heme-containing protein, and its emission from mitochondria into the cytosol triggers more distal apoptotic events, such as the activation of caspases; this action of cytochrome c requires the integrity of its heme prosthetic group. It is possible that up-regulation of HO-1 may impair the heme moiety of cytochrome c; additionally, carbon monoxide, released in increased amounts because of increased HO activity, may impair the heme prosthetic group in cytochrome c, and thus the capacity of cytochrome c to activate subsequent events in apoptosis.

ANTI-APOPTOTIC EFFECTS OF HO-1

Studies in nonrenal cells have also corroborated the anti-apoptotic effect of induced HO-1,[45–47] and provide insights concerning this action of HO-1. For example, in murine lung fibroblasts, conditional overexpression of HO-1 prevents apoptosis induced by tumor necrosis factor-α (TNF-α), an effect reversed by inhibiting HO activity.[45] Tumor necrosis factor-α−induced apoptosis in these cells can also be reduced by exposure to low concentrations of carbon monoxide. Interestingly, carbon monoxide can activate the enzyme, guanylate cyclase, and inhibition of guanylate cyclase reverses the protective effect of overexpression of HO-1 against TNF-α−induced apoptosis in these cells.[45] In aggregate, these findings raise the possibility that the anti-apoptotic effects of HO-1 may reside in carbon monoxide–induced activation of guanylate cyclase. Studies undertaken in vivo also demonstrate the anti-apoptotic effects of a low concentration of carbon monoxide in injured tissue.[46] For example, low concentrations of carbon monoxide reduce inflammatory changes in the lungs and reduce mortality in rats exposed to hyperoxia; such protective effects of carbon monoxide also include the marked reduction in apoptosis in the lungs of hyperoxia-exposed rats.[46]

Tumor necrosis factor-α−induced apoptosis in endothelial cells is also attenuated by induction of HO-1, the latter achieved either by hemin or transfection with HO-1[47]; these protective effects afforded by induction of HO-1 are blocked by inhibiting HO. When HO activity is inhibited in endothelial cells exposed to TNF-α, the concomitant presence of low concentrations of carbon monoxide can restore the resistance to apoptosis. These findings suggest that carbon monoxide may be at least one mechanism through which HO-1 may exert its anti-apoptotic action.[47] These anti-apoptotic effects of HO-1 and carbon monoxide in endothelial cells may involve activation of the p38 MAPK signaling pathways.[47] p38 MAP kinase is induced in endothelial cells exposed to TNF-α, and such activation can be augmented by induction of HO-1 or exposure to carbon monoxide; inhibition of p38 MAP kinase by a pharmacologic approach or by a dominant negative mutant approach prevents the anti-apoptotic effects of HO-1.[47] These observations demonstrate that carbon monoxide may underlie, at least in part, anti-apoptotic effects of induced HO-1 in endothelial cells, and such effects may involve activation of p38 MAP kinase.

Another mechanism by which HO-1 may be anti-apoptotic involves the capacity of induced HO-1 to facilitate the extracellular transport of iron, and thereby minimize the likelihood of iron-driven oxidant stress occurring in the intracellular compartment.[48] For example, apoptosis, induced by different stimuli, is attenuated in cells that overexpress HO-1; in contrast, apoptosis, so induced, is increased in cells with targeted deletion of the HO-1 gene.[48] Assessment of the export of iron from the intracellular compartment in these studies indicates that such export is facilitated to the extent that cells express HO-1; conversely, such export is impaired in cells that are unable to express HO-1. Moreover, in these studies, the propensity towards apoptosis reflects the availability of redox-active iron in the intracellular compartment.[48] These findings led to the conclusion that induced HO-1 facilitates the extracellular transport of iron and thus restrains the elevation in intracellular iron that would otherwise occur; such effects, in turn, reduce the risk of apoptosis that is driven by iron-catalyzed oxidative stress and other iron-dependent pathways.[48]

GENTAMICIN-INDUCED AND MERCURIC CHLORIDE−INDUCED NEPHROPATHY

Heme oxygenase-1 is also induced in other models of acute toxic nephropathy besides cisplatin-induced nephropathy.[8, 9] Gentamicin imposes renal oxidative stress, and gentamicin-induced renal injury is reduced by antioxidants, including iron chelators.[27] Heme oxygenase-1 is significantly induced in this disease model[8];

however, the administration of tin protoporphyrin does not exacerbate renal injury, at least as measured by serum creatinine.[8] Mercuric chloride is another model of ARF that is characterized by precipitous oxidative stress and is accompanied by marked induction of HO-1.[9] When relatively larger amounts of mercuric chloride are used to induce acute renal insufficiency, neither the inhibition of HO nor the prior induction of HO-1 influence renal function.[9] With less severe mercuric chloride−induced renal insufficiency, the prior administration of hemin reduces renal dysfunction[49]; whether this amelioration in renal function specifically reflects the protective effects of induced HO-1 has not been determined at this time.[49]

ACUTE ISCHEMIC RENAL INJURY

HO-1 mRNA and HO activity are induced in the kidney in the clamp model of renal ischemia, as demonstrated in studies undertaken six hours after the release of the clamp,[10, 50] but not in studies undertaken one hour after such ischemic stress.[51] Increased microsomal heme content, as documented in these studies,[10] may contribute to such induction of HO-1. Up-regulation of HO-1 may be functionally significant as observed in some models of ischemic renal injury but not in others.[52] For example, uninephrectomy and ischemic clamping to the remaining kidney one hour after the administration of the inhibitor of heme oxygenase activity, tin mesoprotoporphyrin, were accompanied by worsening of renal function, as evaluated by serum creatinine concentration, in conjunction with exacerbation of tubular epithelial cell injury[52]; such worsening of renal function, structurally and functionally, was also associated with increased microsomal heme content.[52] However, in another model of renal ischemia, the administration of tin protoporphyrin did not affect renal function as evaluated by serum creatinine on sequential days after ischemia.[8] The reasons for these discrepancies in the findings are unclear but may relate to the method of ischemia and the timing of administration of the inhibitor of HO.

Experimental manipulations that induce HO-1 may exert protective effects in ischemic renal injury. For example, the spin trapping agent, N-t-butyl-α-phenylnitrone, massively up-regulates HO-1 when administered before ischemic acute renal injury and reduces lipid peroxidation and deposition of iron that are commonly seen in the medullary rays in the ischemic kidneys.[53] These findings suggest that oxidative stress, at least as reflected by lipid peroxidation and the deposition of iron, imposed by ischemic insults, may be reduced by agents that upregulate among other actions, the expression of HO-1 in the kidney.[53]

Such protection afforded by prior up-regulation of HO-1 may arise not only from direct cytoprotective actions but also from the hemodynamic actions of HO-1. In several vascular beds, a vasodilatory effect of HO-1 and its product, carbon monoxide, is observed.[54–57] This vasorelaxant effect may involve any one or combination of effects: the stimulation of guanylate cyclase, cellular release of preformed nitric oxide, stimulation of potassium channel activity, inhibition of the cytochrome P-450 system, and inhibition of synthesis or expression of vasoconstrictors such as 19-HETE and 20-HETE compounds, endothelin, and PDGF.[54–60] Interestingly, both HO-1 and HO-2 are expressed in the intact kidney, the bulk of such expression occurring in the renal inner medulla with relatively small amounts in the renal cortex[61]: HO-1 mRNA is increased approximately fourfold and threefold in the inner and outer medulla, respectively, when compared with that in the cortex; HO-2 mRNA is also increased in the outer and inner medulla when compared with that in the cortex, albeit to a lesser extent compared with such increments observed with HO-1 mRNA.[61] Inhibition of HO activity in the intact, disease-free kidney reduces medullary blood flow without exerting any effect on cortical blood flow.[61] It is possible that the up-regulation of HO-1 in the ischemic kidney may confer vasodilatory actions that assist in preserving whatever perfusion remains—globally or regionally—in the kidney subjected to ischemia.

Another relevant consideration regarding the induction of HO-1 in ischemic renal injury is the possible interaction between the nitric oxide synthase and HO-1 systems.[62, 63] Inducible nitric oxide synthase (iNOS) is induced in the ischemic kidney, and such availability of iNOS and the attendant generation of large amounts of nitric oxide are incriminated in the pathogenesis of ischemic renal injury.[64, 65] Interestingly, the generation of copious quantities of nitric oxide, as can be achieved by nitric oxide donors, leads to the up-regulation of HO-1.[62, 63] For example, robust induction of HO-1 occurs in renal proximal tubular epithelial cells exposed to the nitric oxide donor, sodium nitroprusside.[63] Such induction of HO-1 is dependent upon alterations in cellular redox: antioxidants such as thiol donors and iron chelators can markedly suppress this up-regulation of HO-1.[63] It is possible that the up-regulated iNOS system may contribute to the induction of HO-1 in the ischemic kidney, and such expression of HO-1 may guard against the injurious effects of large amounts of nitric oxide.

ACUTE INFLAMMATORY NEPHROPATHIES

Up-regulation of HO-1 occurs in models of inflammation in the kidney[11, 12, 66, 67] and other organs.[68–70] A seminal demonstration of the potent anti-inflammatory effects of such up-regulation of HO-1 was provided in a model of acute pleurisy in the rat.[68] Infiltrating leukocytes in this model expressed HO-1, and the inhibition of such HO activity amplified the inflammatory response; conversely, the prior induction of HO-1 by hemin reduced the extent of tissue injury and inflammation.[68] An analogous approach in assessing functionality of HO-1 was subsequently employed in the model of nephrotoxic serum nephritis in the rat,[66] one which resembles antiglomerular basement membrane nephritis. In the heterologous and accelerated forms of this model, there is up-regulation of HO-1 in glomerular macrophages and in renal tubular epithelial cells.[12, 66] The prior induction of HO-1 in rats by the administration of hemin reduced rates of urinary protein excretion in heterologous nephrotoxic serum nephritis and interrupted the infiltration of neutrophils and macrophages in the glomerulus. In addition, in the accelerated form of nephrotoxic serum nephritis, prior treatment with hemin reduced urinary protein excretion, macrophage influx in glomeruli, and the number of microthrombi in the glomerular microcirculation.[66] Subsequent studies in this model have suggested that this protective effect of hemin may involve HO-1–mediated reduction in glomerular expression of iNOS.[67] Nephrotoxic serum nephritis is characterized by co-expression of HO-1 and iNOS, and iNOS is considered a mediator of glomerular injury in this model. The prior induction of HO-1 by hemin in this model leads to a reduction in glomerular expression of iNOS mRNA and decreased NOS activity.[67] Additionally, the expression of iNOS protein and enzyme activity in mesangial cells in response to cytokines is significantly reduced when these mesangial cells are exposed to hemin. These findings led to the conclusion that the protective effect of induction of HO-1 in nephrotoxic serum nephritis may arise from a suppressive effect on the expression of iNOS and iNOS-mediated injury in this model.[67]

Induction of HO-1 occurs in models of tubulointerstitial inflammation. For example, a model of acute tubulointerstitial allograft rejection in the rat is provided by transplanting the kidney from the Brown Norway strain to a Lewis strain. In this model, there is marked expression of HO-1 mRNA and HO-1 protein five days after transplantation of the allograft, and this expression of HO-1 occurs in conjunction with iNOS expression in infiltrating interstitial macrophages.[11] Another model of tubulointerstitial inflammation is provided by ureteral obstruction. This model is associated with prompt inflammatory responses and the occurrence of oxidative stress in the kidney. For example, the marker of oxidative stress, N-carboxymethyl-lysine, is prominently increased in the interstitium of obstructed kidneys. HO-1 mRNA is significantly induced within 12 hours after ureteral obstruction and seems to arise from the peritubular and periglomerular interstitial cells.[14] The functional significance regarding the expression of HO-1 in the kidney following acute obstruction and acute allograft rejection is currently known.

The study of inflammation in other organs and tissues besides the kidney has contributed substantial insights pertaining to the anti-inflammatory actions of HO-1.[69–72] The anti-inflammatory properties of HO-1 are particularly revealing in a model of acute xenotransplant rejection occurring in mouse hearts transplanted into rats.[69] Such rejection can be prevented by the administration of cyclosporin and depletion of complement by cobra venom factor; the efficacy of this pharmacologic manipulation in preventing rejection is critically dependent upon the observed expression of HO-1 that occurs in the endothelium and smooth muscle cells of these xenotransplanted organs.[69] For example, when hearts from HO-1 $-/-$ or HO-1 $+/+$ mice are transplanted into rats treated with cyclosporin and cobra venom factor, the rejection of these hearts from HO-1 $-/-$ mice is markedly increased, and survival is limited to no more than a few days; in contrast, the survival of such xenografts from HO-1 $+/+$ mice is indefinite. The absence of HO-1 in the donor heart is associated with vascular thrombosis in coronary arteries, marked influx of polymorphonuclear leukocytes, monocytes, and macrophages, and prominent apoptosis involving endothelial cells and cardiac myocytes.[69] In another model of inflammation, namely, antibody-induced transplant arteriosclerosis in mouse cardiac allografts, long-term survival and prevention of vascular rejection were effected by the administration of a monoclonal antibody to CD40-ligand and donor cells. Analyses of this phenomenon implicated the up-regulation of HO-1 as a significant mechanism underlying this protection against vascular injury and inflammation[70]; complementary in vitro analyses demonstrated that the induction of HO-1 in endothelial cells markedly attenuated alloantibody-stimulated endothelial activation, the latter assessed by the expression of E-selectin.[70]

Carbon monoxide and bilirubin are two of the products of HO-1 through which HO-1 may exert its anti-inflammatory effects.[71, 72] In analyses of endotoxin-induced inflammation, conducted in vivo and in vitro, carbon monoxide, at relatively low concentrations, attenuated the expression of proinflammatory cytokines such as TNF-α, interleukin-1β, and macrophage inhibitory protein-1β; in contrast, in this model of inflammation, such concentrations of carbon monoxide stimulated expression of interleukin-10, a cytokine that suppresses inflammatory responses.[71] While unable to incriminate nitric oxide or cGMP as the basis for these anti-inflammatory actions of carbon monoxide, these studies uncovered a novel and important effect: these actions of carbon monoxide involved the MAP kinase pathway, specifically, the activation of p38 MAP kinase through mitogen-activated protein kinase kinase 3 (MKK3).[71] In other models of inflammation, carbon monoxide contributes to the anti-inflammatory effects of HO-1, in part, through the suppressive effect of carbon monoxide on proinflammatory cytokines such as endothelin and PDGF.[59] Bilirubin can also contribute to the anti-inflammatory effects of HO-1.[72] For example, studies in mesenteric vessels demonstrate that oxidants such as hydrogen peroxide can induce rolling and adhesion of leukocytes; the prior induction of HO-1 by hemin down-regulates such adhesion, and this anti-inflammatory action of hemin is reversed by inhibition of HO; importantly, bilirubin or biliverdin, in micromolar concentrations, restores the anti-inflammatory actions that are otherwise ablated by inhibition of induced HO activity.[72]

ENDOTOXIN-INDUCED RENAL INJURY

The capacity of HO-1 to down-regulate the inflammatory response and protect against tissue injury is demonstrated in studies of endotoxin-induced injury.[73, 74] Indeed, renal dysfunction and endotoxemia-induced mortality in rats can be reduced by prior induction of HO-1 by hemoglobin[73]; furthermore, HO-1 $-/-$ mice exhibit marked tissue injury and heightened mortality in response to endotoxin.[74] The proinflammatory effects of endotoxin in the kidney, such as the up-regulation of P-selectin and E-selectin, are attenuated when HO is induced by prior treatment with hemin; in contrast, up-regulation of these selectins by endotoxin is amplified when HO activity is inhibited.[75] In these latter studies, the inhibitory effects of HO-1 on the expression of selectins may be mediated through biliverdin or bilirubin since biliverdin was as potent as hemin in suppressing expression of selectins in the kidney following the administration of endotoxin.

ADVERSE EFFECTS OF INDUCED HO-1

While induced HO-1 exerts potent cytoprotective effects in numerous types of acute oxidative and other forms of acute tissue injury, in certain circumstances marked induction of HO-1 fails to protect against oxidative insults.[76] Presumably, in such settings, HO-1 and its products are incapable of safeguarding the specific and critical cellular targets that are injured.[76] Additionally, it is possible that the injurious effects of induced HO-1 may counterbalance or outweigh the protective actions of HO-1. Indeed, in a given setting and in sufficient amounts, the products of induced HO-1—iron, bile pigments, carbon monoxide—can all be harmful.[16] For example, in studies that examined renal proximal tubules harvested from rats subjected to the glycerol model, the inhibition of HO in vitro reduced damage to renal proximal tubules, the latter assessed by the release of LDH[77]; in BSC-1 cells (a renal tubular epithelial cell line), hydrogen peroxide or hemin induces HO-1, and the inhibition of HO improves cellular viability when these cells are exposed to either of these oxidants.[78] An explanation for these adverse effects associated with induction of HO-1 may be found in studies in hamster fibroblasts that were stably transfected with tetracycline-regulatable, rat HO-1 cDNA construct; such transfection afforded HO activity that was increased from 3-fold to 17-fold.[79] Relatively high expression of HO-1 exacerbated oxygen toxicity while lower levels of HO-1 expression reduced oxygen toxicity in these cells.[79] These observations, in conjunction with measurements of heme and nonheme iron, led to the conclusion that beneficial effects of induced HO-1 resided in the degradation of heme; however, such protective effects may be nullified or overwhelmed by the oxidant effects of increasing amounts of iron liberated from the heme, as HO activity progressively increases. If the magnitude of induction of HO-1 does not adequately entrain secondary processes that can safely sequester iron in ferritin or efficiently export iron into the extracellular compartment, or provide some other cytoprotective effect, then iron released from heme may be available in the intracellular compartment in sufficient amounts to stimulate oxidative stress and other pathways of iron-mediated cellular injury. Thus, there may be a range in which the induction of HO-1 is cytoprotective; beyond this range induction of HO-1 may not necessarily be protective and, indeed, may be harmful.

CONCLUSIONS

The recognized biologic actions of HO-1 and its products—actions that affect cellular vitality and its determinants, cell growth and proliferation, inflammation and immune processes, tissue repair, and the regulation of various hemodynamic, homeostatic, and vascular systems—have engendered considerable interest in the induction of HO-1 in acute tissue injury. As outlined, induction of HO-1 occurs in various forms of acute renal insults, and in some of these instances, cytoprotective effects are conferred by HO-1. The biologic actions of HO-1 that appear particularly relevant to acute renal injury are summarized in Table 5–2. While such actions, for the most part, may reduce renal injury, the possibility that induced HO-1 may not be protective needs to be borne in mind; additionally, the effect of HO-1 in retarding cell proliferation, as described in pulmonary epithelial cells[80] and, if applicable to renal epithelial cells, may not necessarily be beneficial in the recovery phase of acute tubular necrosis.

The findings and conclusions regarding the functional significance of HO-1 in acute renal injury, as drawn from relevant disease models, are likely applicable to human renal disease: HO-1 is induced in the human kidney injured by acute insults,[81] and the deficiency of HO-1 in humans leads to kidney disease.[82] The reduction in acute renal injury following the induction of HO-1, the latter achieved by pharmacologic or genetic approaches, raises the possibility that augmenting the expression of HO-1 may offer a therapeutic strategy in acute renal injury; one such approach may involve gene delivery as evidenced by augmentation in HO activity and attendant functional effects in the kidney in rats infused with an adenoviral vector-mediated transfer of human HO-1.[83] Preservation of donor kidneys prior to transplantation represents another avenue in which augmentation in HO may be therapeutically employed.[17] Finally, as is increasingly recognized, the function of the intact, disease-free kidney is influenced by endogenous HO activity[61, 84]; greater understanding of such involvement of HO-1 in physiologic states, in turn, would facilitate attempts to augment and exploit renal expression of HO-1 in the prevention or reduction of acute renal injury.

TABLE 5–2. Actions of HO-1 and Its Products Relevant to Acute Renal Injury

Vasodilatory effects
Cytoprotectant effects
Anti-inflammatory actions
Anti-apoptotic effects
Effects on cell proliferation and cell growth

REFERENCES

1. Tenhunen R, Marver HS, Schmid R: The enzymatic conversion of heme to bilirubin by microsomal heme oxygenase. Proc Natl Acad Sci, USA 1968; 61:748.
2. Maines MD: Heme oxygenase: function, multiplicity, regulatory mechanisms, and clinical applications. FASEB J 1988; 2:2557.
3. Abraham NG, Lin JH-C, Schwartzman ML, et al.: The physiological significance of heme oxygenase. Int J Biochem 1988; 20:543.
4. Nath KA, Agarwal A, Vogt B: Functional consequences of induction of heme oxygenase. In: Goligorsky MS, ed: Contemporary Issues in Nephrology: Acute Renal Failure: Emerging Concepts and Therapeutic Strategies. New York: Churchill Livingstone; 1995:97.
5. Keyse SM, Tyrrell RM: Heme oxygenase is the major 32-kDa stress protein induced in human skin fibroblasts by UVA radiation, hydrogen peroxide and sodium arsenite. Proc Natl Acad Sci, USA 1989; 86:99.
6. Stocker R: Induction of haem oxygenase as a defence against oxidative stress. Free Rad Res Comms 1990; 9:101.
7. Nath KA, Balla G, Vercellotti GM, et al: Induction of heme oxygenase is a rapid, protective response in rhabdomyolysis in the rat. J Clin Invest 1992; 90:267.
8. Agarwal A, Balla J, Alam J, et al: Induction of heme oxygenase in toxic renal injury: a protective role in cisplatin nephrotoxicity in the rat. Kidney Int 1995; 48:1298.
9. Nath KA, Croatt AJ, Likely S, et al: Renal oxidant injury and oxidant response induced by mercury. Kidney Int 1996; 50:1032.
10. Maines MD, Mayer RD, Ewing JF, et al: Induction of kidney heme oxygenase-1 (HSP32) mRNA and protein by ischemia/reperfusion: possible role of heme as both promoter of tissue damage and regulator of HSP32. J Pharmacol Exp Therap 1993; 264:457.
11. Agarwal A, Kim Y, Matas AJ, et al: Gas-generating systems in acute renal allograft rejection in the rat: co-induction of heme oxygenase and nitric oxide synthase. Transplantation 1996; 61:93.
12. Vogt BA, Shanley TP, Croatt AJ, et al: Glomerular inflammation induces resistance to tubular injury in the rat: a novel form of acquired heme oxygenase-dependent resistance to renal injury. J Clin Invest 1996; 98:2139.
13. Vogt BA, Alam J, Croatt AJ, et al: Acquired resistance to acute oxidative stress: possible role of heme oxygenase and ferritin. Lab Invest 1995; 72:474.
14. Kawada N, Moriyama T, Ando A, et al.: Increased oxidative stress in mouse kidneys with unilateral ureteral obstruction. Kidney Int 1999; 56:1004.
15. Maines MD: The heme oxygenase system: a regulator of second messenger gases. Ann Rev Pharmacol Toxicol 1997; 37:517.
16. Platt JL, Nath KA: Heme oxygenase: protective gene or Trojan horse. Nature Medicine, News and Views 1998; 4:1364.
17. Nath KA: Heme oxygenase-1: a redoubtable response that limits reperfusion injury in the transplanted adipose liver. J Clin Invest 1999; 104:1485.
18. Agarwal A, Nick HS: Renal response to tissue injury: lessons from heme oxygenase-1 gene ablation and expression. J Am Soc Nephrol 2000; 11:965.
19. Dong Z, Lavrovsky Y, Venkatachalam MA, et al: Heme oxygenase-1 in tissue pathology: the yin and yang. Am J Pathol 2000; 156:1485.
20. Abraham NG, Drummond GS, Lutton JD, et al: The biological significance and physiological role of heme oxygenase. Cell Physiol Biochem 1996; 6:129.
21. Eisenstein RS, Garcia-Mayol D, Pettingell W, et al: Regulation of ferritin and heme oxygenase synthesis in rat fibroblasts by different forms of iron. Proc Natl Acad Sci, USA 1991; 88:688.
22. Balla G, Jacob HS, Balla J, et al: Ferritin: a cytoprotective antioxidant stratagem of endothelium. J Biol Chem 1992; 267:18148.
23. Barañano DE, Wolosker H, Bae BI, et al: A mammalian iron ATPase induced by iron. J Biol Chem 2000; 275:15166.
24. Hebbel RP, Eaton JW: Pathobiology of heme interaction with the erythrocyte membrane. Semin Hematol 1989; 26:136.

25. Muller-Eberhard U, Fraig M: Bioactivity of heme and its containment. Am J Hematol 1993; 42:59.
26. Balla G, Vercellotti GM, Muller-Eberhard U, et al: Exposure of endothelial cells to free heme potentiates damage mediated by granulocytes and toxic oxygen species. Lab Invest 1991; 64:648.
27. Nath KA: Reactive oxygen species in renal injury. In: Andreucci VE, Fine LG, eds: *International Year Book of Nephrology*. Boston: Kluwer Academic Press; 1991:47.
28. Zager RA: Rhabdomyolysis and myohemoglobinuric acute renal failure. Kidney Int 1996; 49:314.
29. Dhar, GJ, Bossenmaier I, Cardinal R, et al: Transitory renal failure following rapid administration of a relatively large amount of hematin in a patient with acute intermittent porphyria in clinical remission. Acta Med Scan 1978; 203:437.
30. Warden DH, Croatt AJ, Katusic ZS, et al: Physiologic characterization of acute reversible systemic hypertension in a model of heme protein-induced renal injury. Am J Physiol 1999; 277:F58.
31. Nath KA, Balla J, Croatt AJ, et al: Heme protein-mediated renal injury: a protective role for 21-aminosteroids in vitro and in vivo. Kidney Int 1995; 47:592.
32. Moore KP, Holt SG, Patel RP, et al: A causative role for redox cycling of myoglobin and its inhibition by alkalinization in the pathogenesis and treatment of rhabdomyolysis-induced renal failure. J Biol Chem 1998; 273:31731.
33. Nath KA, Grande JP, Croatt AJ, et al.: Intracellular targets in heme protein induced renal injury. Kidney Int 1998; 53:100.
34. Zager RA: Mitochondrial free radical production induces lipid peroxidation during myohemoglobinuria. Kidney Int 1996; 49:741.
35. Stocker R, Yamamoto Y, McDonagh AF, et al.: Bilirubin is an antioxidant of possible physiologic significance. Science 1987; 235:1043.
36. Stocker R, Glazer AN, Ames BN: Antioxidant activity of albumin-bound bilirubin. Proc Natl Acad Sci, USA 1987; 84:5918.
37. Llesuy SF, Tomaro ML: Heme oxygenase and oxidative stress. Evidence of involvement of bilirubin as physiological protector against oxidative damage. Biochim Biophys Acta 1994; 1223:9.
38. Poss KD, Tonegawa S: Heme oxygenase-1 is required for mammalian iron reutilization. Proc Natl Acad Sci, USA 1997; 94:10919.
39. Nath KA, Haggard JJ, Croatt AJ, et al: The indispensability of heme oxygenase-1 (HO-1) in protecting against heme protein-induced toxicity in vivo. Am J Pathol 2000; 156:1527.
40. Abraham NG, Lavrovsky Y, Schwartzman ML, et al: Transfection of the human heme oxygenase gene into rabbit coronary microvessel endothelial cells: protective effect against heme and hemoglobin toxicity. Proc Natl Acad Sci, USA 1995; 92:6798.
41. Nath KA, Croatt AJ, Haggard JJ, et al.: Renal response to repetitive exposure to heme proteins: chronic injury induced by an acute insult. Kidney Int 2000; 57:2423.
42. Nath KA, Vercellotti G, Grande JP, et al: Heme protein-induced chronic renal inflammation: suppressive effect of induced heme oxygenase-1. Kidney Int 2001; 59:106.
43. Shiraishi F, Curtis LM, Truong L, et al: Heme oxygenase-1 gene ablation or express modulates cisplatin-induced renal tubular apoptosis. Am J Physiol 2000; 278:F726.
44. Saikumar P, Dong Z, Mikhailov V, et al: Apoptosis: definition, mechanisms, and relevance to disease. Am J Med 1999; 107:489.
45. Petrache I, Otterbein LE, Alam J, et al: Heme oxygenase-1 inhibits TNF-α–induced apoptosis in cultured fibroblasts. Am J Physiol 2000; 278:L312.
46. Otterbein LE, Mantell LL, Choi AMK: Carbon monoxide provides protection against hyperoxic lung injury. Am J Physiol 1999; 276:L688.
47. Brouard S, Otterbein LE, Anrather J, et al: Carbon monoxide generated by heme oxygenase-1 suppresses endothelial cell apoptosis. J Exp Med 2000; 192:1015.
48. Ferris CD, Jaffrey SR, Sawa A, et al: Haem oxygenase-1 prevents cell death by regulating cellular iron. Nature Cell Biol 1999; 1:152.
49. Yoneya R, Ozasa H, Nagashima Y, et al: Hemin pretreatment ameliorates aspects of the nephropathy induced by mercuric chloride in the rat. Toxicol Lett 2000; 116:223.
50. Raju VS, Maines MD: Renal ischemia/reperfusion up-regulates heme oxygenase-1 (HSP32) expression and increases cGMP in rat heart. J Pharmacol Exp Therap 1996; 277:1814.
51. Paller MS, Nath KA, Rosenberg ME: Heme oxygenase is not expressed as a stress protein after renal ischemia. J Lab Clin Med 1993; 122:341.
52. Shimizu H, Takahashi T, Suzuki T, et al: Protective effect of heme oxygenase induction in ischemic acute renal failure. Crit Care Med 2000; 28:809.
53. Maines MD, Raju VS, Panahian N: Spin trap (N-t-butyl-α-phenylnitrone)-mediated suprainduction of heme oxygenase-1 in kidney ischemia/reperfusion model: role of the oxygenase in protection against oxidative injury. J Pharmacol Exp Therap 1999; 291:911.
54. Suzuki H, Kanamaru K, Tsunoda H, et al: Heme oxygenase-1 gene induction as an intrinsic regulation against delayed cerebral vasospasm in rats. J Clin Invest 1999; 104:59.
55. Motterlini R, Gonzales A, Foresti R, et al: Heme oxygenase-1–derived carbon monoxide contributes to the suppression of acute hypertensive responses in vivo. Circ Res 1998; 83:568.
56. Wang R: Resurgence of carbon monoxide: an endogenous gaseous vasorelaxing factor. Can J Physiol Pharmacol 1998; 76:1.
57. Kozma F, Johnson RA, Zhang F, et al: Contribution of endogenous carbon monoxide to regulation of diameter in resistance vessels. Am J Physiol 1999; 276:R1087.
58. Thorup C, Jones CL, Gross SS, et al: Carbon monoxide induces vasodilation and nitric oxide release but suppresses endothelial NOS. Am J Physiol 1999; 277:F882.
59. Morita T, Kourembanas S: Endothelial cell expression of vasoconstrictors and growth factors is regulated by smooth muscle cell–derived carbon monoxide. J Clin Invest 1995; 96:2676.
60. Levere RD, Martasek P, Escalante B, et al: Effect of heme arginate administration on blood pressure in spontaneously hypertensive rats. J Clin Invest 1990; 86:213.
61. Zou A-P, Billington H, Su N, et al: Expression and actions of heme oxygenase in the renal medulla of rats. Hypertension 2000; 35:342.
62. Foresti R, Motterlini R: The heme oxygenase pathway and its interaction with nitric oxide in the control of cellular homeostasis. Free Rad Res 1999; 31:459.
63. Liang M, Croatt AJ, Nath KA: Mechanisms underlying induction of heme oxygenase by nitric oxide in renal tubular epithelial cells. Am J Physiol 2000; 279:F728.
64. Yu L, Gengaro PE, Niederberger M, et al: Nitric oxide: a mediator in rat tubular hypoxia/reoxygenation injury. Proc Natl Acad Sci, USA 1994; 91:1691.
65. Noiri E, Peresleni T, Miller F, et al: In vivo targeting of inducible NO synthase with oligodeoxynucleotides protects rat kidney against ischemia. J Clin Invest 1996; 97:2377.
66. Mosely K, Wembridge DE, Cattell V, et al: Heme oxygenase is induced in nephrotoxic nephritis and hemin, a stimulator of heme oxygenase synthesis, ameliorates disease. Kidney Int 1998; 53:672.
67. Datta PK, Koukouritaki SB, Hopp KA, et al: Heme oxygenase-1 induction attenuates inducible nitric oxide synthase expression and proteinuria in glomerulonephritis. J Am Soc Nephrol 1999; 10:2540.
68. Willis D, Moore AR, Frederick R, et al: Heme oxygenase: a novel target for the modulation of the inflammatory response. Nature Med 1996; 2:87.
69. Soares MP, Lin Y, Anrather J, et al: Expression of heme oxygenase-1 can determine cardiac xenograft survival. Nature Med 1998; 4:1073.
70. Hancock WW, Buelow R, Sayegh MH, et al: Antibody-induced transplant arteriosclerosis is prevented by graft expression of anti-oxidant and anti-apoptotic genes. Nature Med 1998; 4:1392.
71. Otterbein LE, Bach FH, Alam J, et al: Carbon monoxide has anti-inflammatory effects involving the mitogen-activated protein kinase pathway. Nature Med 2000; 6:422.
72. Hayashi S, Takamiya R, Yamaguchi T, et al: Induction of heme oxygenase-1 suppresses venular leukocyte adhesion elicited by oxidative stress. Circ Res 1999; 85:663.
73. Otterbein L, Chin BY, Otterbein SL, et al: Mechanism of hemoglobin-induced protection against endotoxemia in rats: a ferritin-independent pathway. Am J Physiol 1997; 272:L268.
74. Poss KD, Tonegawa S: Reduced stress defense in heme oxygenase 1–deficient cells. Proc Natl Acad Sci, USA 1997; 94:10925.

75. Vachharajani TJ, Work J, Issekutz AC, et al: Heme oxygenase modulates selectin expression in different regional vascular beds. Am J Physiol 2000; 278:H1613.
76. Nath KA: The functional significance of induction of heme oxygenase by oxidant stress. J Lab Clin Med 1994; 123:461.
77. Zager RA, Burkhart KM, Conrad DS, et al: Iron, heme oxygenase, and glutathione: effects on myohemoglobinuric proximal tubular injury. Kidney Int 1995; 48:1624.
78. da Silva J-L, Morishita T, Escalante B, et al: Dual role of heme oxygenase in epithelial cell injury: contrasting effects of short-term and long-term exposure to oxidant stress. J Lab Clin Med 1996; 128:290.
79. Suttner DM, Dennery PA: Reversal of HO-1 related cytoprotection with increased expression is due to reactive iron. FASEB J 1999; 13:1800.
80. Lee PJ, Alam J, Wiegand GW, et al: Overexpression of heme oxygenase-1 in human pulmonary epithelial cells results in cell growth arrest and increased resistance to hyperoxia. Proc Natl Acad Sci, USA 1996; 93:10393.
81. Ohta K, Yachie A, Fujimoto K, et al: Tubular injury as a cardinal pathologic feature in human heme oxygenase-1 deficiency. Am J Kidney Dis 2000; 35:863.
82. Yachie A, Niida Y, Wada T, et al: Oxidative stress causes enhanced endothelial cell injury in human heme oxygenase-1 deficiency. J Clin Invest 1999; 103:129.
83. Abraham NG, Jiang S, Yang L, et al: Adenoviral vector–mediated transfer of human heme oxygenase in rats decreases renal heme-dependent arachidonic acid epoxygenase activity. J Pharmacol Exp Therap 2000; 293:494.
84. Liu H, Mount DB, Nasjletti A, et al: Carbon monoxide stimulates the apical 70-pS K^+ channel of the rat thick ascending limb. J Clin Invest 1999; 103:963.

CHAPTER 6

Inflammatory Response and Its Consequences in Acute Renal Failure

Hamid Rabb ▪ Robert Star

INTRODUCTION

Despite significant advances in therapeutics over the last 30 years, including the widespread use of dialysis, the mortality and morbidity associated with acute renal failure (ARF) have not appreciably improved.[1, 2] Classically, the pathophysiology of ARF had been thought to consist of mainly vascular derangements, tubular obstruction, and urinary backleak.[3] Because current interventions for clinical ARF have yielded poor results and due to new research tools and concepts in the ARF field, additional paradigms are emerging, including the role of "sublethal" cell injury, apoptosis, and cell repair after injury. Recent developments in immunology and cell biology have demonstrated the importance of inflammation in the pathogenesis of kidney dysfunction. Whereas prolonged ischemia causes anoxic cell death, recent evidence suggests that sublethal injury may be amplified by inflammatory and cytotoxic injury cascades activated during the reperfusion period. In this chapter, studies that have investigated the role of inflammatory mediators in both experimental and human ARF are reviewed. The cellular and humoral components of renal inflammation discovered in animal models are discussed. Clinical data concerning the role of inflammation in allograft and native kidney ARF and in dialysis therapy used to treat ARF are also reviewed. Finally, therapeutic strategies that target the counterproductive effects of inflammation are discussed. In a relatively short period of time, the importance of inflammation has been established in the pathogenesis of ARF, and new therapies are likely to arise from further work in this field.

GENERAL NATURE OF INFLAMMATORY RESPONSE

Inflammation is a basic requirement for human survival that allows living tissues to respond to "hostile" intrusion from their environment.[4] The inflammatory response is meant to destroy or contain injury and pave the path for repair of the damaged tissue. The subsequent repair, which is really a continuum of inflammation, may restore tissue morphology and specialized function. However, the inflammatory-repair process may be harmful, as occurs during a fatal anaphylactic reaction to an insect bite. However, misguided inflammation is usually not as obvious.

Inflammatory responses have many similarities despite the diverse nature of the injury or tissue involved.

Specific characteristic responses occur in blood vessels and neural and inflammatory networks. Blood vessels become congested and permeable to water and plasma proteins. Vascular reflexes are initiated soon after injury but then become intertwined with chemical mediators. Cytokines, chemokines, plasma proteases, complement, clotting factors, prostaglandins, and related products are increased in the local milieu and recruit inflammatory cells into the injured tissue. Leukocytes clump in the microcirculation, thus worsening tissue ischemia ("no-flow"). Leukocytes also emigrate out of the circulation, release a multitude of products, and injure cells. Thus, the study of the role of inflammation in ARF requires both reductionist (single mediator) and integrative (whole-organ) approaches because of the complexity of the body's response to injury. In this context, ARF can be viewed as a form of "nephritis" or "tubulitis," in which the inflammatory response over-reaches its homeostatic mandate and directly worsens the disease.

OVERVIEW OF INFLAMMATORY RESPONSE IN ACUTE RENAL FAILURE

Following acute renal injury, there is a complex orchestrated response that involves an interwoven network of changes in gene expression in renal endothelial and tubular cells and an accumulation of inflammatory cells. These events have been most widely studied using an ischemia-reperfusion model of renal injury. Blood flow to the kidney is completely occluded for 30 to 90 minutes, and then the molecular and cellular events are studied during the reperfusion period. Some of these responses are protective (heat shock proteins, interleukin-10[IL-10]),[5–7] and some lead to a regenerative response (transcription factors, cell cyclin kinases, growth factors).[8–10] There is also an acute inflammatory response that occurs in waves: early induction of adhesion molecules, cytokines, and chemokines in the first hour that induce neutrophil accumulation starting at 2 to 4 hours.[11, 12] Early induction of cytotoxic components involving reactive oxygen radicals or nitric oxide (NO) also occurs.[13, 14] This is followed by later accumulation of monocytes and macrophages and T cells at about 24 hours, which may persist for some time.[15–17] Each wave of injury can potentially set up further injurious cycles.

This chapter reviews data demonstrating that activation of specific components of the inflammatory response following renal injury are maladaptive and can worsen the course of ARF.

ROLE OF SPECIFIC INFLAMMATORY MEDIATORS IN ACUTE RENAL FAILURE

Erythrocytes

The most visible inflammatory response in ARF is the vascular congestion in the microvessels (vasa recta) of the inner stripe of the outer medulla. Erythrocytes aggregate in the venules, as elegantly demonstrated by Mason and coworkers[18] and other studies in animal models of ARF. While capillary congestion is also seen in human ARF, it is not as prominent.[19] The cause of the erythrocyte aggregation is probably multifactorial. First, leukocyte occlusion of the ascending vasa recta in the outer stripe (see later) causes congestion of upstream blood vessels, that is, the ascending vasa recta in the inner stripe. Second, the congestion is probably accentuated by egress of plasma water, because of either high pressure or increased capillary permeability, thus increasing blood viscosity.

A number of observations suggest a pathophysiologic role for erythrocyte congestion in ARF. Patients with sickle cell anemia are particularly vulnerable to renal ischemia,[20] and the accentuation of vascular congestion in these patients could be important in the renal dysfunction. Liberthal and coworkers[21] have elegantly shown that perfusion of the kidney with erythrocytes in addition to artificial plasma is crucial in simulating human tubular injury in the proximal tubule. Pentoxifylline, which has many effects, including altering erythrocyte rheology to facilitate capillary flow, attenuates renal injury after ischemia in rats.[22] In addition, lowering the hematocrit also decreases renal injury in a rat ischemia model.[23]

Leukocytes

NEUTROPHILS

Inflammation is characterized by neutrophil margination to the periphery of blood vessels, emigration into renal tissue, and both phagocytosis and release of destructive enzymes and free radicals. In both the kidneys and numerous other organs, ischemia and subsequent reperfusion causes a prominent accumulation of neutrophils in the postischemic organ. Neutrophils are not easily identified by conventional hematoxylin and eosin staining because the nuclei are squeezed together in the small renal microvessels. Therefore, detection of neutrophils requires special stains (eg, chloroacetate esterase, modified Leder) or other markers (eg, antibodies). Neutrophil accumulation is first noted at 2 to 4 hours,[12, 14, 24] peaks at about 24 hours, then decays over the next 2 to 3 days. Neutrophils are predominantly located in the outer stripe of the outer medulla, particularly between tubules with occasional neutrophils seen in the tubular lumens.

But why does this occur preferentially in this region of the outer stripe? Detailed studies of the renal microcirculation by Kriz[25] and Bankir and coworkers[26] have shown that the outer strip of the outer medulla has only scarce descending (ie, arterial) vasa recta but an abundance of ascending (ie, venous) vasa recta. Hence, oxygen must be supplied by the ascending vasa recta, which is a postcapillary venule, because it has already traversed the inner medulla. This explains why the outer medulla "borders on the edge of hypoxia." Neutrophil accumulation and plugging of the ascending vasa recta leads to red blood cell accumulation and slugging in the outer stripe of the outer medulla (see earlier) in the animal models.

Although neutrophil accumulation is impressive in the animal models of ischemia-reperfusion injury, neutrophils have not been detected to such a degree in human ARF. This difference may be caused by limitations in the human biopsy material. First, clinical biopsies are generally not obtained early in the course of ARF, which is when neutrophils are present in the animal models. Second, medullary sections are usually not obtained. Third, neutrophils tightly squeezed into the vasa recta are not detected by conventional hematoxylin and eosin staining employed in the human biopsy studies. Alternatively, there may be real biological differences between human acute renal failure and the "clamp" model of renal ischemia-reperfusion injury.

Thus, neutrophils were a prime target to evaluate in an attempt to treat experimental ARF. However, studies by different groups have shown either a beneficial role of neutrophil depletion in animal models of ischemia-reperfusion injury[27–29] or no role on outcome.[30–32] With these disparate results by authoritative groups, it is probably that the role of the neutrophil is complex. It is possible that methods to induce neutropenia (eg, neutrophil-depleting serum, cytotoxins), the degree of neutropenia induced, species differences, and subtleties of experimental models could have led to divergent results. The results of other methods of inhibiting neutrophil accumulation (ie, adhesion molecule blockade) are discussed later in this chapter. In sum, it appears that neutrophils have some role in the pathogenesis of reperfusion injury[11] but not as substantial as that in the injury of other organs, such as cardiac injury.[33]

MACROPHAGES

Macrophages are well established to migrate into inflamed tissue but usually in fewer numbers and in a more delayed fashion compared with neutrophils. Macrophage chemoattractants (eg, MCP-1) are up-regulated during experimental renal ischemia-reperfusion injury.[16, 34, 35] Macrophages accumulate in the outer medulla post ischemia in rats, as detected with ED-1 antibody (a macrophage-specific marker).[15] Unlike with neutrophils, no significant increase is seen at 4 hours. However at 24 and 48 hours, macrophage numbers increase greatly and then start to clear by 72 hours. The role of macrophages during the period immediately following injury is unknown. Recently, the use of a macrophage pacifant, CNI 1493, given during renal ischemia-reperfusion injury in rats, decreased the lung injury induced by ARF (injury at a distance) but did not change the course of the renal function.[36] Treatment with an endothelin A or B receptor antagonist reduced infiltration of ED-1–positive cells and reduced matrix accumulation, although there was no effect on renal function (measured by creatinine level).[37] In view of the important role of macrophages in repair, it is important to further explore the role of these cells in early injury during ARF, as well as the possible occurrence of long-term renal fibrosis after ARF in single kidneys.[38]

LYMPHOCYTES

Lymphocytes have not been characteristically associated with the acute phases of inflammation, but an increasing amount of data suggests a prominent role. In human ARF, mononuclear leukocytes are seen in the vasa recta.[19] T cells have also been identified in rat[16] and mouse[17] models of renal ischemia-reperfusion injury when special stains were used. The highly regulatory role of T cells in immune responses suggests that even small numbers may play an important role in directing other processes and amplification of inflammation. Blockade of T cell costimulatory pathway B7-CD28 by CTLA4Ig significantly attenuated renal dysfunction in a rat ischemia-reperfusion model, with decreased cytokine production in the post ischemic kidney.[39] Mice deficient in both CD4[+] and CD8[+] cells have reduced tubular necrosis and neutrophil infiltration and significantly improved renal function at 48 hours after ischemia.[17] However, it is not known which T cell subset is more important in this model or the mechanisms of T cell involvement. Studies from other organs may be revealing, and CD4[+] cells have been shown to be essential for full expression of ischemic liver injury in mice.[40] T cells are also found to regulate adhesion molecule expression in mice, which further regulates leukocyte infiltration into injured tissue.[41] Thus, increasing evidence in ARF, as well as in glomerular diseases,[42] points to an important role for the T cell. Table 6–1[17, 22, 23, 27, 28, 30–32, 36, 39, 46] summarizes studies that evaluate the role of blood cells in experimental ARF.

Leukocyte Adhesion Molecules

Leukocyte adhesion molecules are expressed on leukocytes and regulate many leukocyte functions. In addition, leukocyte adhesion molecules also function in a wide range of normal and abnormal biologic processes, such as development, signaling, inflammation, cancer, and apoptosis. There currently exists a multi-step paradigm of leukocyte migration into inflamed tissue. Leukocytes must initially tether and roll on endothelium via selectins and their ligands.[44, 45] Subsequent activation of leukocytes and endothelium leads to firm activation through integrins and their receptor. Transmigration occurs between endothelial cells, and then diapedesis of leukocytes occurs through matrix to get to the source of the injury, guided by a concentration gradient of cytokines and chemokines. The number of known cell adhesion molecules is rapidly increasing. A framework of these leukocyte adhesive interactions with microvascular endothelium, interstitium, and tubular epithelial cells is shown in Figure 6–1.

The initial studies examining the role of cell adhesion molecules in experimental ARF investigated the role of the leukocyte integrin CD11/CD18 and one of its ligands, intercellular adhesion molecule-1 (ICAM-1). Blockade of CD11/CD18 mitigated experimental ischemia-reperfusion injury in rats with an accompanying decrease in neutrophil infiltration.[43, 46] Blockade of ICAM-1 was also protective in a rat ischemia-reperfusion model, even more so than CD11/CD18 blockade.[43, 47, 48] Perfusion of kidneys with ICAM-1 antisense oligonucleotides inhibits renal ischemia-reperfusion injury in rats.[49] It was important to administer CD11/CD18 or ICAM-1 blockade either during ischemia or soon after in order for it to be effective. ICAM-1–deficient mice also had substantially reduced renal dysfunction after ischemia[29] and reduced mortality at 24 hours in a more severe ischemia-reperfusion model.[50] However, an attempt to block renal injury in rabbits with CD11/CD18 or ICAM-1 antibodies was not successful.[31, 51] Species-selectivity of blocking antibodies may account for this. Small-scale human clinical trials also suggest an important role for CD11a/CD18[52] and

TABLE 6–1. Role of Blood Cells in Experimental Models of ARF

CELL TYPE	MODE OF BLOCKADE	SPECIES	PROTECTION	COMMENTS AND REFERENCE
RBCs	Anemia induction	Rat	yes	Renal cortex also involved[23]
	Pentoxiphylline	Rat	yes	Toxic ARF model[22]
Neutrophils	Anti-serum	Rat	yes	Tubular leakage reduced[27]
	Anti-serum	Rat	yes	LTB4 production by PMNs[28]
	Anti-serum	Rat	no	
	Nitrogen mustard	Rat	yes	Non-specific treatment[30]
	Anti-serum	Rat	no	Both moderate and severe ischemia tested[31]
	Anti-serum	Rat	no	ICAM-1 mediated model[32]
	Anti-serum	Mouse	yes	ICAM-1 mediated model[43]
Macrophages	CNI-1493	Rat	no	Reduced lung injury associated with ARF[36]
T cells	CTLA-4Ig	Rat	yes	Blocked B7 costimulation[39]
	CD4/CD8 knockout	Mouse	yes	Neutrophil infiltration also attenuated[17]
Platelets	Aspirin, heparin	Rat	no	Reference 23

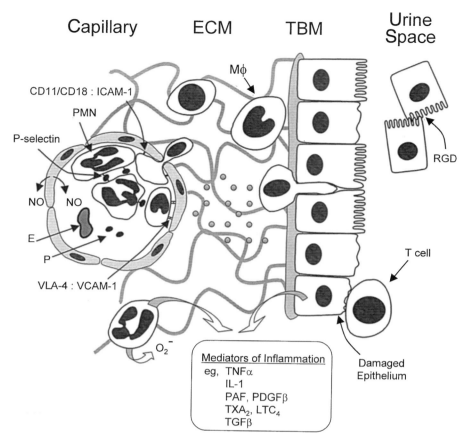

FIGURE 6–1 ▪ Microvascular and tubulointerstitial inflammation in acute renal failure. The initial injury stimulates endothelial cell activation, with resultant dysregulation in vascular tone, enhanced capillary permeability, and microvascular sludging. Activation of leukocytes leads to formation of platelet-leukocyte plugs, which, along with erythrocytes, create a low-flow condition. Production of inflammatory mediators by the tubular cells and interstitium results in a concentration gradient that recruits inflammatory cells from the microvasculature to the matrix, and then through injured tubular basement membrane, allowing interactions with tubular epithelial cells. Tubular epithelial cells that have been sloughed also adhere to each other through RGD and other motifs, leading to increased intraluminal pressure. E, erythrocyte; ECM, extracellular matrix; ICAM-1, intercellular adhesion molecule-1; IL-1, interleukin-1; LTC$_4$, leukotriene C-4; Mϕ, macrophage; NO, nitric oxide; O$_2^-$, oxygen free radical; P, platelet; PAF, platelet activating factor; PDGF-β, platelet derived growth factor-β; PMN, polymorphonuclear leukocyte; RGD, arginine-glycine-aspartic acid; TBM, tubular basement membrane; TNF-α, tumor necrosis factor-α; TXA$_2$, thromboxane A$_2$; TGF-β, transforming growth factor-β; VCAM-1, vascular cell adhesion molecule-1; VLA-4, very late antigen-4.

ICAM-1[53] in ARF. In sum, both the CD11/CD18 and ICAM-1 pathways have been identified as important mediators of ARF that could be useful for therapy.

As selectin engagement of leukocytes precedes CD11/CD18 and ICAM-1, targeting selectins is an attractive way to block inflammation at an even earlier step (Fig. 6–2). In addition, selectin blockade could lead to less susceptibility to bacterial infections than CD11/CD18 blockade.[54] Promising results in heart and ear ischemia-reperfusion injury models further drove studies to evaluate the role of selectins in ARF. P-selectin, found on platelets and endothelium, was initially reported to be an important mediator of renal injury in a rat ischemia model.[55] A subsequent study of experimental renal reperfusion injury in L-selectin–deficient mice, in similar conditions in which ICAM-1 is important, failed to show a role for L-selectin by itself in the course of renal injury or neutrophil infiltration.[24] However, neutrophil migration into peritoneum was diminished in these mice, demonstrating organ specificity for the requirement for L-selectin

in neutrophil emigration out of the microvasculature. Subsequent studies have used the soluble ligand for P-selectin, PSGL-1, which also interferes with L- and E-selectin binding. PSGL-1 significantly decreased renal ischemia-reperfusion injury and inflammation in rats.[16] Alternatively, one can inhibit the sugar residues that are required for selectin binding to ligand.[56] Targeted disruption of the fucosyltransferase IV (but not VII), a key enzyme in carbohydrate processing for ligands for all selectins, led to improved renal function after ischemia in mice.[57] In contrast to panselectin blockade, it is possible to use a small molecule inhibitor that selectively inhibits the sialyl Lewis X (sLeX) moiety on selectin ligands. This approach not only decreased renal injury after moderate renal ischemia in rats but also reduced mortality and renal dysfunction in severe ischemia.[58] Thus, selectins and their ligands are important in the pathogenesis of ARF. Selectin antagonism by sugar-based blockade is attractive because of the promise of oral delivery, the lack of sensitization to host, lower susceptibility to bacterial infections, and

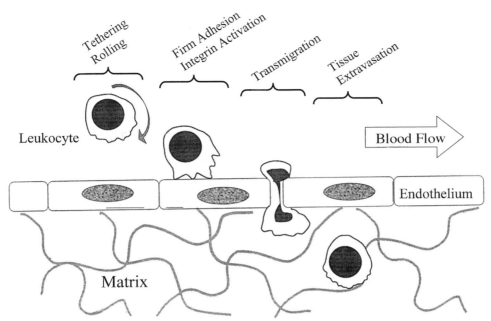

FIGURE 6–2 ■ Current paradigm of multistep process of leukocyte emigration from microvasculature to tissue. Leukocytes normally travel in the inner lumen of blood vessels under conditions of laminar flow. Activation of leukocytes and endothelium leads to slower flow at the periphery of the blood vessels, with subsequent tethering and rolling of leukocytes on endothelium by selectin molecules and their ligands. Adhesion of leukocytes to endothelium leads to further cellular activation, which, in turn, leads to engagement of integrin receptors, including CD11/CD18 and VLA-4. Corresponding ligands on endothelium include ICAM-1 and VCAM-1. Transmigration of leukocytes occurs through less well-defined mechanisms but may include the engagement of CD31. Tissue extravasation and migration through matrix involves complex and rapidly changing interactions between leukocytes and matrix. Migration through matrix probably requires the activation of β1 integrin receptors. It should be noted that there are a growing number of adhesion receptors being discovered, many of which have redundant functions. Thus, actual leukocyte emigration events probably involve many more adhesion molecules and pathways than currently recognized.

potentially lower production costs compared with monoclonal antibodies against CD11/CD18 or ICAM-1.

ARF is characterized by abnormal epithelial cell function, including loss of polarity, detachment from basement membrane, and cast formation that can worsen intratubular pressure and backleak of filtrate.[59, 60] The use of peptides directed to the RGD sequence (arginine-glycine-aspartic acid) of integrins reduces cell-cell interactions and ameliorates the course of experimental ARF.[61] However, RGD peptides also decrease leukocyte endothelial adhesion[62] and, probably, other functions as well. The interplay between infiltrating inflammatory cells and resident kidney cells is largely unknown, but it is probably crucial in the full expression of renal dysfunction in ARF.

Soluble Mediators

CYTOKINES

Cytokines are a diverse group of proteins with pleomorphic cellular functions in inflammation, cell growth, differentiation, and numerous other processes. Cytokines are generally classified as pro-inflammatory (interleukin-1 [IL-1], tumor necrosis factor [TNF], interferon-γ [IFN-γ]) or anti-inflammatory (eg, IL-10, α-melanocyte–stimulating hormone [α-MSH]). Cytokines are increased in the systemic circulation in ARF,[29]

which could be due to enhanced renal production or decreased clearance. The kidney produces many cytokines following ischemia, including IL-1, TNF, IFN-γ, IL-8, and IL-10.[14, 16, 35, 63, 64] To investigate whether pro-inflammatory cytokines have a direct role in ARF, IL-1 receptor–deficient mice were compared with wild-type controls and wild-type mice treated with IL-1 receptor antagonist.[65] Deficiency of the IL-1 receptor accelerated recovery from ischemia-reperfusion injury with fewer neutrophils infiltrating into the kidney, demonstrating a direct role of IL-1 in ARF. However, administration of the IL-1 receptor antagonist SQ, which may not have completely blocked intrarenal IL-1, was not protective. TNF-α also contributes to renal injury, since neutralizing antibodies to TNF decrease neutrophil infiltration and renal injury.[6, 64] The role of the anti-inflammatory cytokine IL-10 as an endogenous protective agent in ischemia-reperfusion injury has been studied by two groups. IL-10 blockade, by either neutralizing antibody or disruption of the IL-10 gene, accentuated renal inflammation and dysfunction after ischemia in mice.[6, 7] Provision of exogenous IL-10 decreased neutrophil infiltration and enhanced renal function after ischemia in Balb/c mice.[7] Thus, both endogenous and exogenous IL-10 have protective roles in renal ischemia-reperfusion injury. The role of other cytokines, such as the profibrotic cytokine transforming growth factor β (TGF-β), is unknown but worthy of further study.

CHEMOKINES

Chemokines are proteins that activate and attract inflammatory cells to a site of inflammation. Most animal models of renal injury have focused on a neutrophil chemokine (IL-8) and a macrophage chemokine (monocyte chemotactic protein-1 [MCP-1]). Both IL-8 and MCP-1 are increased early following experimental renal ischemia-reperfusion injury.[34] The intrarenal location of chemokine production has been evaluated at an mRNA level. MCP-1 is produced primarily in the thick ascending limb[34] and co-localizes with ED-1–staining macrophages.[15] IL-8 induction following ischemia has been localized to the thick ascending limb by laser capture microdissection.[66] However, no studies directly evaluating the role of chemokines using knockout mice or neutralizing antibodies have been performed to our knowledge, but this is likely to be a fruitful area of research.

NITRIC OXIDE

Nitric oxide (NO) is an odorless gas with a broad array of biological properties.[67, 68] All three isoforms of NO synthase and all four isoforms of soluble guanylyl cyclase are expressed in the kidney.[68, 69] NO has both beneficial and harmful effects after ARF.[70] Its beneficial properties include vasodilatation, inhibition of neutrophil adhesion, and inhibition of platelet aggregation. Thus, nonspecific NO inhibitors increase ischemia-reperfusion injury, while NO donors such as nitroprusside decrease injury,[71, 72] although nitroprusside must be given 15 minutes before ischemia.[73] However, at high concentrations produced during inflammation from the inducible isoform of NO synthase (iNOS), NO is a direct cellular toxin. Nitric oxide production is dramatically increased following lipopolysaccharide (LPS) or renal ischemia.[74–76] The trigger may be ischemia itself, because hypoxia increases NO production ex vivo,[74] or as the result of locally high concentrations of pro-inflammatory cytokines.[77, 78] Several studies have shown that iNOS expression and NO production, assessed by its metabolic footprint peroxynitrite, is increased following renal ischemia.[13, 14, 79] Finally, inhibition of NO synthesis protects isolated proximal tubules from hypoxic injury.[74] That the injurious NO is produced by iNOS is suggested by studies using antisense oligonucleotides and knockout mice.[13, 80, 81] Specific inhibition of induction of iNOS protects cultured proximal tubule cells from hypoxic damage in vivo and protects against ischemic injury in vivo.[13, 80] Tubules from iNOS knockout mice are protected from hypoxic injury, whereas tubules from endothelial or neuronal NOS knockout mice are not protected from injury.[81] Finally, a recent study by Ling and coworkers[82] showed that renal ischemia-reperfusion injury was reduced in iNOS knockout mice. Unlike in the studies referenced previously, these authors could not detect any iNOS in ischemic kidneys by the Western blot technique. The reason for this disparity is unknown, but it could be related to differences in mice strains, technical differences in protein isolation, or antibody sensitivity. How-

ever, they did find up-regulation of heat shock protein HSP-72, suggesting a compensatory up-regulation of HSP-72 in the iNOS knockout mice. Thus, the high concentrations of NO produced from iNOS have an injurious role in acute renal failure. This suggests that therapeutic approaches that specifically target iNOS might have beneficial effects in ARF.

COMPLEMENT

Complement is a heat-labile system of highly regulated proteins that carry out many of the effector functions of inflammation.[83] Complement can mediate cytolysis and opsonization to facilitate leukocyte-mediated injury, is chemotactic, and regulates immune complex deposition. The classic pathway for activation is through antibody-antigen complexes, but an alternative pathway can be directly activated. Thus, complement may be important in the inflammatory responses in ARF. Complement has been shown to be an important mediator in cardiac ischemia-reperfusion injury.[84] In addition, studies in transplant models point to an important role for complement component C6 in similar pathways that are involved in ARF.[85] However, the role of complement in renal ischemic injury is only beginning to be evaluated.

α-MELANOCYTE–STIMULATING HORMONE AND IL-10

α-Melanocyte–stimulating hormone (α-MSH) is a potent 13-amino-acid neuropeptide with broad anti-inflammatory effects.[86] α-MSH inhibits neutrophil accumulation at sites of inflammation via direct effects on neutrophils and indirectly by inhibiting production of cytokines, the chemokine IL-8, and the leukocyte adhesion molecule ICAM-1. α-MSH also inhibits cytotoxic events such as the induction of iNOS in macrophages.[87] Chiao and coworkers[14] found that α-MSH enhanced survival and reduced histologic and functional evidence of renal injury. α-MSH also reduced the polyuria that follows mild renal ischemic injury by preventing down-regulation of renal aquaporins (AQP-1 and AQP-2).[88] Furthermore, α-MSH was effective even when started 6 hours after injury. In this model, α-MSH inhibited neutrophil infiltration and induction of renal IL-8, ICAM-1, iNOS, and peroxynitrite (a marker for NO in tissues). α-MSH also inhibited tubular injury in an isolated kidney preparation perfused in the absence of neutrophils and in ICAM-1 knockout mice where neutrophil accumulation is less prominent than in normal mice.[50] These results indicate that α-MSH also acts by pathways that do not involve neutrophils. The broad mechanism of action and the extent of protection afforded even late in the reperfusion period distinguishes α-MSH from other agents that protect against ischemia-reperfusion injury. These results support an interactive cell biology paradigm of ARF, in which release of soluble inflammatory and cytotoxic mediators amplifies sublethal damage into lethal injury. An initial phase 1 safety trial of α-MSH in hemodialysis patients found that α-MSH was safe (up to 600 mg/kg doses tested); the only significant side effect was that α-MSH increased systolic blood pressure.[89] Thus, α-MSH has important hemodynamic effects that may be useful in treating patients with ischemic ARF.

Recent studies have found that α-MSH has effects in renal tubules. Gupta and coworkers[90] have found that α-MSH inhibits LPS-induced transcriptional regulation of iNOS in renal tubule cells via inhibition of the C/EPB transcription factor. This is in marked contrast to inhibition of NF-κB signaling in brain and neuronal cells.[91] Kohda and coworkers[92] recently found that luminal MSH antagonizes the actions of basolateral vasopressin in vivo and in isolated rabbit cortical collecting ducts. Thus, α-MSH has effects on both inflammatory and tubular cells in the kidney.

The actions of α-MSH and IL-10 are similar; both are produced *endogenously* following acute bacterial infection and myocardial infarction. Both inhibit renal injury. Renal IL-10 mRNA increases following renal ischemia. Therefore, Kohda and coworkers[7] hypothesized that IL-10 is a second messenger for α-MSH in renal ischemia-reperfusion injury. They found that α-MSH increased the production of IL-10 and that the protective effect of α-MSH was greatly reduced in mice genetically deficient for IL-10. This suggests that IL-10 is, in part, a second messenger for α-MSH. Table 6–2 summarizes the studies targeting inflammatory pathways in ARF.

CLINICAL EVIDENCE FOR INFLAMMATION IN HUMAN ACUTE RENAL FAILURE

Sepsis is a common predisposing cause of clinical ARF and underlies many of the factors (eg, hypoten-

sion, jaundice, altered sensorium, oliguria) in the clinical scoring systems for determining the severity and predicting the outcome of ARF.[99, 100] Direct evidence for inflammation in human ARF has been difficult to obtain, in part because of the paucity of human biopsy material in early ARF, and because leukocytes are best detected using special stains that are not routinely performed in clinical pathology laboratories. However, there is accumulating evidence that inflammatory processes play an important modulatory role in human ARF.

Inflammation in Allograft Kidney Acute Renal Failure

Acute renal failure occurs in 30% to 40% of cadaveric kidney transplants in the early postoperative period.[101] Early ARF is usually referred to as delayed graft function (DGF). Delayed graft function adds approximately $17,500 to the cost of each kidney transplant.[102] It can predispose to acute rejection, which in turn increases the risk of chronic allograft dysfunction.[101, 103] Although DGF usually resolves, the long-term consequences have been underappreciated until recently. Terasaki and coworkers[104] have demonstrated that ischemic kidney injury following cadaveric kidney transplantation has a worse 3-year graft survival compared with living unrelated kidney transplants. Thus, long-term allograft function can be directly affected by early procurement and storage injury.[105] Experimental data have also shown that, although renal ischemia-reperfusion in the single rat kidney initially resolves, the long-term effect is renal failure.[38] Therefore, ARF is an "antigen-independent" cause of allograft injury that can be a powerful determinant of graft outcome.

Inflammatory changes in human allograft ARF have been demonstrated with an increase in infiltrating leukocytes[106] and up-regulation of leukocyte adhesion molecules.[107, 108] There are important differences between allograft and native kidney ARF. First, it is important to appreciate that the allograft injury starts in the donor. The donor may have preexisting subtle renal changes that are not significant enough to preclude transplantation. In addition, brain death in the donor leads to a myriad of systemic changes in neurotransmitters and neuroimmunomodulators (eg, cytokines). For example, brain death is associated with a systemic catecholamine surge, which itself can induce distant tissue injury.[109] Brain death has been shown to up-regulate renal cytokines and adhesion molecules in a rat model.[110] Thus, brain death may prime the kidney for further ischemic and inflammatory damage. Another important difference between allograft and native kidney ARF is that allograft ARF occurs in the presence of an antigen-directed immune-activated environment, which may further perturb the response to injury. Administration of steroids, cyclosporine and FK506, mycophenolate mofetil, and anti–T-cell antibodies in the early post-transplant state probably modifies inflammation further. Although these immunomodulators affect host responses more than the

TABLE 6–2. ARF Treatment That Targets Inflammatory Pathways

AGENT	COMMENT AND REFERENCE
Cytokines	
IL-1	IL-1 receptor knockout mouse protected from ARF[65]
IL-10	IL-10 functions as a natural antiinflammatory in ARF [6, 7]
TNF	Antibody to TNF protective; TNF receptor knockout mouse not[6, 64, 93]
PAF	Many effects independent of platelet activation[94, 95]
MSH	Works by both blocking inflammation and mediating NO effects[14]
Adhesion molecules	
CD18	Moderate protection in human and rat ARF [46, 43, 96]
ICAM-1	Significant protection in numerous models in humans and animals[29, 43, 46, 48, 49, 50, 53, 97, 98]
Selectin	Protection after blockade by antibody, soluble ligand, fucosylation pathway, or small molecule ligand antagonist[16, 24, 55, 57, 58]
RGD sequence	Cyclic analogs decrease intratubular obstruction[61]

allograft kidney directly, the distinction is not clear, particularly in the case of cyclosporine, with its myriad of renal vascular and cellular effects. Finally, allografted kidneys are also exposed to cold ischemic injury that occurs during transport in organ preservation solutions. This is probably of lesser significance, because important differences in pathophysiology have not yet been shown between cold and warm renal ischemia.[111]

Chronic allograft nephropathy is now the leading cause of allograft loss; thus, it is important to elucidate the early mechanisms that result in ARF-induced long-term graft dysfunction. A possible scenario is that renal injury during allograft procurement and implantation stimulates antigen-independent inflammation in the allograft.[105] Locally elevated levels of free radicals[112] and chemokines[113] stimulate antigen-independent T-cell activation. Finally, the immunologically "primed" kidney undergoes remodeling, which may be imperfect. Continuous waves of injury and remodeling gradually exhaust the ability of the renal cells to heal with fidelity. Halloran and coworkers[114] have recently proposed that the cellular senescence in chronic allograft nephropathy could be caused by progressive defects in the enzyme telomerase, an enzyme that controls the number of divisions that a cell can undergo. Thus, errors in repair and cellular senescence lead to hypo- or nonfunctioning nephrons and tissue fibrosis.

Role of Inflammation as a Result of Dialysis During Acute Renal Failure

It is well established that dialysis stimulates systemic inflammation due to bioincompatibility between dialysis materials and blood.[115] Early studies documented the neutropenia that occurs with a dialysis treatment.[116] Subsequently, sequestration of leukocytes in the pulmonary vasculature with accompanying decreases in pulmonary function were demonstrated.[117] Cellulose-based dialysis membranes activate complement.[118] Complement deposits itself on leukocyte membranes and causes leukocyte adherence. Leukocyte activation then increases expression of surface adhesion molecules such as CD11b/CD18,[119] which predispose to leukocyte sequestration in distant capillary beds and the release of cytokines. Although neutrophils are clearly activated by dialysis, it is unclear whether T cells are also activated by dialysis.[120, 121] CD11b/CD18 activation on neutrophils may be a key component of leukocyte aggregation systemically. Many pro-inflammatory cytokines are increased in dialysis patients. Soluble adhesion molecules, such as ICAM-1, VCAM-1, and L-selectin, are also enhanced in the circulation after dialysis.[122-124]

Although there is little doubt that a single dialysis treatment results in a vigorous inflammatory response with generation of cytokines and activation of leukocytes, the role of these mediators in the dialysis-related neutropenia is unexplored. Dialysis of two Holstein calves with CD11/CD18 deficiency revealed a marked attenuation of the percent drop in leukocytes compared with normal Holsteins, demonstrating that CD11/CD18 is one of the direct mediators of the early neutropenia of dialysis.[125] Re-used dialysis membranes, presumably with a biofilm that adheres to the membrane and interferes with the stimulation of sites on the surface, reduce the inflammatory surge with dialysis.[115, 126] Modified cellulose membranes and newer synthetic substances have been constructed in an attempt to improve biocompatibility. Hakim and coworkers[127] have demonstrated that dialysis with synthetic polymethyl-methacrylate (PMMA) membranes led to the need for fewer dialysis treatments compared with cuprophane and an accelerated improvement in the course of ARF, presumably by decreasing systemic inflammation that perpetuates ARF. A European study also demonstrated a higher survival rate in patients with ARF who were dialyzed with biocompatible membranes than in those dialyzed with cellulose membranes.[128] However, a number of other studies have failed to demonstrate a difference in patient survival or rate of recovery from renal failure based on the type of dialysis membrane used.[129-131]

Recent studies have found that "biocompatible membranes" are not all the same. For example, Gilbert and coworkers[132] found that PMMA membranes, as used in the Hakim trials, caused as much, if not more, neutropenia than did cellulose acetate dialysis membranes. In contrast, polysulfone membranes caused much less neutropenia. Thus, factors other than traditional biocompatibility may be important in selecting dialysis membranes in patients with ARF. Furthermore, these newer membranes are more expensive; however, the cost is probably justified for dialysis in patients with ARF. Continuous dialysis, though not proven to be superior to intermittent dialysis in ARF, may result in less systemic inflammation.

Another approach would be to deliver an anti-inflammatory agent such as α-MSH during dialysis that could be more effective in mitigating the dialysis effect. It should be noted that intermittent hemodialysis for ARF also leads to further ischemic episodes from hypotension, so that the "detrimental" effects of hemodialysis may not be simply due to biocompatibility issues. Perhaps the ability of α-MSH to increase blood pressure might be beneficial. Further work is required in this area to guide clinicians as to the dialytic approach.

THERAPEUTIC APPROACHES TO REDUCING INFLAMMATION IN ACUTE RENAL FAILURE

Currently, there is no specific therapy for ARF. However, adequate nutrition, maintenance of adequate renal perfusion, careful use of diuretics, minimizing nephrotoxins, and dialysis when necessary constitute the standard therapeutic approach. An increasing number of centers are using biocompatible membranes for dialysis during ARF to minimize the deleterious effect of leukocyte activation and cytokine generation on the course of ARF. A clinical trial is under way in transplant patients with delayed graft function to evaluate the efficacy of CD11a/CD18 blockade in

ARF, and the results are anxiously awaited. Promising results from animal experiments that block selectins or their ligands have led to the preparation of a clinical trial. It may be important to modulate inflammation at multiple steps; thus α-MSH is an attractive agent for use in clinical trials. A phase 1 study of α-MSH in stable hemodialysis patients found that α-MSH was safe; the only side effect was that it increased blood pressure.[89] This side effect could be important in the treatment of patients with ischemic ARF. In addition, current anti-inflammatories, such as mycophenolate mofetil, anti-leukocyte antibodies (OKT-3), and anti–IL-2 receptor antibodies that have been developed for transplant resection, may be effective in diminishing the inflammation associated with ARF.

CONCLUSION

Over the last few years, the important role of dysregulated inflammation has been clearly demonstrated in ARF as well as in acute injury to other organs, such as the heart and brain. This has led to the investigation of a whole range of new targets, including cells and soluble mediators. Dramatic advances in immunology, inflammation, and pharmacology now permit us to approach these targets with a solid armamentarium developed by our colleagues in other fields. However, it is becoming increasingly clear that organ-specific injury processes and inflammation occur. Whole-kidney physiology is clearly different from that of heart or lymph node. Recent studies using microarrays have found that 20% of genes are up-regulated following manipulation of serum exposure to cells[133]; therefore, it is likely we have only scratched the surface of the renal response to ARF. Thus, our challenge is only beginning: to develop better animal models of renal injury that more closely mimic human ARF, to understand the inflammatory processes that mediate renal injury in both the ischemic and the nephrotoxic form of ARF, to be able to discern pathways that are deleterious from those required for renal recovery, and to translate these findings into clinical care of the patient with ARF. In addition, the role of inflammation in progressive renal dysfunction and its relationship to hyperfiltration and fibrosis are unknown. Experience has taught us that immunosuppression without specificity is fraught with danger; thus, we need to carefully understand these mechanisms in ARF before we can safely treat our patients. Furthermore, the relationship of dialysis modalities in ARF to inflammation is an area that requires further investigation, particularly because of the implications for the rapid integration of advances into clinical care.

ACKNOWLEDGMENTS

The authors thank Jan Lovick for assistance in manuscript preparation and Frank Daniels for the figures. The work of Hamid Rabb is supported by funds from the American Heart Association, the Hermundslie Foundation, the National Kidney Foundation, and the National Institutes of Health. This work was done during the tenure of an Established Investigatorship from the American Heart Association to Robert Star, and was supported by funds from the National Institutes of Health, the American Heart Association, the U.S. Food and Drug Administration, the National Kidney Foundation, the National Kidney Foundation of Texas, and the Baxter Healthcare Extramural Grant Program.

REFERENCES

1. Thadhani R, Pascual M, Bonventre JV: Acute renal failure. N Engl J Med 1996; 334:1448–1460.
2. Star RA: Treatment of acute renal failure. Kidney Int 1998; 54:1817–1831.
3. Brezis M, Rosen S, Epstein FH: Acute Renal Failure. In: Brenner BM, Rector FC, Jr, eds: The Kidney. Philadelphia: WB Saunders: 1986:735–799.
4. Robbins SL, Angell M, Kumar V: Basic Pathology. 3rd ed. Philadelphia: WB Saunders; 1981:28–61.
5. Van Why SK, Hildebrandt F, Ardito T, et al: Induction and intracellular localization of HSP-72 after renal ischemia. Am J Physiol 1992; 263:F769–F775.
6. Daemen MA, van de Ven MW, Heineman E, Buurman WA: Involvement of endogenous interleukin-10 and tumor necrosis factor-alpha in renal ischemia-reperfusion injury. Transplantation 1999; 67:792–800.
7. Kohda Y, Chiao H, McLeroy P, et al: Anti-inflammatory cascade protects against renal ischemia-reperfusion injury. J Am Soc Nephrol 1998; 9:581A.
8. Safirstein R, DiMari J, Megyesi J, Price P: Mechanisms of renal repair and survival following acute injury. Semin Nephrol 1998; 18:519–522.
9. Hammerman MR, Miller SB: Effects of growth hormone and insulin-like growth factor I on renal growth and function. J Pediatr 1997; 131:S17–S19.
10. Harris RC: Growth factors and cytokines in acute renal failure. Adv Ren Replace Ther 1997; 4:43–53.
11. Rabb H, O'Meara YM, Maderna P, et al: Leukocytes, cell adhesion molecules and ischemic acute renal failure. Kidney Int 1997; 51:1463–1468.
12. Willinger CC, Schramek H, Pfaller K, Pfaller W: Tissue distribution of neutrophils in postischemic acute renal failure. Virchows Arch B Cell Pathol Incl Mol Pathol 1992; 62:237–243.
13. Noiri E, Peresleni T, Miller F, Goligorsky MS: In vivo targeting of inducible NO synthase with oligodeoxynucleotides protects rat kidney against ischemia. J Clin Invest 1996; 97:2377–2383.
14. Chiao H, Kohda Y, McLeroy P, et al: Alpha-melanocyte-stimulating hormone protects against renal injury after ischemia in mice and rats. J Clin Invest 1997; 99:1165–1172.
15. Liu Z, Condon T, Bennett F, Rabb H: Macrophage migration into post-ischemic kidney. J Am Soc Nephrol 1996; 7:1829.
16. Takada M, Nadeau KC, Shaw GD, et al: The cytokine-adhesion molecule cascade in ischemia/reperfusion injury of the rat kidney: inhibition by a soluble P-selectin ligand. J Clin Invest 1997; 99:2682–2690.
17. Rabb H, Daniels F, O'Donnell M, et al: Pathophysiologic role of T lymphocytes in renal ischemia-reperfusion injury in mice. Am J Physiol Renal Physiol 2000; 279:F525–F531.
18. Mason J, Joeris B, Welsch J, Kriz W: Vascular congestion in ischemic renal failure: the role of cell swelling. Miner Electrolyte Metab 1989; 15:114–124.
19. Solez K, Morel-Maroger L, Sraer JD: The morphology of "acute tubular necrosis" in man: analysis of 57 renal biopsies and a comparison with the glycerol model. Medicine (Baltimore) 1979; 58:362–376.
20. Saborio P, Scheinman JI: Sickle cell nephropathy. J Am Soc Nephrol 1999; 10:187–192.
21. Lieberthal W, Stephens GW, Wolf EF, et al: Effect of erythro-

cytes on the function and morphology of the isolated perfused rat kidney. Ren Physiol 1987; 10:14–24.

22. Vadiei K, Brunner LJ, Luke DR: Effects of pentoxifylline in experimental acute renal failure. Kidney Int 1989; 36:466–470.

23. Mason J, Welsch J, Torhorst J: The contribution of vascular obstruction to the functional defect that follows renal ischemia. Kidney Int 1987; 31:65–71.

24. Rabb H, Ramirez G, Saba SR, et al: Renal ischemic-reperfusion injury in L-selectin deficient mice. Am J Physiol 1996; 271:F408–F413.

25. Kriz W: Structural organization of the renal medullary circulation. Nephron 1982; 31:290–295.

26. Bankir L, Bouby N, Trinh TT: Organization of the Medullary Circulation: Functional Implications. In Robinson RR, ed. *Nephrology.* New York: Springer-Verlag; 1994:84–106.

27. Hellberg PO, Kallskog TO: Neutrophil-mediated postischemic tubular leakage in the rat kidney. Kidney Int 1989; 36:555–561.

28. Klausner JM, Paterson IS, Goldman G, et al: Postischemic renal injury is mediated by neutrophils and leukotrienes. Am J Physiol 1989; 256:F794–F802.

29. Kelly KJ, Williams WW, Colvin RB, et al: Intercellular adhesion molecule-1–deficient mice are protected against ischemic renal injury. J Clin Invest 1996; 97:1056–1063.

30. Paller MS: Effect of neutrophil depletion on ischemic renal injury in the rat. J Lab Clin Med 1989; 113:379–386.

31. Thornton MA, Winn R, Alpers CE, Zager RA: An evaluation of the neutrophil as a mediator of in vivo renal ischemic- reperfusion injury. Am J Pathol 1989; 135:509–515.

32. Mendiola C, Dietz J, Saba S, et al: Roles of CD11/CD18 and neutropenia on ischemic acute renal failure. J Am Soc Nephrol 1993; 4:741.

33. Lefer AM, Campbell B, Scalia R, Lefer DJ: Synergism between platelets and neutrophils in provoking cardiac dysfunction after ischemia and reperfusion: role of selectins. Circulation 1998; 98:1322–1328.

34. Safirstein R: Renal stress response and acute renal failure. Adv Ren Replace Ther 1997; 4:38–42.

35. Lemay S, Rabb H, Postler G, Singh AK: Prominent and sustained up-regulation of gp130-signaling cytokines and of the chemokine MIP-2 in murine renal ischemic-reperfusion injury. Transplantation 2000; 69:959–963.

36. Kramer AA, Postler G, Salhab KF, et al: Renal ischemia-reperfusion leads to macrophage-mediated increase in pulmonary vascular permeability. Kidney Int 1999; 55:2362–2367.

37. Forbes JM, Leaker B, Hewitson TD, et al: Macrophage and myofibroblast involvement in ischemic acute renal failure is attenuated by endothelin receptor antagonists. Kidney Int 1999; 55:198–208.

38. Pagtalunan ME, Olson JL, Tilney NL, Meyer TW: Late consequences of acute ischemic injury to a solitary kidney. J Am Soc Nephrol 1999; 10:366–373.

39. Takada M, Chandraker A, Nadeau KC, et al: The role of the B7 costimulatory pathway in experimental cold ischemia-reperfusion injury. J Clin Invest 1997; 100:1199–1203.

40. Zwacka RM, Zhang Y, Halldorson J, et al: CD4(+) T-lymphocytes mediate ischemia-reperfusion–induced inflammatory responses in mouse liver. J Clin Invest 1997; 100:279–289.

41. Horie Y, Chervenak RP, Wolf R, et al: Lymphocytes mediate TNF-α–induced endothelial cell adhesion molecule expression: studies on SCID and RAG-1 mutant mice. J Immunol 1997; 159:5053–5062.

42. Couser WG: Sensitized cells come of age: a new era in renal immunology with important therapeutic implications. J Am Soc Nephrol 1999; 10:664–665.

43. Kelly KJ, Williams WW, Colvin RB, Bonventre JV: Antibody to intercellular adhesion molecule-1 protects the kidney against ischemic injury. Proc Natl Acad Sci USA 1994; 91:812–816.

44. Springer TA: Adhesion receptors of the immune system. Cell 1992; 69:11–25.

45. Lasky LA: Selectins: interpreters of cell-specific carbohydrate information during inflammation. Science 1992; 258:964–969.

46. Rabb H, Mendiola CC, Dietz J, et al: Role of CD11a and CD11b in ischemic acute renal failure in rats. Am J Physiol 1994; 267:F1052–F1058.

47. Rabb H, Mendiola CC, Saba SR, et al: Antibodies to ICAM-1 protect kidneys in severe ischemic reperfusion injury. Biochem Biophys Res Commun 1995; 211:67–73, 1995.

48. Haller H, Dragun D, Miethke A, et al: Antisense oligonucleotides for ICAM-1 attenuate reperfusion injury and renal failure in the rat. Kidney Int 1996; 50:473–480.

49. Chen W, Bennett CF, Wang ME, et al: Perfusion of kidneys with unformulated "naked" intercellular adhesion molecule-1 antisense oligodeoxynucleotides prevents ischemic-reperfusion injury. Transplantation 1999; 68:880–887.

50. Chiao H, Kohda Y, McLeroy P, et al: Alpha-melanocyte–stimulating hormone inhibits renal injury in the absence of neutrophils. Kidney Int 54:765–774, 1998.

51. Brady HR: Leukocyte adhesion molecules and kidney diseases. Kidney Int 1994; 45:1285–1300.

52. LeMauff B, LeMeur Y, Hourmant M, et al: A dose-searching trial of an anti-LFA1 monoclonal antibody in first kidney transplant recipients. Kidney Int Suppl 1996; 53:S44–S50.

53. Haug CE, Colvin RB, Delmonico FL, et al: A Phase I trial of immunosuppression with anti-ICAM-1 (CD54) mAb in renal allograft recipients. Transplantation 1993; 766–773.

54. Sharar SR, Chapman NN, Flaherty LC, et al: L-selectin (CD62L) blockade does not impair peritoneal neutrophil emigration or subcutaneous host defense to bacteria in rabbits. J Immunol 1996; 157:2555–2563.

55. Rabb H, Mendiola C, Saba SR, et al: Antibodies to P-selectin and ICAM-1 protect kidneys from ischemic-reperfusion injury. J Am Soc Nephrol 1994; 5:907A.

56. Maly P, Thall A, Petryniak B, et al: The α(1,3)fucosyltransferase Fuc-TVII controls leukocyte trafficking through an essential role in L-, E-, and P-selectin ligand biosynthesis. Cell 1996; 86:643–653.

57. Rabb H, Haq M, Saba S, et al: Fucosyl transferase IV mediates renal inflammation and dysfunction from ischemia-reperfusion. J Am Soc Nephrol 1998; 9:589A.

58. Nemoto T, Issekutz AC, Berens K, et al: Small molecule inhibition of selectin ligands reduces mortality and improves renal recovery from ischemic reperfusion injury in rats. J Am Soc Nephrol 1999; 10:637A.

59. Molitoris BA, Hoilien CA, Dahl R, et al: Characterization of ischemia-induced loss of epithelial polarity. J Membr Biol 1988; 106:233–242.

60. Kwon O, Nelson WJ, Sibley R, et al: Backleak, tight junctions, and cell-cell adhesion in postischemic injury to the renal allograft. J Clin Invest 1998; 101:2054–2064.

61. Goligorsky MS, DiBona GF: Pathogenetic role of Arg-Gly-Asp–recognizing integrins in acute renal failure. Proc Natl Acad Sci USA 1993; 90:5700–5704.

62. Romanov V, Noiri E, Czerwinski G, et al: Two novel probes reveal tubular and vascular Arg-Gly-Asp (RGD) binding sites in the ischemic rat kidney. Kidney Int 1997; 52:93–102.

63. Goes N, Urmson J, Ramassar V, Halloran PF: Ischemic acute tubular necrosis induces an extensive local cytokine response. Evidence for induction of interferon-gamma, transforming growth factor-beta 1, granulocyte-macrophage colony-stimulating factor, interleukin-2, and interleukin-10. Transplantation 1995; 59:565–572.

64. Donnahoo KK, Meng X, Ayala A, et al: Early kidney TNF-α expression mediates neutrophil infiltration and injury after renal ischemia-reperfusion. Am J Physiol 1999; 277:R922–R929.

65. Haq M, Norman J, Saba SR, et al: Role of IL-1 in renal ischemic reperfusion injury. J Am Soc Nephrol 1998; 9:614–619.

66. Kohda Y, Murakami H, Moe O, Star RA: Analysis of segmental renal gene expression by laser capture microdissection. J Am Soc Nephrol 1999; 10:634.

67. Bredt DS, Snyder SH: Nitric oxide: a physiologic messenger molecule. Annu Rev Biochem 1994; 63:175–195.

68. Kone BC, Baylis C: Biosynthesis and homeostatic roles of nitric oxide in the normal kidney. Am J Physiol Renal Physiol 1997; 272:F561–F578.

69. Star RA: Intrarenal localization of nitric oxide synthase isoforms and soluble guanylyl cyclase. Clin Exp Pharmacol Physiol 1997; 24:607–610.

70. Peer G, Blum M, Iaina A: Nitric oxide and acute renal failure. Nephron 1996; 73:375–381.

71. Lopez-Neblina F, Paez AJ, Toledo-Pereyra LH: Modulation of

neutrophil infiltration through nitric oxide in the ischemic rat kidney. Transplant Proc 1995; 27:1883–1885.

72. Linas S, Whittenburg D, Repine JE: Nitric oxide prevents neutrophil-mediated acute renal failure. Am J Physiol 1997; 272:F48–F54.

73. Lopez-Neblina F, Toledo-Pereyra LH, Mirmiran R, Paez-Rollys AJ: Time dependence of Na-nitroprusside administration in the prevention of neutrophil infiltration in the rat ischemic kidney. Transplantation 1996; 61:179–183.

74. Yu L, Gengaro PE, Niederberger M, et al: Nitric oxide: a mediator in rat tubular hypoxia-reoxygenation injury. Proc Natl Acad Sci USA 1994; 91:1691–1695.

75. Yaqoob M, Edelstein CL, Wieder ED, et al: Nitric oxide kinetics during hypoxia in proximal tubules: effects of acidosis and glycine. Kidney Int 1996; 49:1314–1319.

76. Traylor LA, Proksch JW, Beanum VC, Mayeux PR: Nitric oxide generation by renal proximal tubules: role of nitric oxide in the cytotoxicity of lipid A. J Pharmacol Exp Ther 1996; 279:91–96.

77. Markewitz BA, Michael JR, Kohan DE: Cytokine-induced expression of a nitric oxide synthase in rat renal tubule cells. J Clin Invest 1993; 91:2138–2143.

78. Mohaupt MG, Schwobel J, Elzie JL, et al: Cytokines activate inducible nitric oxide synthase gene transcription in inner medullary collecting duct cells. Am J Physiol 1995; 268:F770–F777.

79. Noiri E, Dickman K, Miller F, et al: Reduced tolerance to acute renal ischemia in mice with a targeted disruption of the osteopontin gene. Kidney Int 1999; 56:74–82.

80. Peresleni T, Noiri E, Bahou WF, Goligorsky MS: Antisense oligodeoxynucleotides to inducible NO synthase rescue epithelial cells from oxidative stress injury. Am J Physiol 1996; 270:F971–F977.

81. Ling H, Ginger PE, Edelstein CL, et al: Effect of hypoxia on proximal tubules isolated from nitric oxide synthase knockout mice. Kidney Int 1998; 53:1642–1646.

82. Ling H, Edelstein C, Gengaro P, et al: Attenuation of renal ischemia-reperfusion injury in inducible nitric oxide synthase knockout mice. Am J Physiol 1999; 277:F383–F390.

83. Abbas AK, Lichtman AH, Pober JS: The Complement System. In Abbas AK, Lichtman AH, Pober JS, eds: Cellular and Molecular Immunology. Philadelphia: WB Saunders; 1991:259–282.

84. Weisman HF, Bartow T, Leppo MK, et al: Soluble human complement receptor type 1: in vivo inhibitor of complement-suppressing postischemic myocardial inflammation and necrosis. Science 1990; 249:146–151.

85. Qian Z, Jakobs FM, Pfaff-Amesse T, et al: Complement contributes to the rejection of complete and class I major histocompatibility complex: incompatible cardiac allografts. J Heart Lung Transplant 1998; 17:470–478.

86. Kohda Y, Chiao H, Star RA: Alpha-melanocyte–stimulating hormone and acute renal failure. Curr Opin Nephrol Hypertens 1998; 7:413–417.

87. Star RA, Rajora N, Huang J, et al: Evidence of autocrine modulation of macrophage nitric oxide synthase by alpha-melanocyte–stimulating hormone. Proc Natl Acad Sci USA 1995; 92:8016–8020.

88. Kwon TH, Knepper MA, Nielsen S: Reduced abundance of aquaporins in rats with bilateral ischemia-induced acute renal failure: prevention by alpha-MSH. Am J Physiol 1999; 277:F413–F427.

89. Star RA, Haynes S, Middelton JP: Phase 1 trial of alpha-melanocyte stimulating hormone. J Am Soc Neph 1998; 9:161A.

90. Gupta AK, Diaz R, Kone BC: Alpha-MSH inhibits LPS induction of the inducible, pro-inflammatory transcription factor CCAAT/enhancer-binding protein (C/ERBP). J Am Soc Nephrol 1997; 8:474.

91. Ichiyama T, Sakai T, Catania A, et al: Systemically administered alpha-melanocyte–stimulating peptides inhibit NF-κB activation in experimental brain inflammation. Brain Res 1999; 836:31–37.

92. Kohda Y, Quigley R, Kong HL, Star RA: Luminal alpha-MSH antagonizes vasopressin-stimulated water permeability in cortical collecting ducts. J Am Soc Nephrol 1999; 10:18A.

93. Haq M, Norman J, Saba S, et al: Increased ICAM-1 and VCAM-1 expression in ischemic kidneys: independence of IL-1 and TNF. J Am Soc Nephrol 1998; 9:578A.

94. Kelly KJ, Tolkoff-Rubin NE, Rubin RH, et al: An oral platelet-activating factor antagonist, Ro-24-4736, protects the rat kidney from ischemic injury. Am J Physiol 1996; 271:F1061–F1067.

95. López-Novoa JM: Potential role of platelet activating factor in acute renal failure. Kidney Int 1999; 55:1672–1682.

96. Le Mauff B, Hourmant M, Rougier JP, et al: Effect of anti-LFA1 (CD11a) monoclonal antibodies in acute rejection in human kidney transplantation. Transplantation 1991; 52:291–296.

97. Linus SL, Whittenburg D, Parsons PE, Repine JE: Ischemia increases neutrophil retention and worsens acute renal failure: role of oxygen metabolites and ICAM-1. Kidney Int 1995; 48:1584–1591.

98. Dragun D, Tullius SG, Park JK, et al: ICAM-1 antisense oligodesoxynucleotides prevent reperfusion injury and enhance immediate graft function in renal transplantation. Kidney Int 1998; 54:590–602.

99. Liano F, Pascual J, Madrid Acute Renal Failure Study Group: Epidemiology of acute renal failure: a prospective, multicenter, community-based study. Kidney Int 1996; 50:811–818.

100. Halstenberg WK, Goormastic M, Paganini EP: Validity of four models for predicting outcome in critically ill acute renal failure patients. Clin Nephrol 1997; 47:81–86.

101. Tilney NL, Guttmann RD: Effects of initial ischemia-reperfusion injury on the transplanted kidney. Transplantation 1997; 64:945–947.

102. Freedland SJ, Shoskes DA: Economic impact of delayed graft function and suboptimal kidneys. Transplant Rev 1999; 13:23–30.

103. Samaniego M, Baldwin WM, Sanfilippo F: Delayed graft function: immediate and late impact. Curr Opin Nephrol Hypertens 1997; 6:533–537.

104. Terasaki PI, Cecka JM, Gjertson DW, Takemoto S: High survival rates of kidney transplants from spousal and living unrelated donors. N Engl J Med 1995; 333:333–336.

105. Lu CY, Penfield JG, Kielar ML, et al: Hypothesis: is renal allograft rejection initiated by the response to injury sustained during the transplant process? Kidney Int 1999; 55:2157–2168.

106. Fuggle SV, Koo DDH: Cell adhesion molecules in clinical renal transplantation. Transplantation 1998; 65:763–769.

107. Solez K, Racusen LC, Abdulkareem F, et al: Adhesion molecules and rejection of renal allografts. Kidney Int 1997; 51:1476–1480.

108. Briscoe DM, Ganz P, Alexander SI, et al: The problem of chronic rejection: influence of leukocyte-endothelial interactions. Kidney Int 1997; 51(suppl 58):S22–S27.

109. Novitzky D, Rose AG, Cooper DK: Injury of myocardial conduction tissue and coronary artery smooth muscle following brain death in the baboon. Transplantation 1988; 45:964–966.

110. Pratschke J, Wilhelm MJ, Kusaka M, et al: Brain death and its influence on donor organ quality and outcome after transplantation. Transplantation 1999; 67:343–348.

111. Molitoris BA: Ischemic acute renal failure: exciting times at our fingertips. Curr Opin Nephrol Hypertens 1998; 7:405–406.

112. Chaudhri G, Clark IA, Hunt NH, et al: Effect of antioxidants on primary alloantigen-induced T cell activation and proliferation. J Immunol 1986; 137:2646–2652.

113. Bacon KB, Premack BA, Gardner P, Schall TJ: Activation of dual T cell signaling pathways by the chemokine RANTES. Science 1995; 269:1727–1730.

114. Halloran PF, Melk A, Barth C: Rethinking chronic allograft nephropathy: the concept of accelerated senescence. J Am Soc Nephrol 1999; 10:167–181.

115. Hakim RM: Clinical implications of hemodialysis membrane biocompatibility. Kidney Int 1993; 44:484–494.

116. Kaplow LS, Goffinet JA: Profound neutropenia during the early phase of hemodialysis. JAMA 1968; 203:1135–1137.

117. Craddock PR, Fehr J, Dalmasso AP, et al: Hemodialysis leukopenia. Pulmonary vascular leukostasis resulting from complement activation by dialyzer cellophane membranes. J Clin Invest 1977; 59:879–888.

118. Cheung AK, Parker CJ, Hohnholt M: Beta2 integrins are required for neutrophil degranulation induced by hemodialysis membranes. Kidney Int 1993; 43:649–660.

119. Arnaout MA, Hakim RM, Todd RF, et al: Increased expression of an adhesion-promoting surface glycoprotein in the granulo-cytopenia of hemodialysis. N Engl J Med 1985; 312:457–462.

120. Chatenoud L, Dugas B, Beaurain G, et al: Presence of preactivated T cells in hemodialyzed patients: their possible role in altered immunity. Proc Natl Acad Sci USA 1986; 83:7457–7461.

121. Rabb H, Agosti S, Pollard S, et al: Activated and regulatory T lymphocyte populations in chronic hemodialysis patients. Am J Kidney Dis 1994; 24:443–452.

122. Gearing AJ, Hemingway I, Pigott R, et al: Soluble forms of vascular adhesion molecules, E-selectin, ICAM-1, and VCAM-1: pathological significance. Ann NY Acad Sci 1992; 667:324–331.

123. Rabb H, Calderon E, Bittle PA, Ramirez G: Alterations in soluble intercellular adhesion molecule-1 and vascular cell adhesion molecule-1 in hemodialysis patients. Am J Kidney Dis 1996; 27:239–243.

124. Rabb H, Agosti SJ, Bittle PA, et al: Alterations in soluble and leukocyte surface L-selectin (CD 62L) in hemodialysis patients. J Am Soc Nephrol 1995; 6:1445–1450.

125. Rabb H, Arnaout MA, Chandran P, Kehrli M: CD18-deficient cows have attenuated leukopenia during hemodialysis. J Am Soc Nephrol 1997; 7:1716.

126. Himmelfarb J, Zaoui P, Hakim R: Modulation of granulocyte LAM-1 and MAC-1 during dialysis: a prospective, randomized controlled trial. Kidney Int 1992; 41:388–395.

127. Hakim RM, Wingard RL, Parker RA: Effect of the dialysis membrane in the treatment of patients with acute renal failure. N Engl J Med 1994; 331:1338–1342.

128. Schiffl H, Lang SM, Konig A, et al: Biocompatible membranes in acute renal failure: prospective case-controlled study. Lancet 1994; 344:570–572.

129. Kurtal H, von Herrath D, Schaefer K: Is the choice of membrane important for patients with acute renal failure requiring hemodialysis? Artif Organs 1995; 19:391–394.

130. Valeri A, Radhakrishnan J, Ryan R, Powell D: Biocompatible dialysis membranes and acute renal failure: a study in postoperative acute tubular necrosis in cadaveric renal transplant recipients. Clin Nephrol 1996; 46:402–409.

131. Jones CH, Goutcher E, Newstead CG, et al: Hemodynamics and survival of patients with acute renal failure treated by continuous dialysis with two synthetic membranes. Artif Organs 1998; 22:638–643.

132. Gilbert P, Toto RD, Star RA: Variability of dialysis-induced neutropenia. J Am Soc Nephrol 1997; 8:236A.

133. Iyer VR, Eisen MB, Ross DT, et al: The transcriptional program in the response of human fibroblasts to serum. Science 1999; 283:83–87.

CHAPTER 7

Growth Factors, Signaling, and Renal Injury and Repair

Takaharu Ichimura ▪ Joseph V. Bonventre

INTRODUCTION

The kidney is exposed to many physical, chemical, and biological agents that can adversely affect its function and lead to glomerular, vascular, epithelial, or interstitial cell activation, injury, and, potentially, death by apoptotic or necrotic mechanisms. In addition, regions of the kidney are particularly susceptible to ischemia because of low basal oxygen tension and high metabolic demand in cells whose mechanism of energy generation is primarily oxidative phosphorylation. After a toxic or ischemic insult, there can be a great deal of anatomic and functional abnormality of the proximal tubules of the kidney; yet proximal tubule epithelial cells are able to undergo repair, regeneration, and proliferation, a feature that distinguishes these cells from heart and brain cells, which do not have the capacity to regenerate. This renal repair capability is a critical factor not only for the organ but also for the organism. Understanding how the kidney manages to repair injured cells and recover from acute renal failure (ARF) is of fundamental importance.

A growing body of knowledge about growth factors has begun to make an impact on the study of kidney physiology, pathology, and development. The kidney is rich in growth factors that act as mitogens, motogens, and morphogens. Growth factors may play an important role in development, homeostasis, and repair. However, growth factors can also produce adverse effects that contribute to the pathogenesis of renal disease. This chapter examines the characteristics of various growth factors that have been implicated in renal injury and repair. The pattern of expression of these growth factors is described for the normal adult kidney and, because renal repair recapitulates ontogeny, for the developing kidney. The regulation of growth factor expression, the effects of these agents on kidney damage and repair, and the current status of the use of growth factor inhibitors or growth factors themselves in models of human disease are also discussed. Finally, there is a discussion of signal transduction as it relates to the injury and repair phases of ARF.

RENAL PROXIMAL TUBULES: ACUTE DAMAGE AND REPAIR

The epithelial cells of the mammalian nephron are especially sensitive to ischemia and a wide variety of nephrotoxic agents.[1-4] The susceptibility to ischemia occurs despite the fact that the kidney receives 20% to 25% of total cardiac output, yet occupies less than 1% of the total body weight. At the same time, the ability of the tubule to concentrate and metabolize chemical species extracted from the blood adds a burden of susceptibility of this organ to toxicants.

Proximal tubules are able to undergo repair, regeneration, and proliferation after ischemic or nephrotoxic damage (see Chapter 3). In the outer cortex, the majority of cells are sublethally injured and undergo repair following the initiation of adequate reperfusion. There are four major phases during this regeneration process[5-11] (Fig. 7-1). The first phase consists of the death and exfoliation of the proximal tubule epithelial cells.[6, 9, 12] While cell death itself is not a regenerative response, in the process of dying, epithelial cells may generate signals that initiate the regenerative response. In this very early phase, stress response gene expression is also observed in renal tubules.[13-17] The accumulation of mononuclear cells becomes evident in this stage as well.[18, 19] Growth factors may play a role in determining the fate of the epithelial cells and may contribute to the generation of signals that result in neutrophil and monocyte infiltration into the tissue.

The second phase of regeneration is initiated with the appearance of poorly differentiated epithelial cells.[6, 9] After both toxin or ischemic injury, these cells possess a morphologically flattened appearance with a poorly differentiated brush border. Cells express vimentin, an embryonic marker for multipotent kidney mesenchyme.[10, 14, 20] This stage is therefore a "dedifferentiation" stage. The expression of vimentin and other proteins is similar to that expressed in the metanephric mesenchyme of the developing kidney and has led to the proposal that regeneration recapitulates aspects of development.[10, 14, 20] Interestingly, this characteristic dedifferentiation response is also recapitulated when differentiated cells are taken from an organ and placed in culture.[10] The change from a differentiated phenotype to a less differentiated one might be important for remodeling of the proximal tubule architecture. Growth factors have been implicated in the control of cell differentiation.[21]

In the third phase, a marked increase in proliferation of the surviving proximal tubule cells is evident.[14, 22] Proliferating cell nuclear antigen or bromodeoxyuridine labeling of newly synthesized DNA, after either ischemic or nephrotoxic damage, indicates extensive cell proliferation adjacent to the damaged area.[14, 22, 23] This is seen primarily in the S3 segment of proximal tubule cells. These proliferating cells are derived from apparently mature proximal tubule cells, which have

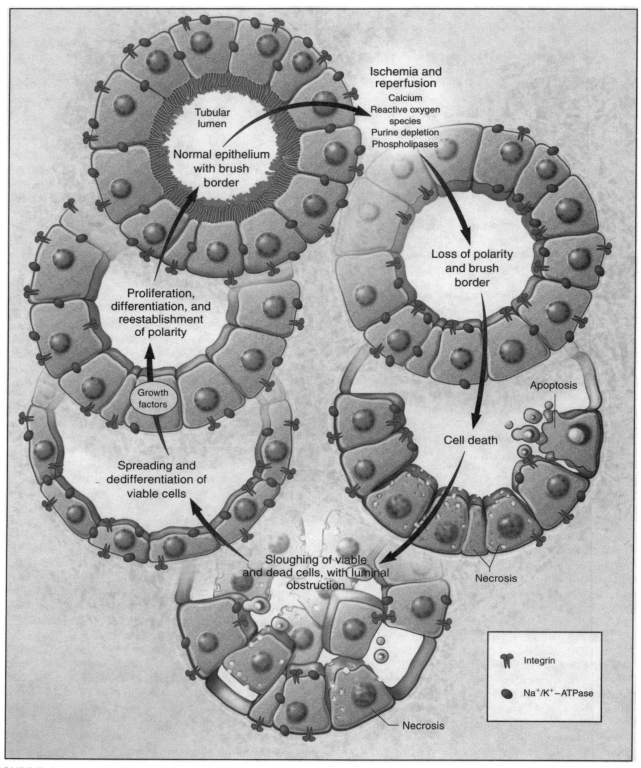

FIGURE 7–1 ■ *(See Color Plate)* Tubular-cell injury and repair in ischemic acute renal failure. After ischemia and reperfusion, morphologic changes occur in the proximal tubules, including loss of the brush border, loss of polarity, and redistribution of integrins and Na+, K+-ATPase to the apical surface. Calcium, reactive oxygen species, purine depletion, and phospholipases probably have a role in these changes in morphology and polarity as well as in the subsequent cell death that occurs as the result of necrosis and apoptosis. There is sloughing of viable and nonviable cells into the tubular lumen, resulting in the formation of casts and luminal obstruction and contributing to the reduction in the glomerular filtration rate. The severely damaged kidney can completely restore its structure and function. Spreading and dedifferentiation of viable cells occur during recovery from ischemic acute renal failure, which duplicates aspects of normal renal development. A variety of growth factors probably contribute to proliferation and the restoration of a normal tubular epithelium. (From Thadhani R, Pascual M, Bonventre JV: Acute renal failure. N Engl J Med 1996; 334:1448–1460; with permission.)

dedifferentiated. Thus differentiated proximal tubule cells retain the ability to dedifferentiate and proliferate. Growth factors may play an important role in this proliferative response.

The last phase of the regeneration process is the stage of redifferentiation.[5, 7] In this late phase, the poorly differentiated regenerative tubular cells regain their differentiated character and produce a normal proximal tubule epithelium. These cells are already in a postmitotic stage when they differentiate.[10] By the end of this phase, most damaged tubules have regained their essential functions and have recovered from the damage.

BIOLOGY OF REGENERATION AND REPAIR

Regeneration is the process through which an organism reconstructs parts of the body that have been lost or injured. Regeneration was first described by the Italian scientist Spallanzani[24] and has been studied for more than two centuries. Perhaps the best known example is the newt limb regeneration model in which an entire limb regenerates.[25] In developmental biology, the concept that regeneration is a form of true development has been accepted for a long time. Although there is diversity in regenerative capability among organisms, the capacity to regenerate is observed throughout the animal kingdom and is one of the most intriguing aspects of the tissue reaction to damage or ablation.[26]

Mammalian regenerative capability is more limited than that of lower vertebrates, and it is perhaps better to use the term *repair*. Both regeneration and repair processes require profound tissue remodeling reactions that are analogous to aspects of development.[26] At the molecular level, these remodeling reactions are regulated by the expression of genes that code for proteins essential to both development and regeneration. For example, ECM proteins and cellular proteins that regulate signal transduction are critical regulators of regenerative and developmental processes.[9, 27–34] Peptide growth factors that regulate mitogenesis, motogenesis, and morphogenesis of various types of cells probably play important roles during regeneration.[35–37] Understanding expression patterns of growth factors, the signaling molecules that regulate growth factor gene expression, and the roles played by growth factors in epithelial cell proliferation, cell-cell interactions, and cell-matrix interactions will greatly improve our comprehension of regeneration and repair processes. With better understanding comes better paradigms for treatment to decrease the injury or hasten the repair.

GROWTH FACTORS IN THE KIDNEY

Polypeptide growth factors are extracellular signaling molecules that are composed of single or multiple polypeptide chains and generate cellular signals by binding to specific cell surface receptors. Generally, growth factors have three types of function, which allow them to act as (1) mitogens that stimulate cell proliferation, (2) motogens that increase cell motility, and (3) morphogens that induce changes in multicellular architecture. Like other organs, the kidney is both a target and a source of polypeptide growth factors. The actions of growth factors in the kidney fall into five categories: endocrine, paracrine, juxtacrine, autocrine, and intracrine. The receptors for polypeptide growth factors are often transmembrane tyrosine or serine-threonine kinases that consist of an extracellular binding domain and an intracellular kinase domain.[38, 39]

Growth factors can have a beneficial effect on the injury and repair processes via a number of mechanisms. They can act as survival factors in the setting of proapoptotic influences.[40, 41] They can protect against a noxious environmental influence by potentiating cellular processes to counteract the impact of that environmental exposure. For example, epidermal growth factor protects gastric epithelial cells against acid-induced damage by activating Na^+/H^+ exchange.[42] Growth factors can promote survival by enhancing cell-cell and cell-ECM interactions.[43] They have been implicated in the production of nitric oxide,[43] which can be protective by enhancing local blood flow.

Growth factors can have a number of beneficial effects on the kidney in the process of repair, from potentiation of adaptive responses to a reduction in functional mass and mediation of the proliferative processes after acute renal injury.[44–47] In addition, growth factors play important roles in angiogenesis. For example, it has been proposed that hepatocyte growth factor (HGF) plays a role in capillary endothelial cell regeneration in the ischemically injured heart.[48] Growth factors are also involved in epithelial cell differentiation,[47] an important step in the restoration of function after injury. They can reestablish cell-ECM and cell-cell interactions, functions that are very important for differentiation and functional integrity of the epithelium.[49] The important roles that growth factors play in renal growth and in development during embryogenesis[50] provide further support for the notion that they play a critical role in ARF.

There are also maladaptive and pathologic effects of growth factors, however, such as those that occur in the fibrotic processes of the glomerulus and interstitium.[51–53] They can increase the synthesis of matrix components and reduce their degradation, may contribute to mesangial cell proliferation and hypertrophy, and can alter the immune response.[54] In the sections of this review that follow, the nature and functions of growth factor actions in the kidney are discussed, with special attention paid to the actions of individual growth factors that may provide insight into the role they play in ARF.

Growth Factors and Kidney Development

Because recovery from ARF recapitulates many aspects of renal development, the actions of growth factors in the two processes may be similar. Therefore, the importance of growth factors in kidney embryogenesis will be discussed. Growth factors can influence cell proliferation and differentiation in kidney development.[31-34, 44, 55] The mechanisms of growth factor actions, however, are complex. Although no single growth factor induces metanephrogenesis in vitro, a mixture of epidermal growth factor (EGF) and pituitary extract in the presence of ECM does induce metanephrogenesis.[56] Insulin-like growth factor-I (IGF-I), IGF-I receptors, IGF-II, and transforming growth factor-α (TGF-α) all are required for metanephrogenesis in vitro.[57-59] In kidney development in vivo, IGF-I, IGF-II, TGF-α, and TGF-βs are all produced by the kidney.[57, 60-62] TGF-βs act to inhibit the differentiation process in cultured metanephroi.[63] Increased renal EGF production is observed after birth in mice, suggesting a possible postpartum effect, because mice kidneys continue to develop after birth.[64] In metanephroi in culture, nerve growth factor (NGF) receptors are transiently expressed and inhibition of NGF expression with antisense oligonucleotides inhibits differentiation.[65] This result suggests that NGF may play a role during kidney development. Both HGF and its receptor c-met are expressed in developing kidneys as well, and HGF stimulates the differentiation of both proximal tubule and distal tubule/collecting duct cell lines.[66-68] Vascular endothelial growth factor (VEGF) and platelet-derived growth factor (PDGF) may also play important roles in renal vascular development. Both VEGF and its receptor are expressed during nephrogenesis, while PDGF and PDGF receptor deletion mutants display malformation of the glomeruli.[69-72] Vascular endothelial growth factor has been implicated in the stimulation of renal endothelial cell mitosis and angiogenesis in the developing kidney.[73]

The critical importance of growth factors for renal development also has been demonstrated by severe abnormalities that result from gene disruption of TGF-β family members, bone morphogenic protein-7 (BMP-7),[74, 75] glial cell line–derived neurotrophic factor (GDNF),[76-78] and c-ret,[79] which is a tyrosine kinase receptor for GDNF.[80, 81] Homozygous c-ret–null mice display renal agenesis due to inhibition of ureteric bud outgrowth.[79] A similar renal phenotype is observed in the GDNF-null mouse.[76-78] Transgenic mice embryos expressing fibroblast growth factor-7 (FGF-7) in serum driven by a liver-specific promoter demonstrated hyperplasia and cystic dilation of the collecting ducts in the kidney.[82] In FGF-7 null mice, when compared with wild-type mice, there is a smaller developing ureteric bud and a mature collecting system with fewer nephrons. In metanephric kidney organ cultures from rat embryos, ureteral bud growth is stimulated by exogenous FGF-7 in vitro.[83] Transgenic mice expressing a soluble dominant-negative mutant FGF receptor-2 IIIb that binds specific subsets of FGFs, including FGF-1 and FGF-7, have defects in the kidney and other organs.[84]

The WT1 gene is expressed in the embryonic kidney and its disruption causes failure of early kidney formation. Deletion of the Wilms' tumor suppressor gene, WT1, causes congenital malignancy of the metanephric blastema.[85] The WT1 gene product is a DNA-binding protein that has been found to repress expression of IGF-II and IGF-I receptor genes by interfering with egr-1 expression.[86-89] The WT1 gene product also represses a regulatory gene Pax-2 in the developing kidney.[90] Growth factors may regulate development via the differential activity of various transcription factors, such as WT1.

ROLES OF SPECIFIC GROWTH FACTORS IN KIDNEY INJURY AND REPAIR

Table 7–1[91-110] lists growth factors and their receptors found in the kidney. Tables 7–2[111-138] and 7–3[139-154] summarize the role of growth factors in kidney hypertrophy, repair, and pathophysiology.

Insulin-Like Growth Factors

The IGF family is composed of two homologous members, IGF-I and IGF-II.[155, 156] Insulin-like growth factor-I is produced in several tissues in a growth hormone–dependent manner. IGF-I is a 70–amino acid single-chain polypeptide, and IGF-II has 67 amino acids. Both share a structural similarity to insulin. In adult kidney, IGF-I is localized to the collecting ducts.[91] Collecting duct IGF-I production is enhanced by growth hormone and EGF.[157, 158] However, glomerular mesangial cells also express IGF-I in vitro.[92] IGF-I is mitogenic for rat proximal tubule epithelial cells (RPTE) in culture.[159] IGF-I, signaling through the IGF receptor, has been shown to have a potent prosurvival capability in the setting of apoptotic stimuli. It has been suggested that the tumor suppressor p53, a critical proapoptotic protein, may mediate some of its apoptotic effects by modulation of the IGF signaling pathway in cells.[160]

Blocking the action of IGF-I or IGF-II with antibodies impairs development of metanephroi in vitro.[161] Circulating IGF-II levels are high in fetal kidney but fall after birth in rodents, observations that suggest a role for IGF-II as a fetal growth factor.[155, 156] Transcription of the IGF-II gene is regulated by the Wilms' tumor gene product, WT1, through its interaction with the Egr-1 transcription factor.[88, 89] Mutations in WT1 prevent down-regulation of Egr-1–driven transcription, resulting in increased production of IGF-II by Wilms' tumors.

The IGF-I receptor is a typical transmembrane receptor tyrosine kinase and is present in glomeruli and the basolateral membranes of proximal tubules.[92, 93] The IGF-II receptor is identical to the mannose-6-phosphate receptor and is found in both the basolateral and the brush border membrane of proximal tubules.[44, 162] Both IGF-I and IGF-II bind to either IGF-I or insulin receptors.

Both IGF-I and IGF-II circulate complexed with carrier proteins of the IGF binding protein family that are also synthesized in the kidney.[163] There are six IGF binding proteins, and the local availability of these

TABLE 7–1. Growth Factors and Their Receptors in Kidney

GROWTH FACTOR	NEPHRON SEGMENT PRODUCING GROWTH FACTOR	LOCATION OF RECEPTOR	REFERENCE
IGF-I	Collecting duct	Proximal tubule	91 92 93
EGF	Distal tubule	Proximal tubule	94 95 96
TGF-α	Proximal tubule Distal tubule Collecting duct	Proximal tubule	97
HGF	Endothelial cell Mesenchymal cell	N/K	98 99
TGF-β1	Distal tubule Collecting duct Glomerulus Proximal tubule in outer medulla	N/K	100 101
PDGF	Glomerulus	Glomerulus Mesenchymal cell	102 103
FGF-1	Glomerulus Distal tubule Thick ascending limb Collecting duct Blood vessel	Papilla Medulla	104 22
FGF-2	Proximal tubule	N/K	104 105
FGF-7	Papilla Mesenchymal cell	Papilla Medulla	106
NGF	Collecting duct	Glomerulus	107 108
VEGF	Glomerulus Collecting duct	Glomerulus Capillary	109
OP-1/BMP-7	Collecting duct	N/K	110

N/K, not known.

proteins may regulate the biological actions of IGF-I and IGF-II. In addition, different binding proteins may mediate different effects of IGFs.[164] Some carrier proteins have been shown to function as both agonists and antagonists for the biological activity of IGF-I in vitro.[44]

IGF-I mRNA and protein levels in the kidney are influenced by the level of both growth hormone and the circulating IGF-I.[165] In hypersomatotropism, both renal hypertrophy and hyperfunction may be mediated by IGF-I.[117, 157] Increased expression of IGF-I in collecting ducts has been shown in conditions characterized by compensatory growth following partial loss of kidney mass, such as occurs with unilateral nephrectomy, partial infarction, or nephron loss associated with a wide variety of glomerular or tubulointerstitial diseases.[111–114, 118] Increased IGF-I is detectable in whole kidney and kidney cortex after damage.[118] Immunoreactive IGF-I is detectable in the collecting ducts and, transiently, in the regenerating cells after ischemic injury to the kidney.[115] In the folic acid–treated rat kidney, mRNA levels of the IGF-I receptor, IGF binding protein (IGFBP)-1 and -2 are increased, whereas mRNA levels of IGF-I, IGFBP-3, and IGFBP-5 are decreased.[116] In the radiocontrast nephropathy model, cortical IGF-I protein and renal IGFBP-1 mRNA increase, whereas medullary IGF-I mRNA and renal IGFBPs decrease.[166] Hepatic IGFBP-2 mRNA increased in IGF-I–treated rats with ischemic ARF.[119] It has been suggested that regulation of IGFBPs may modify IGF-I function during the repair process.

Administration of exogenous IGF-I can accelerate recovery of the postischemic kidney in rats.[139, 140] The beneficial effect of IGF-I is observed when the agent is administered 0.5 hour, 5 hours, or 24 hours after the initiation of reperfusion.[140] The mechanism of the enhanced recovery potentiated by IGF-I administration may be due to its ability to increase glomerular filtration rate (GFR) via altered hemodynamics or to stimulate proximal tubule epithelial repair, regeneration, or proliferation.[44, 139] The effects of IGF-I may be direct or indirect, mediated by proteins whose expression is up-regulated. As an example, osteopontin has been shown to be up-regulated in ischemic models of renal injury[167, 168] and has been shown by a differential display polymerase chain reaction (PCR) technique to be up-regulated in response to IGF-I after ischemic damage.[169] This protein contains an RGD cell adhesion motif and has been implicated in tissue remodeling and repair.

The therapeutic potential of IGF-I for preservation of renal function was tested in humans undergoing surgical procedures involving the suprarenal aorta or the renal arteries.[170] None of the patients in the study developed postoperative severe deterioration in renal function. Although a higher proportion of patients in the placebo group had a decline in renal function

TABLE 7–2. Effect of Growth Factors in Kidney Hypertrophy, Repair, and Pathophysiology

GROWTH FACTOR	CHANGE IN LEVELS	TISSUE RESPONSE	MODEL	REFERENCE
IGF-I	Increase	Hypertrophy	UNX	111
	Increase	Hypertrophy	UNX	112
	Increase	Hypertrophy	UNX	113
	Increase	Hypertrophy	UNX	114
	Increase (in PT)	Repair	Ischemia	115
	Decrease	Repair	Folic acid	116
	Increase	Hypersomatotropism		117
	Increase	Renal mass Reduction	Partial infarction With UNX	118
	Increase	Repair	Radiocontrast	119
IGF-I receptor	Increase	Repair	Folic acid	116
EGF	Increase (in DT)	Hypertrophy	UNX	120
	Increase (as soluble)	Repair	Ischemia	121
	Increase (EGF binding)	Repair	Ischemia	122
	Redistribution (to PT)	Repair	Aminoglycoside	123
	Increase (in PT)	Repair	Ischemia	124
	Decrease	Repair	Ischemia, cisplatin	125
	Decrease	Repair	Ischemia	126
	Decrease	Repair	Aminoglycoside	18
	Decrease		Aminoglycoside	127
HB-EGF	Increased (in CT, CD)	Repair	Ischemia	128
	Increase	Repair	Ischemia	129
	Increase (in G)	Glomerulonephritis		130
EGF receptor	Phosphorylation	Repair	HgCl$_2$	131
HGF	Increase (in M)	Hypertrophy	UNX	98
		Repair	Ischemia, CCl$_4$	
	Increase	Repair	HgCl$_2$	99
	Increase (in serum)	ARF patients		132
HGF receptor	Increase	Hypertrophy	UNX	133
	Increase	Repair	Ischemia	134
	Increase	Repair	Folic acid	135
TGF-β1	Increase (in PT)	Repair	Ischemia	101
TGF-β	Increase	Hypertrophy	UNX	136
TGF-β1	Increase	Glomerulonephritis		137
FGF-1	Increase (in Mø, PT)	Repair	Cysteine conjugate	22
FGF-7	Increase (in M)	Repair	Cysteine conjugate	106
FGF-R2	Increase	Repair	Cysteine conjugate	106
OP-1	Decrease	Repair	Ischemia	138

CD, collecting duct; *DT,* distal tubule; *M,* mesenchymal cell; *PT,* proximal tubule; *unx,* unilateral nephrectomy; *G,* glomerulus; *Mø,* macrophage.

(33% vs 22%), there were no significant differences in level of serum creatinine at discharge, length of hospital stay, length of intubation, or incidence of dialysis or death. In a prospective randomized trial that compared intensive care unit patients with ARF with a placebo-treated group and patients who were administered IGF-I subcutaneously every 12 hours for up to 14 days, there were no differences between the groups in changes from baseline of creatinine clearance, GFR, urine volume, serum blood urea nitrogen, creatinine, albumin, or transferrin, need for dialysis, or mortality.[171] It should be noted, however, that the patient population was very heterogeneous, and the first dose of hormone was administered as long as 6 days after the onset of ARF in some of the patients.

Epidermal Growth Factors

Epidermal growth factor is a mitogen for a broad spectrum of cells,[172] including proximal tubule epithelial cells in culture.[59] EGF and TGF-α belong to the same gene family, and both act on the same EGF receptor.[172, 173] EGF consists of 53 amino acids, and its expression is highest in the salivary gland and kidney in adult mammals. The kidney is the source of urinary EGF, where its concentration (5×10^{-10} M) is higher than in blood ($<10^{-12}$ M).[44] Both EGF and TGF-α precursors contain membrane-spanning regions that anchor them to the plasma membrane.[172, 173] These precursor forms are biologically active. Mature EGF and TGF-α are processed to their circulating forms by proteolytic processing of the extracellular portion of their precursors.[172, 173] There are two possible signaling pathways, depending on whether these factors are soluble or membrane anchored. When EGF and TGF-α are released from the membrane, they can function in an endocrine, paracrine, or autocrine fashion, whereas if EGF and TGF-α are bound to the membrane of a cell adjacent to other cells expressing EGF receptor, they can function in a juxtacrine fashion.[173]

Heparin-binding epidermal growth factor–like growth factor (HB-EGF) is another member of the EGF gene family. This secreted form of the growth factor is a 22-kDa heparin-binding protein originally isolated from conditioned media of a macrophage-like

TABLE 7–3. Effect of Growth Factors in Kidney Hypertrophy, Repair, and Pathophysiology

GROWTH FACTOR	EFFECT	TISSUE RESPONSE	MODEL	REFERENCE
IGF-I	Enhancement of recovery	Repair	Ischemia	139
	Enhancement of recovery	Repair	Ischemia	140
	Preservation of renal function		Postoperative human patients	141
	No effect		Human ARF patients in ICU	142
EGF	Enhancement of recovery	Repair	Ischemia	143
	Enhancement of recovery	Repair	Ischemia	144
	Enhancement of recovery	Repair	HgCl$_2$	145
HGF	Enhancement of recovery	Hypertrophy	UNX	146
	Enhancement of recovery	Repair	Ischemia	146
	Enhancement of recovery	Repair	HgCl$_2$, Cisplatin	147
	Dysfunction prevention		CRF model mice	148
OP-1	Severity reduction	Repair	Ischemia	110
TGF-β1	Suppression of pathogenesis by anti-TGF-β1	Glomerulonephritis		149
	Antibody or inhibitor			150
	Suppression of ECM	Accumulation by dominant-negative receptor		151
FGF-2	Inhibition of cell proliferation of endothelium by anti-FGF-2 antibody	Hypertrophy	UNX	152
FGF-7	Proliferation of urothelium		Normal rat	153
PDGF	Proliferation of interstitium		Normal rat	154

UNX, unilateral nephrectomy.

cell line, U-937 cells.[174] The membrane-bound precursor form migrates at 27 kDa on sodium dodecyl sulfate silver-polyacrylamide gel electrophoresis (SDS-PAGE). It is a potent fibroblast and epithelial cell mitogen that has been implicated in wound healing. HB-EGF is found in the ureteric bud of the developing kidney as early as day 14.5 of gestation, and persists in structures arising from the bud during embryonic development of the kidney.[129]

In the kidney, the precursor form of EGF predominates. Both the EGF protein and mRNA are found in distal tubules and thick ascending limbs in the adult mouse.[94, 175] In distal tubular cells, prepro-EGF is localized in the luminal part of the membrane.[94] TGF-α is expressed largely in the collecting ducts.[97] The EGF receptor (EGFR) is a typical transmembrane tyrosine kinase. EGFRs are expressed in glomeruli, proximal tubules, medullary interstitial cells, and collecting ducts.[96] In these epithelial cells, the EGFR is present on the basolateral membrane.[95]

Immunoreactive EGF production is increased by compensatory renal hypertrophy, and there is redistribution within distal tubule cells.[120] This redistribution of EGF to the basolateral surface may reflect release into the interstitial space, where EGF can interact with receptors on the basolateral part of other cell types. Injection of anti-EGF antibodies inhibited renal tubular cell proliferation, but not hypertrophy, in uninephrectomized mice.[176] In experimental models of membranous and minimal change nephropathy, HB-EGF mRNA and protein were increased in glomerular epithelial cells.[130]

Expression of EGF mRNA and protein decreases rapidly after ischemic injury or gentamicin-induced renal injury; however, the binding capacity of EGF to the proximal tubules, presumably a reflection of an increased number of receptors, increases.[18, 122, 125, 127] Decreased EGF mRNA expression is due to the diminished transcription, rather than instability, of the mRNA.[126] There is an increase of immunoreactive EGF receptors in the proximal tubules of the postischemic rat and rabbit kidney.[124] Phosphorylation of the EGF receptor was observed in the mercuric-chloride–injured rat kidney.[131] Exogenous EGF administration in vivo enhances proliferation and accelerates recovery of damaged proximal tubules after ischemic or mercuric chloride–induced damage.[143–145] Although these observations suggest the involvement of EGF in kidney regeneration, there is a lack of consensus on the role of endogenous EGF.

Induction of HB-EGF mRNA is increased in the outer medulla after ischemia or mercuric chloride damage in rat kidney.[128] The injury-induced increase of HB-EGF may compensate for the deficiency of EGF after damage. HB-EGF protein induction was also observed in gentamicin-damaged rat kidneys.[129] In a segmental infarct model, HB-EGF mRNA was found to be up-regulated in the tubular epithelial cells bordering the infarct area, with maximal in situ hybridization signals observed 5 days after the ischemia.[177]

ProHB-EGF and CD9 co-localize at the cell membrane. Transfection of renal epithelial cells (NRK 52E) with proHB-EGF increased renal epithelial cell survival by promoting cell-cell and cell-ECM interactions.[43] A complex, which includes CD9 and β1 integrin, forms at the site of HB-EGF on the cell membrane.[178] It has been proposed by Takemura and colleagues[43] that coexpression of proHB-EGF and CD9 may render the renal epithelial cells more resistant to disruption of cell-cell and cell-matrix interactions and could accelerate the reestablishment of these attachments.

Transforming Growth Factor-βs

Transforming growth factor-βs are pleiotropic growth regulators that have diverse biological activity, depending on the cell target.[39, 179–181] These growth factors can either promote or inhibit cell proliferation or differentiation. Transforming growth factor-β also stimulates the expression of ECM proteins. These actions suggest that TGF-β might be an important regulator of tissue reconstruction.[179] Indeed TGF-βs have been tested as wound healing agents.[180] These effects on ECM formation, however, also contribute to the negative side of wound repair, ie, excessive fibrosis and sclerotic disease in the kidneys and other organs.[51]

The TGF-βs are a large gene family comprising a homologous group of dimeric polypeptides and another group of more distantly related peptides.[39, 179–181] The first group consists of TGF-β1 to TGF-β5. The second group contains the müllerian-inhibiting substances (MIS), inhibins, activins, bone morphogenic proteins (BMPs), and glial cell line–derived neurotrophic factor (GDNF). These polypeptides are first synthesized as an unprocessed large latent form. The mature form of TGF-β1 is a homodimer of disulfide-linked 112–amino acid subunits.[179] In mouse kidney, TGF-β1 protein is present in the distal tubule.[100] TGF-β1 inhibits proliferation of rat proximal tubule epithelial cells in vitro.[159] Messenger RNA of BMP-7, also known as osteogenic protein-1 (OP-1), is also expressed in mouse kidney.[182]

Unlike other growth factor receptors, TGF-β and activin receptors are membrane serine-threonine kinases, and form heterodimers composed of type 1 receptor and type 2 receptors, which then initiate a signal transduction cascade that is only partially understood.[39, 183, 184] The signaling pathway mediated by TGF-β receptors has been evaluated with the use of both *Xenopus* and mammalian cell systems. The receptors phosphorylate Smad family transcription factor proteins, thereby inducing nuclear translocation.[184, 185] Cardiac Smad-2, -3, and -4 proteins are significantly increased in border and scar tissues 8 weeks after myocardial infarction.[186] Immunofluorescent studies indicate that Smad proteins localize proximal to the cellular nuclei present in the infarct scar. Expression of TGF-β RI (53-kDa) protein was significantly reduced in the scar, whereas the 75-kDa and 110-kDa isoforms of TGF-β RII were unchanged and significantly increased in the scar, respectively. It has been suggested that TGF-β – Smad signaling may be involved in the remodeling of the infarct scar after the completion of wound healing via ongoing stimulation of matrix deposition. TGF-β has been implicated in maladaptive

responses in the kidney.[51, 187] In an acute form of mesangial injury induced by antithymocyte antiserum injection, the expression of TGF-β1 increases.[137] Administration of anti–TGF-β1 antiserum during development of experimentally induced glomerulonephritis in rats suppressed development of disease and ECM formation.[149] The same beneficial effect was observed after administration of decorin, a natural TGF-β inhibitor.[150] In vivo transfection of TGF-β gene into rat kidney induced glomerulosclerosis.[188] Gene transfer by systemic delivery of a soluble dominant-negative TGF-β receptor reduced accumulation of ECM in the rat glomerulosclerosis model.[151] Thus, TGF-βs may play important roles in the progression of glomerulonephritis.

TGF-β levels increase after unilateral nephrectomy in the rat.[136] Renal TGF-β1 mRNA level is up-regulated in regenerating proximal tubules in postischemic kidney.[101] Expression of several genes known to encode proteins that regulate ECM synthesis, such as plasminogen activator inhibitor-1 (PAI-1), tissue inhibitor of metaloproteinase-1 (TIMP-1), α1(IV) collagen, and fibronectin-EIIIA (FN-EIIIA), also increased in a TGF-β1–dependent manner.[189] These results suggest involvement of TGF-β1 in the regulation of ECM synthesis in the postischemic kidney. This growth factor may be important for the development of fibrosis, especially when the ischemia is chronic, as occurs in atherosclerotic and many other forms of renal disease. Acute and chronic rejection of rat renal transplants, which is associated with tissue ischemia and leads to chronic scarring, is associated with an increase in kidney TGF-β1 mRNA levels.[190]

Disruption of BMP-7–OP-1 expression in BMP–7 null mice results in severe abnormalities in kidney development.[74, 75] Bone morphogenic protein-7 is normally expressed at high levels in the embryonic kidney. In the postischemic kidney, medullary OP-1 mRNA expression is decreased, and administration of OP-1 reduces the severity of the postischemic injury.[110, 138, 191]

Glial cell line–derived neurotrophic factor is the ligand for the receptor tyrosine kinase c-*ret* with a coreceptor GDNF receptor α.[80, 81] This is an unusual combination of growth factor and receptor interaction in which TGF-β family member GDNF binds the ret tyrosine kinase.[192]

Platelet-Derived Growth Factor

Platelet-derived growth factor is a heterodimeric polypeptide consisting of A and B chains.[193] The genes for the subunits are localized on different chromosomes, and the dimer is assembled post-transcriptionally.[193] The majority of monomers form heterodimers, but homodimeric complexes exist.[193] The mature PDGF polypeptide is also processed from larger precursors. The target cell types for PDGF are cells of connective tissue (mesenchyme) origin that are involved in wound healing processes in a variety of tissues. Glomerular mesangial cells,[102] renal epithelial cells,[194] Wilms' tumor cells, and human fetal kidney cells express PDGF.[195] PDGF receptors are typical transmembrane tyrosine kinases consisting of two types, type α and type β. Both PDGF α and β receptors are present in the glomerulus and on interstitial cells.[103]

Platelet-derived growth factor has been implicated in maladaptive responses in the kidney.[51, 187] PDGF and its receptor expression increase during experimental as well as human proliferative glomerulonephritis.[103] The infusion of PDGF into rat kidney induces glomerulosclerosis and tubulointerstitial myofibroblast formation.[154, 196] In vivo expression of the PDGF transgene in rat kidney induces glomerulosclerosis.[188] Thus, PDGF may play an important role in the progression of glomerulonephritis. When PDGF-BB is administered to normal rats, there is induction of tubulointerstitial myofibroblasts in the kidney.[154]

Immunostainable PDGF-BB and PDGF-AB is detected in the afferent arterioles and interlobular arteries of kidneys exposed to ischemia or cyclosporin A.[197] Human proximal tubule cells secrete PDGF-AB, and these cells respond to soluble factors generated by cortical fibroblasts by increasing their production of PDGF-AB.[198] It is possible that a positive-feedback process involving PDGF comes into play in the postischemic kidney, especially when the ischemia is prolonged, as may occur during allograft rejection.

Fibroblast Growth Factors

Fibroblast growth factors are mitogenic, angiogenic, and differentiation factors for various types of epithelial and mesenchymal cells.[199] Fibroblast growth factors have been implicated in wound healing, angiogenesis, and cancer. Fibroblast growth factors are expressed in tissues of neuroectodermal and mesodermal origin.[200–202] The FGF gene family is composed of at least 18 structurally related polypeptides. FGF-1 (acidic FGF) and FGF-2 (basic FGF) are the prototypic and best characterized FGFs. These two factors share 50% homology and lack a conventional signal sequence. Fibroblast growth factors 3 through 6 were identified as oncogenes capable of transforming cells in vitro and in vivo. Their expression appears to be limited to transformed cells and the period of development.[200–202] Fibroblast growth factors 7 through 9 were isolated from conditioned medium obtained from various cell lines.[203, 204] Fibroblast growth factor-9 also lacks a conventional signal sequence but is nevertheless actively secreted.[204–206] Fibroblast growth factor-10 was identified from the rat lung by homology-based PCR.[207] Fibroblast growth factor-11 to FGF-14 (FGF homologous factors [FHFs] 1 to 4) were identified from the human retina by a combination of random cDNA sequencing, database searches, and homology-based PCR.[208] FGF-15 was identified as a downstream target of a chimeric homeodomain oncoprotein.[209] Fibroblast growth factor-16 and FGF-17 were identified by homology-based PCR from the rat heart and embryos, respectively.[210, 211] The most recent member of this large family is FGF-18, which was isolated from rat embryos by homology-based PCR.[212]

Kidney expresses several FGFs during both adult and fetal developmental stages. Historically, the metanephric kidney has been a recognized source of angiogenic activities, and embryonic kidney–derived angiogenic activity was characterized as a heparin-binding FGF-like factor.[213, 214] Subsequently, both FGF-1 and FGF-2 proteins and mRNA were identified in adult kidney.[215–217] FGF-1 mRNA is also found in the developing kidney and in Wilms' tumor.[218, 219] Kidney growth factor-1 and FGF-2 are potent mitogens for primary cultures of rat proximal tubule epithelial cells.[159] Immunohistochemical analysis of FGF-1 and FGF-2 in the fetal rat kidney suggests that both factors are localized to the mesenchyme. Fibroblast growth factor-2 is also found in basement membrane.[220, 221] However, FGF-1 is also present in glomeruli, blood vessels, and the urothelium in adult human and rat kidneys, suggesting that developing kidneys and mature kidneys have different FGF-1 expression patterns.[22, 104] Fibroblast growth factor-1 mRNA and protein are found in cultured proximal tubule epithelial cells and regenerating tubules in the damaged kidney.[22, 222] It is interesting that FGFs have been implicated in the regulation of successive rounds of branching that occur during development of the lung branching,[223] a branching process analogous to what happens in the kidney tubule and vascular structures during development.

Fibroblast growth factor-2 is detected in mesangial cells both in vitro and in vivo.[105] Administration of anti–FGF-2 antibody decreased proliferation of endothelial cells during compensatory renal growth.[152] Fibroblast growth factor-7 and FGF-9 mRNA and protein have also been detected in the kidney.[205, 224] Fibroblast growth factor-7 mRNA is expressed in the collecting duct mesenchyme in the embryonic kidney, and at highest levels in the medulla and papilla in the adult rat kidney.[106, 225] Systemic administration of recombinant human FGF-7 to rat and monkey increases cell proliferation in the collecting duct and transitional epithelium of the kidney.[153] The FGFs bind to four closely related receptor tyrosine kinases. Dimerization of receptor monomers leads to activation of kinase domains and transphosphorylation in a manner similar to other growth factor receptors. The FGF-1 receptor has at least seven tyrosine phosphorylation sites. A number of human abnormalities are associated with mutations in the FGF receptors. Fibroblast growth factor receptors (FGFRs) constitute a gene family of four membrane receptor tyrosine kinases. Genes for FGF receptors generate a diversity of mRNAs through alternative splicing.[226, 227] Each receptor and receptor splice variant has an affinity for a different FGF; however, FGF-1 appears to be a universal ligand for all FGF receptors identified to date.

All four FGFR messages are detected in the kidney.[228] FGFR1 is expressed in mesenchyme, Bowman's capsule, and developing tubules in embryonic kidney.[229, 230] FGFR2, including a splice variant specific for FGF-7, is localized to collecting ducts at the same stage of development.[225, 229–231] A similar distribution is also seen within adult rat kidney, where FGFR2 IIIb mRNA is expressed largely in the papilla with weaker expression in the outer medulla.[106] For FGFR1, the β-form is the most dominant splice variant in the developing kidney.[232] FGFR3 mRNA is detected in adult kidney, and FGFR4 mRNA has been localized in collecting ducts in the metanephron.[233, 234]

Because each splice variant of FGFRs possesses a different specificity for each FGF, each receptor variant may play a distinct role in the development and functional response of the kidney to different stimuli. When proximal tubule damage is caused by the nephrotoxicant cysteine conjugate, S-(1,1,2,2-tetrafluoroethyl)-l-cysteine (TFEC), FGF-1 protein expression is increased in invading mononuclear cells at 24 hours after the administration of TFEC. Expression of FGF-1 protein is also increased in poorly differentiated vimentin-positive regenerating epithelial cells.[22] Rat proximal tubule epithelial cells produce FGF-1 in culture, and when rat proximal tubule epithelial cells and pig LLC-PK1 cells are mechanically injured, these cells release autocrine mitotic activity.[222, 235] Expression of FGF-1 persists in the foci of macrophages, interstitial cells, and nephropathic tubules within areas of interstitial expansion 2 weeks after damage.[22] These expression patterns imply that transient FGF-1 expression could play autocrine mitogenic or morphogenic roles during tubular regeneration, whereas persistent expression may be associated with tubular degeneration. The affinity of FGFs for heparin-like molecules, including heparin sulfate proteoglycans, which are located on the cell surface and in the interstitium, probably acts to restrict its diffusion away from the site of production, making the spatial and temporal relationships between FGF and FGF receptors an important regulatory influence.

In the same TFEC nephrotoxic model, FGF-7 (keratinocyte growth factor, KGF) mRNA increased throughout the kidney after 24 hours of toxicant administration, particularly in the outer strip of the outer medulla, the primary site of TFEC-induced damage to proximal tubules, and in the inner medulla.[106] Levels of FGFR2 IIIb, the KGF receptor, mRNA expression are also increased after damage, particularly in the outer stripe of the outer medulla and the inner medulla.[106] These observations suggest involvement of FGFs and their receptors during the repair process. When FGF-7 is administered to normal rats, proliferation of urothelium is observed.[153]

Nerve Growth Factor

Nerve growth factor and other neurotrophic factors function in the regulation of neural development and the maintenance of the neuronal network.[236] The four structurally related members of the neurotrophic factor family are NGF, brain-derived neurotrophic factor (BDNF), neurotrophin-3 (NT-3), and neurotrophin-4/5 (NT-4/5).[236, 237] Another type of neurotrophic factor is called ciliary neurotrophic factor (CNTF).[237] NGF-transgenic mice have reduced brain injury when permanent focal ischemia is imposed by occlusion of the middle cerebral artery.[238] Brain-derived neurotrophic

factor prevents neuronal death and glial activation after global ischemia in the rat.[239] In the kidney, NT-3 mRNA is found,[107, 236] and NGF is localized to the mouse collecting duct principal cell apical and perinuclear cytoplasm.

There are two types of NGF receptors, the high-affinity trk, tyrosine kinase, receptors and the low-affinity p75 receptor.[240] The high-affinity receptor for NGF is trkA; for BDNF and NT-4/5, it is trkB; for NT-3, it is trkC. P75 is a low-affinity receptor without a tyrosine kinase domain and binds all members of the neurotrophin family.[237, 240] P75 is present in the glomerulus and on interstitial cells in human kidney.[108]

Hepatocyte Growth Factor

Hepatocyte growth factor, also known as scatter factor, was originally isolated from partially hepatectomized rats as a serum factor that stimulated growth of hepatocytes.[241] Structurally, HGF is a heterodimer, with a 68-kDa A-chain and a 34-kDa B-chain, with 38% homology to plasminogen.[242] Hepatocyte growth factor is produced by cells of mesenchymal origin, Kupffer cells, and human embryonic lung fibroblasts.[243, 244] In kidney, HGF is localized in peritubular endothelial cells and has mitogenic activity for proximal tubule epithelial cells in vitro.[98, 245, 246] The HGF receptor is the oncogene c-met gene product, which is a transmembrane tyrosine kinase protein.[247]

Hepatocyte growth factor levels increase after unilateral nephrectomy in the rat.[98, 134] Hepatocyte growth factor is another growth factor that is involved in the adaptive response of the damaged kidney. Hepatocyte growth factor and c-met mRNA and HGF activity are increased in chemically or ischemia-damaged kidney.[98, 133, 134] In the damaged kidney, the expression of HGF is localized to interstitial cells and macrophages.[99] In the folic acid–treated rat kidney, renal HGF mRNA, c-met protein, and plasma HGF increase with increased cell proliferation, whereas renal HGF protein decreases.[135] Serum HGF concentration increases in ARF patients compared with chronic renal failure patients.[132] In studies involving the administration of HGF to animals, this growth factor has been shown to protect the tubular epithelium from damage and to accelerate recovery from tubular injury in the postischemic or nephrotoxicant-damaged kidney.[146, 147] Administration of HGF to a mouse in a model of chronic renal disease (ICGN strain) prevented progression of renal dysfunction and fibrosis.[148]

Vascular Endothelial Growth Factor

Vascular endothelial growth factor is a heparin-binding angiogenic factor also known as vascular permeability factor.[248] Four variants of different size are produced from one gene by alternative splicing.[248] Owing to its specificity for endothelial cells, VEGF is a highly specific angiogenic factor and may be involved in neovascularization and the maintenance of blood vessels during development, wound healing, and tumorigenesis. In the kidney, VEGF expression is detected primarily in glomeruli and collecting duct epithelium in embryonic and adult kidneys.[69, 109] Simian virus 40 (SV40) large T-antigen–transformed proximal tubule epithelial cells and other transformed epithelial cells express VEGF.[249, 250]

The VEGF receptors consist of three transmembrane tyrosine kinases: Flk1, FLT1, and FLT4. The Flk1 mRNA is present in both adult and fetal mouse kidney.[251] Flk1 and FLT1 are both co-expressed in glomerular endothelium and peritubular capillaries in fetal and adult human kidneys.[109]

Angiogenesis is an important response to ischemia. Angiogenic factors have been found in lymph draining from postischemic kidneys.[252] In a model of ARF due to glomerular endothelial cell injury, VEGF production was sharply increased in the glomerulus.[253] The role of VEGF and angiogenesis in recovery from ischemic ARF has not been adequately explored.

MITOGEN-ACTIVATED PROTEIN KINASE CASCADES AND TRANSCRIPTION RESPONSES IN RENAL INJURY AND REPAIR

Growth factors exert their actions on cells via a number of different signaling mechanisms. In this chapter, discussion is limited to the mitogen-activated protein (MAP) kinases pathways, for which there are some data from ARF studies. The intracellular signaling events ultimately lead to the transcription of genes whose encoded proteins mediate a response of proliferation, hypertrophy, differentiation, or apoptosis. In vertebrates, many of the stimuli that result in these important cellular responses initiate intracellular signaling events that converge on a set of cellular kinase cascades collectively called the MAP kinase cascades. Three families of MAP kinases have been identified in mammalian cells. These kinase pathways and other cellular signaling pathways are critically important for the regulation of transcriptional events.[254]

The most well characterized of the three MAP kinase cascades is the extracellular signal-regulated kinase (ERK) cascade. Numerous studies have demonstrated that the ERKs are critical to the mitogenic response, to cellular differentiation, and, in some cells, to the induction of hypertrophy.[254] The ERKs are activated by growth factors and many other agonists, including vasoactive peptides, via their receptors and associated molecules, including G-proteins. The two other MAP kinase cascades are activated by cellular stress. One of these is called the p54 MAP kinase, stress-activated protein kinases (SAPKs), or Jun N-terminal kinase (JNK) cascade. Cellular stresses such as oxidant stress, reperfusion of ischemic tissue, mechanical stretch, shear stress, or exposure to the inflammatory cytokines TNF-α or IL-1β, or vasoactive peptides, can activate the SAPK/JNK pathway. P38 and related kinases represent the third cascade and are also stress-response MAP kinases. P38s are activated by many of the same stimuli that activate the SAPK/JNKs, yet the two pathways defined by these two kinases are independently regulated. Some stresses activate the p38 pathway in preference to the SAPK/JNK pathway, and other stresses preferentially activate the SAPK/JNK pathway.

Upon activation, ERK proteins translocate to the nucleus.[255, 256] ERKs phosphorylate and activate several members of the Ets-domain transcription factor family, including Elk-1, SAP1, Ets-1, and Ets-2.[257–259] Elk-1 and the related SAP-1 and SAP-2 are ternary complex factors, which form a complex with SRF (serum response factor) and together bind to the promoter of a number of genes, including c-fos, that contain the serum response element.[260]

The family of rat S6 protein kinases (RSKs), which are substrates of the ERKs, also translocate to the nucleus when the ERK cascade is activated.[261] RSK2 phosphorylates the cAMP response element–binding protein (CREB) at Ser133, which allows it to bind to the co-activator CBP (CREB-binding protein). Phosphorylation of Ser133 is critical for expression of c-fos in response to some growth factors.[262] ERKs also phosphorylate c-Myc in vitro and may play a role in regulation of c-Myc in vivo.[263]

Our laboratory found that the SAPKs are not activated by ischemia alone but are markedly activated by reperfusion of ischemic kidney[15, 264] (Fig. 7–2). Di Mari and colleagues[265] found that administration of N-acetylcysteine inhibited the ischemia-induced increase in SAPK/JNK activity and partially protected the kidney against ischemic injury. Whether the protection was related to the decrease in SAPK/JNK activity or to other antioxidant effects of N-acetylcysteine was not established. In contrast, p38 is activated during the ischemic phase in kidney and heart, but activity declines during reperfusion.[15, 264, 266, 267]

The SAPKs phosphorylate and activate a bZIP transcription factor, ATF-2. The SAPKs are the predominant ATF-2 transactivation domain kinases in the postischemic kidney, suggesting that the SAPKs are physiologically relevant ATF-2 kinases.[260] ATF-2 can form homodimers, or heterodimers with other members of its family, ATF-3 and CREB, or with c-Jun or NF-κB, suggesting it may play a role in the activation of transcription from many promoters. For example, a c-Jun/ATF-2 dimer appears to control induction of c-jun in response to cellular stresses, and it is likely that the SAPKs transduce this signal in the postischemic kidney by phosphorylating both transcription factors.[268]

Di Mari and coworkers[41] have found that whereas JNK is activated in both cortex and inner stripe of the outer medulla, the ERK pathway is activated only in the inner stripe, in which the thick ascending limbs predominate. These results, together with their in vitro data, which showed that proximal tubule cells were more susceptible to oxidant injury than were thick ascending limb cells and ERK activation only occurred in thick ascending limb cells, the authors proposed that cell survival in the postischemic kidney relies on ERK activation.

Conclusion

The kidney is exposed to many physical, chemical, and biological events that can lead to impairment of

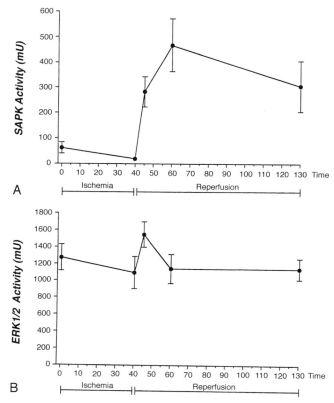

FIGURE 7–2 ■ Effect of ischemia and reperfusion on kidney SAPK and ERK-1 and ERK-2 activities. *A,* Activity of SAPKs. Anesthetized rats were subjected to unilateral renal ischemia (40 min) followed by reperfusion for 5, 20, or 90 minutes. SAPKs were immunoprecipitated, and kinase activity from ischemic-reperfused kidneys was assayed with the use of GST–c-Jun (1–135) as substrate. The value at each time point is the mean ±SE of two experiments. The value at the zero time point is from sham-operated animals. *B,* Activity of ERK-1 and ERK-2. ERK activity from ischemic-reperfused kidneys was assayed in Mono Q fractions, with the use of myelin basic protein as substrate. The values for kinase activity in the two peaks corresponding to ERK-1 and ERK-2 were added together to give a total ERK activity (ERK1/2). The value at each time point is from two experiments. *ERK,* extracellular signal-related kinase; *GST–c-Jun,* glutathione-s-transferase-c-Jun; *SAPK,* stress-activated protein kinases.(From Pombo CM, Bonventre JV, Avruch J, et al: The stress-activated protein kinases are major c-Jun amino-terminal kinases activated by ischemia and reperfusion. J Biol Chem 1994; 269:26546–26551; with permission.)

function in vivo. Proximal tubule epithelial cells are the primary target for these adverse influences. However, proximal tubule cells are able to undergo repair, regeneration, and proliferation after damage to the tissue. This renal repair capability is a critical factor not only for the organ but also for the organism. Understanding how the kidney repairs itself and recovers from ARF is of fundamental biological interest and potentially of great importance therapeutically. If we can identify specific factors responsible for this recovery, then it will be possible to target replacement therapies with the potential to facilitate repair and, by shortening the maintenance phase of human ARF, improve patient outcomes.

A growing body of knowledge has implicated growth factors in many roles in kidney physiology, pathology,

and development. The kidney is rich in growth factors that act as mitogens, motogens, and morphogens. These growth factors may play important beneficial roles in development, homeostasis, and repair. However, they may also be important in the pathogenesis of renal disease, by contributing to fibrosis and other adverse consequences. Thus, for appropriate biological regulation, the production of growth factors and their receptors have to be under strict control. By understanding the mechanisms brought to bear by the kidney during development and repair, we hope to learn how to intervene to improve the outcome in ARF.

ACKNOWLEDGMENT

We would like to thank Dr. James L. Stevens (University of Vermont, Burlington, VT) for critical reading of the preliminary manuscript.

References

1. Hewitt WR, Goldstein RS, Hook JB: Toxic Responses of the Kidney. In: Klasses CD, Doull J, Amdur MO, eds: *Casarett and Doull's Toxicology.* New York: Macmillan; 1990:354–382.
2. Bonventre JV: Mechanisms of ischemic acute renal failure. Kidney Int 1993; 43:1160–1178.
3. Thadhani R, Pascual M, Bonventre JV: Acute renal failure. New Engl J Med 1996; 334:1448–1460.
4. Bonventre JV, Brezis M, Siegel N, et al: Acute renal failure. I. Relative importance of proximal vs. distal tubular injury. Am J Physiol 1998; 275:F623–F632.
5. Cuppage FE, Neagry DR, Tate A: Repair of the nephron following temporary occlusion of the renal pedicle. Lab Invest 1967; 17:660–674.
6. Laurent GG, Toubeau JA, Heuson-Stiennon P, et al: Kidney tissue repair after nephrotoxic injury: biochemical and morphological characterization. Crit Rev Toxicol 1988; 19:147–183.
7. Haagsma BH, Pound AW: Mercuric chloride–induced tubulonecrosis in the rat kidney: the recovery phase. Br J Exp Pathol 1980; 61:229–241.
8. Toback FG: Control of renal regeneration after acute tubule necrosis. In: Robinson RR, ed: *Nephrology.* New York: Springer-Verlag; 1984:748–762.
9. Bacallao R, Fine LG: Molecular events in the organization of renal tubular epithelium: from nephrogenesis to regeneration. Am J Physiol 1989; F913–F924.
10. Wallin A, Zhang G, Jones TW: Mechanism of nephrogenic repair response: studies on proliferation and vimentin expression after ^{32}S-1,2-dichlorovinyl-l-cysteine nephrotoxicity in vivo and in cultured proximal tubule epithelial cells. Lab Invest 1992; 66:474–484.
11. Toback FG: Regeneration after acute tubular necrosis. Kidney Int 1992; 41:226–246.
12. Toback FG, Kartha S, Walsh-Reits MM: Regeneration of kidney tubular epithelial cells. Clin Invest 1993; 71:861–866.
13. Polla BS, Mili N, Bonventre JV: Les proteines de stress: quelles implications en nephrologie. Nephrologie 1991; 12:119–123.
14. Witzgall R, Brown D, Schwarz C, Bonventre JV: Localization of proliferating cell nuclear antigen, vimentin, c-fos, and clusterin in the postischemic kidney: evidence for a heterogeneous genetic response among nephron segments, and a large pool of mitotically active and dedifferentiated cells. J Clin Invest 1994; 93:2175–2188.
15. Pombo CM, Bonventre JV, Avruch J, et al: The stress- activated protein kinases are major c-jun amino-terminal kinases activated by ischemia and reperfusion. J Biol Chem 1994; 269:26546–26551.
16. Safirstein R: Gene expression in nephrotoxic and ischemic acute renal failure. J Am Soc Nephrol 1994; 4:1387–1395.

17. Safirstein R, DiMari J, Megyesi J, Price P: Mechanisms of renal repair and survival following acute injury. Semin Nephrol 1998; 18:519–522.

18. Verstrepen WA, Nouwen EJ, Yue NXS, De Broe ME: Altered growth factor expression during toxic proximal tubular necrosis and regeneration. Kidney Int 1993; 43:1267–1279.

19. Ghielli M, Verstrepen W, Nouwen E, De Broe ME: Regeneration processes in the kidney after acute injury: role of infiltrating cells. Exp Nephrol 1998; 6:502–507.

20. Grone HJ, Weber K, Grone E, et al: Coexpression of keratin and vimentin in damaged and regenerating tubular epithelia of the kidney. Am J Pathol 1987; 129:1–8.

21. Sparks RL, Strauss EE, Manga AV: Regulation of differentiation and protein kinase C expression in 3T3 T proadipocytes: effects of TGF-beta and transformation. Cell Prolif 1994; 27:139–151.

22. Ichimura T, Maier JA, Maciag T: FGF-1 in normal and regenerating kidney: expression in mononuclear, interstitial, and regenerating epithelial cells. Am J Physiol 1995; 269:F653–F662.

23. Abbate M, Brown D, Bonventre JV: Expression of NCAM recapitulates tubulogenic development in kidneys recovering from acute ischemia. Am J Physiol 1999; 277:F454–F463.

24. Spallanzani L: Prodromo sa nu Opera da Imprimersi sopra le Riproduzioni animali. Modena, 1768.

25. Bodemer CW: *Modern Embryology.* Austin, TX: Holt, Reinhart & Winston; 1968:332–348.

26. Weiss P: *Principles of Development: a Text in Experimental Embryoogy.* Darien, CT: Hafner; 1969:458–478.

27. Saxén L: *Organogenesis of the Kidney.* Cambridge: Cambridge University Press; 1987:1–173.

28. Ekblom P: Developmentally regulated conversion of mesenchyme to epithelium. FASEB J 1989; 3:2141–2150.

29. Ekblom P: Renal development. In: Seldin DW, Giebisch G, eds: *The Kidney.* New York: Raven Press; 1992:475–501.

30. Hammerman MR, Rogers SA, Ryan G: Growth factors and metanephrogenesis. Am J Physiol 1992; 262:F523–F532.

31. Kanwar YS, FA Carone, Kumar A, et al: Role of extracellular matrix, growth factors, and proto-oncogenes in metanephric development. Kidney Int 1997; 52:589–606.

32. Vainio S, Muller U: Inductive tissue interactions, cell signaling, and the control of kidney organogenesis. Cell 1997; 90:975–978.

33. Vize PD, Seufert DW, Carroll TJ, Wallingford JB: Model systems for the study of kidney development: use of the pronephros in the analysis of organ induction and patterning. Dev Biol 1997; 188:189–204.

34. Al-Awqati Q, Goldberg MR: Architectural patterns in branching morphogenesis in the kidney. Kidney Int 1998; 54:1832–1842.

35. Jessell TM, Melton DA: Diffusible factors in vertebrate embryonic induction. Cell 1992; 68:257–270.

36. Mercola M, Stiles CD: Growth factor superfamilies and mammalian embryogenesis. Development 1988; 102:451–460.

37. Smith JC: Mesoderm-inducing factors in early vertebrate development. EMBO J 1993; 12:4463–4470.

38. van der Geer P, Hanter T, Lindberg RA: Receptor protein-tyrosine kinases and their signal transduction pathways. Ann Rev Cell Biol 1994; 10: 251–337.

39. Kingsley DM: The TGF-beta superfamily: new members, new receptors, and new genetic tests of function in different organisms. Genes Dev 1994; 8:133–146.

40. Liu Y, Sun AM, Dworkin LD: Hepatocyte growth factor protects renal epithelial cells against apoptotic cell death. Biochem Biophys Res Comm 1998; 29:821–826.

41. Di Mari JF, Davis R, Safirstein RL: MAPK activation determines renal epithelial cell survival during oxidative injury. Am J Physiol 1999; 277:F195–F203.

42. Furukawa O, Matsui H, Suzuki N, Okabe S: Epidermal growth factor protects rat epithelial cells against acid-induced damage through the activation of Na^+/H^+ exchangers. J Pharmacol Exp Ther 1999; 288:620–626.

43. Takemura T, Hino S, Murata Y: Coexpression of CD9 augments the ability of membrane-bound heparin-binding epidermal growth factor-like growth factor (proHB-EGF) to preserve renal epithelial cell viability. Kidney Int 1999; 55:71–81.

44. Hammerman MR, O'Shea M, Miller SB: Role of growth factors in regulation of renal growth. Annu Rev Physiol 1993; 55:305–321.

45. Hammerman MR, Miller SB: Therapeutic use of growth factors in renal failure. J Am Soc Nephrol 1994; 5:1–11.

46. Hammerman M: Potential role of growth factors in the prophylaxis and treatment of acute renal failure. Kidney Int Suppl 1998; 64:S19–S22.

47. Hammerman MR: Growth factors and apoptosis in acute renal injury. Curr Opin Nephrol Hypertens 1998; 7:419–424.

48. Ono K, Matsumori A, Shioi T, et al: Enhanced expression of hepatocyte growth factor/c-Met by myocardial ischemia and reperfusion in a rat model [see comments]. Circulation 1997; 95:2552–2558.

49. Harris RC: Growth factors and cytokines in acute renal failure. Adv Ren Replace Ther 1997; 4(2 Suppl 1):43–53.

50. Cantley LG: Growth factors and the kidney: regulation of epithelial cell movement and morphogenesis. Am J Physiol 1996; 271:F1103–F1113.

51. Border WA, Rouslahti E: Transforming growth factor-beta in disease: the dark side of tissue repair. J Clin Invest 1992; 90:1–7.

52. Border WA, Noble NA: TGF-beta in kidney fibrosis: a target for gene therapy. Kidney Int 1997; 51:1388–1396.

53. Peters H, Noble NA, Border WA: Transforming growth factor-β in human glomerular injury. Curr Opin Nephrol Hypertens 1997; 6:389–393.

54. Shankland SJ, Johnson RJ: TGF-beta in glomerular disease. Miner Electrolyte Metab 1998; 24:168–173.

55. Hammerman MR: Growth factors in renal development. Semin Nephrol 1995; 15:291–299.

56. Perantoni AO, Dove LF, Williams CL: Induction of tubules in the rat metanephrogenic mesenchyme in the absence of an inductive tissue. Differentiation 1991; 48:25–31.

57. Rogers SA, Ryan G, Hammerman MR: Insulin-like growth factors I and II are produced in the metanephros and are required for growth and development in vitro. J Cell Biol 1991; 113:1447–1453.

58. Rogers SA, Ryan G, Hammerman MR: Metanephric transforming growth factor-alpha is required for renal organogenesis in vitro. Am J Physiol 1992; 262:F533–F539.

59. Wada J, Liu ZZ, Alvares K, et al: Cloning of cDNA for a subunit of mouse insulin-like growth factor I receptor and the role of the receptor in metanephric development. Proc Natl Acad Sci USA 1993; 90:10360–10364.

60. Hirvonen H, Sandberg M, Kalino H, et al: The N-myc protooncogene and IGF-II growth factor mRNAs are expressed by distinct cells in human fetal kidney and brain. J Cell Biol 1989; 108:1093–1104.

61. Pelton RW, Saxena B, Jones M, et al:. Immunohistochemical localization of TGF beta 1, TGF beta 2, and TGF beta 3 in the mouse embryo: expression patterns suggest multiple roles during embryonic development. J Cell Biol 1991; 115:1091–1105.

62. Schmid P, Cox D, Bilbe G, et al: Differential expression of TGF b1, b2, and b3 genes during mouse embryogenesis. Development 1991; 111:117–130.

63. Rogers SA, Ryan G, Purchio AF, Hammerman MR: Metanephric transforming growth factor-b1 regulates nephrogenesis in vitro. Am J Physiol 1993; 264:F996–1002.

64. Popliker M, Shatz A, Avivi A, et al: Onset of endogenous synthesis of epidermal growth factor in neonatal mice. Dev Biol 1987; 119:38–44.

65. Sariola H, Saarma M, Sainio K, et al: Dependence of kidney morphogenesis on the expression of nerve growth factor receptor. Science 1991; 254:571–573.

66. Montesano R, Matsumoto K, Nakamura T, Orci L: Identification of a fibroblast-derived epithelial morphogen as hepatocyte growth factor. Cell 1991; 67:901–908.

67. Sonnenberg E, Meyer D, Weidner KM, et al: Scatter factor/hepatocyte growth factor and its receptor, the c-met tyrosine kinase, can mediate a signal exchange between mesenchyme and epithelia during mouse development. J Cell Biol 1993; 123:223–235.

68. Karp SL, Ortiz-Arduan A, Li S, Neilson EG: Epithelial differentiation of metanephric mesenchymal cells after stimulation with hepatocyte growth factor or embryonic spinal cord. Proc Natl Acad Sci USA 1994; 91:5286–5290.

69. Breier G, Albrecht U, Sterrer S, Risau W: Expression of vascular endothelial growth factor during embryonic angiogenesis and

endothelial cell differentiation. Development 1992; 114:521–532.

70. Peters KG, De Vries C, Williams LT: Vascular endothelial growth factor receptor expression during embryogenesis and tissue repair suggests a role in endothelial differentiation and blood vessel growth. Proc Natl Acad Sci USA 1993; 90:8915–8919.

71. Leveen P, Pekny M, Gebre-Medhin S, et al: Mice deficient for PDGF B show renal, cardiovascular, and hematological abnomalities. Genes Dev 1994; 8:1875–1887.

72. Soriano P: Abnormal kidney development and hematological disorders in PDGF beta-receptor mutant mice. Genes Dev 1994; 8:1888–1896.

73. Abrahamson DR, Robert B, Hyink DP, et al: Origins and formation of microvasculature in the developing kidney. Kidney Int Suppl 1998; 67:S7–S11.

74. Dudley AT, Lyons KM, Robertson EJ: A requirement for bone morphogenetic protein-7 during development of the mammalian kidney and eye. Genes Dev 1995; 9:2795–2807.

75. Luo G, Hofmann C, Bronckers ALJJ, et al: BMP-7 is an inducer of nephrogenesis, and is also required for eye development and skeletal patterning. Genes Dev 1995; 9:2808–2820.

76. Moore MW, Klein RD, Farinas I, et al: Renal and neuronal abnormalities in mice lacking GDNF. Nature 1996; 382:76–79.

77. Pichel JG, Shen L, Sheng HZ, et al: Defects in enteric innervation and kidney development in mice lacking GDNF. Nature 1996; 382:73–76.

78. Sanchez MP, Silos-Santiago I, Frisen J, et al: Renal agenesis and the absence of enteric neurons in mice lacking GDNF. Nature 1996; 382:70–73.

79. Schuchardt A, D'Agati V, Larsson-Blomberg L, et al: Defects in the kidney and enteric nervous system of mice lacking the tyrosine kinase receptor Ret. Nature 1994; 367:380–383.

80. Jing S, Wen D, Yu Y, et al: GDNF-induced activation of the ret protein tyrosine kinase is mediated by GDNFR-alpha, a novel receptor for GDNF. Cell 1996; 85:1113–1124.

81. Treanor J, Goodman L, de Sauvage F, et al: Characterization of a multicomponent receptor for GDNF. Nature 1996; 382:80–83.

82. Nguyen HQ, Danilenko DM, Bucay N, et al: Expression of keratinocyte growth factor in embryonic liver of transgenic mice causes changes in epithelial growth and differentiation resulting in polycystic kidneys and other organ malformations. Oncogene 1996; 12:2109–2119.

83. Qiao J, Uzzo R, Obara-Ishihara T, et al: FGF-7 modulates ureteric bud growth and nephron number in the developing kidney. Development 1999; 126:547–554.

84. Celli G, LaRochelle W, Mackem S, et al: Soluble dominant-negative receptor uncovers essential roles for fibroblast growth factors in multi-organ induction and patterning. EMBO J 1998; 17:1642–1655.

85. Schedl A, Hastie N: Multiple roles for the Wilms' tumor suppressor gene, WT1 in genitourinary development. Mol Cell Endocrinol 1998; 140:65–69.

86. Madden SL, Cook DN, Morris JF, et al: Transcriptional repression mediated by the WT1, Wilms tumor gene product. Science 1991; 253:1550–1553.

87. Rauscher III FJ: The WT1 Wilms tumor gene product: a developmentally regulated transcription factor in the kidney that functions as a tumor suppressor. FASEB J 1993; 7:896–903.

88. Drummond IA, Madden SL, Rohwer-Nutter P, et al: Repression of the insulin-like growth factor II gene by the Wilms' tumor suppressor WT1. Science 1992; 257:674–676.

89. Werner H, Re GG, Drummond IA, et al: Increased expression of the insulin-like growth factor I receptor gene, IGF1R, in Wilms tumor is correlated with modulation of IGF1R promoter activity by the WT1 Wilms tumor gene product. Proc Natl Acad Sci USA 1993; 90:5828–5823.

90. Ryan G, Steele-Perkins V, Morris JF, et al: Repression of Pax-2 by WT1 during normal kidney development. Development 1995; 121:867–875.

91. Bortz JD, Rotwein P, DeVol D, et al: Focal expression of insulin-like growth factor I in rat kidney collecting duct. J Cell Biol 1988; 107:811–819.

92. Conti FG, Striker LJ, Elliot SJ: Synthesis and release of insulin-like growth factor I by mesangial cells in culture. Am J Physiol 1988; 255:F1214–F1219.

93. Hammerman MR, Rogers SA: Distribution of IGF receptors in the plasma membrane of proximal tubular cells. Am J Physiol 1987; 253:F841–F847.

94. Salido EC, Yen PH, Shapiro LJ, et al: In situ hybridization of prepro-epidermal growth factor mRNA in the mouse kidney. Am J Physiol 1989; 256:F632–F638.

95. Harris RC, Daniel TO: Epidermal growth factor binding, stimulation of phosphorylation, and inhibition of gluconeogenesis in rat proximal tubule. J Cell Physiol 1989; 139:383–391.

96. Breyer MD, Redha R, Breyer JA: Segmental distribution of epidermal growth factor binding sites in rabbit nephron. Am J Physiol 1990; 259:F553–F558.

97. Walker C, Everitt J, Freed JJ, et al: Altered expression of transforming growth factor-α in hereditary rat renal cell carcinoma. Cancer Res 1991; 51:2973–2978.

98. Nagaike M, Hirao S, Tajima H, et al: Renotropic function of hepatocyte growth factor in renal regeneration after unilateral nephrectomy. J Biol Chem 1991; 266:22781–22784.

99. Igawa T, Matsumoto K, Kanda S, et al: Hepatocyte growth factor may function as a renotropic factor for regeneration in rats with acute renal injury. Am J Physiol 1993; 265:F61–F69.

100. Thompson NL, KC Flanders, Smith JM, et al: Expression of transforming growth factor-β1 in specific cells and tissues of adult and neonatal mice. J Cell Biol 1989; 108:661–669.

101. Basile DP, Rovak JM, Martin DR, Hammerman MR: Increased transforming growth factor-β1 expression in regenerating rat renal tubules following ischemic injury. Am J Physiol 1996; 270:F500–F509.

102. Shultz PJ, DiCorleto PE, Silver BJ, Abboud HE: Mesangial cells express PDGF mRNA and proliferate in response to PDGF. Am J Physiol 1988; 255:F674–F684.

103. Gesualdo L, Di Paolo S, Milani S, et al: Expression of platelet-derived growth factor receptors in normal and diseased human kidney. J Clin Invest 1994; 94:50–58.

104. Hughes SE, Hall PA: Immunolocalization of fibroblast growth factor receptor 1 and its ligands in human tissues. Lab Invest 1993; 69:173–182.

105. Floege J, Eng E, Lindner V, et al: Rat glomerular mesangial cells synthesize basic fibroblast growth factor: release, upregulated synthesis, and mitogenicity in mesangial proliferative glomerulonephritis. J Clin Invest 1992; 90:2362–2369.

106. Ichimura T, Finch PW, Zhang G, et al: Induction of FGF-7 after kidney damage: a possible paracrine machanism for tubule repair. Am J Physiol 1996; 271:F967–F976.

107. Barajas L, Salido EC, Laborde NP: Nerve growth factor immunoreactivity in mouse kidney: an immunoelectron microscopic study. J Neurosci Res 1987; 18:418–424.

108. Alpers CE, Hudkins KL, Ferguson M, et al: Nerve growth factor receptor expression in fetal, mature, and diseased human kidneys. Lab Invest 1993; 69:703–713.

109. Simon M, Grone HJ, Johren O, et al: Expression of vascular endothelial growth factor and its receptors in human renal ontogenesis and in adult kidney. Am J Physiol 1995; 268:F240–F250.

110. Vukicevic S, Basic V, Rogic D, et al: Osteogenic protein-1 (bone morphogenetic protein-7) reduces severity of injury after ischemic acute renal failure in rat. J Clin Invest 1998; 102:202–214.

111. Stiles AD, Sosenko IRS, D'Ercole AJ, Smith BT: Relation of kidney tissue somatomedin-C/insulin-like growth factor I to postnephrectomy renal growth in the rat. Endocrinology 1985; 117:2397–2401.

112. Andersson GL, Scottner A, Jennische E: Immunohistochemical and biochemical localization of insulin-like growth factor 1 in the kidney of rats before and after uninephrectomy. Acta Endocrinol 1988; 119:555–560.

113. Fagin JA, Meland S: Relative increase in insulin-like growth factor I messenger ribonucleic acid levels in compensatory renal hypertrophy. Endocrinology 1987; 120:718–724.

114. Lajara R, Rotwein P, Bortz JD, et al: Dual regulation of insulin-like growth factor I expression during renal hypertrophy. Am J Physiol 1989; 257:F252–F261.

115. Andersson G, Jennische E: IGF-I immunoreactivity is expressed by regenerating renal tubular cells after ischaemic injury in the rat. Acta Physiol Scand 1988; 132:453–457.

116. Hise MK, Li L, Mantzouris N, Rohan RM: Differential mRNA

expression of insulin-like growth factor system during renal injury and hypertrophy. Am J Physiol 1995; 269:F817–F824.

117. Miller SB, Rotwein P, Bortz JD, et al: Renal expression of IGF-I in hypersomatotropic states. Am J Physiol 1990; 259:F251–F257.

118. Rogers SA, Miller SB, Hammerman MR: Enhanced renal IGF-I expression following partial kidney infarction. Am J Physiol 1993; 264:F963–F967.

119. Symon Z, Fuchs S, Agmon Y, et al: The endogenous insulin-like growth factor system in radiocontrast nephropathy. Am J Physiol 1998; 274:F490–F497.

120. Miller SB, Rogers SA, Estes CE, Hammerman MR: Increased distal nephron EGF content and altered distribution of peptide in compensatory renal hypertrophy. Am J Physiol 1992; 262:F1032–F1038.

121. Schaudies RP, Johnson JP: Multiple EGF-containing proteins in rat kidney: increased soluble EGF following ischemia is accompanied by a decrease in membrane associated immunoreactive EGF. Am J Physiol 1993; 264:F523–F531.

122. Safirstein R, Price PM, Saggi SJ, Harris RC: Changes in gene expression after temporary renal ischemia. Kidney Int 1990; 37:1515–1521.

123. Nonclercq D, Toubeau G, Lambricht P, et al: Redistribution of epidermal growth factor immunoreactivity in renal tissue after nephrotoxin-induced tubular injury. Nephron 1991; 57:210–215.

124. Taira T, Yoshimura A, Iizuka K, et al: Expression of epidermal growth factor and its receptor in rabbits with ischemic acute renal failure. Virchows Arch 1996; 427:583–588.

125. Safirstein R, Zelent A, Price P: Reduced preproEGF mRNA and diminished EGF excretion during acute renal failure. Kidney Int 1989; 36:810–815.

126. Price PM, Megyesi J, Saggi S, Safirstein RL: Regulation of transcription by the rat EGF gene promoter in normal and ischemic murine kidney cells. Am J Physiol 1995; 268:F664–670.

127. Nouwen EJ, Verstrepen WA, Buyssens N, et al: Hyperplasia, hypertrophy, and phenotypic alteration of the distal nephron after acute proximal tubular injury in the rat. Lab Invest 1994; 70:479–492.

128. Homma T, Sakai M, Cheng HF, et al: Induction of heparin-binding epidermal growth factor–like mRNA in rat kidney after acute injury. J Clin Invest 1995; 96:1018–1025.

129. Sakai M, Zhang M, Homma T, et al: Production of heparin binding epidermal growth factor–like growth factor in the early phase of regeneration after acute renal injury. Isolation and localization of bioactive molecules. J Clin Invest 1997; 99:2128–2138.

130. Paizis K, Kirkland G, Khong T, et al: Heparin-binding epidermal growth factor–like growth factor is expressed in the adhesive lesions of experimental focal glomerular sclerosis. Kidney Int 1999; 55:2310–2321.

131. Yano T, Yano Y, Yuasa M, et al: The repetitive activation of extracellular signal-regulated kinase is required for renal regeneration in rat. Life Sci 1998; 62:2341–2347.

132. Libetta C, Rampino T, Esposito C, et al: Stimulation of hepatocyte growth factor in human acute renal failure. Nephron 1998; 80:41–45.

133. Ishibashi K, Sasaki S, Sakamoto H, et al: Expressions of receptor gene for hepatocyte growth factor in kidney after unilateral nephrectomy and renal injury. Biochem Biophys Res Commun 1992; 187:1454–1459.

134. Joannidis M, Spokes K, Nakamura T, et al: Regional expression of hepatocyte growth factor/c-met in experimental renal hypertrophy and hyperplasia. Am J Physiol 1994; 267:F231–F236.

135. Liu Y, Tolbert E, Lin L, et al: Up-regulation of hepatocyte growth factor receptor: an amplification and targeting mechanism for hepatocyte growth factor action in acute renal failure. Kidney Int 1999; 55:442–453.

136. Kanda S, Ikawa T, Taida M: Transforming growth factor-β in rat kidney during compensatory renal growth. Growth Reg 1993; 3:146–150.

137. Okuda S, Languino LR, Rusulahti E, Border WA: Elevated expression of transforming growth factor-β and proteoglycan production in experimantal glomerulonephritis. J Clin Invest 1990; 86:453–462.

138. Almanzar M, Frazier K, Dube P, et al: Osteogenic protein-1 (OP-1) mRNA expression is selectively modulated afer acute ischemic renal injury (AIRI) (abstract). J Am Soc Nephrol 1996; 7:1821.

139. Miller SB, Martin DR, Kissane J, Hammerman MR: Insulin-like growth factor I accelerates recovery from ischemic acute tubular necrosis in the rat. Proc Natl Acad Sci USA 1992; 89:11876–11880.

140. Miller SB, Martin DR, Kissane J, Hammerman MR: Rat models for clinical use of insulin-like growth factor I in acute renal failure. Am J Physiol 1994; 266:F949–F956.

141. Franklin S, Moulton M, Sicard GA, et al: Insulin-like growth factor I preserves renal function postoperatively. Am J Physiol 1997; 272:F257–F259.

142. Kopple JD, Hirschberg R, Guler HP, et al: Lack of effect of recombinant human insulin-like growth factor I (IGF-I) in patients with acute renal failure (ARF). (abstract) J Am Soc Nephrol 1996; 7:1375.

143. Humes HD, Cieslinski DA, Coimbra TM, et al: Epidermal growth factor enhances renal tubule cell regeneration and repair and accelerates the recovery of renal function in postischemic acute renal failure. J Clin Invest 1989; 84:1757–1761.

144. Norman J, Tsau YK, Bacay A, Fine LG: Epidermal growth factor accelerates functional recovery from ischemic acute tubular necrosis in the rat: role of the epidermal growth factor receptor. Clin Sci 1990; 78:445–450.

145. Coimbra R, Cieslinski DA, Humes HD: Epidermal growth factor accelerates renal repair in mercuric chloride nephrotoxicity. Am J Physiol 1990; 259:F438–F443.

146. Kawaida K, Matsumoto K, Shimazu H, Nakamura T: Hepatocyte growth factor prevents acute renal failure and accelerates renal regeneration in mice. Proc Natl Acad Sci USA 1994; 91:4357–4361.

147. Miller SB, Martin DR, Kissane J, Hammerman MR: Hepatocyte growth factor accelerates recovery from acute ischemic renal injury in rats. Am J Physiol 1994; 266:F129–F134.

148. Mizuno S, Kurosawa T, Matsumoto K, et al: Hepatocyte growth factor prevents renal fibrosis and dysfunction in a mouse model of chronic renal disease. J Clin Invest 1998; 101:1827–1834.

149. Border WA, Okuda S, Languino LR, et al: Suppression of experimental glomerulonephritis by antiserum against transforming growth factor-β1. Nature 1990; 346:371–374.

150. Border WA, Noble NA, Yamamoto T, et al: Natural inhibitor of transforming growth factor-β protects against scarring in experimental kidney disease. Nature 1992; 360:361–364.

151. Isaka Y, Akagi Y, Ando Y, et al: Gene therapy by transforming growth factor-β receptor-IgG Fc chimera suppressed extracellular matrix accumulation in experimental glomerulonephritis. Kidney Int 1999; 55:465–475.

152. Kanda S, Hisamatsu H, Igawa T, et al: Peritubular endothelial cell proliferation in mice during compensatory renal growth after unilateral nephrectomy. Am J Physiol 1993; 265:F712–F716.

153. Yi E, Shabaik A, Lacey D, et al: Keratinocyte growth factor causes proliferation of urothelium in vivo. J Urol 1995; 154:1566–1570.

154. Tang WW, Ulich TR, Lacey DL, et al: Platelet-derived growth factor-BB induces renal tubulointerstitial myofibroblast formation and tubulointerstitial fibrosis. Am J Pathol 1996; 148:1169–1180.

155. Hammerman MR: The growth hormone–insulin-like growth factor axis in kidney. Am J Physiol 1989; 257:F503–F514.

156. Hammerman MR, Miller SB: The growth hormone insulin-like growth factor axis in kidney revisited. Am J Physiol 1993; 265:F1–F14.

157. Rogers SA, Miller SB, Hammerman MR: Growth hormone stimulated IGF I gene expression in isolated rat collecting duct. Am J Physiol 1990; 259:F474–479.

158. Rogers SA, Miller SB, Hammerman MR: Insulin-like growth factor I gene expression in isolated rat renal collecting duct is stimulated by epidermal growth factor. J Clin Invest 1991; 87:347–351.

159. Zhang GT, Ichimura A, Wallin M: Regulation of rat proximal tubule epithelial cell growth by fibroblast growth factors, insulin-like growth factor-1 and transforming growth factor-B, and analysis of fibroblast growth factors in rat kidney. J Cell Physiol 1991; 148:295–305.

160. Butt AJ, Firth SM, Baxter RC: The IGF axis and programmed cell death. Immunol Cell Biol 1999; 77:256–262.

161. Hammerman MR, Rogers SA, Ryan G: Growth factors and kidney development. Pediatr Nephrol 1993; 7:616–620.

162. Rogers SA, Hammerman MR: Mannose 6-phosphate potentiates insulin-like growth factor II–stimulated inositol triphosphate production in proximal tubular basolateral membranes. J Biol Chem 1989; 264:4273–4276.

163. Kobayashi S, Clemmons DR, Venkatachalam MA: Colocalization of insulin-like growth factor–binding protein with insulin-like growth factor I. Am J Physiol 1991; 261:F22–F28.

164. Powell DR, Durham SK, Brewer ED, et al: Effects of chronic renal failure and growth hormone on serum levels of insulin-like growth factor–binding protein-4 (IGFBP-4) and IGFBP-5 in children: a report of the Southwest Pediatric Nephrology Study Group. J Clin Endocrinol Metab 1999; 84:596–601.

165. Miller SB, Hansen VA, Hammerman MR: Effects of growth hormone and IGF-I on renal function in rats with normal and reduced renal mass. Am J Physiol 1990; 259:F747–F751.

166. Bohe J, Ding H, Qing D, et al: IGF-I binding proteins, IGF-I binding protein mRNA and IGF-I receptor mRNA in rats with acute renal failure given IGF-I. Kidney Int 1998; 54:1070–1082.

167. Kleinman JG, Worcester EM, Beshensky AM, et al: Up-regulation of osteopontin expression by ischemia in rat kidney. Ann NY Acad Sci 1995; 760:321–323.

168. Persy VP, Verstrepen WA, Ysebaert DK, et al: Differences in osteopontin up-regulation between proximal and distal tubules after renal ischemia-reperfusion. Kidney Int 1999; 56:601–611.

169. Padanilam BJ, Martin DR, Hammerman MR: Insulin-like growth factor I–enhanced renal expression of osteopontin after acute ischemic injury in rats. Endocrinology 1996; 137:2133–2140.

170. Franklin SC, Moulton M, Sicard GA, et al: Insulin-like growth factor I preserves renal function postoperatively. Am J Physiol 1997; 272:F257–F259.

171. Hirschberg R, Kopple J, Lipsett P, et al: Multicenter clinical trial of recombinant human insulin-like growth factor I in patients with acute renal failure. Kidney Int 1999; 55:2423–2432.

172. Carpenter G, Cohen S: Epidermal growth factor. J Biol Chem 1990; 265:7709–7712.

173. Massagué J: Transforming growth factor-α. J Biol Chem 1990; 265:21393–21396.

174. Higashiyama S, Abraham JA, Miller J, et al: A heparin-binding growth factor secreted by macrophage-like cells that is related to EGF. Science 1991; 251:936–939.

175. Salido EC, Barajas L, Lechago J, et al: Immunocytochemical localization of epidermal growth factor in mouse kidney. J Histochem Cytochem 1986; 34:1155–1160.

176. Kanda S, Igawa T, Sakai H, et al: Anti-epidermal growth factor antibody inhibits compensatory renal hyperplasia but not hypertrophy after unilateral nephrectomy in mice. Biochem Biophys Res Comm 1993; 187:1015–1021.

177. Kirkland G, Paizis K, Wu LL, et al: Heparin-binding EGF–like growth factor mRNA is upregulated in the peri-infarct region of the remnant kidney model: in vitro evidence suggests a regulatory role in myofibroblast transformation. J Amer Soc Nephrol 1998; 9:1464–1473.

178. Nakamura K, Iwamoto R, Mekada E: Membrane-anchored heparin-binding EGF–like growth factor (HB-EGF) and diphtheria toxin receptor–associated protein (DRAP27)/CD9 form a complex with integrin alpha 3 beta 1 at cell-cell contact sites. J Cell Biol 1995; 129:1691–1705.

179. Massagué J: The transforming growth factor-β family. Annu Rev Cell Biol 1990; 6:597–641.

180. Sporn MB, Roberts AB: Transforming growth factor-beta: recent progress and new challenges. J Cell Biol 1992; 119:1017–1021.

181. Kingsley D: What do BMPs do in mammals? Clues from the mouse short-ear mutation. Trends Genet 1994; 10:16–21.

182. Ozkaynak E, Schnegelsberg PNJ, Oppermann H: Murine osteogenic protein (OP-1): high levels of mRNA in kidney. Biochem Biophys Res Comm 1991; 179:116–123.

183. Zhang Y, Derynck R: Regulation of Smad signalling by protein associations and signalling crosstalk. Trends Cell Biol 1999; 9:274–279.

184. Massague J: TGF-β signaling: receptors, transducers, and Mad proteins. Cell 1996; 85:947–950.

185. Liu F, Hata A, Baker JC, et al: A human Mad protein acting as a BMP-regulated transcriptional activator. Nature 1996; 381:620–623.

186. Hao J, Ju H, Zhao S, et al: Elevation of expression of Smads 2, 3, and 4, decorin and TGF-β in the chronic phase of myocardial infarct scar healing. J Mol Cell Cardiol 1999; 31:667–678.

187. Sharma K, Ziyadeh FN: The emerging role of transforming growth factor-β in kidney diseases. Am J Physiol 1994; 266:F829–F842.

188. Isaka Y, Fujiwara Y, Ueda N, et al: Glomerulosclerosis induced by in vivo transfection of transforming growth factor-β or platelet-derived growth factor gene into the rat kidney. J Clin Invest 1993; 92:2597–2601.

189. Basile DP, Martin DR, Hammerman MR: Extracellular matrix–related genes in kidney after ischemic injury: potential role for TGF-β in repair. Am J Physiol 1998; 275:F894–F903.

190. Paul LC, Saito K, Davidoff A, Benediktsson H: Growth factor transcripts in rat renal transplants. Am J Kidney Dis 1996; 28:441–450.

191. Simon M, Maresh JG, Harris SE, et al: Expression of bone morphogenetic protein-7 in normal and ischemic rat kidney. Am J Physiol 1999; 276:F382–F389.

192. Massague J: Neurotrophic factors: crossing receptor boundaries. Nature 1996; 382:29–30.

193. Ross R, Rains EW, Bowen-Pope DF: The biology of platelet-derived growth factor. Cell 1986; 46:155–169.

194. Kartha S, Toback FG: Purine nucleotides stimulate DNA synthesis in kidney epithelial cells in culture. Am J Physiol 1985; 249:F967–F972.

195. Fraizar GE, Brown-pope DF, Vogel AM: Production of platelet-derived growth factor by cultured Wilms' tumor cells and fetal kidney cells. J Cell Physiol 1987; 133:169–174.

196. Floege J, Eng E, Young BA, et al: Infusion of platelet-derived growth factor or basic fibroblast growth factor induces selective glomerular mesangial cell proliferation and matrix accumulation in rats. J Clin Invest 1993; 92:2952–2962.

197. Shehata M, el Nahas A, Barkworth E, et al: Increased platelet-derived growth factor in the kidneys of cyclosporin-treated rats. Kidney Int 1994; 46:726–732.

198. Johnson DW, Saunders HJ, Baxter RC, et al: Paracrine stimulation of human renal fibroblasts by proximal tubule cells. Kidney Int 1998; 54:747–757.

199. Szebenyi G, Fallon JF: Fibroblast growth factors as multifunctional signaling factors. Int Rev Cytol 1999; 185:45–106.

200. Burgess WH, Maciag T: The heparin-binding (fibroblast) growth factor family of proteins. Annu Rev Biochem 1989; 58:575–606.

201. Goldfarb M: The fibroblast growth factor family. Cell Growth Differ 1990; 1:439–445.

202. Baird A, Klagsbrun M: The fibroblast growth factor family. Cancer Cells 1991; 3:239–243.

203. Rubin JS, Osada H, Finch PW, et al: Purification of characterization of a newly identified growth factor specific for epithelial cells. Proc Natl Acad Sci USA 1989; 86:802–806.

204. Tanaka K, Miyamoto K, Minamoto N, et al: Cloning and characterization of an androgen-induced growth factor essential for androgen-dependent growth of mammary carcinoma cells. Proc Natl Acad Sci USA 1992; 89:8928–8932.

205. Miyamoto M, Naruo K, Seki C, et al: Molecular cloning of a novel cytokine cDNA encoding the ninth member of the fibroblast growth factor family, which has a unique secretion property. Mol Cell Biol 1993; 13:4251–4259.

206. Yamasaki M, Miyake A, Tagashira S, Itoh N: Structure and expression of the rat mRNA encoding a novel member of the fibroblast growth factor family. J Biol Chem 1996; 271:15918–15921.

207. Emoto H, Tagashira S, Mattei M, et al: Structure and expression of human fibroblast growth factor-10. J Biol Chem 1997; 272:23191–23194.

208. Smallwood P, Munoz-Sanjuan I, Tong P, et al: Fibroblast growth factor (FGF) homologous factors: new members of the FGF family implicated in nervous system development. Proc Natl Acad Sci USA 1996; 93:9850–9857.

209. McWhirter J, Goulding M, Weiner J, et al: A novel fibroblast growth factor gene expressed in the developing nervous system is a downstream target of the chimeric homeodomain oncoprotein E2A-Pbx1. Development 1997; 124:3221–3232.

210. Miyake A, Konishi M, Martin F, et al: Structure and expression of a novel member, FGF-16, on the fibroblast growth factor family. Biochem Biophys Res Commun 1998; 243:148–152.

211. Hoshikawa M, Ohbayashi N, Yonamine A, et al: Structure and expression of a novel fibroblast growth factor, FGF-17, preferentially expressed in the embryonic brain. Biochem Biophys Res Commun 1998; 244:187–191.

212. Ohbayashi N, Hoshikawa M, Kimura S, et al: Structure and expression of the mRNA encoding a novel fibroblast growth factor, FGF-18. J Biol Chem 1998; 273:18161–18164.

213. Risau W, Ekblom P: Production of a heparin-binding angiogenesis factor by the embryonic kidney. J Cell Biol 1986; 103:1101–1107.

214. Sariola H, Ekblom P, Lehtonen E, Saxen L: Differentiation and vascularization of the metanephric kidney grafted on the chorioallantoic membrane. Dev Biol 1983; 96:427–435.

215. Gautschi-Sova P, Jiang ZP, Fratoer-Schroder M, Bohlen P: Acidic fibroblast growth factor is present in nonneural tissue: isolation and chemical characterization from bovine kidney. Biochemistry 1987; 26:5844–5847.

216. Baird A, Esch F, Bohlen P, et al: Isolation and partial characterization of an endothelial cell growth factor from the bovine kidney: homology with basic fibroblast growth factor. Regul Pept 1985; 12:201–213.

217. Wang WP, Lehtoma K, Varban ML, et al: Cloning of the gene coding for human class 1 heparin-binding growth factor and its expression in fetal tissues. Mol Cell Biol 1989; 9:2387–2395.

218. Witte DP, Nagasaki T, Stambrook P, Lieberman MA: Identification of an acidic fibroblast growth factor–like activity in a mesoblastic nephroma. Lab Invest 1989; 60:353–359.

219. Sullivan DE, Storch TG: Tissue- and development-specific expression of HBGF-1 mRNA. Biochim Biophys Acta 1991; 1090:17–21.

220. Gonzalez AM, Buscaglia M, Ong M, Baird A: Distribution of basic fibroblast growth factor in the 18-day rat fetus: localization in the basement membranes of diverse tissue. J Cell Biol 1990; 110:753–765.

221. Fu YM, Spirito P, Yu ZX, et al: Acidic growth factor in the developing rat embryo. J Cell Biol 1991; 114:1261–1273.

222. Zhang G, Ichimura T, Maier J, et al: A role for fibroblast growth factor type 1 in nephrogenic repair: autocrine expression in rat kidney proximal tubule epithelial cells in vitro and in the regenerating epithelium following nephrotoxic damage by S-(1,1,2,2-tetrafluoroethyl)-l-cysteine. J Biol Chem 1993; 268:11542–11547.

223. Metzger RJ, Krasnow MA: Genetic control of branching morphogenesis. Science 1999; 284:1635–1639.

224. Finch PW, Rubin JS, Miki T, et al: Human KGF is FGF-related with properties of a paracrine effector of epithelial cell growth. Science 1989; 245:752–755.

225. Finch P, Cunha G, Rubin J, et al: Pattern of keratinocyte growth factor and keratinocyte growth factor receptor expression during mouse fetal development suggests a role in mediating morphogenetic mesenchymal-epithelial interactions. Dev Dyn 1995; 203:223–240.

226. Jaye M, Schlessinger J, Dionne CA: Fibroblast growth factor receptor tyrosine kinases: molecular analysis and signal transduction. Biochim Biophys Acta 1992; 1135:185–199.

227. Givol D, Yayon A: Complexity of FGF receptors: genetic basis for structural diversity and functional specificity. FASEB J 1992; 6:3362–3369.

228. Partonen J, Makela TP, Eerola E, et al: FGFR-4, a novel acidic fibroblast growth factor receptor with a distinct expression pattern. EMBO J 1991; 10:1347–1354.

229. Orr-Urtreger A, Givol D, Yayon A, et al: Developmental expression of two murine fibroblast growth factor receptors, flg and bek. Development 1991; 113:1419–1434.

230. Peters KG, Werner S, Chen G, Williams LT: Two FGF receptor genes are differentially expressed in epithelial and mesenchymal tissues during limb formation and organogenesis in the mouse. Development 1992; 114:233–243.

231. Orr-Urtreger A, Bedford MT, Burakova T, et al: Developmental localization of the splicing alternatives of fibroblast growth factor receptor-2 (FGFR-2). Dev Biol 1993; 158:475–486.

232. Kim EG, Kwon HM, Burrow CR, Ballermann BJ: Expression of rat fibroblast growth factor receptor 1 as three splicing variants during kidney development. Am J Physiol 1993; 264:F66–F73.

233. Peters KG, Ornitz D, Werner S, Williams LT: Unique expression pattern of the FGF receptor 3 gene during mouse organogenesis. Dev Biol 1993; 155:423–430.

234. Stark KL, McMahon JA, McMahon AP: FGFR-4, a new member of the fibroblast growth factor receptor family, expressed in the definitive endoderm and skeletal muscle lineages of the mouse. Development 1991; 113:641–651.

235. Anderson R, Ray C: Potential autocrine and paracrine mechanisms of recovery from mechanical injury of renal tubular epithelial cells. Am J Physiol 1998; 274:F463–F472.

236. Maisonpierre PC, Belluscio L, Squinto S, et al: Neurotrophin-3: a neurotrophic factor related to NGF and BDNF. Science 1990; 247:1446–1451.

237. Thoenen H: The changing scene of neurotrophic factors. Trends Neurosci 1991; 14:165–170.

238. Guegan C, Ceballos-Picot I, Chevalier E, et al: Reduction of ischemic damage in NGF-transgenic mice: correlation with enhancement of antioxidant enzyme activities. Neurobiol Dis 1999; 6:180–189.

239. Kiprianova I, Freiman TM, Desiderato S, et al: Brain-derived neurotrophic factor prevents neuronal death and glial activation after global ischemia in the rat. J Neurosci Res 1999; 56:21–27.

240. Barbacid M: The Trk family of neurotrophin receptors. J Neurobiol 1994; 25:1386–1403.

241. Furlong RA: The biology of hepatocyte growth factor/scatter factor. Bioessays 1992; 14:613–617.

242. Nakamura T, Nishizawa T, Hagiya M, et al: Molecular cloning and expression of human hepatocyte growth factor. Nature 1989; 342:440–443.

243. Tashiro K, Hagiya T, Nishizawa T, et al: Deduced primary structure of rat hepatocyte growth factor and expression of the mRNA in rat tissues. Proc Natl Acad Sci USA 1990; 87:3200–3204.

244. Rubin JS, Chan AM, Bottaro DP, et al:. A broad-spectrum human lung fibroblast-derived mitogen is a variant of hepatocyte growth factor. Proc Natl Acad Sci USA 1991; 88:415–419.

245. Kan M, Zhang GH, Zarnegar R, et al: Hepatocyte growth factor/hepatopoietin A stimulates the growth of rat kidney proximal tubule epithelial cells (RPTE), rat nonparenchymal liver cells, human melanoma cells, mouse keratinocytes, and stimulates anchorage-independent growth of SV-40 transformed RPTE. Biochem Biophys Res Commun 1991; 174:331–337.

246. Igawa T, Kanda S, Kanetake H, et al: Hepatocyte growth factor is a potent mitogen for cultured rabbit renal tubular epithelial cells. Biochim Biophys Res Commun 1991; 174:831–838.

247. Bottaro DP, Rubin JS, Faletto DL, et al: Identification of the hepatocyte growth factor receptor as the c-met proto-oncogene product. Science 1991; 251:802–804.

248. Ferrara N: The vascular endothelial growth factor family of polypeptides. J Cell Biochem 1991; 47:211–218.

249. Zhang G, Sato JD, Herley MT, et al: Stable and temperature transformation of rat kidney epithelial cells suppresses expression of acidic fibroblast growth factor 1 but activates secretion of fibroblast growth factor 3 (int-2) and vascular endothelial growth factor. Cell Growth Differ 1994; 5:349–357.

250. Myoken Y, Kayada Y, Okamoto T, et al: Vascular endothelial growth factor (VEGF) produced by A-431 human epidermoid carcinoma cells and identification of VEGF membrane binding sites. Proc Natl Acad Sci USA 1991; 88:5819–5823.

251. Matthews W, Jordan CT, Gavin M, et al: A receptor tyrosine kinase cDNA isolated from a population of enriched primitive hematopoietic cells and exhibiting close genetic linkage to c-kit. Proc Natl Acad Sci USA 1991; 88:9026–9030.

252. Hollenberg NK, Paskins-Hurlburt AJ, Abrams HL: Collateral arterial formation: lymph draining ischemic kidneys contains a neovascular stimulating agent of high molecular weight. Invest Radiol 1985; 20:58–61.

253. Nangaku M, Alpers CE, Pippin J, et al: A new model of renal microvascular endothelial injury. Kidney Int 1997; 52:182–194.
254. Bonventre JV, Force T: Mitogen-activated protein kinases and transcriptional responses in renal injury and repair. Curr Opin Nephrol Hypertens 1998; 7:425–433.
255. Lenormand P, Sardet C, Pages G, et al: Growth factors induce nuclear translocation of MAP kinases (p42mapk and p44mapk) but not of their activator MAP kinase kinase (p45mapkk) in fibroblasts. J Cell Biol 1993; 122:1079–1088.
256. Gonzalez F, Seth A, Raden D, et al: Serum-induced translocation of mitogen-activated protein kinase to the cell surface ruffling membrane and the nucleus. J Cell Biol 1993; 122:1089–1101.
257. Seger R, Krebs E: The MAPK signaling cascade. FASEB J 1995; 9:726–735.
258. Treisman R: Regulation of transcription by MAP kinase cascades. Curr Opin Cell Biol 1996; 8:205–215.
259. Treisman R: Journey to the surface of the cell: fos regulation and the SRE. EMBO J 1995; 14:4905–4913.
260. Gille H, Sharrocks A, Shaw P: Phosphorylation of transcription factor p62TCF by MAP kinase stimulates ternary complex formation at c-fos promoter. Nature 1992; 358:414–417.
261. Chen R, Sarnecki C, Blenis J: Nuclear localization and regulation of erk- and rsk-encoded protein kinases. Mol Cell Biol 1992; 12:915–927.
262. Xing J, Ginty D, Greenberg M: Coupling of the RAS-MAPK pathway to gene activation by RSK2, a growth factor–regulated CREB kinase. Science 1996; 273:959–963.
263. Gupta S, Davis R: MAP kinase binds to the NH2-terminal activation domain of c-Myc. FEBS Lett 1994; 353:281–285.
264. Morooka H, Bonventre JV, Pombo CM, et al: Ischemia and reperfusion enhance ATF-2 and c-Jun binding to cAMP response elements and to an AP-1 binding site from the c-jun promoter. J Biol Chem 1995; 270:30084–30092.
265. Di Mari J, Megyesi J, Udvarhelyi N, et al: N-Acetyl cysteine ameliorates ischemic renal failure. Am J Physiol 1997; 272:F292–F298.
266. Bogoyevitch M, Gillespie-Brown J, Ketterman A, et al: Stimulation of the stress-activated mitogen-activated protein kinase subfamilies in perfused heart. p38/RK mitogen-activated protein kinases and c-Jun N-terminal kinases are activated by ischemia/reperfusion. Circ Res 1996; 79:162–173.
267. Yin T, Sandhu G, Wolfgang C, et al: Tissue-specific pattern of stress kinase activation in ischemic/reperfused heart and kidney. J Biol Chem 1997; 272:19943–19950.
268. Read MA, Whitley MZ, Gupta S, et al: Tumor necrosis factor-α–induced E-selectin expression is activated by the nuclear factor-κB and c-JUN N-terminal kinase/p38 mitogen-activated protein kinase pathways. J Biol Chem 1997; 272:2753–2761.

CHAPTER **8**

Cytoskeletal Alterations as a Basis of Cellular Injury in Acute Renal Failure

Simon J. Atkinson ▪ Bruce A. Molitoris

Overwhelming evidence now indicates that cytoskeletal alterations occurring in proximal tubule cells (PTCs)during ischemia play a major role in the structural, biochemical, and functional alterations that occur at both the cellular and the organ level. The characteristic structure of the surface membrane of polarized proximal tubule cells is drastically altered by the onset of ischemia. The observed changes are secondary, in large part, to disruption of the cortical actin cytoskeleton. For example, distinctive disruption of apical brush border microvilli occurs rapidly and in a duration-dependent fashion with the onset of ischemia. Microvillar membranes internalize into the cell's cytosol or are shed into the lumen as blebs. The microvillar actin core disassembles concurrent with or preceding these membrane changes. Alterations in the cortical actin cytoskeleton also occur and mediate basolateral membrane changes, including untethering of surface membrane proteins and disruption of junctional complexes. These changes occur during ischemia because actin and its associated binding proteins can no longer interact with the surface membrane to maintain these highly regulated membrane structures. The resultant epithelial cells have a reduced membrane surface area that lacks polarization structurally, biochemically, and physiologically. Furthermore, the changes in the apical microvilli result in tubular obstruction, enhanced and unregulated paracellular flux, and reduced Na^+ absorption. This explains, in part, the reduction in glomerular filtration rate. Recent evidence suggests that these actin surface membrane alterations induced by ischemia are secondary to either activation or inactivation of several actin-associated proteins or actin regulatory proteins, resulting from perturbation of signaling pathways or from the direct biochemical effects of adenosine triphosphate (ATP) depletion or alterations in intracellular pH on cytoskeletal protein-protein interactions. During recovery, the actin-associated proteins reassume their normal cellular localization and function coincident with reformation of the actin surface membrane interactions. Taken together this evidence strongly supports the hypothesis that actin-associated proteins and the actin cytoskeleton play a significant role in ischemic-induced injury in PTCs.

ISCHEMIA

The kidney's primary functions are dependent on the selective reabsorption of water, ions, and macromolecules by tubular cells. This, in turn, requires the structural, biochemical, and physiologic polarization of these cells. A distinctive apical membrane separated from a basolateral membrane domain by cellular junctional complexes structurally characterizes epithelial cells.[1-4] In PTCs, apical membrane microvilli serve to markedly amplify the absorptive surface area, thereby maximizing reabsorptive processes (Fig. 8–1). Junctional complexes form a physical barrier not only to the fluid layer above these cells but also to membrane phospholipids and to proteins such as ion channels, transport proteins, and specific enzymes that make up each of these unique membrane domains. Many studies have demonstrated that the actin cytoskeleton plays a critical role in the establishment and maintenance of these apical microvilli and the cell-cell attachments at these junctional complexes, and in attachment to the extracellular matrix in polarized epithelial cells.[5-7] Thus, the integrity of these polarized cellular membranes and structures is critical to the normal absorptive and secretory functions of these cells.

Severe reductions in renal blood flow result in characteristic rapidly occurring and duration-dependent effects on the apical microvilli and junctional complexes present in these cells[8] (Fig. 8–2). Apical microvillous alterations include formation of membrane-bound vesicles termed "blebs" that either undergo internalization or are released into the lumen.[9-11] These transformations result in a substantial loss of apical membrane surface area, thus reducing effective reabsorption. In addition, the membrane blebs shed into the lumen often aggregate, causing tubular obstruction. Both of these events result in a decrease in the glomerular filtration rate (GFR), a hallmark of ischemic acute renal failure (ARF).[12] Obstruction of the tubule lumen eliminates single nephron GFR by increasing intratubular pressures to levels inconsistent with filtration. Reductions in proximal tubule ion and water reabsorption result in high distal delivery of Na^+, K^+, and Cl^- and high distal flow rates. This, in turn, via tubular glomerular feedback, results in afferent arteriole constriction and its attendant reduction in GFR. Finally, opening of tight junctions results in unregulated paracellular movement of ions and water, resulting in increased backleak, the third mechanism of reduced GFR following ischemic injury.[12] Therefore, ischemia-induced alterations in PTCs account for the reduction in GFR seen following ischemic injury.

In addition to the apical membrane changes, the junctional complex dissociation allows membrane lipids and integral and peripheral membrane proteins to

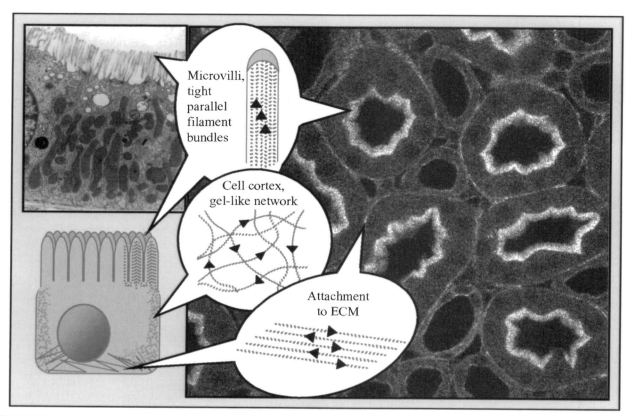

FIGURE 8–1 ■ Schematic representation of the types and intracellular locations of the F-actin cytoskeletal structures in renal proximal tubule cells. Apical microvilli have parallel polarized microfilaments, with their pointed ends facing the terminal web. The cortical actin cytoskeleton consists of short, randomly oriented fibers forming a web-like structure. The basal F-actin cytoskeleton consists of cortical web structures and cables of microfilaments running in alternating fashion that mediate cell–extracellular matrix (ECM) adhesion.

diffuse laterally into the alternative surface membrane domain.[8, 13, 14] This membrane interfusion creates a homogeneous surface membrane outer leaflet no longer unique to the apical or basolateral membrane regions. These now-nonpolarized renal epithelial cells can no longer reabsorb fluid and particles and transport them appropriately.

ACTIN AND ACTIN-BINDING PROTEINS

Basic Properties of Actin

Actin forms helical protein microfilaments (filamentous or F-actin) composed of globular actin monomers (G-actin) that self-assemble spontaneously in physiologic buffers.[15, 16] Actin microfilaments, together with microtubules and intermediate filaments, constitute the cytoskeleton, a framework that gives the cell its shape, allows the components of the cytoplasm to be organized in space, and is used as the machinery to move the cell or organelles within it. The polymerization and depolymerization of actin and the arrangement of actin filaments are controlled by an array of actin-binding proteins (Fig. 8–3).

The actin monomer is a 43-kDa globular protein.[17] The protein folds into a compact globular structure with a cleft dividing the molecule into unequal halves.

This cleft provides binding sites for adenine nucleosides (ATP or ADP) and divalent cations (Ca^{2+} or Mg^{2+}), that are thus placed at the heart of the protein and can influence its conformation and hence its dynamic behavior. Actin is an ATPase, and ATP hydrolysis is activated by polymerization,[18] so that the bulk of actin filament subunits are ADP-bound, whereas (under normal physiologic conditions) most actin monomers are ATP-bound.

Under physiologic conditions of ionic strength and pH, actin monomers spontaneously self-assemble to form filaments.[19] At steady state, the ends of actin filaments exist in equilibrium with a constant monomer concentration, the critical concentration. Below this threshold concentration, actin filaments depolymerize, whereas any increase in actin concentration above the critical concentration results in increased filament formation without an increase in the monomer concentration.

Actin polymerization from monomers exhibits an initial lag in the rate of polymerization that reflects the slower kinetics of polymer nucleation.[20] Actin polymerization that is nucleated by either pre-existing free filament ends or by nucleating factors does not exhibit a lag phase. The rate constants for monomer association and dissociation differ substantially at the two ends of the filament, which are usually designated "barbed" ($+$) and "pointed" ($-$). Rate constants are

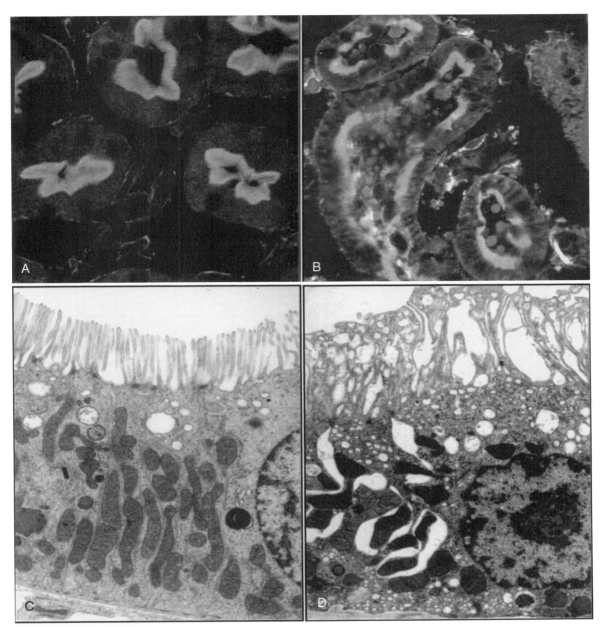

FIGURE 8–2 ■ *(See Color Plate)* Effect of ischemia on proximal tubular cell (PTC) F-actin and ADF localization *(A–D)*. Renal PTCs under physiologic conditions *(A* and *C)* and following 25 minutes of ischemia *(B* and *D)* were stained for F-actin with fluorescein isothiocyanate (FITC)-phalloidin and actin depolymerizing factor (ADF), using a Texas-Red secondary antibody *(A* and *B)*. Ischemia resulted in marked disruption of apical microvillar F-actin and redistribution of ADF to the apical domain and into the lumen in membrane sealed vesicles. Low-power electron micrographs show marked apical damage following mild to moderate ischemic injury with loss of individual microvillar structure, internalization of microvillar membrane, and formation of membrane-bound vesicles in the lumen. (From Schwartz N, Hosford M, Sandoval RM, et al: Ischemia activates actin depolymerizing factor: role in proximal tubule microvillar actin alterations. Am J Physiol 1999; 276:F544–F551; with permission.)

also affected by the availability of ATP, which greatly increases the rate of monomer addition, particularly at the barbed end. In fact, in the presence of ATP, the critical concentrations at the two ends of the filament differ significantly, such that it is possible for there to be net polymerization at barbed ends with simultaneous depolymerization at pointed ends, a behavior known as treadmilling.

Control of Actin Dynamics and Organization by Actin-Binding Proteins

A simple examination of the concentration of actin present in cells (see, for example, Pollard and coworkers[21]) reveals the necessity for actin-binding proteins to control actin polymerization. The total actin concentrations in most cells are typically on the order of

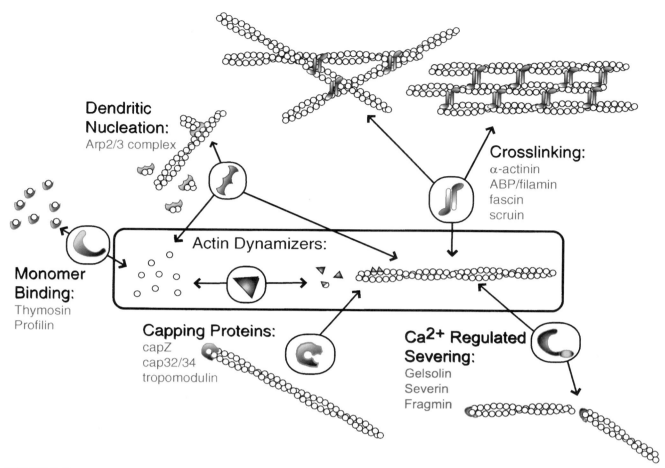

FIGURE 8–3 ▪ Schematic representation of the functional relationships between the major classes of actin-binding proteins that affect the assembly of the cytoskeleton. Not shown are the numerous proteins that show functional overlap between classes and those responsible for the linkage of other cellular components to the cytoskeleton.

30 to 50 μM (much higher in specialized cells, such as neutrophils, and also much higher in particular regions of the cell), far higher than the critical concentration for polymerization (0.2–2 μM).[16] Thus, it is apparent that in the absence of other factors, the bulk of cellular actin would be filamentous; nevertheless, the fraction of polymeric actin in most cells seldom rises above 50%. The actin system is maintained, therefore, in a high potential energy state, which allows rapid polymerization when and where required, but which necessitates the deployment of specific actin-binding proteins to maintain the high concentration of nonfilamentous actin. A consequence is that perturbation of the normal function or regulation of this system can result in excessive and unorganized actin polymerization.

MONOMER:POLYMER EQUILIBRIUM

Two classes of actin-binding proteins modulate the position of the monomer:polymer equilibrium. Sequestering proteins regulate the availability of actin monomers in a polymerizable form, whereas capping proteins regulate the availability of actin filament ends and thus alter the critical concentration (see Fig. 8–3).

Proteins related to thymosin-β[4] bind actin monomers and render them incapable of adding onto actin filament ends.[22] The affinity of thymosins for actin is moderate (0.5 μM for ATP-actin), but they are present at high concentrations in the cytosol of most cell types such that the bulk of nonfilamentous actin exists in complex with thymosin. The affinity of thymosin is 50-fold higher for ATP-actin monomers than for ADP-monomers. Another abundant actin monomer binding protein, profilin, is not a simple sequestering protein, but rather has a more complex effect on actin polymerization that is dependent on the specific cellular context.[23] Actin monomers bound to profilin can add onto actin filament barbed ends (but not pointed ends),[24, 25] unlike those associated with thymosin, which are incapable of polymerization. Perhaps the most important contribution of profilin in controlling actin polymerization is that the presence of a significant concentration of available profilin effectively confines actin polymerization to the barbed ends of preexisting filaments or to Arp2/3 nuclei. This is because profilin-actin complexes cannot add onto filament pointed ends, and cannot contribute to spontaneous filament nucleation.

In the presence of thymosin, it seems most likely that profilin accelerates actin polymerization at actin filament barbed ends, in part by catalyzing nucleotide exchange to recharge actin monomers with ATP,[26] and also by shuttling monomers from the thymosin-bound pool onto actin filament barbed ends.[27] Local signals, therefore, can stimulate rapid polymerization enhanced by profilin in one area in the cell, while the same protein is suppressing spontaneous polymerization elsewhere. Polyphosphoinositides compete with actin for binding to profilin,[28, 29] and so the concentrations of these lipids locally in membranes may provide a means of regulating the activity of profilin. It is also possible that direct regulation of profilin is not required, but that regulation of the availability of barbed ends and nuclei is sufficient. Thymosins appear to be constitutively active.

The heterodimeric capping proteins (also known as CapZ or cap32/34) bind at the barbed ends of actin filaments and inhibit both loss and addition of actin monomers.[30] Capping barbed ends is an effective inhibitor of barbed-end polymerization; hence, profilin (by virtue of suppressing pointed-end polymerization) and capping protein together potently inhibit actin polymerization and contribute to the maintenance of a large monomer pool. Capping protein is removed from actin filament ends by polyphosphoinositide-containing membranes.[31] This mechanism for regulating its activity appears to be significant in platelets,[32] but it has not been demonstrated directly in other cell types. The severing and depolymerizing activity of actin depolymerizing factor (ADF)/cofilin proteins (see later) is another potential mechanism for removing capping protein from filament ends. Gelsolin and related calcium-regulated severing proteins (see later) also cap the barbed ends of severed filaments, ensuring that altering the lengths of existing filaments is not accompanied by a burst of actin polymerization.

Certain heat-shock proteins are also able to bind actin filament ends and alter polymer dynamics in a manner similar to capping proteins (eg, HSP25). The significance of their role in normal cell physiology, where the majority of filament ends are already capped by capping protein, is not established, but they may have more significance in the context of cellular injury.[33, 34]

LENGTH REGULATION

Actin filament length can be regulated to some extent by the position of the monomer:polymer equilibrium, but is also subject to control imposed by the activities of severing proteins and pointed-end capping proteins.

Gelsolin and related proteins from invertebrates sever actin filaments in a calcium-regulated manner, remaining on the barbed end of the severed filament as a cap.[35] These proteins also nucleate filament growth in the pointed-end direction in vitro, but in the presence of profilin or thymosin this activity is unlikely to be of significance in vivo. Therefore, their

activation has a neutral effect with respect to the monomer:polymer equilibrium but does cause an increase in filament number, with a consequent reduction in mean filament length. However, these compounds potentially can have a delayed effect on polymer dynamics, since their activity increases the number of potential barbed ends that could later become sites for monomer addition or loss. Gelsolin is activated by calcium and can be removed from actin filament ends by polyphosphoinositide-containing vesicles.[36] The subtlety of the phenotype of gelsolin knockout mice[37] indicates that gelsolin is not an essential component of the cytoskeleton but rather modulates actin dynamics in a fashion that is most important in motile cells.

Pointed-end capping proteins regulate filament length and stability by capping pointed ends and preventing loss of monomers from this end. Examples include tropomodulin[38] and the Arp2/3 complex (see later). They also influence the ability of ADF/cofilin proteins to depolymerize filaments rapidly, provided that severing by these proteins is not an important factor.

CROSS-LINKING AND BUNDLING

Actin filaments by themselves are thin and flexible, and they break relatively easily.[39] Building rigid structures or structures with any tensile strength requires that the filaments be bundled or cross-linked into higher order assemblies (see Fig. 8–3). Numerous bifunctional actin-binding proteins have been described that are able to promote actin filament association into a variety of gels and bundles. Rheologic studies have demonstrated that the same protein can form either gels or bundles, depending on the concentration of the actin-binding protein and the length and concentration of actin filaments.[40–42] However, many cross-linking proteins are preferential bundlers (examples include scruin),[43] while others are more likely to promote gel formation (eg, ABP280/filamin).[44] Actin-bundling or cross-linking activity is combined with other activities in a number of proteins, of which the best characterized example is the brush border protein villin.[45] This protein has considerable structural similarity to the severing protein gelsolin and also has similar activity in in vitro assays, but it contains an additional "headpiece" domain that allows it to bundle actin filaments. Cross-linking proteins, such as vinculin, can be regulated by interaction with polyphosphoinositides, but in contrast to other actin binding proteins, they promote exposure of the actin binding sites by disrupting internal dimerization.[46] Some α-actinin isoforms are regulated by calcium,[47] but this appears to be exceptional. It may be that most cross-linkers and bundlers are regulated by localizing them to the correct site in the cell and that actin filament assemblies are remodeled by polymerization, depolymerization, severing, and annealing, rather than by altering the activity of these proteins.

POLYMERIZATION AND DEPOLYMERIZATION KINETICS

The importance of specific cellular factors in regulating the kinetics and localization of actin polymerization in cells has only recently been recognized. It is now clear that the observed depolymerization rates for actin in cells can be accounted for only by the action of ADF/cofilin proteins, and that peripheral actin polymerization is largely the result of the activity of Arp2/3 complex (see Fig. 8–3).

Proteins of the ADF/cofilin family have interesting and complex effects on actin filament dynamics.[48] ADF/cofilin proteins bind to actin monomers, and have much higher affinity for ADP monomers than ATP monomers.[49] ADF/cofilin proteins also bind to actin filaments in a nucleotide-dependent manner, with much higher affinity for ADP subunits than for ATP or ADP gamma-phosphate (Pi) subunits in the filament.[50] Dissociation of Pi from the subunits in the filament may provide a timer, rendering older filaments or regions of the filament more sensitive to depolymerization. The affinity for monomer is higher than that for polymer subunits, and this provides the thermodynamic mechanism that drives accelerated depolymerization of the filament, particularly from the pointed end. Moreover, ADF/cofilin proteins are capable of severing filaments, although whether severing has a significant role in the intracellular environment is strongly contested by at least one prominent laboratory.[51] Most ADF/cofilin proteins exhibit strong pH dependence in their filament binding, which is favored at low pH levels and inhibited at high pH levels.[52, 53] The significance of this differential binding under conditions of normal cell physiology is by no means apparent, but in pathologic situations, such as ischemic injury and recovery, in which intracellular pH can fluctuate from 7.5 to 6.0,[54] this property may be very significant. ADF/cofilin proteins are unique among the proteins regulating actin filament dynamics in that most isoforms are directly and negatively regulated by phosphorylation[55, 56] by LIM kinases at a conserved serine residue near the N-terminus.[57, 58] As with other actin-binding proteins, polyphosphoinositides compete with actin for binding.[59] Proteins that bind along actin filament sides, such as tropomyosin, protect these filaments against ADF/cofilin binding; hence, severing and pointed-end depolymerization.[60] This protection may be related to the observation that ADF/cofilin binding changes the twist of the actin filament helix, which may be stabilized by tropomyosin at an unfavorable pitch for ADF/cofilin binding. Not surprisingly, the more stable actin filament assemblies in cells are frequently protected in this way, and dissociation of tropomyosin may initiate destruction of these assemblies following injury (see later).

Arp2/3[61] is a multisubunit protein complex that acts as a nucleus or seed for new filament growth.[62, 63] The complex derives its name from two of the subunits, which are the actin-related proteins Arp2 and Arp3. Structural conservation of actin-actin contact sites indicates that it is these subunits that nucleate actin filaments and allow fila-

ment growth from the barbed end[64] and also allow Arp2/3 to cap pointed ends. The other five subunits in the complex are thought to be regulatory and to confer the ability to bind other ligands, including filament sides. Activation of the complex results in the growth of new filaments at a fixed angle from the sides of existing filaments or the formation of branched structures at filament barbed ends.[65] This leads to formation of a branching structure called a dendritic brush. Binding to members of the SCAR/WASp (Wiskott-Aldrich syndrome protein) family of proteins activates Arp2/3, and binding to pre-existing F-actin is also necessary for maximal activity.[66, 67] Roles for Arp2/3 other than in polymerization of actin filaments at the leading edge of motile cells or in fibroblast membrane ruffles have not yet been described, but it is reasonable to expect Arp2/3 to be an important initiator of filament growth in other cellular contexts.

ACTIN POLYMERIZATION IN ISCHEMIA

Structural Alterations in the Actin Microfilament Network

Both microvillous breakdown and loss of cellular polarity during ischemia are preceded by structural alterations in the actin microfilament network.[5, 68–73] These cytoskeletal changes reflect the severity and duration of the ischemic injury. The microvillous actin cores, the cytoskeletal meshwork of the terminal web, and the cortical actin of the epithelial cell are disrupted. The concentration of F-actin in the cell increases with the formation of F-actin aggregates in the cytoplasm.[74] This aggregation and rearrangement of F-actin implies that ischemia induces depolymerization of F-actin or, perhaps, just disassembly of higher-order structures, followed by extremely rapid re-polymerization in an unregulated fashion.

Regulatory molecules tightly control the interactions of F-actin and G-actin with their associated actin-binding proteins, and during ischemia or ATP depletion, the changes in cellular ATP concentration, pH, ion concentration, and other macromolecules alter this regulation and these associations. The activity of each actin-binding protein is governed by specific cellular conditions affecting the integrity of this association and, therefore, the integrity of structures and activities of the cell. This basic concept can be illustrated by the effect of ischemia or ATP depletion in renal PTCs on the function of specific actin-binding proteins associated with the apical cytoskeleton. During ischemia, dephosphorylation of ezrin inhibits binding of ezrin to the microfilament core, releasing the overlying membrane.[75–77] Also, myosin I alterations may play a role in the actin core breakdown as its localization changes from microvillous to intracytoplasmic aggregates during ischemia.[78] Together, ezrin and myosin I both participate in linking the actin core to the overlying membrane, either directly or through a peripheral or transmembrane protein. Therefore, during ischemia, this finely regulated association is disrupted, resulting in a separation of the actin core from the apical surface membrane.

In addition to losing the connection from the core to the overlying membrane, the microfilament core itself is disrupted. Villin, an actin-severing protein, was initially implicated in this disruption because it was shown that it severed the filaments of the microvillus core in the presence of the Ca^{2+} channel, ionomycin, and increasing concentrations of Ca^{2+}.[79] However, two lines of evidence make this an unlikely scenario in vivo. First, intracellular Ca^{2+} levels would have to reach 10 μM for actin filament severing, and this seems highly unlikely, especially during the early phase of cellular injury. Second, actin alterations are known to occur when intracellular (BAM, unpublished observations) or extracellular Ca^{2+} concentrations are maintained at near physiologic levels.[80] This indicates that the Ca^{2+}-dependent severing by villin or gelsolin is not involved in microfilament severing under in vivo conditions. It is interesting to note that recent evidence suggests that the Ca^{2+}-dependent severing protein, gelsolin, although present in murine PTCs, is not present in human PTCs.[81]

During ischemia and ATP depletion, the complex meshwork of actin filaments beneath the plasma membrane and junctional complexes is also disrupted. The intricate lattice of fodrin is disturbed and dissociates from the cortical actin and its membrane linker, ankyrin.[82, 83] This breakdown results in the loss of specific membrane protein domains and membrane stability. The once-tethered integral membrane proteins are now free to diffuse through the membrane bilayer, which results in the loss of membrane polarity.[82, 83]

Effect of ATP Depletion on Sequestering Protein: Actin Interactions

Many of the effects of ischemia and ATP depletion can be attributed to disruption of the normal regulatory machinery that controls cytoskeletal organization, but recent data,[84] as well as an examination of the in vitro properties of actin and actin-binding proteins, indicate that at least one aspect of cytoskeletal disruption is best explained by a direct biochemical effect of excess ADP-actin on the equilibrium between sequestered and unsequestered actin monomers. Actin itself binds ATP or ADP, and the nature of the bound nucleotide, whether di- or triphosphate, affects the polymerization kinetics of actin monomers.[18] Moreover, the affinity of actin-binding proteins for actin differs, sometimes substantially, depending on the state of the bound nucleotide. For example, thymosin has a higher affinity for ATP- than ADP-bound actin,[85] whereas ADF/cofilin proteins bind preferentially to ADP-bound actin.[49, 86] ATP depletion has been shown to result in the net conversion of G-actin to F-actin.[13] A shift in the cellular concentrations of ATP- and ADP-bound actin may directly cause unregulated polymerization by disturbing the equilibrium between the sequestered and the nonsequestered pools of actin monomers, by means of release of monomers from

thymosin-sequestered pools.[87] These actin monomers can then be driven to polymerize by the action of profilin.[26]

ACTIN ALTERATIONS ASSOCIATED WITH APICAL MEMBRANE DAMAGE: ROLE OF ADF/COFILIN

The role that ADF/cofilin proteins play in ARF has recently been investigated.[88] Indirect immunofluorescent studies of rat kidney cortical sections demonstrated that under physiologic conditions ADF/cofilin proteins were located diffusely in the cytoplasm of all renal cells, with no apparent staining of the nucleus or subcellular compartments and little or no staining of the apical microvillous region. The phosphorylated form of the protein was also distributed throughout the cytoplasm in a homogeneous, fine granular pattern with punctate accumulations. Proximal tubule cells had an apparent higher percentage of the unphosphorylated ADF/cofilin proteins, whereas distal tubule cells had a higher percentage of the phosphorylated form. This evidence suggested that distal tubules have increased amounts of inactive ADF/cofilin proteins, and PTCs had more of the active form. This cytoplasmic protein distribution dramatically changed with renal arterial clamp–induced ischemia. Although the total amount of the ADF/cofilin proteins was not affected by clamping, the concentration of the phosphorylated form in the PTC decreased rapidly in a time-dependent fashion. Since dephosphorylation is associated with activation of the ADF/cofilin proteins, we postulated that ischemia could induce the dramatic actin cytoskeletal changes observed during ischemia through the ADF/cofilin proteins (Fig. 8–4). After 25 minutes of ischemia, the microfilaments present in the apical microvilli were disrupted, and the microvilli broken down. The apical membrane was shed into the lumen of the proximal tubules as membrane vesicles. These intraluminal vesicles or blebs had a high concentration of both G-actin and ADF/cofilin proteins. The high concentration of vesicular G-actin and ADF/cofilin proteins suggested that the microfilaments of the microvilli were depolymerized by the recruitment of activated ADF/cofilin proteins to the apical microvillar surface during ischemia. There was also a loss of total ADF/cofilin and F-actin staining in the ischemic cell, but marked accumulations of ADF and F-actin punctate staining were present. Finally, there are studies[89] that indicate that ischemia resulted in the rapid dissociation of tropomyosin bound to the terminal web actin. This would expose actin filaments to ADF/cofilin binding and pointed-end depolymerization.

The effects of 25 minutes of ischemia followed by a 24-hour reflow recovery period were also investigated. The localization of phosphorylated and unphosphorylated ADF/cofilin proteins was restored to the physiologic distribution. The intraluminal vesicles disappeared, and F-actin staining in the apical microvilli returned to normal, although the microvilli were shorter. Urine from rats exposed to 25 minutes of

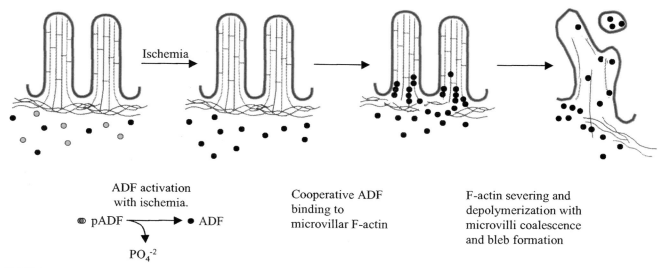

ADF activation
with ischemia.

pADF ⟶ ADF

PO$_4$$^{-2}$

Cooperative ADF
binding to
microvillar F-actin

F-actin severing and
depolymerization with
microvilli coalescence
and bleb formation

FIGURE 8–4 ■ A proposed model for ischemia-induced actin depolymerizing factor (ADF) dephosphorylation, translocation, and binding to apical domain F-actin structures. This results in ADF-mediated severing and depolymerization of F-actin and subsequent apical membrane disruption.

ischemia was analyzed to determine whether the cytoskeletal proteins were excreted. Under physiologic conditions, Western blot analysis of the rat urine did not demonstrate the presence of actin, pADF/cofilin, or ADF/cofilin proteins. However, all three proteins were present in the urine following ischemic cell injury.

These studies suggest alterations in actin-binding proteins, in general, and ADF/cofilin proteins, in particular, play a pivotal role in ischemia-induced injury in PTCs (see Fig. 8–4). Not only were the apical microvilli broken down and shed into the lumen of the tubules following ischemia but also the microfilaments within the microvilli were destroyed. The distribution of the ADF/cofilin proteins, both phosphorylated and unphosphorylated, changed with ischemia from a diffuse localization throughout the cell to enhanced concentrations within vesicles shed from the apical membrane. In kidneys permitted to recover from the ischemic insult, the microvilli re-formed with intact microfilaments, and the distribution of phosphorylated and unphosphorylated ADF/cofilin proteins returned to baseline conditions. Although this evidence is supportive of a role for ADF/cofilin protein during ischemia, there are still many unanswered questions.

REGULATION OF ACTIN ORGANIZATION BY Rho GTPases

The functions of the actin cytoskeleton are integrated and controlled in response to intracellular and extracellular cues and stimuli and are coordinated with other cellular responses, be they mitogenic, apoptotic, or pathologic. Guanosine triphosphatases (GTPases) of the rho family appear to be central to the signaling pathways that accomplish this regulation.[90] Studies in a wide variety of cell types and in many organisms have

confirmed this role. New members of the Rho family are still being identified, but most studies have focused on the three ubiquitous and best studied members of the family, RhoA, Rac, and Cdc42. From the original paradigm of introducing high concentrations of dominant negative or constitutively active mutants into fibroblasts by transfection or microinjection,[91–93] recent experiments have evolved to explore the roles of GTPases in other cell types, and the use of other techniques, such as the use of transgenic animals, is beginning to reveal other more subtle features of their roles.

Mechanism

Rho GTPases are members of the ras superfamily of p21 GTPases. As such, they act as molecular switches (Fig. 8–5), cycling between GTP- and GDP-bound conformations.[94] Transition from the GTP-bound to the GDP-bound state is the result of GTP hydrolysis catalyzed by the GTPase. The intrinsic rate of GTP hydrolysis is typically low and, in the cellular context, is stimulated by GTPase-binding proteins called GAPs (GTPase activating proteins), which therefore act as negative regulators of the pathways downstream of the GTPase. Regeneration of the GTP-bound form requires exchange of the bound GDP for free GTP, which usually predominates in the cytosol.[95] This naturally begs the question of what then is the effect on GTPase pathways of cytosolic GTP depletion.[95] Nucleotide exchange is catalyzed by guanine nucleotide exchange factors (GEFs), the positive regulators of these pathways. The mechanism by which GAPs and GEFs are regulated by upstream signals is a major unanswered question. The three archetypal members of the Rho family are differentially regulated by upstream signaling pathways. In fibroblasts, Rho activation is stimulated by lysophos-

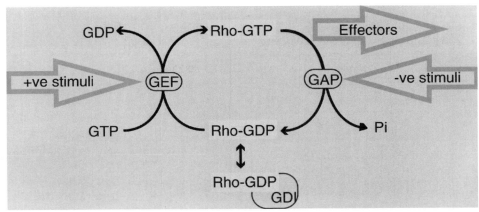

FIGURE 8–5 ■ Schematic representation of the GTPase cycle of Rho and related p21 GTPases. In the GTP-bound form, the GTPase is membrane-associated and can bind and activate downstream effector molecules. In the GDP-bound conformation, the GTPase may be associated with a GDI shuttle molecule. The relative amount of GTP- and GDP-bound GTPase is regulated by the activities of GEF and GAP proteins. *GAP*, guanosine triphosphate activating protein; *GDI*, guanine nucleotide dissociation inhibitor; *GDP*, guanosine diphosphate; *GEF*, guanine nucleotide exchange factor; *GTP*, guanosine triphosphate; *Pi*, inorganic phosphate; *+ve*, positive; *−ve*, negative.

phatidic acid (LPA), Rac activation is stimulated by PDGF and other ligands of tyrosine-kinase–linked receptors, whereas Cdc42 is activated by ligation of heterotrimeric G-protein–coupled receptors.[90] Clearly, the exact signals that result in GTPase activation are cell type–specific. An additional complicating factor is the existence of cross-talk between the activities of the rho GTPases. Early studies in fibroblasts indicated that in this cell type an hierarchical organization operates, in which Cdc42 activation activates Rac, which in turn activates Rho.[93] More recent studies[96] have shown that in other systems Rac activation down-regulates Rho, and our own studies (SJA and DA Williams, et al, submitted) have shown that hematopoietic stem cells lacking Rac2 have hyperactive Cdc42. Moreover, Rho GTPase activity is strongly interdependent with the activity of Ras and related signaling pathways.[97, 98] Moreover, the influence of components of these pathways on one another is fundamentally dependent on the specific cellular context, as illustrated by the discrepant behavior of neutrophils and hematopoietic stem cells from Rac2-deficient mice[99] (and SJA and DA Williams et al, submitted). The degree to which these pathways are influenced by other factors, such as cellular stress or injury, is largely unexplored at present, although there is evidence for activation of rho GTPase-dependent pathways (specifically JUNK/SAPK[100]) in ischemic renal injury.

Effects

The effects of rho GTPase activation have many features in common among different cell types, and there are also significant cell type–specific differences that are related, of course, to the differences in actin organization among the cell types. Activation of RhoA is typically associated with augmentation of cytoskeletal structures involved in cell-substrate adhesion, as typified by focal adhesions and stress fibers in cultured fibroblasts.[91, 92] In epithelial cells, RhoA activation also affects cell-cell adhesion via tight and adherens junctions.[101–106] Rac activation induces actin polymerization to produce membrane ruffles, lamellipodia, or pseudopodia, whose morphology depends on the cell type.[91, 107] In epithelial cells, Rac also induces actin polymerization in association with the adherens junction.[101, 102] Cdc42 induces formation of finger-like filopodia.[93] Studies in a variety of model systems also indicate an important role for this GTPase in setting out and reinforcing polarity in cytoskeletal organization.[108–111] Recent studies have highlighted the effects of rho GTPase activation on processes such as endocytosis and traffic through the secretory pathway,[112, 113] which potentially makes GTPases important in the coordination of morphologic changes and cellular physiology and behavior.

Target Molecules

A number of direct and indirect targets of rho GTPase signaling have been identified. Direct targets, those for which a direct protein-protein interaction with Rho has been demonstrated, are protein serine/threonine kinases, adaptor proteins (ie, proteins with multiple binding sites for other molecules that collect these targets, which are then activated by proximity), and possibly lipid kinases (although recent evidence indicates that activation of lipid kinases may be indirectly mediated via protein kinases[114]). Potentially complete pathways linking GTPase activation to effects on the actin cytoskeleton have been established in a number of cases. Stress fiber assembly induced by RhoA activation, for example, proceeds as the result of activation of two downstream targets, cytoplasmic myosin II and mDia. Of these, mDia, an adaptor protein, is activated directly by binding of RhoA-GTP.[115–117] Its activation results from dissociation of an intramolecular interaction, resulting in exposure of binding sites for a number of proteins, including profilin. Myosin II activation results from activation of the serine/threonine kinase Rock (Rho kinase), a direct target of RhoA.[118-121] This kinase may directly phosphorylate the myosin light chain, but it also is responsible for inhibitory phosphorylation of the myosin light chain phosphatase targeting subunit, also resulting in a net increase in myosin phosphorylation. Cdc42 induction of actin polymerization is mediated by activation of WASP/SCAR adaptor proteins, which bind and activate Arp2/3 complex.[66, 67, 122, 123] Rho, Rac, and Cdc42 all activate LIM kinases, which can phosphorylate ADF/cofilin proteins.[57, 58, 124] In platelets, at least, Rac activation appears to increase the levels of polyphosphoinositides, with resulting uncapping of actin filament barbed ends.[32]

ROLE IN ISCHEMIC ACUTE RENAL FAILURE

Rho family GTPases are obvious candidates for important roles in cytoskeletal disruption in ischemic ARF. This has been explored by expressing constitutively active and dominant negative mutants of RhoA in a proximal tubule–derived cell line.[125] Constitutively active RhoA was found to prevent aspects of cytoskeletal disruption that normally accompany ischemia or ATP depletion, such as stress fiber disassembly and loss of F-actin at the junctional complex. Activated Rho also prevented disruption of tight junctions.[105] A role for Rho GTPases in recovery from ischemic injury is also consistent with the demonstration that there is activation of the JNK/SAPK stress kinase pathways during reflow.[126]

Role in Potential Therapies

The involvement of Rho GTPases in ischemic injury and recovery provides novel pathways that could be targets of therapeutic intervention in the future. Modulation of the activity of these pathways may ameliorate injury or enhance recovery. Growth factors have received attention in the treatment of injury, and in animal models some improvement in renal function was observed in animals to which insulin-like growth factor (IGF), epidermal growth factor (EGF), or human growth factor (HGF) was administered,[127-131] although clinical trials have been disappointing.[132] Therefore, targeting of growth factor receptors known to modulate Rho GTPase activity in specific ways may be a beneficial approach.

THERAPY

As we gain a fuller understanding of the cellular protein-protein interactions regulating the actin cytoskeleton, we can better explain the intracellular protein dynamics under physiologic and ischemic conditions. Many questions remain unanswered, from what events cause the breakdown of the actin structures to how these structures re-form in recovering cells. Answers to these questions may lead to therapeutic applications for the treatment of ARF that minimize injury or accelerate cellular repair and recovery.

REFERENCES

1. Maunsbach AB, Christensen EL: Functional Ultrastructure of the Proximal Tubule. In: Windhager EE, ed: *Handbook of Physiology. Section 8. Renal Physiology.* New York: Oxford University Press; 1992:41–107.
2. Maunsbach AB: Ultrastructure of the Proximal Tubule. In: Orloff J, Berliner RW, Geiger SR, eds: *Handbook of Physiology. Section 8. Renal Physiology.* Baltimore, MD: Waverly Press Inc; 1973:31–70.
3. Sacktor B: Membranes and Cellular Functions. In: Jamieson GA, Robinson DM, eds: *Mammalian Cell Membranes.* Boston, MA: Butterworths; 1977:221–254.
4. Kenny AJ, Booth AG: Microvilli: Their Ultrastructure, Enzymology, and Molecular Organization. In: Campbell PN, Aldridge WN, eds: *Essays in Biochemistry.* New York: Academic Press; 1978:1–44.
5. Molitoris BA: Putting the actin cytoskeleton into perspective: pathophysiology of ischemic alterations. Am J Physiol 1997; 272:F430–F433.
6. Kellerman PS, et al: Role of microfilaments in maintenance of proximal tubule structural and functional integrity. Am J Physiol 1990; 259:F279–F285.
7. Louvard D, Kedinger M, Hauri HP: The differentiating intestinal epithelial cell: establishment and maintenance of functions through interactions between cellular structures. Annu Rev Cell Biol 1992; 8:157–195.
8. Molitoris BA, Falk SA, Dahl RH: Ischemia-induced loss of epithelial polarity: role of the tight junction. J Clin Invest 1989; 84:1334–1339.
9. Venkatachalam MA, et al: Mechanism of proximal tubule brush border loss and regeneration following mild renal ischemia. Lab Invest 1981; 45:355–365.
10. Jones DB: Ultrastructure of human acute renal failure. Lab Invest 1982; 46:254–264.
11. Shanley PF, et al: Hypoxic injury in the proximal tubule of the isolated perfused rat kidney. Kidney Int 1986; 29:1021–1032.
12. Sutton TA, Molitoris BA: Mechanisms of cellular injury in ischemic acute renal failure. Semin Nephrol 1998; 18:490–497.
13. Molitoris BA, Geerdes A, McIntosh JR: Dissociation and redistribution of Na+,K+-ATPase from its surface membrane actin cytoskeletal complex during cellular ATP depletion. J Clin Invest 1991; 88:462–469.
14. Canfield PE, Geerdes AM, Molitoris BA: Effect of reversible ATP depletion on tight-junction integrity in LLC-PK₁ cells. Am J Physiol 1991; 261:F1038–F1045.
15. Feuer G, Straub FB: Studies on the composition and polymerization of actin. Hung Acta Physiol 1948; 1:150–163.
16. Pollard TD, Cooper JA: Actin and actin-binding proteins: a critical evaluation of mechanisms and functions. Annu Rev Biochem 1986; 55:987–1035.
17. Kabsch W, Vandekerckhove J: Structure and function of actin. Annu Rev Biophys Biomol Struct 1992; 21:49–76.
18. Carlier MF: Actin polymerization and ATP hydrolysis. Adv Biophys 1990; 26:51–73.
19. Kasai M, Askura S, Oosawa F: The cooperative nature of G-F transformation of actin. Biochim Biophys Acta 1960; 57:22–30.
20. Frieden C: Actin and tubulin polymerization: the use of kinetic methods to determine mechanism. Annu Rev Biophys Biomol Struct 1985; 14:189–210.
21. Pollard TD, Blanchoin L, Mullins RD: Molecular mechanisms controlling actin filament dynamics in nonmuscle cells. Annu Rev Biophys Biomol Struct 2000; 29:545–576.
22. Safer D, Nachmias VT: Beta thymosins as actin binding peptides. Bioessays 1994; 16:473–479.
23. Machesky LM, Pollard TD: Profilin as a potential mediator of membrane-cytoskeleton communication. Trends Cell Biol 1993; 3:381–385.
24. Pollard TD, Cooper JA: Quantitative analysis of the effect of *Acanthamoeba* profilin on actin filament nucleation and elongation. Biochemistry 1984; 23:6631–6641.

25. Vinson VK, et al: Interactions of *Acanthamoeba* profilin with actin and nucleotides bound to actin. Biochemistry 1998; 37:10871–10880.

26. Goldschmidt-Clermont PJ, et al: The control of actin nucleotide exchange by thymosin beta 4 and profilin: a potential regulatory mechanism for actin polymerization in cells. Mol Biol Cell 1992; 3:1015–1024.

27. Pantaloni D, Carlier MF: How profilin promotes actin filament assembly in the presence of thymosin beta 4. Cell 1993; 75:1007–1014.

28. Lassing I, Lindberg U: Specificity of the interaction between phosphatidylinositol 4,5-bisphosphate and the profilin:actin complex. J Cell Biochem 1988; 37:255–267.

29. Goldschmidt-Clermont PJ, et al: Regulation of phospholipase-C-gamma-1 by profilin and tyrosine phosphorylation. Science 1991; 251:1231–1233.

30. Weeds A, Maciver S: F-actin capping proteins. (Review) Curr Opin Cell Biol 1993; 5:63–69.

31. Schafer DA, Jennings PB, Cooper JA: Dynamics of capping protein and actin assembly in vitro: uncapping barbed ends by polyphosphoinositides. J Cell Biol 1996; 135:169–179.

32. Hartwig JH, et al: Thrombin receptor ligation and activated Rac uncap actin filament barbed ends through phosphoinositide synthesis in permeabilized human platelets. Cell 1995; 82:643–653.

33. Aufricht C, et al: Heat-shock protein 25 induction and redistribution during actin reorganization after renal ischemia. Am J Physiol 1998; 274:F215–F222.

34. Aufricht C, et al: ATP releases HSP-72 from protein aggregates after renal ischemia. Am J Physiol 1998; 274:F268–F274.

35. Yin HL, Stossel TP: Control of cytoplasmic actin gel-sol transformation by gelsolin, a calcium-dependent regulatory protein. Nature 1979; 281:583–586.

36. Yin HL: Gelsolin: calcium- and polyphosphoinositide-regulated actin-modulating protein. Bioessays 1987; 7:176–179.

37. Witke W, et al: Hemostatic, inflammatory, and fibroblast responses are blunted in mice lacking gelsolin. Cell 1995; 81:41–51.

38. Weber A, et al: Tropomodulin caps the pointed ends of actin filaments. J Cell Biol 1994; 127:1627–1635.

39. Janmey PA, et al: Viscoelastic properties of vimentin compared with other filamentous biopolymer networks. J Cell Biol 1991; 113:155–160.

40. Maciver SK, et al: The actin filament severing protein actophorin promotes the formation of rigid bundles of actin-filaments cross-linked with alpha-actinin. J Cell Biol 1991; 115:1621–1628.

41. Wachsstock DH, Schwartz WH, Pollard TD: Affinity of alpha-actinin for actin determines the structure and mechanical properties of actin filament gels. Biophys J 1993; 65:205–214.

42. Wachsstock DH, Schwarz WH, Pollard TD: Cross-linker dynamics determine the mechanical properties of actin gels. Biophys J 1994; 66:801–809.

43. Sanders MC, et al: Characterization of the actin cross-linking properties of the scruin-calmodulin complex from the acrosomal process of *Limulus* sperm. J Biol Chem 1996; 271:2651–2657.

44. Gorlin JB, et al: Human endothelial actin-binding protein (ABP-280, nonmuscle filamin): a molecular leaf spring. J Cell Biol 1990; 111:1089–1105.

45. Friederich E, et al: From the structure to the function of villin, an actin-binding protein of the brush border. Bioessays 1990; 12:403–408.

46. Johnson RP, Craig SW: F-actin binding site masked by the intramolecular association of vinculin head and tail domains. Nature 1995; 373:261–264.

47. Duhaiman AS, Bamburg JR: Isolation of brain alpha-actinin: its characterization and a comparison of its properties with those of muscle alpha-actinins. Biochemistry 1984; 23:1600–1608.

48. Bamburg JR: Proteins of the ADF/cofilin family: essential regulators of actin dynamics. Annu Rev Cell Dev Biol 1999; 15:185–230.

49. Maciver SK, Weeds AG: Actophorin preferentially binds monomeric ADP-actin over ATP-bound actin: consequences for cell locomotion. FEBS Lett 1994; 347:251–256.

50. Blanchoin L, Pollard TD: Mechanism of interaction of *Acanthamoeba* actophorin (ADF/Cofilin) with actin filaments. J Biol Chem 1999, 274:15538–15546.

51. Ressad F, et al: Control of actin filament length and turnover by actin depolymerizing factor (ADF/cofilin) in the presence of capping proteins and ARP2/3 complex. J Biol Chem 1999; 274:20970–20976.

52. Hawkins M, et al: Human actin depolymerizing factor mediates a pH-sensitive destruction of actin filaments. Biochemistry 1993; 32:9985–9993.

53. Hayden SM, et al: Analysis of the interactions of actin depolymerizing factor with G- and F-actin. Biochemistry 1993; 32:9994–10004.

54. Gores GJ, et al: Intracellular pH during "chemical hypoxia" in cultured rat hepatocytes: protection by intracellular acidosis against the onset of cell death. J Clin Invest 1989; 83:386–396.

55. Morgan TE, et al: Isolation and characterization of a regulated form of actin depolymerizing factor. J Cell Biol 1993; 122:623–633.

56. Agnew BJ, Minamide LS, Bamburg JR: Reactivation of phosphorylated actin depolymerizing factor and identification of the regulatory site. J Biol Chem 1995; 270:17582–17587.

57. Arber S, et al: Regulation of actin dynamics through phosphorylation of cofilin by LIM-kinase. Nature 1998; 393: 805–809.

58. Yang N, et al: Cofilin phosphorylation by LIM-kinase 1 and its role in Rac-mediated actin reorganization. Nature 1998; 393:809–812.

59. Yonezawa N, et al: Inhibition of the interactions of cofilin, destrin, and deoxyribonuclease I with actin by phosphoinositides. J Biol Chem 1990; 265:8382–8386.

60. Bamburg JR, Bernstein BW: Actin and actin-binding proteins in neurons. In: Burgoyne RD, ed: *The Neuronal Cytoskeleton.* New York: Wiley-Liss; 1991:121–160.

61. Machesky LM, et al: Purification of a cortical complex containing two unconventional actins from *Acanthamoeba* by affinity chromatography on profilin-agarose. J Cell Biol 1994; 127:107–115.

62. Mullins RD, Heuser JA, Pollard TD: The interaction of Arp2/3 complex with actin: nucleation, high affinity pointed end capping, and formation of branching networks of filaments. Proc Natl Acad Sci USA 1998; 95:6181–6186.

63. Welch MD, et al: Interaction of human Arp2/3 complex and the *Listeria monocytogenes* ActA protein in actin filament nucleation. Science 1998; 281:105–108.

64. Kelleher JF, Atkinson SJ, Pollard TD: Sequences, structural models, and cellular localization of the actin-related proteins Arp2 and Arp3 from *Acanthamoeba.* J Cell Biol 1995; 131:385–397.

65. Blanchoin L, et al: Direct observation of dendritic actin filament networks nucleated by Arp2/3 complex and WASP/Scar proteins. Nature 2000; 404:1007–1011.

66. Machesky LM, Insall RH: Scar1 and the related Wiskott-Aldrich syndrome protein, WASp, regulate the actin cytoskeleton through the Arp2/3 complex. Curr Biol 1998; 31:1347–1356.

67. Machesky LM, et al: Scar, a WASp-related protein, activates nucleation of actin filaments by the Arp2/3 complex. Proc Natl Acad Sci USA 1999; 96:3739–3744.

68. Molitoris BA: New insights into the cell biology of ischemic acute renal failure. J Am Soc Nephrol 1991; 1:1263–1270.

69. Molitoris BA, Wagner MC: Surface membrane polarity of proximal tubular cells: alterations as a basis for malfunction. Kidney Int 1996; 49:1592–1597.

70. Bacallao R, et al: ATP depletion: a novel method to study junctional properties in epithelial tissues. 1. Rearrangement of the actin cytoskeleton. J Cell Sci 1994; 107:3301–3313.

71. Molitoris BA: Ischemia-induced loss of epithelial polarity: potential role of the actin cytoskeleton. (Editorial) Am J Physiol 1991; 260:F769–F778.

72. Leiser J, Molitoris BA: Disease processes in epithelia: the role of the actin cytoskeleton and altered surface membrane polarity. Biochim Biophys Acta 1993; 1225:1–13.

73. Fath KR, Mamajiwalla SN, Burgess DR: The cytoskeleton in development of epithelial cell polarity. J Cell Sci 1993; 17(suppl):65–73.

74. Kellerman PS, Norenberg SL, Jones GM: Early recovery of the actin cytoskeleton during renal ischemic injury in vivo. Am J Kidney Dis 1996; 27:709–714.

75. Chen J, Doctor RB, Mandel LJ: Cytoskeletal dissociation of ezrin during renal anoxia: role in microvillar injury. Am J Physiol 1994; 267:C784–C795.

76. Chen J, Cohn JA, Mandel LJ: Dephosphorylation of ezrin as an early event in renal microvillar breakdown and anoxic injury. Proc Natl Acad Sci USA 1995; 92:7495–7499.

77. Chen J, Mandel LJ: Unopposed phosphatase action initiates ezrin dysfunction: a potential mechanism for anoxic injury. Am J Physiol 1997; 273:C710–C716.

78. Wagner MC, Molitoris BA: ATP depletion alters myosin I beta cellular location in LLC-PK$_1$ cells. Am J Physiol 1997; 272: C1680–C1690.

79. Nurko S, et al: Contribution of actin cytoskeletal alterations to ATP depletion and calcium-induced proximal tubule cell injury. Am J Physiol 1996; 270:F39–F52.

80. Sogabe K, et al: Calcium dependence of integrity of the actin cytoskeleton of proximal tubule cell microvilli. Am J Physiol 1996; 271:F292–F303.

81. Lueck A, Brown D, Kwiatkowski DJ: The actin-binding proteins adseverin and gelsolin are both highly expressed but differentially localized in kidney and intestine. J Cell Sci 1998; 111:3633–3643.

82. Doctor RB, Bennett V, Mandel LJ: Degradation of spectrin and ankyrin in the ischemic rat kidney. Am J Physiol 1993; 264:C1003–C1013.

83. Molitoris BA, Dahl R, Hosford M: Cellular ATP depletion induces disruption of the spectrin cytoskeletal network. Am J Physiol 1996; 271:F790–F798.

84. Molitoris BA, et al: Mechanism of cellular ATP depletion induced actin polymerization. Mol Biol Cell 1996; 7:204a.

85. Carlier MF, et al: Modulation of the interaction between G-actin and thymosin beta 4 by the ATP/ADP ratio: possible implication in the regulation of actin dynamics. Proc Natl Acad Sci USA 1993; 90:5034–5038.

86. Blanchoin L, Pollard TD: Interaction of actin monomers with Acanthamoeba actophorin (ADF/cofilin) and profilin. J Biol Chem 1998; 273:25106–25111.

87. Molitoris BA, Atkinson SJ, Hosford M: Cellular ATP depletion results in reduced ATP–G-actin. Paper presented at 40th American Society for Cell Biology Annual Meeting, 2000; San Francisco, CA.

88. Schwartz N, et al: Ischemia activates actin depolymerizing factor: role in proximal tubule microvillar actin alterations. Am J Physiol 1999; 276:F544–F551.

89. Ashworth SA, et al: Ischemia induces tropomyosin dissociation from the proximal tubule cell terminal web. Paper presented at 40th American Society for Cell Biology Annual Meeting, 2000; San Francisco, CA.

90. Hall A: Rho GTPases and the actin cytoskeleton. Science 1998; 279:509–514.

91. Ridley AJ, et al: The small GTP-binding protein rac regulates growth factor–induced membrane ruffling. Cell 1992; 70:401–410.

92. Ridley AJ, Hall A: The small GTP-binding protein rho regulates the assembly of focal adhesions and actin stress fibers in response to growth factors. Cell 1992; 70:389–399.

93. Nobes CD, Hall A: Rho, rac, and cdc42 GTPases regulate the assembly of multimolecular focal complexes associated with actin stress fibers, lamellipodia, and filopodia. Cell 1995; 81:53–62.

94. Van Aelst L, D'Souza-Schorey C: Rho GTPases and signaling networks. Genes Dev 1997; 11:2295–2322.

95. Dagher PC: Modeling ischemia in vitro: selective depletion of adenine and guanine nucleotide pools. Am J Physiol Cell Physiol 2000; 279:C1270–C1277.

96. Sander EE, et al: Rac downregulates Rho activity: reciprocal balance between both GTPases determines cellular morphology and migratory behavior. J Cell Biol 1999; 147:1009–1022.

97. Zondag GC, et al: Oncogenic Ras downregulates Rac activity, which leads to increased Rho activity and epithelial-mesenchymal transition. J Cell Biol 2000; 149:775–782.

98. Qiu RG, et al: An essential role for Rac in Ras transformation. Nature 1995; 374:457–459.

99. Roberts AW, et al: Deficiency of the hematopoietic cell-specific Rho family GTPase Rac2 is characterized by abnormalities in neutrophil function and host defense. Immunity 1999; 10:183–196.

100. Morooka H, et al: Ischemia and reperfusion enhance ATF-2 and c-Jun binding to cAMP response elements and to an AP-1 binding site from the c-Jun promoter. J Biol Chem 1995; 270:30084–30092.

101. Braga VM, et al: Regulation of cadherin function by Rho and Rac: modulation by junction maturation and cellular context. Mol Biol Cell 1999; 10:9–22.

102. Braga VM, et al: The small GTPases Rho and Rac are required for the establishment of cadherin-dependent cell-cell contacts. J Cell Biol 1997; 137:1421–1431.

103. Jou TS, Schneeberger EE, James Nelson W: Structural and functional regulation of tight junctions by RhoA and rac1 small GTPases. J Cell Biol 1998; 142:101–115.

104. Nusrat A, et al: Rho protein regulates tight junctions and perijunctional actin organization in polarized epithelia. Proc Natl Acad Sci USA 1995; 92:10629–10633.

105. Gopalakrishnan S, et al: Rho GTPase signaling regulates tight junction assembly and protects tight junctions during ATP depletion. Am J Physiol 1998; 275:C798–C809.

106. Takaishi K, et al: Regulation of cell-cell adhesion by rac and rho small G proteins in MDCK cells. J Cell Biol 1997; 139:1047–1059.

107. Allen WE, et al: Rho, Rac and Cdc42 regulate actin organization and cell adhesion in macrophages. J Cell Sci 1997; 110:707–720.

108. Eaton S, Wepf R, Simons K: Roles for Rac1 and Cdc42 in planar polarization and hair outgrowth in the wing of Drosophila. J Cell Biol 1996; 135:1277–1289.

109. Nobes CD, Hall A: Rho GTPases control polarity, protrusion, and adhesion during cell movement. J Cell Biol 1999; 144:1235–1244.

110. Allen WE, et al: A role for Cdc42 in macrophage chemotaxis. J Cell Biol 1998; 141:1147–1157.

111. Drubin DG: Development of cell polarity in budding yeast. Cell 1991; 65:1093–1096.

112. Kroschewski R, Hall A, Mellman I: Cdc42 controls secretory and endocytic transport to the basolateral plasma membrane of MDCK cells. Nat Cell Biol 1999; 1:8–13.

113. Ellis S, Mellor H: Regulation of endocytic traffic by rho family GTPases. Trends Cell Biol 2000; 10:85–88.

114. Oude Weernink PA, et al: Stimulation of phosphatidylinositol-4-phosphate 5-kinase by Rho-kinase. J Biol Chem 2000; 275:10168–10174.

115. Watanabe N, et al: p140mDia, a mammalian homolog of Drosophila diaphanous, is a target protein for Rho small GTPase and is a ligand for profilin. EMBO J 1997; 16:3044–3056.

116. Nakano K, et al: Distinct actions and cooperative roles of ROCK and mDia in Rho small G protein–induced reorganization of the actin cytoskeleton in Madin-Darby canine kidney cells. Mol Biol Cell 1999; 10:2481–2491.

117. Watanabe N, et al: Cooperation between mDia1 and ROCK in Rho-induced actin reorganization. J Cell Biol 1999; 1:136–143.

118. Amano M, et al: Phosphorylation and activation of myosin by Rho-associated kinase (Rho-kinase). J Biol Chem 1996; 271:20246–20249.

119. Kimura K, et al: Regulation of myosin phosphatase by Rho and Rho-associated kinase (Rho-kinase). Science 1996; 273:245–248.

120. Chihara K, et al: Cytoskeletal rearrangements and transcriptional activation of c-fos serum response element by Rho-kinase. J Biol Chem 1997; 272:25121–25127.

121. Amano M, et al: Formation of actin stress fibers and focal adhesions enhanced by Rho-kinase. Science 1997; 275:1308–1311.

122. Ma L, Rohatgi R, Kirschner MW: The Arp2/3 complex mediates actin polymerization induced by the small GTP-binding protein Cdc42. Proc Natl Acad Sci USA 1998; 95:15362–15367.

123. Rohatgi R, et al: The interaction between N-WASp and the Arp2/3 complex links Cdc42-dependent signals to actin assembly. Cell 1999; 97:221–231.

124. Sumi T, *et al: Cofilin phosphorylation and actin cytoskeletal dynamics regulated by rho- and Cdc42-activated LIM-kinase 2. J Cell Biol 1999; 147:1519–1532.

125. Raman N, Atkinson SJ: Rho controls actin cytoskeletal assembly in renal epithelial cells during ATP depletion and recovery. Am J Physiol 1999; 276:C1312–C1324.

126. Pombo CM, et al: The stress-activated protein kinases are major c-Jun amino-terminal kinases activated by ischemia and reperfusion. J Biol Chem 1994; 269:26546–26551.

127. Hirschberg R, Ding H: Mechanisms of insulin-like growth factor-I–induced accelerated recovery in experimental ischemic acute renal failure. Miner Electrolyte Metab 1998; 24:211–219.

128. Hirschberg R, Ding H: Growth factors and acute renal failure. Semin Nephrol 1998; 18:191–207.

129. Vargas GA, Hoeflich A, Jehle PM: Hepatocyte growth factor in renal failure: promise and reality. Kidney Int 2000; 57:1426–1436.

130. Kawaida K, et al: Hepatocyte growth factor prevents acute renal failure and accelerates renal regeneration in mice. Proc Natl Acad Sci USA 1994; 91:4357–4361.

131. Harris RC: Growth factors and cytokines in acute renal failure. Adv Ren Replace Ther 1997; 4(2 suppl 1):43–53.

132. Hirschberg R, et al: Multicenter clinical trial of recombinant human insulin-like growth factor I in patients with acute renal failure. Kidney Int 1999; 55:2423–2432.

Tight Junction and Adherens Junction Dysfunction During Ischemic Injury

James A. Marrs ▪ Shobha Gopalakrishnan ▪ Robert L. Bacallao

INTRODUCTION

Studies of renal ischemia have revealed their significant functional consequences on epithelial cell junctional complexes: tight junctions, adherens junctions, and cell-substrate adhesion complexes. These junctions associate with the actin cytoskeleton, which is severely disrupted during ischemic injury. This chapter focuses exclusively on the biology of cell-cell junctions, specifically adherens and tight junctions and the consequences of renal ischemia on these structures. These two adhesion junctions are located at the apical-most margin of the lateral plasma membrane, with the tight junction located directly apical to the adherens junction. Both the tight junction and the adherens junction associate with the actin cytoskeleton, and there can be coordinate regulation of these two junctions. Some investigators have considered these junctions together as a single unit: the apical junctional complex. However, the two junctions are functionally distinct and can be regulated separately and independently.

Previous reviews have described the morphology of the epithelial cell damage in detail. In pathology specimens, ischemic injury is characterized by cellular necrosis, particularly in the S3 portion of the proximal tubule, tubular obstruction by cellular casts, and cellular swelling.[1] Recent insights from studies of animal and cell culture models have revealed a correlation between the clinical features of acute tubular necrosis and those of cellular injury.[2] For example, junctional complexes and cell polarity break down during ischemic injury.[3] Oliguric acute tubular necrosis can be associated with tubular obstruction, where loss of cell adhesion is a significant contributing factor in inducing cast formation. In addition, cell polarity loss and the accompanying loss of epithelial transport functions could contribute to the oliguric phase of acute tubular necrosis. Recovery from this acute injury requires reconstitution of intracellular energy stores and the reassembly of critical epithelial structures and functional properties.

Structural features of epithelial cells that are lost during ischemic injury are generally actin cytoskeletal structures or are associated with the actin cytoskeleton (Fig. 9–1 *A–C*). Normal organization of filamentous actin is rapidly lost during ischemia. Actin in microvilli, cortical structures, and focal contacts is lost. Paradoxically, filamentous actin levels increase during ischemia. New actin filaments accumulate in unorganized perinuclear aggregates. The dynamics of this reorganization are described in detail elsewhere in this volume

(see Chapter 8). However, it is important to note that cell-cell junctions rely on an intact actin cytoskeleton in order to be properly assembled.[4–6]

Adhesion junctions are membrane-associated protein complexes between transmembrane proteins with adhesive function and peripheral proteins that are linked to the cytoskeleton.[7] Junctional complex assembly requires an intact actin cytoskeleton. Disassembly of the actin cytoskeleton during renal ischemia directly affects the integrity of adhesion junctional complexes.[3] Adherens junction disassembly during ischemia is coupled to loss of cell polarity and tight junction dysfunction (see Fig. 9–1). Tight junction disruption during ischemic injury[8] results in the loss of the paracellular barrier of epithelial cells, giving rise to specific pathophysiologic consequences such as backleak of luminal fluid to interstitial spaces.[8, 9] Cell-cell adhesion junctions actively participate in the establishment and maintenance of normal epithelial cell polarity.[10]

Another junctional complex that associates with the actin cytoskeleton is the integrin-mediated focal adhesion complex that mediates cell adhesion to the extracellular matrix. This chapter does not focus on the effects of ischemia on cell-substrate adhesion. However, studies on the effects of ischemia on focal adhesion complexes have shown that integrin adhesion was disrupted and integrin protein redistributed as a result of ischemia.[11, 12] The disruption of cell-cell and cell-substrate adhesion contributes to the formation of cellular cast obstructions. Goligorsky and colleagues[11, 13] have shown that soluble peptides that block integrin-mediated adhesion also block cellular cast formation following ischemic injury.

TIGHT JUNCTIONS

Tight junctions are located directly apical to adherens junctions,[14–17] producing a gasket-like tight seal between epithelial cells that prevents free diffusion of ions and solutes across cell boundaries (paracellular transport).[18, 19] Tight junctions also block lateral diffusion of apical or basolateral proteins and lipids within the plane of the plasma membrane and prevent them from diffusing into inappropriate plasma membrane domains.[8]

The tight junction is composed of a growing list of proteins that form a multiprotein junctional complex (Fig. 9–2 and Table 9–1). Integral membrane proteins, such as occludin and claudin, are linked to a group of cytoplasmic plaque proteins.[16, 20] Overexpression of

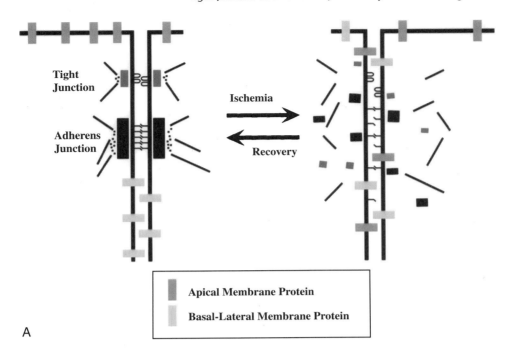

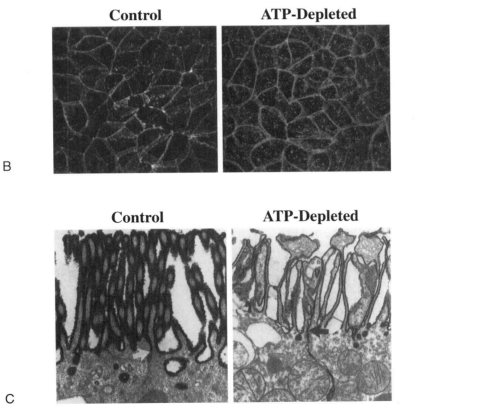

FIGURE 9–1 ■ *(See Color Plate) A,* Ischemia affects epithelial phenotype by disrupting actin cytoskeleton, junctional complexes, and cell polarity. Epithelial cell recovery from ischemic injury requires that these features be re-established. *B,* Extended-focus image of MDCK cells before and after ATP depletion, using fluorescent photomicrography of cultured MDCK cells grown on membrane filter supports, chemically fixed and fluorescence-labeled with anti–E-cadherin antibodies. Each photomicrograph is a stack of 15 image planes obtained from a laser scanning confocal microscope. E-cadherin distribution was altered from the typical adherens junction localization. After ATP depletion, E-cadherin remained localized to the zonula adherens, but a significant proportion of E-cadherin was internalized into punctate vesicular structures distributed throughout the cytoplasm. With longer periods of ATP deprivation, the adherens junction also breaks down. *C,* Rat proximal tubule epithelial cells were labeled using ruthenium red before and after 30 minutes of warm ischemia (cross-clamp model). Ruthenium red–containing fixative solution was directly infused into the kidney to determine the integrity of the tight junctions. Following ischemic injury, the tight junctions were permeable to the ruthenium label, indicating that the tight junction barrier was compromised. *MDCK,* Madin-Darby canine kidney.

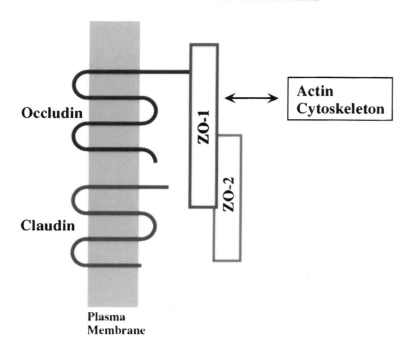

FIGURE 9–2 ■ *(See Color Plate)* Tight junction proteins from a multiprotein complex that controls paracellular permeability. Occludin and claudin are four-pass transmembrane integral membrane proteins. There are numerous members of the claudin family that may create cell type–specific permeability pores. Occludin cytoplasmic domain sequences bind ZO-1 directly. ZO-1 and ZO-2 form a complex with one another, and each of these proteins contains domains that could interact with other tight-junction proteins. ZO-1 also binds actin filaments.

wild-type or mutant occludin increased paracellular transport of small molecules but also increased transepithelial resistance.[21–23] Mutant occludin expression also caused a defect in the lateral diffusion barrier between the apical and the basolateral plasma membrane domains.[21] These studies suggest that the balance of occludin expression affects tight junction function. In embryonic stem cells that have the occludin gene disrupted, tight junctions were still assembled in embryoid bodies.[24] These embryoid bodies formed fluid-filled cavities, demonstrating that a paracellular barrier was established. Therefore, occludin may not be necessary for functional tight junction assembly. Alternatively, there may be other occludin isoforms that can compensate in these embryonic stem cell experiments.

Claudin, another integral membrane protein com-

ponent of the tight junction complex, recruits occludin into the tight junction complex.[25] Several claudins have been discovered,[9, 26, 27] defining a tight junction integral membrane protein gene family.[20] In a landmark study, positional cloning of a gene for an inherited magnesium-wasting disorder revealed that the gene *PCLN-1* encodes a member of the claudin gene family that is expressed in the tight junctions of epithelial cells.[28] The paracellin protein was expressed specifically in the loop of Henle thick ascending limb, where magnesium reabsorption normally occurs. This finding implies that the various claudin family members may form selective ion channels within the tight junction,[29] as had been hypothesized previously.[18] In another study, *Clostridium perfringens* enterotoxin was shown to bind specific claudins in Madin-Darby canine kidney (MDCK) cells, and this toxin disrupts paracellu-

TABLE 9–1. Tight Junction Proteins

PROTEIN	MOLECULAR WEIGHT, kDa	SUPERFAMILY/ISOFORMS	FUNCTION
Occludin	65–80	Series of phosphorylated isoforms	Adhesion and permeability control
Claudin/paracellin	23	Several members	Adhesion and permeability control
ZO-1	210–225	MaGUK	Structural
ZO-2	160	MaGUK	Structural
ZO-3	130	MaGUK	Structural
Symplekin	150		Unknown
Cingulin	140–160		Unknown
			Binds ZO-1, ZO-2, ZO-3, AF-6, and myosin
Protein kinase C	81	α, ζ, and λ	TJ function regulation
Heterotrimeric G protein	41	α I-2	TJ assembly and function regulation
Rab	25–41	13 and 3B	Vesicle targeting/fusion
7H6	155–175		Unknown
AF-6 (afadin)	180–195		Unknown, binds ZO-1

lar barrier functions, demonstrating that claudins are important regulators of paracellular barrier transport.[30]

Other protein components of the tight junction (see Fig. 9–2)[17, 20, 31] may be structural. The first identified component of the tight junction, ZO-1, and the related proteins, ZO-2 and ZO-3, are members of a group of proteins called the membrane-associated guanylate kinase (MAGuK) gene superfamily.[17, 31] There are common structural features among the MAGuK family members, including PDZ domains, an SH3 domain, and a guanylate kinase domain (but this domain lacks critical amino acids for enzyme activity). Proteins containing PDZ domains generally produce a scaffold on the plasma membrane that links several proteins together into a complex structure.[32] The ZO-1 protein also has a large C-terminal proline-rich domain that binds actin filaments directly.[33, 34] The ZO-1 and ZO-2 (or ZO-3) proteins form a molecular complex with one another.[17] ZO-1 binds the cytoplasmic domain of occludin.[31, 35] Therefore, a basic unit of tight junction structure that includes occludin, ZO-1, ZO-2, and actin has been elucidated (see Fig. 9–2).

Linkage of this tight junction structural unit to actin also has important functional consequences. Tension of the actin cytoskeleton on tight junctions regulates paracellular permeability, but specific biophysical details of this regulation remain obscure.[15] The apical junctional complex is intimately associated with a cortical actin belt and with the terminal web of actin that lies directly below the apical microvilli.[7] Myosin contraction can alter epithelial cell shape by constricting the apical junctional complex (like a purse-string).[36] This actinomyosin contraction may physically regulate the tight junction by pulling the junction apart. Evidence for this effect comes from studies using drugs that cause actin cytoskeleton disassembly and disrupt myosin light-chain kinase functions in epithelial cells, thereby altering epithelial cell permeability.[4, 6, 37–40] Regulatory proteins that control actin cytoskeleton assembly, termed Rho-family GTPases, also regulate tight junction assembly.[41–46] Rho-GTPases may regulate tight junctions indirectly through actin assembly changes. Alternatively, Rho-GTPases may directly regulate structural components of the tight junction and influence tight junction protein assembly. For example, Rho-GTPase signaling affects occludin protein phosphorylation states.[40, 41]

ADHERENS JUNCTIONS

Adherens junctions are located directly basal to the tight junction, and they form strong cell-cell adhesion complexes.[47, 48] Cadherin cell-cell adhesion molecules assemble with a large set of membrane-cytoskeletal proteins that link to the actin cytoskeleton.[48] Several signal transduction proteins, including growth factor receptors and tyrosine kinases, also associate with the adherens junction.[49, 50] Adherens junctions integrate signaling pathways that determine cytoskeleton-mediated rearrangements in cell shape.[51] Assembly of adherens junctions is initiated by cadherin molecules binding to one another on neighboring cells, which leads to the formation of a large macromolecular complex with diverse roles in cellular physiology.

Cadherins constitute a large family of proteins that include the calcium-dependent cell adhesion molecules of adherens junctions and desmosomes.[48, 52, 53] Cadherins in the adherens junction were initially named after the tissue where they were first identified, eg, E-cadherin in epithelial tissues and N-cadherin in neural tissues. A typical arrangement of cadherin complexes in the adherens junction is shown in Figure 9–3. Cadherin dimers are thought to be the functional unit having adhesion activity.[48, 54] Extracellular domain repeat sequences (cadherin extracellular repeats) bind calcium and determine homophilic adhesion properties. A single transmembrane domain is followed by a cytoplasmic domain that is highly conserved among different family members. Cytoplasmic domains of adherens junction cadherins associate (directly or indirectly) with membrane-cytoskeletal proteins, such as catenins, ZO-1, vinculin, α-actinin, and actin.[47] Cadherins also mediate intracellular signaling through β-catenin,[55] protein tyrosine phosphatases,[56–58] and, potentially, other mechanisms. Table 9–2 provides a list of some proteins associated with the adherens junction.

E-cadherin is expressed in kidney and most other epithelial cells. Lateral adhesion instructs epithelial cells to organize other adhesion junctional complexes, such as tight junctions, desmosomes, and gap junctions.[48, 53] E-cadherin adhesion in epithelial cells induces a basolateral, polarized Na^+,K^+-ATPase distribution.[59, 60] Therefore, E-cadherin appears to be crucial for normal differentiation of renal epithelial cells.

A ternary complex of the proteins nectin, afadin, and ponsin has recently been described in the adherens junction. The association of these proteins with the adherens junctions is cadherin dependent.[61] Afadin was identified in a screen for actin-binding proteins.[62, 63] It is identical to a gene (AF-6) that formed a translocation fusion with ALL-1,[64] a gene involved in acute leukemia.[65] L-Afadin has one PDZ domain that is thought to mediate recruitment to cell-cell junctions, and it contains proline-rich domains and an actin-binding domain.[63] Afadin's PDZ domain was shown to bind the cytoplasmic domain of Eph receptor tyrosine kinases, which are receptors for the ephrin developmental signaling involved in forming tissue boundaries in the nervous system.[62] L-Afadin binds directly to nectin, an immunoglobulin superfamily cell-cell adhesion molecule,[61] and afadin binds directly to ponsin, an SH3-containing protein that also binds vinculin.[66] The specific roles that the nectin, afadin, and ponsin complexes play in cell adhesion and junctional complex formation are unclear, but a mouse L-afadin knockout was embryonic lethal.[67] These mice show defects during and after gastrulation. Afadin-null mice have disorganized ectodermal layers and defects in mesodermal migration, and fail to form somites and other ectoderm- and mesoderm-derived structures. Afadin-null embryos also show defects in adherens junction and tight junction organization. The afadin-ponsin-nectin

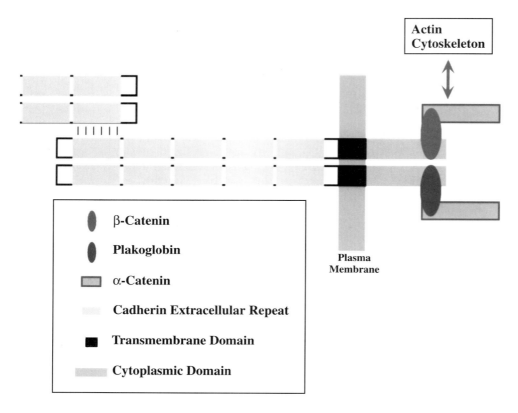

Actin Cytoskeleton

Plasma Membrane

β-Catenin

Plakoglobin

α-Catenin

Cadherin Extracellular Repeat

Transmembrane Domain

Cytoplasmic Domain

FIGURE 9–3 ▪ *(See Color Plate)* Adherens junctions are organized by cadherin cell adhesion molecules. Dimers are probably required for cadherin cell adhesion activity. The extracellular cadherin repeat sequences require calcium binding for proper conformation. The extracellular domain repeats are also responsible for determining homophilic binding activity. Cadherins are single-pass transmembrane integral membrane proteins with a highly conserved cytoplasmic domain that interacts with numerous membrane cytoskeletal proteins and signal transduction molecules. Both β- and γ-catenin bind cadherin cytoplasmic domain sequences, and both of these proteins bind α-catenin. Alpha-catenin is an actin-binding protein that also interacts with other adherens junction components, including vinculin, α-actinin, and IQGAP.

TABLE 9–2. Adherens Junction Proteins

PROTEIN	MOLECULAR WEIGHT	SUPERFAMILY/ISOFORMS	FUNCTION
E-cadherin	120–140 kDa	Classic cadherin superfamily	Homophilic cell-cell adhesion
α-Catenin	102 kDa		Connects E-cadherin complex to actin cytoskeleton
β-Catenin	92 kDa	Armadillo family	Signaling, binds cadherin and LEF/TCF family of transcription factors
Plakoglobin (γ-catenin)	86 kDa	Armadillo family	Binds cadherin
p120ctn	100–120 kDa	Alternatively spliced isoforms	Cell adhesion regulation, binds cadherin and Kaiso (transcription factor)
δ-Catenin	160 kDa	Armadillo family	Cell adhesion, morphology, and motility regulation
Receptor protein tyrosine kinases	180 kDa	eg, EGFR	Signaling
Nonreceptor tyrosine kinases		eg, src family (src, yes)	Signaling
Transmembrane tyrosine phosphatases		PTP1B, LAR	Regulation of cadherin-catenin, complex assembly by signaling
Vinculin	116 kDa		Link to actin cytoskeleton
Afadin (AF-6)	205 kDa		Binds actin
Nectin	60 kDa	Immunoglobulin superfamily	Binds afadin
Ponsin	93 kDa		Binds afadin and vinculin
ERM proteins (ezrin, radixin, moesin)	75–82 kDa	ERM family includes merlin and protein 4.1	Actin binding, bind membrane proteins
α-Actinin	100 kDa		Actin binding, binds α-catenin
IQGAP	170 kDa		Binds β-catenin, signaling response to Rac and Cdc42
Myosin phosphatase	130-kDa (myosin binding subunit), 38-kDa (catalytic), and 20-kDa subunits		Regulates myosin contractility
Phosphatidylinositol-3-kinase	110- and 85-kDa subunits		Associates with E-cadherin complex in response to cell-cell adhesion

complex appears to be a critically important connection between cadherins and the actin cytoskeleton. More studies are needed to examine a potential role for the afadin-ponsin-nectin complex in epithelial injury during ischemia.

DISRUPTION OF JUNCTIONAL COMPLEXES BY ISCHEMIA AND ATP DEPLETION

Disruption of the renal epithelial cell architecture occurs rapidly following the onset of ischemia (see Fig. 9–1). Many investigators have used animal models and ATP depletion of cultured epithelial cells to model human renal epithelial cell damage that occurs during ischemia. These models largely reproduce the pathophysiologic cellular changes occurring during renal ischemia in humans,[2] including indiscriminate actin cytoskeleton rearrangement and junctional complex disruption (see Chapters 1 and 8).

An early response to ischemic injury in vivo and ATP depletion in vitro is the opening of tight junctions.[8, 68] Tight junction components become incorporated into a detergent-insoluble complex during ATP depletion, which may reflect an abnormal assembly state.[69] Epithelial transport functions are dependent on an intact paracellular barrier[15] to prevent the short-circuiting of transport work. Therefore, reestablishment of the normal assembly state during recovery from ischemia is necessary. During this process, there may be alternations in expression levels for specific isoforms or particular tight junction components that are found in recovering tubular epithelial cells. It may be that the proportions of claudin isoforms normally maintained in different nephron segments may be disrupted, and recovery of the appropriate claudin isoform balance would be necessary for appropriate transport functions in tubular epithelial cells.

Breakdown of the plasma membrane lateral diffusion barrier during ischemic injury would prevent epithelial cells from restricting membrane proteins and lipids in their proper plasma membrane domains. Ischemic injury results in relocation of membrane proteins. After injury, Na^+,K^+-ATPase is not restricted to the basolateral plasma membrane but is also redistributed to the apical plasma membrane as well.[70–72] Membrane polarity disruption could occur by passive diffusion of membrane proteins between membrane domains after junctions open.

Cadherins function to organize the lateral membrane in epithelial cells.[8, 70] One specific function of E-cadherin is to determine normal basolateral Na^+,K^+-ATPase distribution.[53, 59, 60] Recovery of normal cell polarity requires the reestablishment of normal E-cadherin function and normal basolateral Na^+,K^+-ATPase distribution. Many features of polarized epithelia may require normal cadherin function.[10] For example, the sec6/sec8 protein complex controls basolateral plasma membrane protein-targeting fidelity, and cadherin adhesion is required for determining normal sec6/sec8 protein complex distribution to the junctional complex.[10, 73]

Specific regulators of junctional complex assembly are not well understood. For example, Rho-GTPase regulates tight junction and adherens junction assembly,[43–46, 74, 75] but this signaling pathway also controls actin cytoskeleton assembly, focal adhesion complex assembly, and growth control.[75] Specific effects of signaling molecules on the junctional complex must be considered in the context of many other cellular events that occur when particular signaling pathways are activated or inhibited.

The consequences of ischemic injury on junctional complexes in humans were examined in reperfused renal allografts.[9, 76–78] As a consequence of acute renal failure, glomerular filtration rate is severely decreased. Backleak of ultrafiltrate into interstitial tissue is one consequence of tight junction disruption.[79] Calculations from several parameters were used to indirectly measure tight junction permeability, and decreased tight junction barrier function was correlated with severity of acute renal failure in reperfused renal allografts.[76] Additional studies showed that normal distributions of tight junction and adherens junction component proteins and Na^+,K^+-ATPase were disrupted in poorly recovering reperfused renal allografts.[77, 78] These studies were seminal, showing that the alterations seen in animal and cell culture models recapitulate important features of the pathophysiology of acute renal failure in humans.

JUNCTIONAL COMPLEX REGULATORY MECHANISMS AND ATP-DEPLETION

Intracellular signaling systems are disrupted by ischemia, which may lead to junctional complex dysfunction. Tyrosine phosphorylation mediated by growth factor receptor stimulation, overexpression of specific tyrosine kinases, or treatment with tyrosine kinase agonists or antagonists correlates with tight junctional complex rearrangement, altered cadherin cell-cell adhesion, and altered paracellular permeability properties in epithelial cells.[80, 81] During ATP depletion, cytoplasmic concentrations of ATP generally fall below the K_m for protein kinase, while protein phosphatases remain active.[82] Thus, junctional complex components, and proteins in general, are dephosphorylated under conditions of ATP depletion.

Serine-threonine phosphorylation mechanisms also control junctional complex assembly and function. For example, sodium permeability in MDCK-cell tight junctions is controlled by protein kinase A.[37] Protein kinase C (PKC) signaling regulates both tight junction and adherens junction assembly.[83, 84] To study junctional complex assembly, many investigators have utilized a calcium-switch protocol, in which epithelial cells are placed in low-calcium medium, causing junctional complex disassembly, then are placed in normal-calcium medium to initiate junctional complex assembly. Various assays (eg, immunofluorescence) can be used to study the assembly process before, during, and after the calcium switch. Including PKC agonists (eg, phorbol esters) in the normal-calcium medium during reassembly increased the rate of tight junction assembly and functional tight junction development.[85, 86] In addition, the treatment of epithelial cells that are held in low-calcium medium with a PKC agonist caused cadherin-independent tight junction assembly and increased barrier function in MDCK-cell monolayers.[87] Paradoxically, the treatment of established epithelial cell monolayers with PKC agonists caused a reduction in tight junction function.[88] Critical targets for PKC phosphorylation have not been identified, but evidence suggests that tight junction and adherens junction proteins, including ZO-1, ZO-2, ZO-3, occludin, vinculin, and p100-p120, are affected by this kinase signaling pathway.[86, 87, 89–91] In an interesting study, van Hengel and colleagues[92] showed that PKC-agonist treatment of a human colon carcinoma that lacks α-catenin expression (which renders the cadherin-catenin complex nonfunctional) induces tight junction and desmosome assembly.[92] These experiments suggest that PKC may activate desmosome adhesive functions. An alternative possibility is that PKC may activate vinculin,[89] which may functionally substitute for α-catenin.[93] Specific PKC isoforms, PKCζ and PKCλ, were localized to the tight junction.[86, 94–96] However, these are termed *atypical PKC isoforms* because they are not regulated by calcium, phorbol esters, or diacylglycerol (unlike the other classes of PKC isoforms).[97] Phorbol ester treatment presumably affects PKC isoforms other than the atypical type. Overexpression of PKCδ in a proximal tubule epithelial cell line caused a breakdown in tight junction barrier function, suggesting that other PKC isoforms regulate tight junction permeability.[98]

Intracellular calcium signals are generated as a part of numerous signaling pathways.[99] Potential effects of intracellular calcium signals on tight junction assembly have been investigated. Buffering calcium changes using the chelator BAPTA-AM slowed assembly of junctions.[86] This effect was confirmed by disrupting normal calcium signaling with the use of thapsigargin.[100] BAPTA-AM also inhibited recovery of transepithelial resistance and reestablishment of normal tight junction assembly state following ATP-depletion in MDCK cells.[101] Calcium regulation may be an important factor in tight junction maintenance and recovery in acute renal failure.

G-protein signaling regulates tight junction and adherens junction functions. Heterotrimeric G-protein subunits have been localized to the tight junction.[102, 103] Expression of mutant heterotrimeric G-protein alpha subunits or treatment with G-protein agonists affected tight junction assembly and function.[102, 103] Heterotrimeric G-protein signaling may facilitate junctional complex assembly during recovery from ischemic injury, and tight junction disruption during ischemia may disrupt normal G-protein signaling.

Rho-GTPase family members regulate adherens junction and tight junction assembly.[40, 41, 43–45, 74] Rho signaling increases tight junction and adherens junction assembly; conversely, blocking Rho signaling significantly inhibits assembly of adherens junctions and tight junctions.[43–45, 74] Upstream and downstream factors of Rho-family GTPase signaling that control junctional complex assembly are being characterized.[104] For example, Tiam-1 is an upstream activator of Rac that controls E-cadherin adhesion, cell migration, and substrate adhesion.[105] Tiam-1–induced activation of Rac prevents MDCK-cell migration in response to hepatocyte growth factor, presumably by activation of E-cadherin adhesion, preventing cells from migrating away from each other.[106] IQGAP is a downstream effector of Rac and Cdc42 GTPase signaling that binds directly to the cadherin-associated protein β-catenin. α-Catenin and IQGAP bind the same domain on the β-catenin molecule.[107] Rac and Cdc42 GTPase signaling decrease IQGAP binding to β-catenin, increasing α-catenin binding and thus increasing cadherin adhesion.[107–109] Integration of many signaling pathways by the cell under various physiologic and pathophysiologic conditions determines the functional assembly states of junctional complexes. However, it is clear that the Rho-family GTPase proteins are positioned at a key control point between signaling input and downstream changes in epithelial cell behavior.

The effects of ischemia and ATP-depletion (cytoskeleton disassembly, cell-substrate adhesion loss, cell-cell junctional complex disruption) are reminiscent of epithelial cells in which Rho-family GTPase signaling was inhibited. Researchers have begun to examine roles of Rho-family GTPase signaling in an in vitro model of renal ischemia.[40] (Gopalakrishnan and Marrs, unpublished observations). Inhibiting Rho in MDCK cells before ATP depletion caused more extensive loss of junctional components from cell contact sites. The junctions of MDCK cells with activated Rho signaling were better maintained during ATP depletion than those in control cells. Thus, activation of Rho signaling protects tight junctions from damage during ATP depletion. In contrast, inhibiting or activating Rho in MDCK cells did not alter adherens junction disassembly during ATP depletion relative to control cells, showing that the protective effects of Rho signaling were specific for the tight junction (Gopalakrishnan and Marrs, unpublished observations). Perhaps Rac or Cdc42 provides a protective signal for the adherens junction during injury. These results suggest an approach to preventing severe disruption of epithelial cell junctional complexes, as well as preventing the consequences of ischemia in epithelial cell and organ function.

Numerous changes in epithelial cells occur in response to ischemia. Alterations in cell-cell junctional complexes may also be a consequence of changes in epithelial cell phenotype. The cadherin-associated protein β-catenin can act as an intracellular signaling molecule as part of the Wnt-signaling pathway (Fig. 9–4).[110] Wnts are secreted glycoprotein signaling molecules that control numerous differentiation processes during development. Wnt receptors inhibit the *disheveled* protein, which inhibits glycogen synthetase kinase-3 (GSK-3) activity. Evidence suggests that GSK-3 directly phosphorylates serine amino acids in the amino terminus of β-catenin. Wnt signals decrease amino-terminus serine phosphorylation of β-catenin, which prevents β-

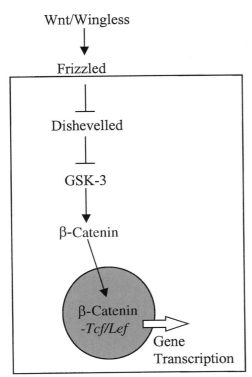

FIGURE 9–4 ▪ Wnt/Wingless signaling pathway. Wnt signals activate the Wnt-receptor *(frizzled),* which down-regulates dishevelled protein. *Dishevelled* down-regulates glycogen synthetase kinase-3 (GSK-3), which can phosphorylate β-catenin. Wnt signals lead to an underphosphorylation of β-catenin, which is the competent for nuclear import. Nuclear β-catenin binds the Tcf/Lef class transcription factors and activates transcription.

catenin ubiquitin conjugation and degradation. This leads to accumulation of β-catenin in the cytoplasm of cells that respond to Wnt. When β-catenin levels increase, β-catenin can translocate to the nucleus and bind to members of the Tcf/Lef class of transcription factors. This complex activates specific target genes. Deleting the amino terminus or mutating specific amino acids in the amino terminus of β-catenin causes the mutant protein to accumulate in the cytoplasm, translocate to the nucleus, and activate genes.[54] The authors have observed that ATP depletion causes a severe reduction in β-catenin phosphorylation (Gopalakrishnan and Marrs, in preparation) that could lead to aberrant transcription activation. It would be interesting to determine whether altered differentiation-factor signaling pathways, such as β-catenin signaling, contribute to the pathophysiologic consequences of ischemic injury.

CONCLUSION

Cell-cell junctional complexes that maintain normal epithelial cell phenotype and physiology are disrupted during ischemic injury and in an in vitro cultured epithelial cell model of ischemic injury. Details of the pathophysiologic consequences of ischemic injury that lead to junctional complex dysfunction are unclear.

However, assembly of the apical adhesion complex determines numerous functional properties of epithelial cells, and regulation of junctional complexes provides a pivotal control point for controlling epithelial cell properties. Conversely, disruption of the apical junctional complex has dramatic downstream effects on the ability of epithelial cells to establish barrier functions and maintain cell polarity.

The various clinical phases of ischemic injury as observed at the whole-organ level can be correlated with cellular alterations in response to ischemia. The initial phase of acute tubular necrosis associated with oliguria correlates with actin cytoskeleton remodeling in renal endothelial and epithelial cells.[2] The extensive changes in the actin organization are accompanied by loss of cell-cell contacts and cell–extracellular matrix contacts as adherens junctions and focal adhesions disassemble.[3, 13] In some cases, the epithelial cells are sloughed off the matrix support, which can aggregate via interactions between E-cadherin or integrins, leading to tubular obstruction[13] that contributes to continuing oliguria-anuria. In the cells that remain attached to the extracellular matrix, cell-cell contacts must be reestablished during the recovery of blood flow to the kidney. Cytoplasmic extensions bridge the gaps in denuded regions of matrix, and epithelial cells must reestablish the adherens junctions, followed quickly by tight-junction assembly. Destruction of junctional complexes during ischemia contributes to tubule back-leak.[8] Sodium reabsorption is limited in the injured cells because of the redistribution of Na^+,K^+-ATPase.[70, 71] The saline diuresis that occurs does not resolve until the polarized distribution of the sodium pump is reestablished.[69] Interventions that inhibit the loss of cell organization or facilitate the reorganization of tight junctions and adhesion junctions could provide an important therapeutic advance for this syndrome.

REFERENCES

1. Lieberthal W, Levinsky NG: Acute Clinical Renal Failure. In: Seldin DW, Giebisch G, eds: The Kidney: Physiology and Pathophysiology. Vol. 3. New York: Raven Press; 1992:3181–3226.
2. Molitoris BA, Weinberg JM, Venkatachalam MA, et al: Acute renal failure. II. Experimental models of acute renal failure: imperfect but indispensable. Am J Physiol 2000; 278:F1–F12.
3. Molitoris BA, Marrs J: The role of cell adhesion molecules in ischemic acute renal failure. Am J Med 1999; 106:583–592.
4. Bentzel CJ, Hainau B, Ho S, et al: Cytoplasmic regulation of tight-junction permeability: effect of plant cytokinins. Am J Physiol 1980; 239:C75–C89.
5. Hirano S, Nose A, Hatta K, et al: Calcium-dependent cell-cell adhesion molecules (cadherins): subclass specificities and possible involvement of actin bundles. J Cell Biol 1987; 105:2501–2510.
6. Madara JL, Moore R, Carlson S: Alteration of intestinal tight junction structure and permeability by cytoskeletal contraction. Am J Physiol 1987; 253:C854–C861.
7. Hirokawa N, Tilney LG: Interactions between actin filaments and between actin filaments and membranes in quick-frozen and deeply etched hair cells of the chick ear. J Cell Biol 1982; 95:249–261.
8. Molitoris BA, Falk SA, Dahl RH: Ischemia-induced loss of epithelial polarity: role of the tight junction. J Clin Invest 1989; 84:1334–1339.

9. Alejandro VS, Nelson WJ, Huie P, et al: Postischemic injury, delayed function and Na⁺, K⁺-ATPase distribution in the transplanted kidney. Kidney Int 1995; 48:1308–1315.

10. Yeaman C, Grindstaff KK, Nelson WJ: New perspectives on mechanisms involved in generating epithelial cell polarity. Physiol Rev 1999; 79:73–98.

11. Goligorsky MS, DiBona GF: Pathogenetic role of Arg-Gly-Asp–recognizing integrins in acute renal failure. Proc Natl Acad Sci USA 1993; 90:5700–5704.

12. Zuk A, Bonventre JV, Brown D, Matlin KS: Polarity, integrin, and extracellular matrix dynamics in the postischemic rat kidney. Am J Physiol 1998; 275:C711–C731.

13. Goligorsky MS, Noiri E, Kessler H, Romanov V: Therapeutic potential of RGD peptides in acute renal injury. Kidney Int 1997; 51:1487–1492.

14. Brown D, Stow JL: Protein trafficking and polarity in kidney epithelium: from cell biology to physiology. Physiol Rev 1996; 76:245–297.

15. Madara JL: Regulation of the movement of solutes across tight junctions. Annu Rev Physiol 1998; 60:143–159.

16. Mitic LL, Anderson JM: Molecular architecture of tight junctions. Annu Rev Physiol 1998; 60:121–142.

17. Stevenson BR, Keon BH: The tight junction: morphology to molecules. Annu Rev Cell Dev Biol 1998; 14:89–109.

18. Cereijido M, Valdes J, Shoshani L, Contreras RG: Role of tight junctions in establishing and maintaining cell polarity. Annu Rev Physiol 1998; 60:161–177.

19. Spring KR: Routes and mechanism of fluid transport by epithelia. Annu Rev Physiol 1998; 60:105–119.

20. Tsukita S, Furuse M: Occludin and claudins in tight-junction strands: leading or supporting players? Trends Cell Biol 1999; 9:268–273.

21. Balda MS, Whitney JA, Flores C, et al: Functional dissociation of paracellular permeability and transepithelial electrical resistance and disruption of the apical-basolateral intramembrane diffusion barrier by expression of a mutant tight junction membrane protein. J Cell Biol 1996; 134:1031–1049.

22. Chen Y, Merzdorf C, Paul DL, Goodenough DA: COOH terminus of occludin is required for tight junction barrier function in early Xenopus embryos. J Cell Biol 1997; 138:891–899.

23. McCarthy KM, Skare IB, Stankewich MC, et al: Occludin is a functional component of the tight junction. J Cell Sci 1996; 109:2287–2298.

24. Saitou M, Fujimoto K, Doi Y, et al: Occludin-deficient embryonic stem cells can differentiate into polarized epithelial cells bearing tight junctions. J Cell Biol 1998; 141:397–408.

25. Furuse M, Sasaki H, Fujimoto K, Tsukita S: A single gene product, claudin-1 or -2, reconstitutes tight junction strands and recruits occludin in fibroblasts. J Cell Biol 1998; 143:391–401.

26. Furuse M, Fujita K, Hiiragi T, et al: Claudin-1 and -2: novel integral membrane proteins localizing at tight junctions with no sequence similarity to occludin. J Cell Biol 1998; 141:1539–1550.

27. Morita K, Furuse M, Fujimoto K, Tsukita S: Claudin multigene family encoding four-transmembrane domain protein components of tight junction strands. Proc Natl Acad Sci USA 1999; 96:511–516.

28. Simon DB, Lu Y, Choate KA, et al: Paracellin-1, a renal tight junction protein required for paracellular Mg²⁺ resorption. Science 1999; 285:103–106.

29. Wong V, Goodenough DA: Paracellular channels! [comment]. Science 1999; 285:62.

30. Sonoda N, Furuse M, Sasaki H, et al: Clostridium perfringens enterotoxin fragment removes specific claudins from tight junction strands: evidence for direct involvement of claudins in tight junction barrier. J Cell Biol 1999; 147:195–204.

31. Mitic LL, Schneeberger EE, Fanning AS, Anderson JM: Connexin-occludin chimeras containing the ZO-binding domain of occludin localize at MDCK tight junctions and NRK cell contacts. J Cell Biol 1999; 146:683–693.

32. Fanning AS, Anderson JM: PDZ domains: fundamental building blocks in the organization of protein complexes at the plasma membrane. J Clin Invest 1999; 103:767–772.

33. Fanning AS, Jameson BJ, Jesaitis LA, Anderson JM: The tight junction protein ZO-1 establishes a link between the transmembrane protein occludin and the actin cytoskeleton. J Biol Chem 1998; 273:29745–29753.

34. Itoh M, Nagafuchi A, Moroi S, Tsukita S: Involvement of ZO-1 in cadherin-based cell adhesion through its direct binding to alpha catenin and actin filaments. J Cell Biol 1997; 138:181–192.

35. Furuse M, Itoh M, Hirase T, et al: Direct association of occludin with ZO-1 and its possible involvement in the localization of occludin at tight junctions. J Cell Biol 1994; 127:1617–1626.

36. Bement WM, Forscher P, Mooseker MS: A novel cytoskeletal structure involved in purse-string wound closure and cell polarity maintenance. J Cell Biol 1993; 121:565–578.

37. Hecht G, Pestic L, Nikcevic G, et al: Expression of the catalytic domain of myosin light chain kinase increases paracellular permeability. Am J Physiol 1996; 271:C1678–C1684.

38. Kovbasnjuk ON, Szmulowicz U, Spring KR: Regulation of the MDCK cell tight junction. J Membr Biol 1998; 161:93–104.

39. Turner JR, Angle JM, Black ED, et al: PKC-dependent regulation of transepithelial resistance: roles of MLC and MLC kinase. Am J Physiol 1999; 277:C554–C562.

40. Turner JR, Rill BK, Carlson SL, et al: Physiological regulation of epithelial tight junctions is associated with myosin light-chain phosphorylation. Am J Physiol 1997; 273:C1378–C1385.

41. Gopalakrishnan S, Raman N, Atkinson SJ, Marrs JA: Rho-GTPase signaling regulates tight junction assembly and protects tight junctions during ATP depletion. Am J Physiol 1998; 275:C798–C809.

42. Hasegawa H, Fujita H, Katoh H, et al: Opposite regulation of transepithelial electrical resistance and paracellular permeability by Rho in Madin-Darby canine kidney cells. J Biol Chem 1999; 274:20982–20988.

43. Jou TS, Nelson WJ: Effects of regulated expression of mutant RhoA and Rac1 small GTPases on the development of epithelial (MDCK) cell polarity. J Cell Biology 1998; 142:85–100.

44. Jou TS, Schneeberger EE, Nelson WJ: Structural and functional regulation of tight junctions by RhoA and Rac1 small GTPases. J Cell Biol 1998; 142:101–115.

45. Nusrat A, Giry M, Turner JR, et al: Rho protein regulates tight junctions and perijunctional actin organization in polarized epithelia. Proc Natl Acad Sci USA 1995; 92:10629–10633.

46. Takaishi K, Sasaki T, Kotani H, et al: Regulation of cell-cell adhesion by rac and rho small G proteins in MDCK cells. J Cell Biol 1997; 139:1047–1059.

47. Farquhar MG, Palade GE: Cell junctions in amphibian skin. J Cell Biol 1965; 26:263–291.

48. Yap AS, Brieher WM, Gumbiner BM: Molecular and functional analysis of cadherin-based adherens junctions. Annu Rev Cell Dev Biol 1997; 13:119–146.

49. Nagafuchi A, Tsukita S, Takeichi M: Transmembrane control of cadherin-mediated cell-cell adhesion. Semin Cell Biol 1993; 4:175–181.

50. Tsukita S, Oishi K, Akiyama T, et al: Specific proto-oncogenic tyrosine kinases of src family are enriched in cell-to-cell adherens junctions where the level of tyrosine phosphorylation is elevated. J Cell Biol 1991; 113:867–879.

51. Adams CL, Nelson WJ: Cytomechanics of cadherin-mediated cell-cell adhesion. Curr Opin Cell Biol 1998; 10:572–577.

52. Kowalczyk AP, Bornslaeger EA, Norvell SM, et al: Desmosomes: intercellular adhesive junctions specialized for attachment of intermediate filaments. [Review] [373 refs]. Int Rev Cytol 1999; 185:237–302.

53. Marrs JA, Nelson WJ: Cadherin cell adhesion molecules in differentiation and embryogenesis. Int Rev Cytol 1996; 165:159–205.

54. Yap AS, Niessen CM, Gumbiner BM: The juxtamembrane region of the cadherin cytoplasmic tail supports lateral clustering, adhesive strengthening, and interaction with p120ctn. J Cell Biol 1998; 141:779–789.

55. Polakis P: The oncogenic activation of beta-catenin. Curr Opin Genet Dev 1999; 9:15–21.

56. Brady-Kalnay SM, Mourton T, Nixon JP, et al: Dynamic interaction of PTPmu with multiple cadherins in vivo. J Cell Biol 1998; 141:287–296.

57. Brady-Kalnay SM, Rimm DI, Tonks NK: Receptor protein tyro-

sine phosphatase PTPmu associates with cadherins and catenins in vivo. J Cell Biol 1995; 130:977–986.

58. Kypta RM, Su H, Reichardt LF: Association between a transmembrane protein tyrosine phosphatase and the cadherin-catenin complex. J Cell Biol 1996; 134:1519–1529.

59. Marrs JA, Andersson-Fisone C, Jeong MC, et al: Plasticity in epithelial cell phenotype: modulation by expression of different cadherin cell adhesion molecules. J Cell Biol 1995; 129:507–519.

60. McNeill H, Ozawa M, Kemler R, Nelson WJ: Novel function of the cell adhesion molecule uvomorulin as an inducer of cell surface polarity. Cell 1990; 62:309–316.

61. Takahashi K, Nakanishi H, Miyahara M, et al: Nectin/PRR: an immunoglobulin-like cell adhesion molecule recruited to cadherin-based adherens junctions through interaction with afadin, a PDZ domain-containing protein. J Cell Biol 1999; 145:539–549.

62. Buchert M, Schneider S, Meskenaite V, et al: The junction-associated protein AF-6 interacts and clusters with specific Eph receptor tyrosine kinases at specialized sites of cell-cell contact in the brain. J Cell Biol 1999; 144:361–371.

63. Mandai K, Nakanishi H, Satoh A, et al: Afadin: a novel actin filament-binding protein with one PDZ domain localized at cadherin-based cell-to-cell adherens junction. J Cell Biol 1997; 139:517–528.

64. Prasad R, Gu Y, Alder H, et al: Cloning of the ALL-1 fusion partner, the AF-6 gene, involved in acute myeloid leukemias with the t(6;11) chromosome translocation. Cancer Res 1993; 53:5624–5628.

65. Cimino G, Moir DT, Canaani O, et al: Cloning of ALL-1, the locus involved in leukemias with the t(4;11)(q21;q23), t(9;11)(p22;q23), and t(11;19)(q23;p13) chromosome translocations. Cancer Res 1991; 51:6712–6714.

66. Mandai K, Nakanishi H, Satoh A, et al: Ponsin/SH3P12: an 1-afadin- and vinculin-binding protein localized at cell-cell and cell-matrix adherens junctions. J Cell Biol 1999; 144:1001–1017.

67. Ikeda W, Nakanishi H, Miyoshi J, et al: Afadin: a key molecule essential for structural organization of cell-cell junctions of polarized epithelia during embryogenesis. J Cell Biol 1999; 146:1117–1132.

68. Mandel LJ, Bacallao R, Zampighi G: Uncoupling of the molecular "fence" and paracellular "gate" functions in epithelial tight junctions. Nature 1993; 361:552–555.

69. Tsukamoto T, Nigam SK: Tight junction proteins form large complexes and associate with the cytoskeleton in an ATP depletion model for reversible junction assembly. J Biol Chem 1997; 272:16133–16139.

70. Fish EM, Molitoris BA: Alterations in epithelial polarity and the pathogenesis of disease states. N Engl J Med 1994; 330:1580–1588.

71. Mandel LJ, Doctor RB, Bacallao R: ATP depletion: a novel method to study junctional properties in epithelial tissues. II. Internalization of Na+,K+-ATPase and E-cadherin. J Cell Science 1994; 107:3315–3324.

72. Molitoris BA, Geerdes A, McIntosh JR: Dissociation and redistribution of Na+,K+-ATPase from its surface membrane actin cytoskeletal complex during cellular ATP depletion. J Clin Invest 1991; 88:462–469.

73. Grindstaff KK, Yeaman C, Anandasabapathy N, et al: Sec6/8 complex is recruited to cell-cell contacts and specifies transport vesicle delivery to the basal-lateral membrane in epithelial cells. Cell 1998; 93:731–740.

74. Braga VM, Machesky LM, Hall A, Hotchin NA: The small GTPases Rho and Rac are required for the establishment of cadherin-dependent cell-cell contacts. J Cell Biol 1997; 137:1421–1431.

75. Hall A: Rho-GTPases and the actin cytoskeleton. Science 1998; 279:509–514.

76. Alejandro V, Scandling JD Jr, Sibley RK, et al: Mechanisms of filtration failure during postischemic injury of the human kidney: a study of the reperfused renal allograft. J Clin Invest 1995; 95:820–831.

77. Kwon O, Corrigan G, Myers BD, et al: Sodium reabsorption and distribution of NA+/K+-ATPase during postischemic injury to the renal allograft. Kidney Int 1999; 55:963–975.

78. Kwon O, Nelson WJ, Sibley R, et al: Backleak, tight junctions, and cell-cell adhesion in postischemic injury to the renal allograft. J Clin Invest 1998; 101:2054–2064.

79. Donohoe JF, Venkatachalam MA, Bernard DB, Levinsky NG: Tubular leakage and obstruction after renal ischemia: structural-functional correlations. Kidney Int 1978; 13:208–222.

80. Aberle H, Schwartz H, Kemler R: Cadherin-catenin complex: protein interactions and their implications for cadherin function. J Cell Biochem 1996; 61:514–523.

81. Anderson JM, Van Itallie CM: Tight junctions and the molecular basis for regulation of paracellular permeability. Am J Physiol 1995; 269:G467–G475.

82. Kobryn CE, Mandel LJ: Decreased protein phosphorylation induced by anoxia in proximal renal tubules. Am J Physiol 1994; 267:C1073–C1079.

83. Madara JL: Tight junction dynamics: is paracellular transport regulated? Cell 1988; 53:497–498.

84. Mullin JM, O'Brien TG: Effects of tumor promoters on LLC-PK1 renal epithelial tight junctions and transepithelial fluxes. Am J Physiol 1986; 251:C597–C602.

85. Citi S, Denisenko N: Phosphorylation of the tight junction protein cingulin and the effects of protein kinase inhibitors and activators in MDCK epithelial cells. J Cell Sci 1995; 108:2917–2926.

86. Stuart RO, Nigam SK: Regulated assembly of tight junctions by protein kinase C. Proc Natl Acad Sci USA 1995; 92:6072–6076.

87. Balda MS, Gonzalez-Mariscal L, Matter K, et al: Assembly of the tight junction: the role of diacylglycerol. J Cell Biol 1993; 123:293–302.

88. Ojakian GK: Tumor promoter–induced changes in the permeability of epithelial cell tight junctions. Cell 1981; 23:95–103.

89. Perez-Moreno M, Avila A, Islas S, et al: Vinculin but not alpha-actinin is a target of PKC phosphorylation during junctional assembly induced by calcium. J Cell Sci 1998; 111:3563–3571.

90. Ratcliffe MJ, Rubin LL, Staddon JM: Dephosphorylation of the cadherin-associated p100/p120 proteins in response to activation of protein kinase C in epithelial cells. J Biol Chem 1997; 272:31894–31901.

91. Ratcliffe MJ, Smales C, Staddon JM: Dephosphorylation of the catenins p120 and p100 in endothelial cells in response to inflammatory stimuli. Biochem J 1999; 338:417–478.

92. van Hengel J, Gohon L, Bruyneel E, et al: Protein kinase C activation upregulates intercellular adhesion of alpha-catenin–negative human colon cancer cell variants via induction of desmosomes. J Cell Biol 1997; 137:1103–1116.

93. Hazan RB, Kang L, Roe S, et al: Vinculin is associated with the E-cadherin adhesion complex. J Biol Chem 1997; 272:32448–32453.

94. Dodane V, Kachar B: Identification of isoforms of G proteins and PKC that colocalize with tight junctions. J Membr Biol 1996; 149:199–209.

95. Izumi Y, Hirose T, Tamai Y, et al: An atypical PKC directly associates and colocalizes at the epithelial tight junction with ASIP, a mammalian homologue of Caenorhabditis elegans polarity protein PAR-3. J Cell Biol 1998; 143:95–106.

96. Saxon ML, Zhao X, Black JD: Activation of protein kinase C isozymes is associated with post-mitotic events in intestinal epithelial cells in situ. J Cell Biol 1994; 126:747–763.

97. Nishizuka Y: Protein kinase C and lipid signaling for sustained cellular responses. Faseb J 1995; 9:484–496.

98. Mullin JM, Kampherstein JA, Laughlin KV, et al: Overexpression of protein kinase C-delta increases tight junction permeability in LLC-PK1 epithelia. Am J Physiol 1998; 275:C544–C554.

99. Tsien RW, Tsien RY: Calcium channels, stores, and oscillations. Annu Rev Cell Biol 1990; 6:715–760.

100. Stuart RO, Sun A, Bush KT, Nigam SK: Dependence of epithelial intercellular junction biogenesis on thapsigargin-sensitive intracellular calcium stores. J Biol Chem 1996; 271:13636–13641.

101. Ye J, Tsukamoto T, Sun A, Nigam SK: A role for intracellular calcium in tight junction reassembly after ATP depletion-repletion. Am J Physiol 1999; 277:F524–F532.

102. Denker BM, Saha C, Khawaja S, Nigam SK: Involvement of a heterotrimeric G protein alpha subunit in tight junction biogenesis. J Biol Chem 1996; 271:25750–25753.

103. Saha C, Nigam SK, Denker BM: Involvement of Galphai2 in the maintenance and biogenesis of epithelial cell tight junctions. J Biol Chem 1998; 273:21629–21633.
104. Ridley AJ: Rho: theme and variations. Curr Biol 1996; 6:1256–1264.
105. Michiels F, Collard JG: Rho-like GTPases: their role in cell adhesion and invasion. Biochem Soc Symp 1999; 65:125–146.
106. Hordijk PL, ten Klooster JP, van der Kammen RA, et al: Inhibition of invasion of epithelial cells by Tiam1-Rac signaling. Science 1997; 278:1464–1466.
107. Fukata M, Kuroda S, Nakagawa M, et al: Cdc42 and Rac1 regulate the interaction of IQGAP1 with beta-catenin. J Biol Chem 1999; 274:26044–26050.
108. Kuroda S, Fukata M, Nakagawa M, et al: Role of IQGAP1, a target of the small GTPases Cdc42 and Rac1, in regulation of E-cadherin-mediated cell-cell adhesion. Science 1998; 281:832–835.
109. Kuroda S, Fukata M, Nakagawa M, Kaibuchi K: Cdc42, Rac1, and their effector IQGAP1 as molecular switches for cadherin-mediated cell-cell adhesion. Biochem Biophys Res Commun 1999; 262:1–6.
110. Wodarz A, Nusse R: Mechanisms of Wnt signaling in development. Annu Rev Cell Dev Biol 1998; 14:59–88.

CHAPTER 10

Heat Shock Proteins: Role in Prevention and Recovery From Acute Renal Failure

Scott K. Van Why ▪ Norman J. Siegel

INTRODUCTION

In recent years there have been progressive interest and advances in the understanding of the cellular mechanisms of renal tubular cell injury. The goal of these many investigations is to identify therapeutic maneuvers that either ameliorate the injury or speed the recovery from acute renal failure (ARF). Processes that contribute to tubule injury include increases in intracellular calcium, production of reactive oxygen molecules, and activation of phospholipases and proteases.[1, 2] Precipitating each of these events and central to injury from ischemia is a prompt and profound fall in cellular adenosine triphosphate (ATP) level. Progressive renal hypoperfusion causes tubular necrosis and functional impairment only when significant ATP depletion occurs.[3, 4] Moreover, cellular energetics affect not only survival but also function of the sublethally injured cell. When challenged with a diminished supply of ATP, the transport functions of renal cells are sacrificed and energy is conserved for functions essential for survival of the injured epithelium.[5, 6]

These mediators of epithelial injury in ischemia-induced ARF cause distinct structural and functional alterations in the sublethally injured cell, as described elsewhere in this book. Central to the disorganization of cellular architecture is the breakdown of organized subcellular domains, with the loss of cytoskeletal integrity. Among the several manifestations of this cytoskeletal breakdown is loss of the normal polar distribution of integral membrane proteins. In particular, Na^+,K^+-ATPase, normally restricted to the basolateral domain, redistributes to the apical domain, thereby reducing solute reabsorptive ability, which does not recover until cell polarity is restored.[7–10] Furthermore, it appears that the recycling of misplaced Na^+,K^+-ATPase is the means by which proximal tubule cells regain normal enzyme distribution after an ischemic insult, rather than through increased biosynthesis of new subunits.[11, 12] Study results from several groups of investigators have begun to provide insight into intrinsic mechanisms that may prevent injury from ischemic or toxic insults and into the way in which injured cells may recycle disrupted enzymes and cytoskeletal elements during recovery. What the cell requires is an efficient mechanism for preserving structure and for restoring normal cell architecture and function by resurrecting disrupted proteins, shuttling misplaced proteins back to their correct location, and disposing of irreparably damaged proteins. All of these vital functions would need to be accomplished in a confused cellular milieu. In addition, with an ischemic injury, the essential mediators of protection and recovery would need to compete successfully for the residual pool of cellular ATP at a time when energy sources are depressed.

GENERAL CHARACTERISTICS OF HEAT SHOCK PROTEINS

The candidates ideally suited for this role are the stress proteins, or heat shock proteins (HSPs). Members of each HSP family assist intracellular protein trafficking and have been termed *protein chaperones.* The individual HSPs have different but complementary functions in providing overall chaperoning of an individual protein substrate. Some of the stress proteins may prevent inappropriate peptide interactions in unfolding proteins, some can unfold protein substrates, and some can assist in the folding of polypeptides into their correct conformation. The discrete activity of each HSP allows the protein chaperones to cooperate in the disassembly of protein aggregates, the translocation of proteins across intracellular membranes, and the reconfiguration of denatured or improperly folded proteins. The separate classes of HSPs are organized according to size and apparent function. Certain members within each family can be induced in response to cellular injury; the pattern of stress protein induction depends on the cell type and the specific insult.[13] The rapid induction of stress proteins in response to an insult occurs via activation of the preformed heat shock transcription factor (HSF) that trimerizes and binds to the consensus sequences contained within the heat shock element (HSE) (Fig. 10–1). The activity of HSF appears to be modulated by constitutively expressed HSP-90 and HSP-70 proteins, which are themselves affected by levels of denatured proteins within the cell.[14, 15] These features allow for detection of the stress response at its earliest event, activation of HSF.

Members of the 70-kDa HSPs (HSP-70) were initially the primary focus of study as general protein chaperones and in injured renal cells. They are highly inducible in mammalian cells, can provide cytoprotection following heat shock, and have chaperone activity that contributes to proper protein folding by preventing deleterious peptide interactions and aggregation.[13, 16] Furthermore, HSP-70 proteins have the demonstrated ability to reactivate denatured proteins.[17] The activity of HSP-70 proteins for the reconstitution of denatured

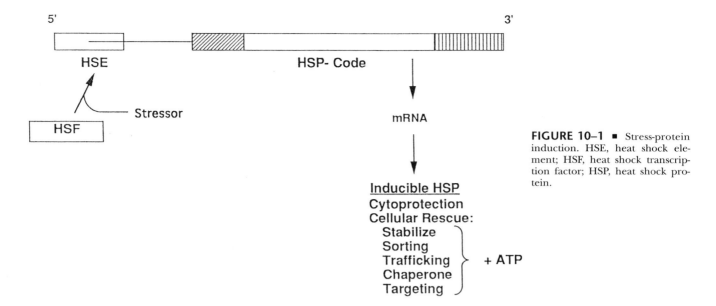

FIGURE 10–1 ■ Stress-protein induction. HSE, heat shock element; HSF, heat shock transcription factor; HSP, heat shock protein.

proteins is highly dependent on the hydrolysis of ATP, which has been used to define functional activity of HSP-70. Fortunately, these protein chaperones have a high affinity for ATP,[13] which would be of particular value in competing for diminished cellular ATP after an ischemic insult. HSP-70 proteins, then, could use the residual ATP for the critical processes necessary to assist in cellular stabilization and repair. Since disruption of the actin-fodrin–based cytoskeleton is central to the structural derangement in cells injured by energy depletion, prevention of this derangement and reconstitution of the cytoskeletal array would be a necessary component of cellular reorganization. The HSP-70 proteins are potentially pivotal elements in the protection and restructuring of the cytoskeleton. HSP-70 proteins have been implicated as cross linkers between cytoskeletal proteins, in particular actin, and other cellular proteins during their translocation through the cell.[18] Furthermore, HSP-70 has been co-localized with spectrin (fodrin) both by double immunofluorescence and by co-immunoprecipitation from lymphocytes.[19] Activation of the lymphocytes resulted in repositioning of HSP-70 congruent with spectrin. Addition of ATP, which typically releases HSP-70 from its substrate, abolished the co-immunoprecipitation of HSP-70 with the spectrin. Therefore, HSP-70 can have direct interaction with cytoskeletal proteins and could be instrumental in reconstituting the array after ischemic injury.

Although most of the attention has been on HSP-70 proteins because of their abundance, inducibility, and cytoprotectant effects, interest has developed regarding the role of other stress proteins in general chaperoning and in cell injury. It has become apparent that each of the HSPs, though having separate characteristics, cooperate with members of other classes of stress proteins in assisting peptides to their final conformation, location, and activity. The integrated view of cooperation between different protein chaperones was first demonstrated by the sequential interaction of DnaK, DnaJ, and GroEL (the prokaryotic homologues of HSP-70 and HSP-60) with a folding peptide in a reaction coupled by a small HSP (GrpE) in an ATP-dependent reaction.[20] This concept of separate but complementary roles of the chaperones has been confirmed, wherein a series of denatured enzymes have been reconstituted to full activity by the sequential addition of the prokaryotic homologues of HSP-70, HSP-60, and the small HSPs, along with ATP.[21–25] Eukaryotic stress proteins HSP-90, HSC-70, and Hdj-1 also have been shown to have distinct but cooperative roles in reconstituting the enzymatic activity of denatured β-galactosidase in vitro.[17] By sequentially adding purified stress proteins individually and in combination to the denatured substrate, these investigators demonstrated that no individual chaperone reactivated the denatured enzyme. HSP-90 maintained the denatured substrate in a folding competent state but did not participate in active refolding. Purified HSP-70, in conjunction with Hdj-1 actively refolded the enzyme in a process requiring ATP. It appeared, then, that HSP-90 maintained the enzyme in a configuration on which the other stress proteins could act to reconstitute the protein to its native form.[17] Similar in vitro studies have shown the small HSP, HSP-25, to have action analogous to HSP-90, that is, to trap unfolding proteins in a folding competent state. This function allowed the cooperative action of HSP-70 to refold the denatured enzyme and reconstitute its activity. Therefore, HSP-25 may complex with aggregating proteins to create a reservoir of non-native proteins to be reactivated by other protein chaperones once cellular metabolism is restored.[26] Finally, it has been shown that the eukaryotic stress protein HSP-104 can act in concert with HSP-70 and HSP-40 to reactivate proteins that previously have been denatured and allowed to aggregate. This action is different from that shown for HSP-25 and HSP-90, in which the function seems to be to prevent aggregation of denatured proteins. In contrast, in the case of HSP-104, the remodeling activity occurs through action on proteins that have already been trapped within aggregates and are refractory to the action of other chaperones. HSP-104 appears to produce a peptide intermediate that can then be refolded by the other protein chaperones.[27] In an analogous manner, different classes of stress proteins probably cooperate in restoring injured eukaryotic cells and, in particular, injured renal epithelium.

Study of the role of HSPs in renal cell injury has been guided thus by the knowledge of specific processes that occur in injured renal epithelium, of the protective role of HSPs in other models of cell injury, and of specific functions of individual HSPs. Models of osmotic, toxic, heat-induced, and energy deprivation energy have broadened the understanding of HSPs and their role in injured renal epithelium. The remainder of this chapter describes how these studies have expanded our knowledge of (1) the signals, processes, and pattern of induction of stress proteins following an insult to renal epithelium; (2) the role of stress proteins in cytoprotection in renal epithelium; and (3) the function of HSPs in assisting cellular recovery following the injury.

INDUCTION OF THE STRESS RESPONSE IN INJURED RENAL EPITHELIA

The genes for inducible HSPs have in common sequences called HSEs upstream from the coding regions for the particular HSPs (see Fig. 10–1). These elements consist of a series of complementary nGAAn repeats that are recognized and bound by activated HSF. Several heat shock factors have been identified, but the best studied and apparently the most active HSF in models of cell stress is HSF1. This transcription factor is preformed and maintained in an inactive monomeric state that has no DNA binding activity in unstressed cells. However, once cells undergo physiologic stress, HSF1 activates to form a trimer that binds the HSE. This event then initiates active transcription of heat shock genes in preference to other cellular proteins.[13, 28] A series of HSPs then can be induced rapidly and preferentially. In fact, one of the most highly inducible of these stress proteins, the HSP-70 family, is unique among eukaryotic genes in having no introns and therefore no need for RNA processing prior to translation. This allows for rapid elaboration of this stress protein in response to a cellular insult. Overall, then, the HSP system essentially is poised to respond to a variety of stresses. HSF can be bound by both 70- and 90-kDa HSPs, and it appears that this interaction between HSF and constitutively expressed HSPs maintains the HSF in its inactive monomeric state.[14, 15] Several cellular events may contribute to HSF activation, but evidence suggests that the central signal for HSF activation is the accumulation of denatured or aggregated proteins.[15, 28] With an increased demand for their protein chaperone function, the constitutively expressed HSPs release HSF to trimerize and bind to the HSE in HSP genes. The subsequent elaboration of inducible HSPs can then supplement the action of

their constitutively expressed cognates. Once sufficient protein chaperones are produced, HSF is inactivated and production of inducible HSPs is reduced to baseline levels.

A series of studies in injured renal epithelium have examined both potential signals for HSP induction and the pattern of HSP elaboration following a specific insult. In large part, these studies have supported the general model of HSP induction and suggest that accumulation of abnormal cellular protein is the crucial signal for the stress response in injured renal epithelium. Activation of HSF not only is the initial event in stress protein induction but also can be used as the first indicator of the stress response. Activation of transcription factor to bind the HSE, along with HSP mRNA elaboration, has been used to examine potential signals for stress response induction in models of both ischemic and toxic renal cell injury. ATP depletion is a principal event in the ischemic injury; thus the relationship of specific decrements in cellular ATP to initiation of the stress response was examined in rat kidneys subjected to regulated partial vascular occlusion.[29] Renal cortex ATP levels were monitored during the partial occlusion with the use of in situ NMR spectroscopy. Activation of HSF was not present, and HSP-70 mRNA induction did not occur in renal cortex when ATP levels were maintained above 60% of control levels. Reduction in ATP levels in the renal cortex to below 50% of control values resulted in both HSF activation and low-level expression of inducible HSP-70 mRNA. More profound decrements in cellular ATP resulted in greater activation of HSF and greater HSP-70 mRNA elaboration. In addition, HSF was activated by as little as 15 minutes of total vascular occlusion. Reflow was not required for activation of HSF after ischemia. Therefore, it appeared that cellular ATP or some metabolic consequence associated with ATP depletion could be a threshold factor for initiation of the stress response in the kidney. In addition, once the threshold was crossed, HSP induction appeared to be a graded response that was modulated by the degree of energy deprivation.[29]

A separate study also suggests that a cellular consequence of ATP depletion, rather than oxidant injury, is the inducer of the stress response in renal ischemia. Folic acid induces ischemic renal injury and rapidly induces HSP-70. Pretreatment of animals with a combination of antioxidants (allopurinol and DMSO [dimethyl sulfoxide]) before folic acid treatment did not alter HSP-70 gene expression but did alter the expression of other early response genes.[30] Combined with the previous findings that ischemia activated HSF without the establishment of reperfusion, this study indicates that HSP-70 induction does not depend on oxidative stress or reactive oxygen species.

Energy deprivation causes many perturbations within renal epithelium that could be signals for activation of the stress response. Studies using cultured renal epithelium have begun to elucidate some of the intracellular events that may contribute to HSF activation and stress response induction. Cellular perturbations in kidney epithelium examined as potential signals for the stress response include changes in the intracellular free calcium [Ca]ᵢ that could modulate HSF activity and stress protein induction,[31–34] disruption of cell architecture that accompanies an ischemic injury,[38] the oxidative state of the cell,[30, 35, 36] and the accumulation of abnormal cellular proteins.[35–38] Many of these events are rapid and reversible in sublethally injured cells.

In a model of energy deprivation in cultured proximal tubule cells (LLC-PK₁), the degree of HSF activation, changes in intracellular calcium, and the degree of disruption of membrane protein–cytoskeletal interactions were determined relative to specific decrements in cellular ATP. In a striking correspondence to the previous study of rat kidney in vivo, HSF was first activated when cellular ATP was reduced below a threshold of 50% of control, and further decrements in cellular ATP resulted in progressive activation of HSF (Fig. 10–2). Changes in free [Ca]ᵢ and Na^+,K^+-ATPase attachment to the cytoskeleton were detectable before HSF activation. Therefore, alterations in cell architecture and calcium homeostasis appeared to be instrumental in activating or modulating the stress response in cells deprived of energy. HSF activation by

ATP depletion was not associated with any increase in cell death, indicating that the stress response in renal epithelium is not merely a manifestation of lethal injury. Progressive decrements in cellular ATP below the respective thresholds caused incremental increases in [Ca]ᵢ, Na^+,K^+-ATPase detachment from the cytoskeleton, and HSF activation.[38] Thus, the degree to which the stress response is activated appears to be tightly linked to the severity of the insult. In renal epithelium injured by energy depletion, the stress response is not an all-or-nothing affair. It seems to be an adaptive response that is measured to the severity of the injury. In renal epithelium injured by ischemia, it is likely that neither ATP depletion itself nor changes in intracellular calcium are sufficient to induce the stress response, though both may modulate the response once it is induced.

The principal trigger for the stress response in energy-depleted renal epithelium is most probably the accumulation of disrupted, non-native, or denatured cellular proteins. ATP depletion alone causes denaturation and aggregation of proteins in mammalian cells.[39] Two separate research groups have shown that accumulation of abnormal cellular proteins is an important signal for stress-response induction in renal epithelium.[35–37] Inhibitors of the proteasome block the degradation of both normal cytosolic and endoplasmic reticulum (ER)–associated proteins. Madin-Darby canine kidney (MDCK) cells treated with proteasome inhibitors accumulate normally short-lived proteins and have a concomitant increase in mRNAs that encode cytosolic HSPs, HSP-70 and polyubiquitin, as well as the ER chaperones BiP, Grp-94, and ERp-72.[37] The efficacy of the separate proteasome inhibitors in inducing the HSPs and ER chaperones correlated with each inhibitor's potency in inhibiting the proteasome. In addition, the inhibitors did not appear to affect total protein synthesis or ER morphology and function at the time when the chaperones were induced. Stress response initiation by proteasome inhibition could occur either from accumulation of abnormal proteins that would have been degraded by the proteasome or from prevention of the degradation of HSFs. In fact, HSF2 has been shown in other, nonrenal cell lines to be regulated by the ubiquitin-proteasome pathway. Inhibition of the proteasome in these cells prevents the normal rapid turnover of HSF2, causing induction of the stress response in erythroid cell lines.[40] Since the proteasome plays a large part in ATP-dependent proteolysis, reduced proteasome activity secondary to ATP depletion during ischemia could contribute to stress protein induction. The profile of HSF activation in LLC-PK₁ cells in response to ATP depletion was compared with the profile in the same cells in response to isolated proteasome inhibition. Each insult activated both HSF1 and HSF2 in the same pattern. The study did not separate the relative contribution of decreased clearance of abnormal proteins from the contribution of increased disruption of proteins to the total initiation of the stress response during ATP depletion. However, it is clear that induction of HSPs during ischemia-

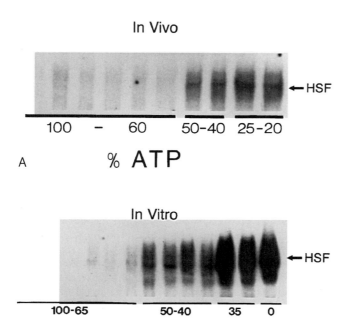

In Vivo

A   **% ATP**

In Vitro

B   **%ATP**

FIGURE 10–2 ■ Gel retardation assays showing activation of heat shock transcription factor (HSF) as a function of cellular ATP depletion. The *dark bands* indicate activated HSF. *A*, Activation of HSF in renal cortex in vivo during graded ATP depletion by partial vascular occlusion. *B*, HSF activation in cultured renal epithelium during graded ATP depletion from substrate depletion and mitochondrial inhibition. Both in vivo and in vitro, HSF is activated in renal epithelium when the level of cellular ATP falls below a threshold of 50% control. Further decrements in cellular ATP level cause additional activation of HSF. (*A* from Van Why SK, Mann AS, Thulin G, et al: Activation of heat-shock transcription factor by graded reductions in renal ATP, in vivo, in the rat. J Clin Invest 1994; 94:1518; with permission. *B* from Van Why SK, Kim SA, Geibel J, et al: Thresholds for cellular disruption and activation of the stress response in renal epithelia. Am J Physiol 1999; 277:F227; with permission.)

induced ARF is multifactorial and that reduced proteasome activity may play a prominent role.[38]

The signal for induction of the stress response in renal injury from toxins also appears to be the accumulation of abnormal proteins. In LLC-PK$_1$ cells treated with reactive electrophiles, 70-kDa HSPs are rapidly induced. Blocking the rise in intracellular calcium and lipid peroxidation prevented injury of these cells but did not alter HSP-70 induction in response to the reactive electrophiles.[35] Reducing disulfide bonds with dithiothreitol (DTT), however, did prevent HSP-70 transcription. Therefore, it appeared that the reactive electrophiles caused a change in protein conformation within the LLC-PK$_1$ cells that was the primary signal for transcriptional activation of HSP-70.

This group also has provided evidence that, as in ischemic injury, induction of the stress response in toxin-induced renal cell injury is not mediated by oxidative stress. Iodoacetamide is an alkylating agent that has several effects that injure proximal tubule cells. It causes protein alkylation, a decrease in cellular glutathione that contributes to oxidative stress and lipid peroxidation. Iodoacetamide activated HSF1 and increased HSP-70 transcription in LLC-PK$_1$ cells. Treating these cells with antioxidants and iron or calcium chelators prevented cell death but did not prevent either HSF1 activation or HSP-70 transcription. Furthermore, treating the cells exposed to iodoacetamide with DTT, to break disulfide bonds, blocked both HSF1 activation and HSP-70 transcription. The results of this study showed that oxidant injury is not involved in activation of HSF or HSP-70 elaboration in this form of injury. However, alteration of protein conformation by formation of disulfide-linked aggregates seems to be a signal for induction of the stress response in this toxin-induced renal injury.[36] These series of studies, then, suggest that the accumulation of abnormal intracellular proteins is the critical event leading to stress protein induction in renal epithelia from a variety of insults, including energy depletion, proteasome inhibition, and other toxin-induced injury.

HEAT SHOCK PROTEIN EXPRESSION AFTER RENAL INJURY

The pattern of HSP elaboration after an injury to the kidney has given initial clues to the function of these chaperones. The focus has been on the inducible HSP-70 proteins in ischemic injury in vivo, although an expanding array of other stress-inducible proteins in other forms of renal injury are being studied. As outlined previously, renal ischemia in vivo rapidly activates HSF, the initial event in the stress response. Even greater HSF activation is found during early reflow, at 15 minutes, but activated HSF has begun to decline by 2 hours of reflow.[29] Messenger RNA for inducible HSP-70 is found within minutes of the ischemic insult and HSF activation. HSP-70 mRNA peaks within the first 6 hours of reflow after 45 minutes of ischemia.[30, 41, 42] Inducible HSP-70 mRNA thereafter progressively declines. HSP-72, the inducible protein, appears shortly after the message increases, accumulates up to 24 hours, and can persist for days.[30, 41–43] This pattern of stress response induction shortly followed by down-regulation coinciding with the accumulation of the inducible protein is consistent with the current general model of heat shock gene regulation. The inducible HSP suppresses general HSP gene expression by deactivating HSF trimers once enough of the inducible chaperone has accumulated.

The pattern of HSP-72 protein expression within the kidney following ischemia has suggested that it is involved in the process of recovery after the injury. This inducible HSP-70 is, at best, barely detectable in uninjured renal cortex from rats and humans.[41–44] Following ischemic injury in rat kidney, HSP-72 is rapidly detectable in the cortex and outer medulla.[41–43] In diseased human kidneys, the pattern of HSP-72 expression varied but was most strongly related to the activity and location of the disease process.[44] In particular, HSP-72 was found in proximal tubules and collecting ducts of kidneys that had suffered an ischemic insult or acute tubular necrosis. Likewise, in the rat kidney, HSP-72 was found in proximal tubules after an ischemic injury.[41] Therefore, it appears that this stress protein is induced most markedly in the cells that have sustained the most significant injury following ischemia. When one examines injured proximal tubules after ischemia, the pattern of HSP-72 distribution and redistribution is even more striking. Early after ischemia in rat kidney, at 15 minutes of reperfusion, HSP-72 is found almost exclusively in the apical domain of proximal tubule cells. The same area undergoes the most striking morphologic changes at this time. The brush border has characteristic alterations, including retraction of microvilli and associated cytoskeletal proteins, along with blebbing and shedding of the brush border into the lumen. The cytoskeleton in the apical terminal web is disrupted, with coincident generalized loss of cell polarity, including redistribution of Na^+, K^+-ATPase into the apical membrane. Later during reperfusion, at 2 and 6 hours after ischemia, HSP-72 is found throughout the cytoplasm in a coarse aggregated pattern. By 24 hours of reperfusion, HSP-72 has migrated away from the apical domain, coincident with restoration of cellular architecture.[41] The pattern of HSP-70 induction, then, indicates that the cells are poised to respond to an insult by rapidly producing this protein chaperone, which goes to the area of most intense injury within a cell. These chaperones then appear to migrate to different subcellular compartments as repair progresses.

Several other stress proteins, which probably have functions different from but complementary to those of the HSP-70 chaperones, have been examined following renal cell injury. One group of chaperones, called the small-stress proteins, include the HSP 27 (HSP-27) in humans and its closely related analog HSP-25 in rodents.[45] Because these small HSPs are involved in regulation of actin dynamics and because disorganization of the actin cytoskeleton is a prominent feature in the ischemic injury, the expression of HSP-25 in rat kidneys after ischemia was examined by several investigators.[42, 46, 47] HSP-25 expression in control-rat cortex was low, similar to that for HSP-72. Ischemia induced HSP-25 expression in cortex as rapidly as and to a degree similar to that of HSP-72.[41, 42, 46] Increased levels of HSP-25 were detectable as early as 2 hours of reflow after ischemia, had peaked by 6 hours, and then persisted for days. Ischemia caused a dramatic shift of HSP-25 within subcellular compartments separate from the overall increased expression. During and shortly after ischemia, constitutive HSP-25 shifted from a predominantly soluble protein fraction to an insoluble fraction that traditionally is associated with cytoskeletal elements. By the time that total HSP-25 expression had increased, its distribution had reverted to a predominantly soluble, non–cytoskeleton-associated pattern.[42, 46] As discussed in more detail later, this shift in detergent extractability of HSP-25 suggested that this small-stress protein may be involved in the early cytoskeletal alterations that accompany ischemic renal injury.

An entirely separate class of stress proteins, in a subcellular compartment different from HSP-70 and HSP-25, are also induced following renal ischemia. Both acute renal ischemia in the rat and ATP depletion in cultured MDCK cells cause a marked increase in mRNA levels for the ER chaperones grp-78, BiP, grp-94, and ERp-72. Because increased expression of these stress proteins is typically associated with the accumulation of misfolded or misassembled secretory proteins in the ER, their induction following energy depletion suggests that the normal maturation of secretory proteins in the ER may be impaired during renal ischemia.[48] The ER chaperone grp-78 is also induced in LLC-PK$_1$ cells subjected to toxic injury from the disulfide reducing agent DTT.[49]

Other forms of toxic renal injury also increase HSP expression in renal epithelium. In cisplatin-induced ARF, HSP-90 expression is increased in the S3 segment of the proximal tubule.[50] Rats with acute proximal tubule injury from gentamicin have increased expression of the constitutive 70-kDa HSP, HSC-73. The increase in HSC-73 occurred as soon as 36 hours after treatment with gentamicin and persisted for days. In addition, HSC-73 redistributed from a predominantly nuclear to a granular pattern within the cytoplasm, which appeared to coincide with enlarged lysosomes. As the kidneys recovered, HSC-73 localization returned to the pattern seen in normal kidneys.[51] Finally, nephrotoxic injury from mercuric chloride caused an increase in the expression of HSP-72, HSP-90, and a 110-kDa protein that has not been characterized but may, in fact, be HSP-110. These proteins were preferentially induced over other proteins concomitant with a generalized alteration in protein synthesis after treatment with mercuric chloride.[52] These findings are quite similar to observations in ischemia-induced ARF. Ischemia causes a decreased expression and transcription for the majority of constitutively expressed proteins in the kidney but a marked increase in expression of the stress proteins.[11, 41, 53] Therefore, the generalized increase in stress proteins described in this section does not represent a nonspecific response of the injured renal epithelium. Rather, the increased expression of stress proteins appears to be a specific and highly regulated response whereby transcription and production of proteins involved in the normal day-to-day function of the renal epithelium are down-regulated, and proteins that may be crucial for the survival and restructuring of injured cells are preferentially synthesized.

Finally, osmotic stress also induces HSP expression. Treating MDCK cells with hyperosmotic NaCl increased HSP-70 mRNA expression.[54] The hyperosmotic-induced stress response occurred at the same time that total RNA transcription and total protein synthesis was suppressed, indicating that, as with ischemia, the HSP-70 induction by osmotic stress is a regulated response. Subsequent to this first description of osmotic stress induction of HSPs, several HSPs were identified within various regions of mammalian kidney, including HSP-70, HSP-60, and HSP-25/27.[55] Furthermore, recognition that renal medullary cells face routine osmotic stress provided researchers with the opportunity to discover novel eukaryotic stress proteins. Osmotic stress protein 94 (Osp-94) was identified first in medullary cells from mouse kidney.[56] Sequence analysis showed Osp-94 to have 65% homology to HSP-110 and 30% homology to 70-kDa HSPs, placing Osp-94 in the HSP-110 gene subfamily of the HSP-70 superfamily. The sequence homology gives Osp-94 an amino-terminal ATP-binding domain and a putative C-terminal peptide-binding domain similar to its related protein chaperones. As expected, the expression of this novel stress protein increased in the inner medulla when animals were water-restricted. Inflicting hyperosmotic and heat or toxic stress with cadmium chloride on cultured inner medulla collecting duct cells induced Osp-94 mRNA expression.[57] Therefore, the newly identified Osp-94 probably acts as a protein chaperone, similar to other members of the HSP-70 superfamily, as indicated by the sequence analysis of this novel stress protein and by its induction by toxic, osmotic, and heat stress.

When a similar approach was used, four putative molecular chaperones with estimated molecular weights of 46, 60, 78, and 200 kDa have been isolated from inner medulla collecting duct cells in hyperosmolar conditions. Each of these proteins have typical chaperone features, such as being up-regulated under hypertonic conditions, binding to denatured proteins, and being released upon the addition of ATP. One protein was identified as the mitochondrial chaperone mtHSP-70 and a second appears to be similar to β-actin.[58]

In sum, stress proteins in several subcellular compartments, in different renal epithelial cells, and in separate regions of the kidney have been shown to be induced by ischemic, osmotic, and toxic stress. Induction of stress proteins is regulated and occurs in preference to production of other proteins at times of cellular stress. The pattern of individual HSP elaboration is distinct and varies according to the cell and the specific stress. The particular pattern of HSP induction and elaboration of individual stress proteins has provided the initial insight into the role of stress proteins in cytoprotection and recovery from renal cell injury.

ROLE OF STRESS PROTEINS IN RENAL EPITHELIAL CYTOPROTECTION

Heat shock proteins have long been recognized to be responsible for the phenomenon of thermotolerance in a variety of prokaryotic and eukaryotic organisms. Individual HSPs have been confirmed as having cytoprotectant effects in a variety of plant, animal, and mammalian cells in heat-induced injury. In addition, the stress proteins have been implicated in cross-tolerance to separate injury, particularly ischemia in the brain and heart.[59–61] Likewise, HSPs seem to be ideal candidates for involvement in protecting renal epithelia from a variety of injuries, including insults from osmotic stress, toxins, and ischemia.

Among human tissues, the renal medulla is unique in being challenged routinely with as much as 10-fold variations in osmolarity. The rapidity and magnitude of this osmotic stress would be lethal to most mammalian cells, but renal medullary cells can readily accumulate intracellular organic osmolytes for protection. However, the speed of organic osmolyte accumulation and discharge may not keep pace with the osmotic fluctuations in medullary cells. Additional cytoprotectants, then, would seem helpful if not necessary for supplementing the organic osmolytes on a routine basis. This concept led to the examination of HSP expression within different regions of the kidney related to medullary tonicity and volume state in vivo and in response to osmotic stress in cultured renal epithelial cells in vitro.

It is possible that a variety of stress proteins may cooperate in providing cytoprotection against osmotic stress to the renal medulla; thus, the distributions of several HSPs have been examined in different regions of the kidney. Under constitutive conditions the inducible HSP-72 is barely detectable in the cortex but is easily detectable in the medulla and especially in the renal papilla.[43, 55] Likewise, many other HSPs are more prominently expressed in the medulla than in the cortex under constitutive conditions. HSP-25, Osp-94, HSP-110, and HSP-70RY occur in higher amounts in the medulla than in cortex.[55, 57] Exceptions to this rule include higher levels of HSP-60 found in renal cortex and a uniform distribution of HSC-73 throughout the kidney.[55] A series of studies have examined whether physiologic changes in medullary tonicity or inhibition of organic osmolyte regulation could alter the expression of stress proteins both in cultured cells and in medullary tissue in vivo. The prior accumulation of organic osmolytes in MDCK cells attenuates subsequent induction of HSP-70 in response to acute hypertonic and heat stress.[62] This suggested that the 70-kDa HSPs may supplement the cytoprotection provided by organic osmolytes. The finding that HSP-70 is induced in the renal medulla in response to changes in medullary sodium and urea concentration showed that the previous in vitro finding can be translated to the kidney in vivo.[63] Furthermore, kidneys from water-restricted rats displayed increased mRNA expression for HSP-25 and HSP-60 in the papilla. However, in this case, neither water diuresis nor water restriction appeared to alter HSP-70 mRNA levels.[64] Nevertheless, support for the notion that HSP-70 chaperones engage in osmoprotection in vivo is provided by a study of vasopressin administration in rats.[65] This maneuver activated the heat shock factor and increased HSP-70 mRNA and protein within the kidney. No similar changes were found in tissues outside of the kidney. The vasopressin-mediated, kidney-specific, stress response induction was prevented by V_2 receptor blockade, suggesting that the HSP-70 induction was caused by osmotic changes.[65] Strengthening the case for osmotic changes being a signal for stress-protein induction is a study in which rats underwent long-term diuresis from chronic furosemide administration.[66] Treating these rats with ketoconazole increased the efflux of organic osmolytes from the medullary cells and further increased the expression of HSP-25 and HSP-72.[66] The augmented osmotic stress placed on the medullary cells when ketoconazole disrupts their normal osmotic adaptation thus seems to call for additional protein chaperones to compensate for the lost organic osmolytes. Furthermore, expression of both of these HSPs in the medulla has been linked to urea concentration, implying that the level of urea present might contribute to regulation of overall HSP content in the renal medulla.[67]

Separate from the distribution of these proteins within the kidney and the changes in their expression in response to water loading or deprivation is the direct evidence of their role in protection against osmotic injury that is just emerging. Pretreatment with sublethal heat stress protected cultured mouse inner medulla collecting duct cells from subsequent lethal osmotic stress.[57] MDCK cells pretreated with hypertonic sodium chloride were more likely to survive subsequent exposure to urea, which correlated with increased HSP-72 expression.[68] Treatment of preconditioned MDCK cells with a p38 kinase inhibitor reduced HSP-72 content in the cells and reduced survival following urea treatment.[68] Finally, clones of MDCK cells stably transfected with DNA antisense to HSP-72 had inhibited HSP-72 induction by hypertonic media. The degree that HSP-72 induction was inhibited in each clone by the antisense HSP-72 transfection correlated with reduced survival following treatment with urea.[69] In sum, the search into whether HSPs can be cytoprotective against osmotic stress so far indicates that these protein chaperones probably complement the cytoprotection provided by organic osmolytes. HSP-mediated cytoprotection may be crucial, particularly at times when organic osmolyte regulation is delayed, insufficient, or impaired.

Whether stress proteins are instrumental in protecting the kidney against ischemic injury has been a more controversial issue. When HSPs were examined in the intact rat kidney or in proximal tubules isolated from the injured kidney, minimal cytoprotection against ischemia or hypoxia could be attributed to

HSPs. Preconditioning ischemia did protect proximal tubules from subsequent hypoxic injury, but the post-ischemic HSP synthesis correlated poorly with the observed cytoresistance. In addition, when HSP expression was induced by hyperthermia, there was only trivial protection against subsequent hypoxic injury in isolated tubules.[70] Likewise, preconditioning heat stress in rats increased the expression of several HSPs in the kidney but provided no evident protection against subsequent ischemic injury as manifested by either functional or morphologic parameters.[71] However, protection against injury from either subsequent heat shock or ATP depletion could be correlated with the prior accumulation of HSP-72 in several different cultured renal epithelial cell lines.[72–74] The discrepancy between the in vivo and in vitro studies may be explained in part by the complexity of injury in the intact kidney compared with cells in culture. Also, as described previously, stress protein induction and distribution varies between regions of the kidney, between cells within a region, and between subcellular compartments according to the specific stress applied. Quite simply, cytoprotection attributable to stress proteins in the intact kidney may be difficult to demonstrate with the use of a cross-tolerance approach, because the distribution of the HSPs resulting from the inducing stress may be quite different from the sites most susceptible to the subsequent insult. The use of cross-tolerance studies to demonstrate the effects of stress proteins suffers from a more fundamental problem; it requires the attribution of cytoprotection to HSPs induced by one insult against injury from a different insult that may have quite varied qualitative and quantitative effects. Delineating the function of induced HSPs in this setting thus is confounded by the cell's having been previously injured by a different insult. The stress proteins induced by the first insult may be fully engaged in a subcellular compartment separate from the injury caused by the second insult. Despite these problems, the lure of discovering a role for stress protein–mediated cytoprotection in the kidney remains. Therefore, studies of cross-tolerance continue, and more refined studies are providing convincing evidence that stress proteins do indeed play a role in providing cytoprotection to renal epithelia in specific forms of cell injury.

Most of these studies now use culture models of cell injury to remove the complexity of in vivo injury as a confounding factor. Preconditioning with sublethal heat shock or cyclosporine exposure protected LLC-PK$_1$ cells against subsequent toxic doses of cyclosporine. The observed cytoprotection was correlated with both the timing and the level of HSP-70 induction.[75] In proximal tubule opossum kidney cells, prior heat stress improved survival from subsequent ATP depletion, which was correlated again with accumulation of HSP-72.[74] Preconditioning heat stress also protected primary cultures of proximal tubules from winter flounder against subsequent heat shock injury.[76] Of particular interest in the latter study is the fact that the protection was manifested by improved transepithelial transport and preservation of microvillus structure,

both prominent features in ischemic injury to the proximal tubule. Proteasome inhibitors reduced the clearance of short-lived proteins, caused an accumulation of abnormal proteins within MDCK cells, and induced mRNA expression for ER and cytosolic chaperones.[37] The prior induction of protein chaperones by proteasome inhibitors was associated with improved survival following severe heat shock. Treatment of MDCK cells with tunicamycin or the compound A23187 induced ER, but not cytosolic chaperones, and was associated with protection from ATP-depletion–induced injury. Cycloheximide did not completely block the protective effect from pretreating the cells with these compounds, indicating that not all of the protection may be attributable to induction of the stress proteins. Nevertheless, this study does suggest that ER chaperones may be involved in protecting renal epithelium from ATP depletion.[77] Conversely, protection from cisplatin-induced injury to rat kidneys by concomitant administration of glycine could not be attributed to HSP-70 induction.[78] In light of the recent cell culture work just described and detailed later, this in vivo study[78] does not eliminate HSP-70 as a player in providing cytoprotection in the kidney. Rather, it is consistent with the earlier in vivo and in vitro studies, showing that cytoprotection is a complex process that is affected by the individual cellular milieu created by both the preconditioning stress and the subsequent injury.

Several recent studies in renal epithelia directly show the complexity of attributing cytoprotective cross-tolerance to stress proteins. LLC-PK$_1$ cells subjected to reductive stress caused increased transcription for the stress response genes GADD-153 and Grp-78 but did not increase transcription for HSP-70. On the other hand, oxidative stress to these same cells strongly induced HSP-70 but had only a weak effect on GADD-153 and Grp-78 transcription. Preconditioning of the cells with reductive stress induced tolerance to toxin-induced cell injury.[49] Therefore, the regulated gene expression for individual stress proteins within a single type of cell is specific to the type of insult. Cytoprotection may be present and attributable to the specific set of stress proteins induced when the preceding conditioning insult is similar to the subsequent toxic insult. When medullary collecting duct cells were conditioned with hypertonic media, a series of stress proteins were overexpressed.[79] These preconditioned cells were resistant to injury from heat shock, ATP depletion, and cyclosporine, but not cadmium chloride. In fact, preconditioning the cells with hypertonic media had the opposite effect and caused increased cell death from cadmium chloride treatment.[79] Nevertheless, there was cross-tolerance demonstrated between hypertonic injury and heat shock injury by preconditioning with a sublethal level of the converse insult.[57] Therefore, these studies in composite are complementary and show that the profile of stress proteins induced in cells is specific to the particular insult, and that stress proteins induced by one insult do not confer uniform protection against all other potential forms of injury.

Transfected overexpression of specific HSPs in renal

epithelial cells has provided the best evidence of the role of HSPs in cytoprotection. COS cells transiently transfected with *Drosophila* HSP-27 were less sensitive to injury from heat stress and hydrogen peroxide.[80] Parallel transfection of the COS cells with sequential deletion mutants of the HSP-27 protein showed that the protective effect was preserved as long as the last 42 amino acids in the conserved α-crystallin domain of HSP-27 was retained. In the transfectants that were protective, the effect appeared to be at the level of the nucleus.[80] LLC-PK$_1$ cells with transfected overexpression of labeled HSP-25 had less detachment of Na$^+$,K$^+$-ATPase from the cytoskeleton during ATP depletion and recovered more rapidly.[81] LLC-PK$_1$ cells also have been stably transfected to overexpress HSP-72, which did not affect the expression of other HSPs. The HSP-72 transfectants were resistant to lethal injury from hydrogen peroxide and cisplatin.[82] In an innovative study, LLC-PK$_1$ cells were transiently co-transfected with HSP-70 and with luciferase. Luciferase activity was used as a reporter for normal cell protein conformation and function. Both heat and hypoxia decreased luciferase activity. Compared with control co-transfectants that did not include the HSP-70 insert, the HSP-70 transfectants protected against the heat-induced decrease in luciferase activity but did not protect against the hypoxia-induced decrease in luciferase activity.[83] This study does not prove that HSPs have no role in hypoxic injury but is a strong argument for the specific action of an individual HSP that varies according to the cellular insult.

Studies of several forms of toxin-induced injury in LLC-PK$_1$ cells have shown that ER protein chaperones can play a role in cytoprotection. Pretreatment with the ER stressors DTTox, thapsagargin, or tunicamycin increased the expression of the ER chaperones Grp-78 and Grp-94 and rendered the cells tolerant to injury from the alkylating chemical iodoacetamide. However, prior heat shock did not protect the cells against iodoacetamide. LLC-PK$_1$ cells transfected to produce mRNA antisense to Grp-78 had an impaired up-regulation of Grp-78 and Grp-94 in response to the ER stressors, and the antisense transfection caused attenuation of protection against iodoacetamide.[84] Prior treatment of LLC-PK$_1$ cells with DTTox, to increase levels of Grp-78 and other stress proteins, rendered the cells tolerant to TFEC, a potent nephrotoxic cysteine conjugate.[49] Again, prior ER stress using the various inducers of ER chaperones increased levels of Grp-78, Grp-94, and another ER chaperone, calreticulin, and was associated with resistance against oxidant injury from tBHP, a prototypical organic oxidant(terbutyl hydroperoxide).[85] To show that this was a specific effect from an ER chaperone, cells were transfected with a construct to produce mRNA antisense to Grp-78, which prevented the induction of this stress protein. Compared with the transfectants that contain the vector without the Grp-78 antisense insert, the Grp-78 antisense transfectants were sensitized to the oxidative injury from tBHP. Therefore, these studies demonstrate that stress proteins located in the ER can be instrumental in providing cytoprotection against toxic

insults and also confirm that cross-tolerance against injury attributable to HSPs is neither generalized nor uniform.

Ultimately, the intent of studying whether stress proteins can provide cytoprotection is to harness this function for clinical benefit. Induction of the chaperones by a prior insult complicates the study of cytoprotection and is not a preferred therapeutic maneuver. Ideally, pharmacologic modulation of stress protein levels might be used therapeutically. Since salicylates might change the threshold for stress response induction, the potential for their use in enhancing the stress response in vivo has been studied. In response to heat, rats receiving aspirin had a more than three-fold induction of HSP-70 above the level in animals that did not receive aspirin. However, the enhanced HSP-70 expression was correlated with a more prominent hyperthermic response in the salicylate-treated animals, an indication that the enhanced stress response in vivo from salicylate treatment may be neither pharmacologic nor beneficial.[86, 87] Both hyperthermia and hypothermia have been shown to activate HSF and increase HSP-70 mRNA levels in several tissues within the mouse, including the kidney.[88] This raises the intriguing possibility that cytoprotection of organs for transplantation through cold preservation may not result solely from a reduction in metabolic activity but also may be a function of HSP induction.

FUNCTION OF STRESS PROTEINS IN PREVENTING RENAL EPITHELIAL CELL INJURY AND IN PROMOTING RECOVERY

Although the beneficial effects of stress proteins in renal epithelia have now been established, the specific function that each stress protein provides in each form of injury is just beginning to be discovered. The distribution of each HSP both before and after the injury has provided initial clues to particular functions, especially since the distribution of HSPs (most notably the cytosolic HSPs) following an injury is not static. Certainly, the function of the stress proteins in cytoprotection and cell recovery is multifaceted, because members of each major class of HSPs are located in most subcellular compartments and because cells face a plethora of insults that have different manifestations of injury. The function of an individual stress protein, then, depends on its location, the potential substrates on which it can act, and the particular mechanism of injury.

The role of stress proteins in renal injury appears to be to preserve or restore normal cellular architecture and function. The evidence is provided by the distribution of HSPs during the injury and redistribution during recovery and by the functional effects resulting from modulating stress protein expression. Proximal tubule injury in rats from acute gentamicin toxicity and other forms of lysosomal insults causes an accumulation of HSC-73 and HSP-90 in the injured lysosomes.[51, 89] Heat shock proteins may be involved in the preservation of cellular ATP levels in injured renal

epithelium. ATP depletion is a central feature in ischemic injury and can be a feature of heat stress injury.[72]
Preconditioning medullary collecting duct cells with a
sublethal heat stress preserved the state III mitochondrial respiration and the glycolytic rate in cells subsequently subjected to a heat stress more severe than
that in nonpreconditioned cells.[73] Likewise, in opossum kidney cells subjected to ATP depletion, recovery
of maximal mitochondrial ATP production and cell
ATP content was improved if the cells were previously
exposed to heat stress.[74] Conversely, agents that cause
covalent modifications of mitochondrial HSPs are
nephrotoxic when administered to rats. [90] Therefore,
HSP-mediated preservation or restoration of cellular
metabolism and ATP levels may assist cellular repair
following both toxic and ischemic renal injury.

During recovery from renal ischemia, the cytosolic
stress proteins HSP-72 and HSP-25/27 appear to help
restore cell architecture by acting on several proteins
disrupted by the ischemic insult. These stress proteins
may interact with units of Na^+,K^+-ATPase, tight junction proteins, or elements of the actin-based cytoskeleton, which normally organize cell architecture. In uninjured proximal tubule cells, a low level of HSP-72 is
distributed diffusely throughout the cytoplasm. However, early in recovery, at 15 minutes of reflow after
ischemia, HSP-72 redistributes in a distinct pattern to
a subapical localization in the injured proximal tubule
cells.[41] This is the area in the cell that suffers the
most striking injury at this time. HSP-72 could be
chaperoning disrupted elements of the cytoskeleton to
assist the restructuring of the terminal web. In addition, a portion of the subapical HSP-72 co-localizes
with Na^+,K^+-ATPase, which is displaced to the apical
membrane (Fig. 10–3). Thus, early in recovery after
an ischemic injury, this protein chaperone may be
helping to restore both the structure of the apical
cytoskeleton and the correct localization of Na^+,K^+-
ATPase. Later in recovery, HSP-72 is distributed in

coarse cytoplasmic aggregates.[41] A significant portion
of this HSP-72 co-localizes with Na^+,K^+-ATPase within
the aggregates at 2 hours of recovery, but by 6 hours
of recovery most of the HSP-72 no longer co-localizes
with Na^+, K^+-ATPase (see Fig. 10–3). The pattern of
redistribution later in recovery suggests that the stress
protein may be providing additional restorative functions by chaperoning other proteins disrupted by the
ischemic injury.

Protein aggregates have been isolated from injured
renal cortex following ischemia to study putative interactions between HSP-72 and Na^+,K^+-ATPase or actin.
Mg-ATP was added to cortical homogenates to enhance ATP-dependent HSP-72 activity and to release
the chaperone from its substrates. The addition of Mg-
ATP reduced HSP-72, Na^+,K^+-ATPase, and actin in
the protein aggregates subsequently isolated from the
cortical homogenates. Purifying aggregates from the
homogenates first and then alternately enhancing or
inhibiting ATP hydrolysis had different effects. Inhibiting ATP hydrolysis preserved HSP-72 association with
the aggregates but allowed release of a portion of the
Na^+, K^+-ATPase present in the aggregates. Enhancing
ATP hydrolysis had the converse effect. HSP-72 was
released from the aggregates and Na^+,K^+-ATPase binding to the aggregates was preserved. There was no
effect on actin under either condition. At later intervals of recovery, when cell architecture was largely
restored, addition of Mg-ATP caused a similar release
of HSP-72 from the aggregates but had little effect
on Na^+,K^+-ATPase.[91] This study showed that HSP-72
complexes with aggregated, non-native cellular proteins from injured renal cortex in an ATP-dependent
manner. HSP-72 very possibly may be interacting with
proteins other than Na^+,K^+-ATPase or actin in the
aggregates, because it has been shown that tight junction proteins redistribute to large complexes associated with cytoskeletal proteins during ATP depletion.[92]
It may be that enhancing HSP-72 function after an

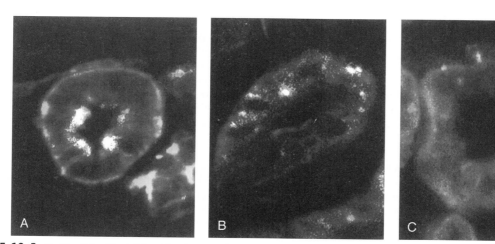

FIGURE 10–3 ■ *(See Color Plate)* After 45 minutes of ischemia and reflow of 15 minutes *(A)*, 2 hours *(B)*, and 6 hours *(C)*, rat kidneys
were perfusion-fixed in situ. Proximal tubules were examined by fluorescence microscopy after treatment with separately labeled antibodies
to HSP-72 (in *orange*) and Na^+,K^+-ATPase (in *green*). Co-localization appears in *yellow.* At 15 minutes of reflow, HSP-72 co-localizes with
Na^+,K^+-ATPase in the apical domain of proximal tubules. At 2 hours of reflow, the two proteins have redistributed and co-localize in an
aggregated pattern. By 6 hours of reflow, HSP-72 remains in an aggregated pattern in the cytoplasm, but Na^+,K^+-ATPase has returned to
the basolateral domain. Minimal co-localization is present.

ischemic renal injury could assist in refolding disrupted Na+, K+-ATPase or aggregated elements of the cytoskeleton and tight junction to help the sublethally injured cell return to a more organized state.

Two preconditioning studies also have indicated that cytosolic HSPs may protect the cytoskeleton and secure cell architecture organized by the cytoskeleton. Prior heat stress preserved the structure of actin stress fibers in ATP-depleted mouse proximal tubule cells. Protection of the actin stress fibers preserved tight junction integrity as measured by transepithelial electrical resistance and dye flux through tight junctions.[93] In addition, preconditioning ischemia associated with HSP-72 induction preserved Na+,K+-ATPase attachment to the cytoskeleton and the normal basolateral distribution of Na+,K+-ATPase during a subsequent ischemic insult.[94] Therefore, cytosolic HSPs may help secure epithelial cell polarity during an ischemic insult by maintaining the integrity of the cytoskeleton and its interaction with tight junction and integral membrane proteins. The preservation of cell architecture could then help maintain renal transport function after an ischemic injury similar to the preservation of function demonstrated after heat shock injury.[76]

HSP-72 does not seem to be alone in interacting with the cytoskeleton to preserve and restore cell architecture after an ischemic renal injury. The small-stress proteins play a significant role in regulating actin dynamics.[45] HSP-27 is distributed throughout the human kidney, and its rodent cognate HSP-25 has been examined in rat kidneys following ischemia.[42, 46, 95] As described previously, ischemia induced the production of HSP-25 in renal cortex and caused an initial shift of HSP-25 from a predominantly soluble cytoplasmic fraction to an insoluble cytoskeletal fraction.[42, 46] Furthermore, the distribution of HSP-25 within injured proximal tubules changed as recovery progressed. In uninjured tubules, HSP-25 was found predominantly in the subapical area in a pattern that suggests interaction with the cytoskeleton in the terminal web. Early after ischemia, HSP-25 is dispersed throughout the cytoplasm in a distribution that coincides with fragmented DNase-reactive actin. Later in reflow, HSP-25 accumulates in the cytoplasm in coarse aggregates.[46] The redistribution of HSP-25 within the injured cells and the shift from a soluble to an insoluble cytoskeletal-associated fraction suggests that HSP-25 interacts with fragmented actin during the early postischemic reorganization of the cytoskeleton. Later in recovery, when HSP-25 shifts back to a predominantly soluble cytoplasmic distribution (which does not coincide significantly with either filamentous or fragmented actin), HSP-25 may be performing a function separate from regulating actin dynamics. The particular role that it plays later in recovery after ischemia is not currently known, but an in vitro protein reconstitution study indicates that HSP-25 can act cooperatively with HSP-70 to trap unfolding proteins in a folding-competent state.[26] A general chaperone function separate from regulating actin dynamics may be the primary activity of HSP-25 later in recovery. For example, later in reflow, when HSP-25 is highly induced and in an aggre-

gated pattern, the stress protein may be complexing with other aggregated proteins to create a reservoir of non-native proteins that can be reactivated once cellular metabolism is restored. This chaperone function of HSP-25 could promote the recycling of a variety of disrupted cellular proteins after renal ischemia.

The principal function of HSP-25 early in the injury, however, appears to be to interact with actin in order to preserve cell architecture. In LLC-PK₁ cells transfected and overexpressing labeled HSP-25, Na+,K+-ATPase attachment to the cytoskeleton was preserved during ATP depletion. The protection was coincident with direct interaction of HSP-25 with actin during ATP depletion. With the use of fluorescence energy transfer, the labeled HSP-25 was seen to interact with actin during ATP depletion, but only minimally in control cells and in cells that had recovered from ATP depletion injury. This is consistent with the in vivo co-localization of these two proteins after ischemia and indicates that HSP-25 is involved in the regulation of actin dynamics during the disruption and remodeling of the cytoskeleton that is an integral part of this injury.[81] Cytosolic HSP-72, HSP-25, and HSP-27 appear, then, to interact with several different proteins in different areas of the cell to preserve and restore architecture.

An additional subcellular compartment where stress proteins act during renal cell injury is in the ER. Renal ischemia and ATP depletion in cultured cells induce several ER chaperones.[48] Depleting thyroid epithelial cells of ATP inhibited the maturation and secretion of thyroglobulin, which formed large macromolecular complexes retained in the ER. The retained proteins stably associated with the ER chaperones BiP, Grp-94, and ERp-72. The implication is that energy depletion from renal ischemia causes misfolding of secretory proteins, which induces the ER chaperones. This event could contribute to cellular injury and require additional stress proteins in the ER to restore normal processing of newly formed proteins. Results from renal cells treated with several other toxins indicate that this is only one function that ER chaperones have in injured renal epithelia. A more significant role may be to prevent injury in a cellular compartment outside of the ER, the cytosol.

Not surprisingly, stress proteins in other cellular compartments appear to function differently from the cytoplasmic stress proteins in protecting the renal epithelium from injury. As discussed earlier, prior induction of ER stress proteins in LLC-PK₁ cells prevents injury from the alkylating agent iodoacetamide and the oxidizing agent tBHP.[84, 85] Both of these agents cause an increase in intracellular calcium and lipid peroxidation as part of the injury process. Inducing the expression of Grp-78 and Grp-94, overexpressing calreticulin, and inhibiting the induction of Grp-78 showed that these ER chaperones prevent the increase in intracellular calcium and lipid peroxidation that normally would result from iodoacetamide.[84] Likewise, these same maneuvers prevented the expected increase in intracellular calcium following treatment with the oxidant tBHP but did not prevent lipid peroxidation. Nevertheless, cell death was prevented.[85] The ER, and particularly the ER chaperones, appear then to be important regulators of intracellular calcium homeostasis during oxidative stress. Induction of these ER stress proteins could prevent disturbances in intracellular calcium homeostasis and thus limit the oxidative stress and cell death from these toxins. Preventing calcium disturbances within the cell may be a general mechanism by which the ER and its stress proteins protect renal epithelium against injury. Recalling that increased intracellular calcium is a prominent mechanism in ischemia-induced injury to renal epithelia (through activation of degradative proteolytic and lipolytic enzymes, by stimulation of oxidant production, and by contributing to signals for apoptotic cell death), the ER stress proteins very well may help prevent or promote recovery from ischemic renal injury. By limiting increases in intracellular calcium or helping to restore cell calcium homeostasis following an ischemic insult, the ER chaperones could limit calcium-mediated injury or help restore calcium homeostasis so that other cytoplasmic repair processes can be effective. In this manner, the ER chaperones would complement their cytosolic counterparts that would be directly involved in restoring protein conformation to repair cell architecture.

CONCLUSION

There is now compelling evidence that a series of stress proteins distributed throughout the cell in several compartments cooperate to prevent injury or promote recovery from a variety of insults to renal epithelia. They do so by the limiting processes of injury such as perturbations in calcium homeostasis, enhancing cell metabolism, and preserving or restoring cell architecture to ensure cell survival. We hope that this knowledge eventually gives direction to how these protein chaperones can be harnessed to prevent the onset of renal injury and to improve the outcome of patients who suffer from ARF.

ACKNOWLEDGMENTS

The work by the authors included in this chapter was done with support from grants from the American Heart Association and the National Institutes of Health DK 44336 and HD 32573.
We are grateful to all who have given excellent assistance with the studies included here, and especially to Michael Kashgarian and Tom Ardito, who provided the immunofluorescence micrographs, and to Marie Campbell for her secretarial support.

References

1. Weinberg JM: The cell biology of ischemic renal injury. Kidney Int 1991; 39:476.

2. Epstein FH, Mandel LJ: Forefronts in nephrology: summary of the newer aspects of renal cell injury. Kidney Int 1992; 42:523.
3. Zager RA: Partial aortic ligation: a hypoperfusion model of ischemic acute renal failure and comparison to renal artery occlusion. J Lab Clin Med 1987; 110:396.
4. Ratcliffe PJ, Moonen CTW, Holloway PAH, et al: Acute renal failure in hemorrhagic hypotension: cellular energetics and renal function. Kidney Int 1986; 30:355.
5. Gaudio KM, Thulin G, Ardito T, et al: Redistribution of cellular energy following renal ischemia. Pediatr Nephrol 1991; 5:591.
6. Sakarean A, Aricheta R, Baum M: Intracellular cystine loading causes proximal tubule respiratory dysfunction: effect of glycine. Pediatr Res 1992; 32:710.
7. Molitoris BA: New insights into the cell biology of ischemic acute renal failure. J Am Soc Nephrol 1991; 1:1263.
8. Kashgarian M, Van Why SK, Hildebrandt F, et al: Regulation of Expression and Polar Distribution of Na+,K+,-ATPase in Renal Epithelium During Recovery From Ischemic Injury. In: Kaplan JH, De Weer P, eds: *The Sodium Pump: Recent Developments*. New York: Rockefeller University Press; 1991:573.
9. Spiegel DM, Wilson PD, Molitoris BA: Epithelial polarity following ischemia: a requirement for normal cell function. Am J Physiol 1989; 256:F430.
10. Molitoris BA, Chan LK, Shapiro JL, et al: Loss of epithelial polarity: a novel hypothesis for reduced proximal tubule Na+ transport following ischemic injury. J Membr Biol 1989; 107:117.
11. Van Why SK, Mann AS, Ardito T, et al: Expression and molecular regulation of Na+,K+-ATPase after renal ischemia. Am J Physiol 1994; 267:F75.
12. Bodziak KA, Fish E, Molitoris BA: Reutilization and reinsertion of Na+,K+-ATPase into the surface membrane following cellular ATP depletion. J Am Soc Nephrol 1993; 4:732.
13. Nover L, ed: Heat Shock Response. Boca Raton, FL: CRC Press, 1991:1–499.
14. Zou J, Guo Y, Guettouche T, et al: Repression of heat shock transcription factor HSF1 activation by HSP90 (HSP90 complex) that forms a stress-sensitive complex with HSF1. Cell 1998; 94:471.
15. Mifflin LC, Cohen RE: HSC 70 moderates the heat shock (stress) response in *Xenopus laevis* oocytes and binds to denatured protein inducers. J Biol Chem 1994; 269:15718.
16. Frydman J, Hartl FU: Molecular Chaperone Functions of HSP-70 and hsp60 in Protein Folding. In: Morimoto RI, Tissieres A, Georgopoulos C, eds: *The Biology of Heat Shock Proteins and Molecular Chaperones*. New York: Cold Spring Harbor Laboratory Press; 1994:251.
17. Freeman BC, Morimoto RI: The human cytosolic molecular chaperones hsp-90, hsp-70 (hsc-70), and hdj-1 have distinct roles in recognition of a non-native protein and protein refolding. EMBO J 1996; 15:2969.
18. Tsang TC: New model for 70 kDa heat-shock proteins' potential mechanisms of function. FEBS Lett 1993; 323:1.
19. Di YP, Repasky E, Laslo A, et al: HSP-70 translocates into a cytoplasmic aggregate during lymphocyte activation. J Cell Physiol 1995; 165:228.
20. Langer T, Lu C, Echols H, et al: Successive action of DnaK, DnaJ, and Gro EL along the pathway of chaperone mediated protein folding. Nature (London) 1992; 356:683.
21. Hutchinson JP, el-Thaher TS, Miller AD: Refolding and recognition of mitochondrial malate dehydrogenase by *Escherichia coli* chaperonins cpn 60 (GroEL) and cpn 10 (Gro ES). Biochem J 1994; 302:405.
22. Hartman DJ, Surin BP, Dixon NE, et al: Substoichiometric amounts of the molecular chaperones GroEL and GroES prevent thermal denaturation and aggregation of mammalian mitochondrial malate dehydrogenase in vitro. Proc Natl Acad Sci USA 1993; 90:2276.
23. Zheng X, Rosenberg LE, Kalousek F, et al: Gro EL, Gro ES, and ATP-dependent folding and spontaneous assembly of ornithine transcarbamylase. J Biol Chem 1993; 268:7489.
24. Hwang DS, Crooke E, Kornberg A: Aggregated Dna A protein is dissociated and activated for DNA replication by phospholipase or dnaK protein. J Biol Chem 1990; 265:19244.
25. Fisher MT: On the assembly of dodecameric glutamine synthe-

tase from stable chaperonin complexes. J Biol Chem 1993; 268:13777.

26. Ehrnsperger M, Graber S, Gaestel M, et al: Binding of non-native protein to HSP-25 during heat shock creates a reservoir of folding intermediates for reactivation. EMBO J 1997; 16:221.

27. Glover JR, Lindquist S: Hsp104, Hsp70, and Hsp40: a novel chaperone system that rescues previously aggregated proteins. Cell 1998; 94:73.

28. Wu C: Heat shock transcription factors: structure and regulation. Annu Rev Dev Biol 1995; 11:441.

29. Van Why SK, Mann AS, Thulin G, et al: Activation of heat-shock transcription factor by graded reductions in renal ATP, in vivo, in the rat. J Clin Invest 1994; 94:1518.

30. Bardella L, Comolli R: Differential expression of c-jun, c-fos, and hsp 70 mRNAs after folic acid and ischemia-reperfusion injury: effect of antioxidant treatment. Exp Nephrol 1994; 2:158.

31. Ding XZ, Smallridge RC, Galloway RJ, et al: Increases in HSF1 translocation and synthesis in human epidermoid A-431 cells: role of protein kinase C and $[Ca^{2+}]_i$. J Invest Med 1996; 44:144.

32. Gu H, Smith MW, Phelps PC, et al: H-ras transfection of the rat kidney cell line NRK-52E results in increased induction of c-fos, c-jun, and hsp70 following sulofenur treatment. Cancer Lett 1996; 106:199.

33. Kiang JG, Carr FE, Burns MR, et al: HSP-72 synthesis is promoted by increase in $[Ca^{2+}]_i$ or activation of G proteins but not pHi or cAMP. Am J Physiol 1994; 36:C104.

34. Price BD, Calderwood SK: Ca^{2+} is essential for multistep activation of the heat shock factor in permeabilized cells. Mol Cell Biol 1991;11:3365.

35. Chen Q, Yu K, Stevens JL: Regulation of the cellular stress response by reactive electrophiles: the role of covalent binding and cellular thiols in transcriptional activation of the 70-kilodalton heat shock protein gene by nephrotoxic cysteine conjugates. J Biol Chem 1992; 267:24322.

36. Liu H, Lightfoot R, Stevens JL: Activation of heat shock factor by alkylating agents is triggered by glutathione depletion and oxidation of protein thiols. J Biol Chem 1996; 271:4805.

37. Bush KT, Goldberg AL, Nigam SK: Proteasome inhibition leads to a heat-shock response, induction of endoplasmic reticulum chaperones, and thermotolerance. J Biol Chem 1997; 272:9086.

38. Van Why SK, Kim SA, Geibel J, et al: Thresholds for cellular disruption and activation of the stress response in renal epithelia. Am J Physiol 1999; 277:F227.

39. Nguyen VT, Bensaude O: Increased thermal aggregation of proteins in ATP-depleted mammalian cells. Eur J Biochem 1994; 220:239.

40. Mathew A, Mathur SK, Morimoto RI: Heat shock response and protein degradation: regulation of HSF2 by the ubiquitin-proteasome pathway. Mol Cell Biol 1998; 18:5091.

41. Van Why SK, Hildebrandt F, Ardito T, et al: Induction and intracellular localization of HSP-72 after renal ischemia. Am J Physiol 1992; 263:F769.

42. Schober A, Muller E, Thurau K, et al: The response of heat shock proteins 25 and 72 to ischemia in different kidney zones. Pflugers Arch 1997; 434:292.

43. Emami A, Schwartz JH, Borkan SC: Transient ischemia or heat stress induces a cytoprotectant protein in rat kidney. Am J Physiol 1991; 260:F479.

44. Dodd SM, Martin JE, Swash M, et al: Expression of heat shock protein epitopes in renal disease. Clin Nephrol 1993; 39:239.

45. Arrigo AP, Landry J: Expression and Function of the Low-Molecular-Weight Heat Shock Proteins. In: Morimoto RI, Tissieres A, Georgopoulos C, eds: *The Biology of Heat Shock Proteins and Molecular Chaperones*. New York: Cold Spring Harbor Laboratory Press, 1994:335.

46. Aufricht C, Ardito T, Thulin G, et al: Heat-shock protein 25 induction and redistribution during actin reorganization after renal ischemia. Am J Physiol 1998; 274:F215.

47. Smoyer WE, Harris RC, Ransom R, et al: Differential renal expression of HSP-27 and αβ-crystallin in rats following acute ischemia. J Am Soc Nephrol 1997; 8:595A.

48. Kuznetsov G, Bush KT, Zhang PL, et al: Perturbations in maturation of secretory proteins and their association with endoplasmic reticulum chaperones in a cell culture model for epithelial ischemia. Proc Natl Acad Sci USA 1996; 93:8584.

49. Halleck MM, Liu H, North J, et al: Reduction of trans-4,5-dihydroxy-1,2-dithiane by cellular oxidoreductases activates gadd 153/chop and grp78 transcription and induces cellular tolerance in kidney epithelial cells. J Biol Chem 1997; 272:21760.

50. Satoh K, Wakui H, Komatsuda A, et al: Induction and altered localization of 90-kDa heat-shock protein in rat kidneys with cisplatin-induced acute renal failure. Ren Fail 1994; 16:313.

51. Komatsuda A, Wakui H, Satoh K, et al: Altered localization of 73-kilodalton heat-shock protein in rat kidneys with gentamicin-induced acute tubular injury. Lab Invest 1993; 68:687.

52. Goering PL, Fisher BF, Chaudhary PP, et al: Relationship between stress protein induction in rat kidney by mercuric chloride and nephrotoxicity. Toxicol Appl Pharmacol 1992; 113:184.

53. Rosenberg ME, Paller MS: Differential gene expression in the recovery from ischemic renal injury. Kidney Int 1991; 39:1156.

54. Cohen DM, Wasserman JC, Gullans SR: Immediate early gene and HSP-70 expression in hyperosmotic stress in MDCK cells. Am J Physiol 1991; 261:C594.

55. Muller E, Neuhofer W, Ohno A, et al: Heat shock proteins HSP25, HSP60, HSP72, HSP73 in isoosmotic cortex and hyperosmotic medulla of rat kidney. Pflugers Arch 1996; 431:608–617.

56. Kojima R, Randall J, Brenner BM, et al: Osmotic stress protein 94 (Osp94). A new member of the Hsp110/SSE gene subfamily. J Biol Chem 1996; 271:12327.

57. Santos BC, Chevaile A, Kojima R, et al: Characterization of the Hsp110/SSE gene family response to hyperosmolality and other stresses. Am J Physiol 1998; 274:F1054.

58. Rauchman RL, Pullman J, Gullans SR: Induction of molecular chaperones by hyperosmotic stress in mouse inner medullary collecting duct cells. Am J Physiol 1997; 273:F9.

59. Parsell DA, Linquist S: Heat Shock Proteins and Stress Tolerance. In: Morimoto RI, Tissieres A, Georgopoulos C, eds: *The Biology of Heat Shock Proteins and Molecular Chaperones*. New York: Cold Spring Harbor Laboratory Press, 1994:457.

60. Benjamin IJ, Williams RS: Expression and Function of Stress Proteins in the Ischemic Heart. In: Morimoto RI, Tissieres A, Georgopoulos C, eds: *The Biology of Heat Shock Proteins and Molecular Chaperones*. New York: Cold Spring Harbor Laboratory Press, 1994:533.

61. Nowak TS, Abe H: Postischemic Stress Response in Brain. In: Morimoto RI, Tissieres A, Georgopoulos C, eds: *The Biology of Heat Shock Proteins and Molecular Chaperones*. New York: Cold Spring Harbor Laboratory Press, 1994:553.

62. Sheikh-Hamad D, Garcia-Perez A, Ferraris JD, et al: Induction of gene expression by heat shock versus osmotic stress. Am J Physiol 1994; 267:F28.

63. Cowley BD Jr, Muessel MJ, Douglass D, et al: In vivo and in vitro osmotic regulation of HSP-70 and prostaglandin synthase gene expression in kidney cells. Am J Physiol 1995; 269:F854.

64. Medina R, Cantley L, Spokes K, et al: Effect of water diuresis and water restriction on expression of HSPs-27, -60, and -70 in rat kidney. Kidney Int 1996; 50:1191.

65. Xu Q, Ganju L, Fawcett TW, et al: Vasopressin-induced heat shock protein expression in renal tubular cells. Lab Invest 1996; 74:178.

66. Ohno A, Muller E, Fraek ML, et al: Ketoconazole inhibits organic osmolyte efflux and induces heat shock proteins in rat renal medulla. Kidney Int Suppl 1996; 57:S110.

67. Ohno A, Muller E, Fraek ML, et al: Solute composition and heat shock proteins in rat renal medulla. Pflugers Arch 1997; 434:117.

68. Santos BC, Chevaile A, Hebert MJ, et al: A combination of NaCl and urea enhances survival of IMCD cells to hyperosmolality. Am J Physiol 1998; 274:F1167.

69. Neuhofer W, Muller E, Burger-Kentischer A, et al: Inhibition of NaCl-induced heat shock protein 72 expression renders MDCK cells susceptible to high urea concentrations. Pflugers Arch 1999; 437:611.

70. Zager RA, Iwata M, Burkhaut KM, et al: Postischemic acute renal failure protects proximal tubules from O_2 deprivation injury, possibly by inducing uremia. Kidney Int 1994; 45:1760.

71. Joannidis M, Cantley LG, Spokes K, et al: Induction of heat-

shock proteins does not prevent renal tubular injury following ischemia. Kidney Int 1995; 47:1752.

72. Nissam I, Hardy M, Pleasure J, et al: A mechanism of glycine and alanine cytoprotective action: stimulation of stress-induced HSP-70 mRNA. Kidney Int 1992; 42:775.

73. Borkan SC, Emami A, Schwartz JH: Heat stress protein–associated cytoprotection of inner medullary collecting duct cells from rat kidney. Am J Physiol 1993; 265:F333.

74. Wang YH, Borkan SC: Prior heat stress enhances survival of renal epithelial cells after ATP depletion. Am J Physiol 1996; 270:F1057.

75. Yuan CM, Bohen EM, Musio F, et al: Sublethal heat shock and cyclosporine exposure produce tolerance against subsequent cyclosporine toxicity. Am J Physiol 1996; 40:F571.

76. Brown MA, Upender RP, Hightower LE, et al: Thermoprotection of a functional epithelium: heat stress effects on transepithelial transport by flounder renal tubule in primary monolayer culture. Proc Natl Acad Sci USA 1992; 89:3246.

77. Bush KT, George SK, Zhang PL, et al: Pretreatment with inducers of ER molecular chaperones protects epithelial cells subjected to ATP depletion. Am J Physiol 1999; 277:F211.

78. Musio F, Carome MA, Bohen EM, et al: Effect of glycine on cisplatin nephrotoxicity and heat-shock protein 70 expression in the rat kidney. Ren Fail 1997; 19:33.

79. Santos BC, Pullman J, Chevaile A, et al: Chronic hyperosmolality induces robust, constitutive expression of stress proteins and confers enhanced tolerance of nephrotoxins and ischemic injury. J Am Soc Nephrol 1997; 8:130A.

80. Mehlen P, Briolay J, Smith L, et al: Analysis of the resistance to heat and hydrogen peroxide stresses in COS cells transiently expressing wild type or deletion mutants of the *Drosophila* 27-kDa heat-shock protein. Eur J Biochem 1993; 215:277.

81. Maldonado A, Mann AS, Ardito T, et al: Overexpression of HSP-25 provides cytoprotection through direct interactions with the cytoskeleton. J Am Soc Nephrol 1999; 10:636A.

82. Komatsuda A, Wakui H, Oyama Y, et al: Overexpression of the human 72 kDa heat shock protein in renal tubular cells confers resistance against oxidative injury and cisplatin toxicity. Nephrol Dial Transplant 1999; 14:1385.

83. Turman MA, Rosenfeld SL: Heat shock protein 70 overexpression protects LLC-PK₁ tubular cells from heat shock but not hypoxia. Kidney Int 1999; 55:189.

84. Liu H, Bowes RC 3rd, van de Water B, et al: Endoplasmic reticulum chaperones GRP78 and calreticulin prevent oxidative stress, Ca^{2+} disturbances, and cell death in renal epithelial cells. J Biol Chem 1997; 272:21751.

85. Liu H, Miller E, van de Water B, et al: Endoplasmic reticulum stress proteins block oxidant-induced Ca^{2+} increases and cell death. J Biol Chem 1998; 273:12858.

86. Jurivich DA, Sistonen L, Kroes RA, et al: Effect of sodium salicylate on the human heat shock response. Science 1992; 255:1243.

87. Fawcett TW, Xu O, Holbrook NJ: Potentiation of heat stress–induced hsp 70 expression in vivo by aspirin. Cell Stress Chaperones 1997; 2:104.

88. Cullen KE, Sarge KD: Characterization of hypothermia-induced cellular stress response in mouse tissues. J Biol Chem 1997; 272:1742.

89. Komatsuda A, Wakui H, Ohtani H, et al: Intracellular localization of HSP73 and HSP90 in rat kidneys with acute lysosomal thesaurismosis. Pathol Int 1999; 49:513.

90. Bruschi SA, West KA, Crabb JW: Mitochondrial HSP60 (P1 protein) and a HSP70-like protein (mortalin) are major targets for modification during S-(1,1,2,2-tetrafluoroethyl)-ı-cysteine–induced nephrotoxicity. J Biol Chem 1993; 268:23157.

91. Aufricht C, Lu E, Thulin G, et al: ATP releases HSP-72 from protein aggregates after renal ischemia. Am J Physiol 1998; 274:F268.

92. Tsukamoto T, Nigam SK: Tight junction proteins form large complexes and associate with the cytoskeleton in an ATP depletion model for reversible junction assembly. J Biol Chem 1997; 272:16133.

93. Borkan SC, Wang YH, Lieberthal W, et al: Heat stress ameliorates ATP-depletion–induced sublethal injury in mouse proximal tubule cells. Am J Physiol 1997; 272:F347.

94. Aufricht C, Bidmon B, Regele H, et al: Ischemic conditioning prevents Na^+,K^+-ATPase dissociation from the cytoskeletal fraction after repeat renal ischemia. 2000; in press.

95. Khan W, McGuirt JP, Sens MA, et al: Expression of heat shock protein 27 in developing and adult human kidney. Toxicol Lett 1996; 84:69.

Section II
THE CLINICAL SPECTRUM OF ACUTE RENAL FAILURE

CHAPTER 11

Clinical and Laboratory Diagnosis of Acute Renal Failure

Robert J. Anderson

INTRODUCTION

Acute renal failure (ARF) is an abrupt decrease in renal function sufficient to result in retention of nitrogenous waste.[1–5] While there is uniform agreement on this general definition, there is no consensus concerning the specific quantification of the decline in renal function (ie, magnitude of rise of serum creatinine [S_{Cr}] concentration) sufficient to allow the clinician to ascribe a diagnosis of ARF.[3] Moreover, in individuals with normal renal function, ARF resulting in large reductions in glomerular filtration rate (GFR) often initially produces only small (0.1–0.3 mg/dL) increments in S_{Cr} concentration.[6] Thus, the prudent clinician thoroughly evaluates each occurrence of even mild increases in S_{Cr} concentration.

A powerful rationale underlies such a timely and thorough approach to evaluating each case of ARF. In contemporary medical practice, especially hospital practice, ARF is encountered with high frequency.[7–15] Moreover, diverse pathophysiologic events encountered in multiple clinical settings produce an identical clinical picture of ARF.[1–7, 9–19] Alleviation or attenuation of ARF requires identification and therapy directed at the underlying pathophysiologic state. Also, mild forms of ARF are often reversible, and several studies have demonstrated a direct relationship between the magnitude of the rise in S_{Cr} level and ARF mortality.[1, 7–14, 20] Finally, all causes and degrees of severity of ARF are potentially associated with significant morbidity and mortality.[1, 6–13, 18–20] This chapter reviews the clinical and laboratory features of the various causes of ARF and suggests a stepwise approach to timely diagnosis.

PRESENTING MANIFESTATIONS OF ACUTE RENAL FAILURE

Most commonly, ARF is diagnosed when there is an increased concentration of S_{Cr} or blood urea nitrogen (BUN). Generally, the BUN/S_{Cr} ratio is about 15:1, and the BUN and S_{Cr} levels increase by 10 to 15 mg/dL per day and 1.0 to 1.5 mg/dL per day, respectively, in the absence of GFR. There are, however, several clinical situations that disproportionately affect either the BUN or the S_{Cr} (Fig. 11–1) thereby altering the BUN/S_{Cr} ratio.[21] Moreover, as is apparent in Figure 11–1, factors other than a reduction in GFR can be associated with increased concentrations of BUN (eg, catabolic state with enhanced urea nitrogen formation) and S_{Cr} (eg, medication effects that impair renal tubular secretion of creatinine and that chemically interfere with creatinine measurements).

The S_{Cr} concentration is usually a better marker of GFR than is the BUN. In a steady state setting, a reasonable approximation is that each time the GFR halves, the S_{Cr} concentration doubles. Thus, steady-state GFRs of 100, 50, 25, 12.5, and 6.25 mL/min are associated with S_{Cr} concentrations of about 1.0, 2.0, 4.0, 8.0, and 16.0 mg/dL, respectively. However, ARF usually occurs in a non–steady-state condition in which the three determinants of S_{Cr} concentration (production, volume of distribution, and renal elimination) fluctuate.[22] Computerized models derived from ARF patients demonstrate that several patterns of change in GFR occur during development and recovery from ARF, and often these GFR changes are poorly reflected by daily changes in S_{Cr} concentration.[22] Moreover, the rise in S_{Cr} that occurs in ARF is a post-facto finding. Unfortunately, although real-time, noninvasive monitoring of GFR can be done in seriously ill patients, these techniques currently are expensive and not widely available.[23]

The second way in which ARF is clinically recognized is by the development of oligoanuria.[16] The presence of either oliguria (<400 mL/24 h) or anuria (no urine output) always signifies the presence of some form of ARF.[16] However, most cases of ARF encountered in current medical practice are nonoliguric in nature.[1, 9] Recent clinical studies find that the urine flow rate in ARF patients correlates strongly and directly with residual GFR and poorly with tubular function.[24] These observations, coupled with a large body of data from experimental models of ARF, support the contention that it is the level of GFR that is the primary determinant of urine flow in ARF. The higher level of residual GFR in nonoliguric patients is compatible with less severe renal failure and lower mortality and morbidity than is seen in oliguric ARF.[1, 9]

A third, less common manner in which ARF comes to the attention of the clinician is through evaluation of either a laboratory result (eg, anemia, hyperka-

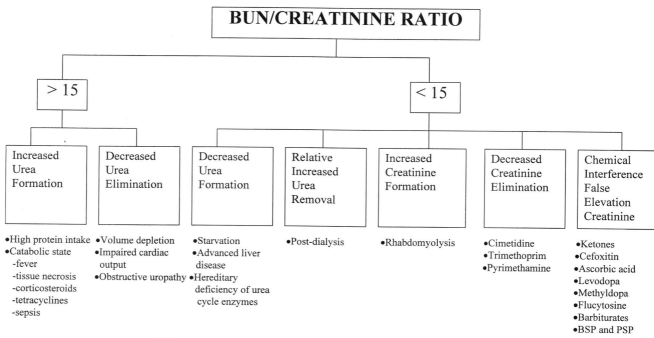

FIGURE 11-1 ■ The causes of abnormalities in the BUN/creatinine ratio.

lemia, acidemia, hypocalcemia, hyperphosphatemia, hypermagnesemia, hyperuricemia) or a clinical (fluid overload; mental status alterations; anorexia, nausea, vomiting; pericarditis) finding that occurs as a consequence of ARF.

Sometimes, it is not clear whether an elevated BUN or S_{Cr} level is due to an acute or to a chronic process. In this setting, review of previous records is helpful. In the absence of previous values, the measurement of carbamylated hemoglobin can be helpful. Nonenzymatic carbamylation of the terminal valine of hemoglobin occurs in direct relationship to the magnitude and duration of the increase in BUN.[25, 26] Precise "cut-off" values of carbamylated hemoglobin that allow clear-cut differentiation between acute and chronic renal failure remain to be determined, however, and overlap between the acute and the chronic forms of renal failure is common.[25, 26] The presence of small kidney size on an imaging study strongly supports a diagnosis of chronic renal disease. Because reversible factors are often operative in both acute and chronic renal failure, the clinician should assume the presence of potentially treatable conditions in all cases of renal failure.[27]

CAUSES OF ACUTE RENAL FAILURE

A time-honored classification of the causes of ARF is outlined in Figure 11-2.[1, 2] Prerenal factors refer to conditions associated with renal hypoperfusion as the cause of filtration failure. Prerenal events are the most commonly encountered causes of ARF.[1, 2, 5, 7-9, 11-15] If left untreated, prerenal ARF can progress to ischemic acute tubular necrosis (ATN). In prerenal ARF, a vasomotor factor such as decreased renal perfusion pressure, afferent arteriolar constriction, or efferent arteri-

olar dilation acts to decrease glomerular hydrostatic pressure.[28] Prerenal events that can decrease renal perfusion pressure include loss of extracellular fluid (eg, vomiting, nasogastric suctioning, diarrhea, gastrointestinal hemorrhage, burns, heat stroke, diuretics, glycosuria), sequestration of extracellular fluid (eg, muscle crush injury, intra-abdominal surgery, pancreatitis, interferon therapy, early sepsis), impaired cardiac output, and antihypertensive medications. Afferent arteriolar constriction caused either by enhanced vasoconstrictor influences (eg, circulating norepinephrine, angiotensin II, endothelin, enhanced renal adrenergic neural traffic) or by a decrease in vasodilators (eg, eicosanoids, nitric oxide, bradykinin) occurs in many cases of prerenal ARF. Such constriction can be due to medications such as nonsteroidal anti-inflammatory agents (NSAIDs), cyclosporine, radiocontrast medium, and amphotericin,[29, 30] and seen with the postoperative state, early sepsis, advanced liver disease, edematous disorders, and volume-depleted states. Efferent arteriolar dilation occurs in the context of angiotensin-converting enzyme inhibitors or angiotensin receptor antagonists.

A relatively unusual "prerenal" form of ARF is that due to a hyperoncotic state.[31-33] Infusion of either osmotically active substances such as mannitol and dextran or of protein can lead to high oncotic pressure, which exceeds glomerular capillary hydrostatic pressure.[31-33] This stops glomerular filtration and produces an anuric form of ARF, which is usually rapidly alleviated by removal of the offending substance.

Postrenal (after the formation of glomerular filtrate) causes of ARF are less commonly encountered, but they are nearly always treatable.[1, 7, 8, 11, 12, 34-36] Postrenal forms of ARF obstruct flow of either tubular (intrarenal) fluid or formed (extrarenal) urine. Since several

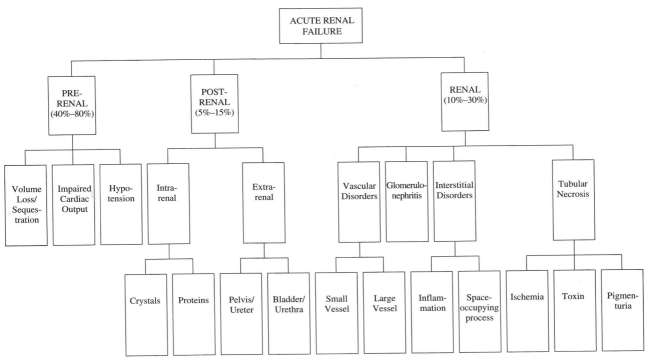

FIGURE 11–2 ■ The differential diagnosis of acute renal failure.

proximal tubules drain into a single collecting tubule, intra–collecting tubular precipitation of either relatively insoluble crystals (methotrexate, acyclovir, sulfonamides, indinavir, uric acid, triamterene, oxalic acid)[37–43] or protein (plasma cell dyscrasia)[44] can increase intratubular pressure. If sufficiently high, the intratubular pressure opposes glomerular filtration pressure (glomerular hydrostatic pressure minus plasma colloid oncotic pressure) sufficiently to decrease GFR. Similarly, obstruction of the extrarenal collecting system at any level (pelvis, ureters, bladder, and urethra), can lead to postrenal ARF.

Once prerenal and postrenal causes have been considered, attention should focus on the kidney itself, that is, on the renal causes of ARF. From an organizational view, it is helpful to consider renal causes in terms of the anatomic compartments of the kidney. Disorders of the renal vasculature, including the small arteries (eg, vasculitis, thrombotic thrombocytopenic purpura [TTP], hemolytic-uremic syndrome [HUS], malignant hypertension, eclampsia, scleroderma, disseminated intravascular coagulation [DIC]), the large arteries (eg, thrombosis, emboli), and the renal veins (acute occlusion) all can result in ARF.[45–56] All forms of acute glomerulonephritis can, if severe, present as ARF.[57] Acute inflammation and space-occupying processes of the renal interstitium (eg, drug-induced, infectious, and autoimmune disorders, leukemia or lymphoma, sarcoidosis) can also result in ARF.[58] Finally, tubular damage or ATN, which usually results from renal ischemia due to prolonged prerenal ARF, nephrotoxins (eg, radiocontrast medium, aminoglycosides, pentamidine, foscarnet, cisplatin, amphotericin, NSAIDs, heavy metals, hydrocarbons), and pig-

menturia (eg, intravascular hemolysis, rhabdomyolysis) are relatively common causes of ARF.[1–7, 9–15, 37]

DIAGNOSTIC APPROACH TO ACUTE RENAL FAILURE

History and Record Review

A suggested sequential diagnostic approach to patients with ARF is shown in Figure 11–3. General information gleaned from the clinical setting in which the ARF has occurred may be helpful. For example, community-acquired ARF can often be attributed to a single cause (often prerenal or postrenal or medication-induced; occasionally due to bacteremia) and generally has a good prognosis.[1, 3, 8, 11, 12, 59, 60] Acute renal failure acquired on a hospital ward often occurs in the setting of underlying comorbidity, has more than a single cause, and is associated with higher mortality.[1–5, 7–11, 60, 61] Acute renal failure acquired in the intensive care unit almost always is multifactorial, is associated with sepsis and multiple organ failure, and results in high mortality.[1, 3, 4, 9, 10, 13, 14, 20]

Causes of ARF can also be considered within the context of the underlying setting in which it occurs (Fig. 11–4). Thus, a spectrum of unique causes of ARF can be seen in the setting of malignancy, with immunodeficiency virus (HIV) infection, pregnancy, intensive care, and the postoperative state.[1, 3, 7–9, 13–15, 20, 37, 43, 44, 53–55, 62–64] Two settings, not shown in Figure 11–4, in which ARF is frequently encountered are the elderly population and patients with liver disease. The effect of advancing age in decreasing renal reserve and the

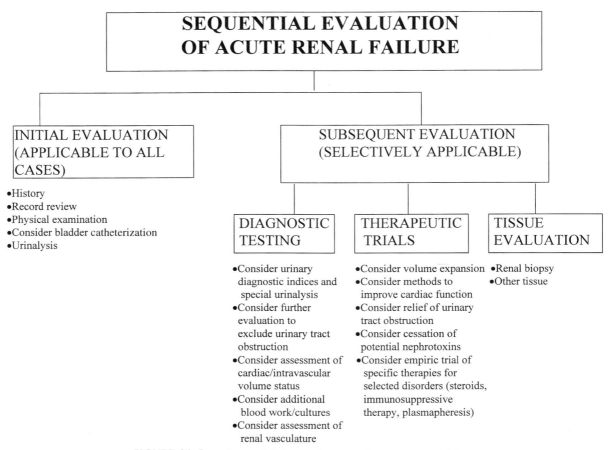

FIGURE 11–3 ■ Sequential diagnostic approach to acute renal failure.

associated comorbid conditions of elderly patients would be expected to increase the risk of ARF. Indeed, Feest and coworkers[11] demonstrated that there is a dramatic (three- to eight-fold), progressive, age-dependent increase in the frequency of development of community-acquired ARF in patients older than 60 years of age. Also, the mean age of patients with ARF has increased by 5 to 15 years over the past quarter of a century.[14, 65] The frequency of prerenal and postrenal causes of ARF appears to be especially high in the elderly, although all causes of ARF are encountered in this age group.[66–68]

Patients with liver disease are susceptible to several renal insults, including those of prerenal (aggressive diuresis, large-volume paracentesis, gastrointestinal hemorrhage, sepsis) and renal (glomerulopathy, ischemic and toxic ATN, acute interstitial nephritis) origins.[69] In addition, a significant percentage of patients with advanced liver disease develop intense vasoconstriction and a form of ARF (the hepatorenal syndrome) that responds poorly to treatment and is associated with high mortality.[70]

A careful history, record review, and physical examination remain the cornerstone of evaluation of ARF. The history with regard to clinical events associated with intravascular volume loss or sequestration and impaired cardiac function is important. A history of thirst, orthostatic lightheadedness, and symptoms of

congestive heart failure supports a prerenal cause of ARF. Postrenal causes of ARF are common in the very young and the very old with a history of changes in the size and force of the urine stream; the presence of bladder, prostate, or pelvic cancer; the use of anticholinergic and α-adrenergic medications; the presence of anuria, suprapubic pain, or urolithiasis; and a history of medication use associated with crystalluria.[37–43, 71] The presence of either a single kidney or a significant decrease in the function of one kidney should make the clinician even more concerned about the possibility of postrenal ARF, because a single lesion may obstruct the good kidney. A history of factors that predispose to vascular disease (smoking, hypertension, diabetes mellitus, hyperlipidemia, claudication, stroke, myocardial infarction, arterial catheterization involving the aorta, known abdominal aortic aneurysm, atrial fibrillation, and selected medication use) is compatible with vascular events leading to ARF. A history of systemic infections and the presence of systemic symptoms may support a glomerular cause of ARF. Medication exposure, symptoms of systemic infection, and a history suggestive of acute pyelonephritis may point to acute interstitial nephritis as the cause of ARF. The presence of disorders known to be associated with either rhabdomyolysis or intravascular hemolysis suggests the possibility of pigmenturia contributing to the ARF.[1, 37, 72, 73] In all cases of ARF,

```
┌─────────────────────────────────────┐
│         ACUTE RENAL FAILURE:         │
│      ETIOLOGY BY CLINICAL SETTING    │
└─────────────────────────────────────┘
```

| Malignancy | HIV | Pregnancy | ICU/Post-operative states |

Malignancy

Prerenal
- Vomiting
- Pericardial tamponade
- Drug-induced
- Cardiac dysfunction

Postrenal
- Ureteric blockade (metastasis, retroperitoneal fibrosis)
- Bladder neck blockade (prostatic/bladder cancers)
- Crystalluria (uric acid, methotrexate)
- Protein deposition (plasma cell dyscrasia)

Renal
- Toxins (chemotherapeutic agents, antimicrobials, contrast, NSAIDs)
- Sepsis
- Tumor-lysis/hyperuricemia
- Hypercalcemia
- Tumor infiltration
- Tumor glomerulopathy
- Light chain toxicity
- Thrombotic microangiopathy

HIV

Prerenal
- Anorexia/hypodipsia
- Diarrhea

Postrenal
- Ureteric blockage (lymphoma)
- Crystalluria (sulfonamides, acyclovir, protease inhibitors)
- Protein deposition (B-cell lymphoma)

Renal
- Toxins (aminoglycosides, foscarnet, pentamidine, amphotericin B, vancomycin, contrast, NSAIDs)
- Sepsis
- HIV-associated glomerulopathy
- Thrombotic microangiopathy
- Interstitial nephritis

Pregnancy

Prerenal
- Hyperemesis gravidarum

Postrenal
- Gravid uterus blocking ureters

Renal
- Sepsis
- HELLP syndrome/eclampsia
- Post-partum hemorrhage
- Thrombotic microangiopathy
- Cortical necrosis

ICU/Post-operative states

Prerenal
- Volume depletion
- Volume sequestration
- Impaired cardiac output

Postrenal
- Bladder outlet obstruction
- Ureteric ligation (surgery)

Renal
- Sepsis
- Toxins (aminoglycosides, contrast, vancomycin, amphotericin, NSAIDs, CEIs)
- Multiple organ failure
- Rhabdomyolysis

FIGURE 11–4 ▪ Causes of acute renal failure by clinical setting.

a meticulous review of medication and toxin exposure is critical. Several studies demonstrate that up to 25% of all cases of ARF can be attributed to nephrotoxin exposure.[7–9, 11–15, 29, 30, 43, 58, 62, 74, 75]

Physical Examination

Physical examination remains an important diagnostic tool for determining the cause of ARF. Assessing the volume status of patients with ARF is sometimes difficult. A recent meta-analysis suggests that 1-minute orthostatic tachycardia (>30 beats/min) or a decrease in systolic blood pressure (>20 mm Hg), dry axillae, dry oral mucous membranes, and longitudinal tongue furrows, but not decreased skin turgor or impaired capillary refill time, are of diagnostic value in detecting the presence of hypovolemia.[76]

On eye examination, the presence of Hollenhorst plaques is suggestive of atheroemboli,[49] and there may be other findings compatible with bacterial endocarditis, vasculitis, or malignant hypertension. Neck examination for jugular venous pressure and carotid pulses and sounds may be helpful in detecting the presence of heart failure, aortic valve disease, and vascular disease. Cardiac examination for rate, rhythm, murmurs, gallops, and rubs may be of help in detecting the presence of heart failure and possible sources of emboli (eg, atrial fibrillation, endocarditis). Lung exami-

nation can assist in determining the presence of either heart failure or a pulmonary-renal syndrome associated with ARF. Abdominal examination can reveal possible sources of bacteremia, evidence of liver disease (eg, ascites, collateral venous pattern, hepatosplenomegaly), findings compatible with vascular disease (bruits, palpable abdominal aortic aneurysm), masses that could be malignant, and a distended bladder, which can be indicative of outlet obstruction. Extremity examination for pulses (vascular disease), embolic phenomena (eg, gangrene), and edema can be helpful. Skin examination can reveal palpable purpura (vasculitis), a fine maculopapular rash (drug-induced interstitial nephritis), and livido reticularis (atheroemboli). If neurologic findings are present, systemic disorders such as vasculitis, TTP, subacute bacterial endocarditis, and malignant hypertension could be present. Peripheral neuropathy in the setting of ARF raises the possibility of neural compression caused by rhabdomyolysis, ischemia, heavy metal intoxication, and plasma cell dyscrasia. Pelvic examination in females and rectal examination may help ascertain whether a cause of obstructive uropathy is present.

Laboratory Data

A review of the hemogram can be helpful in evaluating the cause of ARF. The presence of disproportionate anemia could point to either recent hemorrhage or intravascular hemolysis as factors contributing to ARF. A microangiopathic state (thrombocytopenia, reticulocytosis, elevated lactic acid dehydrogenase (LDH), deformed red blood cells on peripheral smear) with ARF occurs in the setting of TTP, HUS, eclampsia of pregnancy, vasculitis, HIV infection, malignant hypertension, and selected medications.[43, 46, 52, 55, 56] Anemia with rouleaux formation in the ARF setting suggest a plasma cell dyscrasia. Acute renal failure with eosinophilia is compatible with atheroemboli, acute interstitial nephritis, and polyarteritis nodosa.[1] Leukopenia is common in patients with systemic lupus erythematosus (SLE) and ARF.[1] Thrombocytopenia in the setting of ARF is compatible with a thrombotic microangiopathy, SLE, DIC, rhabdomyolysis, advanced liver disease with hypersplenism, and "white clot syndrome" resulting from heparin administration as causes of the ARF.[1, 43, 46, 52, 55, 56, 77-81] The presence of coagulation abnormalities, such as prolongation of the international normalized ratio (INR) and partial thromboplastin time (PTT), suggests underlying liver disease (increased INR), DIC (increased INR and PTT), and antiphospholipid syndrome (increased PTT), all of which can be associated with ARF.[69, 70, 77-81]

Hyperkalemia of modest degree (<5.5 mEq/L) is a common accompaniment of ARF. More marked hyperkalemia suggests the possibility of rhabdomyolysis, tumor lysis syndrome, intravascular hemolysis, or the use of NSAIDs as contributors to ARF.[1, 37, 72, 73] Mild metabolic acidosis occurs frequently as a consequence of ARF and is often associated with a modest (5–10 mEq/L) increase in anion gap. Marked acidosis with large anion gaps in the setting of ARF should raise the suspicion of ethylene glycol poisoning, marked rhabdomyolysis, and lactic acidosis resulting from sepsis as contributors to ARF.[1, 37, 82] Modest hyperuricemia (<10 mg/dL) usually accompanies ARF.[1] Much higher levels of uric acid occur when tumor lysis syndrome, rhabdomyolysis, and heat stroke are associated with ARF.[83] Elevations in creatinine kinase, serum glutamic-oxaloacetic transaminase, and LDH often occur in the setting of tumor-lysis and rhabdomyolysis.[1, 37]

Urine Flow and Urinalysis

Analysis of the quantity and quality of urine is a key step in the evaluation of ARF(Fig. 11–5). Anuria should suggest either complete urinary tract obstruction or a vascular-glomerular disorder associated with cessation of glomerular filtration (eg, rapidly progressive glomerulonephritis, acute cortical necrosis, or renal arterial occlusion). Brief (<24–48 h) episodes of severe oliguria (<100 mL/day) occur in some cases of ATN, especially those seen in the context of heat stroke.[83] Prerenal forms of ARF nearly always present with oliguria (<400 mL/day), although nonoliguric forms have been reported.[84] Postrenal and renal forms of ARF can present with any pattern of urine flow ranging from anuria through polyuria. As noted previously, most cases of ARF seen in contemporary medi-

cal practice that result from ATN are nonoliguric in nature.[1, 9]

Routine dipstick and microscopic analysis of urine is often helpful in determining the cause of ARF. In one older study,[7] diagnostically useful information was obtained from routine urinalysis in about 75% of ARF cases. Generally speaking, a normal urinalysis in the setting of ARF suggests a prerenal or, rarely, a postrenal cause. An abnormal urinalysis suggests a renal cause. Two studies,[7, 85] but not a third,[86] suggest a direct relationship between the presence and the degree of abnormalities seen on routine urinalysis and the prognosis in ARF. In the study of ARF patients by Hou and coworkers,[7] a normal urinalysis (probable prerenal cause) was associated with a mortality of 15%, and an abnormal urinalysis (probable renal cause) had a mortality of 35%. More recent studies indicate, however, that patients with a clinical course typical of prerenal forms of ARF can have a significant number of casts and cellular elements on microscopic examination of their urine.[85]

The "dipstick" orthotoluidine reaction for blood is sensitive for about three red blood cells/high-power field. If no red blood cells are present, this reaction is positive in the presence of either myoglobinuria (clear plasma as a result of rapid clearance) or hemoglobinuria (sometimes pink plasma resulting from less rapid clearance). The dipstick protein measurement detects only albumin. Acid precipitation (sulfosalicylic acid or Exton's reagent) detects all types of protein. Thus, small amounts of protein found by dipstick measurement, with larger amounts found by acid precipitation, suggest the presence of light chains. If the dipstick reaction for protein is moderately or strongly positive in the setting of ARF, quantification (timed sample or spot urine albumin/creatinine ratio) is indicated. The presence of more than 1 to 2 g/d of urine protein suggests a glomerular or vascular cause of ARF.

Examination of the urine sediment is of great value in ARF. The presence of gross or microscopic hematuria suggests a glomerular, vascular, interstitial, or other structural renal cause (stone, tumor, infection, trauma) of the ARF and can rarely be seen with ATN.[87] Recently, considerable attention has focused on urinary red blood cell (RBC) morphology as a clue to the cause of hematuria. Initially, dysmorphic urinary RBCs found with phase-contrast microscopy, scanning or electron microscopy, or Coulter counter were felt to be diagnostic of a glomerular process. More recently, routine bright-field microscopy was found to be capable of demonstrating so-called G_1 RBCs (doughnut-shaped RBCs with one or more circular blebs or protrusions), which are highly suggestive of a glomerular process.[88] There are, however, no data examining the morphology of urinary RBCs in the setting of ARF of diverse causes. The presence of a large number of white blood cells (WBCs) on urinalysis in ARF suggests the presence of either pyelonephritis or interstitial nephritis. Recently, cytodiagnostic quantitative assessment of urine demonstrated that patients with ARF due to ATN have significantly more collecting duct cells and total casts on urinalysis than those of patients

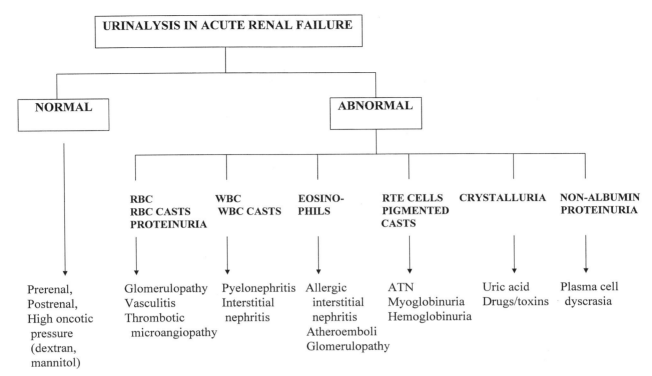

FIGURE 11–5 ■ Routine and microscopic urinalysis in acute renal failure.

with ARF resulting from a variety of other causes. However, a large overlap was seen, which limits sensitivity, specificity, and predictive power.[85] Transmission electron microscopy of urine sediment clearly appears capable of differentiating ATN from other causes of ARF, but practical considerations limit applicability.[89]

Eosinophiluria in the setting of ARF is an area of great interest. Hansel's stain is clearly superior to Wright's stain in detecting eosinophiluria.[90, 91] The presence of eosinophiluria (>1% urine WBCs) is clearly nonspecific inasmuch as it occurs with acute interstitial nephritis, many forms of glomerulonephritis, including rapidly progressive glomerulonephritis, atheroembolic disease, urinary tract infections, prostatitis, acute rejection of renal allografts, and obstructive uropathy.[49, 90, 91] However, when ARF occurs in a setting compatible with either allergic interstitial nephritis (drug exposure, fever, rash, peripheral eosinophilia[58]) or atheroembolic disease (vascular catheterization, Hollenhorst plaques, livedo reticularis, purple toes[48, 49]), eosinophiluria may be diagnostically helpful.

The presence of RBC casts strongly suggests a glomerular or vascular cause of ARF but has occasionally been reported with acute interstitial nephritis. White blood cell casts may indicate the presence of either pyelonephritis or other forms of acute interstitial nephritis.[58, 92]

Examination of the urinary sediment for crystals in patients with ARF may yield diagnostic clues.[29, 30, 37–43, 71] Such evaluation is maximized with the use of fresh warm urine, polarizing microscopy, knowledge of the urine pH, and an experienced microscopist.[71] The presence of a large number of uric acid crystals suggests acute uric acid nephropathy, tumor lysis syndrome, or catabolic ARF. Oxalate crystals are compatible with ethylene glycol, jejunoileal bypass, or massive doses of vitamin C underlying the ARF.[29, 30, 40, 71] Pharmacologic-agent crystals from the use of sulfonamides, indinavir, and triamterene may suggest a role for these substances in the etiology of ARF.[29, 30, 37–43, 71]

Urinary Chemical Indices and Other Markers

Randomized, prospective studies have clearly established the diagnostic helpfulness of measurement of selected urinary concentrations of electrolytes, uric acid, and creatinine in the setting of ARF (Fig. 11–6).[1, 93] The major use of such spot urine chemistries is to differentiate prerenal from renal (especially ATN) forms of ARF. Basically, prerenal disorders are characterized by intact tubular function with avid reabsorption of filtered salts and water and selective organic acids, resulting in relatively low urine concentrations of sodium, chloride, lithium, and uric acid and relatively high urine/plasma (U/P) ratios of osmolality, urea nitrogen, and creatinine.[1, 2, 93, 96] By contrast, ATN is associated with impaired tubular function, with resultant higher urinary concentrations of sodium, chloride, trace lithium, and uric acid and lower U/P ratios of osmolality, urea nitrogen, and creatinine (see Fig. 11–6). In general, the fractional excretion of sodium ($FE_{Na} = [U/P_{Na} \div U/P_{Cr} \times 100]$) appears to be the most sensitive urinary index for differentiating prerenal ARF from ATN.[93] Studies in animal models

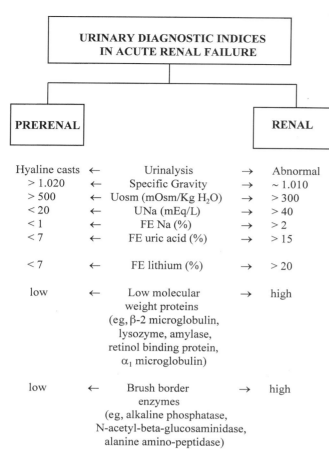

		URINARY DIAGNOSTIC INDICES IN ACUTE RENAL FAILURE		
	PRERENAL			**RENAL**
Hyaline casts	←	Urinalysis	→	Abnormal
> 1.020	←	Specific Gravity	→	~ 1.010
> 500	←	Uosm (mOsm/Kg H_2O)	→	> 300
< 20	←	UNa (mEq/L)	→	> 40
< 1	←	FE Na (%)	→	> 2
< 7	←	FE uric acid (%)	→	> 15
< 7	←	FE lithium (%)	→	> 20
low	←	Low molecular weight proteins (eg, β-2 microglobulin, lysozyme, amylase, retinol binding protein, α_1 microglobulin)	→	high
low	←	Brush border enzymes (eg, alkaline phosphatase, N-acetyl-beta-glucosaminidase, alanine amino-peptidase)	→	high

FIGURE 11–6 ▪ Urinary diagnostic indices in acute renal failure.

of ARF have clarified the mechanisms whereby tubular injury is associated with the relative increase in urine salt excretion in ATN.[97–99] Thus, loss of epithelial cell polarity with translocation of the Na^+,K^+-ATPase pump from basolateral to apical location could contribute to this process.[97] Also, a major Na^+ exchanger in the proximal tubule, NHE-3, is transcriptionally down-regulated with ischemic injury, as are other, more distal transport systems that regulate tubular sodium reabsorption, such as the bumetanide-sensitive Na-K-2Cl cotransporter and the thiazide-sensitive Na-Cl cotransporter.[98, 99]

The use of urinary biochemical indices to assist in the differential diagnosis of ARF requires the application of several caveats. First, there is no "gold standard" for ATN, which makes definitive conclusions about sensitivity and specificity of indices difficult. Second, despite routine use, no study has demonstrated that these indices alter either management or outcome of ARF. Third, nearly all studies have been based on indices obtained at a single time point relatively late in the course of ARF. The process of ARF is undoubtedly dynamic in nature.[28, 100, 101] For example, the early phases of the prerenal forms of ARF are associated with intact tubular function. If the cause or causes of the prerenal insult cannot be readily reversed, then ischemic ATN can intervene with impaired tubular function. Such a sequence of events has been clearly

documented in experimental ARF settings[102] and may explain the low FE_{Na} reported early in the course of ARF accompanying rhabdomyolysis, sepsis, administration of radiocontrast medium, nonoliguric forms of ARF, and NSAID exposure. [103–107] Fourth, the specificity of urinary biochemical indices is limited.

Thus, early in the course of urinary tract obstruction, glomerulonephritis, and thrombotic microangiopathies, the FE_{Na} can resemble that seen in prerenal ARF.[1, 108, 109] Acute interstitial nephritis and acute renal artery occlusion can result in indices indistinguishable from those of ATN.[110, 111] Also, indices identical to those seen with ATN occur when prerenal forms of ARF are associated with impaired renal tubular reabsorption of sodium, as occurs in the setting of diuretic use, bicarbonaturia, glycosuria, mineralocorticoid deficiency, and salt-wasting nephropathy.[1, 112] Finally, while the fractional excretion of trace lithium appears to be a reliable index for differentiating prerenal from some renal forms of ARF, the special analytical techniques required (atomic absorption spectrophotometry) limited usage. Many of the urinary diagnostic indices depicted in Figure 11–6 are used as an aid in determining the cause of ARF and also provide prognostic data on outcome in ARF patients. They may also help predict response to diuretic and vasoactive therapies in ARF patients.[1, 113, 114]

Two additional types of urinary markers have been applied as diagnostic aids in ARF. The first type is urinary excretion of enzymes found in the brush borders of nephron segments (eg, intestinal form of alkaline phosphatase, N-acetyl-β-glucosaminidase, alanine aminopeptidase). The second type is urinary excretion of small-molecular-weight proteins (eg, β-2 microglobulin, amylase, lysozyme, retinol-binding protein, α_1-macroglobulin) that are readily filtered and usually reabsorbed by the proximal tubule. If tubular damage is present, then increased urinary excretion of enzymes and small molecular weight proteins would be anticipated to occur. While this generally happens, the urinary excretion of selected enzymes and small proteins has not been sufficiently sensitive or specific to warrant their routine use in delineating the cause of ARF.[115, 116]

Examination of urine may also provide diagnostic clues if a monoclonal gammopathy is suspected as the cause of the renal failure. Urinary electrophoresis for light chains may be diagnostically helpful. Immunofluorescence of urine sediment with antisera to light-chain immunoglobulins appears to be a sensitive and specific noninvasive method of diagnosing light-chain nephropathy.[117]

Preliminary data suggest that urinary excretion of growth factors is of potential diagnostic benefit in ARF.[118, 119] For example, urine levels of epidermal growth factor are reduced in ATN.[118] By contrast, urinary excretion of hepatocyte growth factor is increased in ATN.[119] Clearly, more work is indicated to ascertain whether such growth factor markers are helpful in delineating the various causes of ARF.

Two magnetic resonance (MR) spectroscopy studies of experimental models of ARF have suggested possible diagnostic utility.[120, 121] In the first, ^{31}P MR spectroscopy of kidneys with a ligated ureter revealed a reproducible, unique inorganic phosphorus peak that appeared in the urine.[120] In the second, ^{3}H MR spectroscopy of human urine revealed unique peaks in patients with prerenal and ATN forms of ARF.[121] Confirmation and extension of these studies in large numbers of patients with various forms of ARF are needed.

Possible Urinary Tract Obstruction

A postrenal form of ARF is especially common in an aging population and in community-acquired ARF.[1, 11, 12, 34] Bladder catheterization and ultrasonography are commonly done in many patients with ARF to screen for obstructive uropathy. Postrenal forms of ARF that either are especially acute or are associated with extensive retroperitoneal disease may have no or minimal collecting-system dilation detectable by ultrasonography as well as by other methods, including computed tomography (CT) scanning, isotopic methods, and magnetic resonance imaging (MRI).[34, 36]

Other Testing

Sometimes, review of the medical record, physical examination, and available laboratory findings are insufficient to accurately assess intravascular volume status and cardiac output. In such cases, noninvasive tests such as chest radiography, echocardiography, and gated blood-pool scan may be helpful. There is currently great debate as to whether invasive pulmonary artery catheterization, when broadly applied, is helpful in the management of seriously ill patients.[122] In selected cases of ARF, this procedure may be diagnostically helpful in assessing volume states and left ventricular filling pressure.

When either systemic disorders or a glomerular cause of ARF is suspected, additional diagnostic testing may be indicated. Blood cultures, heart valve echocardiography, and CT imaging may help detect the presence and source of sepsis. Measurement of antineutrophil cytoplasmic antibodies, anti-DNA antibodies, antibodies to glomerular basement membrane, and anti-streptolysin O titers may be diagnostically helpful in selected cases, as well as tests for detecting the presence of hepatitis viruses and tests for complement components and circulating immune complexes (eg, cryoglobulins, rheumatoid factor, and C1q binding). If there are questions regarding a possible vascular cause of ARF, duplex Doppler ultrasonography and MR angiography can be diagnostically helpful and are less invasive than angiography.[45–47]

Therapeutic Trials

The response to therapeutic interventions can provide diagnostic information in the ARF setting. Improvement in renal function either with fluid replacement or with improvement in cardiac index (eg,

dobutamine, afterload and preload reduction, other inotropes) supports a prerenal cause. Improved renal function after relief of obstructive uropathy (eg, bladder catheterization, ureteric stenting, percutaneous nephrostomy) suggests a postrenal cause.[1, 11, 12, 34–36] Improved renal function after cessation of selected pharmacologic agents (eg, NSAIDs, converting enzyme inhibitors) suggests a role for these agents in causing ARF.[29, 30] When mechanical (eg, angioplasty, bypass surgery, stenting) and pharmacologic (eg, thrombolytic agents) therapy results in improved renal blood flow, it lends support to vascular occlusion as the cause of ARF.[45–47] In selected circumstances, when renal function improves in response to corticosteroid therapy and other strategies for treating immune-mediated processes, it may indicate a diagnosis of allergic interstitial nephritis or glomerulonephritis.

Analysis of Renal Tissue

Sometimes, despite thorough evaluation, the cause of ARF cannot be ascertained with a reasonable degree of certainty. Older observations suggest that the clinical evaluation discussed previously is capable of establishing a diagnosis of the cause of ARF in 75% to 80% of cases.[123] When doubt exists as to the cause of ARF after careful evaluation, it is appropriate to consider obtaining renal biopsy material.[123–128] Indications for renal biopsy in the setting of ARF have not been firmly established. Many nephrologists strongly consider a biopsy when prerenal and postrenal factors have been excluded, and the clinical setting and laboratory data do not support a diagnosis of ATN.[123–128] The presence of extrarenal manifestations that suggest a systemic disorder, heavy proteinuria, and RBC casts would also strongly support obtaining renal biopsy material in the ARF setting.

Several studies have examined the role of renal biopsy in the diagnosis and management of ARF.[123–128] In an older series, Wilson and coworkers[127] obtained renal biopsy material from 84 ARF patients who were thought to have features atypical for ATN. Of these patients, 52% were found to have a glomerular disorder, 30% a tubulointerstitial disorder, and 18% a vascular disorder. A clinical diagnosis of acute tubulointerstitial disease was 77% sensitive and 86% specific, while a clinical diagnosis of acute glomerular disease was 56% sensitive and 66% specific.[127] Mustonen and coworkers[123] obtained renal biopsy material from 91 consecutive patients believed to have a renal cause for ARF. Overall, about 20% of these patients had a glomerular cause of ARF. Clinical diagnosis was about 86% sensitive for identifying an acute tubulointerstitial disorder and 67% sensitive for identifying an acute glomerular disorder as the cause of the ARF.[123] Taken together, these two studies suggest that the likelihood ratio for a clinical diagnosis of acute tubulointerstitial disease is about 4, and for acute glomerular disease it is about 1.5.

A study by Cohen and coworkers[126] found that about 20% of all renal biopsies performed in their urban

Southern California pathology referral practice were done for ARF of unclear cause. Of 21 biopsies done for ARF, a correct prebiopsy diagnosis was present in only one third of cases, and the biopsy resulted in a significant change of therapy in more than 50% of these cases. Occasionally, a renal biopsy in the setting of ARF reveals a potentially treatable, completely unexpected finding.[129]

In addition to indications for performing a renal biopsy in ARF, two other issues are of concern. The first is safety. Recent developments in treating the coagulopathy associated with renal failure plus improvements in biopsy techniques (eg, biopsy guided by real-time ultrasonography or CT imaging, use of smaller needles and biopsy guns) have improved safety. Indeed reasonable safety has been demonstrated in the setting of uncooperative patients in intensive care who required mechanical ventilation.[130] In this small study, percutaneous renal biopsy procedure performed on critically ill patients in intensive care undergoing mechanical ventilation was compared with an open biopsy procedure. Sufficient renal tissue for diagnosis was obtained in all seven patients undergoing percutaneous biopsy, and the rate of complications was roughly comparable to the patients undergoing open biopsy.[130] The timing of biopsy in ARF remains a key issue. In the past, a lack of recovery of renal function and anuria persisting after several days were considered indicators for ARF biopsy. At the present time, concerns about the irreversible nature of many forms of severe glomerulopathy and of acute interstitial disorders, if left untreated, have led to a much more timely approach to ARF biopsy when the cause is not clear.

SUMMARY

Early detection and prompt, thorough evaluation of ARF can potentially lead to therapy that attenuates the renal failure. Careful analysis of the patient's medical record and review of the history, physical examination, urinalysis, and routine laboratory data often (40%–60% of cases) establishes the cause of ARF. Sometimes (20%–30% of cases), additional diagnostic testing and therapeutic trials are needed. In a smaller but significant number of cases of ARF (5%–20%), histologic examination of renal tissue is required for accurate diagnosis.

REFERENCES

1. Anderson RJ, Schrier RW: Acute Tubular Necrosis: Clinical Settings, Diagnosis, Treatment, and Outcome. In: Schrier RW, Gottshalk CW, eds: *Diseases of the Kidney*. 6th ed. Boston: Little, Brown; 1997:1069.
2. Thandani R, Pascual M, Bonventre JV: Acute renal failure. N Engl J Med 1996; 334:1448.
3. Elasy T, Anderson RI: Changing demography of acute renal failure. Semin Dial 1996, 9:438.
4. Nolan CR, Anderson RJ: Hospital-acquired acute renal failure. J Am Soc Nephrol 1998; 9:711.
5. Stewart CL, Barnen R: Acute renal failure in infants, children, and adults. Crit Care Clin 1997; 13:575.
6. Couchoud C, Pozet N, Labeeuw M, et al: Screening early renal failure cut-off values for serum creatinine as an indicator of renal impairment. Kidney Int 1999; 55:1878.
7. Hou SH, Bushinsky DA, Wish JB, et al: Hospital-acquired renal insufficiency: a prospective study. Am J Med 1983; 74:243.
8. Liano F, Pascual J: Epidemiology of acute renal failure: a prospective, multicenter, community-based study. Kidney Int 1996, 50:811.
9. Anderson RJ, Linas SL, Berns AS, et al: Nonoliguric acute renal failure. N Engl J Med 1977; 296:1134.
10. Levy EM, Viscoli CM, Horwitz RI: The effect of acute renal failure on mortality. JAMA 1996; 275:1489.
11. Feest TG, Round A, Hamad S: Incidence of severe acute renal failure in adults: results of a community-based study. BMJ 1993; 306:481.
12. Kaufman J, Dhakal M, Patel B, et al: Community-acquired acute renal failure. Am J Kidney Dis 1991; 17:191.
13. Brivet FG, Kleinknecht Di, Loirat P, et al: Acute renal failure in intensive care units: causes, outcome, and prognostic factors of hospital mortality: a prospective, multicenter study. Crit Care Med 1996; 24:192.
14. McCarthy JT: Prognosis of patients with acute renal failure in the intensive care unit: a tale of two eras. Mayo Clin Proc 1996, 71:117.
15. Shusterman N, Strom BL, Murray TG, et al: Risk factors and outcome of hospital-acquired acute renal failure. Am J Med 1987; 83:65.
16. Klahr S, Miller SB: Acute oliguria. N Engl J Med 1998; 338:671.
17. Humes HD: Limiting acute renal failure. Hosp Pract 1999; 34:31.
18. Mindell JA, Chertow GM: A practical approach to acute renal failure. Med Clin North Am 1997; 81:731.
19. Zand MS, Steinman TI: Identifying the cause of acute renal failure. Contemp Intern Med 1997; 9:20.
20. Hamel MB, Phillips RS, Davis RB, et al: Outcomes and cost-effectiveness of initiating dialysis and continuing aggressive care in seriously ill hospitalized adults. Ann Intern Med 1997; 127:195.
21. Jurado R, Mattix H: The decreased serum urea nitrogen–creatinine ratio. Arch Intern Med 1998; 158:2509.
22. Moran SM, Meyers BD: Course of acute renal failure studied by a model of creatinine kinetics. Kidney Int 1985; 27:928.
23. Rabito CA, Panico F, Rubin R, et al: Noninvasive, real-time monitoring of renal function during critical care. J Am Soc Nephrol 1994; 4:1421.
24. Rahman SN, Conger JD: Glomerular and tubular factors in urine flow ratios of acute renal failure patients. Am J Kidney Dis 1994; 23:788.
25. Han JS, Kim YS, Chen HJ, et al: Temporal changes and reversibility of carbamylated hemoglobin in renal failure. Am J Kidney Dis 1997; 30:36.
26. Smith J, Shaykh M, Anwar F, et al: Factors determining hemoglobin carbamylation in renal failure. Kidney Int 1995; 48:1605.
27. Rabman M, Smith MC: Chronic renal insufficiency. Arch Intern Med 1998; 158:1473.
28. Back KF, Ichikawa I: Prerenal failure: a deleterious shift from renal compensation to decompensation. N Engl J Med 1988; 319:623.
29. Choudhury D, Ahmed Z: Drug-induced nephrotoxicity. Med Clin North Am 1997; 81:705.
30. Bennett WM: Drug nephrotoxicity: an overview. Ren Fail 1997; 19:221.
31. Moran M, Kapsner C: Acute renal failure associated with elevated plasma oncotic pressure. N Engl J Med 1987; 317:150.
32. Dorfman HR, Sandheim JH, Candnapapornchai P: Mannitol-induced acute renal failure. Medicine 1990; 69:153.
33. Cayco AV, Perazella MA, Harplett JP: Renal insufficiency after intravenous immune globulin therapy: a report of two cases and an analysis of the literature. J Am Soc Nephrol 1997; 8:1788.
34. Klahr S: Urinary tract obstruction. In: Schrier RW, Gottshalk CW, eds: *Diseases of the Kidney*. 6th ed. Boston: Little, Brown; 1997:709.
35. Chapman ME, Reid JH: Use of percutaneous nephrostomy in malignant ureteric obstruction. Br J Radiol 1991; 64:318.

36. Bhandari S, Johnston P, Fowler RC, et al: Non-dilated bilateral ureteric obstruction. Nephrol Dialysis Transplant 1995; 10:2337.
37. Don BR, Rodriguez RA, Humphreys MA: Acute Renal Failure Associated With Pigmenturia or Crystal Deposits. In: Schrier RW, Gottshalk CW, eds: *Diseases of the Kidney*. 6th ed. Boston: Little, Brown; 1997:49.
38. Becker BN, Schulman G: Nephrotoxicity of antiviral therapies. Curr Opin Nephrol Hypertens 1996; 5:375.
39. Roy LF, Villeneuve JP, Dumont A, et al: Irreversible renal failure associated with triamterene. Am J Nephrol 1991; 11:486.
40. Ramaswamy CR, Williams JD, Griffiths DF: Reversible acute renal failure with calcium oxalate cast nephropathy: possible role of ascorbic acid. Nephrol Dial Transplant 1993; 8:1387.
41. Berns JS, Cohen RM, Silverman M, Turner J: Acute renal failure due to indinavir crystalluria: report of two cases. J Kidney Dis 1997; 30:558.
42. Kopp JB, Miller KD, Mican JA, et al: Crystalluria and urinary tract abnormalities associated with indinavir. Ann Intern Med 1997; 127:119.
43. Rao TK: Acute renal failure in human immunodeficiency virus infection. Semin Nephrol 1998; 10:378.
44. Blade J, Ferenandez-Llama P, Basch F, et al: Renal failure in multiple myeloma. Arch Intern Med 1998; 158:1889.
45. Hays SR: Ischemic acute renal failure. Am J Med Sci 1992; 304:93.
46. Abuelo O: Diagnosing vascular causes of acute renal failure. Ann Intern Med 1995; 123:601.
47. Sandy D, Vidt DO: How to identify and limit ischemic nephropathy: presentation, screening tests, therapeutic approaches. J Crit Illness 1998; 13:503.
48. Bell SP, Frinkel A, Brown EA: Cholesterol emboli: uncommon or unrecognized. J R Soc Med 1997; 90:543.
49. Wilson DM, Salazer TL, Farkouh ME: Eosinophiluria in athero-embolic renal disease. Am J Med 1991; 91:186.
50. Rudnick MR, Berns JS, Cohen RM, Goldfarb S: Nephrotoxic risks of renal angiography contrast media–associated nephrotoxicity and atheroembolism: a critical review. Am J Kidney Dis 1994; 24:713.
51. McCullough PA, Wolyn R, Rocher LL, et al: Acute renal failure after coronary intervention: incidence, risk factors, and relationship to mortality. Am J Med 1997; 103:368.
52. Remuzzi U, Ruggenenti P: The hemolytic-uremic syndrome. Kidney Int 1998; 66:554.
53. Marwah D, Howe S: Renal disease in pregnancy. Curr Opin Nephrol Hypertens 1996; 5:147.
54. Benedetto C, Hollo S, Sigolini GP: Is pregnancy-related acute renal failure a disappearing entity? Ren Fail 1996; 18:575.
55. Sibai BM, Kustermann L, Velasco J: Current understanding of severe preeclampsia, pregnancy-associated hemolytic uremic syndrome, thrombotic thrombocytopenic purpura, hemolysis, elevated liver enzymes, and low platelet syndrome and postpartum acute renal failure. Curr Opin Nephrol Hypertens 1994; 3:436.
56. Gordon LI, Kewan HC: Cancer- and drug-associated thrombotic thrombocytopenic purpura and hemolytic uremic syndrome. Semin Hematol 1997; 34:140.
57. Hricik DE, Chung-Park M, Sedar JR: Glomerulonephritis. N Engl J Med 1998; 339:888.
58. Eknoyan G: Acute tubulointerstitial nephritis. In: Schrier RW, Gottshalk CW, eds: *Diseases of the Kidney*. 6th ed. Boston: Little, Brown; 1997:1249.
59. Rayner BL, Willeox PA, Pascoe MD: Acute renal failure in community-acquired bacteremia. Nephron 1990; 54:32.
60. Welage LS, Walawander CA, Timm EG, Grasela TH: Risk factors for acute renal insufficiency in patients with suspected or documented bacterial pneumonia. Ann Pharmacother 1994; 28:515.
61. Mattana J, Singhal PC: Prevalence and determinants of acute renal failure following cardiopulmonary resuscitation. Arch Intern Med 1993; 153:235.
62. Liano F, Junco E, Pascual J, et al: The spectrum of acute renal failure in the intensive care unit compared with that seen in other settings. The Madrid Acute Renal Failure Study Group. Kidney Int Suppl 1998; 66:S16.
63. Weinman EJ, Patak RV: Acute renal failure in cancer patients. Oncology 1992; 6:47.
64. Harris KP, Hattersley JM, Feehally J, Walls J: Acute renal failure associated with malignancies: a review of 10 years experience. Eur J Haematol 1991; 47:119.
65. Turney JH, Marshall DH, Brownjohn AM, et al: The evolution of acute renal failure. QJM 1990; 74:83.
66. Macias-Nunez JF, Lopez-Novoa JM, Martinez-Maldonado M: Acute renal failure in the aged. Semin Nephrol 1996; 16:330.
67. Andreucci YE, Fuiano G, Russo D, et al: Vasomotor nephropathy in the elderly. Nephrol Dial Transplant 1998; 13:17.
68. Pascual J, Liano F: Causes and prognosis of acute renal failure in the very old. J Am Geriatr Soc 1998; 46:721.
69. Gines P, Rodes J: Clinical Disorders of Renal Function in Cirrhosis With Ascites. In: Arroyo V, Gines P, Rodes J, Schrier RW, eds: *Ascites and Renal Dysfunction Liver Disease*. Malden, MA: Blackwell Science; 1999:36.
70. Bataller R, Sort P, Gines P, et al: Hepatorenal syndrome: definition, pathophysiology, clinical features, and management. Kidney Int 1998; 53:47.
71. Fogazzi GB: Crystalluria: a neglected aspect of urinary sediment analysis. Nephrol Dial Transplant 1996; 11:379.
72. Zager RA: Rhabdomyolysis and myohemoglobinuria in acute renal failure. Kidney Int 1996; 49:314.
73. Abassi ZA, Hoffman A, Belter OS: Acute renal failure complicating muscle crush. Semin Nephrol 1998; 18:558.
74. Abuelo JG: Renal failure caused by chemicals, foods, plants, animal venoms and misuse of drugs. Arch Intern Med 1990; 150:505.
75. Davidman M, Olson P, Kohen J, et al: Iatrogenic renal disease. Arch Intern Med 1991; 151:1809.
76. McGee S, Abernathy WB, Timel DL: Is this patient hypovolemic? JAMA 1999; 281:1022.
77. Rysava R, Zabka J, Peregrin JH, et al: Acute renal failure due to bilateral renal artery thrombosis associated with primary antiphospholipid syndrome. Nephrol Dial Transplant 1998; 13:2645.
78. Rainfray M, Hamon-Vilcot B, Nasr A, et al: A 90-year-old woman with acute renal failure revealing an antiphospholipid syndrome. J Am Geriatr Soc 1997; 45:200.
79. Hughson MD, Nadasedy T, McCarty GA: Renal thrombotic microangiopathy in patients with systemic lupus erythematosus and the antiphospholipid syndrome. Am J Kidney Dis 1992; 20:150.
80. Somers DL, Sotolongo C, Bertolatus IA. White clot syndrome associated with acute renal failure. J Am Soc Nephrol 1993; 4:137.
81. Roth D, Alarcon FJ, Fernandez JA, et al: Acute rhabdomyolysis with cocaine intoxication. N Engl J Med 1988; 319:673.
82. Oster JR, Sanger I, Contreras GN, et al: Metabolic acidosis with extreme elevation of anion gap: case report and literature review. Am J Med Sci 1999; 317:38.
83. Schrier RW, Henderson HS, Tisher CC, Tannen RL: Nephropathy associated with heat stress and exercise. Ann Intern Med 1967; 67:356.
84. Miller PD, Krebs RA, Neal BJ, McIntyre DO: Polyuric prerenal failure. Arch Intern Med 1980; 140:907.
85. Mareussen N, Schumann J, Campbell P, Kjellstrand C: Cytodiagnostic urinalysis is very useful in the differential diagnosis of acute renal failure and can predict severity. Renal Fail 1995; 17:721.
86. Minuth AN, Terrell YB, Suki WN: Acute renal failure. Am J Med Sci 1976; 271:317.
87. Duflat J, Cohen AN, Adler S: Macroscopic hematuria as the presenting manifestation of acute renal failure. Am J Kidney Dis 1993; 22:607.
88. Dinda AK, Saxena S, Guleria S, et al: Diagnosis of glomerular haematuria: role of dysmorphic red cell, G1 cell, and bright-field microscopy. Scand J Clin Lab Invest 1997; 57:203.
89. Mandal AK, Sklar AH, Hudson JB: Transmission electron microscopy of urine sediment in human acute renal failure. Kidney Int 1985, 38:58.
90. Nolan CR, Anger MS, Kelleher SP: Eosinophiluria: a new method of detection and definition of the clinical spectrum. New Engl J Med 1986; 315:1516.
91. Nolan CR, Kelleher SP: Eosinophiluria. Clin Lab Med 1988; 8:555.

92. Jones BE, Nanra RS, White KH: Acute renal failure due to acute pyelonephritis. Am J Nephrol 1991; 11:257.
93. Miller TR, Anderson RI, Linas SL, et al: Urinary diagnostic indices in acute renal failure: a prospective study. Ann Intern Med 1978; 88:47.
94. Rabb H: Evaluation of urinary markers in acute renal failure. Curr Opin Nephrol Hypertens 1998; 7:681.
95. Fushimi N, Shechin M, Mariano F: Decreased fractional excretion of urate as a predictor of prerenal azotemia. Am J Nephrol 1990; 10:489.
96. Steinhausen F: Fractional excretion of trace lithium and uric acid in acute renal failure. J Am Soc Nephrol 1994; 4:1429.
97. Spiegal DM, Wilson PD, Molitans BA: Epithelial polarity following ischemia: a requirement for normal cell function. Am J Physiol 1989; 256:430.
98. Wang Z, Rabb H, Craig T, et al: Ischemic-reperfusion injury in the kidney: overexpression of colonic H+-K+-ATPase and suppression of NHE-3. Kidney Int 1997; 51:1106.
99. Wang Z, Rabb H, Haq M, et al: A possible molecular basis of natriuresis during ischemic-reperfusion injury in the kidney. J Am Soc Nephrol 1998; 9:605.
100. Bock HA: Pathophysiology of acute renal failure in septic shock failure. Kidney Int 1998; 53:15.
101. Lam M, Kaufman CE: Fractional excretion of sodium as a guide to volume depletion during recovery from acute renal failure. Am J Kidney Dis 1985; 6:18.
102. Reinek HJ, O'Connor GT, Lifschitz MD, et al: Sequential studies on the pathophysiology of glycerol-induced acute renal failure. J Lab Clin Med 1980; 96:356.
103. Fang LS, Siroa RA, Ebert TH, Lichtenstein NS: Low fractional excretion of sodium with contrast-media–induced acute renal failure. Arch Intern Med 1980; 140:531.
104. Steiner RW: Low fractional excretion of sodium in myoglobinuric renal failure. Arch Intern Med 1982; 142:1216.
105. Vaz AJ: Low fractional excretion of urinary sodium in acute renal failure due to sepsis. Arch Intern Med 1983; 143:738.
106. Corwin HL, Schrieber MI, Fang LS: Low fractional excretion of sodium: occurrence with hemoglobinuric- and myoglobinuric-induced acute renal failure. Arch Intern Med 1984; 144:981.
107. Diamond IR, Yoburn DC: Nonoliguric acute renal failure associated with a low fractional excretion of sodium. Ann Intern Med 1982; 96:596.
108. Hoffman LM, Suki WN: Obstructive uropathy mimicking volume depletion. JAMA 1976; 236:2096.
109. Hilton PJ, Jones NF, Barraclough MA, Lloyd-Davies RW: Urinary osmolality in acute renal failure due to glomerulonephritis. Lancet 1969; 2:655.
110. Lins RL, VeTooten GA, DeClerk DS, et al: Urinary indices in acute interstitial nephritis. Clin Nephrol 1986; 26:131.
111. Liano F, Gamey C, Pascual I, et al: Use of urinary parameters in the diagnoses of total acute renal artery occlusion. Nephron 1994; 66:170.
112. Anderson RI, Gross PA, Gabow PA: Urinary chloride concentration in acute renal failure. Miner Electrolyte Metab 1984; 10:92.
113. Graziani G, Cantaluppi A, Casati S: Dopamine and furosemide in oliguric acute renal failure. Nephron 1984; 27:39.
114. Luke RG, Briggs JD, Allison MI: Factors determining response to mannitol in acute renal failure. Am J Med Sci 1970; 259:168.
115. Chew SL, Lins RL, Daelemans R, et al: Urinary enzymes in acute renal failure. Nephrol Dial Transplant 1993; 8:507.
116. Hoffmann W, Regenbogen C, Edel H, et al: Diagnostic strategies in urinalysis. Kidney Int 1994; 46S:111.
117. Fogazzi GB, Pazzi C, Passenni P, et al: Utility of immunofluorescence of urine sediment for identifying patients with renal disease due to monoclonal gammopathies. Am J Kidney Dis 1991; 17:211.
118. Di Paolo S, Gesualdo L, Stallone G, et al: Renal expression and urinary concentration of EGF and IL-6 in acutely dysfunctioning kidney transplanted patients. Nephrol Dial Transplant 1997; 12:2687.
119. Taman M, Liu Y, Talbert E, et al: Increased urinary hepatocyte growth factor excretion in human acute renal failure. Clin Nephrol 1997; 48:241.
120. Panvar F, Barker PB, Chan L, et al: Image-guided localized 31P MRI of acute urinary obstruction in the pig kidney. Kidney Int 1990; 37:461.
121. Malhoutra D, Shapiro JI, Chan LU: H-I nuclear magnetic resonance spectroscopy of urine. Kidney Int 1990; 37:280.
122. Connors AF, Speroif T, Dawson NV: The effectiveness of right heart catheterization in the initial care of critically ill patients. JAMA 1996; 276:889.
123. Mustonen J, Pasternak A, Helm H, et al: Renal biopsy in acute renal failure. Am J Nephrol 1984; 4:27.
124. Andreucci VE, Fuiano G, Stanzcate P, et al: Role of renal biopsy in the diagnosis and prognosis of acute renal failure. Kidney Int 1998; 53:91.
125. Racuson LC: Pathology of acute renal failure structure/function correlates. Adv Ren Replace Ther 1997; 4:3.
126. Cohen AH, Nast CC, Adler SG, Kopple JD: Clinical utility of kidney biopsies in the diagnosis and management of renal disease. Am J Nephrol 1989; 9:309.
127. Wilson DM, Turner DR, Cameron JS, et al: Value of renal biopsy in acute intrinsic renal failure. BMJ 1976; 2:459.
128. Richards NT, Darby S, Howie AJ, et al: Knowledge of renal histology alters patient management in over 40% of cases. Nephrol Dial Transplant 1994; 9:1255.
129. Border WA, Cohen AH: Renal biopsy diagnosis of clinically silent multiple myeloma. Ann Intern Med 1980; 93:43.
130. Conlon PJ, Kovalik E, Schwab SJ: Percutaneous renal biopsy of ventilated intensive care unit patients. Clin Nephrol 1995; 43:309.

CHAPTER **12**

Metabolic and Electrolyte Disturbances: Secondary Manifestations

Emmanuel A. Burdmann ▪ Luis Yu

INTRODUCTION

This chapter begins with a review of the definition of acute renal failure (ARF) found in recent publications on this syndrome. Most of them state that ARF is a sudden and generally reversible impairment of kidney function that causes accumulation of nitrogenous waste products and may ultimately progress to "uremic syndrome," a clearly undisputed concept.[1–3] However, besides this effect on nitrogenous metabolism, the abrupt disruption of normal renal function also has a deep impact on homeostasis of salt, water, electrolytes, and acid radicals and interferes with many hormonal pathways that involve renal regulation.[4] So, renal dysfunction, in addition to its primary effect on uremia development, also frequently induces a complex constellation of secondary manifestations that includes volume overload, hyponatremia, hyperkalemia, hypermagnesemia, acidosis, hypocalcemia, hyperphosphatemia, anemia, coagulation disorders, hypercatabolism, glucose intolerance, and other systemic changes (Table 12–1).

Another important point to consider is which patients are likely to develop ARF. Most cases of ARF develop in older individuals with acute tubular necrosis (ATN) and comorbid diseases (mainly cardiovascular), who are being treated in the intensive care unit in a setting of multiple organ failure[5, 6] (Table 12–2). The combination of these characteristics with uremia and the panel of ARF-induced systemic manifestations described previously makes these patients extremely vulnerable and difficult to treat. This is probably related to the high morbidity and mortality seen in ARF,[7] as well as to the importance of ARF as an independent death factor.[8, 9]

This chapter focuses on the mechanisms, clinical

TABLE 12–2. Some Epidemiologic Characteristics of a Series of 393 Patients With ARF*

PARAMETER	PERCENT OCCURRENCE
Patient location in hospital	
Intensive care units	54.8
Emergency ward	23.6
Nonemergency wards	21.6
Presence of comorbid diseases	85
Most usual comorbid diseases	
Heart disease	52
Hypertension	25
Presence of multiple organ failure	56
(ARF plus one or more organ failure)	—

Patients followed throughout 1993 by the Acute Renal Failure Unit at the Medical School, University of São Paulo, Brazil; age mean ± SD = 55 ± 18 years.

importance, prevention, and available treatment options for the most important secondary manifestations of ARF.

VOLUME OVERLOAD

Volume overload resulting from salt and water accumulation due to decreased glomerular filtration rate (GFR) is usually the first clinical problem of ARF, occurring when blood urea nitrogen (BUN) and creatinine serum levels are still relatively low. The majority of ARF patients become volume-overloaded in the first days of disease because of inadvertent maintenance of fluid intake during the unrecognized phase of renal injury or aggressive attempts to restore diuresis in oliguric patients. Moreover, as already mentioned, many ARF patients are critically ill individuals, requiring obligatory interventions such as intravenous medications and enteral or parenteral nutrition, which may make limitation of fluid administration unfeasible even after the diagnosis of ARF is made (Fig. 12–1). In addition, because most of the ARF patients seen at the present time are nonoliguric,[6, 10] fluid overload is frequently neglected in the early stages of renal dysfunction, and the problem is acknowledged only when there are already definite clinical findings that support it, such as edema, hypertension, and heart failure.

When one considers that many patients are old and have heart disease, it is easy to understand that volume overload could be particularly dangerous in this population. In fact, it has been shown that ARF patients

TABLE 12–1. Most Usual Secondary Manifestations in a Series of 393 Patients With ARF*

MANIFESTATION	PREVALENCE (%)
Anemia (hemoglobin level < 12 g/L)	65
Acidosis (pH < 7.35)	63
Hyperkalemia (potassium level > 5 mEq/L)	57
Hyponatremia (sodium level < 135 mEq/L)	56
Infection	15
Overt hypervolemia	13
Acute digestive bleeding	6
Other bleeding	6

Patients followed throughout 1993 by the Acute Renal Failure Unit at the Medical School, University of São Paulo, Brazil.

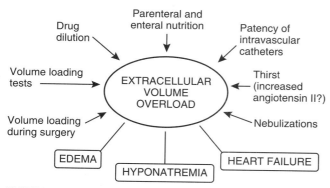

FIGURE 12–1 ■ Possible causes and consequences of volume overload in ARF.

who began dialysis as the result of hypervolemia had a higher mortality rate than that of patients who started dialysis because of uremia (56% versus 48.5%),[11] suggesting that fluid overload may be an important factor in adverse outcome in ARF. However, a multivariate analysis in 879 ARF patients did not confirm these data, suggesting instead that there was a worse prognosis for dialysis treatment given for uremia (odds ratio for death, 1.64).[10]

Prevention

The primary objective in ARF is to keep the patient euvolemic, because volume contraction could aggravate renal ischemia, causing more injury and retarding recovery of tubular cells.[12] After normal intravascular volume is ensured, a careful daily evaluation of volume status should be done in order to prevent or minimize fluid overload. Thus, daily assessment of supine and standing (if feasible) blood pressure, and heart rate, evaluation of skin turgor and mucous membrane condition, and evaluation of signs of pulmonary or peripheral edema are obligatory for these patients. However, the best way to perform an early diagnosis of volume overload is the daily evaluation of the patient's weight. ARF is a catabolic condition,[13, 14] so if the patient is in zero balance of fluid, he or she should lose approximately 200 to 300 g of body weight per day.[15] Weight gain in an ARF patient certainly means positive fluid balance and deserves attention. Another way of keeping track of volume status is the daily measurement of hydric balance. For this, both the intake and the output records and the insensible water losses and the generation of endogenous water should be considered. A resting, afebrile person usually experiences fluid losses of 0.5 to 0.6 mL/kg of body weight per hour (around 850 to 1000 mL/day in a 70-kg individual) through the skin and expired air. Fever increases this loss by nearly 13% for each centigrade degree increase. Conversely, the metabolic oxidation of carbohydrate, protein, and fat generates about 400 to 450 mL of endogenous water a day or even more in hypercatabolic status as ARF.[15] It is obvious that these figures can be highly variable and imprecise. If we also con-

sider the possibility of minor inaccuracies in the daily records of water intake and output, it is clear that the results for cumulative water balances should be used with caution, because they may roughly misstate the real volume condition of the patient. This is most likely to occur if the patient is under normal supervision in a non–intensive care setting. Invasive monitoring measurements, such as central venous pressure or pulmonary capillary wedge pressure, have little value as isolated parameters, but their variation can suggest volume changes if heart function is stable. Finally, when clinical signs of volume overload, such as peripheral edema, pleural effusion, ascites, jugular vein distention, hypertension, and tachycardia or pulmonary crackles, are evident, it means that there is already extensive fluid accumulation, and the risk of heart failure and pulmonary edema is high.

In order to prevent volume overload–induced complications, the daily volume of fluid intake should be similar to the daily volume of urine produced plus 400 mL (approximately the difference between insensible water losses and endogenous water production). It should be emphasized again that the best method for checking whether this objective is being achieved is to measure body weight variation. If there is volume accumulation in patients eating and drinking spontaneously, it is important to reduce fluid ingestion as well as the amount of dietary salt.

Treatment

Unfortunately, fluid and salt restriction is often insufficient to keep ARF patients free from volume overload. In this case, the administration of diuretics should be considered. Thiazide diuretics and loop diuretics are weak organic acids that bind largely to serum albumin and are secreted by the organic anion transport system in the proximal tubule. Thiazide diuretics do not work well when GFR is below 30 mL/min, so loop diuretics are generally the most appropriate option in severe oliguric ARF.[16–18]

Loop diuretics act at the luminal membrane of the cells of the thick ascending limb of the loop of Henle, inhibiting the $Na^+/2Cl^-/K^+$ transporter, and can increase the fractional excretion of sodium up to 20%. The most studied diuretic of this class in ARF treatment is probably furosemide. This drug has a bioavailability of up to 69% and binds extensively to albumin (91% to 99%). The main route of furosemide elimination is a probenecid-sensitive transport in the proximal tubule, but small amounts of the drug are also metabolized in the gut and liver.[16] The half-life of furosemide increases significantly in renal failure.[19] Furosemide should be used as early as possible, preferably in the first 24 to 48 hours of ARF development. The ceiling dose (dose that produces the maximal increase in the excreted fraction of filtered sodium [FE_{Na}]) in severe ARF is 500 mg IV.[20] Doses of 2 g/day have been used.[20] Furosemide can cause significant side effects. The most usual are metabolic: hyponatremia, hypokalemia, hypomagnesemia, hypocalcemia, metabolic alkalosis, and thiamine deficiency.[16, 17, 21, 22] Deafness can occur, is generally transitory, but sometimes permanent.[16, 20] Rapid infusions or high serum peak levels of the diuretic, hypoalbuminemia, and the concomitant use of other ototoxic drugs such as aminoglycoside increase the risk of this injury.[23–26] More rarely, furosemide can induce idiosyncratic reactions, such as cutaneous rash, Stevens-Johnson syndrome, pancreatitis, bone marrow dyscrasias, renal interstitial nephritis, and fever.[16, 17, 23, 27–37]

Several factors can cause diuretic resistance in ARF: decreased drug delivery to peritubular capillaries due to reduced renal blood flow, increased amount of organic acids competing for proximal tubule transporters, and increased extrarenal furosemide metabolism caused by decreased serum albumin.[17, 19] When optimal doses of bolus loop diuretics fail to improve urinary output, continuous diuretic infusion might be successful. Continuous furosemide infusion has been associated with higher efficacy, with bypass of diuretic resistance and with fewer diuretic-induced side effects.[17, 18, 20, 38–41] Another maneuver that might succeed when furosemide alone does not is the concomitant use of a thiazide and furosemide.[16, 18, 20, 23, 42, 43] However, this combination can significantly potentiate diuretic-induced metabolic side effects.[16, 20] In the same way, the use of low doses of dopamine (1 to 3 µg/kg/min) has a synergistic effect with furosemide, potentially increasing diuresis in a significant way, compared with furosemide alone.[20, 44, 45] Nevertheless, dopamine is a vasoactive drug that can cause significant vasoconstriction and life-threatening arrhythmias even in modest doses, so its use should be carefully evaluated, comparing risks with potential benefits for each patient.[45] When furosemide alone does not work in the setting of blood albumin values lower than 2 mg/dL, the administration of furosemide with albumin in the same vial may increase diuresis substantially, as well as the renal excretion of the diuretic.[18, 20, 46, 47] The goal of this approach is not to increase serum albumin levels, but to allow furosemide that is already bound to albumin to reach the peritubular capillary. A tentative step-by-step schedule for the use of furosemide in ARF is summarized in Table 12–3.

There is no consistent evidence proving that increased diuresis in ARF reduces patient mortality.[16, 17, 48, 49] An analysis of 19 published results of the use of diuretics in ARF (18 used furosemide) failed to show improvement in prognosis, although some authors found decreases in the necessity of dialysis and an increase in GFR (Table 12–4).[50] The same picture is true for dopamine: no studies showed conclusive evidence of the benefits of its use.[45, 48–50] A recent prospective randomized, double-blind placebo-controlled study assessed the use of torasemide and furosemide in ARF and did not find evidence of changes in renal recovery, of the need for dialysis, or of a decrease in mortality rate, although the loop diuretics increased significantly the urinary flow.[51]

This inconsistency between increases in diuresis volume and improvements in morbidity and mortality in ARF might be related to the value used for oliguria

TABLE 12–3. Possible Alternatives for the Use of Furosemide in ARF*

1. Single dose: Start with 20 mg; increase to 500 mg IV. Doses higher than 500 mg have little, if any, additional effect. Do not exceed infusion rate of 4–15 mg/min.
2. Continuous therapy: Starting bolus of 20–80 mg IV. Continuous infusion rate: 2–70 mg/h. Do not use more than 2 g/day. Monitor for ototoxicity.
3. Combination therapy: Ceiling dose of furosemide plus hydrochlorothiazide, 25 to 100 mg/day PO, or chlorothiazide, 500 to 1000 mg 1 to 2 times/day IV. Monitor carefully for metabolic adverse effects.
4. Dopamine: Ceiling dose of furosemide or optimal continuous infusion plus dopamine 1 µg/kg/min. Carefully monitor for tachycardia, cardiac arrhythmias, inadequate blood pressure increase, ischemia in extremities, and mesenteric ischemia.
5. Albumin: If plasma albumin <2.0 g/dL, add 60 mg of furosemide to 50 mL of 25% albumin (or 5 mg of furosemide/g infused albumin) and infuse via IV.

*Start with single-dose or continuous therapy approaches and, if neither works, use clinical judgment to choose the next step that best suits the patient characteristics.

definition. The "classic" limit for oliguria is based on the concept that the minimal urinary volume necessary for excretion of the usual daily amount of solute produced is 400 mL, if maximal renal concentration capacity is activated.[3] However, it is evident that this urinary volume is frequently inadequate for the maintenance of volume homeostasis in critically ill patients with ARF, which suggests revision of 400 mL as the borderline of oliguria. In fact, we have recently demonstrated that ARF patients with urinary flow rates above 1000 mL/day had a significantly lower mortality rate (38%) than that of the group with daily urinary volume of 400 to 1000 mL (mortality rate of 59%). From this finding, it appears that the urinary flow rate is an independent variable for ARF prognosis, with urinary volume over 1000 mL/24 h associated with a significantly lower odds ratio for mortality[10] (Fig. 12–2). It is reasonable that when we look for diuresis induction in ARF, the answer is not as simple as reaching a value above a fixed limit, but it matters what value is reached for a specific patient in order to fit his or her needs of volume accommodation. Studies about the prognosis for ARF patients that assess the results of diuretic-induced elevation of diuresis as a continuous variable are urgently needed.

TABLE 12–4. Effects of Diuretic Administration on Established ARF: A Summary of 19 Studies

	FAVORABLE ACTION	NO IMPROVEMENT	EQUIVOCAL
Renal function (18 reports)	7	9	2
Need for dialysis (14 reports)	7	5	2
Mortality (15 reports)	1	14	

From Levinsky NG, Bernard DB: Mannitol and Loop Diuretics in Acute Renal Failure. In: Brenner BM, Lazarus JM, eds: *Acute Renal Failure*. 2nd ed. New York: Churchill Livingstone; 1988:841.

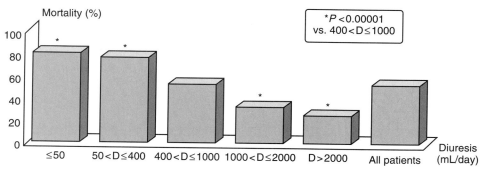

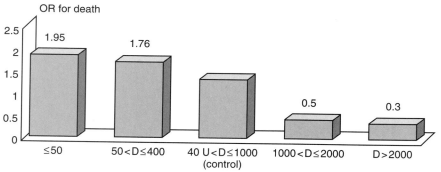

FIGURE 12–2 ■ Influence of diuresis volume on mortality in 864 patients with ARF. (Data from Avila MO, Zanetta DM, Yu ALF, et al: Is diuresis important in acute renal failure mortality? How much is enough? J Am Soc Nephrol 1997; 8:122A.)

If volume overload is not being satisfactorily controlled by preventive measures or by optimized pharmacologic-induced natriuresis, an early dialytic approach should be strongly considered. It should be emphasized again that when peripheral edema is visible, there is already a significant extracellular fluid excess probably affecting most of the vital organs, a condition that should definitely be avoided. The form of dialytic therapy (isolated ultrafiltration, intermittent dialysis, or continuous renal replacement therapy) should be selected on the basis of the patient's needs: dialysis has to meet the patient's needs and not vice versa.[52, 53]

HYPONATREMIA

Hyponatremia is an electrolyte disturbance frequently found in ARF. For instance, more than 50% of ARF patients followed in a university hospital had, at some point, a serum sodium level below 135 mEq/L (see Table 12–2).[5] Normal kidneys have an enormous capacity to excrete free water, allowing a subject to drink as much as 15 L of water a day without metabolic derangements, if his or her urinary diluting mechanism is working appropriately. For this, three key functions have to be competent in renal function[54, 55]:

1. Normal GFR, delivering appropriate water and solute load to distal tubules,
2. Perfect functioning of sodium reabsorption in Henle's thick ascending loop (diluting segment) in order to produce hypotonic intraluminal fluid and interstitial hypertonicity, and
3. Normal regulation of antidiuretic hormone (ADH) in the collecting duct.

In ARF, the decrease in GFR and the tubular injury impair the production of free water clearance, and so if the patient receives more free water than he or she is able to excrete, hyponatremia develops. This is true even for nonoliguric patients. As a model, a patient with ARF and a GFR of 5 mL/min can be considered. This patient filters 7200 mL of water in 24 hours and 70% of it is reabsorbed in the proximal tubules. The remaining approximately 2 L will reach the distal segments of the nephron. Even if the diluting segment is working normally and the collecting duct is impermeable to ADH, no more than 2 L of urine free from solutes may be produced, and free water ingestion above this value produces hyponatremia.[56] In fact, impairment of free water clearance occurs very early in the course of ARF, preceding oliguria and elevations of creatinine and BUN.[57, 58]

Usually, ARF-associated hyponatremia is hypervolemic (retention of sodium and water, total body water increase > total body sodium increase) and less frequently euvolemic (increased total body water with normal total body sodium). Although most of ARF-associated hyponatremia is dilutional, ARF occurring simultaneously with or caused by excessive gastrointestinal, renal, or "third space" electrolyte losses (eg, vomiting, diarrhea, drugs, leptospirosis, burns, pancreatitis, and muscle injury) can present with hypovolemic hyponatremia (loss of both water and sodium, sodium > water).[54, 55, 59, 60]

When faced with a patient with hyponatremia, we should also rule out pseudohyponatremia. If plasma sodium is measured by flame photometry, substances occupying a large fraction of the plasma volume cause artificially decreased sodium concentration. This phenomenon can be caused by excessive anomalous proteins, as in multiple myeloma or high amounts of lipids, as in severe hyperlipidemias. In these cases, the serum osmolality is normal. Another circumstance that can induce hyponatremia without excessive intake of exogenous free water is the presence of plasmatic osmotically active solutes, such as glucose or mannitol, that translocate water from the intracellular to the extracellular space. In these cases, a low plasma sodium level is caused by water redistribution. There is no real hypotonic condition, and serum osmolality actually is increased. The correction of hyperglycemia or withdrawal of mannitol normalizes plasma sodium.[54, 55]

The clinical picture of true hyponatremia is related largely to cell swelling caused by the hypotonic environment. Most of the symptoms are neurologic: lethargy, ataxia, headache, behavior disturbances, and seizures. This clinical picture can progress to coma, respiratory depression, and death due to tentorial herniation. Gastrointestinal and muscular symptoms, such as nausea, vomiting, muscular weakness, and cramps, are also frequent. One problem here is that most of these signs and symptoms can also be present in uremic syndrome, making the early clinical diagnosis of hyponatremia difficult in ARF. Patients with hypovolemic hyponatremia are generally asymptomatic for hyponatremia, probably because the concomitant loss of water and solute limits the development of brain edema.[54, 55, 61, 62]

For therapeutic purposes, hyponatremia is considered to be acute (known duration less than 48 hours) or chronic (unknown duration or more than 48 hours). Acute and chronic symptomatic hyponatremia are medical emergencies that can be particularly difficult to treat. If treatment is too slow, there can be significant cerebral morbidity and mortality; if it is too fast, it can precipitate demyelination syndrome.[63, 64] Acute symptomatic hyponatremia should be aggressively treated with hypertonic saline (3% NaCl) and furosemide. Saline should be given at 1 to 2 mL/kg per hour until symptoms are abolished or plasma sodium reaches 130 mEq/L, without exceeding a correction rate of 2 mEq/L per hour.[54, 55, 62] Chronic symptomatic hyponatremia should also be treated with 3% saline at 1 to 2 mL/kg per hour and furosemide until serum sodium increases 10% or symptoms resolve. After initial correction, serum sodium should not increase more than 1.5 mEq/h or more than 8 (safer) to 12 mEq/L per day.[54, 55, 62]

Obviously, these therapeutic approaches are even more difficult to follow in ARF, particularly in oliguric patients. These patients have a serious limitation in producing free water, because GFR is severely decreased, so infusion of saline could be disastrous, leading to heart failure and pulmonary edema, if it is not followed by proportional diuresis. Mild to moderate asymptomatic hyponatremia in hypervolemic ARF patients can be initially managed with water restriction if patients are euvolemic, or water and sodium restriction and the use of loop diuretics if they are hypervolemic. It is important to remember that for this approach to be effective the sum of urinary sodium and urinary potassium should be lower than the plasma sodium, ie, the patient is excreting electrolyte-free water.[55] Patients

who do not respond to this approach and are severely hyponatremic or who have symptomatic hyponatremic ARF should be treated by dialysis, preferably continuous replacement therapies.[52] In patients with moderate or severe chronic hyponatremia, it is advisable to set the dialysis sodium concentration at levels no higher than 15 to 20 mEq/L above the plasma level, and correct hyponatremia over a period of days, avoiding rapid changes. Peritoneal dialysis is an efficient, gentle, and slow way of correcting hyponatremia.[65]

Treatment of hypovolemic hyponatremia should include the administration of isotonic saline and measures to achieve resolution of the trigger condition. In hypovolemic hyponatremia with marked reduction of plasma sodium, alternate isotonic saline (0.9% NaCl) and half isotonic saline (0.45% NaCl) should be used in order to produce a more gradual and safer correction.[62]

HYPERKALEMIA

Potassium, the most abundant intracellular cation, has a pivotal role in many cellular functions and in cell volume regulation. A normal 70-kg adult has about 4000 mEq of total body potassium, mostly (2300 to 3000 mEq) in the muscle cells. Only 1.5% to 2.5% of total body potassium (around 60 mEq) is found in the extracellular compartment. So, the intracellular fluid (ICF) has a potassium concentration of 150 mEq/L, which is 38-fold higher than the extracellular fluid (ECF) concentration (about 4 mEq/L). This potassium gradient generates the resting membrane potential (RMP) that is essential for muscle contraction, neuronal transmission, and several cellular signaling mechanisms.[56, 66–70]

The acute control of potassium homeostasis is carried out by a moment-to-moment, delicate, and precise set of mechanisms that keep this cation ECF level in a narrow and safe range, despite wide variations in dietary intake, promoting fast potassium shifts across the cellular membrane. The main components that maintain this critical balance are the RMP itself, the enzyme Na^+, K^+-ATPase, hormones (insulin, catecholamines, aldosterone), the acid-base balance, and serum tonicity. The kidneys are the main organ responsible for long-term homeostasis by adjusting excretion of potassium to match daily dietary intake. The usual Western diet provides about 100 mEq of potassium per day. In normal balance conditions, about 10 mEq/day are excreted in the stool and the remaining 90 mEq should be excreted by the kidneys. Approximately 65% of the filtered potassium is reabsorbed in the proximal tubule, 20% by Henle's loop, and therefore, only 15% of the filtered load reaches the distal nephron. If we consider a serum potassium concentration of about 3 to 4 mEq/L, 60 to 90 mEq of potassium reach the distal nephron. There, mainly in the cortical collecting duct (CCD), the fine modulation of potassium balance takes place as the result of secretion, when dietary intake is excessive, or reabsorption, when the diet is potassium deficient. The [K^+] secretion in the distal tubule is dependent on lumen-negative transepithelial voltage generated by sodium reabsorption, the presence of [K^+] channels, and high fluid flow through terminal CCDs.[56, 66–70]

Hyperkalemia is a common complication of ARF (see Table 12–1), and renal failure is one of the principal predisposing factors for the development of hyperkalemia.[71] Decreased GFR, low CCD flow rate, distal tubular damage, and decreased distal sodium load can significantly reduce the renal excretory capacity during an ARF episode, leading to abrupt and sharp increases in the serum potassium level.[66–69] It has been experimentally demonstrated that ATN down-regulates CHIF, a gene related to [K^+] homeostasis, in renal medulla and papilla, whereas it up-regulates this gene in the colon.[72] Many of the situations that cause ATN also increase the release of endogenous potassium as the result of cell destruction by processes such as rhabdomyolysis and hemolysis (Table 12–5). It is not unusual that acute deterioration of renal function is provoked by or occurs concomitantly with nephrotoxic drugs that impair potassium excretion, such as nonsteroidal anti-inflammatory drugs, angiotensin-converting enzyme inhibitors, and many others (Table 12–6).[73–82] Finally, ARF patients are frequently acidotic and hypercatabolic, which causes shifts of potassium from the ICF to the ECF, leading to the development of hyperkalemia.

The possibility of pseudohyperkalemia should also be considered in an ARF patient. The most usual causes of this phenomenon are the prolonged use of a tourniquet or a tourniquet that is too tight, excessive fist clenching (mainly in cachectic patients), hemolysis of drawn blood, leukemia-induced marked leukocytosis (> $10^5/mm^3$), and megakaryocytosis (> $10^6/mm^3$).[66, 69]

TABLE 12–5. Hyperkalemia: Possible Endogenous and Exogenous Sources Contributing to Increase of Serum Potassium in ARF Patients

Endogenous
 Rhabdomyolysis
 Hemolysis
 Tumoral lysis
 Hematoma reabsorption
 Gastrointestinal bleeding
 Prolonged fasting

Exogenous
 Food (eg, potatoes, beans, peas, nuts, bananas, cantaloupe, oranges, chocolate, beef, chicken)
 Salt substitute (contains around 13 mEq [K^+]/g)
 Urinary alkalinization (potassium citrate)
 Potassium oral supplements
 Fluoride-rich water
 Water softeners
 Stored blood (1 U of blood stored for 10 or more days contains ~30 mEq [K^+]/L)
 Drugs (eg, potassium penicillin contains 1.7 mEq [K^+]/million U)
 Parenteral replacement
 Renal allograft preservation solution
 Potassium cardioplegia in cardiac surgery

TABLE 12–6. Drugs That Can Cause Hyperkalemia and Their Mechanisms of Action

DRUGS	MECHANISM OF ACTION
Beta blockers α-Adrenergic agonists Insulin antagonists (somatostatin, diazoxide) Digitalis Depolarizing agents (eg, succinylcholine, suxamethonium) Arginine hydrochloride	Potassium shift from the intracellular fluid to the extracellular fluid
Heparin Ketoconazole Nonsteroidal anti-inflammatory drugs Beta blockers Angiotensin-converting enzyme blockers Angiotensin II receptors inhibitors	Decreased aldosterone biosynthesis
Amiloride Triamterene Trimethoprim Pentamidine	Blockade of sodium channel in the cortical collector duct
Spironolactone	Decreased aldosterone binding to its receptor
Cyclosporine	Chloride shunt disorder in the cortical collector duct

Clinical Manifestations

The signs and symptoms of hyperkalemia are related to the changes in the ratio of intracellular to extracellular [K^+] concentration in muscle and myocardial cells. The increased serum potassium level decreases the ICF/ECF [K^+] ratio, and RPM becomes less negative than normal and closer to the membrane excitability threshold. The cell is partially depolarized, and as a result there is a decrease in the conduction velocity and an increase in the depolarizing rate.[56, 69]

The most dangerous effect of hyperkalemia is cardiac arrhythmias. The first electrocardiographic (ECG) sign of hyperkalemia is an increase in T-wave amplitude, which becomes tall, thin, peaked, and symmetrical. Further increases in serum [K^+] concentration delay ventricular and His-Purkinje system conduction, causing prolongation of the PR interval, depressed ST segment, and widening of the QRS complex.[83] With progressive hyperkalemia, the P wave flattens and finally disappears, and the QRS broadens even more, ultimately merging with the T wave, producing a sine wave pattern. The most feared arrhythmias complicating hyperkalemia are ventricular tachycardias and asystole, which usually follow shortly after P-wave disappearance or QRS widening.[66–69] Electrocardiography is a fast and noninvasive method for assessing whether changes in serum [K^+] are affecting heart cells. However, there is not a straight correlation between the ECG changes and the severity of hyperkalemia,[84] and life-threatening arrhythmias or cardiac arrest can occur suddenly without previous ECG abnormalities. Acute hyperkalemia induces changes in heart rhythm at lower potassium levels, and many dysfunctions, such as acidosis, hyponatremia, hypocalcemia, and pre-existing heart disease, that are usually present in a patient with ARF significantly potentiate potassium heart toxicity. On the other hand, infants or super-marathon runners are better able to tolerate a slow increase in serum potassium or hyperkalemia.[56, 66–69]

At the neuromuscular level, severe hyperkalemia may cause paresthesias, muscular weakness, and ultimately depressed deep tendon reflexes. These muscular changes can progress to flaccid paralysis, beginning in the limbs and extending up to the trunk and to the phonation and respiratory muscles, sometimes causing mechanical respiratory failure.[66–69, 85, 86]

Prevention and Treatment of Mild Asymptomatic Hyperkalemia

Hyperkalemia is a preventable cause of sudden death. Oliguric ARF patients are more prone to developing hyperkalemia, but even nonoliguric ARF can induce significant serum $[K^+]$ increase, mainly in the presence of tissue cell damage, excessive exogenous load, or drugs that impair potassium homeostasis. The guidelines for treatment of hyperkalemia have been extensively reviewed in recent publications.[66–69, 87, 88]

The first step in the prevention or early management of mild asymptomatic hyperkalemia (serum $[K^+]$ < 6.5 mEq/L and no ECG changes) is to decrease the exogenous potassium load. The dietary intake should be reduced to 50 mEq/day or less. Potential exogenous sources of potassium or the presence of elements that alter potassium balance should be carefully scrutinized in the patient's habits and in the medical office or hospital prescription, and interrupted, if possible (see Table 12–5).[88–92] Sometimes these sources are not obvious, such as fluoride-rich water,[89] water softeners,[90] or decreased insulin levels due to prolonged fasting.[93, 94] Drugs that impair potassium homeostasis should be avoided or discontinued as soon as possible.[73–82] A summary of these drugs and their mechanisms of action is offered in Table 12–6.

Urinary excretion can be used for nonemergency removal of body potassium excess. Thus, the use of loop diuretics may extend kaliuresis through the increase of flow rate in the CCD (try furosemide, 40 to 120 mg IV).[67–69, 87, 88]

Another way of extending potassium wasting is the use of cation exchange resins by the gastrointestinal route. These resins are made of a polystyrene framework to which is bound an unabsorbable and nonmetabolizable anion that is counterbalanced by an exchangeable and absorbable cation. These cations are exchanged for potassium, mainly in the colon. Sodium polystyrene sulfonate (Kayexalate) exchanges sodium for potassium, at an approximate rate of 1 mEq of K^+ per gram of resin. There are no fixed doses. When used by the oral route, doses of 15 g (4 level teaspoons) to 50 g are given diluted in water, 10% glucose, or 20% sorbitol to avoid constipation (use approximately 1.25 g/5 mL) and repeated every 4 to 6

hours as necessary. If the oral route is not feasible, the resin may be given by enema. Doses of 50 to 100 g of Kayexalate are diluted in 100 to 200 mL of sorbitol 20%, instilled by rectum, and retained in colon for at least 30 to 60 minutes (preferably more). The continuous use of this approach is able to eliminate 25 to 50 mEq of potassium or to induce a 0.5 to 1.0 mEq/L decrease in serum potassium level in an interval of 4 to 6 hours.[67–69, 87, 88] The main side effects potentially caused by Kayexalate are volume overload (each gram contains 4.1 mEq of sodium) and colonic necrosis or gastrointestinal ulcers.[67–69, 87, 88] This resin-induced severe side effect occurred in postoperative patients, probably because of an increased contact of hypertonic sorbitol with gastrointestinal mucous membrane caused by decreased intestinal motility.[95–98] Calcium polystyrene sulfonate (Sorcal) exchanges calcium for potassium, at an approximate rate of 1.3 mEq of K^+/g. This resin is provided in 30 g folders, and each gram contain 3.3 mEq of calcium. The method of administration is similar to that for Kayexalate: 15 to 30 g PO, diluted in 20 to 100 mL of water every 4 to 6 hours, or 30 g of resin in 200 mL of methylcellulose, or 100 mL of sorbitol 20% by enema. It should be stressed that the use of cation exchange resins is rational only when there is no need for an urgent decrease in potassium levels. In fact, a recent paper pointed out that a single dose of resin-cathartic therapy did not reduce serum potassium concentrations in chronic renal failure (CRF) patients.[99]

Treatment of Moderate to Severe Hyperkalemia or Symptomatic Hyperkalemia

There are some circumstances in which hyperkalemia should be considered as a medical emergency and treated as such.[67–69, 87, 88] These circumstances include the following:

1. Hyperkalemia and ECG changes (any level of serum potassium)
2. Serum potassium ≥ 6.5 mEq/L (even with normal ECG)
3. Sudden rise in serum potassium combined with continuous cellular lysis or the presence of drugs that impair potassium homeostasis

These conditions are associated with an elevated risk of lethal arrhythmia and demand immediate treatment to antagonize potassium effects on cellular membrane potential, promote acute shift of potassium from the ECF to the ICF, and rapidly remove potassium from the body. It should be emphasized again that the ECG is not a reliable predictor of severe arrhythmias and that rapid deterioration of cardiac rhythm can occur at any potassium level during hyperkalemia.

ANTAGONIZING CARDIAC EFFECTS

This is the first procedure to be done in emergency treatment of hyperkalemia and can be achieved by intravenous infusion of calcium salts. Calcium does not change serum potassium concentrations but is able to acutely decrease membrane excitability. There is no correct dose; the cation should be titrated under ECG monitoring. It starts to work within 1 to 3 minutes, and its effect persists for 30 to 60 minutes. If there is no effect, the dose can be repeated after 5 to 10 minutes. As an initial approach, 10 mL of 10% calcium gluconate can be given intravenously in 10 minutes. Each mL of this solution contains 9.0 mg of elemental calcium or 0.5 mEq of Ca^{2+}. Conversely, 3 to 4 mL of 10% calcium chloride can be given (each mL has 27 mg of elemental calcium). Special care should be exerted in patients taking digitalis, because a serum calcium increase may precipitate digitalis intoxication.[67–69, 87, 88]

PROMOTING RAPID INTRACELLULAR SHIFTING OF POTASSIUM

Insulin and Glucose

This is the best, least controversial, and most consistent way of quickly decreasing serum potassium. It could have dramatic effects when the patient is severely hyperglycemic or in low aldosterone diabetic subjects.[88] When the patient has normal or mildly increased serum glycemia, 4 to 5 g of glucose should be given for each unit of insulin infused. It starts to work within minutes, with detectable effects in approximately 15 minutes (mean decrease of 0.6 to 1.0 mEq of potassium after 1 hour) and has a duration of action of about 4 to 6 hours.[67–69] Start treatment with 10 units of insulin, IV as a bolus, plus infusion of 50 g of glucose or continuous infusion of 10 U of insulin/h in a 20% glucose solution.[67–69, 88] If the patient has diabetes mellitus and is hyperglycemic, give only 10 U of insulin IV.[68, 88] The main side effect is delayed hypoglycemia, which can occur in as many as 75% of the patients.[67–69]

Sodium Bicarbonate

The efficacy of this time-honored intervention in lowering potassium is questioned when it is used in CRF patients.[100] If metabolic acidosis is present (serum bicarbonate < 20 mEq/L), it should be tried.[67–69] It is better used as an isotonic solution: 50 to 150 mEq should be given IV over 15 to 30 minutes.[68, 69, 88] It starts to act within 5 to 15 minutes, and its effects last for 1 to 2 hours. It can be repeated after 30 minutes, if necessary.[68, 69, 88] It may act synergistically with insulin plus glucose infusion.[67, 68, 88] Solutions of 10% sodium bicarbonate contain 1.2 mEq of HCO_3^-/mL, and 3% sodium bicarbonate solutions contain 0.4 mEq of HCO_3^-/mL. The main side effects of sodium bicarbonate are volume overload, hypernatremia (use of hypertonic solutions), a decrease in ionized Ca^{2+} due to excessive Ca binding to albumin and causing tetany, metabolic alkalosis, and an increase in CO_2.[67–69, 88]

β₂-Adrenergic Agonists

Studies in CRF patients showed that the administration of β₂-agonists by nebulization or by the intravenous route was able to reduce serum potassium levels in as many as 60% to 80% of these individuals. The effect is detectable within minutes and lasts for 2 to 4 hours. Reductions in serum potassium from 0.6 to 1.5 mEq have been observed. The doses used by nebulization are 10 or 20 mg of albuterol or salbutamol in 4 mL of saline over 10 minutes. These dosages are 4 to 8 times higher than the usual amount of β₂-agonists given for asthma treatment, and their peak of action is up to 90 minutes. Dosages of 0.5 mg of salbutamol can also be given by parenteral route, its peak action occurring in 30 minutes. The main potential side effects of these drugs are tachycardia, cardiac arrhythmias, myocardial ischemia in patients with baseline coronary disease, palpitations, tremor, nausea, and headache.[67–69, 101–105] Insulin plus glucose and β₂-agonists act synergistically to decrease potassium levels.[106]

REMOVING POTASSIUM RAPIDLY

All the measures previously recommended for emergency treatment of hyperkalemia are merely palliative, intended to avoid serious cardiac arrhythmias and buy some time in order to correct the causal disease. However, there are many times when a rapid recovery of renal function is not achieved and/or correction of coadjuvant factors for hyperkalemia are not feasible, and rapid removal of body potassium by dialysis is mandatory. Therefore, when symptomatic or moderate to severe ARF-related hyperkalemia occurs in the presence of oliguria not responsive to diuretics or volume infusion, or with drugs impairing potassium homeostasis, or when continuous release of intracellular potassium is anticipated (severe rhabdomyolysis, tumor cell lysis), dialysis therapy is strongly advised as soon as possible.[52] Classic intermittent hemodialysis is significantly more efficient than peritoneal dialysis for the rapid removal of potassium and should be the method of choice in hyperkalemia emergencies.[53, 65, 67, 69, 88] Actually, the speed of potassium removal by peritoneal dialysis can be similar to that achieved by cation exchange resins. The efficacy of hemodialysis in removing potassium is approximately five times greater than that of peritoneal dialysis, being capable of removing 30 to 50 mEq/h.[88] Potassium concentration in the dialysis bath should be maintained at 2 mEq/L to avoid cardiac arrhythmias resulting from excessively fast serum potassium reductions.[69, 107] Besides the characteristics of membrane and blood flow, the main factor influencing potassium withdrawn by dialysis is the potassium serum concentration. So infusion of glucose-insulin should stop when dialysis begins, and the dialysate glucose should be kept as low as possible, without causing hypoglycemia, in order to decrease the ICF shift of potassium and allow more potassium to be removed.[65, 67–69, 88]

A practical summary of the emergency treatment of hyperkalemia can be found in Table 12–7.

ACIDOSIS

The kidneys are responsible for the final preservation of acid balance throughout the excretion of non-

TABLE 12–7. Emergency Treatment of Hyperkalemia

1. Decrease membrane excitability in heart cells. Give 10 mL of calcium gluconate 10% (or 3.3 mL of calcium chloride 10%) in 10 min. Should work in 3 min and last for at least 30 min. If not effective, repeat after 5 to 10 min. It can be repeated many times. Be careful with patients taking digitalis (possibility of intoxication).
2. Shift potassium to the intracellular fluid.
   A. Give 10 U regular insulin in bolus, plus 50 g glucose (500 mL of glucose 10% or 200 mL glucose 25% via IV in 1 to 2 h). Alternatively, use continuous infusion of 10 U regular insulin in 20% glucose solution. If the patient is hyperglycemic, use only 10 U regular insulin. Should have detectable effects in 15 min and last for at least 4 h. Watch for late hypoglycemia.
   B. If serum bicarbonate is lower than 20 mEq/L, give 100 mEq sodium bicarbonate IV in 30 min. It should start to work in no more than 15 min and last for at least 1 h. It can be repeated after 30 min. Be careful with volume overload, hypernatremia, and tetany.
   C. If insulin plus glucose had an effect lower than expected, give 10 to 20 mg albuterol or salbutamol in 4 mL of saline in 10 min by nebulization or 0.5 mg salbutamol IV. The effect should be in min and lasts for at least 2 h. Watch for tachycardia and cardiac arrhythmias. Avoid use in patients with coronary disease.
3. Remove potassium by dialysis: Make urgent arrangements for hemodialysis. Use "classic" intermittent procedure (bath with 2 mEq/L of potassium and low glucose).

volatile acids and the tubular reabsorption and regeneration of bicarbonate. Most of the daily production of nonvolatile acids comes from ingestion and metabolism of proteins and amino acids. The metabolism of cysteine and methionine generates sulfuric acid, and the metabolism of lysine, arginine, and cysteine yields hydrochloric acid. Other sources of nonvolatile acids are the metabolism of fat and carbohydrates and substances from the diet, as ingested phosphate. In fact, the production of nonvolatile acids is strongly influenced by the everyday diet. Normally, an adult who consumes the average Western diet produces 1 mEq/kg per day of hydrogen ion. To maintain normal acid balance, the kidneys have to excrete this acid production, reabsorb filtered HCO_3^-, and regenerate it to replace the HCO_3^- used for buffering ECF fixed acids or HCO_3^- lost in stools and urine. When an acid load occurs, the kidneys react by increasing titratable acid and NH_4^+ excretion (and consequently regenerating new base) and promoting maximal reabsorption of filtered HCO_3^-. If there is not enough renal function to excrete the acid produced daily and to regenerate bicarbonate, or if there is an increased (exogenous or endogenous) acid load that overrides renal excretion or an exaggerated renal or gastrointestinal loss of bicarbonate, metabolic acidosis follows. This brief introduction about renal control of acid balance would not be complete without taking into consideration that evaluations of acid-base disorders should always include a calculation of the anion gap, ie, the amount of unmeasured anions present in plasma. If one assumes that normal values for albumin exist, the anion gap (AG) is equal to $[Na^+ - (Cl^- + HCO_3^-)]$ and normally has a value of 10 ± 2 mEq/L.[108–111]

Clinical Manifestations

Moderate renal dysfunction results in a normal AG metabolic acidosis, caused, in part, by decreased proximal tubule reabsorption of HCO_3^-, but mainly by failure of the damaged renal tissue to produce enough ammonia and consequently regenerate the amount of bicarbonate that is required. With a progressive fall in GFR, there is an accumulation of organic acids such as sulfate and phosphate, so patients with severe renal failure present with an increased AG metabolic acidosis. In CRF patients, acidosis is usually seen only when 80% or more of the renal mass is lost.[108–111] These patients rarely have an HCO_3^- concentration below 15 mEq/L and an AG over 15 to 20 mEq/L.[108–112] They have stable pH and bicarbonate levels (mostly due to buffering by bone alkaline salts) over long periods of time and are asymptomatic or oligosymptomatic until the very late stages of renal disease.[108–111]

In a patient with "pure" ARF, without exacerbated catabolism, one should expect a serum bicarbonate decrease of 1 to 2 mEq/day, considering a daily production of 1 mEq/kg of hydrogen.[15] However, it is clear that this kind of ARF is rather an exception to the rule in today's patients. They are usually hypercatabolic, have multiple organ failure, and have multifactorial ARF associated with trauma or sepsis. These patients can often have a rapid consumption of serum bicarbonate, which can be as much as 15 to 20 mEq/day, and very elevated AG caused by an impressive cell release of organic acids.[53, 113, 114] Moreover, not infrequently, lactic or ketotic acidosis, as well as respiratory acidosis induced by permissive hypercapnia ventilatory techniques, can be present in critically ill ARF patients, compounding renal failure–induced acidosis and causing severe acidemias.[52]

Metabolic acidosis is generally the least of the early electrolyte abnormalities in ARF, except when it is part of the causal or comorbid disease. The clinical picture of metabolic acidosis is multisystemic, comprising changes in the respiratory, cardiac, gastrointestinal, and nervous systems, and in vascular reactivity, and is related to the intensity and pace of development. Thus, CRF patients who had a slow and gradual development of acidosis can be asymptomatic, with levels of pH and bicarbonate substantially lower than the levels in symptomatic ARF patients. Metabolic acidosis causes a typical respiratory pattern characterized by deep inspiration and increased respiratory rate, the so-called Kussmaul respiration. This increased ventilation is directly linked to the fall in serum HCO_3^-. Acidosis, especially when pH is lower than 7.20, has a negative effect on myocardial contractility and can induce life-threatening arrhythmias. Moreover, it causes peripheral vasodilation, venous vasoconstriction, and resistance to vasopressor agents. At the gastrointestinal level, it induces abdominal pain, nausea, and vomiting. Acidosis affects the central nervous system, causing signs and symptoms ranging from headache and lethargy to stupor and coma.[108–111, 115] At the metabolic level, it produces insulin resistance and impairs carbohydrate utilization (can cause hyperglycemia), reduces

ATP production, induces or aggravates hyperkalemia, and enhances catabolism.[114, 115] It can also provoke a leukemoid reaction, with white blood cell counts over 25,000 to 40,000. Finally, acidosis might have adverse effects on ARF induced by myoglobinuria and hemoglobinuria or related to Bence Jones protein, probably as a result of worsening of tubular obstruction by casts or pigment-induced tubular injury.[116, 117] The main systemic and metabolic consequences of acidosis are summarized in Table 12–8.

Treatment

There are still controversies about metabolic acidosis treatment in ARF. Some authors state that usually a case of "noncomplicated" ARF does not cause a serum bicarbonate decrease below 16 to 18 mEq/L, so treatment is rarely necessary.[15] However, the experience of a group devoted to ARF treatment in a tertiary hospital showed that more than 70% of the ARF cases followed were made up of critically ill patients and more than 63% had metabolic acidosis (see Tables 12–1 and 12–2).[5] As already stated, these patients frequently have comorbid conditions that significantly aggravate acidosis. Moreover, because renal mechanisms for correction of both hyperchloremic and high anion-gap acidosis are deeply impaired in the presence of ARF, these patients usually do need to receive exogenous alkali therapy in order to maintain HCO_3^- at an acceptable level.[110]

ARF-induced moderate acidosis with normal AG can be managed by oral sodium bicarbonate (if one assumes the existence of a bicarbonate volume of distribution of 50% of the body weight) to maintain serum bicarbonate between 20 and 22 mEq/L and pH over 7.20.[110, 111] Adequate amounts of nonprotein calories should be given in order to decrease catabolism. Renal bicarbonaturia induced by acetazolamide use or intestinal waste of HCO_3^- by diarrhea or laxative administration should be prevented. Excessive intake of acid radicals through parenteral nutrition or free ECF

TABLE 12–8. Main Systemic and Metabolic Features of Severe Acidosis

Kussmaul respiration (potential for muscle fatigue)
Nausea and vomiting
Abdominal pain
Body ache
Fatigue
Headache, lethargy, stupor, and coma
Decreased myocardial contractility ⎫
Peripheral arteriolar vasodilation and ⎬ Heart failure
  venous vasoconstriction ⎪
Increased pulmonary vascular resistance ⎪
Centralization of blood volume ⎭
Cardiac arrhythmias
Resistance to vasopressor drugs
Hyperkalemia, hyperphosphatemia, and hyperuricemia leukocytosis
Insulin resistance (hyperglycemia)
Hypercatabolism
Inhibition of anaerobic glycolysis and decrease in ATP synthesis

expansion with bicarbonate free isotonic saline should be avoided.[111]

Severe metabolic acidosis (defined as pH ≤ 7.10) in an ARF patient should be treated with intravenous $NaHCO_3$. Acidosis of this magnitude can cause severe derangements in enzymatic cellular mechanisms, resistance to the effects of vasopressor drugs, myocardial depression, and ominous arrhythmias, and the use of intravenous $NaHCO_3$ removes the immediate danger of death.[111, 115, 118] The amount of bicarbonate to be given can be estimated with the use of the following formula (using 70% as the space of distribution for HCO_3^- in severe metabolic acidosis) and should be enough to raise serum bicarbonate over 10 mEq/L and systemic pH to 7.20[108, 115]:

$$NaHCO_3 \text{ required (mEq/L)} = \text{Body weight (kg)} \times 0.7 \times (\text{Desired } [HCO_3^-] - \text{Current } [HCO_3^-])$$

Worsening of acidosis extends the binding of H^+ to intracellular proteins and consequently the bicarbonate apparent space of distribution also increases, which ultimately means that more infusion of bicarbonate is needed in order to raise serum HCO_3^-.[108, 111, 115] Administration of sodium bicarbonate is far from being an innocuous therapy. It can cause significant volume overload, hypernatremia, worsening of lactic acidosis, and life-threatening decreases of ionized calcium.[108, 111, 115, 119] Sodium bicarbonate therapy also augments CO_2 production and consequently raises ICF and ECF partial pressure of carbon dioxide (P_{CO_2}), an obviously undesirable effect.[108, 115] Before sodium bicarbonate is given, the serum calcium level must always be checked and corrected, if necessary, electrolytes must be monitored, and minute ventilation must be adjusted in patients on mechanical respiration in order to compensate for P_{CO_2} elevation.[108, 111] The risks of sodium bicarbonate therapy have spurred the search for other effective and safer buffering agents. Carbicarb, a mixture of 1:1 of $NaHCO_3$ and Na_2CO_3 is an attractive buffer alternative for metabolic acidosis because it does not produce the increase in P_{CO_2} observed with the use of sodium bicarbonate. However, clinical experience with this drug is still limited, and the risks of hypervolemia and hypertonicity associated with its use are similar to those observed with $NaHCO_3$.[115, 119, 120] THAM, a sodium-free solution of 0.3N tromethamine, is a CO_2-consuming buffer that can be used in both metabolic and respiratory acidosis. Although the fact that it is sodium free and limits CO_2 formation makes it potentially very appropriate, results with its use were not better than results with $NaHCO_3$, and it actually was associated with some severe adverse effects, such as hyperkalemia, hypoglycemia, ventilatory depression, local injury associated with solution extravasation, and liver necrosis in neonates.[115]

Besides sodium bicarbonate infusion, some basic and general procedures are obligatory in the treatment of severe metabolic acidosis. The patient has to have a proper airway in order to be able to hyperventilate. Optimization of blood flow rate to vital organs and tissue oxygen delivery is necessary. Other causes of acidosis occurring concomitantly with ARF have to be ruled out (eg, methanol, salicylate intoxication, and lactic acidosis), and if present, they must be specifically treated. If the patient is on mechanical respiration, the ventilation rate should be increased in order to decrease P_{CO_2}. Similarly, drugs that depress the respiratory system should be avoided.[108, 110, 111]

Severe acidosis in oliguric ARF, acidosis in hemodynamically unstable ARF patients requiring vasoactive drug support, or acidosis characterized by an increasing demand for intravenous bicarbonate to maintain acceptable serum HCO_3^- levels is better controlled by dialytic therapy. Hemodialysis is far more efficient than peritoneal dialysis in controlling ARF-related acidosis. Besides an increase in pH and bicarbonate levels, hemodialysis is also effective for the correction of changes in calcium and potassium levels, commonly associated with severe acidosis. The use of acetate as a buffer in dialysis baths is now very unusual and is totally contraindicated in ARF because of its adverse effects on ventilation, the cardiovascular system, and biocompatibility. Critically ill, hemodynamically unstable, or vasopressor drug–dependent patients should be preferentially treated with continuous renal replacement therapy (CRRT) methods, as slow, continuous hemodialysis or venovenous hemofiltration. The dialysates and replacement fluids for CRRT generally use lactate as a buffer, because of its greater stability compared with bicarbonate. In fact, the latter precipitates as an insoluble salt when sterilized with calcium or magnesium. Usually, lactate-buffered solutions are well tolerated and as effective as bicarbonate-buffered substitution solutions for acidemia control. However, patients with severe multiple organ failure, lactic acidosis, or liver failure can have difficulties in metabolizing lactate. In such patients, the use of bicarbonate as a buffer in dialysate and replacement solutions is advisable.[52, 53, 108, 121–123]

CALCIUM, PHOSPHORUS, AND MAGNESIUM ABNORMALITIES

ARF-related divalent ion homeostatic changes occur in most patients soon after renal injury and are especially frequent in oliguric patients. ARF patients are usually hypocalcemic, hyperphosphatemic, and hypermagnesemic, but, depending on the comorbid disease or ARF etiology, or both, hypercalcemia, metastatic calcifications, hypophosphatemia, and hypomagnesemia can occur.

Hypocalcemia

Calcium balance is maintained by the interplay of the gastrointestinal tract, the kidneys, and bone turnover. The fine regulation of serum calcium is mostly dependent on parathyroid hormone (PTH) and 1,25-dihydroxycholecalciferol ($[1,25-(OH_2)D_3]$). Despite the fact that hypocalcemia is commonly found in ARF, it is rarely symptomatic or severe enough to require

treatment. The etiopathogenesis of this disorder in ARF is not totally understood, and it is has been related to increased serum phosphate levels caused by reduced GFR, skeletal resistance to PTH, decreased synthesis of 1,25-$(OH_2)D_3$, and deposition of calcium in injured tissue.[124] The combination of retained phosphate with calcium would be the most direct explanation for serum calcium reduction in ARF. However, the occurrence of a significant calcium decrease in the presence of normal serum phosphate level has been described in ARF patients.[125, 126] Although an early increase in PTH levels has been consistently described in ARF, skeletal resistance to the hormone action blunts serum calcium elevation.[126–128] Altered vitamin D metabolism caused by tubular lesions and worsened by hyperphosphatemia and acidosis is also considered an important factor for serum calcium depression. Decreased levels of 1,25-$(OH)_2D_3$ impair calcium bone mobilization and calcium intestinal absorption.[124, 126, 129] Significant tissue calcium deposition can contribute to decreased serum calcium levels, particularly in rhabdomyolysis-induced ARF.[130–135] Indeed, muscle calcium sequestration associated with rhabdomyolysis has been described even in the absence of renal failure.[130] The use of blood derivatives or CRRT with citrate anticoagulation potentiates hypocalcemia in ARF patients because of the calcium chelation caused by sodium citrate, especially in patients with liver disease who may have impaired hepatic metabolism of citrate.[136–138] Similarly, sodium bicarbonate infusion can induce an acute decrease in serum calcium and consequent tetany. A decrease in serum calcium can potentiate hyperkalemia-induced arrhythmias and cause prolongations of the QT interval and nonspecific T-wave changes on the ECG. Hypocalcemia associated with rhabdomyolysis or pancreatitis can be particularly severe,[131, 139] even though neuromuscular irritability and seizures are unusual in ARF patients, probably because acidosis counterbalances calcium effects on neuromuscular excitability.[124] ARF-related hypocalcemia should be cautiously treated only if clear symptoms are present. Inadequate calcium supplementation or high calcium levels in dialysate or replacement fluid for CRRT can enhance metastatic calcifications, induce or worsen late hypercalcemia during ARF recovery, and be harmful for ATN recovery.[107, 124, 132, 140, 141]

Hypercalcemia

Hypercalcemia is unusual in the early phases of ARF. When present, it is indicative of comorbid diseases such as myeloma, lymphoma, leukemia and other tumors, sarcoidosis, or milk-alkali syndrome.[142–147] It can cause hypertension and intensify the vasoconstriction and tubular injury frequently found in ARF.[141, 148, 149] Significant hypercalcemia can be seen in about 30% of the patients during the diuretic recovery phase of ARF-induced rhabdomyolysis.[150] This electrolyte disorder has been attributed to mobilization of $CaPO_4$ accumulated in damaged tissue, to an increase in calcitriol levels (note that low calcitriol levels have also been reported), and, more inconsistently, to a return of bone response to high serum levels of PTH.[130, 131, 135, 150]

Hyperphosphatemia

Approximately 80% of total body phosphorus is present in bone mineral, 19% in the intracellular space, and only 1% in the ECF. Hyperphosphatemia is almost invariably seen in ARF patients, but rarely are phosphate levels higher than 8 mg/dL.[124] The causal mechanisms for serum phosphate increase in ARF are impaired renal excretion, release from injured tissue, and ICF-to-ECF shifts caused by acute acidosis and hypercatabolism. When severe hyperphosphatemia occurs in an ARF patient, there is a high possibility that active tissue necrosis is taking place. Very elevated levels of phosphate have been reported in tumor lysis syndrome, rhabdomyolysis, bowel ischemia, malignant hyperthermia, and hemolysis.[151–155] An unusual cause of severe ARF-related hyperphosphatemia recently reported is the use of phosphate-containing bowel-cleansing preparations.[156–158] Hyperphosphatemia may contribute to the increased PTH levels seen in ARF, probably through the direct stimulation of PTH release by phosphorus.[159] Phosphate also inhibits renal 1α-hydroxylase activity, decreasing generation of 1,25-$(OH_2)D_3$, and thus contributing to the hypocalcemia found in ARF.[154] Calcium X phosphate product exceeding 70 may cause metastatic calcifications in soft tissues, lowering serum calcium levels even more.[154] The best way to treat or prevent hyperphosphatemia is the use of intestinal phosphate binding salts. In ARF patients, treatment should be done with calcium carbonate 0.5 to 1.0 g with meals. If calcium X phosphate product is high, aluminum hydroxide, 15 to 30 mL with meals, can be used alternatively.[15] Magnesium-containing binding salts should be avoided in ARF patients.

Hypophosphatemia

Hypophosphatemia is infrequently found in ARF patients. It is related to burns, alcoholism, hyperalimentation, and inadequate reposition in CRRT, or with tubular injury induced by nephrotoxic drugs such as aminoglycoside, cisplatin, ifosfamide, and foscarnet.[107, 160–165] Usually, as renal failure progresses, phosphate levels increase to normal or supranormal values. The need for replacement therapy is very rare, but when it is necessary, the oral route is preferred, if possible.

Hypermagnesemia

Magnesium is the most abundant intracellular divalent cation, and most of the 2000 mg of total body magnesium is located in bone and soft tissues. Mild asymptomatic hypermagnesemia is commonly found in ARF patients and can be exacerbated by magnesium-containing cathartics or antacids. Hypermagnesemia can lead to hypocalcemia. When severe (levels > 5 mg/dL), hypocalcemia may induce nausea, hypotension, bradycardia, ECG changes (increases in PR, QRS, and QT intervals), respiratory depression, neurologic abnormalities (somnolence and lethargy), and even complete heart block and cardiac arrest. Treatment of mild to moderate asymptomatic hypermagnesemia consists of avoiding magnesium intake. Severe or symptomatic hypermagnesemia should be corrected by hemodialysis. As in hyperkalemia, palliative treatment with calcium and glucose or insulin intravenously should be carried out unless dialysis is needed in order to avoid life-threatening arrhythmias.[154, 166, 167]

Hypomagnesemia

Hypomagnesemia, normally asymptomatic, may occur in ARF caused by or existing concomitantly with the intake of drugs that affect tubular transport of magnesium, such as cisplatin,[168–170] amphotericin,[171, 172] aminoglycosides,[173, 174] cyclosporine,[175, 176] tacrolimus,[176, 177] foscarnet,[161] and pentamidine.[178] It may also be associated with ARF in alcoholic or malnourished patients.[179, 180] The clinical picture may include neuromuscular irritability (tremor, cramps, seizures), muscular weakness, ECG abnormalities (prolonged PR and QT intervals), ventricular and supraventricular arrhythmias, and resistant hypokalemia or hypocalcemia.[154, 167, 169, 180, 181]

ANEMIA

Anemia in the absence of hemorrhage or hemolytic diseases has been recognized as a frequent complication of ARF syndrome for a long time.[182] It has a high prevalence, ranging from 65% (hematocrit [Hct] < 12.0 g/L, see Table 12–1) to 95% (Hct < 35) or 77% (Hct < 30).[5, 183] ARF-induced anemia was described as more pronounced in oliguric than in nonoliguric patients.[183]

A decreased Hct level occurs a few days after renal dysfunction, reaches a nadir in about 10 to 14 days, and only recovers late, that is, weeks after normalization of renal function.[184–188] Experimental studies demonstrated that hemoglobin and Hct can decrease as early as 2 to 48 hours after ARF induction.[189, 190] Characteristically, ARF-associated anemia is normochromic-normocytic, there is no iron deficiency, ferritin serum levels are normal or even increased, and peripheral reticulocytes do not increase significantly.[184, 187, 188, 191] The bone marrow demonstrates normal cellularity or is slightly hypercellular.[184]

The mechanisms behind hemodilution and subclinical or iatrogenic hemorrhagic losses that cause the initial and rapid fall in Hct are not totally understood. Increased erythrocyte fragility, putatively due to a "uremic" environment, has already been demonstrated[184, 192] and can account for the increased rate of red blood cell destruction.[189] Assessment of heme biosynthesis disclosed abnormalities that did not explain the early anemia development.[190] On the other hand, a robust body of evidence strongly suggests that the sustained anemia and the lack of compensatory reticulocytosis seen in established and recovery ARF phases are due to inappropriate levels of serum erythropoietin (EPO). In fact, it has been consistently shown that EPO levels are low or in the normal range despite the presence of significant anemia in clinical or experimental ARF, and that adequate EPO levels are achieved only weeks after normalization of renal function.[185–189, 192–195] This low EPO serum level is caused by decreased synthesis, but not by increased EPO catabolism.[187, 188] Recently, an elegant experimental study evaluated the role of EPO in ARF-induced anemia, using the renal artery occlusion model. The authors induced left kidney ischemia and preserved the contralateral kidney. The injured kidney lost the sensitivity of EPO response to blood oxygen availability, and the normal contralateral kidney and liver did not increase EPO levels in response to anemia.[189] It is important to point out that EPO response is also blunted in critically ill patients without ARF, arguing against the uremic milieu as the only factor generating dysfunction of EPO production.[196] Finally, although PTH has been incriminated in the pathogenesis of CRF-induced anemia, no correlation was found between PTH and EPO levels in ARF.[193]

A sudden drop in hemoglobin level in an ARF population composed mostly of critically ill individuals with comorbid cardiovascular disease can bring serious consequences. ARF-induced anemia can cause or exacerbate heart failure and symptomatic coronary disease, cause central nervous system symptoms, impair oxygenation, prevent weaning of the patient from mechanical ventilation, impair wound healing, and worsen bleeding tendency.[184, 197] It may also aggravate renal ischemic injury and hamper tubular regeneration, resulting from tissue hypoxia, abnormal regional hemodynamics, increased lipid peroxidation, and free radical generation.[198] Thus, in order to prevent these complications, it is advisable to maintain hemoglobin at levels greater than 10 to 11 g/L in this patient group.[199, 200] Iatrogenic losses caused by dialysis or by excessive blood sampling for laboratory examinations should be avoided. Iron stores should be checked and restored if necessary. The use of drugs affecting hemoglobin synthesis as angiotensin-converting enzyme inhibitors and angiotensin II receptor blockers should be discontinued.[201, 202] Blood transfusions should be administered as necessary. However, because transfusion therapy is expensive and not free from risks, the use of exogenous recombinant human EPO has been considered an appealing alternative. Erythropoietin administration increased red blood cell count and hemoglobin levels in experimental gentamicin-induced and cisplatin-induced ARF.[192, 195, 198] Moreover, EPO enhanced renal functional and tubular recovery after experimental cisplatin-induced ARF.[198] The role of parenteral EPO in clinical ARF is less clear, with some reports of positive erythropoietic response in ARF-induced anemia after ATN, acute crescentic glomeru-lonephritis, and total bilateral renal cortical necrosis.[187, 188]

In order to assess the role of EPO in the correction of ARF-related anemia, the authors performed a pilot study with 10 ARF patients whose serum creatinine (SCr) was greater than 5 mg/dL and whose serum hemoglobin was less than 10 g/L (or Hct level < 30%). The treated group (five patients) received EPO, 100 U/kg IV three times a week, and the control group (five patients) received only the same volume of saline intravenously. Both groups received as many blood transfusions as necessary, with a target hemoglobin level of at least 10 g/L. Although the mean number of blood transfusions were similar in the two groups (2.6 vs 2.8 transfusions), the patients treated with EPO reached a significantly higher hemoglobin level compared to baseline, whereas control patients did not. These results are shown in Figure 12–3. There were no EPO-related adverse effects.

BLEEDING DISORDERS

Advanced renal dysfunction induces a hemorrhagic diathesis in which the basic abnormality is a platelet qualitative dysfunction. If there are no comorbid diseases that are consuming platelets, the platelet count is usually normal or in the low normal range.[203, 204] Most of the studies that assessed the mechanisms of the renal failure–associated bleeding tendency were performed in CRF patients. Several biochemical and functional abnormalities were described in platelets during uremia, such as decreased availability of platelet factor 3; decreased intracellular platelet content of ADP, ATP, ATPase, β-thromboglobulin, platelet factor 4, and serotonin; increased activity of adenylate cyclase; increased content of cAMP; impaired function of membrane glycoprotein IIb–IIIa; impaired platelet-endothelium adhesion; reduced aggregation after appropriated stimulus; and inadequate release reaction.[203–207] Because dialysis improves substantially and

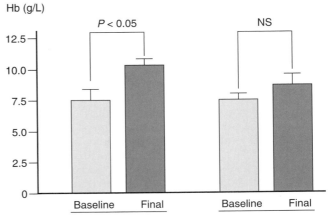

FIGURE 12–3 ■ Effects of exogenous recombinant erythropoietin administration plus blood transfusion (n = 5) vs. blood transfusion alone (n = 5) in ARF-induced anemia. *NS*, not significant.

renal transplantation totally corrects renal failure–acquired platelet dysfunction, it has been suggested that accumulation of yet unknown "uremic toxins" is responsible for the majority of changes observed. In fact, incubation of normal platelets with uremic plasma results in decreased aggregation, and incubation of platelets from uremic patients with normal plasma induces partial recovery of aggregation capacity. Some of the candidates for this toxin are urea, creatinine, phenols, and guanidinosuccinic acid.[203, 204, 208] Another important factor related to bleeding diathesis in ARF is anemia. The effect of red blood cells is mediated by the release of platelet agonist and ADP and by rheologic changes influencing platelet movement to the vessel wall.[203, 204] Correction of anemia by EPO in CRF improved platelet function.[209] Other possible determinants of platelet dysfunction in uremia are increased endothelial production of nitric oxide and prostaglandin I_2, abnormalities in von Willebrand factor, and increased serum PTH.[203, 204, 207, 210] Besides the bleeding dysfunction related to uremia, patients with ARF frequently have additional hemostatic defects caused by comorbid diseases causing platelet dysfunction and thrombocytopenia (eg, hemolytic-uremic syndrome, thrombotic thrombocytopenic purpura, HELLP syndrome, sepsis, and systemic inflammatory response syndrome), massive transfusion, blood exposure to artificial surfaces (eg, cardiopulmonary bypass, dialysis), liver disease, and use of drugs (eg, β-lactam antibiotics, nonsteroidal anti-inflammatory drugs, aspirin, and heparin).[203, 204]

The most sensitive test result for the diagnosis of uremia-induced platelet dysfunction is an increased bleeding time.[203, 205] It has a better correlation with hemorrhagic complications than with BUN level, creatinine level, or in vitro platelet aggregation tests.[205] The clinical consequences of the abnormal platelet homeostasis in ARF may range from mild mucous membrane, skin, and wound bleeding to life-threatening hemorrhages, especially in the gastrointestinal tract.[205]

Dialytic Treatment of Bleeding Disorders

The best way of preventing or reducing hemorrhagic complications in ARF patients is the performance of optimal dialysis therapy (in terms of efficiency and amount), a task that is not always easy to accomplish.[203–205] Moreover, anticoagulation for hemodialysis may start or intensify bleeding and induce thrombocytopenia.[205, 211–214] Several approaches to overcoming this limitation can be found in recent reviews.[211, 215, 216] The use of peritoneal dialysis was demonstrated as a suitable alternative for some patients.[217] Efficient hemodialysis without anticoagulant can be done with high blood flow and 200 mL of saline to flush the filter every 20 minutes.[215, 218] Priming of the circuit with 2 L of saline containing 20,000 U of heparin for 1 to 4 hours before the beginning of treatment, followed by low doses of heparin (20 U/kg/h) with bedside coagulation monitoring, is another possible

maneuver.[211, 215, 219] Regional citrate anticoagulation is probably the method associated with the lowest risk of bleeding.[211, 220] However, it requires a special low-sodium and alkali- and calcium-free dialysate and intravenous calcium infusion. Moreover, special care is necessary for the avoidance of hypocalcemia or hypercalcemia, hypernatremia, and metabolic alkalosis.[211, 215, 221, 222] Prostacyclin is a potent inhibitor of platelet aggregation, with a short half-life, but it can cause significant hypotension, making it inadequate for critically ill patients. Furthermore, its effect on platelets is difficult to monitor, it may still persist up to 2 hours after stopping infusion, with no known way of reversing it, and the drug is expensive.[211, 215] Low-molecular-weight heparin causes less thrombocytopenia than does regular heparin,[223] but it has a prolonged half-life (18 hours) and is not neutralized by protamine. Regional heparinization with the use of heparin and protamine is no longer favored, because heparin rebound can occur up to 10 hours after dialysis.[211, 215] Nafamostat mesilate and r-hirudin[222, 224–226] are new alternatives, but more clinical experience is needed with them.

Nondialytic Treatment of Bleeding Disorders

Anemia must be corrected until Hct is greater than or equal to 30%, because of its strong influence on bleeding. Drugs that impair platelet homeostasis should be avoided. Desmopressin acetate (1-deamino-8-D-arginine vasopressin, DDAVP), conjugated estrogen, and cryoprecipitate can be used as ancillary or palliative measures for correcting the bleeding tendency, probably acting on von Willebrand factor.[15, 203–205, 227]

DDAVP should be used in doses of 0.3 to 0.4 μg/kg. The drug should be diluted in 50 to 100 mL of saline and infused IV over 15 to 30 minutes. It has a fast effect (less than 1 hour) that persists for 4 to 24 hours. If necessary the initial load can be repeated 1 to 2 times, with an interval from 6 to 12 hours. Its continued use is associated with tachyphylaxis.[15, 203, 205] Potential side effects of DDAVP are facial flushing, headache, tachycardia, and a decrease in systolic blood pressure. Usually, these effects are mild and transitory and do not occur if doses of 0.3 μg/kg are infused over 30 minutes.[228] Conjugated estrogens have a more long-lasting action (about 2 to 4 weeks). The onset of action occurs in about 6 hours but takes several days (up to 5) to be effective. Conjugated estrogens should be administered intravenously in a dose of 25 mg; their main side effects are liver failure and hypertension.[15, 203, 205, 229] Cryoprecipitate should be administered intravenously in a dosage of 10 U. It has a peak effect from 1 to 12 hours after administration, and its action vanishes after 24 to 36 hours.[15, 203, 205]

Gastrointestinal bleeding is an especially severe bleeding complication associated with significant mortality in ARF patients. Gastroduodenal mucous protection can be accomplished with the use of aluminum hydroxide or sucralfate PO (15 to 60 mL 4 to 6 times per day) or the use of an H_2-receptor antagonist, such as ranitidine (150 mg PO or 50 mg IV once a day).[15, 230] The use of proton pump blockers in gastrointestinal bleeding is still a matter of study, but a recent paper showed a positive result with omeprazole (initial dose 40 mg, followed by another dose of 40 mg 6 to 8 hours later, and then 20 mg daily).[231] In high-risk patients, early prophylactic dialysis should be strongly considered.[15]

Recommendations for the prevention and treatment of uremic bleeding diathesis are summarized in Table 12–9.

INFECTIOUS COMPLICATIONS

Infection has been considered a usual complication and a most important cause of death for ARF patients in most of the series published from 1953 to the present.[182, 232–235] In a recent survey of 879 ARF cases in a tertiary hospital, 79% of the patients had infection at some point in their clinical course (Ávila and Burdmann, unpublished results). Clearly, breakdown of mucocutaneous barriers after trauma or surgery and invasive procedures, such as the placement of intravenous lines, or tracheal tubes, and bladder catheterization, account, in great part, for this complication. Development of malnutrition or a low nutritional status at the beginning of an ARF episode is another important factor that predisposes to infection.[236, 237] However, the uremic environment itself has also been identified as inducing an immunosuppressive state.[238–240] Again, most of the studies were performed in CRF patients. Polymorphonuclear leukocyte (PMNL) dysfunction has been consistently shown in uremic patients. Impaired PMNL chemotaxis, oxidative metabolism, phagocyte activity, degranulation, intracellular killing, and carbohydrate metabolism have been reported.[241–244] Published results indicate that uremic neutrophils undergo accelerated apoptosis in vitro and that uremic plasma induces accelerated apoptosis in normal neutrophils, causing a dysfunctional pattern similar to that found in uremia.[245] The presence of low- and high-molecular-weight inhibitors such as granulocyte inhibitory proteins and PMNL chemotactic movement inhibitors were confirmed in blood and peritoneal fluid from uremic patients.[243, 244, 246–248] Similarly, changes in complement activation, T-cell function, expression of adhesion molecules, and production of cytocrines have been observed.[243, 249, 250] There is also strong clinical evidence of deficient behavior of T lymphocytes and impaired specific antibody responses in uremic patients.[237] The use of activating-complement membranes in hemodialysis has also been incriminated as a potential cause of PMNL malfunction and an increased rate of infections in advanced renal failure.[243, 251–253]

The most usual sites of infection are the respiratory tract, surgical or post-trauma wounds, the urinary tract, intravascular catheter sites, and the peritoneum. The best procedure available for ARF-associated infection is prevention. A possible infection focus should be meticulously scrutinized when the patient arrives, including sinuses, oral cavity, upper and lower respiratory tract, heart valves, abdomen, urogenital tract, and skin. Urine catheters should be placed only if really necessary, and should be removed as soon as the patient is able to void. Respiratory physiotherapy should be done in patients susceptible to respiratory infections. Intravenous catheters used for dialysis require extraordinarily special care in ARF patients, and curatives must be administered under rigorous aseptic technique. If fever, chills, or other signs and symptoms of infection develop and no evident focus is found, the withdrawal of the intravascular dialysis catheter should be strongly considered. Prophylactic antibiotics are useless and probably dangerous in ARF. Early detection of infection and conscious antibiotic therapy are crucial for improvement of the outcome of these patients. Prolonged antibiotic use may cause superinfection with resistant bacteria or opportunistic agents, such as *Candida*. Nephrotoxic drugs should be avoided when possible.

NUTRITION

ARF is associated with significant catabolism.[13, 14] Moreover, many times these patients are already malnourished when renal dysfunction occurs.[237] This extremely important issue is discussed in Chapter 37.

HORMONAL CHANGES

It has been well established that the presence of renal failure affects several hormonal pathways. The majority of studies exploring this issue were carried out in the setting of CRF, and there is little information about ARF-related hormonal dysfunction. Changes in PTH and EPO regulation were discussed early in this chapter. Some information about glucagon, insulin, plasma renin activity (PRA) and aldosterone, thyroid

TABLE 12–9. Measures for Prevention and Correction of Uremic-Related Bleeding Disorders in ARF Patients

1. Correct anemia. Keep hematocrit level >30%.
2. Avoid use of drugs that impair platelet homeostasis (eg, aspirin, NSAIDs, beta-lactam antibiotics).
3. DDAVP: Use 0.3 to 0.4 µg/kg IV in 50–100 mL of saline. Infuse over 15 to 30 min. Repeat 1 to 2 times after 6 to 12 h, if necessary. Effect starts in 1 h and persists for 4 to 24 hours. It can induce tachyphylaxis.
4. Conjugated estrogens (eg, Premarin [Wyeth-Ayerst]): Use 25 mg IV. Repeat after 6 to 12 h, if necessary. It may be effective only after some days, effect persists for 2 to 4 wk. It may cause hypertension and liver failure.
5. Cryoprecipitate: Use 10 U IV. Effect peaks between 1 and 12 h and ends after 24 to 36 h.
6. Protect gastrointestinal tract: aluminum hydroxide or sucralfate, 15 to 60 mL every 4 to 6 h or ranitidine, 150 mg PO or 50 mg IV once a day.
7. In high-risk or bleeding patients: start dialytic therapy.

hormones, and sexual hormones is presented in the paragraphs that follow (Table 12–10).

Glucose Intolerance, Glucagon, and Insulin

Glucose intolerance is an acknowledged complication of ARF. The role of glucagon and the liver in the pathogenesis of this dysfunction has been explored, with conflicting results. Proglucagon products and glucagon are elevated in plasma from uremic patients and in experimental ARF.[254–256] Enhanced hepatic amino acid uptake, urea synthesis, and gluconeogenesis have been described in experimental ARF,[257, 258] but decreased liver glycogen synthesis has been reported as well.[259] ARF-induced gluconeogenesis was reversed by the administration of RU 38486, an antiglucocorticoid compound, suggesting that glucocorticoids have an important role in the altered hepatic production of urea and glucose in acute uremia.[260] Finally, hepatic glucose output has been reported as increased,[257, 261] normal,[262] or decreased,[263–265] and glucagon-induced glycemic response as either decreased[263, 264] or increased in uremia.[261]

On the other hand, a well-documented status of early resistance to insulin certainly contributes to carbohydrate intolerance in ARF.[264, 265] Consistent experimental data indicate the skeletal muscle as the primary site of ARF-induced insulin peripheral resistance.[124, 266] Muscle glucose uptake, glycogen synthesis, and protein turnover are impaired, whereas glycolysis and glucose oxidation are normal.[124, 255, 264, 265, 267–271] The defect apparently is located after the insulin-binding receptor.[124, 262, 269, 272] Glucose intolerance, insulin sensitivity, and glycemic response to glucagon improved after dialysis, suggesting that a factor present in the uremic blood is responsible for the abnormal carbohydrate metabolism.[124]

Plasma Renin Activity and Aldosterone

ARF patients usually present with a high plasma renin activity (PRA) level, even in the presence of volume overload, and normal or moderately elevated levels of serum aldosterone and normal serum cortisol levels.[273–278] Aldosterone levels do not correlate with PRA, angiotensin II, or serum potassium levels.[124, 275] This dissociation between PRA and aldosterone might be caused by an increased release of atrial natriuretic factor, inhibiting the expected increase in aldosterone

after angiotensin II stimulation or by impaired feedback between those two hormones.[60, 124]

Thyroid Hormones

Decreased levels of free and total triiodothyronine (T_3) and thyroxine (T_4) have been observed in the early phase of clinical or experimental ARF.[279–283] These hormone levels correlated negatively with SCr.[279, 282] Plasma thyroid stimulating hormone (TSH) levels were normal, and there were no clinical signs or symptoms of hypothyroidism.[279, 282, 283] Decreased T_3 levels have also been reported in renal transplant recipients with delayed graft function due to ATN or acute rejection.[284] The mechanisms of these changes in thyroid function are not clear yet. Patients suffering from exertional heat stroke with or without ARF showed a decrease in T_3, T_4, and free T_4 that normalized after recovery, suggesting a role for stress in thyroid dysfunction, although a negative correlation was demonstrated between SCr and T_4.[280, 282] Recently, low plasma selenium levels paralleling thyroid hormone concentration were found in CRF and ARF. Selenium is important for thyroid function; thus, it is possible that selenium deficiency plays a role in ARF-induced changes in T_3 and T_4.[283] Although the administration of thyroid hormone showed beneficial effects in experimental ARF,[285, 286] there is not enough evidence to support its use in clinical ARF at the moment.

Sex Hormones

Renal failure has been associated with disturbances of the hypothalamic-pituitary-gonadal (HPG) axis[287] that can also occur early in ARF. A marked decrease in serum testosterone levels and increased concentrations of prolactin have been observed in the oliguric phase of clinical ARF[288, 289] or after 3 days in an ARF experimental model.[290] There is an abnormal response of follicle-stimulating hormone (FSH), luteinizing hormone (LH), prolactin, estradiol, and testosterone to exogenous administration of gonadotropin-releasing hormone (GnRH) and thyrotropin-releasing hormone (TRH).[124, 288, 289] Normal or elevated levels of LH and decreased or normal levels of FSH have been reported.[288, 289] Both free and total testosterone are decreased with normal function of binding proteins, suggesting that the problem is due to reduced production or release by the testes.[124, 289] The mechanisms of an ARF-induced decrease in testosterone level have been related to hyporesponsiveness of Leydig cells to LH and to increased PTH levels.[124, 288, 289] In fact a direct correlation between prolactin and PTH has already been demonstrated in ARF patients.[289] Infusion of exogenous PTH increased prolactin in healthy volunteers,[291] and prior parathyroidectomy prevented testosterone decrease in a model of ARF.[290] This latter study also showed that acute uremia increased calcium levels in the hypothalamus, pituitary glands, and testes of animals.[290] All of the abnormalities just described in

---

TABLE 12–10. Hormonal Abnormalities in ARF

Increased parathyroid hormone
Inadequate erythropoietin levels
Increased glucagon
Peripheral insulin resistance
Increased plasma renin activity and aldosterone
Decreased T_3 and T_4
Decreased testosterone

the HPG axis normalize with recovery of renal function.[124] A recent study carried out in experimental CRF found elevated levels of 17α-hydroxy progesterone and androstenedione and low levels of testosterone, providing evidences that gonadal dysfunction in uremia may be related to 17β-hydroxysteroid oxidoreductase activity.[292] Finally, it is interesting to note that orchiectomy-induced decreases in LH and testosterone prevented renal dysfunction in the mercury-chloride ARF model, suggesting that hypogonadism may be a defensive mechanism in ARF.[293]

OTHER METABOLIC AND ELECTROLYTE DISTURBANCES

Hypokalemia

Occasionally, hypokalemia can be seen in the early phase of ARF. This may occur in nephrotoxic injury caused by aminoglycoside,[294] cisplatin,[295, 296] or amphotericin[172, 297] or in leptospirosis-induced ARF.[60, 298] If potassium levels are significantly low, a cautious correction should be done in order to avoid cardiac arrhythmias and worsening of tubular injury.[299–301] Usually, potassium retention and increased potassium levels develop as GFR decreases further.

Hyperuricemia

The main routes of elimination of uric acid are via glomerular filtration and proximal tubular cell secretion. Usually, ARF patients develop asymptomatic elevations of serum uric acid levels that do not exceed 10 mg/dL. Severe hyperuricemia in ARF is indicative of tumor lysis syndrome, rhabdomyolysis, or some other causes of rapid nucleic acid turnover or tissue destruction.[302–304] In this situation, the combination of acidosis and overproduction of uric acid may precipitate intrarenal urate, mainly in the distal tubules, collecting ducts, and renal pelvis, aggravating renal dysfunction. Adequate hydration and careful systemic alkalinization should be done in order to prevent this disorder. As an initial approach, oral bicarbonate or the addition of 50 mEq of sodium bicarbonate to each liter of fluid infused (preferably 0.45% saline) may be tried.[305] However, as previously stated in this chapter, inadequate bicarbonate load can cause or aggravate a decrease in ionized calcium levels. Moreover, if urinary output is not sufficient, volume overload and hypernatremia can result. Use of allopurinol may not prevent hyperuricemia acutely and can be associated with a severe and life-threatening hypersensitivity syndrome characterized by fever, eosinophilia, hepatic failure, severe cutaneous reaction, and acute interstitial nephritis. This syndrome occurred more frequently in patients with increased SCr and is likely caused by allopurinol metabolites.[306] A new and attractive alternative for prevention and treatment of hyperuricemia is the use of recombinant urate oxidase, a naturally occurring proteolytic enzyme that degrades uric acid

to allantoins. Allantoins are also excreted by the kidneys but are many times more soluble than uric acid. Preliminary clinical results confirmed that the drug (SR29142) is highly efficient, but cases of acute hypersensitivity have been reported.[307, 308] Hemodialysis is very effective in uric acid reduction. Six hours of classic intermittent hemodialysis reduces plasma levels of uric acid in 50% of cases. If high-flow, high-efficiency membranes and a blood flow of 300 mL/min are used, the uric acid average clearance is 150 to 230 mL/min, in sharp contrast with the clearance of 15 mL/min obtained in peritoneal dialyses.[305]

Hyperlipidemia

Hypertriglyceridemia may be observed in the early stages of ARF.[309–311] The mechanisms of disturbed lipid metabolism in acute uremia have been ascribed to an increased hepatic triglyceride synthesis,[309] decreased clearance of triglyceride,[312, 313] decreased lipoprotein lipase activity (LPL),[310, 311, 314] impaired lipolysis caused by metabolic acidosis,[315] the presence of an LPL inhibitor in the uremic serum,[316] increased PTH levels,[317] and decreased levels of apoprotein C-II, the most important LPL activator.[318]

Vitamin Deficiencies

Deficiencies in serum levels of fat-soluble vitamins (vitamin A, vitamin D_3, vitamin E) and folate, and elevated serum levels of vitamin K, have been described in ARF patients.[319, 320]

ACKNOWLEDGMENTS

The authors wish to thank Lívia Cais Burdmann for the careful grammar review of this text.

REFERENCES

1. Brady HG, Brenner BM, Lieberthal W: Acute Renal Failure. In: Brenner BM, ed: *The Kidney*. Vol. 2. 5th ed. Philadelphia: WB Saunders; 1996:1200.
2. Short A, Cumming A: Renal support. BMJ 1999; 319:41.
3. Nissenson A: Acute renal failure: definition and pathogenesis. Kidney Int Suppl 1998; 66:S7.
4. Thadhani R, Pascual M, Bonventre JV: Acute renal failure. N Engl J Med 1996; 334:1448.
5. Burdmann EA, Oliveira MB, Ferraboli R, et al: Epidemiologia. In: Schor N, Boim MA, dos Santos OFP, eds: *Insuficiência Renal Aguda: Fisiopatologia, Clínica e Tratamento*. São Paulo: Sarvier; 1997:1.
6. Liaño F, Pascual J: Epidemiology of acute renal failure: a prospective, multicenter, community-based study. The Madrid Acute Renal Failure Study Group. Kidney Int 1996; 50:811.
7. Star RA: Treatment of acute renal failure. Kidney Int 1998; 54:1817.
8. Levy EM, Viscoli CM, Horwitz RI: The effect of acute renal failure on mortality: a cohort analysis. JAMA 1996; 275:1489.
9. Chertow GM, Levy EM, Hammermeister KE, et al: Independent association between acute renal failure and mortality following cardiac surgery. Am J Med 1998; 104:343.

10. Ávila MO, Zanetta DM, Yu ALF, et al: Is diuresis important in acute renal failure mortality? How much is enough? J Am Soc Nephrol 1997; 8:122A.
11. Mehta R, McDonald B, Gabbai F, et al: Indication for dialysis influences outcome from acute renal failure in the ICU: results from a randomized multicenter trial. J Am Soc Nephrol 1997; 8:144A.
12. Bersten AD, Holt AW: Prevention of Acute Renal Failure in the Critically Ill Patient. In: Bellomo R, Ronco C, eds: *Acute Renal Failure in the Critically Ill.* Berlin: Springer-Verlag; 1995: 122.
13. Leverve X, Barnoud D: Stress metabolism and nutritional support in acute renal failure. Kidney Int Suppl 1998; 66:S62.
14. Druml W, Mitch WE: Nutritional Management of Acute Renal Failure. In: Brady HR, Wilcox CS, eds: *Therapy in Nephrology and Hypertension.* Philadelphia, WB Saunders; 1999:65.
15. Barri YM, Shah SV: Prevention and Nondialytic Management of Acute Renal Failure. In: Glassock RJ, ed: *Current Therapy in Nephrology and Hypertension.* 4th ed. St. Louis: Mosby; 1998:240.
16. Wilcox CS: Diuretics. In: Brenner BM, ed: *The Kidney.* Vol. 2. 5th ed. Philadelphia: WB Saunders; 1996:2299.
17. Unwin RJ, Capasso G, Wilcox CS: Therapeutic Use of Diuretics. In: Brady HR, Wilcox CS, eds: *Therapy in Nephrology and Hypertension.* Philadelphia: WB Saunders; 1999: 654.
18. Kellun JA: Use of diuretics in the acute care setting. Kidney Int Suppl 1998; 66:S67.
19. Ritz E, Fliser D, Nowicki M, et al: Treatment with high doses of loop diuretics in chronic renal failure. Nephrol Dial Transplant 1994; 9(suppl 3):40.
20. Ellison DH, Wilcox CS: Diuretic Resistance. In: Brady HR, Wilcox CS, eds: *Therapy in Nephrology and Hypertension.* Philadelphia: WB Saunders; 1999:665.
21. Shimon I, Almog S, Vered Z, et al: Improved left ventricular function after thiamine supplementation in patients with congestive heart failure receiving long-term furosemide therapy. Am J Med 1995; 98:485.
22. Pepersack T, Garbusinsky J, Robberecht J, et al: Clinical relevance of thiamine status among hospitalized elderly patients. Gerontology 1999; 45:96.
23. Suki WN: Use of diuretics in chronic renal failure. Kidney Int Suppl 1997; 59:S33.
24. Rybak LP: Ototoxicity of loop diuretics. Otolaryngol Clin North Am 1993; 26:829.
25. Rybak LP, Whitworth C, Scott V: Furosemide ototoxicity is enhanced in analbuminemic rats. Arch Otolaryngol Head Neck Surg 1993; 119:758
26. Rybak LP: Pathophysiology of furosemide ototoxicity. J Otolaryngol 1982; 11:127.
27. Hendricks WM, Ader RS: Furosemide-induced cutaneous necrotizing vasculitis. Arch Dermatol 1977; 113:375.
28. Thestrup-Pedersen K: Adverse reactions in the skin from antihypertensive drugs. Dan Med Bull 1987; 43(suppl 1):3.
29. Cerottini JP, Ricci C, Guggisberg D, et al: Drug-induced linear IgA bullous dermatosis probably induced by furosemide. J Am Acad Dermatol 1999; 41:103.
30. Stenvinkel P, Alvestrand A: Loop diuretic–induced pancreatitis with rechallenge in a patient with malignant hypertension and renal insufficiency. Acta Med Scand 1988; 224:89.
31. Lankisch PG, Droge M, Gottesleben F: Drug-induced acute pancreatitis: incidence and severity. Gut 1995; 37:565.
32. Wilmink T, Frick TW: Drug-induced pancreatitis. Drug Saf 1996; 14:406.
33. Kelly JP, Kaufman DW, Shapiro S: Risks of agranulocytosis and aplastic anemia in relation to the use of cardiovascular drugs: The International Agranulocytosis and Aplastic Anemia Study. Clin Pharmacol Ther 1991; 49:330.
34. Wiholm BE, Emanuelsson S: Drug-related blood dyscrasias in a Swedish reporting system, 1985–1994. Eur J Haematol 1996; 60(suppl):42.
35. Magil AB: Drug-induced acute interstitial nephritis with granulomas. Hum Pathol 1983; 14:36.
36. Jennings M, Shortland JR, Maddocks JL: Interstitial nephritis associated with frusemide. J R Soc Med 1986; 79:239.
37. Clegg HW, Riopel DA: Furosemide-associated fever. J Pediatr 1995; 126:817.
38. Rudy DW, Voelker JR, Greene PK, et al: Loop diuretics for chronic renal insufficiency: a continuous infusion is more efficacious than bolus therapy. Ann Intern Med 1991; 115:360.
39. Krasna MJ, Scott GE, Scholz PM, et al: Postoperative enhancement of urinary output in patients with acute renal failure using continuous furosemide therapy. Chest 1986; 89:294.
40. Van Meyel JJM, Smits P, Dormans T, et al: Continuous infusion of furosemide in the treatment of patients with congestive heart failure and diuretic resistance. J Intern Med 1994; 235:329.
41. Dormans TP, Van Meyel JJM, Gerlag PG, et al: Diuretic efficacy of high-dose furosemide in severe heart failure: Bolus injection versus continuous infusion. J Am Coll Cardiol 1996; 28:376.
42. Fliser D, Schroter M, Neubeck M, et al: Coadministration of thiazides increases the efficacy of loop diuretics even in patients with advanced renal failure. Kidney Int 1994; 46:482.
43. Knauf H, Mutschler E: Functional state of the nephron and diuretic dose-response—rationale for low-dose combination therapy. Cardiology 1994; 84(suppl 2):18.
44. Lindner A: Synergism of dopamine and furosemide in diuretic-resistant, oliguric acute renal failure. Nephron 1983; 33:121.
45. Denton MD, Chertow GM, Brady HR: "Renal-dose" dopamine for the treatment of acute renal failure: scientific rationale, experimental studies and clinical trials. Kidney Int 1996; 50:4.
46. Inoue M, Okajima K, Itoh K, et al: Mechanism of furosemide resistance in analbuminemic rats and hypoalbuminemic patients. Kidney Int 1987; 32:198.
47. Mattana J, Patel A, Ilunga C, et al: Furosemide-albumin complexes in refractory nephrotic syndrome and chronic renal failure. Nephron 1996; 73:122.
48. Shilliday I, Allison MEM: Diuretics in acute renal failure. Renal Fail 1994; 16:3.
49. Conger JD: Interventions in clinical acute renal failure: what are the data? Am J Kidney Dis 1995; 26:565.
50. Levinsky NG, Bernard DB: Mannitol and Loop Diuretics in Acute Renal Failure. In: Brenner BM, Lazarus JM, eds: *Acute Renal Failure.* 2nd ed. New York: Churchill Livingstone; 1988:841.
51. Shilliday I, Quinn KJ, Allison MEM: Loop diuretics in the management of acute renal failure: a prospective, double-blind, placebo-controlled, randomized study. Nephrol Dial Transplant 1997; 12:2592.
52. Bellomo R, Ronco C: Indications and criteria for initiating renal replacement therapy in the intensive care unit. Kidney Int Suppl 1998; 66:S106.
53. Lameire N, Biesen WV, Vanholder R, et al: The place of intermittent dialysis in the treatment of acute renal failure in the ICU patient. Kidney Int Suppl 1998; 66:S110.
54. Halperin MD, Goldstein MB: Hyponatremia. In: *Fluid, Electrolyte, and Acid-Base Physiology.* 3rd ed. Philadelphia: WB Saunders; 1999:283.
55. Halterman RK, Berl T: Therapy of Dysnatremic Disorders. In: Brady HR, Wilcox CS, eds: *Therapy in Nephrology and Hypertension.* Philadelphia: WB Saunders; 1999:257.
56. Seguro AC, Magaldi AJB, Helou CMB: Distúrbios eletrolíticos no paciente crítico. In: Cruz J, Barros RT, eds: *Atualidades em Nefrologia.* São Paulo: Sarvier; 1996:28.
57. Baek SM, Makabali GG, Brown RS, et al: Free-water clearance patterns as predictors and therapeutic guides in acute renal failure. Surgery 1975; 77:632.
58. Brown R, Babcock R, Talbert J, et al: Renal function in critically ill postoperative patients: sequential assessment of creatinine osmolar and free water clearance. Crit Care Med 1980; 8:68.
59. Berghmans T: Hyponatremia related to medical anticancer treatment. Support Care Cancer 1996; 4:341.
60. Abdulkader RC, Seguro AC, Malheiros PS, et al: Peculiar electrolyte and hormonal abnormalities in acute renal failure due to leptospirosis. Am J Trop Med Hyg 1996; 54:1.
61. Gross P, Reimann D, Neidel J, et al: The treatment of severe hyponatremia. Kidney Int Suppl 1998; 64:S6.
62. Halperin ML, Oh SM: The Dysnatremias: Hyponatremia and Hypernatremia. In: Glassock RJ, ed: *Current Therapy in Nephrology and Hypertension.* 4th ed. St. Louis: Mosby; 1998:1.
63. Berl T: Treating hyponatremia: Damned if we do and damned if we don't. Kidney Int 1990; 37:1006.

64. Verbalis JG: Adaptation to acute and chronic hyponatremia: implications for symptomatology, diagnosis, and therapy. Semin Nephrol 1998; 18:3.

65. Ross EA, Nissenson AR: Acid-base and electrolyte disturbances. In: Daugirdas JT, Ing TS, eds: *Handbook of Dialysis*. 2nd ed. Boston: Little, Brown & Company; 1994:401.

66. Halperin ML, Kamel SK: Potassium. Lancet 1998; 352:135.

67. Kamel SK: The Dyskalemias: Hypokalemia and Hyperkalemia. In: Glassock RJ, ed: *Current Therapy in Nephrology and Hypertension*. 4th ed. St. Louis: Mosby; 1998:9.

68. Kamel SK, Halperin ML: Treatment of Hypokalemia and Hyperkalemia. In: Brady HR, Wilcox CS, eds: *Therapy in Nephrology and Hypertension*. Philadelphia: WB Saunders; 1999:270.

69. Kamel KS, Halperin ML, Faber MD, et al: Disorders of Potassium Balance. In: Brenner BM, ed: *The Kidney*. 5th ed. Vol. 2. Philadelphia: WB Saunders; 1996:999.

70. Halperin MD, Goldstein MB, eds: Potassium Physiology. In: *Fluid, Electrolyte, and Acid-Base Physiology*. 3rd ed. Philadelphia: WB Saunders; 1999:371.

71. Acker CG, Johnson JP, Palevsky PM, et al: Hyperkalemia in hospitalized patients: causes, adequacy of treatment, and results of an attempt to improve physician compliance with published therapy guidelines. Arch Intern Med 1998; 158:917.

72. Shustin L, Wald H, Popovtzer MM: Role of down-regulated CHIF mRNA in the pathophysiology of hyperkalemia of acute tubular necrosis. Am J Kidney Dis 1998; 32:600.

73. Siamopoulos KC, Elisaf M, Katopodis K: Iatrogenic hyperkalemia: points to consider in diagnosis and treatment. Nephrol Dial Transplant 1998; 13:2402.

74. Preston RA, Hirsh MJ, Oster JR, et al: University of Miami Division of Clinical Pharmacology Therapeutic Rounds: drug-induced hyperkalemia. Am J Ther 1998; 5:125.

75. Chiu TF, Bullard MJ, Chen JC, et al: Rapid life-threatening hyperkalemia after addition of amiloride HCl/hydrochlorothiazide to angiotensin-converting enzyme inhibitor therapy. Ann Emerg Med 1997; 30:612.

76. Hansen D: Suxamethonium-induced cardiac arrest and death following 5 days of immobilization. Eur J Anaesthesiol 1998; 15:240.

77. Berkahn JM, Sleigh JW: Hyperkalaemic cardiac arrest following succinylcholine in a long-term intensive care patient. Anaesth Intensive Care 1997; 25:588.

78. Marinella MA: Trimethoprim-sulfamethoxazole associated with hyperkalemia. West J Med 1997; 167:356.

79. Alappan R, Buller GK, Perazella MA: Trimethoprim-sulfamethoxazole therapy in outpatients: is hyperkalemia a significant problem? Am J Nephrol 1999; 19:389.

80. Albareda MM, Corcoy R: Reversible impairment of renal function associated with enalapril in a diabetic patient. CMAJ 1998; 159:1279.

81. Fenton F, Smally AJ, Laut J: Hyperkalemia and digoxin toxicity in a patient with kidney failure. Ann Emerg Med 1996; 28:440.

82. Hottelart C, Achard JM, Moriniere P, et al: Heparin-induced hyperkalemia in chronic hemodialysis patients: comparison of low molecular weight and unfractionated heparin. Artif Organs 1998; 22:614.

83. Brady WJ, Skiles J: Wide QRS complex tachycardia: ECG differential diagnosis. Am J Emerg Med 1999; 17:376.

84. Martinez-Vea A, Bardaji A, Garcia C, et al: Severe hyperkalemia with minimal electrocardiographic manifestations: a report of seven cases. J Electrocardiol 1999; 32:45.

85. Nielsen EH: Hyperkalaemic muscle paresis side-effect of prostaglandin inhibition in a haemodialysis patient. Nephrol Dial Transplant 1999; 14:480.

86. Freeman SJ, Fale AD: Muscular paralysis and ventilatory failure caused by hyperkalaemia. Br J Anaesth 1993; 70:226.

87. Greenberg A: Hyperkalemia: treatment options. Semin Nephrol 1998; 18:46.

88. Halperin MD, Goldstein MB, eds: Hyperkalemia. In: *Fluid, Electrolyte, and Acid-Base Physiology*. 3rd ed. Philadelphia: WB Saunders; 1999:447.

89. Nicolay A, Bertocchio P, Bargas E, et al: Hyperkalemia risks in hemodialysed patients consuming fluoride-rich water. Clin Chim Acta 1999; 281:29.

90. Graves JW: Hyperkalemia due to a potassium-based water softener. N Engl J Med 1998; 339:1790.

91. Myles PS, Buckland MR, Pastoriza-Pinol JV, et al: Massive hyperkalemia during combined heart-lung transplantation: inadvertent contamination with modified Euro-Collins solution. J Cardiothorac Vasc Anesth 1992; 6:600.

92. Sato K, Kondo T, Iwao H, et al: Sodium and potassium in red blood cells of premature infants during the first few days: risk of hyperkalaemia. Acta Paediatr Scand 1991; 80:899.

93. Gifford JD, Rutsky EA, Kirk KA, et al: Control of serum potassium during fasting in patients with end-stage renal disease. Kidney Int 1989; 35:90.

94. Allon M, Takeshian A, Shanklin N: Effect of insulin plus glucose infusion with or without epinephrine on fasting hyperkalemia. Kidney Int 1993; 43:212.

95. Gerstman BB, Kirkman R, Platt R: Intestinal necrosis associated with postoperative orally administered sodium polystyrene sulfonate in sorbitol. Am J Kidney Dis 1992; 20:159.

96. Rashid A, Hamilton SR: Necrosis of the gastrointestinal tract in uremic patients as a result of sodium polystyrene sulfonate (Kayexalate) in sorbitol: an underrecognized condition. Am J Surg Pathol 1997; 21:60.

97. Gardiner GW: Kayexalate (sodium polystyrene sulphonate) in sorbitol associated with intestinal necrosis in uremic patients. Can J Gastroenterol 1997; 11:573.

98. Roy-Chaudhury P, Meisels IS, Freedman S, et al: Combined gastric and ileocecal toxicity (serpiginous ulcers) after oral Kayexalate in sorbital therapy. Am J Kidney Dis 1997; 30:120.

99. Gruy-Kapral C, Emmett M, Santa Ana CA, et al: Effect of single-dose renin-cathartic therapy on serum potassium concentration in patients with end-stage renal disease. J Am Soc Nephrol 1998; 9:1924.

100. Blumberg A, Weidman P, Ferrari P: Effect of prolonged bicarbonate administration on plasma potassium in terminal renal failure. Kidney Int 1992; 41:369.

101. Montoliu J, Lens XM, Revert L: Potassium-lowering effect of albuterol for hyperkalemia in renal failure. Arch Intern Med 1987; 147:713.

102. Allon M, Dunlay R, Copkney C: Nebulized albuterol for acute hyperkalemia in patients on hemodialysis. Ann Intern Med 1989; 110:426.

103. McClure RJ, Prasad VK, Brocklebank JT: Treatment of hyperkalemia using intravenous and nebulized salbutamol. Arch Dis Child 1994; 70:126.

104. Mandelberg A, Krupnik Z, Houri S, et al: Salbutamol metered-dose inhaler with spacer for hyperkalemia: how fast? How safe? Chest 1999; 115:617.

105. Wong SL, Maltz HC: Albuterol for the treatment of hyperkalemia. Ann Pharmacother 1999; 33:103.

106. Allon M, Copkney C: Albuterol and insulin for treatment of hyperkalemia in hemodialysis patients. Kidney Int 1990; 38:869.

107. Locatelli F, Pontoriero G, Di Filippo S: Electrolyte disorders and substitution fluid in continuous renal replacement therapy. Kidney Int Suppl 1998; 66:S151.

108. Bushinsky DA: Metabolic Acidosis. In: Glassock RJ, ed: *Current Therapy in Nephrology and Hypertension*. 4th ed. St. Louis: Mosby; 1998:34.

109. DuBose TD Jr: Metabolic Acidosis. In: Brady HR, Wilcox CS, eds: *Therapy in Nephrology and Hypertension*. Philadelphia: WB Saunders; 1999:279.

110. DuBose TD Jr, Cogan MG, Rector Jr FC: Acid-Base Disorders. In: Brenner BM, ed: *The Kidney*. Vol. 2. 5th ed. Philadelphia: WB Saunders; 1996:929.

111. Halperin MD, Goldstein MB: Metabolic Acidosis. In: *Fluid, Electrolyte, and Acid-Base Physiology*. 3rd ed. Philadelphia: WB Saunders; 1999:73.

112. Caravaca F, Arrobas M, Pizarro JL, et al: Metabolic acidosis in advanced renal failure: differences between diabetic and nondiabetic patients. Am J Kidney Dis 1999; 33:892.

113. Oster JR, Singer I, Contreras GN, et al: Metabolic acidosis with extreme elevation of anion gap: case report and literature review. Am J Med Sci 1999; 317:38.

114. Knochel JP: Biochemical, Electrolyte, and Acid-Base Disturbances in Acute Renal Failure. In: Brenner BM, Lazarus JM, eds: *Acute Renal Failure*. 2nd ed. New York: Churchill Livingstone; 1988:677.

115. Adrogue HJ, Madias NE: Management of life-threatening acid-base disorders: first of two parts. N Engl J Med 1998; 338:26.

116. Bank N, Better OS: Acid-base balance and acute renal failure. Miner Electrolyte Metab 1991; 17:116.

117. Zager RA: Rhabdomyolysis and myohemoglobinuric acute renal failure. Kidney Int 1996; 49:314.

118. Halperin FA, Cheema-Dhadli S, Chen CB, et al: Alkali therapy extends the period of survival during hypoxia: studies in rats. Am J Physiol 1996; 271:R381.

119. Rhee KH, Toro LO, McDonald GG, et al: Carbicarb, sodium bicarbonate, and sodium chloride in hypoxic lactic acidosis: effect on arterial blood gases, lactate concentrations, hemodynamic variables, and myocardial intracellular pH. Chest 1993; 104:913.

120. Shapiro JI: Pathogenesis of cardiac dysfunction during metabolic acidosis: therapeutic implications. Kidney Int Suppl 1997; 61:S47.

121. Kierdorf H, Leue C, Heintz B, et al: Continuous venovenous hemofiltration in acute renal failure: is a bicarbonate- or lactate-buffered substitution better? Contrib Nephrol 1995; 116:38.

122. Bret M, Hurot JM, Mercatello A, et al: Acetate-free biofiltration for acute renal failure. Ren Fail 1998; 20:493.

123. Feriani M, Dell'Aquila R: Acid-base balance and replacement solutions in continuous renal replacement therapies. Kidney Int Suppl 1998; 66:S156.

124. May RC, Stivelman JC, Maroni BJ: Metabolic and Electrolyte Disturbances in Acute Renal Failure. In: Lazarus JM, Brenner BM, eds: *Acute Renal Failure*. 3rd ed. New York: Churchill Livingstone; 1993:107.

125. Massry SG, Arieff AI, Coburn JW, et al: Divalent ion metabolism in patients with acute renal failure: studies on the mechanism of hypocalcemia. Kidney Int 1974; 5:437.

126. St. John A, Davis TM, Binh TQ, et al: Mineral homeostasis in acute renal failure complicating severe falciparum malaria. J Clin Endocrinol Metab 1995; 80:2761.

127. Massry SG, Stein R, Garty J, et al: Skeletal resistance to the calcemic action of parathyroid hormone in uremia: role of 1,25 $(OH)_2 D_3$. Kidney Int 1976; 9:467.

128. Somerville PJ, Kaye M: Evidence that resistance to the calcemic action of parathyroid hormone in rats with acute uremia is caused by phosphate retention. Kidney Int 1979; 16:552.

129. Shieh SD, Lin YF, Lin SH: A prospective study of calcium metabolism in exertional heat stroke with rhabdomyolysis and acute renal failure. Nephron 1995; 71:428.

130. Akmal M, Bishop JE, Telfer N, et al: Hypocalcemia and hypercalcemia in patients with rhabdomyolysis with and without acute renal failure. J Clin Endocrinol Metab 1986; 63:137.

131. Hadjis T, Grieff M, Lockhat D, et al: Calcium metabolism in acute renal failure due to rhabdomyolysis. Clin Nephrol 1993; 39:22.

132. Wada A, Nakata T, Tsuchihashi K, et al: Massive myocardial calcification of right and left ventricles following acute myocarditis complicated with rhabdomyolysis-induced acute renal failure. Jpn Circ J 1993; 57:567.

133. Saito T, Tsuboi Y, Fujisawa G, et al: An autopsy case of licorice-induced hypokalemic rhabdomyolysis associated with acute renal failure: special reference to profound calcium deposition in skeletal and cardiac muscle. Nippon Jinzo Gakkai Shi 1994; 36:1308.

134. Chapman DM, Boskey AL, Tesch M, et al: Subcutaneous microvascular (capillary) calcification: another basis for livedo-like skin changes? Clin Exp Dermatol 1995; 20:213.

135. Sperling LS, Tumlin JA: Case report: delayed hypercalcemia after rhabdomyolysis-induced acute renal failure. Am J Med Sci 1996; 311:186.

136. Chernow B, Zaloga G, McFadden E, et al: Hypocalcemia in critically ill patients. Crit Care Med 1982; 10:848.

137. Niven MJ, Zohar M, Shimoni Z, et al: Symptomatic hypocalcemia precipitated by small-volume blood transfusion. Ann Emerg Med 1998; 32:498.

138. Meier-Kriesche HU, Finkel KW, Gitomer JJ, et al: Unexpected severe hypocalcemia during continuous venovenous hemodialysis with regional citrate anticoagulation. Am J Kidney Dis 1999; 33:E8.

139. Agarwal N, Pitchumoni CS: Acute pancreatitis: a multisystem disease. Gastroenterologist 1993; 1:115.

140. Thyssen EP, Hou SH, Alverdy JC, et al: Temporary loss of limb function secondary to soft tissue calcification in a patient with rhabdomyolysis-induced acute renal failure. Am J Kidney Dis 1990; 16:491.

141. Edelstein CL, Alkhunaizi AA, Schrier RW: The role of calcium in the pathogenesis of acute renal failure. Ren Fail 1997; 19:199.

142. Casella FJ, Allon M: The kidney in sarcoidosis. J Am Soc Nephrol 1993; 3:1555.

143. Abreo K, Adlakha A, Kilpatrick S, et al: The milk-alkali syndrome: a reversible form of acute renal failure. Arch Intern Med 1993; 153:1005.

144. Muldowney WP, Mazbar SA: Rolaids-yogurt syndrome: a 1990s version of milk-alkali syndrome. Am J Kidney Dis 1996; 27:270.

145. Irish AB, Winearls CG, Littlewood T: Presentation and survival of patients with severe renal failure and myeloma. QJM 1997; 90:773.

146. Antunovic P, Marisavljevic D, Kraguljac N, et al: Severe hypercalcaemia and extensive osteolytic lesions in an adult patient with T cell acute lymphoblastic leukaemia. Med Oncol 1998; 15:58.

147. Lam KK, Kuo CY: Bone marrow examinations as final clue to diagnosis of hypercalcemia: report of two cases. Ren Fail 1999; 21:101.

148. Karpati RM, Mak RH, Lemley KV: Hypercalcemia, hypertension and acute renal insufficiency in an immobilized adolescent. Child Nephrol Urol 1991; 11:215.

149. Bedani PL, Gilli P: Hypertensive emergency due to hypercalcemia after acute renal failure secondary to rhabdomyolysis. Nephron 1995; 69:120.

150. Meneghini LF, Oster JR, Camacho JR, et al: Hypercalcemia in association with acute renal failure and rhabdomyolysis: case report and literature review. Miner Electrolyte Metab 1993; 19:1.

151. Thatte L, Oster JR, Singer I, et al: Review of the literature: severe hyperphosphatemia. Am J Med Sci 1995; 310:167.

152. Jones DP, Mahmoud H, Chesney RW: Tumor lysis syndrome: pathogenesis and management. Pediatr Nephrol 1995; 9:206.

153. Abassi ZA, Hoffman A, Better OS: Acute renal failure complicating muscle crush injury. Semin Nephrol 1998; 18:558.

154. Weisinger JR, Bellorin-Font E: Magnesium and phosphorus. Lancet 1998; 352:391.

155. Haas M, Ohler L, Watzke H, et al: The spectrum of acute renal failure in tumour lysis syndrome. Nephrol Dial Transplant 1999; 14:776.

156. Ahmed M, Raval P, Buganza G: Oral sodium phosphate catharsis and acute renal failure. Am J Gastroenterol 1996; 91:1261.

157. Vukasin P, Weston LA, Beart RW: Oral Fleet Phospho-Soda laxative-induced hyperphosphatemia and hypocalcemic tetany in an adult: report of a case. Dis Colon Rectum 1997; 40:497.

158. Orias M, Mahnensmith RL, Perazella MA: Extreme hyperphosphatemia and acute renal failure after a phosphorus-containing bowel regimen. Am J Nephrol 1999; 19:60.

159. Slatopolsky E, Finch J, Denda M, et al: Phosphorus restriction prevents parathyroid gland growth: high phosphorus directly stimulates PTH secretion in vitro. J Clin Invest 1996; 97:2534.

160. Keating MJ, Sethi MR, Bodey GP, et al: Hypocalcemia with hypoparathyroidism and renal tubular dysfunction associated with aminoglycoside therapy. Cancer 1977; 39:1410.

161. Gearhart MO, Sorg TB: Foscarnet-induced severe hypomagnesemia and other electrolyte disorders. Ann Pharmacother 1993; 27:285.

162. Ferrari S, Zolezzi C, Bacci G, et al: A prospective study on nephrotoxicity induced by continuous infusion of high-dose ifosfamide (15/m²). Minerva Pediatr 1997; 49:29.

163. Funabiki Y, Tatsukawa H, Ashida K, et al: Disturbance of consciousness associated with hypophosphatemia in a chronically alcoholic patient. Intern Med 1998; 37:958.

164. Berger MM, Rothen C, Cavadini C, et al: Exudative mineral losses after serious burns: a clue to the alterations of magnesium and phosphate metabolism. Am J Clin Nutr 1997; 65:1473.

165. Druml W, Kleinberger G: Hypophosphatemia in patients with chronic renal failure during total parenteral nutrition. JPEN 1999; 23:45.

166. Clark BA, Brown RS: Unsuspected morbid hypermagnesemia in elderly patients. Am J Nephrol 1992; 12:336.

167. Monk RD, Bushinsky DA: Treatment of Calcium, Phosphorus, and Magnesium Disorders. In: Brady HR, Wilcox CS, eds: *Therapy in Nephrology and Hypertension*. Philadelphia: WB Saunders; 1999:303.

168. Safirstein R, Winston J, Goldstein M, et al: Cisplatin nephrotoxicity. Am J Kidney Dis 1986; 8:356.

169. Rodriguez M, Solanki DL, Whang R: Refractory potassium repletion due to cisplatin-induced magnesium depletion. Arch Intern Med 1989; 149:2592.

170. Lajer H, Daugaard G: Cisplatin and hypomagnesemia. Cancer Treat Rev 1999; 25:47.

171. Barton CH, Pahl M, Vaziri ND, et al: Renal magnesium wasting associated with amphotericin B therapy. Am J Med 1984; 77:471.

172. Sawaya BP, Briggs JP, Schnermann J: Amphotericin B nephrotoxicity: the adverse consequences of altered membrane properties. J Am Soc Nephrol 1995; 6:154.

173. Akbar A, Rees JH, Nyamugunduru G, et al: Aminoglycoside-associated hypomagnesaemia in children with cystic fibrosis. Acta Paediatr 1999; 88:783.

174. Wu B, Atkinson AS, Halton JM, et al: Hypermagnesiuria and hypercalciuria in childhood leukemia: an effect of amikacin therapy. J Pediatr Hematol Oncol 1996; 18:86.

175. Burdmann EA, Andoh TF, Lindsley J, et al: Effects of oral magnesium supplementation on acute experimental cyclosporin nephrotoxicity. Nephrol Dial Transplant 1994; 9:16.

176. de Mattos AM, Olyaei AJ, Bennett WM: Pharmacology of immunosuppressive medications used in renal diseases and transplantation. Am J Kidney Dis 1996; 28:631.

177. Andoh TF, Burdmann EA, Fransechini N, et al: Comparison of acute rapamycin nephrotoxicity with cyclosporine and FK506. Kidney Int 1996; 50:1110.

178. Shah GM, Alvarado P, Kirschenbaum MA: Symptomatic hypocalcemia and hypomagnesemia with renal magnesium wasting associated with pentamidine therapy in a patient with AIDS. Am J Med 1990; 89:380.

179. Vamvakas S, Teschner M, Bahner U, et al: Alcohol abuse: potential role in electrolyte disturbances and kidney diseases. Clin Nephrol 1998; 49:205.

180. al-Ghamdi SM, Cameron EC, Sutton RA: Magnesium deficiency: pathophysiologic and clinical overview. Am J Kidney Dis 1994; 24:737.

181. Agus ZS: Hypomagnesemia. J Am Soc Nephrol 1999; 10:1616.

182. Swann RC, Merril JP: The clinical course of acute renal failure. Medicine 1953; 32:215.

183. Hales M, Solez K, Kjellstrand C: The anemia of acute renal failure: association with oliguria and elevated blood urea. Ren Fail 1994; 16:125.

184. Steinman TI, Lazarus JM: Organ-System Involvement in Acute Renal Failure. In: Brenner BM, Lazarus JM, eds: *Acute Renal Failure*. 2nd ed. New York: Churchill Livingstone; 1988:705.

185. Lipkin GW, Kendall R, Haggett P, et al: Erythropoietin in acute renal failure. Lancet 1989; 1:1029.

186. Lipkin GW, Kendall RG, Russon LJ, et al: Erythropoietin deficiency in acute renal failure. Nephrol Dial Transplant 1990; 5:920.

187. Nielsen OJ, Thaysen JH: Erythropoietin deficiency in acute tubular necrosis. J Intern Med 1990; 227:373.

188. Thaysen JH, Nielsen OJ, Brandi L, et al: Erythropoietin deficiency in acute crescentic glomerulonephritis and in total bilateral renal cortical necrosis. J Intern Med 1991; 229:363.

189. Tan CC, Tan LH, Eckardt KU: Erythropoietin production in rats with postischemic acute renal failure. Kidney Int 1996; 50:1958.

190. Fontanellas A, Herrero JA, Trobo JI, et al: Abnormalities of heme biosynthesis in experimental acute renal failure. J Am Soc Nephrol 1996; 7:628.

191. Mavromatidis K, Fytil C, Kynigopoulou P, et al: Serum ferritin levels are increased in patients with acute renal failure. Clin Nephrol 1998; 49:296.

192. Nagano N, Koumegawa J, Arai H, et al: Effect of recombinant human erythropoietin on new anaemic model rats induced by gentamicin. J Pharm Pharmacol 1990; 42:758.

193. Kokot F, Wiecek A, Grzeszczak W: Plasma parathyroid hormone and erythropoietin levels in patients with noninflammatory acute renal failure. Int Urol Nephrol 1993; 25:89.

194. Morgera S, Heering P, Szentandrasi T, et al: Erythropoietin in patients with acute renal failure and continuous veno-venous haemofiltration. Int Urol Nephrol 1997; 29:245.

195. Baldwin MD, Zhou XJ, Ing TS, et al: Erythropoietin ameliorates anemia of cisplatin induced acute renal failure. ASAIO J 1998; 44:44.

196. Rogiers P, Zhang H, Leeman M, et al: Erythropoietin response is blunted in critically ill patients. Intensive Care Med 1997; 23:159.

197. Kraus P, Lipman J: Erythropoietin in a patient following multiple trauma. Anaesthesia 1992; 47:962.

198. Vaziri ND, Zhou XJ, Liao SY: Erythropoietin enhances recovery from cisplatin-induced acute renal failure. Am J Physiol 1994; 266:F360.

199. Druml W: Nondialytic management of the patient with acute renal failure. Nephrol Dial Transplant 1996; 11:1517.

200. Breen D, Bihari D: Acute renal failure as a part of multiple organ failure: the slippery slope of critical illness. Kidney Int Suppl 1998; 66:S25.

201. Gossmann J, Thurmann P, Bachmann T, et al: Mechanism of angiotensin converting enzyme inhibitor-related anemia in renal transplant recipients. Kidney Int 1996; 50:973.

202. Macdougall IC: The role of ACE inhibitors and angiotensin II receptor blockers in the response to epoetin. Nephrol Dial Transplant 1999; 14:1836.

203. Andrassy K: Bleeding in Acute Renal Failure. In: Bhiari D, Neild G, eds: *Acute Renal Failure in the Intensive Care Unit*. London: Springer-Verlag; 1990:243.

204. Schetz MRC: Coagulation disorders in acute renal failure. Kidney Int Suppl 1998; 66:S96.

205. Weigert AL, Schafer AI: Uremic bleeding: pathogenesis and therapy. Am J Med Sci 1998; 316:94.

206. Gawaz MP, Dobos G, Spath M, et al: Impaired function of platelet membrane glycoprotein IIb–IIIa in end-stage renal disease. J Am Soc Nephrol 1994; 5:36.

207. Malyszko J, Malyszko JS, Pawlak D, et al: Hemostasis, platelet function and serotonin in acute and chronic renal failure. Thromb Res 1996; 83:351.

208. Zwaginga JJ, IJsseldijk MJ, de Groot PG, et al: Defects in platelet adhesion and aggregate formation in uremic bleeding disorder can be attributed to factors in plasma. Arterioscler Thromb 1991; 11:733.

209. Zwaginga JJ, IJsseldijk MJ, de Groot PG, et al: Treatment of uremic anemia with recombinant erythropoietin also reduces the defects in platelet adhesion and aggregation caused by uremic plasma. Thromb Haemost 1991; 66:638.

210. Noris M, Benigni A, Boccardo P, et al: Enhanced nitric oxide synthesis in uremia: implications for platelet dysfunction and dialysis hypotension. Kidney Int 1993; 44:445.

211. Manns M, Sigler MH, Teehan BP: Continuous renal replacement therapies: an update. Am J Kidney Dis 1998; 32:185.

212. van de Wetering J, Westendorp RG, van der Hoeven JG, et al: Heparin use in continuous renal replacement procedures: the struggle between filter coagulation and patient hemorrhage. J Am Soc Nephrol 1996; 7:145.

213. Freedman MD: Pharmacodynamics, clinical indications, and adverse effects of heparin. J Clin Pharmacol 1992; 32:584.

214. Yamamoto S, Koide M, Matsuo M, et al: Heparin-induced thrombocytopenia in hemodialysis patients. Am J Kidney Dis 1996; 28:82.

215. Kaplan AA: Dialysis and Other Extracorporeal Therapy for Acute Renal Failure. In: Glassock RJ, ed: *Current Therapy in Nephrology and Hypertension*. 4th ed. St. Louis: Mosby; 1998: 249.

216. Davenport A: The coagulation system in the critically ill patient with acute renal failure and the effect of an extracorporeal circuit. Am J Kidney Dis 1997; 30(5 suppl 4):S20.

217. Hajarizadeh H, Rohrer MJ, Herrmann JB, et al: Acute peritoneal dialysis following ruptured abdominal aortic aneurysms. Am J Surg 1995; 170:223.

218. Romao JE Jr, Fadil MA, Sabbaga E, et al: Haemodialysis without anticoagulant: haemostasis parameters, fibrinogen kinetic, and dialysis efficiency. Nephrol Dial Transplant 1997; 12:106.

219. Gretz N, Quintel M, Ragaller M, et al: Low-dose heparinization for anticoagulation in intensive care patients on continuous hemofiltration. Contrib Nephrol 1995; 116:130.

220. Ward DM, Mehta RL: Extracorporeal management of acute renal failure patients at high risk of bleeding. Kidney Int Suppl 1993; 41:S237.

221. Mehta RL, McDonald BR, Ward DM: Regional citrate anticoagulation for continuous arteriovenous hemodialysis. An update after 12 months. Contrib Nephrol 1991; 93:210.

222. Mehta RL: Anticoagulation strategies for continuous renal replacement therapies: what works? Am J Kidney Dis 1996; 28(suppl 3):S8.

223. Warkentin TE, Levine MN, Hirsh J, et al: Heparin-induced thrombocytopenia in patients treated with low molecular weight heparin or unfractionated heparin. N Engl J Med 1995; 332:1330.

224. Ohtake Y, Hirasawa H, Sugai T, et al: Nafamostat mesilate as anticoagulant in continuous hemofiltration and continuous hemodiafiltration. Contrib Nephrol 1991; 93:215.

225. Kubota T, Miyata A, Maeda A, et al: Continuous haemodiafiltration during and after cardiopulmonary bypass in renal failure patients. Can J Anaesth 1997; 44:1182.

226. Steuer S, Boogen C, Plum J, et al: Anticoagulation with r-hirudin in a patient with acute renal failure and heparin-induced thrombocytopenia. Nephrol Dial Transplant 1999; 14(suppl 4):45.

227. DeLoughery TG: Management of bleeding with uremia and liver disease. Curr Opin Hematol 1999; 6:329.

228. Sutor AH: Desmopressin (DDAVP) in bleeding disorders of childhood. Semin Thromb Hemost 1998; 24:555.

229. Heunisch C, Resnick DJ, Vitello JM, at al: Conjugated estrogens for the management of gastrointestinal bleeding secondary to uremia of acute renal failure. Pharmacotherapy 1998; 18:210.

230. Tryba M, Cook D: Current guidelines on stress ulcer prophylaxis. Drugs 1997; 54:581.

231. Phillips JO, Metzler MH, Palmieri MT, et al: A prospective study of simplified omeprazole suspension for the prophylaxis of stress-related mucosal damage. Crit Care Med 1996; 24:1793.

232. Woodrow G, Turney JH: Cause of death in acute renal failure. Nephrol Dial Transplant 1992; 7:230.

233. Brivet FG, Kleinknecht DJ, Loirat P, et al: Acute renal failure in intensive care units: causes, outcomes, and prognostic factors of hospital mortality; a prospective, multicenter study. French Study Group on Acute Renal Failure. Crit Care Med 1996; 24:192.

234. Weisberg LS, Allgren RL, Genter FC, et al: Cause of acute tubular necrosis affects its prognosis. The Auriculin Anaritide Acute Renal Failure Study Group. Arch Intern Med 1997; 157:1833.

235. Chrysopoulo MT, Jeschke MG, Dziewulski P, et al: Acute renal failure in severely burned adults. J Trauma 1999; 46:141.

236. Haag-Weber M, Dumann H, Horl WH: Effect of malnutrition and uremia on impaired cellular host defense. Miner Electrolyte Metab 1992; 18:174.

237. Fiaccadori E, Lombardi M, Leonardi S, et al: Prevalence and clinical outcome associated with preexisting malnutrition in acute renal failure: a prospective cohort study. J Am Soc Nephrol 1999; 10:581.

238. Haag-Weber M, Horl WH: Uremia and infection: mechanisms of impaired cellular host defense. Nephron 1993; 63:125.

239. Vanholder R, Van Loo A, Dhondt AM, et al: Influence of uraemia and haemodialysis on host defense and infection. Nephrol Dial Transplant 1996; 11:593.

240. Cohen G, Haag-Weber M, Horl WH: Immune dysfunction in uremia. Kidney Int Suppl 1997; 62:S79.

241. Vanholder R, Ringoir S: Polymorphonuclear cell function and infection in dialysis. Kidney Int Suppl 1992; 38:S91.

242. Vanholder R, Dell'Aquila R, Jacobs V, et al: Depressed phagocytosis in hemodialyzed patients: in vivo and in vitro mechanisms. Nephron 1993; 63:409.

243. Haag-Weber M, Horl WH: The immune system in uremia and during its treatment. New Horiz 1995; 3:669.

244. Horl WH: Neutrophil function and infections in uremia. Am J Kidney Dis 1999; 33: xlv.

245. Cendoroglo M, Jaber BL, Balakrishnan VS, et al: Neutrophil apoptosis and dysfunction in uremia. J Am Soc Nephrol 1999; 10:93.

246. Haag-Weber M, Mai B, Horl WH: Isolation of a granulocyte inhibitory protein from uraemic patients with homology of β2-microglobulin. Nephrol Dial Transplant 1994; 9:382.

247. Haag-Weber M, Horl WH: Are granulocyte inhibitory proteins contributing to enhanced susceptibility to infections in uraemia? Nephrol Dial Transplant 1996; 11(suppl 2):98.

248. Cohen G, Rudnicki M, Horl WH: Isolation of modified ubiquitin as a neutrophil chemotaxis inhibitor from uremic patients. J Am Soc Nephrol 1998; 9:451.

249. Ryan J, Beynon H, Rees AJ, et al: Evaluation of the in vitro production of tumour necrosis factor by monocytes in dialysis patients. Blood Purif 1991; 9:142.

250. Shu KH, Lu YS, Cheng CH, Lian JD: Soluble interleukin-2 receptor in dialyzed patients. Artif Organs 1998; 22:142.

251. Himmelfarb J, Hakim RM: Biocompatibility and risk of infection in hemodialysis patients. Nephrol Dial Transplant 1994; 9(suppl 2):138.

252. Schiffl H, Sitter T, Lang S, et al: Bioincompatible membranes place patients with acute renal failure at increased risk of infection. ASAIO J 1995; 41:M709.

253. Vanholder R: Relationship between biocompatibility and neutrophil function in hemodialysis patients. Adv Ren Replace Ther 1996; 3:312.

254. Lefebvre PJ, Luyckx AS: Effect of acute kidney exclusion by ligation of renal arteries on peripheral plasma glucagon levels and pancreatic glucagon production in the anesthetized dog. Metabolism 1975; 24:1169.

255. Perez G, Carteni G, Ungaro B, et al: Influence of nephrectomy on the glucoregulatory response to insulin administration in the rat. Can J Physiol Pharmacol 1980; 58:301.

256. Lacy WW: Uptake of individual amino acids by perfused rat liver: effect of acute uremia. Am J Physiol 1970; 219:649.

257. Frohlich J, Scholmerich J, Hoppe-Seyler G, et al: The effect of acute uraemia on gluconeogenesis in isolated perfused rat livers. Eur J Clin Invest 1974; 4:453.

258. Orskov C, Andreasen J, Holst JJ: All products of proglucagon are elevated in plasma from uremic patients. J Clin Endocrinol Metab 1992; 74:379.

259. Laouari D, Jurkovitz C, Burtin M, et al: Uremia-induced disturbances in hepatic carbohydrate metabolism: enhancement by sucrose feeding. Metabolism 1994; 43:403.

260. Schaefer RM, Riegel W, Stephan E, et al: Normalization of enhanced hepatic gluconeogenesis by the antiglucocorticoid RU 38486 in acutely uraemic rats. Eur J Clin Invest 1990; 20:35.

261. Horl WH, Stepinski J, Heidland A: Carbohydrate metabolism and uraemia-mechanisms for glycogenolysis and gluconeogenesis. Klin Wochenschr 1980; 58:1051.

262. Smith D, DeFronzo RA: Insulin resistance in uremia mediated by postbinding defects. Kidney Int 1982; 22:54.

263. Mondon CE, Reaven GM: Evaluation of enhanced glucagon sensitivity as the cause of glucose intolerance in acutely uremic rats. Am J Clin Nutr 1980; 33:1456.

264. Mondon CE, Marcus R, Reaven GM: Role of glucagon as a contributor to glucose intolerance in acute and chronic uremia. Metabolism 1982; 31:374.

265. Cianciaruso B, Bellizzi V, Napoli R, et al: Hepatic uptake and release of glucose, lactate, and amino acids in acutely uremic dogs. Metabolism 1991; 40:261.

266. Mondon CE, Dolkas CB, Reaven GM: The site of insulin resistance in acute uremia. Diabetes 1978; 27:571.

267. Horl WH, Heidland A: Glycogen metabolism in muscle in uremia. Am J Clin Nutr 1980; 33:1461.

268. Clark AS, Mitch WE: Muscle protein turnover and glucose uptake in acutely uremic rats. Effects of insulin and the duration of renal insufficiency. J Clin Invest 1983; 72:836.

269. Palmer TN, Caldecourt MA, Gossain S, et al: Impaired muscle glucose metabolism in acute renal failure. Biosci Rep 1985; 5:433.

270. May RC, Clark AS, Goheer MA, et al: Specific defects in insulin-mediated muscle metabolism in acute uremia. Kidney Int 1985; 28:490.

271. Druml W: Protein metabolism in acute renal failure. Miner Electrolyte Metab 1998; 24:47.

272. Davis TA, Klahr S, Karl IE: Glucose metabolism in muscle of sedentary and exercised rats with azotemia. Am J Physiol 1987; 252:F138–F145.

273. Tu WH: Plasma renin activity in acute tubular necrosis and other renal diseases associated with hypertension. Circulation 1965; 31:686.

274. Paton AM, Lever AF, Oliver NW, et al: Plasma angiotensin II, renin, renin-substrate and aldosterone concentrations in acute renal failure in man. Clin Nephrol 1975; 3:18.

275. Kokof F: Endocrine System in Acute Renal Failure. In: Andreucci VE, ed: *Acute Renal Failure: Pathophysiology, Prevention, and Treatment.* Boston: Martinus Nijhoff; 1984:167.

276. Hilgenfeldt U, Kienapfel G, Kellermann W, et al: Renin-angiotensin system in sepsis. Clin Exp Hypertens A 1987; 9:1493.

277. Panos MZ, Anderson JV, Forbes A, et al: Human atrial natriuretic factor and renin-aldosterone in paracetamol induced fulminant hepatic failure. Gut 1991; 32:85.

278. Cruz C, Ibarra-Rubio ME, Pedraza-Chaverri J: Circulating levels of active, total and inactive renin (prorenin), angiotensin I and angiotensinogen in carbon tetrachloride-treated rats. Clin Exp Pharmacol Physiol 1993; 20:83.

279. Hronek I, Hronkova B, Davenport A, et al: Thyroid hormone levels in acute renal failure. Ren Fail 1993; 15:47.

280. Bogicevic M, Ilic S, Djordjevic V, et al: Thyroid hormone profiles in experimental acute renal failure. Ren Fail 1993; 15:173.

281. Rogers SA, Miller SB, Hammerman MR: Altered EGF expression and thyroxine metabolism in kidneys following acute ischemic injury in rat. Am J Physiol 1996; 270:F21.

282. Chen WL, Huang WS, Lin YF, et al: Changes in thyroid hormone metabolism in exertional heat stroke with or without acute renal failure. J Clin Endocrinol Metab 1996; 81:625.

283. Makropoulos W, Heintz B, Stefanidis I: Selenium deficiency and thyroid function in acute renal failure. Ren Fail 1997; 19:129.

284. Reinhardt W, Misch C, Jockenhovel F, et al: Triiodothyronine (T_3) reflects renal graft function after renal transplantation. Clin Endocrinol 1997; 46:563.

285. Johnson JP, Grillo FG: Thyroid hormone induction of ornithine decarboxylase in ischemic acute renal failure. Ren Fail 1994; 16:435.

286. Seiken G, Grillo FG, Schaudies RP, et al: Modulation of renal EGF in dichromate-induced acute renal failure treated with thyroid hormone. Kidney Int 1994; 45:1622.

287. Palmer BF: Sexual dysfunction in uremia. J Am Soc Nephrol 1999; 10:1381.

288. Kokot F, Mleczko Z, Pazera A: Parathyroid hormone, prolactin, and function of the pituitary-gonadal axis in male patients with acute renal failure. Kidney Int 1982; 21:84.

289. Levitan D, Moser SA, Goldstein DA, et al: Disturbances in the hypothalamic-pituitary-gonadal axis in male patients with acute renal failure. Am J Nephrol 1984; 4:99.

290. Akmal M, Goldstein DA, Kletzky OA, et al: Hyperparathyroidism and hypotestosteronemia of acute renal failure. Am J Nephrol 1988; 8:166.

291. Isaac R, Merceron RE, Caillens G, et al: Effect of parathyroid hormone on plasma prolactin in man. J Clin Endocrinol Metab 1978; 47:18.

292. Adachi Y, Nakada T: Effect of experimentally induced renal failure on testicular testosterone synthesis in rats. Arch Androl 1999; 43:37.

293. Nomura K, Kikuchi C, Ogasawara M, et al: LH and testosterone modulate mercuric chloride-induced acute renal failure in male rats: the implication of stress-induced hypogonadism. J Endocrinol 1996; 148:553.

294. Landau D, Kher KK: Gentamicin-induced Bartter-like syndrome. Pediatr Nephrol 1997; 11:737.

295. Bjornson DC, Stephenson SR: Cisplatin-induced massive renal tubular failure with wastage of serum electrolytes. Clin Pharm 1983; 2:80.

296. Elisaf M, Milionis H, Siamopoulos KC: Hypomagnesemic hypokalemia and hypocalcemia: clinical and laboratory characteristics. Miner Electrolyte Metab 1997; 23:105.

297. Dorea EL, Yu L, De Castro I, et al: Nephrotoxicity of amphotericin B is attenuated by solubilizing with lipid emulsion. J Am Soc Nephrol 1997; 8:1415.

298. Seguro AC, Lomar AV, Rocha AS: Acute renal failure of leptospirosis: nonoliguric and hypokalemic forms. Nephron 1990; 55:146.

299. Emery C, Young RM, Morgan DB, et al: Tubular damage in patients with hypokalaemia. Clin Chim Acta 1984; 140:231.

300. Cronin RE, Thompson JR: Role of potassium in the pathogenesis of acute renal failure. Miner Electrolyte Metab 1991; 17:100.

301. Bernardo JF, Murakami S, Branch RA, et al: Potassium depletion potentiates amphotericin-B-induced toxicity to renal tubules. Nephron 1995; 70:235.

302. Larsen G, Loghman-Adham M: Acute renal failure with hyperuricemia as initial presentation of leukemia in children. J Pediatr Hematol Oncol 1996; 18:191.

303. Visweswaran P, Guntupalli J: Rhabdomyolysis. Crit Care Clin 1999; 15:415.

304. Steele TH: Hyperuricemic nephropathies. Nephron 1999; 81(suppl 1):45.

305. Richards JM, Weinman EJ: Acute and Chronic Hyperuricemic Nephropathy. In: Glassock RJ, ed: *Current Therapy in Nephrology and Hypertension.* 4th ed. St. Louis: Mosby; 1998:94.

306. Lupton GP, Odom RB: The allopurinol hypersensitivity syndrome. J Am Acad Dermatol 1979; 1:365.

307. Pui CH, Relling MV, Lascombes F, et al: Urate oxidase in prevention and treatment of hyperuricemia associated with lymphoid malignancies. Leukemia 1997; 11:1813.

308. Mahmoud HH, Leverger G, Patte C, et al: Advances in the management of malignancy-associated hyperuricaemia. Br J Cancer 1998; 77(suppl 4):18.

309. Nitzan M: Abnormalities of carbohydrate and lipid metabolism in experimentally induced acute uremia. Nutr Metab 1973; 15:187.

310. Druml W, Laggner A, Widhalm K, et al: Lipid metabolism in acute renal failure. Kidney Int Suppl 1983; 16:S139.

311. Gupta KL, Majumdar S, Sakhuja V: Postheparin lipolytic activity in acute and chronic renal failure. Ren Fail 1994; 16:609.

312. Gregg R, Mondon CE, Reaven EP, et al: Effect of acute uremia on triglyceride kinetics in the rat. Metabolism 1976; 25:1557.

313. Savdie E, Gibson JC, Crawford GA, et al: Impaired plasma triglyceride clearance as a feature of both uremic and posttransplant triglyceridemia. Kidney Int 1980; 18:774.

314. Ransom J, Garfinkel AS, Nikazy J, et al: Metabolic studies of adipose tissue in acute uremia. Metabolism 1981; 30:1165.

315. Zimmermann E, Hohenegger M: Lipid metabolism in uremic and nonuremic acidosis. Nephron 1979; 24:217.

316. Crawford GA, Savdie E, Stewart JH, et al: Inhibition of normal plasma lipases by serum from chronic renal failure patients. Trans Am Soc Artif Intern Organs 1979; 25:426.

317. Massry SG, Akmal M: Lipid abnormalities, renal failure, and parathyroid hormone. Am J Med 1989; 87:42N.

318. Rapoport J, Aviram M, Chaimovitz C, et al: Defective high-density lipoprotein composition in patients on chronic hemodialysis. A possible mechanism for accelerated atherosclerosis. N Engl J Med 1978; 299:1326.

319. Geerlings SE, Rommes JH, van Toorn DW, et al: Acute folate deficiency in a critically ill patient. Neth J Med 1997; 51:36.

320. Druml W, Schwarzenhofer M, Apsner R, et al: Fat-soluble vitamins in patients with acute renal failure. Miner Electrolyte Metab 1998; 24:220.

CHAPTER **13**

Imaging Techniques in Acute Renal Failure

Richard L. Clark ▪ Steven W. Falen ▪ Andrew I. Choi

There is no real difference between structure and function; they are the two sides of the same coin. If structure does not tell us anything about function, it means we have not looked at it correctly.

Albert Szent-Gyorgyi, 1950

INTRODUCTION

In managing the patient with acute renal failure (ARF), there are a number of imaging techniques from which to choose.[1] Not surprisingly, the pragmatic clinical question often becomes what specific modality gives the most information for the least cost not only in financial terms but also in terms of patient comfort and risk. The purpose of this chapter, therefore, is to summarize the current status of each technique as it aids in the diagnosis and treatment of the many etiologies and clinical manifestations of ARF and to present a number of illustrations that demonstrate the utility of these modalities in clinical practice. No attempt is made to present a detailed atlas of imaging findings. The interested reader is encouraged to consult standard genitourinary radiology texts and other recent reviews.[2–8]

Table 13–1 lists the current techniques that should be available in all tertiary care centers. Most modalities or procedures are also available in radiology departments in community hospitals and outpatient imaging centers.

Chapter 29 presents a discussion of the effects of various intravascular contrast media on renal physiology. The reader is urged to review this material as well as other recent publications[9] to gain a better perspective regarding the additional danger that contrast medium contributes to many imaging techniques.

TABLE 13–1. Imaging Techniques in Acute Renal Failure

Abdominal plain film radiography (KUB) with or without
 tomography
Intravenous urography (excretory urography or IVP)
Computed tomography without or with contrast media
Ultrasonography (preferably with Doppler capability)
Radionuclide techniques, including diuretic renography and cortical
 scintigraphy
Magnetic resonance imaging, including MR angiography
Conventional and digital angiography
Interventional techniques, including percutaneous nephrostomy and
 stent placement
Retrograde pyelography and other related urologic interventional
 procedures
Voiding cystourethrography (VCUG)

KUB, supine film including the kidneys, ureters, and bladder. IVP, intravenous pyelography.

ABDOMINAL PLAIN FILM RADIOGRAPHY

Much useful information can be obtained from a careful examination of the "low-tech" and thus inexpensive abdominal plain film of a patient presenting with ARF. A good KUB (supine film to include the kidneys, ureters, and bladder) should be obtained with relatively low kVp (60–65) to enhance radiographic contrast, thus facilitating the visualization of subtle calcifications, renal outlines, possible urinary tract gas shadows, and bony structures. Proper collimation that excludes the flanks also improves resolution and contrast by eliminating image degradation and scattered and unnecessary primary radiation. It is well known to experienced radiologists that the properly exposed "scout" film for an intravenous urogram often demonstrates far more information than the typical abdominal film obtained in the emergency room, which is usually lower in contrast and, by design, includes the whole abdomen.

Although information about renal size, shape, and position is often obtained from the KUB, ultrasound is definitely more reliable in this regard (see later). Nevertheless, renal length as seen on plain films or tomography (see later) continues to be helpful, as long as one is aware of the variations of normal size, depending on body habitus, age, and to a lesser extent, hydration. We use the well-accepted internal standard of the combined heights of three to four lumbar vertebral bodies as a rough indicator of normal renal length. Kidneys longer than the combined heights of four and a half vertebral bodies definitely are considered to be enlarged, and those less than two and a half vertebral bodies in length definitely are considered to be small.

Generally, kidneys are normal in size in prerenal causes of ARF (notable exceptions being acute shock and acute renal ischemia, conditions in which they are often small) and are increased in size in acute tubular necrosis and acute glomerulonephritis. Other causes of bilateral nephromegaly include bilateral papillary necrosis, pyelonephritis, sickle cell nephropathy, multiple myeloma, amyloidosis, rhabdomyolysis-myoglobinuria, urate nephropathy, HIV (human immunodeficiency virus) nephropathy, and diabetes. Postrenal causes of ARF, such as acute bilateral obstruction or bilateral renal vein thrombosis, also may be associated with nephromegaly, depending on the stage of each condition.

The presence, character, and distribution of renal or other urinary tract calcifications are often easily determined with plain films. However, most pathologic conditions that exhibit characteristic cortical calcification patterns are associated with chronic renal failure, not ARF. Examples of these conditions are cortical necrosis, chronic glomerulonephritis, and oxalosis. However, the presence of diffuse collecting system or medullary calcifications in patients with ARF may suggest bilateral obstruction caused by stones passing from kidneys with papillary necrosis (sloughed calcified papillae), renal tubular acidosis (Fig. 13–1) or medullary sponge kidneys, or more commonly from patients with bilateral stone disease associated with infection, hyperoxaluria, or hypercalcemia.

Thus, the distribution patterns of renal calcification together with the determination of renal size often enable the clinician not only to distinguish between acute and chronic forms of renal failure but also to differentiate more precisely between entities in each category. Recognizing the difference among the typical diffuse medullary calcifications of type 2 renal tubular acidosis and medullary sponge kidney or between the

papillary calcifications of analgesic nephropathy and renal tuberculosis is more than an intellectual exercise limited only to radiology conferences.

The KUB can also provide an assessment of the bony skeleton for the presence of metastatic disease, renal osteodystrophy, or even some rare congenital anomaly, such as iliac horns, a sign that is seen in onycho-osteodysplasia (nail-patella syndrome or Fong's disease) and that frequently is associated with renal failure.

Occasionally, such as in the circumstance of a patient with diabetes and urosepsis, the prompt recognition of characteristic gas shadows of emphysematous pyelonephritis on the KUB can provide lifesaving information.

The addition of retroperitoneal tomography or laminography to plain film assessment of factors such as renal size and presence of calcifications increases diagnostic accuracy with only a minimal increase in cost

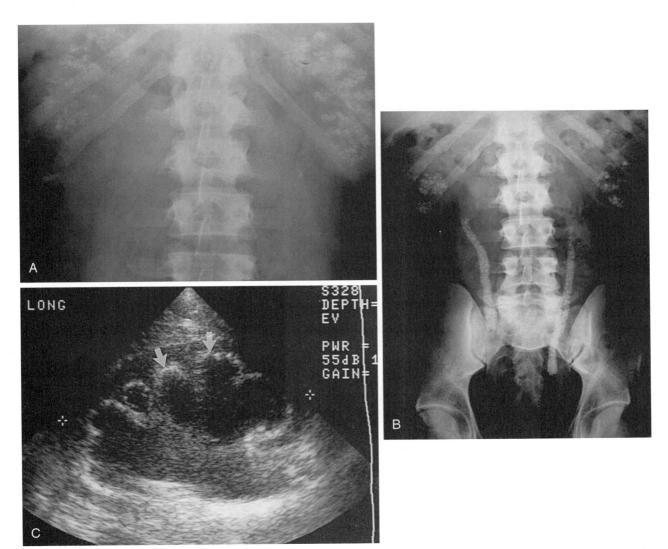

FIGURE 13–1 ■ Renal tubular acidosis. *A,* 34-year-old man with type 2 (distal) renal tubular acidosis. Characteristic diffuse and very extensive medullary calcifications are seen on radiograph. *B,* Same patient as in *A* 3 years earlier, when he presented with extensive ureteral calcifications requiring bilateral stenting. *C,* Ultrasound appearance of medullary calcifications. Note the extensive pericalyceal echogenic foci *(arrows).*

and radiation exposure and no significant added risk. Tomography is the radiographic technique whereby tissue planes in front of and behind a selected level (usually 1 cm thick) are blurred, thus clarifying the particular tissue slice of interest (by means of opposing movements of the x-ray tube and the film during the exposure). Tomograms are almost universally obtained during intravenous urography (IVU) in adults but are in the authors' opinion underutilized in association with KUBs. They are particularly helpful when there is a large amount of overlying stool and bowel gas obscuring the kidneys and have proved particularly useful in the evaluation of subtle renal calcifications. Unfortunately, equipment for performing tomography is not usually available in standard radiographic rooms where most of the KUBs are obtained.

INTRAVENOUS UROGRAPHY (INTRAVENOUS PYELOGRAPHY OR EXCRETORY UROGRAPHY)

While the development of cross-sectional imaging modalities, such as ultrasound, computed tomography (CT), and magnetic resonance imaging (MRI) has greatly decreased the use of IVU, in general, and in patients with renal failure, in particular, note should be made of the contribution of nephrographic analysis to our understanding of the way the kidney handles contrast medium during different pathophysiologic conditions. Technically, the nephrogram is the increased density produced by iodine atoms in renal tubules following the intravascular administration of contrast medium. The degree of enhancement de-

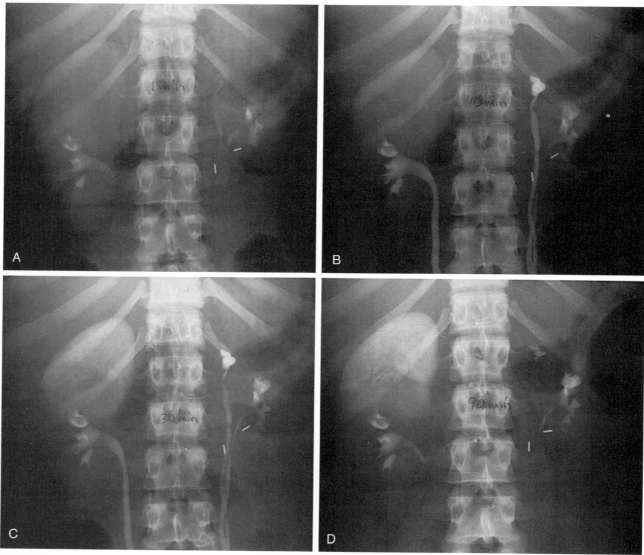

FIGURE 13–2 ■ Nephrogram of obstruction. Gradual increasing segmental nephrographic density due to a distal right ureteral calculus, producing acute obstruction of the upper moiety. *A,* Soon after injection; *B,* 10 minutes after injection; *C,* 30 minutes after injection; *D,* 90 minutes after injection.

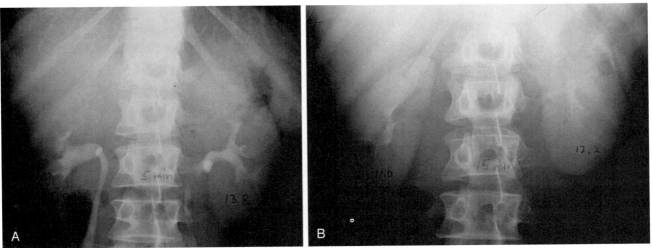

FIGURE 13–3 ■ Contrast medium–induced shock. A young woman experienced chills and hypotension during an intravenous urogram. Note the increase in nephrographic density between the 5-minute *(A)* and 15-minute *(B)* films. Also note the decrease in renal size (12.0 to 11.0 cm on the right and 13.8 to 12.2 cm on the left) during shock.

pends on a number of factors, including the total dose of iodine in the contrast medium, the rate of injection and thus the peak plasma concentration of contrast medium, the state of hydration, and the glomerular filtration rate (GFR). Fry and Cattell[10] first described the ability to distinguish between different causes of acute or chronic renal failure by carefully evaluating the nephrogram over time during IVU. They reported that there were three different patterns that were encountered in patients with renal failure, as follows:

• Type I: Immediate, faint, persistent nephrogram seen in patients with chronic glomerular disease.
• Type II: Increasingly dense nephrogram, seen classically in patients with acute extrarenal obstruction, and less often, in patients with hypotension, ischemia, acute glomerular disease, intratubular block, acute renal vein thrombosis, or ARF.
• Type III: Immediate dense, persistent nephrogram, seen most frequently in patients with ATN or acute suppurative pyelonephritis.

This now classic article by Fry and Cattell[10] discusses the pathophysiologic reasons and their hypotheses that account for the three distinct nephrographic patterns observed. In type I, the nephrogram is immediate, faint, and persistent because of a reduction in the number of functioning nephrons and in the ability of the kidney to concentrate urine, together with an increase in diuresis associated with azotemia. In type II, the nephrogram becomes increasingly dense over time (Fig. 13–2) and is usually seen in acute obstruction, often by a ureteric calculus. Despite the severity of the acute obstruction, there is still continued glomerular filtration of contrast medium that cannot be normally passed from the kidney. This results in tubular dilatation and an increase in the concentration of contrast medium, because of increased water and salt resorption. However, any cause of sluggish tubular flow, such as that which occurs in shock (Fig. 13–3), interstitial edema due to renal vein thrombosis, or

intratubular precipitation of protein may produce an increasingly dense nephrogram, as the result of the mechanisms just described. In type III, the nephrogram is immediately dense and persistent. This pattern is seen most often in ATN or acute suppurative pyelonephritis (Figs. 13–4 and 13–5). Although the pathophysiology of this pattern is still not well understood, it is probable that continued renal blood flow with filtration in the presence of some degree of tubular obstruction with chronic leakage and recirculation of contrast medium plays a role in producing this nephrographic finding. Fry and Cattell[10] admitted that there is often an overlap in these patterns, and in the authors' own experience it is very difficult to distinguish

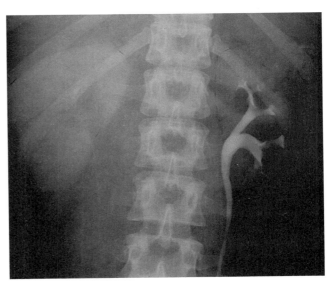

FIGURE 13–4 ■ Acute pyelonephritis. Acute right suppurative pyelonephritis in a young woman. Note the dense appearance on the nephrogram that was immediate and persistent. There is some excretion of contrast medium, but it is markedly diminished because of renal edema and tubular obstruction. There is no extrarenal obstruction.

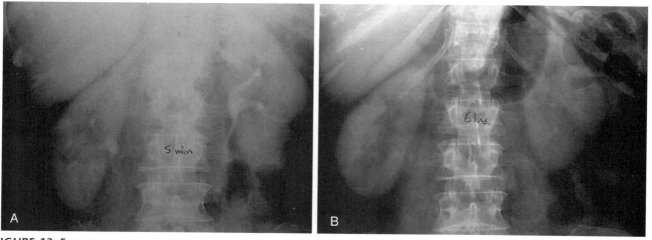

FIGURE 13-5 ▪ Acute pyelonephritis. *A* and *B*, A 61-year-old woman with acute pyelonephritis, who tested positive for *Proteus* and *E. coli* organisms at culture. Pyuria, fever, and bilateral flank pain were present. Note that both kidneys demonstrate a persistent nephrogram at 6 hours *(B)* despite the disappearance of the normal pyelogram phase seen at 5 minutes in *A*.

between type II and type III. Nevertheless, it is still useful to try to understand how the kidney handles contrast medium in different clinical settings and to correlate pathophysiology with radiologic observations.

Striated Nephrogram

In certain situations, the nephrogram, which is usually of homogeneous density, may be finely or coarsely striated. Most coarsely striated nephrograms indicate either the presence of multiple small parenchymal infarcts, such as those occurring in polyarteritis nodosa, or scattered areas of focal acute bacterial pyelonephritis. Finely striated nephrograms usually are associated with renal edema or acute obstruction. Ordinarily, the medullary rays (bundles of collecting ducts that extend from the cortex to the medulla) are not resolved with urography. However, interstitial edema and lymphatic engorgement separate these bundles of tubules, and, under ideal imaging conditions, fine linear opaque lines alternating with non-opaque linear shadows (Fig. 13–6) are seen. Acute obstruction is the most frequently associated renal pathology that produces fine striations. These kidneys are edematous, and the tubular and collecting duct contrast medium may be denser because of tubular stasis and increased water resorption. Other causes of fine medullary ray visualization are acute renal vein thrombosis, acute interstitial nephritis, and contrast medium–induced tubular protein precipitation.

Vicarious Excretion of Contrast Medium

Occasionally in patients with ARF to whom contrast medium was administered for other studies (eg, head computed tomography), the large bowel or gallbladder can be visualized on a KUB 12 to 24 hours after contrast administration.[11] Although most of the contrast

medium is filtered and excreted by normal kidneys, in instances where there is an extremely low GFR, the iodinated molecules are bound by plasma proteins and processed by the liver, with resultant excretion into the bile, which becomes concentrated in the gallbladder and thus visible on radiography. Additionally, contrast medium can also be excreted directly by the large and small bowel, with resulting colonic visualization following large-bowel water resorption.

Despite the dangers of contrast medium–induced nephrotoxicity, high-dose IVU was used in the past to visualize, albeit poorly, the urinary tract in patients with ARF, particularly in cases of suspected bilateral obstruction. However, there is absolutely no indication for its use today with the universal availability of ultrasound as well as vastly improved non–contrast-enhanced CT and MRI techniques.

COMPUTED TOMOGRAPHY

Recent engineering advances, such as the development of higher resolution and rapid acquisition spiral techniques, have facilitated the use of CT in the evaluation of renal failure.[4] Even without contrast medium–enhanced techniques, hydronephrosis can be diagnosed and parenchymal thinning or irregularity and stones are easily seen in most patients. Although ultrasound remains the study of choice for convenience, safety, and economic reasons (see later), CT is invaluable when ultrasound is equivocal, particularly in obese patients or in individuals with marked oliguria in whom collecting system distention may be minimized. Computed tomography also has the advantage of being useful in quickly evaluating other abdominal organs for possible associated pathology. For example, bilateral renal arterial obstruction or segmental infarcts could be the result of an abdominal aortic aneurysm (dissecting or purely atherosclerotic) that might be the source of emboli.

Because of the inherent ability of CT to resolve

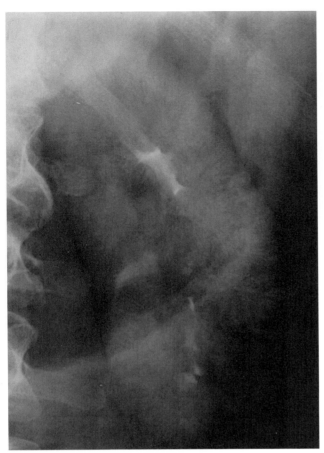

FIGURE 13–6 ■ Renal vein thrombosis. A 60-year-old man with renal edema thought to be due to chronic partial renal vein thrombosis. Note the fine striations in the nephrogram and the attenuated appearance of the pyelogram 20 minutes following injection. The striations are due to thousands of bundles of tubules (medullary rays), containing slowly moving concentrated contrast medium that are being separated and rendered more visible by interstitial edema, dilated lymphatics, and interlobular veins.

subtle differences in tissue density within 3- to 5-mm slices, all clinically significant stones and other renal calcifications are visualized, acute hemorrhage is identified, and most diffuse cystic diseases and tumors are also seen. Nearly the same nephrographic analyses can be made with CT as with IVU, with doses of contrast medium that are lower than those usually required for IVU (Fig. 13–7). In fact, the coarsely striated and persistent nephrogram so typical of acute pyelonephritis (and less often present in contrast medium–induced nephrotoxicity; Fig. 13–8) is seen much more frequently with CT than with IVU (Fig. 13–9). In addition, other findings, such as the highly reliable "rim sign" in acute cortical necrosis[12] (Fig. 13–10) or acute renal artery occlusion, can be seen and very accurate distinctions between some types of renal masses can be made (Fig. 13–11).

Complications of specific causes of renal failure, such as perinephric hemorrhage in patients with autosomal dominant polycystic renal disease or polyarteritis nodosa, multiple renal infarcts also in patients with polyarteritis nodosa (Fig. 13–12), or the develop-

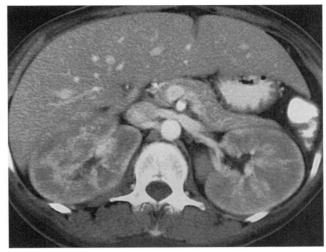

FIGURE 13–7 ■ Lupus nephritis. This patient with systemic lupus erythematosus had recently begun dialysis for ARF. Note that on this contrast-enhanced CT, the kidneys appear swollen and there is very poor enhancement of the medullary pyramids and some reduction in the cortical nephrogram. One would expect the cortical enhancement to be persistent. Compare with Figure 13–28. (From Kenney PJ, McClennan BL: The Kidney. In Lee JKT, Sagel SS, Stanley RJ, et al, eds: Computed Body Tomography with MRI Correlation. Vol. II. 3rd ed. Philadelphia: Lippincott-Raven; 1998:1158; with permission.)

ment of renal cell carcinoma in patients with acquired renal cystic disease, are easily identified. In patients with renal transplants, decreased allograft function may be due to lymphocele formation and associated

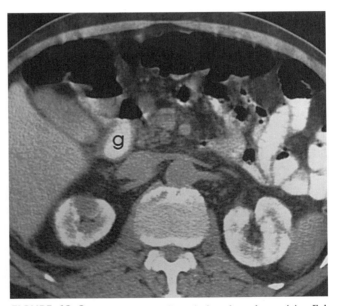

FIGURE 13–8 ■ Contrast medium–induced nephrotoxicity. Following a coronary angiogram, this patient's creatinine level rose from 3.0 to 8.0 mg/dL over a period of 8 days. Note the persistent nephrograms, typical of contrast nephrotoxicity and gallbladder opacification from vicarious excretion of contrast medium by the liver. (From Kenney PJ, McClennan BL: The Kidney. In Lee JKT, Sagel SS, Stanley RJ, et al, eds: Computed Body Tomography with MRI Correlation. Vol. II. 3rd ed. Philadelphia: Lippincott-Raven; 1998:1159; with permission.)

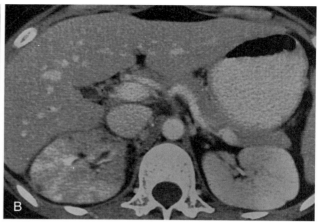

FIGURE 13–9 ▪ Acute pyelonephritis. Two patients with acute pyelonephritis, whose study results demonstrate coarse, wedge-shaped defects in the nephrograms. The process is bilateral in *A* and unilateral in *B*. The cortical enhancement would also be persistent. Compare with Figures 13–4 and 13–5. (From Kenney PJ, McClennan BL: The Kidney. In Lee JKT, Sagel SS, Stanley RJ, et al, eds: Computed Body Tomography with MRI Correlation. Vol. II. 3rd ed. Philadelphia: Lippincott-Raven; 1998:1146; with permission.)

ureteral obstruction. Computed tomography is also a very accurate way of evaluating the perinephric space in these patients, particularly if ultrasound findings are equivocal.

Thus, CT is a very valuable and powerful tool that often plays an important role in the management of patients with ARF.

ULTRASOUND TECHNIQUES

Ultrasound has proved extremely useful as the initial imaging modality for most patients with ARF. Although prerenal and renal causes often result in nonspecific findings, the ultrasound examination can be used to identify easily correctable causes, mainly hydronephrosis and obstruction. The advantages of ultrasound include (1) portable units, permitting bedside

scans; (2) no need for contrast agents; (3) no ionizing radiation; and (4) relatively low cost.

However, the reproducibility and quality of the examination depends heavily on the person who performs the scan. The body habitus of the patient also influences the results. Specifically, the larger the patient, the more difficult it is for the beam to penetrate into the kidneys.

The normal kidney on an ultrasonogram (Fig. 13–13) typically measures 9 to 12 cm long by 4 to 6 cm transverse dimension by 2.54 cm in anteroposterior diameter.[13] The more peripheral renal cortex has lower echogenicity (ie, it is darker) than the echogenic (bright) renal sinus fat centrally. The cortex has echotexture similar to or slightly less bright than that of the liver and spleen. Small, punctate echogenic dots may occasionally be seen, usually representing the arcuate vessels.

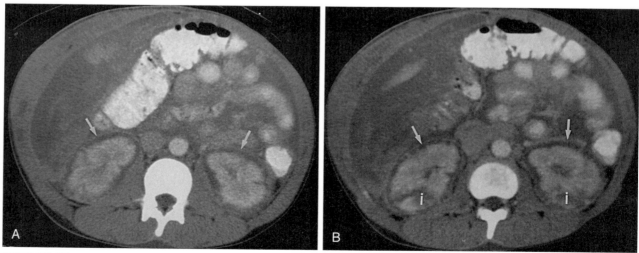

FIGURE 13–10 ▪ Cortical necrosis. A 19-year-old man with sickle cell disease presented with intraperitoneal hemorrhage and extensive renal cortical infarcts that were confluent and consistent with the diagnosis of acute cortical necrosis. In both *A* and *B*, note the thin rim of outer cortical tissue *(arrows)* still perfused by capsular collaterals. In *B*, there are larger areas of decreased perfusion due to infarcts *(i)* extending into the medullary areas.

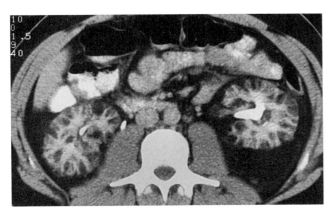

FIGURE 13–11 ■ Tuberous sclerosis with angiomyolipomas. This contrast-enhanced CT scan demonstrates numerous small fat attenuation masses in both kidneys, all of which are angiomyolipomas. (From Kenney PJ, McClennan BL: The Kidney. In Lee JKT, Sagel SS, Stanley RJ, et al, eds: Computed Body Tomography with MRI Correlation. Vol. II. 3rd ed. Philadelphia: Lippincott-Raven; 1998:1110; with permission.)

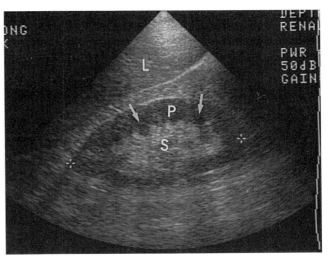

FIGURE 13–13 ■ Normal renal ultrasound. Ultrasonographic image of a normal right kidney in the longitudinal plane. Note the relatively less echogenic appearance of the renal parenchyma (P) compared to the adjacent liver (L) and the markedly echogenic central area produced by the collecting system and renal sinus (S) fat. The sonolucent renal pyramids can also be seen (arrows). (Courtesy of Carol A. Mittelstaedt, MD.)

Hypoechoic structures, each with a nearly triangular shape, lie between the renal sinus fat and the cortex. These represent the medullary pyramids. Within the central renal sinus fat is the renal pelvis and infundibulum. Normally, these structures are decompressed and rarely seen.

In the presence of hydronephrosis caused by obstruction or other etiologies, the calyces and renal pelvis become dilated (Fig. 13–14) and appear as nearly anechoic (dark) structures within the renal sinus fat that connect to the proximal ureter. When visualized, the obstruction can be relieved by antegrade or retrograde approaches.[14] False-negative and false-positive findings on ultrasonography are not uncommon.[15–18] There is a delay between the onset of

obstruction and the appropriate findings on ultrasonography that can extend to 24 hours or more. Sometimes hydronephrosis may not even be evident. This may be secondary to decompression from a ruptured fornix, but distal obstructing lesions that interfere with ureteral peristalsis, such as retroperitoneal fibrosis or tumors in the retroperitoneum, can also give a falsely negative ultrasound appearance.[19]

Ultrasonography in the setting of ARF is fairly nonspecific. In most patients, the kidneys can appear normal sonographically.[1] Decreased size and cortical thinning suggest chronic nephropathy. Eventually, the kidneys become small, echogenic structures—the typical appearance of chronic renal failure.[6] Sometimes,

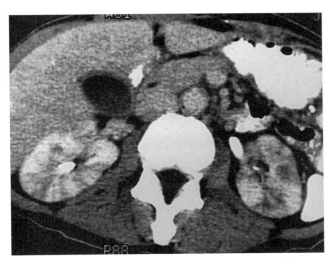

FIGURE 13–12 ■ Polyarteritis. This contrast-enhanced CT scan demonstrates the typical coarse, wedge-shaped defects in the cortical nephrogram produced by numerous small parenchymal infarcts associated with a vasculitis. Compare with Figure 13–27. (From Kenney PJ, McClennan BL: The Kidney. In Lee JKT, Sagel SS, Stanley RJ, et al, eds: Computed Body Tomography with MRI Correlation. Vol. II. 3rd ed. Philadelphia: Lippincott-Raven; 1998:1153; with permission.)

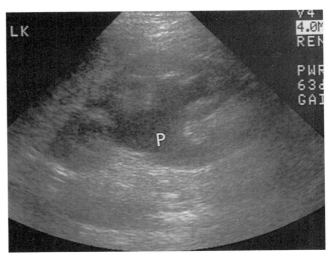

FIGURE 13–14 ■ Hydronephrosis. In this sagittal plane, the dilated proximal ureter, renal pelvis (P), and calyces can be seen as hypoechoic areas with associated decreased parenchymal thickness. (Courtesy of Carol A. Mittelstaedt, MD.)

the kidneys may increase in size in patients with acute glomerular nephritis and ATN. The presence of large, smooth, and often echogenic kidneys without hydronephrosis (Fig. 13–15) suggests an acute, potentially reversible event.

Occasionally, a more patchy distribution of wedge-shaped lesions can be seen. This was initially described on delayed contrast-enhanced CT and has subsequently been seen on ultrasonography.[20] The findings are thought to be due to areas of patchy vasoconstriction.

Doppler Ultrasonography

Doppler studies have been suggested as a means of distinguishing prerenal cause of ARF from renal ones. This is done by analyzing the waveforms of arterial vessels within the kidneys, specifically at the level of the interlobar and arcuate arteries. Partly as the result of intrarenal vasoconstriction, ATN usually produces a significant reduction in renal blood flow. A threshold value of 0.70 has been suggested as a useful upper normal limit for the resistance index (RI). The RI is the peak systolic frequency minus the end diastolic frequency divided by the peak systolic frequency.[21] Resistance indices greater than 0.75 have been described in 91% of kidneys with ATN, compared with less than 0.75 in 80% of kidneys with acute prerenal failure.[22] However, the RI results can overlap between these two major causes. Additionally, patients with hepatorenal syndrome can have elevated RIs (>0.75) with minimal intrarenal changes.[23, 24] More normal RIs can be seen in reversible ARF.

Elevated RIs can also be seen in acute obstruction. False-negative results may be obtained in scans performed less than 6 hours after the onset of obstruction.[25] A specific threshold value (eg, >0.70) may not be reliable in patients with superimposed medical renal disease (diffusely echogenic kidneys on ultra-sound). A more useful method is to compare the RIs between the two kidneys in cases of unilateral obstruction. A difference of greater than 0.10 has proved to be more predictive for unilateral obstruction than the use of a threshold value.[21]

The findings obtained for differential diagnosis based on ultrasound and Doppler ultrasound are nonspecific enough that renal biopsies are the only way of establishing a specific diagnosis. Via a posterior approach, a needle can be inserted into the cortex of the lower pole, with few complications under continuous real-time guidance.

RADIONUCLIDE TECHNIQUES

Radionuclide imaging can provide a combination of both anatomic and functional evaluation of the kidneys in patients with ARF. Imaging can provide help not only in establishing the cause of renal failure but also in determining prognosis. Radiopharmaceuticals used for the evaluation of kidney morphology and function fall into three main categories: glomerular filtration agents, tubular secretion agents, and tubular fixation agents.

Glomerular Filtration Agents

The radionuclides used for the measurement of GFR are ^{99m}Tc diethylenetriamine pentaacetic acid (DTPA) and ^{51}Cr ethylenediaminetetraacetic acid (EDTA). The plasma clearance of ^{51}Cr EDTA corresponds closely with the GFR determined by inulin clearance.[26] Measurement of GFR with ^{99m}Tc DTPA correlates very well with levels of both ^{51}Cr EDTA and inulin. However, renal clearance of both ^{99m}Tc DTPA and ^{51}Cr EDTA is slightly lower than inulin.[27, 28] There are disadvantages to the use of ^{51}Cr EDTA in that it cannot be used for imaging, and it is not readily available. ^{99m}Tc DTPA is commonly used to estimate the GFR because it is readily available and inexpensive, can be used for gamma camera imaging, and gives a low radiation dose to the patient. Gamma camera imaging is useful in that it can be used to estimate the differential GFR.

Tubular Secretion Agents

The second category of renal radiopharmaceuticals is the tubular secretion agents. This group consists of either ^{123}I- or ^{131}I-labeled orthoiodohippurate (^{123}I or ^{131}I OIH) and ^{99m}Tc mercaptoacetyl triglycine (^{99m}Tc MAG3). ^{131}I OIH, which was introduced in 1960, was one of the first radiotracers to be used to evaluate renal failure.[29] Chemically similar to para-aminohippuric acid (PAH), it can be used not only to image the kidneys using a gamma camera but also to determine the plasma clearance or effective renal plasma flow (ERPF).[30] OIH is secreted primarily by the proximal tubular cells (80%) with only 20% being filtered by the glomeruli.[31]

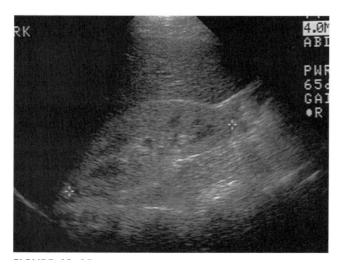

FIGURE 13–15 ■ Acute renal failure. Note the increased echogenicity of the renal parenchyma compared with the liver in this sagittal image of an otherwise normal-appearing right kidney. (Courtesy of Carol A. Mittelstaedt, MD.)

There are some drawbacks to the use of both [131]I- and ^{123}I-labeled OIH. [131]I has a high photon energy of 364 keV that is not ideal for imaging and a long physical half-life ($t_{1/2}$) of 8 days. It also decays by beta emission. Even though ^{131}I OIH is rapidly cleared by the kidneys, the absorbed dose can be high in renal failure, resulting in a high radiation dose to the patient. As a result, only a small amount of this agent can be administered for imaging, usually 7.4 to 11.1 MBq ^{131}I OIH. A larger amount of radiolabeled OIH can be administered if ^{123}I is used, usually 14.8 to 18.5 MBq. [123]I also has a better photon energy for imaging, 159 keV, and no particulate radiation. Unfortunately, it is expensive and not as readily available as [131]I.

Because of the high radiation dose to the patient when ^{131}I OIH is used, ^{99m}Tc MAG3 is the current tubular secretion agent of choice. [99m]Tc MAG3 is used to evaluate renal blood flow and function. It also can be used to evaluate plasma clearance or ERPF.[30, 32] Once administered intravenously, it clears from the blood in a biphasic pattern. The first component has a $t_{1/2}$ of 3.18 minutes, and the second component has a $t_{1/2}$ of 16.9 minutes.[33] [99m]Tc MAG3 is highly protein bound and is predominantly secreted by the proximal tubular cells.[34]

Technetium 99m has very good photon energy for imaging (140 keV), a short physical half-life of only 6 hours, no beta emission, and is readily available by generator. Because of these characteristics, a greater amount of activity can be administered (111.0 MBq), which results in better imaging. Even in renal failure, the absorbed dose is limited by the 6-hour $t_{1/2}$ of ^{99m}Tc compared with the 8-day $t_{1/2}$ of [131]I. Both ^{99m}Tc MAG3 and ^{123}I or ^{131}I OIH can be used for renography.

Tubular Fixation Agents

The last category of renal radiopharmaceuticals consists of the tubular fixation agents. These agents are used to image the renal parenchyma. The two agents currently in use are ^{99m}Tc dimercaptosuccinic acid (DMSA) and ^{99m}Tc glucoheptonate (GH). They are excreted by both tubular secretion and glomerular filtration. The uptake in the renal parenchyma is related to the relative amount of functioning renal tissue. Uptake in the renal cortex is prolonged with good clearance from the background and urine, which results in good imaging of the cortex and allows for the determination of differential function. Single photon emission computed tomography (SPECT) can also be obtained for higher resolution imaging of the renal parenchyma (Fig. 13–16).

Renography

Nuclear medicine renography provides functional information about the kidneys. Renography refers to calculation of renal time-activity curves after administration of the radiopharmaceutical. A renogram graphically displays the uptake and clearance of the radiotracer within the kidneys over time. Renal time-activity curves are produced by obtaining multiple serial images of the kidneys during a specified time interval. Regions of interest (ROIs) are drawn around the kidneys, the renal cortices, and renal pelves in each of the images to calculate the amount of activity in the structures of interest. Activity in these regions is then plotted against time. In general, renography is per-

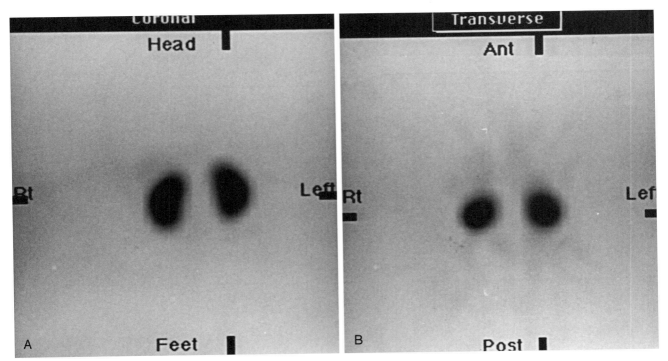

FIGURE 13–16 ■ Normal kidneys in a 4-year-old patient. Coronal *(A)* and transverse *(B)* SPECT images of the kidneys. Note the diffuse, homogeneous radiotracer uptake in the renal parenchyma in this normal ^{99m}Tc DMSA scan.

formed to evaluate suspected ureteral obstruction, renal artery stenosis, acute tubular necrosis, and rejection in transplant kidneys.

Once hydronephrosis has been established through another imaging method such as ultrasound, nuclear medicine evaluation of the dilated upper urinary tract is usually accomplished with diuresis renography to differentiate between obstructive and nonobstructive hydronephrosis. A ^{99m}Tc MAG3 renogram is shown in Figure 13–17. Regions of interest were drawn around the kidneys on the computer screen, and time-activity curves calculated for each kidney. The normal renogram has three segments. The first segment represents the vascular phase during which radiotracer in the blood first arrives in the kidneys. This usually only lasts

about 30 seconds. The second phase represents the uptake of the radiotracer in the kidney prior to any excretion. Normally, the time to peak accumulation of the renal radiopharmaceutical in the renal cortex is between 3 and 5 minutes. The third phase is the clearance phase, representing clearance of the radiotracer from the kidneys into the urine. In obstruction, there is a delay in the time to peak activity in the renal cortex, followed by delayed clearance from the kidney. If the obstruction is functional, there is typically a good response to administration of a diuretic, usually furosemide, 40 mg in an adult patient. If the obstruction is mechanical, there will be no response or a poor response to diuretic administration (Fig. 13–18).

Renal ischemia continues to be a major cause of

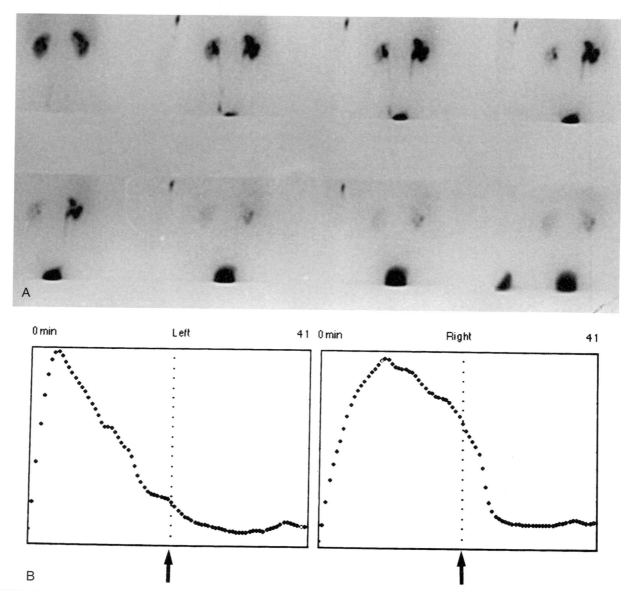

FIGURE 13–17 ▪ ^{99m}Tc MAG3 diuretic renogram. *A,* Posterior 5-minute-per-frame images demonstrate delayed clearance of the right kidney with prominence of the right collecting system. *B,* The left renal time-activity curve demonstrates a normal appearance with a rapid upslope (vascular phase), good accumulation of the radiotracer in the renal cortex, and good clearance from the collecting system. The time to peak activity is delayed on the right side, with some delay in clearance. There was a prompt response to the administration of a diuretic 20 minutes into the study *(arrows),* which was consistent with nonobstructive hydronephrosis in the right kidney.

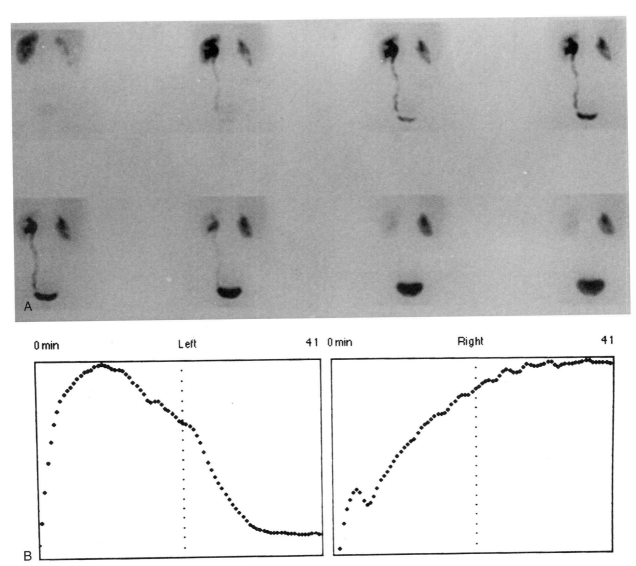

0 min   Left   41 | 0 min   Right   41

FIGURE 13–18 ▪ Obstructive and nonobstructive hydronephrosis. A ⁹⁹ᵐTc MAG3 diuretic renogram. Posterior 5-minute-per-frame images *(A)* and renal time-activity curves *(B)* demonstrating obstruction in the right kidney and nonobstructive hydronephrosis in the left kidney.

ARF and occurs in two different clinical situations: (1) when it is anticipated, as in elective surgery, and (2) during unplanned ischemic events (including crush injuries, severe sepsis, or obstructive uropathy).[35] Scintigraphically, ATN demonstrates relatively preserved renal blood flow with delayed uptake of the radiotracer along with delayed clearance (Fig. 13–19).

Cortical Scintigraphy

Renal cortical scintigraphy using a tubular fixation agent has been shown to be a sensitive technique for the diagnosis of acute pyelonephritis in the appropriate clinical setting. Decreased uptake of ⁹⁹ᵐTc DMSA is demonstrated in the renal parenchyma as the result of both ischemia and tubular cell dysfunction.[36] Patchy renal cortical defects can be seen in Figure 13–20 in a child with acute pyelonephritis. This can be compared

with the homogeneous radiotracer uptake seen in a normal ⁹⁹ᵐTc DMSA renal scan (see Fig. 13–16).

MAGNETIC RESONANCE IMAGING

Magnetic resonance imaging can be useful in the evaluation of renal disease. Although not usually used for initial evaluation of ARF, it can provide functional and anatomic information (Fig. 13–21), especially in situations in which the risk-benefit ratio of using iodinated contrast material is high. In fact, techniques of MR urography that require no contrast medium are beginning to rival even ultrasound (Fig. 13–22).

In patients with elevated serum creatinine concentration, the renal cortex shows changes on MRI examination (Fig. 13–23). One study showed loss of corticomedullary differentiation on precontrast T1-weighted fat-suppressed images in all patients with

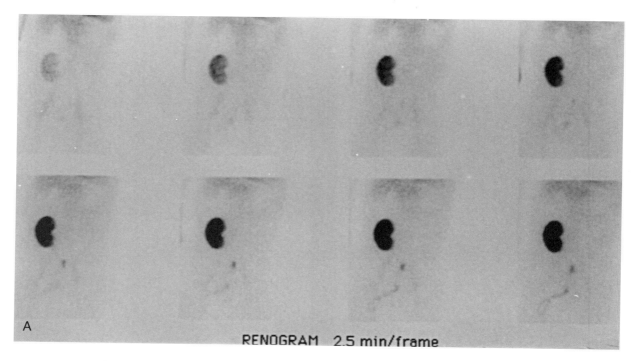

RENOGRAM 2.5 min/frame

0 min   Transplant   21

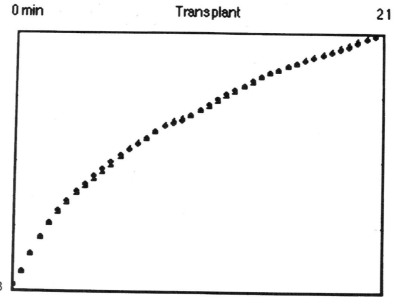

FIGURE 13–19 ■ Acute tubular necrosis. A ⁹⁹ᵐTc MAG3 renogram. Anterior 2.5-minute-per-frame images *(A)* and renal time-activity curve *(B)* demonstrating markedly delayed time-to-peak radiotracer uptake, with no clearance seen in a postoperative day 2 renal transplant patient. The results are consistent with acute tubular necrosis.

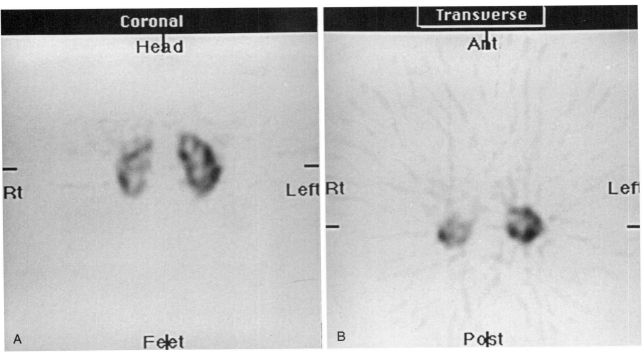

FIGURE 13–20 ■ Acute pyelonephritis. ^{99m}Tc DMSA SPECT images show associated coronal *(A)* and transverse *(B)* sections through the kidneys. There are patchy cortical defects seen in both kidneys, most prominent in the right upper pole in this eight-year-old patient with acute pyelonephritis.

serum creatinine concentrations greater than 3.0 mg/dL.[37] About half the patients with creatinine levels between 1.5 and 2.9 mg/dL showed similar findings. On postcontrast scans, these changes were not apparent until creatinine levels exceeded 8.5 mg/dL. This finding is not as useful in the immediate acute setting. In patients in whom creatinine levels have been elevated for less than a week, corticomedullary differentiation may still be maintained on precontrast scans.[38]

The cortical thickness and relative vascularity are easily demonstrated on immediate postcontrast MR scans because of the 5 to 10 times greater blood flow to the cortex relative to the medulla.[39] Cortical thinning is therefore readily detectable without resorting to iodinated contrast. The pattern of thinning or reduction in enhancement may be helpful in assessing possible causes of renal failure (Fig. 13–24). The pattern is similar to that seen on CT examination and angiography and is probably related to the distribution of parenchymal involvement or the vessels involved.[37, 38] A more regular pattern can be seen in diseases that can affect the entire kidney or the main renal artery alone, such as glomerular or tubulointerstitial disease, or that occur as the result of chemotherapeutic agents. A more irregular pattern can be seen in hypertension or diabetes mellitus from microvascular involvement progressing to irreversible scarring. Infectious and obstructive nephropathy can produce similar findings.

Renal Vein Thrombosis

Renal vein thrombosis can be easily visualized on MRI scans. Catheter venography has limited diagnostic

use because of the contrast medium used and the possibility of dislodging a thrombus, creating a pulmonary embolus. Although the diagnosis can be inferred on ultrasound in a patient with a diffusely hypoechoic, edematous, enlarged kidney, the clot may not be visible, and flow in nonobstructed renal veins, let alone in renal vein thrombosis, may be too slow to visualize on color Doppler ultrasound.[40] Nevertheless, assessment of RIs to infer renal vein thrombosis has some utility in the transplanted kidney, specifically, the absence or reversal of end-diastolic flow. However, this has not proved to be useful in native kidneys.[42] By comparison, postcontrast MRI almost always shows a filling defect within a contrast-opacified renal vein. Other noncontrast sequences can also be used to directly visualize the thrombus.[37, 42]

Renal Artery Stenosis

The gold standard for assessing renal artery stenosis (RAS) continues to be catheter angiography. Attempts to use Doppler ultrasound (Fig. 13–25) to evaluate for RAS have yielded varying results, with the accuracy-of-detection rate ranging from as high as 90% to considerably lower. Assessing tortuous vessels and limited visualization in some patients (eg, body habitus, overlying bowel gas) contribute to the wide variation in these statistics. In one study analyzing Doppler waveform patterns, there was interobserver correlation in analyzing waveforms in terms of normal or abnormal flow patterns. However, angiographic correlation based on waveform analysis was poor.[43] Color flow images can

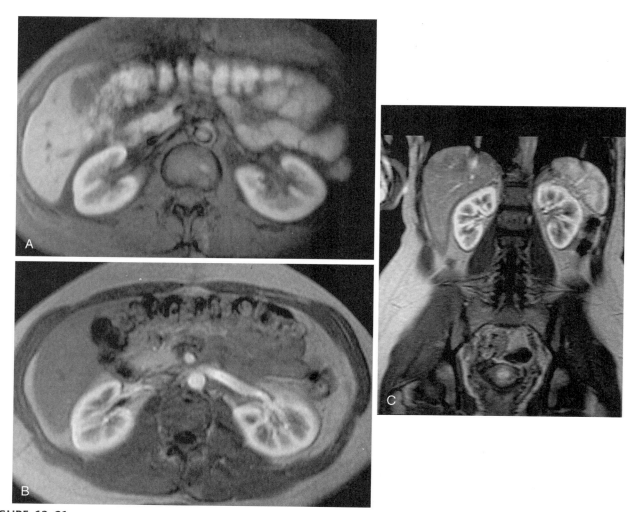

FIGURE 13–21 ■ Normal renal MRI. *A,* non–contrast-enhanced T1-weighted, fat-suppressed axial image. Note the excellent cortical medullary differentiation. *B,* Immediately following administration of gadolinium contrast medium, there is intense signal enhancement of the aorta, renal veins, and cortex in this T1-weighted axial image. *C,* Coronal image through the kidneys immediately following gadolinium contrast enhancement. (Courtesy of Richard C. Semelka, MD.)

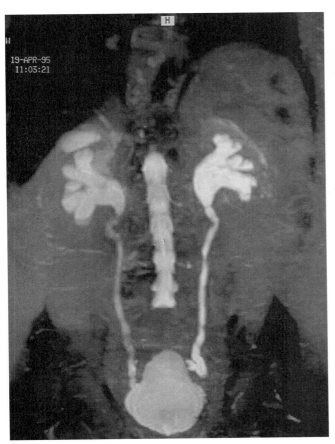

FIGURE 13–22 ■ Hydronephrosis demonstrated with MR urography. Heavily T2-weighted coronal image without contrast enhancement. Prostate carcinoma had invaded the bladder, producing outlet obstruction. (Courtesy of Richard C. Semelka, MD.)

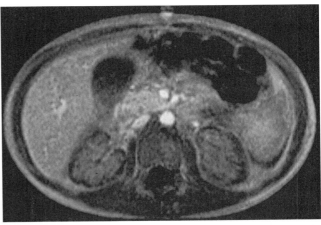

FIGURE 13–24 ■ Acute cortical necrosis. Post–gadolinium contrast T1-weighted axial image shows markedly decreased cortical signal intensity (compare with Fig. 13–10). (Courtesy of Richard C. Semelka, MD.)

be suboptimal owing to various technical factors, including the angle of the imaged vessel relative to the ultrasound beam. Power Doppler ultrasound, because of its greater sensitivity to flow and less dependence on angles, has shown promise in improving assessment and visualization of renal vessels. However, more stud-

ies are needed to determine its usefulness as a screening tool.[44]

Contrast-enhanced MR angiography (Fig. 13–26) has improved the quality of the images and shortened acquisition times to about 3 to 5 minutes for each plane acquired (coronal or axial).[45] When compared with iodinated contrast angiograms, specificities and sensitivities of 87% to 100% have been reported.[14, 46] In a recent study independently comparing magnetic resonance angiography (MRA) with angiography, there was similar interobserver variability for each modality. Although there was slightly better concordance for angiography than for MRA when assessing for clinically important disease (50% or greater stenosis), the differences were not statistically significant.[47] The results have not been as satisfactory for disease in the more distal vessels,[14] limiting assessment for such diseases as fibromuscular dysplasia. Furthermore, accessory renal vessels can be missed on MRA when compared with angiography.[46]

ANGIOGRAPHIC AND INTERVENTIONAL TECHNIQUES

Although conventional and even newer and safer digital subtraction renal angiography techniques have been replaced largely by other less invasive ones to evaluate renal blood flow, such as Doppler ultrasound and MRA, there still is the occasional situation when direct visualization of the renal artery and its branches or veins is essential for optimal patient management (Figs. 13–27 to 13–29).

A case of ARF in a previously healthy patient is not often caused by an acute arterial compromise, because both kidneys are only rarely affected at the same time. This is in contrast with acute renal vein thrombosis that often involves both kidneys, particularly if there is underlying glomerular disease. Obviously, in patients with renal allografts, the onset of ARF very much could be due to either acute arterial or venous obstruction,

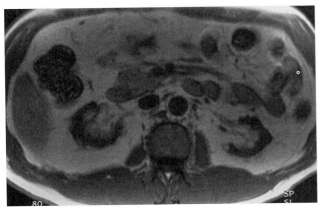

FIGURE 13–23 ■ Renal failure due to membranous glomerulopathy. Non–contrast-enhanced T1-spoiled gradient echo technique. Decreased parenchymal thickness was observed, and no cortical medullary differentiation was evident. (Courtesy of Richard C. Semelka, MD.)

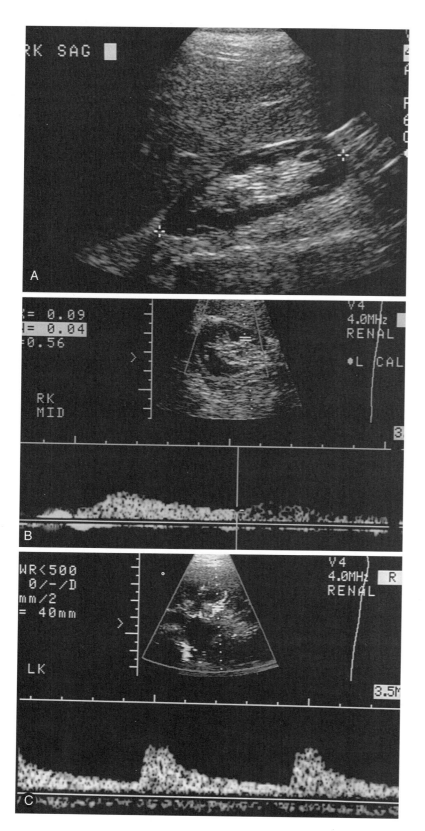

FIGURE 13–25 ■ Renal artery stenosis. This small (7.2 cm) right kidney was evaluated with Doppler ultrasound (A). Note the markedly decreased resistance index (RI = 0.56) with a tardus-parvus waveform manifesting a slowed systolic acceleration (SAT), with a low amplitude of the systolic peak (B). In contrast, the normal left kidney demonstrates a normal RI of 0.70 with a normal waveform and normal SAT (C). (Courtesy of Carol A. Mittelstaedt, MD.)

and optimal renovascular visualization is usually required. Modern vascular interventional techniques, including balloon angioplasty, stent-grafting, and thrombolysis are then employed with often dramatic organ salvage.

Vascular interventional procedures are not limited to the correction of arterial or venous occlusions, stenoses, or thromboses. Acute posttraumatic organ-threatening hemorrhage or even neoplastic lesions can be treated with various embolotherapies. However, patients with these conditions rarely have ARF, unless they have a solitary kidney or a transplant.

The management of acute obstruction with or without associated ARF is now routinely facilitated by interventional techniques. Percutaneous nephrostomy is often a lifesaving procedure in patients with acute pyohydronephrosis, and an antegrade nephrostogram often precisely defines the cause and location of obstruction.[48] The special case of renal allograft failure may demand antegrade interventional radiologic skills

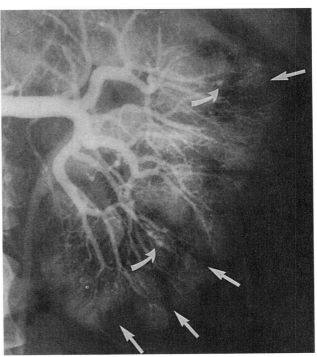

FIGURE 13–27 ■ Polyarteritis nodosa. A 21-year-old woman with malignant hypertension, rising creatinine level, gross and microscopic hematuria, and proteinuria underwent bilateral selective magnification renal angiography. A representative image demonstrates numerous cortical perfusion defects (straight arrows) and microaneurysms (curved arrows), typical of polyarteritis nodosa. (From Putman CE, Raven CE: Textbook of Diagnostic Imaging. 2nd ed. Philadelphia: WB Saunders; 1994:1133; with permission.)

once acute rejection, ATN, and cyclosporine nephrotoxicity have been excluded with the use of less invasive imaging modalities.

RETROGRADE PYELOGRAPHY AND OTHER UROLOGIC TECHNIQUES

Although a discussion of retrograde urologic techniques is beyond the scope of this chapter, the clinician is reminded of the many recent advances in cystoscopic and ureteroscopic equipment that greatly facilitate the investigation and treatment of obstructing urinary tract lesions from a bladder approach.[49, 50] Occasionally in the setting of ARF and gross hematuria, retrograde pyelography may be the only remaining imaging technique for reliably evaluating the urothelium and calyces. For example, the radiologic diagnosis of fulminant bilateral renal papillary necrosis can be made only with retrograde pyelography (Fig. 13–30).

VOIDING CYSTOURETEROGRAPHY (VCUG)

Although not usually considered a frontline procedure for evaluating patients with ARF, a voiding cystoureterography (VCUG) should be considered if bilateral vesicoureteral reflux is thought to be contributing

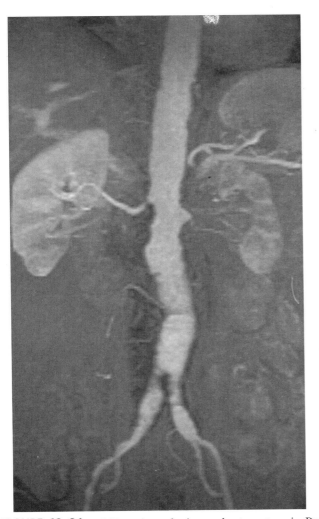

FIGURE 13–26 ■ MR angiography in renal artery stenosis. Dynamic gadolinium-enhanced three-dimensional coronal image demonstrates right renal artery stenosis and occlusion of the left renal artery as well as atherosclerotic changes of the abdominal aorta and both iliac vessels. (Courtesy of Richard C. Semelka, MD.)

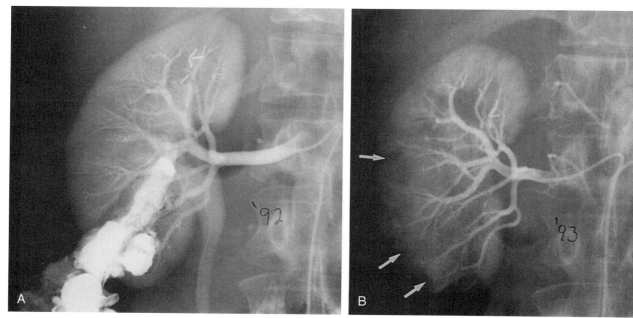

FIGURE 13–28 ■ Lupus vasculitis. *A* and *B*, Middle-aged woman with systemic lupus erythematosus demonstrated the development of renal vasculitis and renal failure over the course of 1 year. Although no microaneurysms were seen on selective renal angiography, numerous cortical infarcts were demonstrated *(arrows in B)* as well as generalized decreased cortical perfusion and irregular small renal arteries. Note the difference between the two studies (*A*, 1992, normal; *B*, 1993, renal vasculitis).

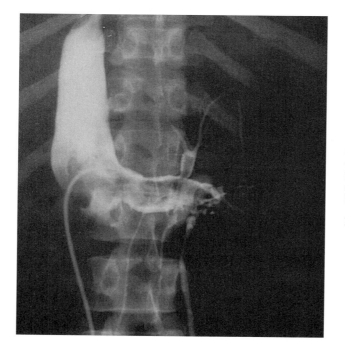

FIGURE 13–29 ■ Renal vein thrombosis. A 33-year-old woman with diabetes mellitus and systemic lupus erythematosus presented with proteinuria, edema, hypertension, and an increasing creatinine level. Renal biopsy revealed diffuse glomerusclerosis, and there was clinical suspicion of pulmonary emboli. Selective renal venography demonstrated bilateral renal vein thrombi with extension of clot into the vena cava. (From Putman CE, Ravin CE: Textbook of Diagnostic Imaging. 2nd ed. Philadelphia: WB Saunders; 1994:1137; with permission.)

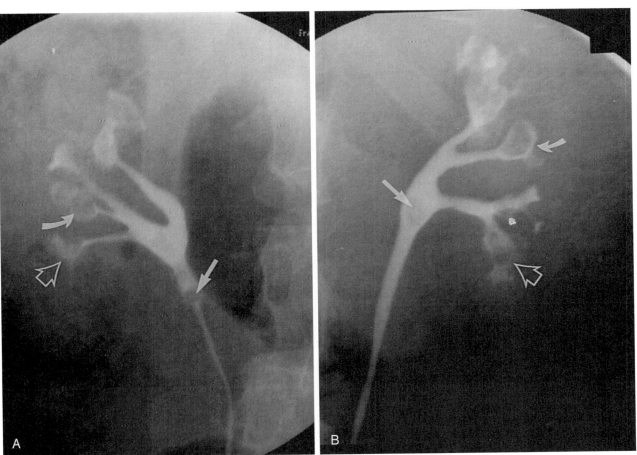

FIGURE 13–30 ■ Papillary necrosis. A 55-year-old man with diabetes mellitus and chronic renal failure presented with gross hematuria. Note on this bilateral retrograde pyelography the classic signs of papillary necrosis. Sloughed papillae that remain in the calyces produce the "ring" signs *(curved arrows)* and those that pass may be seen as filling defects in the pelvis *(straight arrows)*. Irregular shaggy calyces are also present *(open arrows)*.

TABLE 13–2. American College of Radiology Appropriateness Criteria*

RADIOLOGIC EXAMINATION PROCEDURE	APPROPRIATENESS RATING†	COMMENTS
Ultrasound techniques	9	Preferably with Doppler
Radionuclide techniques (renal scintigraphy)	4	Global and differential function
		Assess recoverability; distinguish from chronic
Abdominal plain film radiography (KUB)	3	Assess for calculi
Computed tomography (CT)	3	Potentially helpful in trauma
Arteriography, DSA	3	Potentially helpful in trauma; evaluation for renal artery occlusion
Voiding cystourethrography	2	(see exceptions)
Magnetic resonance imaging	1	
Renal phlebography	1	(see exceptions)
Body coil magnetic resonance imaging	1	(see exceptions)
Intravenous urography (IVP)	1	Problem of contrast nephrotoxicity

*Clinical Condition: Renal Failure; Variant 1: Acute (Acute Renal Failure, Unspecified)
†Appropriateness Criteria Scale: 1 2 3 4 5 6 7 8 9; 1 = Least appropriate 9 = Most appropriate

to the renal failure. An example of this situation might include a patient with mild azotemia due to bilateral pyelonephritis (reflux nephropathy) who has undergone antirefluxing procedures and now presents with superimposed ARF. The VCUG may also be indicated in patients with already marginal renal function but who are now manifesting ARF as the result of recent reflux secondary to new bladder outlet or urethral obstruction.

THE AMERICAN COLLEGE OF RADIOLOGY APPROPRIATENESS CRITERIA

Over the past several years, the American College of Radiology (ACR) has sponsored an extensive project that has reviewed the appropriateness of the various imaging modalities in the evaluation of many common clinical conditions. The task force included an expert panel in the genitourinary field made up of radiologists, urologists, and nephrologists. One of the conditions evaluated was renal failure (variant 1—ARF, unspecified). Their conclusions provide a helpful and clinically useful summary of much of material in this chapter (Table 13–2).[51] The entire report is available from the ACR.

CONCLUSION

The many available imaging techniques in ARF challenge the clinician to understand their widely divergent diagnostic efficacies in different clinical settings. Economic considerations[52] and availability of various modalities also influence management decisions. Consultation with knowledgeable renal imaging specialists, together with the information provided in this chapter, should permit a rational approach to diagnostic imaging in patients with ARF.

REFERENCES

1. Mucelli R, Bertolotto M: Imaging techniques in acute renal failure. Kidney Int 1998; 53(suppl 66):S102.

2. Becker JA, Carvlin M, Choyke PL, et al: Imaging of Renal Failure. In: Pollack HM, ed: *Clinical Urography: An Atlas and Textbook of Urological Imaging.* Vol. III. Philadelphia: WB Saunders; 1990:2595.

3. Davidson AJ, Hartman DS, Choyke PL, et al: *Radiology of the Kidney and Genitourinary Tract.* 3rd ed. Philadelphia: WB Saunders; 1999.

4. Kenney PJ, McClennan BL: The Kidney. In Lee JKT, Sagel SS, Stanley RJ, et al, eds: *Computed Body Tomography with MRI Correlation.* Vol II. 3rd ed. Philadelphia: Lippincott-Raven; 1998:1087.

5. Curry NS: Genitourinary Tract. In: Griffiths HJ, ed: *Radiology of Renal Failure.* 2nd ed. Philadelphia: WB Saunders; 1990:1.

6. Barbaric ZL: Renal Failure. In: *Principles of Genitourinary Radiology.* 2nd ed. New York: Thieme Medical Publishers; 1994: 251.

7. Dunnick NR, Sandler CM, Amis ES, Newhouse JH: Renal Failure and Medical Renal Disease. In: *Textbook of Uroradiology.* 2nd ed. Baltimore: Williams & Wilkins; 1997:225.

8. Levine E: Acute renal and urinary tract disease. Radiol Clin North Am 1994; 32:989.

9. Katzberg RW: Urography into the 21st century: new contrast media, renal handling, imaging characteristics, and nephrotoxicity. Radiology 1997; 204:297.

10. Fry IK, Cattell WR: The nephrographic pattern during excretion urography. Br Med Bull 1972; 28:227.

11. Becker JA, Gregoire A, Berdon W, et al: Vicarious excretion of urographic media. Radiology 1968; 90:243.

12. Badiola-Varela CM: Acute renal cortical necrosis: contrast-enhanced CT and pathologic correlation. Urol Radiol 1992; 14:159.

13. Curry RA, Tempkin BB, Shepherd GW: The Urinary System. In: *Ultrasonography: An Introduction to Normal Structure and Functional Anatomy.* Philadelphia: WB Saunders; 1995:114.

14. Bush WH: Radiologic Investigation of Causes of Renal Failure. American College of Radiology Appropriateness Criteria. Reston, VA: American College of Radiology; 1995:UR10.1.

15. Maillet PJ, Pelle-Francoz D, Laville M, et al: Nondilated obstructive acute renal failure: diagnostic procedures and therapeutic management. Radiology 1986; 160:659.

16. Curry NS, Gobien RP, Schabel SI: Minimal dilatation obstructive nephropathy. Radiology 1982; 143:531.

17. Naidich JB, Rackson ME, Mossey RT, et al: Nondilated obstructive uropathy: percutaneous nephrostomy performed to reverse renal failure. Radiology 1986; 160:653.

18. Kamholtz RG, Cronan JJ, Dorfman GS: Obstruction and the minimally dilated renal collecting system: US evaluation. Radiology 1989; 170:51.

19. Spital A, Valvo JR, Segal Al: Nondilated obstructive uropathy. Urology 1988; 31:478.

20. Sakemi T, Ikeda Y, Matsuo Y, et al: Renal wedge-shaped lesions on computed tomography and ultrasonography in two patients who developed acute renal failure with severe loin pain after exercise. Nephron 1996; 73:679.

21. Platt JF: Duplex Doppler evaluation of native kidney dysfunction: obstructive and nonobstructive disease. AJR 1992; 158:1035.

22. Platt JF, Rubin JM, Ellis JH: Acute renal failure: possible role of duplex Doppler US in distinction between acute prerenal failure and acute tubular necrosis. Radiology 1991; 179:219.

23. Epstein M: Renal failure in the patient with cirrhosis: the role of active vasoconstriction. Am J Med 1970; 49:175.

24. Platt JF: Doppler ultrasound of the kidney. Semin Ultrasound CT MRI 1997; 18:22.

25. Platt JF, Rubin JM, Ellis JH: Acute renal obstruction: evaluation with intrarenal duplex Doppler and conventional US. Radiology 1993; 196:685.

26. Brochner-Mortenson J, Giese J, Rossing N: Renal inulin clearance versus total plasma clearance of Cr-51 EDTA. Scand J Clin Lab Invest 1969; 23:301.

27. Rehling M, Moller ML, Tramdrup B, et al: Simultaneous measurement of renal clearance and plasma clearance of technetium-99m-diethylenetriaminepenta-acetate: ^{51}Cr-labeled ethylenediaminetetra-acetate and inulin in man. Clin Sci 1984; 66:613.

28. Fleming JS, Wilkinson J, Oliver RM, et al: Comparison of radionuclide estimation of glomerular filtration rate using technetium-99m-diethylenetriaminepenta-acetic acid and chromium-51 ethylenediaminetetra-acetic acid. Eur J Nucl Med 1991; 18:391.

29. Tubis M, Posnich E, Nordyke RA: Preparation and use of ^{131}I-labeled sodium iodohippurate in kidney function tests. Proc Soc Exp Biol Med 1960; 103:497.

30. Blaufox MD, Mattias A, Bubeck B, et al: Report of the Radionuclides in Nephrourology Committee on Renal Clearance. In: Taylor A, Nally J, Thomsen H, eds: *Radionuclides in Nephrourology.* Reston, VA: Society of Nuclear Medicine; 1997:22–36.

31. Saha GB: *Fundamentals of Nuclear Pharmacy.* 4th ed. New York: Spinger-Verlag; 1998:271.

32. O'Reilly P, Aurell M, Britton K, et al: Consensus on Diuresis Renography for Investigating the Dilated Upper Urinary Tract. In: Taylor A, Nally J, Thomsen H, eds: *Radionuclides in Nephrourology.* Reston, VA: Society of Nuclear Medicine; 1997:1–7.

33. Taylor A Jr, Eshima D, Fritzberg A, et al: Comparison of iodine-131 OIH and technetium-99m MAG3 renal imaging in volunteers. J Nucl Med 1986; 27:795.

34. Taylor AJ, Nally JV: Clinical applications of renal scintigraphy. AJR 1995; 164:31.

35. McDougal WS: Renal perfusion/reperfusion injuries: review article. J Urol 1988; 140:1325.

36. Majd M, Rushton HG: Renal cortical scintigraphy in the diagnosis of acute pyelonephritis. Semin Nucl Med 1992; 12:98.

37. Semelka RC, Corrigan K, Ascher SM, et al: Renal corticomedullary differentiation: observation in patient with differing serum creatinine levels. Radiology 1994; 190:149.

38. Kettritz U, Semelka RC, Brown ED, et al: MR findings in diffuse renal parenchymal disease. J Magn Reson Imaging 1996; 6:136.

39. Brezis M, Rosen S, Epstein FH: Acute Renal Failure. In: Brenner BM, Rector FC, eds: *The Kidney.* 4th ed. Philadelphia: WB Saunders; 1991:993.

40. Thurston W, Wilson SR: The Urinary Tract. In: Rumack CM, Wilson SR, Charboneau JW, eds: *Diagnostic Ultrasound.* 2nd ed. St. Louis: Mosby; 1998:329.

41. Platt JF, Ellis JH, Rubin JM: Intrarenal arterial Doppler sonography in the detection of renal vein thrombosis of the native kidney. AJR 1994; 162:1367.

42. Tempany CMC, Morton RA, Marshall FF: MRI of the renal veins: assessment of nonneoplastic venous thrombosis. JCAT 1992; 16:929.

43. Kliewer MA, Tupler RH, Hertzberg BS, et al: Doppler evaluation of renal artery stenosis: interobserver agreement in the interpretation of waveforms morphology. AJR 1994; 162:1371.

44. Helenon O, Corteas J, Chabriais J, et al: Renal vascular Doppler imaging: clinical benefits of power mode. Radiographics 1998; 18:1441.

45. Borello JA: Renal MR angiography. MRI Clin North Am 1997; 5:83.

46. Postina CT, Joosten FB, Rosenbusch O, Thien T: Magnetic resonance angiography has a high reliability in the detection of renal artery stenosis. Am J Hypertension, 1997; 10:957.

47. Gilfeather M, Yoon HC, Siegelman ES, et al: Renal artery stenosis: evaluation with conventional angiography versus gadolinium-enhanced MR angiography. Radiology 1999; 210:367.

48. Clayman RV, McDougall EM, Nakada SY: Endourology of the upper urinary tract: percutaneous renal and ureteral procedures. In: Walsh PC, Retik AB, Vaughn D, et al, eds: *Campbell's Urology.* 7th ed. Philadelphia: WB Saunders; 1998: 2789.

49. Huffman JL: Ureteroscopy. In: Walsh PC, Retik AB, Vaughn D, et al, eds: *Campbell's Urology.* 7th ed. Philadelphia: WB Saunders; 1998:2755.

50. Carter HB: Instrumentation and Endoscopy. In: Walsh PC, Retik AB, Vaughn D, et al, eds: *Campbell's Urology.* 7th ed. Philadelphia: WB Saunders; 1998:159.

51. Amis ES, Bush WH: Renal Failure. In: *American College of Radiology Appropriateness Criteria.* Reston, VA: American College of Radiology; 1995:UR10.1.

52. Grossman ZD, Katz DS, Santelli ED, et al: Renal Failure. In: *Cost-Effective Diagnostic Imaging: The Clinician's Guide.* 3rd ed. St. Louis: Mosby-Yearbook; 1995:107.

CHAPTER 14

Hemoglobinuria

Karl A. Nath

INTRODUCTION

Hemoglobinuria describes the presence in urine of hemoglobin that has undergone filtration in the kidney and has escaped uptake or degradation by the renal tubular epithelium. When red blood cell destruction occurs, hemoglobin that is released from red cells is avidly bound to haptoglobin, the latter present in the serum at a concentration of 50 to 300 mg/dL. Haptoglobin can bind up to 200 mg/dL of hemoglobin. This hemoglobin-haptoglobin complex is sufficiently large such that it cannot be filtered at the glomerular filtration barrier; this complex subsequently undergoes uptake and degradation by the reticuloendothelial system.[1] The release of hemoglobin from lysed erythrocytes in quantities that swamp the binding capacity of haptoglobin leads to the presence of free hemoglobin in serum. Free hemoglobin in serum exists not only in tetrameric form (2α and 2β globin chains, molecular weight 68 kDa) but also in dimeric form (1α and 1β globin chains, molecular weight 32 kDa). For example, it is estimated that in a solution of hemoglobin at a concentration of 100 mg/dL, and studied under physiologic conditions, 25% of hemoglobin is in the dimeric state.[1–3] Dimeric hemoglobin is readily filtered at the glomerular filtration barrier, and such filtered hemoglobin is taken up by the renal tubular epithelium and metabolized.[1–3] Tetrameric hemoglobin is also filtered into the urine, albeit to a very much reduced extent as compared with dimeric hemoglobin. However, tetrameric hemoglobin is filtered more readily than a similarly sized protein such as albumin (68 kDa), and such preferential filtration may reflect the isoelectric point of hemoglobin (approximately 6.8 to 7.1) or the shape of tetrameric hemoglobin.[4]

Filtered hemoglobin is taken up by the renal proximal tubule and undergoes scission into the heme and globin moieties.[1–3] The heme moiety of hemoglobin is degraded by the rate-limiting enzyme, heme oxygenase.[1] Normally, the activity of heme oxygenase in the kidney is quite low, but it is readily induced in circumstances in which the kidney is subjected to large amounts of heme proteins.[5, 6] Heme oxygenase facilitates the opening of the heme ring and the conversion of heme to biliverdin. During this conversion, iron is released from the heme ring. Biliverdin is subsequently converted to bilirubin by the enzyme biliverdin reductase. The iron that is released from the heme ring may be stored as ferritin-hemosiderin, recycled back into the intracellular iron pool, or utilized in the synthesis of iron-containing proteins. In hemoglobinuric states, hemosiderin may be detected in tubular epithelial cells

that are shed into urine, and such hemosiderinuria may be employed as a diagnostic aid.

In health, the tissues that express the greatest amounts of heme oxygenase activity are those of the reticuloendothelial system involved with the culling of senescent red blood cells from the circulation; heme oxygenase is needed in these tissues to degrade heme as these senescent red blood cells are destroyed.[1] In diseased states in which there is extravascular hemolysis, hemoglobin so released usually can be metabolized by the reticuloendothelial system such that heme is converted to biliverdin and, subsequently, to bilirubin. In these circumstances, the kidney is not exposed to large quantities of hemoglobin. In contrast, intravascular hemolysis of sufficient severity may impose such a large burden of hemoglobin that the binding capacity of haptoglobin and the degradative capacity of heme oxygenase are overwhelmed: large amounts of hemoglobin thus reach the kidney. In such circumstances, hemoglobinemia leads to hemoglobinuria and, in certain settings, may precipitate acute renal insufficiency. Hemoglobinuric acute renal insufficiency thus usually reflects intravascular, not extravascular, hemolysis, which subjects the kidney to copious amounts of heme proteins.

PATHOGENESIS OF HEMOGLOBINURIC ACUTE RENAL FAILURE

The pathogenesis of hemoglobinuric acute renal failure (ARF) is only briefly reviewed in this chapter, because a more detailed description is provided in Chapter 9. Current understanding of the pathogenesis of hemoglobinuric ARF is derived from clinical observations of this disorder, from studies using the glycerol myohemoglobinuric model and those employing direct infusion of hemoglobin, and from a sizable literature based on attempts to develop safe hemoglobin-based red blood cell substitutes.[4, 6–8] From such multiple lines of evidence, it is clear that the pathogenesis of hemoglobinuric ARF represents the confluence and commingling of three pathogenetic mechanisms[6–8]: renal vasoconstriction, direct cytotoxicity of hemoglobin, and nephron cast formation. The likelihood that hemoglobin induces marked renal injury in the unperturbed state is low; however, in certain settings (see later), the risk of hemoglobin-induced renal injury increases appreciably. Renal vasoconstriction induced by hemoglobin arises, at least in part, from scavenging of nitric oxide from the renal vasculature by hemoglobin; additionally, increased renal production of vasoconstrictors such as endothelin, thromboxanes, and isoprostanes may be stimulated by hemoglobin. Renal vasoconstriction predisposes toward renal ischemia, and the metabolic and other consequences of ischemia, in turn, render the kidney prone to the toxicity of heme proteins. The toxicity of hemoglobin arises partly from its heme moiety. Heme is toxic to cellular organelles, either directly or through its released iron, and by mechanisms that involve the generation of reactive oxygen species. Hemoglobin may directly generate reactive oxygen species as its heme-iron cycles between ferric and ferryl oxidation states of iron.[9] The third pathway involves tubular cast formation, which represents the interaction of heme proteins with Tamm-Horsfall protein, and one that is accentuated by reduced urinary pH. Tubular cast formation not only occludes nephrons but also, by inhibiting the urinary egress of heme proteins, prolongs exposure of renal tubular epithelium to denatured hemoglobin, thereby increasing the risk of cellular toxicity from the latter. Renal ischemia provoked by hemoglobin-induced vasoconstriction predisposes toward tubular injury and the sloughing of epithelial cells into the urinary space. In turn, such cellular debris would promote cast formation and obstruction of nephrons. Thus, these three major pathways all interact and accentuate the nephrotoxic actions of each other.

CLINICAL CONDITIONS THAT PREDISPOSE TOWARD ACUTE RENAL FAILURE DURING HEMOGLOBINURIA

A number of factors predispose toward acute renal insufficiency during hemoglobinuria. These include the severity and precipitancy of intravascular hemolysis, volume depletion, systemic hypotension, acidosis, and concurrent sepsis.[8] Conditions such as volume depletion and systemic hypotension impair renal perfusion, predispose to renal ischemia, decrease urinary output, and promote tubular cast formation. Acidosis promotes the oxidation of hemoglobin and thereby the formation of methemoglobin, hemichromes, and the likelihood that free heme would be liberated; such oxidative denaturation of hemoglobin increases its nephrotoxicity. Acidosis also promotes tubular cast formation and thus the obstruction of nephrons.[8]

Sepsis heightens the nephrotoxicity of heme proteins.[10] For example, the concomitant administration of endotoxin worsens renal function induced either by the glycerol model of heme protein injury or by the direct administration of heme proteins.[10] Specific cytokines are incriminated in this exacerbatory effect of sepsis. For example, tumor necrosis factor-α (TNF-α) levels are increased during experimental rhabdomyolysis, and the administration of an antibody to TNF-α protects against renal injury.[11] Thus, it is possible that high circulating levels of cytokines such as TNF-α during sepsis may exacerbate that component of hemoglobinuric renal disease that is dependent on TNF-α. Other mechanisms by which sepsis may accentuate the risk of hemoglobinuric ARF include the generation of cytokines such as endothelin, the latter copiously produced by the kidney during sepsis. The vasoconstrictive effect of this cytokine may predispose toward ARF in hemoglobinuric conditions. Like sepsis, conditions such as multiorgan failure and those characterized by extensive tissue ischemia and infarction may also be associated with elevated circulating levels of assorted cytokines; such cytokines, in conjunction with hemoglobinuria, may exert adverse effects on the kidney.

Hemoglobinuric acute renal disease may be seen in microangiopathic disorders. These conditions diminish tissue perfusion, impose renal ischemia, and thus increase the risk of hemoglobinuric renal insufficiency. Additionally, these conditions may be associated with endothelial injury that leads to "activation" of the endothelium: a proinflammatory and a procoagulant phenotype of the endothelium thus emerges. Such alteration in the endothelium provides sources of cytokines and other inflammatory mediators that accentuate the nephrotoxicity of heme proteins.

DIFFERENTIAL DIAGNOSIS OF HEMOGLOBINURIA

Hemolysis that is severe enough to induce hemoglobinuria may originate from pathogenetic lesions intrinsic or extrinsic to the red blood cell (Table 14–1). Erythrocytic membrane disorders include conditions such as paroxysmal nocturnal hemoglobinuria, in which there is an underlying abnormality in the glycosylphosphatidylinositol (GPI) anchor in the cytoskele-

TABLE 14–1. Differential Diagnosis of Hemoglobinuria

Mechanisms intrinsic to red blood cells
  Abnormalities in erythrocyte membrane or cytoskeleton, eg, paroxsymal nocturnal hemoglobinuria
  Abnormalities in erythrocyte metabolism, eg, glucose-6-phosphate dehydrogenase
  Abnormalities in hemoglobin, eg, sickle cell disease
Mechanisms extrinsic to red blood cells
  Immune-mediated
    Transfusion reactions
    Autoimmune hemolytic anemia
  Drugs and chemicals
    Oxidant stressors
    Immune injury
    Other agents
  Osmotic stressors
    Hypotonic solutions
    Hypertonic solutions
  Mechanical and traumatic injury
    Cardiovascular prostheses
    March hemoglobinuria
  Microangiopathies
    Disseminated intravascular coagulation
    TTP/HUS
    Vasculitides
  Infections
    Parasitic
    Bacterial
  Venoms and toxins
  Burn injury
  Bone marrow transplantation
  Hemoglobin-based red blood cell substitutes

ton of the erythrocyte.[12] This, in turn, leads to the loss of several proteins that normally reside on the plasma membrane, and these include anticomplementary proteins, such as CD55 and CD59.[12] CD55 inhibits the activation of complement component C3, while CD59 interrupts the distal steps in complement activation that culminate in the formation of polymeric C9.[12] The absence of these proteins in the plasma membrane of the erythrocyte in patients with this disorder thus predisposes toward complement-induced lysis of red blood cells. Acute hemolysis can occur spontaneously in this disorder or may be induced by bacterial or viral infections or by blood transfusions; acute reversible renal failure is a recognized complication of such hemolytic episodes.[13–15]

Abnormalities in erythrocyte metabolism that predispose to hemoglobinuria include disturbances in the hexose monophosphate shunt.[16–18] This pathway provides reducing equivalents, such as NADPH, and includes the enzyme glucose-6-phosphate dehydrogenase (G-6-PD). NADPH assists in maintaining glutathione largely in its reduced form. Reduced glutathione provides important antioxidant functions, such as the scavenging of hydrogen peroxide and the prevention of oxidation of hemoglobin.[19] Oxidation of hemoglobin yields methemoglobin, an unstable derivative, which can be oxidatively denatured to hemichromes. The heme moiety may be released from hemichromes.[19] Hemichromes, or heme, can directly destabilize the cytoskeleton and plasma membrane, leading to lysis. Thus, maintenance of adequate levels of NADPH and reduced glutathione is a critical requirement in safeguarding against the oxidation of hemoglobin. Individuals that are deficient in G-6-PD, especially when exposed to drugs (quinine) or conditions (sepsis) that foster oxidant stress, may develop hemolysis and hemoglobinuria.[16–18] Hemoglobinuria may also occur in assorted hemoglobinopathies and is well described, especially after exercise, in patients with sickle cell disease.[20, 21]

Extrinsic causes of hemoglobinuria are diverse and include immune-mediated mechanisms. Hemolytic transfusion reactions are less common than previously observed because of the rigor of current blood-banking practices. The acute reactions result from lysis of the transfused cells by preformed antibodies in the recipient, and could give rise to precipitous and overwhelming intravascular hemolysis, hemoglobinuria, and ARF.[22] In addition to the potentially nephrotoxic actions of hemoglobin, red cell stroma may exert injurious effects on the kidney.[23] Delayed hemolytic transfusion reactions occur several days after transfusion and are usually associated with extravascular hemolysis, and thus a lesser likelihood of hemoglobinuric ARF; however, ARF may also occur with delayed transfusion reactions.[24] Posttransfusion acute intravascular hemolysis may also arise from the transfusion of ABO incompatible platelets.[25] Not all posttransfusion hemoglobinuria, however, is immune-mediated; for example, hemoglobinuria may be induced by white cell filters and a pressure infusion system employed in the reduction of leukocytes during transfusions.[26] Inadvertent or

excessive warming of blood may also give rise to injury to red cells and hemoglobinuria.[27]

Autoimmune hemolytic anemia may be caused by warm- or cold-associated antibodies.[28] The former may be caused by hematologic malignancies, connective tissue diseases, or assorted medications. Cold agglutinin syndrome is a form of autoimmune hemolytic anemia that is secondary to an underlying hematologic malignancy. This disorder may also be induced by infections with such agents as *Mycoplasma* and Epstein-Barr virus.[28] Paroxysmal cold hemoglobinuria represents a form of autoimmune hemolytic anemia that is precipitated by exposure to the cold; it may occur as an idiopathic disorder or as a complication of congenital or latent syphilis[29, 30]; it occurs in children after viral syndromes and usually spontaneously remits.[29, 30]

A diverse range of drugs and chemicals used in clinical practice can induce hemolysis and hemoglobinuria, and these include antibiotics,[31–34] nonsteroidal agents,[35] α-interferon therapy,[36] fluorescein,[37] ethanolamine oleate used for sclerotherapy of varicose veins,[38] and intravenous immunoglobulin.[39] Such drugs may induce hemolysis by oxidant stress and by immune mechanisms, as well as by pathways that have not yet been elucidated.[28] Drug-induced hemolysis may give rise to fulminant ARF[31] and can be fatal.[32] Immunologically mediated, drug-induced hemolytic anemia may reflect autoantibody production, immune complex formation, or hapten formation.[28] Hemolysis and attendant hemoglobinuric acute renal insufficiency are recognized complications resulting from immune complex formation incurred by rifampicin[34] and minocycline[33] and from hapten formation induced by penicillin.[31] For example, rifampicin provokes the formation of IgG and IgM antibodies that are directed against the I antigen on the red blood cell, which leads to hemolysis and hemoglobinuria.[34]

A wide range of chemicals with industrial and other uses—benzene, phenol, other organic solvents, naphthalene, copper and mercuric salts, sodium chlorate—are quite toxic to red blood cells and may induce hemoglobinuric acute renal insufficiency.[40] Toxic injury to red blood cells may also be induced by assorted venoms derived from certain species of snakes, spiders, scorpions, and jellyfish.[41]

Osmotic stress can also induce hemolysis and hemoglobinuria. For example, hypotonic solutions used for irrigation of the genitourinary tract[42, 43] or inadvertently used in plasmapheresis could give rise to intravascular hemolysis.[44] Conversely, hemolysis may be induced by hypertonic stress following the use of contrast agents in dehydrated patients,[45] and following the use of hypertonic saline employed as an abortifacient.[46] Hypertonic glycerol has been used to reduce intracranial pressure, and its use can be complicated by hemoglobinemia, hemoglobinuria, and ARF.[47] Propylene glycol, used as a vehicle for medications, may give rise to solutions with high osmolality that contributes to hemolysis and hemoglobinuria.[48]

Hemoglobinuria also arises from traumatic injury to red cells incurred by prosthetic heart valves and synthetic material used for repairing cardiac and vascular defects[49–51] and following percutaneous rotational atherectomy.[52] Prosthetic heart valves may give rise to hemoglobinuria severe enough to suggest gross hematuria.[51] March hemoglobinuria (footstrike hemolysis), initially described in soldiers, is now recognized in diverse forms of trauma and activity that involve repetitive injury to red blood cells.[53–59] In certain instances, it may reflect an underlying red blood cell abnormality that predisposes to lysis. For example, anecdotal reports link the occurrence of such hemoglobinuria to deficiencies in red blood cell enzymes such as glutathione peroxidase and glutathione reductase, which assist in scavenging peroxides and in maintaining glutathione in its reduced state, respectively.[55] Additionally, a predisposition to march hemoglobinuria may arise in individuals with reduced hemoglobin-binding capacity due to unexplained chronic reduction in haptoglobin levels or in those with genetic haptoglobin variants.[57]

Fragmentation of erythrocytes and attendant hemoglobinemia is also a recognized manifestation of microangiopathic diseases such as hemolytic-uremic syndrome/thrombotic thrombocytopenic purpura (HUS/TTP), disseminated intravascular coagulation (DIC), assorted vasculitides, and allograft rejection.[28, 60] In these disorders, endothelial injury, activation of coagulation, deposition of platelet-fibrin thrombi on damaged endothelium, and inflammatory processes, promote injury to, and fragmentation of, erythrocytes as they traverse the microcirculatory beds. Hemoglobinemia and hemoglobinuric renal insufficiency may ensue.

Infectious causes of hemoglobinuric ARF include falciparum malaria.[61] Complications stemming from ARF significantly contribute to mortality in severe falciparum infections.[61, 62] In this disorder, hemolysis occurs in the extravascular compartment because of rheologic and biochemical alterations in parasitized and nonparasitized cells, in conjunction with alterations in splenic structure and function and activation of monocytes.[61] Intravascular hemolysis can also occur especially in the setting of G-6-PD deficiency and antimalarial agents that are pro-oxidant.[61–63] Fulminant hemolysis leading to marked hemoglobinuria and dark urine is described as blackwater fever. Quinine and other pro-oxidant anti-malarial therapies may be implicated in such hemolysis if patients are deficient in the enzyme G-6-PD. In recent studies of blackwater fever in southern Vietnam, 56% of cases reviewed were associated with quinine ingestion, 54% with G-6-PD deficiency, and 32% with concurrent malaria infection.[63] Parasitization of red blood cells, as occurs in babesiosis, may also give rise to hemoglobinuria.[64] Other forms of infections associated with hemolysis include bacterial infections from organisms, such as Clostridium perfringens, that produce hemolysins.[65]

ARF commonly complicates extensive burn injury, occurring either within days of the insult or several weeks after the burn injury.[66, 67] The early form of ARF is commonly associated with intravascular hemolysis and depletion of extracellular fluid volume, while the more delayed form of ARF is associated with sepsis, multisystem dysfunction, and DIC.[66, 67] Thermal insults activate complement and stimulate leukocytes to produce copious amounts of reactive oxygen species. Such oxidant stress, in conjunction with thermal injury, damages red blood cells, thereby giving rise to hemoglobinemia and hemoglobinuria.[66, 67]

Hemoglobinuria is a recognized, early-onset complication of bone marrow transplantation.[68] Hemoglobinemia reflects hemoglobin released from red cells lysed during cryopreservation and red cell lysis induced by DMSO, the latter used as a cytoprotectant during cryopreservation.[68] Hemoglobinuria may occur several weeks after bone marrow transplantation because of microangiopathic injury to red cells resulting from HUS/TTP.[68]

Hemoglobin-based red blood cell substitutes can themselves give rise to hemoglobinuria as a consequence of alterations in the glomerular filtration barrier induced by the hemoglobin preparations, or the effects of such hemoglobin preparations on tubular reabsorptive processes.[69–71] Much of the focus of the large industry centered around the development of safe, hemoglobin-based red blood cell substitutes is directed toward the prevention of renal clearance of hemoglobin (and thereby preservation of its retention time in the systemic circulation) and the reduction in the nephrotoxic actions of these red blood cell substitutes.

LABORATORY FINDINGS IN HEMOGLOBINURIA

Hemoglobinuria is usually associated with laboratory evidence of hemolysis. Thus, elevations in serum lactate dehydrogenase and unconjugated bilirubin occur in conjunction with diminished serum levels of haptoglobin and elevated free hemoglobin concentrations. The reticulocyte count is increased, and the peripheral smear may demonstrate fragmented erythrocytes and spherocytes, depending on the underlying cause, and other abnormal red blood cell morphology. The serum exhibits a pink discoloration because of the binding of hemoglobin to haptoglobin and the retention of hemoglobin in serum. The latter finding serves to distinguish hemoglobinuria from myoglobinuria, because the rapid excretion of myoglobin in urine does not permit accumulation of myoglobin in serum in myoglobinuric states.

Hemoglobinuria and myoglobinuria are associated with pigmented urine. Appropriate clinical and laboratory findings serve to exclude causes other than those due to heme proteins—drugs (eg, certain laxatives, phenazopyridine, metronidazole, methyldopa), disease (eg, porphyria), and dietary intake (eg, rhubarb, beets)—that can induce such discoloration of the urine. Examination of a spun urinary sample allows further differentiation, in that a red sediment is suggestive of hematuria, whereas a supernatant that is red and exhibits blood on testing by dipstick is indicative of myoglobinuria or hemoglobinuria. Myoglobinuria can be directly demonstrated, and the concentration of myoglobin determined, by immunoassays that use antibodies to myoglobin.[72]

Acute renal insufficiency occurs less commonly with hemoglobinuria than it does with myoglobinuria. Additionally, the pentad of electrolyte-metabolite disturbances observed with myoglobinuria—hyperkalemia, acidosis, hyperphosphatemia, hypocalcemia, hyperuricemia—occurs much less frequently in hemoglobinuria.

TREATMENT AND PREVENTION OF HEMOGLOBINURIC ACUTE RENAL INSUFFICIENCY

The risk of renal insufficiency occurring in hemoglobinuric patients is heightened by concomitant extracellular volume contraction, systemic acidosis, and concomitant sepsis. Thus, it is important to maintain expansion of the extracellular fluid and adequate renal perfusion by administration of isotonic saline and other intravenous fluids, as appropriate. Because acidosis predisposes toward the nephrotoxicity of heme proteins, while alkalosis antagonizes such injury, attempts should be made to alkalinize the urine with the administration of bicarbonate so that the urine pH is maintained above 6.5. One method that may provide effective prophylaxis against hemoglobinuric renal insufficiency is the administration of an isotonic fluid prepared by adding sodium bicarbonate (100 mEq HCO_3) and mannitol (25 g mannitol) to 5% dextrose; such fluid can be infused at a rate of 250 mL/h, and additional bicarbonate may be given so as to maintain alkalinization of the urine.[73] In addition to attention to volume expansion and alkalinizing the urine, attention also should be directed toward effective therapy for any underlying or associated infection.

Whenever possible, specific therapies targeted at the underlying mechanism accounting for the destruction of red blood cells should be applied: for example, cessation of exposure to the offending drug or agent, employment of appropriate protocols for transfusion reactions, and surgical correction for cardiovascular prostheses. In some instances, innovative therapies have met with success in certain settings: for example, the risk of hemoglobinuric acute renal insufficiency may be reduced by the administration of haptoglobin after extensive burns.[74, 75] Deferoxamine B may protect against hemolysis in patients with G-6-PD deficiency,[76] while exchange transfusion may be helpful following *Plasmodium falciparum* hyperparasitemia.[77]

The occurrence of ARF may require dialytic support for several weeks. Recovery from ARF usually occurs. Expertise in the management of renal failure clearly improves outcome in hemoglobinuric ARF. For example, in tropical areas where falciparum malaria is endemic, the establishment of teams dedicated to the management of malaria complicated by renal failure has resulted in a decline in mortality from malaria-associated ARF from 75% to 26%.[62]

REFERENCES

1. Pimstone NR: Renal degradation of hemoglobin. Semin Hematol 1972; 9:31.
2. Bunn HF, Esham WT, Bull RW: The renal handling of hemoglobin. I. Glomerular filtration. J Exp Med 1969; 129:909.
3. Bunn HF, JandI JH: The renal handling of hemoglobin. II. Catabolism. J Exp Med 1969; 129:925.
4. Simoni J, Simoni G, Hartsell A, et al: An improved blood substitute. In vivo evaluation of its renal effects. ASAIO J 1997; 43:M714.
5. Nath KA, Balla G, Vercellotti GM, et al: Induction of heme oxygenase is a rapid, protective response in rhabdomyolysis in the rat. J Clin Invest 1992; 90:267.
6. Nath KA, Balla J, Croatt AJ, et al: Heme protein–mediated renal injury, a protective role for 21-aminosteroids in vitro and in vivo. Kidney Int 1995; 47:592.
7. Nath KA, Grande JP, Croatt AJ, et al: Intracellular targets in heme protein–induced renal injury. Kidney Int 1998; 53:100.
8. Zager RA: Rhabdomyolysis and myohemoglobinuric acute renal failure. Kidney Int 1996; 49:314.
9. Moore KP, Holt SO, Patel RP, et al: A causative role for redox cycling of myoglobin and its inhibition by alkalinization in the pathogenesis and treatment of rhabdomyolysis-induced renal failure. J Biol Chem 1998; 273:31731.
10. Vogt BA, Alam J, Croatt AJ, et al: Acquired resistance to acute oxidative stress: possible role of heme oxygenase and ferritin. Lab Invest 1995; 72:474.
11. Shulman LM, Yuhas Y, Frolkis I, et al: Glycerol-induced ARF in rats is mediated by tumor necrosis factor-α. Kidney Int 1993; 43:1397.
12. Rosse WF: Paroxysmal nocturnal hemoglobinuria as a molecular disease. Medicine 1997; 76:63.
13. Jackson OH, Noble RS, Maung ZT, et al: Severe haemolysis and renal failure in a patient with paroxysmal nocturnal hemoglobinuria. J Clin Pathol 1992; 45:176.
14. Zeidman A, Chagnac A, Wisnovitz M, et al: Hemolysis-induced acute renal failure in paroxysmal nocturnal hemoglobinuria. Nephron 1994; 66:112.
15. Mooraki A, Boroumand B, Mohammad Zadeh F, et al: Acute reversible renal failure in a patient with paroxysmal nocturnal hemoglobinuria. Clin Nephrol 1998; 50:255.
16. Owusu SK, Addy JH, Foli AK, et al: Acute reversible renal failure associated with glucose-6-phosphate-dehydrogenase deficiency. Lancet 1972; 1:1255.
17. Agarwal RK, Moudgil A, Kishore K, et al: Acute viral hepatitis, intravascular haemolysis, severe hyperbilirubinemia and renal failure in glucose-6-phosphate dehydrogenase deficient patients. Postgrad Med 1985; 61:971.
18. Sarkar S, Prakash D, Marwaha RK. et al: Acute intravascular haemolysis in glucose-6-phosphate dehydrogenase deficiency. Ann Trop Paediatr 1993; 13:391.
19. Zerez CR, Tanaka KR: Erythrocyte Metabolism. In: Embury SH, Hebbel RP, Mohandas N, Steinberg MN, eds: *Sickle Cell Disease: Basic Principles and Clinic Practice.* New York: Raven Press; 1994:153.
20. Crosby WH, Dameshek W: The significance of hemoglobinemia and associated hemosiderinuria, with particular reference to various types of hemolytic anemia. J Lab Clin Med 1951; 38:829.
21. Platt OS: Exercise-induced hemolysis in sickle cell anemia: shear sensitivity and erythrocyte dehydration. Blood 1982; 59:1055.
22. Sloop ID, Friedberg RC: Complications of blood transfusion: how to recognize and respond to noninfectious reactions. Postgrad Med 1995; 98:159.
23. Schmidt PJ, Holland PV: Pathogenesis of the acute renal failure associated with incompatible transfusion. Lancet 1967; 2:1169.
24. Meltz D, Bertles J, David D, et al: Delayed haemolytic transfusion reaction with renal failure. Lancet 1971; 2:1348.
25. McManigal S, Sims KL: Intravascular hemolysis secondary to ABO-incompatible platelet products. An underrecognized transfusion reaction. Am J Clin Pathol 1999; 111:202.
26. Ma SK, Wong KF, Siu L: Hemoglobinemia and hemoglobinuria complicating concomitant use of a white cell filter and a pressure infusion device. Transfusion 1995; 35:180.

27. Phillips WA, Pottenger LA, DeWald R: Extracorporeal hemolysis in orthopedic patients. Clin Orthop 1989; 238:241.

28. Tabbaral A: Hemolytic anemias: diagnosis and management. Med Clin North Am 1992; 76:649.

29. Heddle NM: Acute paroxysmal cold hemoglobinuria. Transfus Med Rev 1989; 3:219.

30. Escoda L, Pereira A, Macna A, et al: Paroxysmal cold hemoglobinuria: only in the textbooks? Med Clin (Barc) 1991; 96:419.

31. Ries CA, Rosenbaum TJ, Garratty G, et al: Penicillin-induced immune hemolytic anemia: occurrence of massive intravascular hemolysis. JAMA 1975; 233:432.

32. Garratty G, Nance S, Lloyd M, et al: Fatal immune hemolytic anemia due to cefotetan. Transfusion 1992; 32:269.

33. Kudob T, Nagata N, Suzuki N, et al: Minocycline-induced hemolytic anemia. Acta Paediatr Japonica 1994; 36:701.

34. DeVriese AS, Robbrecht DL, Vanholder RC, et al: Rifampicin-associated acute renal failure: pathophysiologic, immunologic, and clinical features. Am J Kidney Dis 1998; 31:108.

35. van Dijk BA, Rico PB, Hoitsma A, Kunst VA: Immune hemolytic anemia associated with tolmetin and suprofen. Transfusion 1989; 29:638.

36. Yanaihara H, Nakazono M, Tsunoda S: A case of drug-induced immune hemolytic anemia during α-interferon therapy for renal cell carcinoma. Nippon Hinyokika Gakkai Zasshi 1996; 87:714.

37. Munizza M, Kavitsky D, Schainker BA, et al: Hemolytic anemia associated with injection of fluorescein. Transfusion 1993; 33:689.

38. Ohta M, Hashizume M, Ueno K, et al: Albumin inhibits hemolysis of erythrocytes induced by ethanolamine oleate during endoscopic injection sclerotherapy. Hepatogastroenterology 1993; 40:65.

39. Kim HC, Park CL, Cowan JH III, et al: Massive intravascular hemolysis associated with intravenous immunoglobulin in bone marrow transplant recipients. Am J Pediatr Hematol Oncol 1988; 10:69.

40. Dubrow A, Flamenbaum W: Acute Renal Failure Associated With Myoglobinuria and Hemoglobinuria. In: Brenner BM, Lazarus JM, eds: Acute Renal Failure. 2nd ed. New York: Churchill Livingstone; 1988:279.

41. Warrell DA: Venomous bites and stings in the tropical world. Med J Aust 1993; 159:773.

42. Goldberg SD, Gray RR, St. Louis EL, et al: Nonoperative management of complications of percutaneous renal nephrostomy. Can J Surg 1989; 32:192.

43. Bell MD: Sudden death due to intravascular hemolysis after bladder irrigation with distilled water. J Forensic Sci 1992; 37:1401.

44. Danielson C, Parker C, Watson M, Thelia A: Immediate gross hemolysis due to hypotonic fluid administration during plasma exchange: a case report. J Clin Apheresis 1991; 6:161.

45. Cohen LS, Kokko JP, Williams WH: Hemolysis and hemoglobinuria following angiography. Radiology 1969; 92:329.

46. Carvallo A, Currier CB Jr: Acute renal failure as a complication of hypertonic saline abortion in a kidney allograft recipient. Clin Nephrol 1977; 8:491.

47. Hkgnevik K, Gordon E, Lins L-E, et al: Glycerol-induced haemolysis with haemoglobinuria and acute renal failure. Lancet 1974; 1:75.

48. Van de Wide B, Rubinstem E, Peacock W, et al: Propylene glycol tonicity caused by prolonged infusion of etomidate. J Neurosurg Anesthesiol 1995; 7:259.

49. Park CH, Maytin O, Rubmi I: Postperfusion and macroangiopathic hemolytic syndromes after cardiac surgery. South Med J 1969; 62:348.

50. Okita Y, Miki S, Kusuhara K, et al: Intractable hemolysis caused by perivascular leakage following mitral valve replacement with St. Jude Medical prosthesis. Ann Thorac Surg 1988; 46:89.

51. Lander EB: Severe hemoglobinuria masquerading as gross hematuria following mitral valve replacement. J Urol 1995; 153:1639.

52. Dorros G, Iyer S, Zaitoun R, et al: Acute angiographic and clinical outcome of high speed percutaneous rotational atherectomy (Rotablator®). Catheter Cardiovasc Diag 1991; 22:157.

53. Pollard TD, Weiss IW: Acute tubular necrosis in a patient with march hemoglobinuria. N Engl J Med 1970; 283:803.

54. Schwartz KA, Flessa HC: March hemoglobinuria: report of a case after basketball and congo drum playing. Ohio State Med J 1973; 69:448.

55. Bernard IF, Galand C, Boivin P: March hemoglobinuria: one case with erythrocyte glutathione peroxidase deficiency. Nouvelle Press Med 1975; 4:1117.

56. Rimer RL, Roy S III: Child abuse and hemoglobinuria. JAMA 1977; 238:2034.

57. Baker BA, Schwartz KA, Segan DJ, et al: Hemoglobinuria after fraternity hazing. Kidney Dis 1982; 2:268.

58. Blaser S, Macknin ML: Head-banging with subsequent hemoglobinuria and acute renal failure. Cleve Clin Q 1983; 50:347.

59. Jones GR, Newhouse I: Sport-related hematuria: a review. Clin J Sport Med 1997; 7:119.

60. Singh N, Gayowski T, Marino LK: Hemolytic uremic syndrome in solid-organ transplant recipients. Transpl Int 1996; 9:68.

61. Etam-Ong S, Sitpnja V: Falciparum malana and the kidney: a model of inflammation. Am J Kidney Dis 1998; 32:361.

62. Trang TT, Phu NH, Vinh H, et al: Acute renal failure in patients with severe falciparum malaria. Clin Infect Dis 1992; 15:874.

63. Tran TH, Day NP, Ly VC, et al: Blackwater fever in Southern Vietnam: a prospective descriptive study of 50 cases. Clin Infect Dis 1996; 23:1274.

64. Brasseur P, Gorenflot A: Human babesiosis in Europe. Mem Inst Oswaldo Cruz 1992; 87:131.

65. Rogstad B, Ritland S, Lunde S, Hagen AG: Clostridium perfringens septicemia with massive hemolysis. Infection 1993; 21:54.

66. Hatherill JR, Till GO, Bruner LH: Thermal injury, intravascular hemolysis, and toxic oxygen products. J Clin Invest 1986; 78:629.

67. Aikawa N, Wakabayashi O, Ueda M, et al: Regulation of renal function in thermal injury. J Trauma 1990; 305:174.

68. Zager RA: Acute renal failure in the setting of bone marrow transplantation. Kidney Int 1994; 46:1443.

69. Savitsky JP, Doczi J, Black J, Arnold JD: A clinical safety trial of stroma-free hemoglobin. Clin Pharmacol Therap 1978; 23:73.

70. Lieberthal W: Renal Effects of Hemoglobin-Based Blood Substitutes. In: Rudolph AS, Rabinovici R, Feuerstein GZ, eds: Red Blood Cell Substitutes. Basic Principles and Clinical Applications. New York: Marcel Dekker; 1998:189.

71. Alayash AI: Hemoglobin-based blood substitutes: oxygen carriers, pressor agents, or oxidants? Nat Biotechnol 1999; 17:545.

72. Hamilton RW, Hopkins MB III, Shihabl ZK: Myoglobinuria, hemoglobinuria, and acute renal failure. Clin Chem 1989; 35:1713.

73. Eneas JE, Schoenfeld PY, Humphreys MB: The effect of infusion of mannitol-sodium bicarbonate on the clinical course of myoglobinuria. Arch Intern Med 1979; 139:801.

74. Yoshioka T, Sugimoto T, Ukai T, et al: Haptoglobin therapy for possible prevention of renal failure following thermal injury, a clinical study. J Trauma 1985; 25:281.

75. Imaizumi H, Tsunoda K, Ichimiya N, et al: Repeated large-dose haptoglobin therapy in an extensively burned patient: case report. J Emerg Med 1994; 12:33.

76. Khalifa AS, el-Alfy MS, Mokhtar G, et al: Effect of desferrioxamine B on hemolysis in glucose-6-phosphate dehydrogenase deficiency. Acta Haematol 1989; 82:113.

77. Looareesuwan S, Phillips RE, Karbwang J, et al: Plasmodium falciparum hyperparasitaemia: use of exchange transfusion in seven patients and a review of the literature. QJM 1990; 75:471.

CHAPTER 15

Nontraumatic Rhabdomyolysis

James P. Knochel

INTRODUCTION

Rhabdomyolysis is a term defining injury to skeletal muscle cells sufficient to result in leakage of their contents into the blood and their appearance in the urine. Clinically, myalgias, muscle tenderness, swelling, stiffness, weakness, or even paralysis may result. The physical findings may include tender, firm muscles that are painful when moved. Paradoxically, some patients, especially those with nontraumatic rhabdomyolysis, may present with very meager physical findings despite grossly abnormal laboratory findings.

Laboratory findings in acute rhabdomyolysis include elevation of the total creatine kinase (CK) level, which may reach approximately 2 million or more IU/L in severe cases. Ninety-four percent of CK in skeletal muscle is the CK-MM species, 6% or less is CK-MB.[1] Accordingly, an elevated CK-MB level does not imply myocardial damage in the presence of a substantially elevated total CK level. There is no troponin 1 in skeletal muscle.[2] In most cases of rhabdomyolysis, the CK-MM peak in serum occurs after 24 to 48 hours. Its half-life generally ranges between 36 and 48 hours.[3] Persistent or rising levels portend ongoing muscle damage. Other enzymes that may become markedly elevated include lactate dehydrogenase (LDH), aspartate transaminase (AST), alanine transaminase (ALT), and aldolase, but they lack specificity for skeletal muscle cell injury. Carbonic anhydrase III is reported to be specific for skeletal muscle but is seldom employed clinically.

Many patients with myoglobinuria show a positive result on urine dipstick testing for glucose in the absence of hyperglycemia. This occurs very early in the course of myoglobinuria and generally disappears after 12 hours. This apparent renal glycosuria presumably reflects impaired glucose resorption in the proximal tubule as the result of pigment-induced injury.

It is common to observe a disproportionate elevation of the ratio of serum creatinine to urea nitrogen in early rhabdomyolysis. This increase probably reflects a creatine leak from muscle cells, because any creatine released into extracellular fluid would spontaneously become dehydrated to creatinine. In some instances, the first time that the serum creatinine concentration is measured, it may be 3 or 4 mg/dL in the presence of a normal urea nitrogen level. This finding usually disappears after 24 hours.

Since the molecular weight of myoglobin is only 17,800 Da, its fractional clearance is 0.75 of creatinine, and thus it is cleared rapidly by the glomerulus. For practical purposes, there is no protein binding of myoglobin in serum. If the myoglobin concentration in the urine exceeds 100 mg/dL, it becomes visible and usually imparts a root beer color to the urine, because the pigment has undergone oxidation. The serum remains clear except in patients with massive rhabdomyolysis. Myoglobinuria is frequently transient and often missed by the patient and physician alike. Since it is a heme pigment, myoglobin causes a positive dipstick reaction for blood. It is seldom necessary to measure myoglobin specifically in urine. In almost all instances, the clinical findings, the elevated CK-MM, and the positive result for heme pigment in the urine dipstick test are sufficient to make a clinical diagnosis of rhabdomyolysis and myoglobinuria. Nonetheless, there are specific immunoassay methods for quantitating myoglobin that are not subject to interference by hemoglobin in the same sample.[4]

THE MECHANISM OF RHABDOMYOLYSIS

Studies on cellular injury from many disciplines have facilitated a general understanding of the mechanism by which rhabdomyolysis occurs.[5] Theoretically, the initiating insults, including trauma, toxins and drugs, physical agents (heat), immunologic reaction, enzymes (snake venom), or substances that alter ion transport, must alter sarcolemmal permeability. For example, an increase in sodium permeability of sufficient magnitude, by activating the Na^+, K^+-ATPase pump, could lead to exhaustion of the ATP supply, which would impair virtually every active transport process in the cell. The next step, which is regarded as critical, is calcium overload.[6] Indeed, experimental exposure of a healthy muscle cell to a calcium ionophore allows the cytosolic calcium concentration to rise.[7] This activates a variety of lytic enzymes that destroy the cell. A calcium channel blocker, such as verapamil, can block this process. Reduction of ATP stores in the cell opens potassium channels and independently blocks calcium uptake by the sarcoplasmic reticulum, which is one of the major regulators of myoplasmic calcium concentration. In skeletal muscle, like all excitable tissues, there exists another mechanism for controlling myoplasmic calcium, the $2Na^+/Ca^{2+}$ exchanger in the plasma membrane.[8] This transporter is driven by the high concentration gradient of Na^+ in the extracellular fluid, and the electronegative interior of the cell, which favors Na^+ uptake. As sodium ions enter the cell by this process, each pair is exchanged for a single Ca^{2+} ion, which is extruded. The Na^+ ions entering the cell are pumped out by the Na^+, K^+-ATPase at a rate exceeding their exchange for inwardly moving K^+ ions, by a ratio of 3:2, thus maintaining electronegativity of the cell interior, which sustains the $2Na^+/Ca^{2+}$ exchanger. When these processes fail, Ca^{2+} floods the cell, explaining in a major way how serum calcium concentration falls to such low levels in cases of severe rhabdomyolysis. Calcium-damaged mitochondria may generate superoxide with the resultant oxidant stress.[6] Infiltrating monocytes and neutrophils release their toxic products, which create additional inflammation and injury. Obviously, damage must also occur to capillary endothelium (endotheliopathy?), which would be necessary to permit access into the circulation of myoplasmic macromolecules such as myoglobin and creatine kinase, with molecular weights of 17,800 and 82,000 Da, respectively.[9] The important role of endothelial activation and associated injury has generally been ignored as a critical factor associated with rhabdomyolysis.[10]

CAUSES OF RHABDOMYOLYSIS

The causes of rhabdomyolysis are shown in Table 15–1. The most common cause of rhabdomyolysis is physical exertion. Repetitious, exhaustive exercise is a particularly prominent cause. Examples are violent calisthenics such as squat-thrusts, wind sprints by football players, weightlifting, pushups, and other similar activities. Long-distance running, especially in hot weather, is a common cause. Heat exaggerates muscle injury. A normal person shows elevated CK-MM levels after strenuous exercise but lesser degrees after exercise training. Eccentric muscle contractions (walking downhill or down stairs) are much more damaging to muscle tissue than concentric exercise (walking uphill or up stairs). For any given level of exercise, men develop more extensive rhabdomyolysis than women do.

Direct trauma to skeletal muscle with rhabdomyolysis is discussed separately in Chapter 16. Ischemic rhabdomyolysis occurs in arterial occlusion, in comatose patients lying on hard surfaces with limb compression, or during prolonged operative procedures, especially in the lithotomy position. Overdose with heroin or barbiturates probably causes rhabdomyolysis by this mechanism. Chronic congestive heart failure is often associated with modest elevations of CK-MM as the result of hypoxia and poor tissue perfusion.

Metabolic causes of rhabdomyolysis may be hereditary or acquired.[11] Examples of hereditary causes are shown in Table 15–2. Patients with McArdle's syndrome often give a history of repeated episodes of muscle cramps followed by myoglobinuria. Characteris-

TABLE 15–1. Causes of Rhabdomyolysis

Physical exertion	Infection
Direct trauma	Sepsis/hyperthermia
Ischemia	Drugs
Metabolic	Toxins
Hereditary	Immunologic
Acquired	

TABLE 15–2. Hereditary Metabolic Abnormalities Causing Rhabdomyolysis

Myophosphorylase deficiency (McArdle's disease)
Carnitine palmitoyltransferase deficiency (CPT)
Myoadenylate deaminase deficiency (MAD)
Phosphofructokinase deficiency (Tarui's disease)
Phosphorylase kinase deficiency
Phosphoglycerate kinase deficiency
Phosphoglycerate mutase deficiency
Lactate dehydrogenase deficiency
Combined CPT and MAD deficiencies
Malignant hyperthermia

tically, exercise performance is improved following a period of warm-up, the so-called second-wind phenomenon. Muscular work under conditions of ischemia (ischemic arm test) does not result in elevations of venous lactate, because these patients lack myophosphorylase and cannot convert glycogen to glucose, thus there is no lactate production in muscle. Malignant hyperthermia is a rare, often familial disorder of calcium transport in skeletal muscle, which is usually precipitated by administration of halothane or depolarizing substances.[12] It is characterized by the rapid development of rigidity, hyperpyrexia, increased oxygen consumption with hypoxia, increased CO_2 production, lactic acidosis, and rhabdomyolysis often resulting in acute renal failure (ARF). The specific prophylaxis and treatment of this condition is dantrolene, which acts specifically on calcium transport in the muscle cell. A number of studies have shown that this defect results from an abnormality in the Ca^{2+} release channel (ryanodine receptor).[13]

Examples of acquired metabolic defects causing rhabdomyolysis include chronic alcoholism, potassium deficiency, and phosphorus deficiency. Potassium deficiency causes rhabdomyolysis by two mechanisms. First, glycogen synthesis is reduced in skeletal muscle, which limits energy production, and second, potassium deficiency prevents the normal release of potassium ions from muscle cells during contraction. This, in turn, prevents the normal rise of blood flow during exercise, resulting in ischemia.[14] Specific conditions, drugs, and substances causing rhabdomyolysis as the result of potassium deficiency are listed in Table 15–3. Chronic alcoholics develop a myopathy characterized, in particular, by muscle phosphorus depletion and accumulation of salt, water, and calcium in their muscle cells.[15, 16] Because their muscle integrity is already tenuous,[17] a withdrawal seizure may result in frank rhabdomyolysis. In addition, they commonly become severely hypophosphatemic during hospitalization when they are given intravenous glucose or as a result of their characteristic respiratory alkalosis during withdrawal. Superimposition of acute hypophosphatemia on the preexisting myopathy induced by alcohol can provoke acute rhabdomyolysis. Hypomagnesemia, which also occurs commonly in alcoholics, has been reported to cause rhabdomyolysis in patients receiving cyclosporine. Magnesium deficiency and hypomagnesemia can cause potassium deficiency and hypoka-

TABLE 15–3. Causes of Rhabdomyolysis in Association with Potassium Deficiency

Glue sniffing (toluene)
Chinese herbs
Distal renal tubular acidosis
Liqueur absinthe
Amphotericin B
Bartter's syndrome
Gitelman's syndrome
Hyperemesis gravidarum
Carbenoxolone
Licorice (Glycyrrhiza glabra)
Diuretics (metolazone, chlorthalidone)
Terbutaline
Heat acclimatization
Conn's syndrome
Magnesium deficiency

lemia. Selective magnesium depletion can produce rhabdomyolysis in dogs.[18]

Certain infectious diseases may directly affect skeletal muscle and cause rhabdomyolysis (Table 15–4) or, alternatively, may provoke rhabdomyolysis in patients with a subclinical myopathy due to a metabolic defect, such as carnitine palmitoyltransferase (CPT-ase) deficiency.[19] The most common viral infections include influenza A and B and coxsackie viruses.[20] Other less common viral and bacterial infections are also listed in Table 15–4. HIV infections are well described.[21] In falciparum malaria, the black water fever may be the result of myoglobinuria, rather than hemoglobinuria.[22]

Patients who are septic as the result of bacteremia with gram-negative organisms commonly show modest elevations of CK-MM. The mechanism may involve impaired muscle perfusion secondary to hypovolemia and shock, hyperpyrexia, or the effects of cytokines such as interleukin-6 (IL-6). Severe hyperthermia in patients with heatstroke, especially of the exertional

TABLE 15–4. Infectious Diseases Causing Rhabdomyolysis

Viral Infections
   Influenza A and B
   Coxsackievirus
   Human immunodeficiency virus
   Epstein-Barr virus
   Cytomegalovirus
   Adenovirus
   Herpes simplex
   Varicella-zoster viruses
   Parainfluenza
Bacterial Infections
   Legionella pneumonia
   Brucellosis
   Tularemia
   Streptococcal pneumonia
   Salmonella species
   Staphylococcus aureus
   Streptococcus pyogenes
   Listeriosis
   Falciparum malaria
Ehrlichiosis
Leptospirosis
Q fever
Sepsis

variety, may show pronounced rhabdomyolysis, which often plays a major role in their morbidity.[23]

Drugs and Rhabdomyolysis

Although physical exertion is the most common overall cause of rhabdomyolysis in the general population, the most common cause among hospitalized patients is drugs (Table 15–5). Abuse of cocaine, "ecstasy" (methylenedioxymethamphetamine, MDMA), and "eve" (methylenedioxyethylamphetamine, MDEA) cause the majority of cases. Amphetamine and its relatives, such as methadrine (methamphetamine), have become less popular. Cocaine toxicity is multifactorial. First, in vitro, cocaine is directly toxic to muscle cells, causing leakage of both CK-MM and myoglobin.[24] In addition, the leakage of these substances is reduced by dantrolene, suggesting that the mechanism of injury implicates loss of calcium regulation in the myoplasm. Cocaine also increases the level of physical activity and heat production to such a degree that many patients develop exertional heatstroke. The vasoconstrictive properties of cocaine implicate ischemia as an additional cause of injury. Exertional heatstroke has been observed following overdosage with amphetamines as well.

Of great interest at the present time are the 3-hydroxy-3-methylglutaryl coenzyme A (HMG-CoA) reductase inhibitors employed to reduce cholesterol synthesis. Although the prevalence of myotoxicity pre-

TABLE 15–5. Drugs as Established Causes of Rhabdomyolysis

Cocaine
Crack cocaine
Amphetamine derivatives
   Methylenedioxymethyamphetamine (ecstasy, MDMA)
   Methylenedioxyethylamphetamine (eve, MDEA)
   Methadone
   Methamphetamine
Colchicine
Ergot derivatives
Diphenhydramine
Ethanol
Aminocaproic acid
Propylthiouracil
Phenytoin
Isoniazide
HMG-CoA reductase inhibitors
   Lovastatin
   Simvastatin
   Atorvastatin
   Pravastatin
   Cerivastatin
   Fluvastatin
Drugs that provoke rhabdomyolysis when used in conjunction with HMG-CoA reductase inhibitors
   Niacin
   Nicotinic acid
   Gemfibrozil
   Fibric acid derivatives
   Erythromycin
   Cyclosporin A I
   Itraconazole

dicted to occur with these important drugs has not materialized, nevertheless there have been serious instances of frank rhabdomyolysis. This is especially the case when the HMG-CoA reductase inhibitors are employed in conjunction with other medications.[25] These include other lipid-lowering drugs, such as niacin, nicotinic acid, gemfibrozil, and fibric acid derivatives, and unrelated drugs, including erythromycin, cyclosporin A, and itraconazole. Myopathy defined as muscle pain, tenderness, or weakness with CK-MM values at least 10 times that of normal occur less often with pravastatin, cerivastatin, and fluvastatin than with lovastatin, simvastatin, or atorvastatin. The reduced toxicity of the first three statins as well as reduced interaction with other drugs appears to be the result of less dependence on renal excretion, lower blood levels, and lesser distribution into skeletal muscle. In a study comparing pravastatin and lovastatin, the in vitro toxicity of the statin drugs appears to be directly related to the propensity of the HMG-CoA reductase inhibitors to cause depletion of mevalonate, fomesol, and geranylgeraniol, which are necessary for synthesis of the essential regulatory proteins of the myocyte.[26]

Convulsive seizures are a well-known cause of rhabdomyolysis, even in persons without muscle disease. Conditions or drugs that cause seizures, severe muscle spasms, or rigidity, which essentially represent exertional rhabdomyolysis in the absence of direct myotoxicity, are shown in Table 15–6.

Among this group of disorders is the relatively common neuroleptic malignant syndrome. This has been provoked by a number of neuroleptic drugs, by antipsychotic medications, or by withdrawal of medications employed for the treatment of Parkinson's disease. It is characterized by mental confusion, symptoms of autonomic instability, including tachycardia, hypertension, diaphoresis, fever, dystonia, and grimacing; and parkinsonian-like symptoms. The severity of hyperpyrexia and rhabdomyolysis in severe cases can probably be related to the severity of muscular contractions.

Although the drugs discussed previously are well established as causes of muscle injury with plausible mechanisms, others are associated with the condition only on the basis of anecdotal evidence, and accord-

TABLE 15–7. Anecdotal Reports of Drugs or Other Substances Causing Rhabdomyolysis

2, 4-Dichlorophenoxyacetic acid (2,4-D)	Ibuprofen
Diclofenac	Paraphenylenediamine
β-Blockers (propranolol, labetalol, pindolol)	Pyrazinamide
	Glutethemide
Acyclovir	Ethylene glycol
Isopropyl alcohol	Chromium picolinate
Isoretinoin	Gasoline distillate
Organophosphate (fenthion)	Interferon
Anti-C22 antibody (RFB4) for cancer	Cyclohexanone
Bradifacoum (super-warfarin)	Propofol
Amantadine	Lamivudine
Melperone	Calcium polysulfide
Loxapine	Azathioprine
Risperidone	Uranium acetate
Olanzapine	Tetrabenazine
Venlafaxine	Cyclophosphamide
Lamotrigine	Fenoverine
Tacrolimus	Chloropicrin
Naltrexone	

ingly, their relationship to rhabdomyolysis could be purely coincidental.[27] These are listed in Table 15–7.

Toxins, Venoms, and Rhabdomyolysis

Toxins and venoms are well-established causes of life-threatening rhabdomyolysis (Table 15–8). Historically, there have been epidemics of Haff disease (acute rhabdomyolysis) in persons who have consumed fish (icthyosarcotoxin) that contain an unidentified myotoxin.[28] The term *Haff disease* is derived from its appearance on Königsberg Haff in East Prussia. It occurred in both men and animals that consumed eels and burbot. The fish also died. More recently, cases of rhabdomyolysis following consumption of buffalo fish in the United States have been described[29] but, again, without identifying a specific toxin. Another report

TABLE 15–6. Conditions and Drugs Causing Muscle Contractions or Seizures and Secondary Rhabdomyolysis

Seizures	Muscle Spasm/Contractions
Classic epilepsy	Tetanus
Electroshock therapy	Tetany
Hypomagnesemia	Hypocalcemia
Alcoholic withdrawal	Hypomagnesemic tetany
Amoxapine	Malignant hyperthermia
Paint thinner inhalation	Neuroleptic malignant syndrome
Theophylline	Haloperidol
Pemoline	Strychnine
Thiodan (endosulfan)	Suxamethonium
Phencyclidine	Pancuronium
Barbiturate withdrawal	
Benzodiazepine withdrawal	

TABLE 15–8. Toxins, Venoms, and Rhabdomyolysis

SOURCE	AGENT
Fish poisoning	
Haff disease	Unidentified myotoxin in fish
Buffalo fish (*Ictiobus cyprinellus*)	Unidentified myotoxin in fish
Blue humphead parrotfish	Palytoxin
Quail poisoning	Myotoxin from *Galeopsis laudanum* seeds
	Hemlock seeds
Food poisoning	*Bacillus cereus* toxin
Envenomization	
Spiders	
Black widow	α-Latrotoxin
Brown recluse	Proteases, esterases, sphingomyelinase B
Bark scorpion	Neurotoxin
Africanized honeybee	Mellitin, hyaluronidase, and phospholipases
Snakes	Lipases, phospholipases, neurotoxins, hemorrhagins, proteolytic enzymes, myocardial depressants

describes rhabdomyolysis following consumption of the blue humphead parrotfish, its toxicity ascribed to palytoxin.[30] Rhabdomyolysis following consumption of quail has been reported from the Mediterranean coast, Greece, and Spain. In the reports from Spain,[31] *Galeopsis laudanum* seeds consumed by quail are metabolized to the toxin stachydrine, which is stored in muscle. When consumed by humans, fatal cases of rhabdomyolysis have followed. In the reports from Algeria and Greece,[32] the quail consumed hemlock (*Conium maculatum*) or hellebore seeds, which are also metabolized to an alkaloid, coniine, which accumulates in muscle of the quail. In both instances, the disease can be experimentally replicated by feeding either of these seeds to quail, then feeding the quail to rats or dogs, which then develop rhabdomyolysis. Some interesting speculation has been published regarding the biblical description of "the quails" and deaths of the Israelites during the Exodus when they were led by Moses through the Sinai desert.[33]

Envenomization by a variety of spiders and snakes may cause serious cases of rhabdomyolysis. In the United States, rhabdomyolysis following the sting of the black widow spider has been related to α-latrotoxin. Muscle spasms could be a cause of rhabdomyolysis in this condition. The brown recluse spider produces a variety of proteases and esterases, and sphingomyelinase B. The bark scorpion in the Southwestern United States may cause rhabdomyolysis. Finally, rhabdomyolysis has occurred in patients who have received 100 or more bites from the Africanized honeybee. A number of snakes produce venom that can cause massive rhabdomyolysis, hemolysis, and often neurotoxicity. The names of these snakes and their locations are shown in Table 15–9. In the United States, severe cases of rhabdomyolysis have occurred after bites from various species of rattlesnakes.

COMPLICATIONS OF RHABDOMYOLYSIS

Acute Renal Failure

Factors favoring the development of ARF in patients with rhabdomyolysis include the severity of muscle injury, the quantity of myoglobin retained in nephrons, the presence of an acidic highly concentrated urine,

TABLE 15–9. Snakebites Causing Rhabdomyolysis and Their Geographic Origin

SNAKE	ORIGIN
King brown snake (*Pseudechis australis*)	Singapore
Viper (*Agkistrodan halys blomhoffi*)	India
Russell's viper (*Vipera russelli formogenesis*)	China
Jararacucu (*Bothrops jararacucu*)	Brazil
Sea snake (*Colloselasma rhodostonn*)	Malaya
Canebrake rattler	United States
Diamond back rattler	United States
European viper	Europe
Tiger snake	Australia

and delay in the recognition of the disease. The specific mechanisms underlying heme pigment toxicity to the nephron and preventive measures are detailed in the first part of this chapter.

Metabolic Acidosis

At least six factors contribute toward the severity of metabolic acidosis in patients with severe rhabdomyolysis. First, sulfate from amino acids and phosphoric acid from injured muscle cells are major factors. Second, nucleic acids are also released from injured muscle that are converted to uric acid in the liver and account for the extreme hyperuricemia seen in these patients. Third, increased permeability of injured muscle cells possibly allows entrance of bicarbonate into the inside of the cell, where it may precipitate as calcium carbonate or calcium phosphate. This could explain the enlarged volume of bicarbonate distribution seen in patients with rhabdomyolysis.[34] Fourth, in patients with circulatory obstruction of a limb, upon reperfusion there may occur a washout of lactate that had accumulated in the ischemic muscle. Fifth, if rhabdomyolysis is sufficiently severe to impair diaphragm or intercostal muscle function, respiratory acidosis can complicate the metabolic acidosis. Finally, renal failure per se prevents excretion of protons.

Hyperkalemia

Because muscle cell injury is associated with increased sarcolemmal permeability, impaired Na^+/K^+ exchange, muscle cell electrical depolarization, and opening of potassium channels, hyperkalemia must be anticipated and is often a cause of death in these patients. Patients should be monitored very carefully for this complication. Hyperkalemia is aggravated markedly by the prevailing level of ionized calcium, which often demands administration of calcium salts and intensive dialysis therapy. Studies[35, 36] suggest that administration of sodium bicarbonate or potassium-binding resins provides no favorable improvement in hyperkalemia. Similarly, the potential arrhythmogenicity of β-agonists limits their employment for hyperkalemia. Infusions of glucose and insulin are often useful but may be less effective because of the associated muscle-cell and hepatic injury that is often associated with this condition.

Calcium Metabolism

Disorders of calcium metabolism occur early in the course of rhabdomyolysis. Derangements of ion transport in the injured muscle cell allow ionized calcium and calcium salts to accumulate in injured skeletal muscle cells. Pronounced hypocalcemia may occur with levels as low as 2.3 mg/dL.[37] Of interest, tetany seldom appears despite this degree of hypocalcemia, suggesting that the high calcium levels in injured muscle cells may impair contractility. The major effects of hypocalcemia are on the heart, because it directly aggravates hyperkalemic cardiotoxicity and also augments the myocardial depressant effects of hyperkalemia. Nonetheless, treatment of hypocalcemia in ARF is a double-edged sword. Calcium salts must be given for urgent hyperkalemic toxicity, but large infusions of calcium lead to additional accumulation of calcium in injured muscle. If these patients survive the initial phases of rhabdomyolysis, they become hypercalcemic later in the course of this illness, as the calcium salts become mobilized.

Hyperphosphatemia

Phosphate is the predominant anion in skeletal muscle cells, and as a result injury is associated with release of phosphorus in large quantities, which explains hyperphosphatemia. Hyperphosphatemia may promote precipitation of calcium phosphate in vital organs, although this process is mitigated by the presence of metabolic acidosis.

Hyperuricemia

Release of nucleic acids from injured muscle cells results in the formation of large quantities of uric acid in the liver. This explains the hyperuricemia seen in patients with rhabdomyolysis.[38] Instances in which serum uric acid levels exceed 30 mg/dL have been observed in patients whose serum urea concentration may be only 20 mg/dL. There is no solid evidence that hyperuricemia in this situation contributes to ARF.

Disseminated Intravascular Coagulation

Endothelial activation[10] is a major component of overall cellular injury in patients with rhabdomyolysis, and as a result intravascular coagulation occurs and explains the reduction in platelets and the occurrence of hemorrhage. Thrombocytopenia appears early in cases of severe rhabdomyolysis and can become extremely severe. Administration of platelet packs is not helpful because of ongoing platelet consumption. The associated reduction in clotting factors necessitates that hemorrhage be treated with packed red cells and fresh-frozen plasma.

A late complication of rhabdomyolysis is ischemic necrosis of involved skeletal muscles that are encased by a fibrous sheath, such as the anterior tibial muscle. The thigh muscles, the gluteus maximus muscles, and the deltoids can also become involved in this process. Degradation of muscle proteins inside the surrounding capsule increases osmotic forces, which, in turn, cause water uptake from the adjacent circulation. Recall that 1 mOsm/kg H_2O resulting from an impermeable protein molecule exerts a hydrostatic pressure of 19.5 mm Hg. Thus, it requires very little degradation of large proteins to increase pressure inside the muscle com-

partment to block arterial blood flow. This mechanism results in a second wave of muscle necrosis. One must be vigilant for this complication by measuring tissue pressure and performing fasciotomy as necessary. The potential beneficial effects of mannitol as prophylaxis against compartment syndromes are discussed in Chapter 12.

REFERENCES

1. Lang H, ed: *Creatine Kinase Isoenzymes: Pathophysiology and Clinical Application.* New York: Springer-Verlag; 1981:4–5.
2. Muller-Bardorff M, Hallermayer K, Schroder A, et al: Improved troponin T ELISA specific for cardiac troponin T isoform: assay development and analytical and clinical validation. Clin Chem 1997; 43:458–466.
3. Wakabayashi Y, Kikuno T, Ohwada T, Kikawada R: Rapid fall in blood myoglobin in massive rhabdomyolysis and acute renal failure. Intensive Care Med 1994; 20:109–112.
4. Loun B, Astles R, Copeland KR, Sedor FA: Adaptation of a quantitative immunoassay for urine myoglobin: predictor in detecting renal dysfunction. Am J Clin Pathol 1996; 105:479–486.
5. Knochel JP: Mechanisms of rhabdomyolysis. Curr Opin Rheumatol 1993; 5:725–731.
6. Zager RA: Rhabdomyolysis and myohemoglobinuric acute renal failure. Kidney Int 1996; 49:314–326.
7. Duncan CJ, Jackson MJ: Different mechanisms mediate structural changes and intracellular enzyme efflux following damage to skeletal muscle. J Cell Sci 1987; 87:183–188.
8. Saccheto R, Margreth A, Pelosi M, Carafoli E: Colocalization of the dihydropyridine receptor, the plasma membrane ATPase isoform 1 and the sodium/calcium exchanger to the junctional-membrane domain of transverse tubules of rabbit skeletal muscle. Eur J Biochem 1996; 237:483–488.
9. Orth HD: The Cytoplasmic Creatine Kinase Isoenzyme From Human Tissues. In: Lang H, ed: *Creatine Kinase Isoenzymes.* New York: Springer-Verlag; 1981:15.
10. Ballerman BJ: Endothelial cell activation. Kidney Int 1998; 53:1810–1826.
11. Haller RG, Knochel JP: Metabolic Myopathies. In: Johnson RT, Griffin JW, eds: *Current Therapy in Neurologic Disease.* New York: BC Decker; 1993:397–402.
12. Loke J, MacLennan DH: Malignant hyperthermia and central core disease: disorders of Ca^{2+} release channels. Am J Med 1998; 104:470–486.
13. Mickelson JR, Gallant EM, Litterer LA: Abnormal sarcoplasmic ryanodine reception on malignant hyperthermia. J Biol Chem 1988; 263:9310–9315.
14. Knochel JP: Clinical Effects of Potassium Deficiency on Skeletal Muscle. In: Whelton P, Whelton A, Walker W, eds: *Potassium in Cardiovascular and Renal Medicine.* New York: Marcel Dekker; 1986:97–109.
15. Agarwal R, Knochel JP: Fluids and Electrolytes. In: Kokko JP, Tannen RL, eds: *Fluid and Electrolyte Disorders Associated With Alcoholism and Liver Disease.* 3rd ed. Philadelphia: WB Saunders; 1996:449–485.
16. Knochel JP: Hypophosphatemia and rhabdomyolysis. Am J Med 1992; 92:455–457.
17. Ferguson E, Blachley J, Carter N, Knochel JP: Derangements of muscle composition, ion transport and oxygen consumption in chronically alcoholic dogs. Am J Physiol 1984; 246:F700–F709.
18. Cronin RE, Ferguson ER, Shannon WA, Jr, Knochel JP: Skeletal muscle injury after magnesium deficiency in the dog. Am J Physiol 1982; 243:F113–F120.
19. Katzir Z, Hochman B, Biro A, et al: Carnitine palmitoyltransferase deficiency: an underdiagnosed condition? Am J Nephrol 1996; 16:162–166.
20. Singh U, Scheld WM: Infectious etiologies of rhabdomyolysis: three case reports and review. Clin Infect Dis 1996; 22:642–649.
21. Ytterberg SR: Infectious agents associated with myopathies. Curr Opin Rheumatol 1996; 8:507–513.
22. Moore G, Knochel JP: Blackwater fever due to myoglobinuria in

a patient with falciparum malaria. N Engl J Med 1993; 329:1206–1207.

23. Knochel JP, Reed G: Disorders of Heat Regulation. In: Narins R, ed: *Clinical Disorders of Fluid and Electrolyte Metabolism.* 5th ed. New York: McGraw-Hill; 1994.

24. Pagala M, Amaladevi B, Bernstein A, et al: Dantrolene sodium reduces the enhanced leakage of creatine kinase caused by ethanol, cocaine, and electrical stimulation in isolated fast and slow muscles of rat. Alcohol Clin Exp Res 1997; 21:63–67.

25. Pogson GW, Kindred LH, Carper BG: Rhabdomyolysis and renal failure associated with cerivastatin-gemfibrozil combination therapy. Am J Cardiol 1999; 83:1146.

26. Flint OP, Masters BA, Gregg RE, Durham SK: HMG CoA reductase inhibitor–induced myotoxicity: pravastatin and lovastatin inhibit the geranylgeranylation of low-molecular-weight proteins in neonatal rat muscle cell culture. Toxicol Appl Pharmacol 1997; 145:99–110.

27. National Library of Medicine, Pub Med Web site. (1966–). Bethesda, MD: National Library of Medicine Available at: http://www.ncbi.nlm.nih.gov/PubMed/medline.html. Accessed July 14, 1999.

28. Kagen L: Myoglobin: Biochemical, Physiological and Clinical Aspects. New York: Columbia University Press; 1973:109–110.

29. Haff disease associated with eating buffalo fish—United States 1997. MMWR Morb Mortal Wkly Rep 1998; 47:1091–1093.

30. Okano H, Masuoka H, Kamei S, et al: Rhabdomyolysis and myocardial damage induced by palytoxin, a toxin of blue humphead parrotfish. Intern Med 1998; 37:330–333.

31. Aparicio R, Onate JM, Arizcun A: Epidemic rhabdomyolysis due to the eating of quail: a clinical, epidemiological and experimental study. Med Clin 1999; 112:143–146.

32. Ouzounellis TI: Myoglobinuries par ingestion de cailles. Presse Med 1968; 76:1863–1864.

33. Rutecki GW, Ognibene AJ, Geib JD: Rhabdomyolysis in antiquity: from ancient descriptions to scientific explication. Pharos 1998; 61:18–22.

34. Garella S, Dana C, Chazan JA: Severity of metabolic acidosis as a determinant of bicarbonate requirements. N Engl J Med 1973; 289:121–126.

35. Kim HJ: Combined effect of bicarbonate and insulin with glucose in acute therapy of hyperkalemia in end-stage renal disease patients. Nephron 1996; 72:476–482.

36. Emmett M, Hootkins RE, Fine KD: Effect of three laxatives and a cation exchange resin on fecal sodium and potassium excretion. Gastroenterology 1995; 108:752–760.

37. Knochel JP: Pigment Nephropathy. In: Greenberg A, Cheung AK, Coffinann TM, et al, eds: *Primer on Kidney Diseases.* 2nd ed. San Diego: Academic Press; 1998:273–276.

38. Knochel JP, Dotin LN, Hamburger RJ: Heat stress, exercise, and muscle injury: effects on urate metabolism and renal function. Ann Intern Med 1974; 81:321–328.

CHAPTER 16

Post-Traumatic Acute Renal Failure With Emphasis on the Muscle Crush Syndrome

Ori S. Better ▪ Irit Rubinstein

INTRODUCTION

As long ago as the beginning of the last century, it was noted that combat casualties characteristically complained of intense thirst and were oliguric. These features suggest to the modern observer that the victims suffered from the consequences of circulatory underfill (hypovolemia) and were therefore susceptible to the development of acute renal failure (ARF). Although a relationship was noted between sustained blunt trauma to the muscles and the development of ARF in casualties of World War I,[1] the first systematic search for the cause of post-traumatic oliguria was made by the Spanish military orthopedic surgeon Joseph Trueta during the Spanish civil war (1936–1939) and again during World War II.[2–4] Trueta extended his observations using an experimental rabbit model of induced ischemic myopathy. In this model, the myopathy caused extreme renal cortical vasospasm and ischemia.[3]

The observations of Trueta on post-traumatic cortical renal ischemia in the rabbit were confirmed 20 years later in humans by renal perfusion studies utilizing radioisotopes and angiography.[5] Retrospective studies of patients undergoing open heart or aortic surgery during the 1950s and 1960s revealed that post-surgical ARF occurred in approximately 20% of these patients.[6] This type of post-traumatic ARF was also attributed to renal cortical vasospasm. In the late 1980s, the incidence of ARF following cardiac and aortic surgery was reduced to 5% or less with the introduction of intraoperative volume replacement, the use of mannitol,[6] and advances in anesthesia.

It is interesting to note that post-traumatic renal cortical ischemia in humans has a physiologic parallel in the diving reflex of marine mammals. For example, in the Weddell seal, during the anoxic stress of a 70-minute dive, regional blood supply is maintained only to the brain, spinal cord, and retina. This occurs at the expense of all other organs, including the kidneys, which undergo vasoconstriction.[7, 8] Thus, it may be teleologically argued that during existential anoxic stress the brain, with a "warm ischemic time" of approximately 4 minutes, is generously perfused with blood diverted from other organs, such as the kidney, that have a "warm ischemic time" of approximately 1 hour. Functional temporary suppression of urine flow has also been considered advantageous during volume depletion and in land mammals.

Rambam Hospital at the Technion Faculty of Medicine admits some 3000 civilian and military[9] trauma casualties annually. Also, at Haifa, the distance from the frontline in Southern Lebanon is only approximately 50 miles. With the extensive use of helicopters, the evacuation time is often less than 1 hour, enabling an early evaluation and management of mass disaster and combat casualties. The purpose of this chapter is to review the authors' experience with the prevention and management of post-traumatic ARF, with an emphasis on trauma to the limbs.

Mass disasters, such as the "blitz" of London in the autumn of 1940,[10, 11] or following the major earthquake in Armenia on December 7, 1988,[12] inflict a heavy loss of lives and leave in their wake hundreds of casualties suffering myoglobinuric ARF as the result of renal involvement in the muscle crush syndrome (MCS). Although both MCS and myoglobinuric ARF were described early this century and a prophylactic regimen for the prevention of this type of ARF was suggested in 1944[11] and implemented in 1982[13], the general acceptance of this protocol by the world medical community has been slow.[1, 11] Thus, during the course of the rescue of casualties of the earthquake in Kobe, Japan,[14] on January 17, 1995, there were 372 casualties suffering from myoglobinuric ARF secondary to MCS. Apparently, these survivors did not benefit from adequate early volume replacement, because the rescuers, by their own account, were not familiar with MCS and its current management.[14] As a result, these casualties in Kobe were more susceptible to the excessive dangers of hypovolemic shock, hyperkalemia, and myoglobinuric ARF than they might otherwise have been.[14] These lethal complications were potentially preventable. It is, therefore, timely to review recent advances in the understanding of the profound circulatory collapse accompanying MCS, the attendant derangement of electrolyte and acid-base metabolism, and the causation and prevention of the associated pigment nephropathy. For more detailed background information, readers are referred to three review articles.[13, 15, 16]

THE SKELETAL MUSCLES AND THEIR SUSCEPTIBILITY TO RHABDOMYOLYSIS

The muscles constitute the largest organ of the body (approximately 40%–50% of total body weight). Unlike the brain and the vital internal organs, the skeletal muscles lack extensive bony protection and are highly exposed to mechanical trauma. In addition to their sheer bulk, the muscles contain the largest single pool of body water (approximately 30 L in an adult) and of body potassium (approximately 75%) and the largest concentration of membranal Na^+,K^+-ATPase pumps. It is therefore not surprising that widespread skeletal muscle injury may result in extreme disturbances in plasma electrolyte concentrations and in the size of body fluid compartments. These extreme metabolic perturbations, particularly hyperkalemia, may be lethal within 1 to 2 hours of injury, and yet they are potentially reversible with vigorous early medical intervention.[10, 13]

Under normal conditions, the sarcolemma (the membrane of muscle cells) is almost entirely impermeable to extracellular fluid (ECF) and its cations and thus protects the relatively hyperoncotic cytosol from being flooded by the ECF and its solutes down their steep electrochemical gradients.[13] Any minor physiologic sarcolemmal leak is compensated for by the Na^+,K^+-ATPase sarcolemmal cationic pumps, which maintain cytosolic electronegativity, sequester potassium intracellularly, and extrude sodium ions into the ECF. Sarcolemmal damage caused by mechanical injury, stretch,[13, 17] excessive physical exertion, hyperthermia, or metabolic lesions interferes with sarcolemmal integrity and impermeability and causes a two-way overwhelming leak: calcium and sodium, followed by water, penetrate the cytosol and possibly the interstitium, causing depletion of the ECF and hypovolemic hypocalcemic shock. Potassium, phosphate, proteins, purines (precursors of urate), and myoglobin leak into the ECF.[13] With the exception of potassium, these metabolites or their derivatives are highly nephrotoxic, particularly against the background of hypovolemic shock, renal vasoconstriction, aciduria, and increased urinary concentration. All of the preceding are invariably seen in casualties with hypovolemic shock due to trauma to the muscles.

Entry of calcium into the cytosol of damaged myocytes and, ultimately, into the mitochondria causes damage that interferes with mitochondrial function and with their ability to generate ATP, a function that is vital to all normal cellular functions. In this respect, muscle mitochondrial dysfunction secondary to stretch occurs much earlier than mitochondral impairment secondary to ischemia (3–4 hours).[17]

Nitric Oxide Involvement

In the last decade, a new regulator of skeletal muscle function and blood supply has been described. This regulator is the nitric oxide (NO) system. It has been demonstrated that NO, the small gaseous molecule, regulates contractility of skeletal muscle,[18, 19] blood vessel tone, and blood flow.[20–22] Under normal conditions, human skeletal muscle contains the two constitutive types of nitric oxide synthase (NOS), the enzyme that regulates NO metabolism. The two constitutive types of NOS are brain (neuronal) NOS (bNOS) and endothelial NOS (eNOS).[23] Human skeletal muscle lacks the inducible form of NOS (iNOS). Brain NOS immunoreactivity has been found in the sarcolemma and cytoplasm of all human skeletal muscle fibers. It is present in all fiber types, adjacent to the cellular locations of mitochondria. Endothelial NOS immunoreactivity has been observed in the endothelium of blood vessels—large vessels as well as microvessels of the muscles. This isoform has also been detected in the cytoplasm of mitochondria-rich muscle fibers.[19]

A major known function of NO is regulation of blood vessel tone and therefore of blood flow.[20, 23] Studies in humans and animals[24, 25] have shown that NO is involved in skeletal muscle perfusion through its vasodilatory action. The stimulus for NO release from vascular endothelial cells in skeletal muscle may be shear stress resulting from increased blood flow.[26] Another function of NO is to regulate the contractile force of skeletal muscles.[18, 19] Myocyte function is sensitive to redox modulation under basal conditions. Reactive oxygen intermediates (ROIs) and NO molecules are two classes of molecules that modulate muscle function under physiologic conditions.[27] The ROIs promote excitation-contraction coupling and appear to be obligatory to optimal contractile function.[27, 28] Nitric oxide opposes the action of ROI. The dynamic balance between production and inactivation of ROI and NO maintains redox homeostasis within the cell. Nitric oxide synthase activity has a decisive influence on the effectiveness of excitation-contraction coupling. Inhibitors of NOS increase twitch and submaximal tetanic force production in skeletal muscles, whereas NO donors decrease force production.[18]

Following endotoxin administration, mouse skeletal muscle shows the ability to induce the macrophage (inducible) form of iNOS mRNA and protein and has iNOS activity as well.[29] Rubinstein and coworkers[25] have found an excessive induction of iNOS and increased immunoreactivity following muscle crush injury in the rat model. Inducible NOS is responsible for the excess generation of NO. It is induced by macrophages, by certain cytokines, such as tumor necrosis factor (TNF) and interleukins, and by lipopolysaccharides (LPS), which act through the release of cytokines. Cytokines regulate iNOS, some promoting and others inhibiting the induction of the enzyme.[30] Mechanically crushed muscle contains macrophages[25] and therefore has the potential to induce iNOS. The NO that is produced by iNOS may exert an autocytotoxic effect, as well as a cytotoxic effect, on other cells in the vicinity.[23, 30] The induction of iNOS in the macrophages results in the sustained production of NO. There, the NO combines with iron-sulfur centers in key enzymes of both the mitochondrial respiratory cycle and the DNA synthesis pathway. In normal situations, NO is capable of rapidly and reversibly inhibiting the mitochondrial respiratory chain, but when NO is generated by iNOS, it may change the pattern of the inhibition to a prolonged one.[31, 32] Such enzymatic inhibition may cause cellular hypoxia, despite intact circulation. The end result of mitochondrial failure is myocytic anoxia and acidosis, which may be lethal. Furthermore, uncontrolled excessive NO production in crushed muscle could conceivably cause, propagate, and aggravate rhabdomyolysis. The impact of excess NO production on muscle perfusion might have a further influence on muscle function and possibly on systemic hemodynamics. Extreme vasodilatation, caused by sustained vascular NO production, may result in hemodynamic-hypovolemic shock, which is the hallmark of the crush syndrome in humans. Increased NO formation (by induction of iNOS) may also cause devastating damage to the muscular tissue[33] on its own or via its metabolite, the oxidant peroxynitrite, and thus aggravate and possibly propagate rhabdomyolysis. Inducible NOS is similarly responsible for the sustained increased levels of NO in septic shock, characteristically often complicated by ARF. In view of the clear evidence that mechanical trauma to muscles induces NO production, it can be speculated that NO is involved in the pathogenesis of acute compartment syndrome (ACS).

Acute Compartment Syndrome

Acute compartment syndrome often complicates trauma to the blood vessels and muscles of the limb. It can cause myoglobinuric ARF,[34, 35] yet ACS is hardly mentioned in the nephrology literature. It is the authors' opinion that a nephrologist should be consulted in the management of the ACS.

Acute compartment syndrome is a devastating local complication of post-traumatic or postexertional rhabdomyolysis. Its clinical manifestation is a rapid painful turgid swelling of the affected limb. In extreme cases, ACS may be accompanied by local neurologic motor or sensory deficits and by myoglobinuric ARF.[34, 35] The etiologic hallmark of ACS is a steep increase in the intracompartmental interstitial pressure from the normal of 0.0 ± 2.0 mm Hg to pressures that may exceed the mean arterial pressure.

The cause of the intracompartmental "hypertension" in ACS is massive interstitial edema and hyperoncotic swelling of myocytes within muscle compartments covered by tight sheaths of fibrous fascia with relatively low compliance. In subacute compartment syndrome, further increases in intracompartmental pressure may conceivably be due to hyperperfusion secondary to stimulation of local production of NO and vasodilatation.[25] The increase in intracompartmental pressure tends to block the venous drainage out of the compartment. This imbalance between blood inflow and outflow to the affected compartment leads to its swelling and ultimately to turgidity and tamponade. Thus, within hours to days following injury, ACS is superimposed on the ischemic damage to muscles already undergoing traumatic rhabdomyolysis.

It is obvious that management of ACS is immediate decompression. The prevailing textbook view is that early fasciotomy is mandatory in ACS.[36] Before 1982, the treatment of ACS with fasciotomy in combat casualties from the South Lebanon arena yielded poor results, with prohibitory loss of limbs and even lives.[13] As a result, starting in 1982, surgeons from the authors' institution became conservative with the indications for fasciotomy and now perform it only rarely. Moreover, nonsurgical decompression of the ACS has been

achieved with intravenous hypertonic mannitol in ACS in humans,[37] in dogs,[38] and in rabbits.[39] The authors suggest that casualties with ACS who are candidates for fasciotomy should first be given a trial of intravenous mannitol (20%). If intravenous mannitol results in symptomatic relief and reduction of the circumference of the affected swollen limb, then fasciotomy can be postponed or pre-empted altogether. It is interesting to note that fasciotomy for ACS was associated with increased mortality and morbidity in victims of the extensive earthquake in Iran in 1990, which claimed 43,390 casualties.[40] These authors therefore question, on the basis of their vast personal experience, the advisability of fasciotomy in the management of ACS. Furthermore, fasciotomy increased the incidence of sepsis from 13% to 18% ($P < 0.001$, n = 518) following the August 17, 1999 earthquake in Turkey (MS Sever, E Erek, Istanbul Medical Faculty. Personal communication).

Another promising nonsurgical approach to the management of ACS comes from experimental studies in the dog that use hyperbaric oxygen treatment.[41] Also, preliminary experimental results in the rat model of crush injury suggest that hyperbaric oxygen treatment has a protective effect on the crushed muscle. In the future, hyperbaric oxygen treatment may serve as a therapeutic adjunct in severe cases of crush syndrome and ACS in humans.

Plasma Electrolyte Disorder in Muscle Crush Syndrome

Within 2 hours of extrication of casualties that have been buried, the clinical condition may be marked by hyperkalemia, hypocalcemia, hyperphosphatemia, hyperuricemia, and metabolic acidosis ("extrarenal uremic pattern"). The hypocalcemia aggravates the cardiotoxicity of hyperkalemia and has a suppressive effect on the entire cardiovascular tree. Hyperphosphatemia intensifies the hypocalcemia and further undermines kidney function.[42]

Circulatory Failure in Muscle Crush Syndrome

Casualties suffering from MCS usually are in a profound state of hemodynamic shock. The main reason for this circulatory collapse is uptake of ECF by the crushed muscle. Almost all of the 14 L of the ECF can be sequestered in the crushed muscles within hours of injury. The depleted circulation is further depressed by the combination of hyperkalemia and hypocalcemia, which are negatively inotropic and chronotropic. The hyperkalemia of MCS may reach extreme levels of well above 10 mEq/L in casualties suffering from the combined effects of exertional and traumatic rhabdomyolysis[43] (Table 16–1). Even excessive muscle damage caused by marathon-type exertion in normal trained athletes may cause hyperkalemia approaching 9.0 mEq/L.[44] Furthermore, the volume depletion and ar-

TABLE 16-1. Causes of Hemodynamic Shock in the Compartmental Syndrome[13]

Internal volume losses resulting from sequestration of fluid and solute in traumatized muscles ("third spacing") may reach 10–18 L/d.

External volume losses caused by dehydration (eg, from excessive sensible and insensible losses; exertion or prostration in hot, arid environments; hyperthermia; vomiting and diarrhea).

Cardiovascular depression caused by the combination of hyperkalemia and hypocalcemia and the action of cytokines and endotoxin.

Vasodilatation in crushed muscles as a result of excesive increase in the activity of inducible NO synthase and NO production.[25]

NO, nitric oxide.

terial hypotension of MCS would probably be aggravated by profuse vasodilatation in the crushed muscles. Such crush-induced vasodilation has been demonstrated in the authors' laboratory in experimental animals and was due to an increase in iNOS generation and NO production in the muscle.[25]

The circulatory collapse in untreated MCS triggers the release, via the baroreceptors, of powerful systemic vasoconstrictors, such as norepinephrine, angiotensin II, endothelin (ET), and thromboxane, which tend to cause renal cortical vasoconstriction and hypoperfusion, hypofiltration, and ischemia. Such renal vasoconstriction is intensified by myoglobin, which chelates renal vasodilatory NO.[42] It is interesting to note that extreme renal cortical ischemia following extensive muscle injury may occur even in animals, such as the rabbit, whose muscles lack myoglobin.[2] Thus, the nephrotoxicity of myoglobinuria is not a prerequisite for renal failure caused by trauma to muscles.

There are two main components of myoglobinuric ARF: a vasomotor response, with renal vasoconstriction and renal ischemia, and direct nephrotoxicity. In addition, intrarenal obstruction caused by tubular cast formation containing muscle metabolites (myoglobin, urate, and phosphate) can be demonstrated. These metabolites are leaked from disintegrating muscle into the circulation and thence to the kidneys. The aciduria and hyperosmolarity of the urine potentiate the nephrotoxicity of both myoglobin and urate in myoglobinuric ARF.

MORPHOLOGIC ALTERATIONS IN THE KIDNEYS

Myoglobinuric ARF in humans and experimental animals is characterized by striking morphologic changes that include (1) formation of heme casts in the distal nephron and (2) proximal tubular necrosis and detachment of epithelial cells from the basement membrane.[42] These tubular casts obstruct the luminal flow and thus impair kidney function.[45, 46] Tubular obstruction apparently occurs in the first few hours after the induction of pigment nephropathy, whereas the established phase of ARF is associated with collapsed tubules.[47, 48] Thus, the relative importance of the neph-

rotoxic versus the obstructive elements in the pathogenesis of ARF is still being debated.

Zager and Gamelin[49] suggested that heme-protein cytotoxicity plays a critical role in tubular epithelial damage during myoglobinuria. In this condition, formation of casts causes luminal obstruction and stasis. Such stasis further enhances cast formation and allows increased cast contact with tubular epithelium. Urinary concentration and acidity in the MCS aggravate not only the nephrotoxicity of myoglobin and of urate but also of the myoglobin–Tamm-Horsfall polymers in the distal tubules.[42]

MECHANISMS OF RENAL IMPAIRMENT FOLLOWING ACUTE MYOPATHY

Two factors are considered to play a pivotal role in the initiation of renal impairment following acute myopathy: renal ATP depletion and oxidant stress (Fig. 16–1).[42, 49]

Ischemic Damage and ATP Depletion

As in other forms of ARF, the available evidence suggests that myoglobinuric renal injury is largely secondary to the ischemic as well as toxic renal insults induced by heme proteins. A reduction in renal perfusion has been consistently reported in experimental models of myohemoglobinuric ARF.[50] This effect is attributed to heme protein–induced renal vasoconstriction and hypoperfusion. Trifillis and coworkers[51] have demonstrated that the ATP content in the renal cortex of rats with glycerol-induced myoglobinuric ARF is decreased. Renal ATP depletion is due not only to ischemia but also, in large part, to leak of ATP precursors (adenosine, inosine, and hypoxanthine within hours of glycerol injection) resulting from the increased permeability of the injured tubular cells. This drain of precursors renders the generation of ATP more costly and slower.[52] Therefore, the provision of ATP or its precursors, or inhibitors of the enzymes that convert nucleotides to nucleosides and bases, accelerates recovery of this type of ARF.[53] Depletion of cellular ATP, which usually accompanies ischemia, impairs energetic metabolism and the function of sarcolemmal ionic pumps.[42] The end result is an increase in cytosolic calcium as a result of the following mechanisms: (1) failure of Ca^+-ATPase–driven calcium efflux due to ATP depletion; (2) interference with intracellular Ca^+ sequestration; and (3) increased Na^+/Ca^+ exchange following intensive Na^+ influx, which further depletes the precariously low cytosolic ATP content.

Interestingly, when myoglobin was infused into rats in the presence of iron chelator, ATP levels[54] remained intact. Similar results were obtained when free iron—a low-molecular-weight protein (~17 kDa)—was infused into experimental animals, indicating that iron plays a critical role in heme-protein ATP depletion.

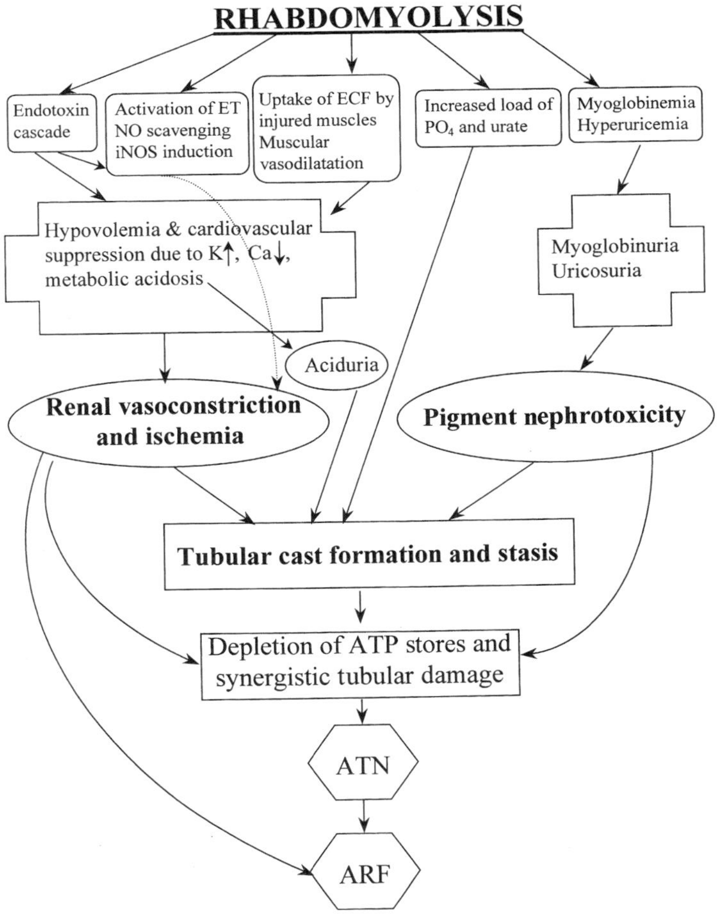

FIGURE 16–1 ▪ Pathogenesis of rhabdomyolysis-induced nephrotoxicity. On the *left side* are shown the factors leading to renal vasoconstriction via activation of the baroreceptor system located mainly in the great intrathoracic vessels. Chelators of intrarenal nitric oxide (NO) by myoglobin further intensify this renal vasoconstriction. Along with the renal hypoperfusion, there is increased sensitivity to the nephrotoxicity of muscle metabolites (right side). These metabolites (myoglobin and urate) cause toxic intratubular obstruction. Acute hyperphosphatemia, also due to leakage of phosphate from the muscles, can lead to acute renal failure (ARF) and metastatic renal calcification. It is interesting to note that the devastating pattern of myoglobinuric ARF resolves completely and spontaneously in survivors of the crush syndrome.[83] *ATN*, acute tubular necrosis; *ECF*, extracellular fluid; *iNOS*, inducible nitric oxide synthase.

Oxidant Tissue Stress

Heme proteins appear to be toxic to the proximal tubular cells.[42] This notion stems from the observation that pretreatment of rats prior to renal artery occlusion with nontoxic doses of myoglobin or hemoglobin potentiates the induction of ischemic ARF.[55–57] The mechanisms underlying this phenomenon are incompletely understood. However, because non–iron-containing proteins were also able to intensify the cytotoxicity of ischemia, Zager and coworkers[58] concluded that endocytic protein uptake, and not necessarily cell iron loading, per se, is largely responsible for the nephrotoxicity of the heme protein. These authors have further supported their theory by experimental data involving in vitro incubation of proximal tubule segments (PTS), derived from either normal or heme-infused mice or rats, with exogenous phospholipase A$_2$ (PLA$_2$), a critical determinant of ischemia-induced cellular damage. Although normal PTSs were not affected by this enzyme, heme-loaded PTSs were severely damaged. This indicates that heme proteins directly sensitize these cells to lethal injury.

Reactive oxygen and non–oxygen-based radicals have been implicated in the pathogenesis of a variety of renal diseases, including myoglobinuric ARF.[42] The first step in this pathway is proximal tubular cell trans-port and accumulation of poryphrin rings. Within the proximal epithelial cells, the rings undergo degradation, resulting in iron release, which is eliminated within several weeks.[59] The extension and site of iron release are critically dependent on the concentration of heme protein in the lumen of proximal tubules.[59, 60] For example, when the filtered load of either myoglobin or hemoglobin exceeds the absorptive capacity of proximal tubules, they congest the tubules, and subsequently iron is released into the lumen.[59] Regardless of the controversy about the nephrotoxicity of iron, the fact that iron is an intermediate accelerator in the generation of free radicals, and could itself become a free radical, contributes to the pathogenesis of ARF. This notion, termed "iron-induced oxidant stress," is supported by numerous studies in which administration of iron chelators, such as deferoxamine, or scavengers of reactive oxygen metabolites, such as glutathione, can protect against hemoglobinuric ARF.[42, 60–63] Moreover, the production of H$_2$O$_2$ in rat kidney increased following myohemoglobinuric procedures.[63, 64] Considering that hydrogen peroxide constitutes an important source for radical formation and that it may itself promote the release of iron from intracellular sites, these findings indicate that hydroxyl radical formation (most likely in the mitochondria) plays a critical role in heme-induced nephrotoxicity.

Renal Vasoconstriction

Renal perfusion is regulated by the interaction of vasoactive endothelial metabolites. Chief among these are vasoconstrictors, such as endothelin, and vasodilators, such as prostacyclin and NO.[21, 65]

ENDOTHELIN

Endothelin plays an important role in the pathophysiology of the ischemic and myoglobinuric types of ARF.[65, 66] Intrarenal administration of ET leads to a steep reduction in renal blood flow (RBF) and glomerular filtration rate (GFR), resembling the early ischemic pattern of experimental ARF. Furthermore, ET-1 level and its renal binding sites are increased in the rat ischemic ARF model.[67] Similarly, Karam and coworkers[68] reported that plasma ET-1 levels and urinary ET excretion were increased 24 hours after intramuscular glycerol injection in rats (myoglobinuric model). The increased ET-1 immunoreactivity and that of ET mRNA following these renal insults are considered to be secondary to renal hypoxia and exaggerated production of oxygen radicals. Most ET-receptor antagonists were able to ameliorate the renal hypoperfusion-hypofiltration and excretory function in the rat myohemoglobinuric ARF and ischemic ARF models. Pretreatment with Bosentan, a novel potent nonpeptide ETA/ETB receptor antagonist, restored RBF almost completely in myoglobinuric rats.[68] Taken together, these findings indicate that activation of the systemic and renal ET system contributes to renal vasoconstriction in myoglobinuric and other types of rat ARF.

NITRIC OXIDE

Originally described as the endothelial-derived relaxing factor, NO is a diffusable gaseous molecule produced in endothelial cells of renal and nonrenal vasculature, as well as in tubular epithelial and mesangial cells, from its precursor, L-arginine.[20, 69–72] Nitric oxide exerts a tonic vasodilatory action on renal microcirculation, primarily in the afferent arteriole and mediates the renal vasorelaxant action of acetylcholine and bradykinin. In addition to its vascular effects, NO also affects renal function by modulating tubuloglomerular feedback, renin release, and tubular salt reabsorption.[20, 71, 72] In addition, NO is capable of inhibiting the migration and proliferation of vascular smooth muscle cells (VSMCs) and the aggregation of platelets.[20, 71, 72] Given the importance of NO in the defense of RBF, the role of the NO system in myoglobinuric ARF should be examined. Indeed, renal NO production is impaired in response to many renal insults, including ischemia and exposure to heme proteins.[51, 73] Renal ischemia can impair vasodilator generation and can stimulate production of vasoconstrictors. Furthermore, the ischemic kidney is almost exclusively dependent on NO synthesis for maintenance of RBF, GFR, and medullary oxygenation.[74] This protective role of NO against renal vasoconstriction can be augmented by providing L-arginine that is metabolically an NO donor.[75] Heme proteins derived from disintegrating muscles are powerful NO scavengers. In the kidney, they deplete NO stores and undermine renal ability to counteract ET-induced vasoconstriction. Moreover, there is growing evidence that NO and its metabolic product peroxynitrite (ONOO) are involved in the pathophysiology of both toxic- and hypoxia-reperfusion–induced injury.[76] Lieberthal[77] showed that suppression of tubular NO pro-

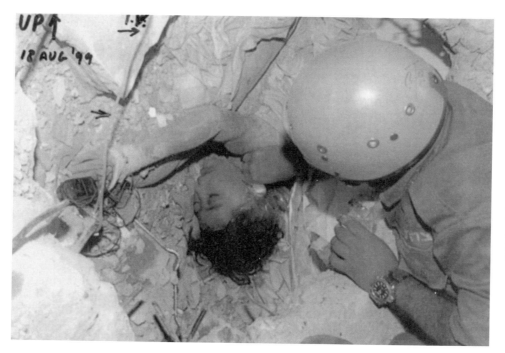

FIGURE 16–2 ■ Rescue of a Turkish girl who was buried during the major earthquake in Turkey on August 17, 1999. Note the intravenous line *(arrow)* for early volume replacement during the hours prior to complete extrication of the victim. Such an infusion may contribute to the prevention of myoglobinuric ARF in those suffering from crush syndrome.[13] (Courtesy of the spokesman of the Israeli Defense Forces, to whom we are indebted.)

duction aggravates ischemic nephrotoxicity. The locally produced NO in the tubular cells is most likely generated via iNOS activity. It should be emphasized that both free myoglobin and hemoglobin are toxic and may induce iNOS production.[77] Most recently, Schwartz and coworkers[78] have demonstrated that NO generated by iNOS after LPS administration inhibited eNOS, a renal vasodilator. Selective inhibition of iNOS prevents the decrease in GFR following LPS administration, suggesting that excess iNOS is detrimental to kidney function, probably via suppressing the "good" isoform of NOS. Furthermore, NOS is strongly induced by several cytokines, including TNF.[79] Plasma levels of TNF are increased in rats during glycerol-induced ARF, suggesting a role for TNF, probably through iNOS, in the pathogenesis of this experimental form of ARF.[79] Infusion of neutralizing anti–TNF-α antiserum immediately prior to glycerol injection significantly protected kidney function.[80] Similarly anti–TNF-α improves myocardial recovery after ischemia and reperfusion.[81] In summary, as in other forms of ARF, rhabdomyolysis-induced ARF is associated with reduced endothelium-derived NO production, which causes vasoconstriction. Furthermore, increased NO generation in the tubular cells by iNOS exacerbates the deleterious effects of ischemia and endotoxin. This may explain the controversial reports about the role of NO donors and NOS inhibitors in the prevention of ARF. Therefore, any future modulation of NO activity in ARF must be directed toward preservation of eNOS activity, while suppressing iNOS action, to protect the kidney against ischemia.

MANAGEMENT OF CASUALTIES WITH IMPENDING MYOGLOBINURIC ARF (POST-TRAUMATIC AND POSTEXERTIONAL)

Casualties with massive muscle crushing commonly seen following earthquakes suffer from profound hypovolemic shock (see Table 16–1). Therefore, the mainstay of management of these casualties is early massive volume replacement, starting preferably in the field (Fig. 16–2). This step is followed in the hospital stage by forced solute (mannitol)-alkaline diuresis (Table 16–2), which alkalizes the urine and protects the kidney against the nephrotoxicity of myoglobin and urate. During this regimen, the mild metabolic alkalosis and the increase in blood bicarbonate by themselves may ameliorate the hyperkalemia, which is an early, potentially lethal complication of the MCS. Furthermore, the hyperosmotic effect of mannitol may decompress edematous muscles and protect them against further rhabdomyolysis. This presumed "muscle-sparing" effect of mannitol would decrease the muscular leak of myoglobin, purines, and phosphate and lower the burden of these nephrotoxic metabolites on the kidney. Mannitol diuresis increases intratubular pressure and flow and flushes toxic tubular pigment plugs. Thus, by increased urinary elimination and suppression of leak from muscles, mannitol reduces plasma pooling of nephrotoxic muscle metabolites. If the regi-

TABLE 16–2. Suggested Volume Replenishment During Extrication of Young Adults From Under Collapsed Buildings[13] or Resuscitation From Prolonged Coma

When a limb is extricated, start immediately with IV saline at a rate of 1 L/h. The entire extrication stage may last 4–8 h. Once the patient is freed, monitor arterial blood pressure, central venous pressure, and urinary output.

Following extrication, continue IV infusion with 500 mL saline, alternating with 5% glucose, 1 L/h.

Once the patient is admitted to hospital, add sodium bicarbonate ampules of 50 mEq/L to each second or third bottle of glucose, so that the pH of the urine is maintained above 6.5 (usual requirement for bicarbonate, 200–300 mEq for the first day).

Once there is evidence of urine flow, add a 20% solution of mannitol at a rate of 1–2 g/kg body weight over 4 h.

Keep urine flow to at least 8 L/d. This will generally require a fluid infusion of 12 L/d. The positive balance of 4 L/d is due to edema, mainly in the limbs, which is an acceptable risk in young adults. Elderly traumatized patients may require lower and slower volume replacements.

The amount of mannitol required to maintain a urinary flow of 8 L/d should not exceed 200 g/d. Plasma osmolar gap should remain below 55 mOsm/kg, corresponding to 1000 mg/dL of mannitol in the blood.[81]

If bicarbonate administration has produced metabolic alkalosis (arterial blood pH above 7.45), use acetazolamide as a bolus IV of 500 mg. The above regimen should be continued until urinary myoglobin has disappeared, usually by the third day.

If the patient is anuric, a bolus of 20 g mannitol combined with 120 mg furosemide may be tried to initiate urinary output. If these measures do not result in urinary flow, dopamine infusion will not reverse the situation. Yet some authorities suggest administration of a "renal dose" of dopamine, 1–2 μg/kg body weight/min.

Mannitol should *not* be given to casualties with established anuria.[81]

As an antihyperkalemic defense, the following may be considered: inhalation of β-2 agonists (eg, albuterol), IV 10% glucose and insulin and/or IV calcium 1 g as 10% solution.

men suggested in Table 16–2 is started within less than six hours following extrication of trapped casualties, myoglobinuric ARF can be completely prevented, even in those buried for up to 32 hours. This salvage rate is in contrast with the 100% mortality associated with myoglobinuric ARF in casualties buried for 3 to 4 hours in London in 1940.[10] The therapeutic potential of mannitol in the prevention of myoglobinuric ARF as well as its limitations and contraindications have recently been reviewed.[82] Interestingly, the predominant majority of survivors with established myoglobinuric ARF have spontaneous ultimately full recovery of renal function even following prolonged dialysis treatment. Complete resolution of myoglobinuric ARF in practically all reported cases has also been noted by others.[83]

REFERENCES

1. Better OS: History of the crush syndrome: from the earthquakes of Messina, Sicily 1909 to Spitak, Armenia 1988. Am J Nephrol 1997; 17:392–394.
2. Trueta J: *The Principles and Practice of War Surgery.* London: Hamilton Medical Books and Heinemann Medical Books; 1943.
3. Trueta J, Barclay AE, Daniel PM, et al: *Studies of the Renal Circulation.* Oxford: Blackwell; 1947.

4. Better OS: Josep Trueta (1897–1977): military surgeon and pioneer investigator of acute renal failure. Am J Nephrol 1999; 19:343–345.
5. Hollenberg NK, Epstein M, Rosen SM, et al: Acute oliguric renal failure in man: evidence for preferential cortical ischemia. Medicine (Baltimore) 1968; 47:455–474.
6. Myers BD: Nature of Postischaemic Renal Injury Following Aortic or Cardiac Surgery. In: Bihari D, Neild G, (eds): *Acute Renal Failure in the Intensive Therapy Unit.* New York: Springer-Verlag; 1989.
7. Zapol WM: Diving adaptations of the Weddell seal. Sci Am 1987; 255:100–105.
8. Butter PJ, David RJ: Physiology of diving of birds and mammals. Physiol Rev 1997; 77:837–899.
9. Better OS: Rescue and salvage of casualties suffering from the crush syndrome after mass disasters. Mil Med 1999; 164:366–369.
10. Bywaters EGL, Beal D: Crush syndrome with impairment of renal function. BMJ 1941; 1:427–432.
11. Bywaters EGL: 50 years on: the crush syndrome. BMJ 1990; 301:1412–1415.
12. Collins AJ: Kidney dialysis treatment for victims of the Armenian earthquake. N Engl J Med 1989; 320:1291–1292.
13. Better OS, Stein JH: Early management of shock and prophylaxis of acute renal failure in traumatic rhabdomyolysis. N Engl J Med 1990; 322:825–829.
14. Oda J, Tanaka H, Yoshioka T, et al: Analysis of 372 patients with crush syndrome caused by the Hanshin-Awaji earthquake. J Trauma 1997; 42:470–476.
15. Knochel JP: Rhabdomyolysis and myoglobinuria. Semin Nephrol 1981; 1:75–86.
16. Better OS, Rubinstein I, Winaver J: Recent insights into the pathogenesis and early management of the crush syndrome. Semin Nephrol 1992; 12:217–222.
17. Heppenstall RB, Scott R, Sapega A, et al: A comparative study of the tolerance of skeletal muscle to ischemia. J Bone Joint Surg 1986; 68-A:820–828.
18. Kobzik L, Reid MB, Bredt DS, et al: Nitric oxide in skeletal muscle. Nature 1994; 372:546–548.
19. Kobzik L, Stringer B, Balligand JL, et al: Endothelial-type nitric oxide synthase in skeletal muscle fibers: mitochondrial relationships. Biochem Biophys Res Commun 1995; 211:375–381.
20. Moncada SR, Palmer RM, Higgs EA: Nitric oxide: physiology, pathophysiology, and pharmacology. Pharmacol Rev 1991; 43:109–142.
21. Moncada S, Higgs A: Endogenous nitric oxide: physiology, pathology, and clinical relevance. Eur J Clin Invest 1991; 21:361–374.
22. Moncada S, Higgs A: The L-arginine–nitric oxide pathway. N Engl J Med 1993; 329:2002–2012.
23. Frandsen U, Lopez-Figueroa M, Hellsten Y: Localization of nitric oxide synthase in human skeletal muscle. Biochem Biophys Res Commun 1996; 227:88–93.
24. Vallance P, Collier J, Moncada S: Effects of endothelium-derived nitric oxide on peripheral arteriolar tone in man. Lancet 1989; 2:997–1000.
25. Rubinstein I, Abassi Z, Coleman R, et al: Involvement of nitric oxide system in experimental muscle crush injury. J Clin Invest 1998; 101:1325–1333.
26. Pohl U, Herlan K, Huang A, Bassenge E: Platelet inhibition by an L-arginine–derived substance released by IL-1–treated vascular smooth muscle cells. Am J Physiol 1991; 261:H2016–H2023.
27. Reid MB: Reactive oxygen and nitric oxide in skeletal muscle. News Physiol Sci 1996; 11:114–119.
28. Reid MB, Khawli FA, Moody MR: Reactive oxygen in skeletal muscle. III. Contractility of unfatigued muscle. J Appl Physiol 1993; 75:1081–1087.
29. Thompson ML, Becker DB, Williams G, et al: Expression of the inducible nitric oxide synthase gene in diaphragm and skeletal muscle. J Appl Physiol 1996; 81:2415–2420.
30. Moncada S, Higgs A: Molecular mechanisms and therapeutic strategies related to nitric oxide. FASEB J 1995; 9:1319–1330.
31. Cleeter MWJ, Cooper CE, Drley-Usmar VM, et al: Reversible inhibition of cytochrome c oxidase, the terminal enzyme of the mitochondrial respiratory chain, by nitric oxide: implications for neurodegenerative disease. FEBS Lett 1994; 345:50–54.
32. Brown GC, Cooper CE: Nanomolar concentrations of nitric oxide reversibly inhibit synaptosomal respiration by competing with oxygen at cytochrome oxidase. FEBS Lett 1994; 356:295–298.
33. Anggard E: Nitric oxide: mediator, murderer, and medicine. Lancet 1994; 343:1199–1206.
34. Blick SS, Brumback RJ, Poka A, et al: Compartment syndrome in open tibial fractures. J Bone Joint Surg 1986; 68A:1348–1353.
35. Schwartz JT Jr, Brumback RJ, Lakatos R, et al: Acute compartment syndrome of the thigh. J Bone Joint Surg 1989; 71A:392–400.
36. Mubarak SJ, Hargens AR: Compartment Syndrome and Volkmann's Contracture. In: *Saunders Monographs in Clinical Orthopaedics.* Vol. III. Philadelphia: WB Saunders; 1981:106.
37. Daniels M, Reichman J, Brezis M: Mannitol treatment for acute compartment syndrome. Nephron 1998; 79:492–493.
38. Better OS, Zinman C, Reis DN, et al: Hypertonic mannitol ameliorates intercompartmental tamponade in model compartment syndrome in the dog. Nephron 1991; 58:344–346.
39. Oredsson S, Plate G, Qvarfordt P: The effect of mannitol on reperfusion injury and postischemic compartment pressure in skeletal muscle. Eur J Vasc Surg 1994; 8:326–331.
40. Nadjafi I, Atef MR, Broumand B, et al: Suggested guidelines for treatment of acute renal failure in earthquake victims. Ren Fail 1997; 19:655–664.
41. Strauss MB, Hargens AR, Gershuni DH, et al: Reduction of skeletal muscle necrosis using intermittent hyperbaric oxygen in a model compartment syndrome. J Bone Joint Surg 1983; 65:656–662.
42. Zager RA: Rhabdomyolysis and myohemoglobinuric acute renal failure. Kidney Int 1996; 49:314–326.
43. Schaller MD, Fischer AP, Perret CH: Hyperkalemia: a prognostic factor during hypothermia. JAMA 1990; 264:1842–1845.
44. McKechnie JK, Leary WP, Joubert SM: Some electrocardiographic and biochemical changes recorded in marathon runners. S Afr Med J 1967; 41:722–725.
45. Baker SL, Dodds EC: Obstruction of the renal tubules during the excretion of haemoglobin. Br J Exp Pathol 1925; 6:247–260.
46. Jaenike JR: Micropuncture study of methemoglobin-induced acute renal failure in the rat. J Lab Clin Med 1969; 73:459–468.
47. Ruiz-Guninazu A, Coelho JB, Paz RA: Methemoglobin-induced acute renal failure in the rat. Nephron 1967; 4:257–275.
48. Jaenike JR: The renal lesion associated with hemoglobinuria: a study of the pathogenesis of the excretory defect in the rat. J Clin Invest 1967; 46:378–387.
49. Zager RA, Gamelin LM: Pathogenetic mechanisms in experimental hemoglobinuric acute renal failure. Am J Physiol 1989; 256:F446–F455.
50. Vetterlein R, Hoffmann F, Pedina J, et al: Disturbances in renal microcirculation induced by myoglobin and hemorrhagic hypotension in anesthetized rat. Am J Physiol 1995; 268:F839–F846.
51. Trifillis AL, Kahng MW, Trump BF: Metabolic studies of glycerol-induced acute renal failure in the rat. Exp Mol Pathol 1981; 35:1–13.
52. Simon E: New aspects of acute renal failure. Am J Med Sci 1995; 310:217–221.
53. Rischereder M, Trick W, Nath KA: Therapeutic strategies in the prevention of acute renal failure. Semin Nephrol 1994; 14:41–52.
54. Zager RA: Myoglobin depletes renal adenine nucleotide pools in the presence and absence of shock. Kidney Int 1991; 39:111–119.
55. Badenoch AW, Darmady EM: The effect of stroma free hemoglobin on the ischemic kidney of the rabbit. Br J Exp Pathol 1948; 29:215–223.
56. Yuile CL, Gold MA, Hinds EG: Hemoglobin precipitation in renal tubules. J Exp Med 1945; 82:361–374.
57. Lowe MB: Effects of nephrotoxins and ischemia in experimental hemoglobinuria. J Pathol Bacteriol 1966; 92:319–323.
58. Zager RA, Teubner EJ, Adler S: Low molecular weight proteinuria exacerbates experimental ischemic renal injury. Lab Invest 1987; 56:180–188.
59. Bunn HF, Jandl JH: The renal handling of hemoglobin. II. Catabolism. J Exp Med 1969; 129:925–934.
60. Bunn HF, Eshman WT, Bull RW: The renal handling of hemoglobin. I. Glomerular filtration. J Exp Med 1969; 129:909–924.

61. Shah SV, Walker PD: Evidence suggesting a role for hydroxyl radical in glycerol-induced acute renal failure. Am J Physiol 1988; 255:F438–F443.

62. Abul-Ezz SR, Walker PD, Shah SV: Role of glutathione in an animal model of myoglubinuric acute renal failure. Proc Natl Acad Sci USA 1991; 88:9833–9837.

63. Paller MS: Hemoglobin- and myoglobin-induced acute renal failure in rats: role of iron in nephrotoxicity. Am J Physiol 1988; 255:F539–F544.

64. Guidet B, Shah SV: Enhanced in vivo H_2O_2 generation by rat kidney in glycerol-induced acute renal failure. Am J Physiol 1989; 257:F440–F445.

65. Kohan DE: Endothelin in the normal and diseased kidney. Am J Kidney Dis 1997; 29:2–26.

66. Brooks DP: Endothelin: "the prime suspect" in kidney disease. News Physiol Sci 1997; 12:83–89.

67. Firth JD, Ratcliffe PJ: Organ distribution of the three rat endothelin messenger RNAs and the effects of ischemia on renal gene expression. J Clin Invest 1992; 90:1023–1031.

68. Karam H, Bruneval P, Clozel JP, et al: Role of endothelin in acute renal failure due to rhabdomyolysis in rats. J Pharmacol Exp Ther 1995; 274:481–486.

69. Baylis C, Harton P, Engels K: Endothelial-derived relaxing factor controls renal hemodynamics in the normal rat kidney. J Am Soc Nephrol 1990; 1:875–881.

70. King AJ, Brenner BM: Endothelium-derived relaxing factor and renal vasculature. Am J Physiol 1991; 260:R653–R662.

71. Luscher TF, Bock HA, Yang Z, et al: Endothelium-derived relaxing and contracting factors: perspectives in nephrology. Kidney Int 1991; 39:575–590.

72. Bachmann S, Mundel P: Nitric oxide in the kidney: synthesis, localization, and function. Am J Kidney Dis 1994; 24:112–129.

73. Peters H, Noble NA: Dietary L-arginine in renal disease. Semin Nephrol 1996; 16:567–575.

74. Agmon Y, Peleg H, Greenfeld Z, et al: Nitric oxide and prostanoid protect the renal outer medulla from radiocontrast toxicity in the rat. J Clin Invest 1994; 94:1069–1075.

75. Wakabayashi Y, Kikawada R: Effect of L-arginine on myoglobin-induced acute renal failure in the rabbit. Am J Physiol 1996; 270:F784–F789.

76. Noiri E, Peresleni T, Miller F, et al: In vivo targeting of inducible NO synthase with oligodeoxynucleotides protects rat kidney against ischemia. J Clin Invest 1996; 97:2377–2383.

77. Lieberthal W: Biology of acute renal failure: therapeutic implications. Kidney Int 1997; 52:1102–1115.

78. Schwartz D, Mendonca M, Schwartz I, et al: Inhibition of constitutive nitric oxide synthase (NOS) by nitric oxide generated by inducible NOS after lipopolysaccharide administration provokes renal dysfunction. J Clin Invest 1997; 100:439–448.

79. Kone BC: Nitric oxide in renal health and disease. Am J Kidney Dis 1997; 30:311–333.

80. Shulman LM, Yuhas Y, Frolkis I, et al: Glycerol-induced ARF in rats mediated by tumor necrosis factor-alpha. Kidney Int 1993; 43:1397–1401.

81. Gurevitch J, Frolkis I, Yuhas Y, et al: Anti–tumor necrosis factor alpha improves myocardial recovery after ischemia and reperfusion. J Am Coll Cardiol 1997; 30:1554–1561.

82. Better OS, Rubinstein I, Winaver JM, et al: Mannitol therapy revisited (1940–1997). Kidney Int 1997; 51:886–894.

83. Szeweczyk D, Ovadia P, Abdullah F, et al: Pressure-induced rhabdomyolysis and ARF. J Trauma 1998; 44:384.

CHAPTER 17

Renal Failure in Disasters

An S. De Vriese ▪ Ravindra Mehta ▪ Raymond Vanholder ▪ Norbert H. Lameire

INTRODUCTION

The management of renal failure in a disaster setting requires an understanding of the events associated with a disaster that contribute to acute renal failure (ARF) and the impact of the disaster on patients with known chronic end-stage renal disease (ESRD). ARF induced by traumatic rhabdomyolysis and crush syndrome is a well-known complication occurring in the wake of natural or man-made disasters. Early recognition of the crush syndrome and rapid initiation of fluid replacement can dramatically reduce the incidence of ARF. However, because of surrounding damage or overwhelmed local medical capabilities, extrication of the victims and initiation of prophylactic measures may be delayed, leading to the development of ARF. In addition, existing dialysis facilities may be destroyed, leaving many chronic dialysis patients without treatment. The medical community may thus be confronted with a request to institute renal replacement therapy (RRT) in tens to hundreds of patients. A rapid, appropriate, and effective international response can be achieved only by rational planning and the establishment of an infrastructure composed of trained personnel, equipment, supplies, and transportation that can be mobilized at a few hours' notice. When a devastating earthquake struck Armenia in 1988, the international community responded with an unprecedented relief action, including extensive dialysis support.[1–5] Valuable lessons were learned from the Armenian experience about disaster relief, in general, and management of ARF, in particular. In 1989, this experience led to the formation within the International Society of Nephrology (ISN) of the Renal Disaster Relief Task Force (RDRTF) to provide a coordinated international response to the problem of renal failure following major disasters.[6] This chapter describes the epidemiology of ARF in disasters, the medical approach to ARF and chronic renal failure in disaster victims, and the organization of the international response.

EPIDEMIOLOGY OF ACUTE RENAL FAILURE IN DISASTERS

Acute renal failure is a well-recognized complication of natural and man-made disasters and has also been described in the setting of an epidemic (Table 17–1). Rational planning of a potential intervention must be based on valid assumptions derived from the study of experiences in past disasters. Knowledge of the incidence and determinants of ARF in these circumstances is essential to the estimation of the immediate medical needs. Unfortunately, little is known regarding the epidemiology and natural history of ARF in disasters.

Bywaters and Beall[7] described the crush syndrome in victims of the London Blitz in 1940 and linked the development of ARF to the release of myoglobin from damaged muscles. Casualties with rhabdomyolysis leading to ARF have since been reported in catastrophes such as earthquakes, volcanic eruptions, mine collapses, bombings, and train accidents. The most important source of crush syndrome leading to ARF remains, however, major earthquakes (Table 17–2). The incidence of crush syndrome after earthquakes varies widely, because of the unique character of each disaster. Earthquakes occurring in densely populated areas, with collapse of multistory buildings and trapping of many victims under the fallen masonry, typically lead to high numbers of crush syndrome. In the Mexico City earthquake of 1985, ARF from crush injury was noted in 24.7% of the hospitalized patients.[8] The devastating Armenian earthquake in 1988 caused crush syndrome in several thousand victims. A detailed epidemiologic analysis indicated building height and construction weaknesses as main determinants of death and injury in Armenia.[9] The poor quality of the buildings was also an important factor in the 1999 earthquake in Marmara, Turkey. In the 1980 earthquake in Southern Italy, death and injury rates were significantly associated with the number of floors in the buildings.[10] In contrast, in earthquakes occurring in rural areas with collapse of wooden or adobe buildings, crush injury is not a major problem. In the most recent earthquakes in Nicaragua, El Salvador, and Guatemala, rhabdomyolysis or ARF was rarely diagnosed.[11, 12] In the 1990 earthquake on the Philippine island of Luzon, there were 1283 deaths, but no cases of myoglobinuric ARF were reported.[13] After the Tangshan earthquake in China, an estimated 2% to 5% of the victims

TABLE 17–1. Types of Disasters

DISASTER TYPE	EXAMPLE	REPORTED RENAL PROBLEMS
Natural	Earthquake Hurricanes Tornados Volcanoes Floods	Armenia, Mexico, Japan, Iran, Turkey
Man-made	War Nuclear leaks Civil unrest	Lebanon, Kosovo
Epidemic	DEG toxicity Plague Cholera	Haiti

TABLE 17–2. Epidemiologic Data From the Most Recent Major Earthquakes

DATE	LOCALIZATION	RS	DEATH	INJURED	CRUSH	ARF	RRT
1976	Tanshan, China	7.8	242,769	164,851	2%–5%		
1976	Guatemala	7.5	22,778	76,504			
1980	Campania-Irpinia, Italy		3000	87*	19*	12*	10*
1985	Mexico City	8.1	5000–10,000			24.7% of those hospitalized	
1987	Whittier Narrows, California	5.9		1349			
1988	Spitak, Armenia	6.9	24,944 (official) 60,000 (estimate)	130,000 injured; 14,000 hospitalized	Several thousand	Several hundred	323
1989	Loma Prieta, California	7.1	62	3757		1	
1990	Iran	7.8	13,888 (official) 40,000–50,000 (estimate)	43,390 (official)			156
1990	Luzon, Philippines	7.7	1283	2786			
1992	Erzincan, Turkey	6.8	683	3500			
1994	Northridge, California	6.7	33	8000–11,000			
1995	Hanshin, Japan	7.2	5500	41,000	372	202	123
1999	Marmara, Turkey	7.4	>17,000	35,000		699	491

ARF, acute renal failure; *RRT*, renal replacement therapy; *RS*, Richter scale.
*Data only for the Second Policlinic of the University of Naples.

developed crush syndrome,[14] and in the 1990 Iranian earthquake 0.5% of the hospitalized patients required dialysis.[15, 16] One should be aware that these figures may be an underestimation, because of poor diagnosis and early death from hyperkalemia. Earthquakes that occur in cities where modern engineering and building techniques have led to buildings with high seismic safety are associated with a low incidence of death and crush syndrome. No crush syndrome was seen after the recent large California earthquakes, and only one case was reported after the earthquake in Loma Prieta, California, in 1989.[17, 18]

The timing of the earthquake may also play a role: seisms occurring during the night or early morning, when everybody is at home, usually result in more victims. This was dramatically illustrated in Turkey, where the Marmara earthquake struck at 3 AM. Because houses in California are designed with potential earthquakes in mind, most casualties during the Loma Prieta earthquake occurred in people on the road. The earthquake took place at 5:00 PM, when the roads are normally crowded. Fortunately, on that day, many people were watching a World Series baseball game at home.[19]

Another important determinant of the incidence of ARF is the presence of intact local medical and support facilities. After the collapse of an eight-story building during the Lebanon War in 1982, rescue teams administered prophylactic fluid therapy to the trapped victims even before they were fully extricated from under the rubble, and patients were transported by helicopter to a fully functional intensive care unit.[20, 21] None of these patients developed ARF, although all of them had serious crush injury. In contrast, the Mexico City earthquake severely damaged major hospitals, with loss of many health care workers.[8] In Armenia, none of the hospitals in the earthquake region was left standing, and 80% of the medical personnel were either killed or injured.[22] More than 95% of the trapped people

were rescued by local inhabitants with no first-aid training or knowledge. Of the injured persons who required medical care, 48% did not receive any first aid until at least 5 hours after rescue.[22] A considerable number of victims died of hyperkalemia in the hours following extrication.[23] An unknown number developed ARF, of which several hundreds required dialytic support.[4] The 1999 earthquake in Turkey struck a densely populated area and a large number of victims were trapped under the debris of multistory buildings. Although preventive fluid administration was initiated rapidly, a large fraction of the patients admitted with crush syndrome appeared to be dehydrated. Because hospitals had been declared unsafe, patients were treated outside in the extreme heat. The need to transport patients to major cities such as Istanbul, Bursa, and Ankara, located at more than 80 km from the damaged area, further complicated the situation. An unprecedented number of patients (491) could nevertheless be treated with dialysis.

In summary, the incidence of crush injury and ARF following an earthquake reflects a complex interplay among factors such as the severity and timing of the earthquake, the population density of the area, the construction materials and engineering techniques of the buildings, the availability of intact health care services, and the efficiency of the initial therapeutic approach, making comparisons very difficult.

Between November 1995 and June 1996, an epidemic of 109 cases of toxic ARF was seen in children aged 3 months to 13 years in Haiti. Of 87 patients with follow-up information who remained in Haiti for treatment, 85 (98%) died; 3 (27%) of 11 patients transported to the United States for intensive care unit management died before hospital discharge. The epidemic was subsequently traced to contamination of acetaminophen syrup with an industrial solvent diethylene glycol (DEG).[24, 25] The solvent was found to have contaminated glycerin, which is used in the manufacture of the syrup.[26] The identification of the offending agent involved multiple agencies, including the US Agency for International Development (USAID) office, the Centers for Disease Control and Prevention (CDC), and the Red Cross, and led to the removal of the contaminated brands of the drug from the market. There were no further cases. The incident was subsequently linked to previous episodes of contamination with the same agent (Table 17–3), the first having occurred in 1937 in the United States and having led to the formation of the US Food and Drug Administration (FDA).[27]

MEDICAL MEASURES

Crush syndrome must be rapidly recognized, and its severity evaluated. The first measures should be directed at preventing ARF by immediately replacing volume losses and inducing forced mannitol-alkaline diuresis. In some patients, ARF is already established by the time of treatment or has evolved despite adequate hydration, requiring the subsequent institution of RRT. For detailed information on prevention and treatment of ARF in patients with rhabdomyolysis and crush syndrome, the reader is referred to Chapter 16. This chapter focuses on features relevant for management of rhabdomyolysis and ARF in the disaster setting.

Recognition of Patients at Risk for Acute Renal Failure

The reported incidence of ARF in the large series of patients with rhabdomyolysis varied from 0% to 100%.[28] Given this wide range, several investigators have attempted to predict those at highest risk for renal failure at the time of presentation. The value of laboratory parameters such as peak serum creatinine kinase, venous bicarbonate, serum myoglobin, and myoglobin clearance and of formulas using clinical as well as laboratory data is discussed in other chapters. However, none of this information is useful in the rapid initial triage of victims in a disaster setting.

On-site emergency care workers should be trained to recognize crush syndrome, to evaluate the extent of injury, and to consider indications for transferring patients to hospitals. Attention should be drawn to clinical signs such as low urinary volume, the presence

of dark-brown or red urine, limb swelling, and paralysis. In studies performed in earthquake victims, no significant correlation was found between the amount of time that the victim was trapped and the severity of the crush syndrome[29] and the incidence of ARF.[14, 15] Massive volume resuscitation has been effective in preventing ARF in patients who were trapped for up to 28 hours.[20] Indeed, it is well known that the sequence of events leading to shock and ARF is not initiated before the patient is extricated and the damaged muscle is reperfused. The extent of muscle damage is significantly associated with the incidence of ARF in most,[15, 29, 30] but not all,[14] studies. The number of crushed limbs may serve as an initial estimation of the extent of the underlying muscle damage. In the victims of the Hanshin-Awaji earthquake in Japan, the incidence of ARF was 50.5%, 74.7%, and 100% for those with one, two, and three crushed extremities, respectively.[29] The most important predictor of the development of ARF in patients with rhabdomyolysis, however, is the time delay before the initiation of fluid resuscitation.[20–22, 28–30] It should be emphasized that the general condition of the patients may initially be reasonably good and that they may at first be dismissed as minor casualties. Patients may need primarily surgical care, and the necessity to institute massive fluid resuscitation may be overlooked. Delays in transport and extrication by inexperienced workers contribute to the incidence of ARF in victims with crush syndrome.[22]

Prevention of Acute Renal Failure in Patients With Rhabdomyolysis and Crush Syndrome

Measures for preventing ARF in patients with traumatic rhabdomyolysis and crush syndrome are not different from those in patients with rhabdomyolysis due to other causes. Although it is clear that early vigorous fluid resuscitation and forced alkaline diuresis are the cornerstone of management of patients with crush syndrome in the disaster setting, no controlled clinical data are available for the formulation of valid guidelines on the optimal timing, rate, and amount of fluid therapy.

It has been repeatedly suggested that ARF may be prevented if massive fluid therapy is initiated within 6 hours of extrication.[15–17, 31–33] These recommendations were originally based on the retrospective analysis of data from two noncontrolled series of patients with severe traumatic rhabdomyolysis that was gathered during the Lebanon War. The first group in 1979 received initial fluid resuscitation at least 6 hours after extrication, and all seven patients developed ARF despite appropriate volume replacement.[34] In the second group in 1982, crystalloids were administered before extrication and throughout the transport to the hospital, where massive volume replacement was continued in seven patients.[20, 21] Fluid therapy was aimed at achieving a diuresis of more than 300 mL/h, which necessitated the infusion of an average of 568 mL/h. None of the patients that were treated with this regi-

TABLE 17–3. Epidemics of ARF Traced to Diethylene Glycol Contamination

SITE	YEAR	DEATHS, n
USA	1937	76
South Africa	1969	7
Netherlands	1985	21
India	1986	14
Bangladesh	1990	65
Nigeria	1990	47
Haiti	1996	86

men had ARF or even a transitory rise in renal function parameters. The eighth patient was transferred to another ward, accidentally received little fluid therapy, and developed ARF that required dialysis.[20, 21] Although the outcome of these patients is striking and may serve to formulate guidelines, it should be kept in mind that these series are noncontrolled and involve only a small number of patients. Furthermore, the implementation of massive fluid replacement may prove to be unrealistic in the setting of a natural disaster with large numbers of injured patients. Too liberal fluid administration may even be dangerous in older patients or victims with already established ARF and anuria. In a series of earthquake victims from Iran, a more conservative fluid regimen of 3 L/d apparently prevented ARF in a number of people.[15, 16] However, treatment was started on arrival at the hospital, 14 to 36 hours after injury, making comparison with the Lebanon series difficult. In a group of victims from the Hanshin-Awaji earthquake, 8 of 14 patients with crush syndrome developed ARF.[30] ARF was associated with fluid administration of less than 5 L/d, but no adjustments were made for the delay in treatment and the extent of muscle damage.

In summary, in the absence of controlled studies, it is difficult to make firm recommendations on fluid resuscitation in earthquake victims, and one needs to rely on common sense. Hydration should probably be started as early as possible, preferably on-site and, if possible, before extrication of the victim. Extracellular volume should be rapidly corrected, followed by a forced alkaline diuresis if urine flow is established. The optimal urine flow rate is unknown but may not be as high as the 300 mL/h recommended by Better and coworkers.[31–33] The addition of mannitol may be beneficial, as discussed in other chapters.

Hyperkalemia

Within a few hours of extrication, when urea and creatinine are still normal, potentially lethal hyperkalemia, hypocalcemia, hyperphosphatemia, and metabolic acidosis may be present in crush injury, and hyperkalemic cardiac arrest is an important cause of early death in these patients.[28, 31, 32, 35] In Armenia, a considerable number of patients died suddenly a few hours after extrication and stabilization while they were waiting for transport to the hospital, most probably as a result of hyperkalemia.[23] Early on-site identification of hyperkalemia may occur with a portable battery-powered electrocardiographic apparatus. In a study challenging the predictive value of an electrocardiographic diagnosis of hyperkalemia, the physicians were confounded by the high prevalence of left ventricular hypertrophy and bundle branch block in their study population.[36] In a disaster population, largely unaffected by cardiac disease, however, an electroencephalographic (ECG) reading probably remains a practical and reliable means of diagnosing hyperkalemia. More recently, point-of-care devices using biosensor chips have become available and may permit more rapid recognition of hyperkalemia. These devices use preconfigured cartridges which, using a few drops of blood, can give rapid measurements of blood electrolyte and hematocrit levels. Appropriate management of hyperkalemia with calcium gluconate, bicarbonate, hypertonic glucose with insulin, inhaled β2-adrenergic agonists, kayexalate, and, if necessary, blood purification should follow. It is important to emphasize that the magnitude of hyperkalemia initially may be underestimated, and it may become manifest only when volume repletion has occurred in conjunction with the release of pressure over the crushed area. The massive release of cellular contents often requires aggressive and prolonged management of hyperkalemia and is an indication for dialysis.

Other Causes of Acute Renal Failure in Disasters

Often, ARF complicates the course of a disaster victim in the absence of a crush syndrome. In these cases, the ARF occurs as the result of multiorgan failure, typically from sepsis or an unrelated event (eg, myocardial infarction). Important causes of sepsis are infected wounds or fasciotomies. In these circumstances, the course and management of ARF is similar to that seen in nondisaster situations. Recognition of the potential for ARF and appropriate intervention with RRT is required.

Treatment of Acute Renal Failure in Disasters: Renal Replacement Therapy

The need for dialytic support in ARF patients may be immediate to manage life-threatening hyperkalemia and acidosis or may be required a few days after the injury for support of patients with ARF secondary to rhabdomyolysis or sepsis. Ideally, patients should be transferred to a facility where dialysis is available. Often, this may not be feasible immediately, and dialysis may need to be initiated in less than favorable circumstances. Dialyzing patients in damaged and unsafe hospitals, where intensive care and surgical facilities are lacking, however, should be discouraged. In the great Hanshin earthquake in Japan, fatalities were more frequent in crush syndrome patients treated in damaged hospitals. The 491 ARF patients in need of dialysis in the Marmara earthquake all were dialyzed in well-equipped dialysis units, which probably explains the low mortality (20%).

The standard modality of therapy utilized worldwide is intermittent hemodialysis (IHD), although peritoneal dialysis (PD) and continuous RRT have also been used. The choice of RRT needs to be determined in the light of the local needs and circumstances. A key determinant is whether dialysis facilities and trained personnel are available locally. In the damaged area, personnel may be killed or wounded or temporarily absent because of problems with their houses or family members. Local power and water supplies and hygienic conditions are other important elements to consider, although in principle dialysis aid should be fully self-supporting. A skilled team, comprising dialysis technicians, nurses, and physicians, must accompany the equipment to ensure its adequate functioning. The team should be experienced in treating both adult and pediatric patients.

Intermittent hemodialysis has the advantage of being a routine procedure with high clearance. It allows the efficient treatment of a large number of patients with a limited amount of supplies. However, disaster patients are likely to be hypercatabolic and require daily dialysis for several hours per day to control acid-base and electrolyte abnormalities, uremia, and fluid overload. Hence, the demands for IHD may be significantly greater. As many as five ARF patients can be treated per position per day, if chronic dialysis patients are transferred to other units. If chronic patients are maintained in the unit, two ARF patients per position per day can be treated, when some rearrangements are made (eg, two chronic dialysis sessions per week).

Hemodialysis requires sophisticated technical support. Simple mechanical-based machines are preferable to heavily computerized equipment. The machines should be adaptable to local electric supply or emergency power. The set-up of appropriate water treatment, including charcoal filtration, softening, and reverse osmosis, may be a problem. In Armenia, a dialysis team from the United Kingdom circumvented the problem by using the portable REDY sorbent system (SORB, Oklahoma City, OK).[3, 5] The system operates with a small volume of unprepared water that circulates in a closed loop between the dialyzer and a sorbent cartridge.

Peritoneal dialysis is an alternative, particularly for pediatric patients, but is often not sufficient to meet the catabolic needs of the adult patient. The advantages of the use of PD in the disaster setting are its simplicity and its independence of water and power supplies. However, the delivery and distribution of large volumes of sterile solutions may not be manageable by the available transport facilities. In practice, PD has not been easy to utilize. Unhygienic local conditions, the presence of infected wounds or abdominal trauma, and the necessity to rapidly correct fluid and electrolyte disorders may preclude the safe and effective use of PD in disaster conditions.

Continuous arteriovenous hemofiltration with and without dialysis (CAVH, CAVHD) are alternatives to deliver blood purification in disaster situations, because they can be assembled without the need for technicians and also do not depend on water supply.[37] In addition, substantial removal of myoglobin by CAVHD has been reported.[38] Newer methods of continuous RRT using pumped systems have not been utilized in disaster settings, although they may have an inherent advantage in providing continuous solute and electrolyte control, even for catabolic patients. The need for continuous heparinization may be a concern, eg, in patients with abdominal trauma or fasciotomy. However, alternative methods of anticoagulation using regional citrate have been developed and can be uti-

lized.[39] A disadvantage is the requirement for sterile dialysate and replacement fluid and electric power for the pumps. Additionally, these therapies require some experience and training for their use and are less likely to be available than IHD.

Emergency Provision of Dialysis: The Experiences in Armenia, Haiti, and Turkey

If dialysis facilities are not available locally or existing facilities have been destroyed or are overwhelmed, the choice of RRT is based on what can be provided as part of an external relief effort. Our experience over the last few disasters has clearly highlighted some of the issues.

The international relief effort for the Armenian earthquake pointed out some major problems with the provision of dialysis equipment and supplies as part of a relief effort.[1–5, 22] Several different dialysis machines, supplies, and blood lines were sent to Armenia utilizing different modes of transportation. Heavy equipment was difficult to transport and was inoperative on arrival. Local conditions were unable to permit the sophisticated pieces of equipment to be utilized, and it is thus not surprising that of the 163 dialysis machines donated to Armenia in December 1988, only 32 were ever used and only 28 were still functioning by February 1989.[17]

During the 1995–1996 Haiti epidemic, there were no existing dialysis facilities in the country and no trained nephrologists or nurses. Because the pediatric population was affected, PD was considered to be the logical choice. The US component of the RDRTF organized a relief effort, through Fresenius USA and Baxter International, to transport PD supplies from the Fresenius warehouse in Newburg, New York, and Baxter's supplies in the Dominican Republic. More than 3700 bags of PD fluid (19,200 lb) were air-lifted by a US Army plane to Port-au-Prince in Haiti, and Baxter supplies were transported across the Dominican Republic border. Unfortunately, despite these massive efforts, the supplies were largely unutilized, because there was a lack of basic infrastructure for the life-support systems that were required in addition to dialysis. Furthermore, there were no trained personnel in the area. Even when a team of pediatric nephrologists went to the Port-au-Prince hospital and tried to establish PD, they were unable to provide this therapy.

For the Marmara earthquake in Turkey, dialysis facilities were available in Istanbul, Bursa, and Ankara. The international response was initiated and coordinated by the European branch of the RDRTF. After reorganization of the chronic-dialysis patient shifts, and the importation of extra machines, dialyzers, and catheters, it became possible to cope with the patient load. This necessitated early intervention (arrival and assessment within 24 hours) and a day-to-day follow-up in order to anticipate patient needs. Six nephrologists and 29 nurses volunteered to offer labor support when the workload became too stringent.

The Nephro Crash Cart Concept

The experience in Armenia, Haiti, and, more recently, in Turkey has served to emphasize that provision of dialysis equipment and supplies as part of an external relief effort also requires a consideration of transport facilities. In general, most dialysis equipment and solutions are bulky and weigh several hundreds of pounds, which makes transport difficult. One must take into account available air-freight space, local airport unloading capabilities, and ground transportation. The transport process needs to ensure that the equipment and supplies are not damaged en route. Often the primary transport from the donor is uneventful, but subsequent local transport from the airport to the hospital and the setup of the equipment may be problematic because of a lack of familiarity on the part of personnel with the equipment and supplies.

Given the limitations and expense of transporting dialysis equipment and supplies to disaster areas, it may be useful to develop a standard method of delivering dialysis as part of a relief effort. The "Nephro Crash Cart" concept envisions a self-sufficient system to provide dialytic support using previously assembled components that are adaptable for adults and children, easily transportable, and easy to use regardless of the environment.[40] The main elements of this cart are a standard air-cargo container, which is equipped with a generator for power, a water-purification system to produce water suitable for dialysis, dry concentrate that can be mixed with the water at the site to produce dialysate or replacement solutions, and compact blood pumps for individual use. The container is preconfigured with all the necessary filters and machines, as well as the supplies for vascular access. The unit has a standard method of packaging for transport, is compact, and weighs significantly less than conventional equipment. It can support multiple patients, is not dependent on local power supply, and can use limited quantities of water to provide dialysis and replacement solutions. While this is still a concept, the authors hope that the unit will be developed in the near future for application in future disasters as required.

ORGANIZATION OF DISASTER RELIEF ACTION

To deliver rapid, appropriate, and effective relief in a major disaster, the international medical community must deploy a graded and coordinated response. In 1989, the ISN Commission on ARF founded the RDRTF to initiate and coordinate an international relief action following major disasters. Its purposes are to deliver prophylactic treatment in patients at risk for ARF, to provide RRT in victims with established ARF, and to support damaged local dialysis facilities.[6] Originally, three divisions were established for disaster relief in the corresponding areas of the globe: North and South America, the Far East and Australia, and Europe. The European branch is responsible for Europe, the Middle East, and North Africa and has, at least to date, the most elaborate structure and organization.[41] The organizational plan for intervention of the European Branch of RDRTF is shown in Figure 17–1.

The ARF commission of the ISN, in conjunction with the National Kidney Foundation, organized a conference on Disaster Relief in Macedonia in May 1996. At this conference, criteria were developed for the intervention of the Task Force based on the level of support required in different countries. Level I countries are those that have already well established dialysis programs and do not require any external assistance. Level II countries are those that would potentially benefit from support of the Task Force and education from the ISN. In level III countries, no established dialysis programs are present. Currently, efforts are underway to construct a data base of the dialysis services available in the different countries, with details on the number and location of the dialysis units, the personnel and equipment available at the facilities, and their resources and support. One of the aims of this effort is to update a list of key persons from all countries represented in the ISN, to interact with the Task Force leaders and to establish contacts with the responsible health and government authorities of their respective countries.[6] They have the responsibility of drawing up lists of physicians, nurses, and technicians who can volunteer to participate in a disaster relief mission and who are available to leave their commitments at short notice.

Supplies, Equipment, and Funding

Financial support has been negotiated from governmental and nongovernmental relief organizations and corporate sources. The European branch of the RDRTF has agreements with the European Community Humanitarian Office (ECHO), a department of the European Commission that has the task of managing and allocating funds from the European Union for humanitarian purposes.[41] ECHO collaborates with international governmental and nongovernmental organizations or other bodies involved in humanitarian aid. To obtain the financial support of ECHO, the RDRTF participates in a joint venture with Médecins Sans Frontières (MSF, Doctors without Borders).[41] It was agreed that MSF would add the additional costs incurred by the RDRTF for the renal relief action to the overall budget. A further benefit of the collaboration with MSF is the facilitated access to and communications with foreign governments for the purpose of quickly obtaining visas, landing rights, and various other authorizations. MSF also has a contract with the Belgian Air Force for the transportation of personnel and equipment.[41] The involvement of the military has important advantages, since they have extensive experience with problems inherent in disaster management.

The Baxter Healthcare Corporation, in the United States and abroad, has agreed to support the effort financially by providing the necessary equipment for initial relief.[6, 41] However, other companies such as Fresenius Medical Care and Gambro have in the past

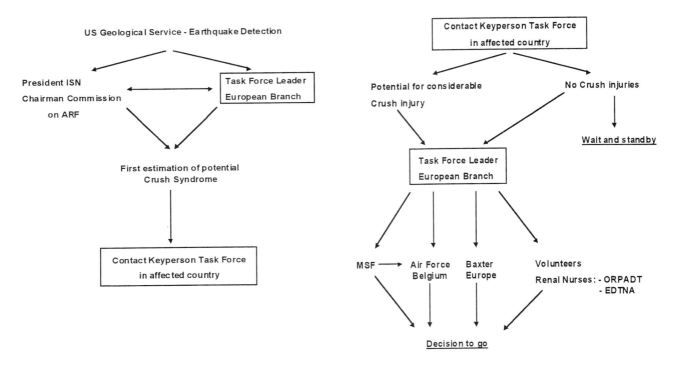

FIGURE 17–1 ■ Flow chart of the organization and planning of the Renal Disaster Relief Task Force (RDRTF): European Branch.

greatly supported different actions of the Task Force. Requirements for drugs, fluids, and dialysis machines have been listed. For the European branch, equipment that is primarily intended for prevention of ARF, such as rehydration fluids, plasma expanders, mannitol, and bicarbonate, is stockpiled at the MSF warehouse, whereas dialysis equipment is stockpiled at the Baxter warehouse.[41] The stock is checked regularly by the logistics experts of MSF and Baxter, and the material is constantly turned over. As noted previously, dialysis teams should be self-sufficient. Therefore, the need for other equipment, such as communication devices, portable generators, water purification systems, portable blood analyzers, and portable ECG machines, has also been foreseen. The collaboration of the RDRTF with MSF and the medical service of the Belgian Army is crucial in this area.

In the US region, no stockpiling of supplies or equipment currently exists. The Task Force leader has established contacts with all of the major dialysis providers, who have agreed to provide equipment and supplies as needed at the time of a disaster. While this arrangement is less formal than that in Europe, supplies and equipment have been provided when required. At the current time, this model is being examined further to see if it would be beneficial to enhance it in a manner similar to the European model.

Action Plan

ASSESSMENT OF NEED

In the event of an actual disaster, the president of the ISN Commission on ARF and the RDRTF leaders communicate with the key person of the affected country. The key person makes a rough estimation of the number of possible crush injuries and collaborates with the RDRTF leaders to compose relief teams and to coordinate transportation and communication.[6] Attempts are made to communicate with the local key contacts in the region of the disaster and with disaster relief teams already in place. If required, an advance nephrologic team is sent to the disaster region to evaluate and treat crush injuries and to assess the need for RRT. They would need to explore whether transportation, communications, and electric and power supplies have been destroyed or incapacitated by the catastrophe and to assess the capabilities of the local hospitals and dialysis facilities, if present.

The European branch of the RDRTF has an agreement with MSF that the advance dialysis team will be transported to the disaster area by the Belgian Air Force or another carrier together with the pilot MSF team within the first 12 to 24 hours.[41] In other instances, members of MSF or Médecins du Monde themselves may be able to perform the initial evaluation and treatment of crush injury and assessment of the need for dialysis support. When assessment teams arrive on the spot, they are coupled to local aid providers, to avoid misunderstandings based on linguistic or cultural differences.

MOBILIZATION OF RESOURCES

The primary information is relayed back to the Task Force leaders, who can rapidly mobilize additional teams and supplies as needed. If dialysis support is required, it has to be deployed in a matter of no more than 3 to 4 days to be effective. It is important that the staff and the equipment arrive together in the disaster area, without the need to rely on local transport facilities, which may be completely overwhelmed. A permanent communication with the national key person and the Task Force leaders is established. A leader for the nephrology team is identified, and this person assumes the responsibility for coordinating the disaster relief effort locally.

RELIEF EFFORTS DURING THE DISASTER

The team leader at the site takes responsibility to triage the victims and to coordinate the distribution of resources. It is imperative that the team leader coordinate the care with other disaster relief teams already in the area. If the demand for dialysis is overwhelming, patients with life-threatening hyperkalemia, acidosis, or fluid overload receive priority. Appropriate triage is one of the most important and difficult medical acts in a disaster setting. The medical team must alter its philosophy of care: it is no longer centered on the individual patient but must be readjusted to deliver the greatest good to the greatest number of people.[42] Local authorities have ultimate control of the patient, and in every stage of the process, the local medical community should be involved as much as possible. Flexibility and sensitivity to the local customs, conditions, and political situation are essential to the success of the relief operation.

SUPPORT OF CHRONIC DIALYSIS PATIENTS DURING DISASTERS

One of the problems faced by the disaster relief team is support of chronic dialysis patients in the vicinity of a disaster. If the dialysis facility providing dialysis is destroyed or damaged during the disaster, as happened in the Tokyo and Los Angeles earthquakes, patients need to be accommodated at other centers that are still functioning. In the United States, the National Kidney Foundation has developed a set of guidelines for dialysis facilities for preparedness for disasters.[43] These include sharing agreements with neighboring dialysis facilities. Patients on PD pose special problems because the availability of PD solutions and supplies may be compromised by the disaster. During the Tokyo earthquake, patients were unable to get normal delivery of supplies because there was ma-

jor destruction of the highway system. Support was provided by an ingenious system using motorcycle delivery personnel who could maneuver around the areas of road damage to deliver supplies.[44] Often, chronic dialysis patients require long-term transfer to other facilities if their primary dialysis center is destroyed. Having a plan for managing these patients is crucial for each facility.

In countries where chronic dialysis is not routinely available or is limited to a subgroup of patients, disaster relief efforts are faced with a different set of problems. To avoid overload of the existing systems, patients may need to be accommodated at alternative locations. An example of this approach is the recent experience of the RDRTF during the Kosovo War. Since late April 1999, the European RDRTF has been approached by the United Nations High Commissioner for Refugees in the Former Yugoslavian Republic of Macedonia, which is responsible for the refugees from Kosovo. Among the thousands of refugees, numerous chronic hemodialysis patients, who had been treated in Pristina and other dialysis centers in Kosovo, were admitted to the Macedonian dialysis centers for urgent dialysis. These centers could not cope with this unexpectedly high number of new patients. The RDRTF coordinated the transfer of dialysis patients and their families to several European countries. Important quantities of dialysis equipment and drugs (eg, erythropoietin and vitamin D) were donated to Macedonia and Albania by several industries. The RDRTF acted as an intermediate in all the negotiations necessary for the correct transport and distribution of this equipment.

POSTDISASTER MANAGEMENT

Short-Term Interventions

Although the prognosis of myoglobinuric ARF is good and the majority of the patients recover renal function, some continue to require dialytic treatment. This latter problem is particularly relevant in countries without dialysis infrastructure. The introduction of new technology in a country with previous limited experience with RRT changes the expectations toward medical care. Patients with ESRD may be discovered who would otherwise not have been dialyzed. Efforts to provide educational and technical support to the local staff to ensure continued operation of the equipment must be an integral component of the relief action. Arrangements should be made to ensure a continuous flow of material, once the donated supplies have run out. Restoration of damaged infrastructure should be organized.

Long-Term Interventions

One of the opportunities offered by the involvement of the RDRTF in a disaster is a hands-on appraisal of existing infrastructure in the region affected by the disaster. As part of the postdisaster management plan, it is relevant to enhance the infrastructure to better enable the region to cope with subsequent events. In this respect, a key issue is to establish training programs for personnel in the region.

In this regard, the efforts of the renal division of the University Hospital of Antwerp should be mentioned. Following the Armenian earthquake, 24 Armenian health care workers (10 medical doctors, 10 nurses, 2 technicians, and 2 administrative workers) have received a training in the renal division at Antwerp University Hospital during the years 1988 to 1995. Between the years 1996 and 1998, an ISN Renal Sister Program was established between the Uro-Nephrology center of Yerevan and the University of Antwerp. The collaboration focused on the organization of a renal transplant program, the introduction of dialysis in children, and the organization of the transfer of dialysis machines and disposables from Belgium to Armenia. Furthermore, 10 Armenian children undergoing hemodialysis have been prepared for transplantation. In April 1999, two living related donor transplantations were performed in Armenia by an Antwerp surgeon, assisted by his Armenian colleagues (M. De Broe and JP Van Waeleghem, personal communication). Another example is the effort made by the European RDRTF, together with the ISN Commission on Informatics and Commission for the Global Advancement of Nephrology (COMGAM) to commence a teaching and training program in dialysis in Kosovo.

CONCLUSION

Over the last decade, our knowledge of disaster relief efforts targeted to the management of renal failure has been significantly enhanced. We have made progress in defining the key areas for intervention immediately following a disaster. Our experience over the last several disasters has permitted reappraisal of the organizational structure required to deal with disasters. This chapter provides a framework for future development in this area. It is the authors' hope that, with the continued involvement and further development of the RDRTF, renal complications related to disasters will be better managed.

REFERENCES

1. Collins AJ: Kidney dialysis treatment for victims of the Armenian earthquake. Kidney Int 1989; 320:1291–1292.
2. van der Reijden HJ: Ervaringen met nierdialyse in het rampgebied van Armenië. Ned Tijdschr Geneeskd 1989; 133:567–570.
3. Richards NT, Tattersall J, McCann M, et al: Dialysis for acute renal failure due to crush injuries after the Armenian earthquake. BMJ 1989; 298:443–445.
4. Eknoyan G: Acute renal failure in the Armenian earthquake. Ren Fail 1992; 14:214–244.
5. Tattersall JE, Richards NT, McCann M, et al: Acute hemodialysis during the Armenian earthquake disaster. Injury 1990; 21:25–28.
6. Solez K, Bihari D, Collins AJ, et al: International dialysis aid in earthquakes and other disasters. Kidney Int 1993; 44:479–483.
7. Bywaters EG, Beall D: Crush injuries with impairment of renal function. BMJ 1941; 1:427–432.
8. Villazon-Sahagun A: Mexico City earthquake: medical response. J World Assoc Disaster Med 1986; 1:15–20.
9. Armenian HK, Melkonian A, Noji EK, Hovanesian AP: Deaths and injuries due to the earthquake in Armenia: a cohort approach. Int J Epidemiol 1997; 26:806–813.
10. De Bruycker M, Greco D, Lechat MF, et al: The 1980 earthquake in Southern Italy: morbidity and mortality. Int J Epidemiol 1985; 14:113–117. (Erratum in Int J Epidemiol 1985; 14:504.)
11. Glass RI, Urrutia JJ, Sibony S, et al: Earthquake injuries related to housing in a Guatemalan village. Science 1977; 197:638–643.
12. Whittaker R, Fareed D, Green P, et al: Earthquake disaster in Nicaragua: reflections on the initial management of mass casualties. J Trauma 1974; 14:37–43.
13. Roces MC, White ME, Dayrit MM, Durkin ME: Risk factors for injuries due to the 1990 earthquake in Luzon, Philippines. Bull World Health Organ 1992; 70:509–514.
14. Zhi-Yong S: Medical support in the Tangshan earthquake: a review of the management of mass casualties and certain major injuries. J Trauma 1987; 27:1130–1135.
15. Atef MR, Nadjatfi I, Boroumand B, Rastegar A: Acute renal failure in earthquake victims in Iran: epidemiology and management. QJM 1994; 87:35–40.
16. Nadjafi I, Atef MR, Broumand B, Rastegar A: Suggested guidelines for treatment of acute renal failure in earthquake victims. Ren Fail 1997; 19:655–664.
17. Noji EK: Acute renal failure in natural disasters. Ren Fail 1992; 14:245–249.
18. Shoaf KI, Sareen HR, Nguyen LH, Bourque LB: Injuries as a result of California earthquakes in the past decade. Disasters 1998; 22:218–235.
19. Pointer JE, Michaelis J, Saunders C, et al: The 1989 Loma Prieta earthquake: impact on hospital patient care. Ann Emerg Med 1992; 21:1228–1233.
20. Ron D, Taitelman U, Michaelson M, et al: Prevention of acute renal failure in traumatic rhabdomyolysis. Arch Intern Med 1984; 144:277–280.
21. Michaelson M, Taitelman U, Bshouty Z, et al: Crush syndrome: experience from the Lebanon war, 1982. Isr J Med Sci 1984; 20:305–307.
22. Noji EK, Armenian HK, Oganessian A: Issues of rescue and medical care following the 1988 Armenian earthquake. Int J Epidemiol 1993; 22:1070–1076.
23. Collins AJ, Burzstein S: Renal failure in disasters. Crit Care Clin 1991; 7:421–435.
24. Mehta R, Bunchman T, Parekh R, et al: Epidemic of acute renal failure. J Am Soc Nephrol 1997; 8:128A.
25. O'Brien KL, Selanikio JD, Hecdivert C, et al: Epidemic of pediatric deaths from acute renal failure caused by diethylene glycol poisoning. Acute Renal Failure Investigation Team. JAMA 1998; 279:1175–1180.
26. Fatalities associated with ingestion of diethylene glycol-contaminated glycerin used to manufacture acetaminophen syrup—Haiti, November 1995–June 1996. MMWR Morb Mortal Wkly Rep 1996; 45:649–650.
27. Woolf AD: The Haitian diethylene glycol poisoning tragedy: a dark wood revisited. JAMA 1998; 279:1215–1216.
28. Slater MS, Mullins RJ: Rhabdomyolysis and myoglobinuric renal failure in trauma and surgical patients: a review. J Am Coll Surg 1998; 186:693–716.
29. Oda J, Tanaka H, Yoshioka T, et al: Analysis of 372 patients with crush syndrome caused by the Hanshin-Awaji earthquake. J Trauma 1997; 42:470–476.
30. Shimazu T, Yoshioka T, Nakata Y, et al: Fluid resuscitation and systemic complications in crush syndrome: 14 Hanshin-Awaji earthquake patients. J Trauma 1997; 42:641–646.
31. Better OS, Stein JH: Early management of shock and prophylaxis of acute renal failure in traumatic rhabdomyolysis. N Engl J Med 1990; 322:825–829.
32. Better OS: Acute renal failure in casualties of mass disasters. Kidney Int 1993; 43:S235–S236.
33. Abassi ZA, Hoffman A, Better OS: Acute renal failure complicating muscle crush injury. Semin Nephrol 1998; 18:558–565.
34. Reis ND, Michaelson M: Crush injury to the lower limbs: treatment of the local injury. J Bone Joint Surg [Am] 1986; 68:414–418.
35. Allister C: Cardiac arrest after crush injury. BMJ 1983; 287:531–532.
36. Wrenn KD, Slovis CM, Slovis BS: The ability of physicians to

predict hyperkalemia from the ECG. Ann Emerg Med 1991; 20:1229–1232.

37. Omert L, Reynolds HN, Wiles CH: Continuous arteriovenous hemofiltration with dialysis: an alternative to hemodialysis in the mass casualty situation. J Emerg Med 1991; 9(suppl 1):51–56.

38. Berns JS, Cohen RM, Rudnick MR: Removal of myoglobin by CAVH-D in traumatic rhabdomyolysis. Am J Nephrol 1991; 11:73.

39. Mehta RL: Anticoagulation strategies for continuous renal replacement therapies: what works? Am J Kidney Dis 1996; 28(suppl 3):S8–S14.

40. Mehta RL, Schlaeper C, Manns M, Sax A: Advances in renal replacement therapy for acute renal failure in disaster settings: the Nephro Crash Cart. J Am Soc Nephrol 1996; 7:1414.

41. Lameire N, Vanholder R, Clement J, et al: The organization of the European Renal Disaster Relief Task Force. Ren Fail 1997; 19:665–671.

42. Waeckerle JF: Disaster planning and response. N Engl J Med 1991; 324:815–821.

43. Letteri JM, Adams MB, Duffy M, et al: Disaster preparedness for renal facilities and patients. Ren Fail 1997; 19:673–685.

44. Naito H: Renal replacement therapy in a disaster area: the Hanshin earthquake experience. Nephrol Dial Transplant 1996; 11:2135–2138.

CHAPTER **18**

Acute Renal Failure in Burns

Emaad M. Abdel-Rahman ▪ A. Vishnu Moorthy

Burn remains a devastating problem with significant complications and a high mortality rate. Reports from burn centers from throughout the world show the magnitude of the problem, with hospital admissions for burn-related causes as high as 1500 burn admissions per million populations per year.[1–13] There were 156,000 global deaths related to fires alone in 1995.[5] In 1992, there were 1.25 million patients who suffered from burn injuries in the United States, requiring more than 50,000 hospital admissions,[5] with an average cost of $3000 to $5000 per day per patient,[14] and 5500 annual deaths related to fire and burn.[15]

Following a global trend, the annual burn-related deaths have decreased in the United States.[14] This can be attributed to several changes in the management practices. Increased emphasis has been placed on primary prevention of all causes of burns through several precautionary measures. Immediate actions to minimize the area burned, applying cold water to burned areas, and immediate admission to the care of a specialized burn team when necessary have been among the most helpful measures taken. Once admitted, fluid resuscitation, the use of topical antibiotics, and excision of the burn eschar of large burns have been among the pivotal factors in the global improvement in burn-associated mortality over the past decade.[9, 13] Other important factors that have contributed to the increased survival of burned patients have been early enteral feeding and prevention and management of comorbid conditions, along with the recent improvement in clinical and technical skills in patient care.

PATHOPHYSIOLOGY OF BURNS

Burns may be caused by thermal, chemical, inhalation, and electrical injuries. The pathophysiology of burn injuries may vary according to the cause.

Thermal and Chemical Injuries

Thermal and chemical injuries, partial or full-thickness, can cause coagulative necrosis of the skin and underlying subcutaneous tissue, eliciting a series of responses (Fig. 18–1). Release of mediators, both local and systemic, along with changes in hormonal and immunologic responses, plays a major role in the pathophysiology of burn injuries.

CIRCULATING AND LOCAL MEDIATORS

Several circulating and local mediators are released following major burns. These include cytokines such as interleukin-1, interleukin-2, interleukin-6, and tumor necrosis factor produced by the mononuclear phagocytic cells. Local mediators produced include nitric oxide, prostaglandins, bradykinin, and leukotrienes. Both local and circulating mediators can aggravate organ failure through immunosuppression, hypermetabolism, or proteolysis.[16, 17]

The initial release of prostaglandin leads to arteriolar and venular vasodilation and accumulation of neutrophils at the site of burn. Prostaglandin, together with leukotrienes, can also increase microvascular permeability. Increased microvascular permeability in conjunction with direct cutaneous injury can cause significant fluid loss with subsequent decrease in extracellular fluid and circulatory plasma, leading to hypovolemic shock.[18–20]

Vasoconstrictor thromboxane A_2 (TXA_2) may also be released, leading to neutrophil migration, vascular stasis, and tissue damage in burn wounds. The release of local TXA_2 can also cause vasoconstriction to the gut, increasing mesenteric vascular resistance and de-

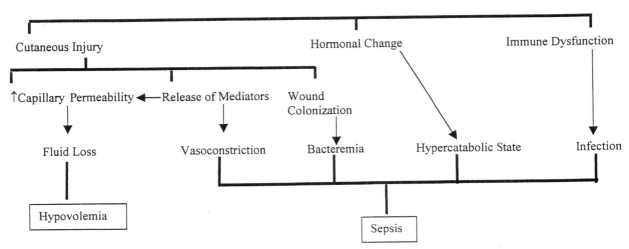

FIGURE 18–1 ▪ Pathophysiology of burns.

247

creasing gut perfusion and gut immune function. This can lead to gut bacterial translocation and sepsis. Wound colonization and infections, leading to circulating endotoxemia, can potentiate sepsis further.[18–20]

HORMONAL CHANGES

Hormonal changes can also occur as a consequence of burn injury. Increased levels of cortisol, glucagon, and catecholamines can affect several metabolic functions. On the one hand, the increased levels of hormones can elevate serum glucose by gluconeogenesis and glycogenolysis. On the other hand, they can cause negative nitrogen and calcium balance and lipolysis, with resultant loss of tissue protein, peripheral muscle wasting, and hepatic fat deposition. This catabolic state can be a factor responsible for delayed wound healing, decreased host resistance, and predisposition to life-threatening sepsis.[21]

IMMUNOLOGIC RESPONSE

The immunologic response is also impaired in a patient with burns and protein-energy malnutrition. There is a decrease in macrophage and neutrophil phagocytic activity and decreased production of opsonins, immunoglobulin, chemotactic factors, and protease inhibitors.[18–20] This predisposes the patient to develop infections as well as being unable to eradicate them.

Inhalation Injury

Inhalation injury and the associated chemicals in smoke, through various mediators such as thromboxane and neuropeptides, can cause bronchoconstriction and moderate-sized airway obstruction. This may result in progressive respiratory distress. Smoke inhalation injury remains a major cause of death in burn patients, increasing mortality further by 50%.[18–20]

Electric Injury

Electric injury can cause tissue destruction at the point of contact and along the current pathway. Cardiac arrhythmia, neurologic complications, and musculoskeletal injury have been reported in patients suffering from electrical injury. Acute renal failure (ARF) has also been reported in that setting and can be secondary to muscle crush injury and rhabdomyolysis.[12, 22]

COMPLICATIONS OF BURNS

In patients with extensive second- and third-degree burns, the outcome is often determined by the extent and severity of the complications that may develop. Multiorgan failure complicating the course of burns

accounts for one third[11] to two thirds of burn-related death.[23] Heart failure, anemia, intravascular hemolysis, hepatic dysfunction, encephalopathy, pulmonary embolism, acute respiratory distress syndrome, and renal diseases are among the complications noted in these patients.[24] The lungs are the first organ to be affected, followed by the gastrointestinal tract, central nervous system, heart, hematologic system, and liver, with the kidneys being the last organ to fail.[23]

Identifying risk factors for mortality in burned patients can help in adopting a more vigorous approach in managing those patients with the highest mortality risks. The patient's age, the percentage of total body surface area (TBSA) burned, and the presence of multiorgan dysfunction were found to correlate with mortality.[3, 6, 13]

Mortality complicating burn injury could be secondary to multiple causes. In a recent study, Sheridan and coworkers[23] reviewed causes of all burn-related deaths in their unit between 1989 and 1994 and found that two thirds of their patients died of multiorgan failure. The lungs were the most common organs affected (100%), followed by the gut and kidneys (68%). Cardiac, hematologic, central nervous system, and hepatic complications occurred in 50%, 45%, 38%, and 36%, respectively, of their cohorts. Withdrawal of support, resuscitation failure, and isolated pulmonary death accounted for 21%, 6%, and 6% of burn-related deaths, respectively.[23]

BURNS AND THE KIDNEY

Burns are associated with several functional and anatomic changes in the kidneys (Table 18–1).

Changes in Glomerular Filtration Rate and Renal Blood Flow

Almost 40 years ago, Graber and Sevitt noted that glomerular filtration rate (GFR) fluctuates following burn injury.[25] The change in GFR following burns has been controversial, with some studies showing a

TABLE 18–1. Renal and Electrolyte Abnormalities in Patients with Burns

Increased mean kidney weight
GFR alterations
Increased renal blood flow
Acute renal failure
Hematuria
Hyponatremia or hypernatremia
Hyperaldosteronism with sodium and water retention and hypokalemia
Hypocalcemic hypoparathyroidism
Hypercalcemia
Hypomagnesemia
Hemolytic-uremic syndrome
End-stage renal failure

GFR, glomerular filtration rate.

decreased GFR, whereas others noted an increased GFR.[26]

Goodwin and coworkers[27] measured renal blood flow (RBF) 71 to 112 days after 24.5% to 61% TBSA burn in seven convalescing burn patients. They also reviewed autopsy records of patients dying less than 2 days or more than 2 months following burn injury. They observed that RBF in the convalescent group, and the mean kidney weight in patients dying 2 or more months after burn injury, were increased as compared with normal healthy volunteers ($P < 0.001$), and patients dying within two days ($P < 0.001$), respectively. Their findings suggest an association between the increase in both RBF and kidney weight.[27] The changes in GFR, RBF, and kidney weight may have been secondary to the metabolic and circulatory changes that follow severe burn.

The assessment of renal function in a patient with burns can pose a challenge to the clinician. The serum creatinine level may not correlate with the creatinine clearance. Serum creatinine may be minimally elevated despite considerable decline in GFR. This is due to considerable catabolism and muscle wasting that can occur quite rapidly in the patient with extensive burns. The urine volume may also be an inadequate measure of renal function. Nonoliguric ARF is common in this setting. The blood urea nitrogen (BUN) levels generally are a better index of renal function in the patient with burns. However, BUN levels may at times be elevated considerably due to gastrointestinal bleeding, increased protein intake in enteral or parenteral nutrition, or sepsis.

Proximal Renal Tubular Abnormalities

Several studies have described proximal renal tubular dysfunction in the presence of normal or abnormal GFR complicating the postburn course.[25, 28] Lindquist and colleagues[28] studied proximal renal tubular function in 11 patients with severe burns and normal GFR. They noted increased clearance of lysozyme and β_2-microglobulin and increased fractional excretion of uric acid and amylase, suggesting proximal renal tubular dysfunction.

Electrolyte Abnormalities

Several electrolyte abnormalities can develop and complicate the patients' course following burn injuries. Both hyponatremia and hypernatremia may develop, the former due to use of hypotonic replacement fluids and the latter due to use of replacement fluids rich in sodium such as normal saline, fresh frozen plasma, and sodium bicarbonate. Although urinary sodium and chloride excretion are decreased after burn injury, urinary potassium excretion is increased. This could be due to increased secretion of aldosterone after the burn injury.[24]

Klein and associates studied 10 children with more than 30% TBSA burn and noted that serum calcium, magnesium, and parathyroid hormone levels were decreased in all patients studied.[29] No change in serum calcium level was noted following synthetic parathyroid hormone infusion. The decrease in magnesium level noted could be explained by magnesium loss through the burn wound exudate, urinary magnesium loss, and intracellular shift of magnesium.[29, 30] Because the lowest serum calcium levels were associated with low serum magnesium concentrations, they concluded that hypomagnesemia could be a contributing factor to the pathogenesis of hypocalcemic hypoparathyroidism seen in burn patients.[29] Hypercalcemia may also be noted in the patient with burns. This is often seen after several weeks of hospitalization and is likely due to prolonged immobilization and demineralization of the skeleton. Hypercalcemia may also develop in patients with burns and renal failure. In this setting along with elevation of serum inorganic phosphorus levels, metastatic calcification becomes a risk. Use of dialysate containing lower levels of calcium and agents such as calcitonin and bisphosphates such as pamidronate may be required to lower serum calcium levels.

Hematuria

Tweddell and coworkers[31] found hematuria in 91 patients from a total of 1785 children (5.1%) who suffered from burning injury. Urinary tract infection was the cause of hematuria in 54.9%, followed by renal stones (15.4%), catheter-related trauma (7.7%), renal vein thrombosis (5.5%), and acute tubular necrosis (ATN) (4.4%). The mortality in burned patients with hematuria was 21.25%. Although no patients with hematuria secondary to renal stones or catheter-related trauma died, all patients with hematuria and ATN died,[31] suggesting that hematuria with ATN carries an ominous prognosis.

Hemolytic-Uremic Syndrome

Recently, Emil and colleagues published a case report of hemolytic-uremic syndrome (HUS) in a 1-year-old child occurring as a complication of second-degree burn.[32] Infection with Escherichia coli 0157:H7 might have been responsible for HUS in this patient.

ACUTE RENAL FAILURE IN THE PATIENT WITH BURNS

The course of patients with burn injury, whether the source was thermal, electrical, inhalation, or chemical injury, can be further complicated by ARF. Although there have been several reports on the development of ARF in patients with burns, these reports vary considerably in criteria used to define ARF. Wilkins and Faragher[33] showed that burn injuries were the most common cause for ARF in their very sick patients treated in the intensive care unit. They further demonstrated that ARF increased the mortality of their patients from 39% in presence of normal kidney functions to 88% when the course of their patients was further complicated by ARF. They were successful in predicting ARF in 79% of their patients based on increased age or the presence of either hypotension or sepsis.

Although, fortunately, ARF complicating burn injuries is uncommon, the mortality rate associated with this complication is high, ranging between 73% and 100%.[33–42] Several investigators studied the impact of ARF, complicating burn injuries, on patients' survival. Until 1967, only three burn patients with ARF were reported in the literature as survivors.[35] Davies and coworkers[34] reviewed the published data obtained from five sources from 1953 until 1979 and found that ARF developed in 119 patients from a total of 7126 patients (1.6%) who suffered from burn injury during that period. The mortality of their patients with ARF complicating burn injury was extremely high, with 111 (93.2%) of 119 patients dying. In agreement, Cameron and Miller-Jones studied 110 patients with burn injury and showed that ARF in severely burned patients is almost always a fatal event, with a mortality of 95.4% when the BUN level exceeded, at any time, the level of 100 mg/dL.[35] Sawada and coworkers[36] shared this observation. On reviewing the literature, they found reports of only 20 patients with severe burn and ARF who survived up to 1984.

Management of patients with burn injuries in general, and in patients with burn injury complicated by ARF, has advanced in recent years. In a more recent study, Jeschke and coworkers[37] reported 100% mortality in 24 children treated for burn injuries between 1966 to 1983. Mortality improved to 56% in a second cohort of 36 children treated for burn injuries between 1984 and 1997 ($P < 0.001$). Several factors may have contributed to the increase in survival noted in the more recent patients' cohort. The time from the burn injury to both intravenous fluid resuscitation and wound excision has decreased markedly in the recent period as compared with the earlier period ($P < 0.005$ and $P < 0.001$, respectively). Better infection control might also have been a factor to explain decreased mortality, with the incidence of sepsis decreasing from 71% before 1984 to 44% after 1984 ($P < 0.5$).[37]

The report by Chrysopoulo and coworkers was in agreement with these findings.[38] They reviewed records of 1404 acutely burned patients, of whom 76 developed ARF (5.4%). They reported a lesser incidence of sepsis and lesser delay in initiating fluid resuscitation in the subgroup that survived compared with the nonsurvivors ($P < 0.001$).

PATHOGENESIS OF ACUTE RENAL FAILURE IN BURN PATIENTS

ARF complicating burn injury can occur in a bimodal pattern. It can occur early within the first few days after burn injuries or be delayed to 1 or more weeks later.[38, 39] Early ARF is usually secondary to hypotension and renal hypoperfusion. Later cases are usually secondary to hemodynamic changes associated with other burn complications such as sepsis and other organ damage, and/or secondary to iatrogenic causes such as use of nephrotoxic drugs (Fig. 18–2).

Renal hypoperfusion occurs consequent to extensive fluid loss from the burn wound, causing hypovolemia and a decrease in cardiac output. Glomerular afferent vessel vasoconstriction with increased sympathetic nervous system tone, renin-angiotensin-aldosterone system activation, and vasopressin secretion in response to stress[38, 43, 44] further complicate the hypovolemia. Glomerular microthrombi have been noted in some patients with burns and may account for ARF in these patients.[43]

Renal tubular damage can result from a combination of factors, including prolonged renal hypoperfusion and nephrotoxic drugs.[38, 43, 44] Rhabdomyolysis following both electrical and thermal burns may be another mechanism responsible for ARF.[45, 46]

Increased levels of the potent vasoconstrictor endothelin-1 (ET-1) and the vasodilatory prostaglandin E_2 (PGE$_2$) have been noted by Huribal and colleagues.[47] They suggested that these agents play a role in organ damage and ARF found in patients suffering from burn injuries. Support for a role for these factors in the pathogenesis of renal impairment is provided by a case report showing transient renal function impairment in a patient suffering from burn injury after the

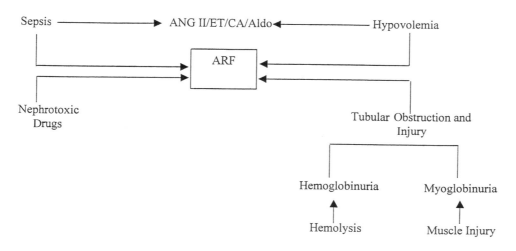

FIGURE 18–2 ■ Pathogenesis of acute renal failure following burns. *ANG II*, angiotensin; *ET*, endothelin; *CA*, catecholamines; *Aldo*, aldosterone; *ARF*, acute renal failure.

use of a nonsteroidal anti-inflammatory drug (NSAID). The renal impairment was considered secondary to the NSAID-induced inhibition of prostaglandins synthesis.[48]

MANAGEMENT OF PATIENTS WITH BURNS AND ACUTE RENAL FAILURE

Early and highly skilled management of patients suffering from burn injuries is crucial for both preventing and treating further complications in these patients. Management can be classified into general measures for managing burns and specific measures in the management of ARF occurring in the postburn period.

General Measures

FLUID RESUSCITATION

Early and adequate fluid resuscitation has been associated with a decrease in the incidence of fatal ARF occurring in the first week following burn injury. Presence of concomitant injuries as inhalation and thermal injuries together necessitates even larger volume for resuscitation. Several formulas for intravenous fluid resuscitation have been proposed, including crystalloid and colloid preparations and hypertonic saline infusions.[18–20] After large burns, there is a marked loss of plasma protein from the circulation due to increased capillary permeability and decreased hepatic albumin synthesis. Although human albumin or plasma protein substitutes can maintain oncotic pressure, this has not been proven to be superior.[18]

MANAGEMENT OF SEPSIS

Although the incidence of sepsis has declined, it remains a major cause of death following burn injury. Causes of sepsis are multifactorial. Wound colonization and breakdown in gut mucosal integrity with reduced gut oxygenation, allowing bacteria and toxins to pass through the barrier, can lead to sepsis. The catabolic state resulting from hormonal changes associated with burns can further contribute to sepsis.[18–20] In the management of patients with burns and sepsis, care should be paid to the selection of antimicrobial agents. Avoiding agents with potential for nephrotoxicity, adjusting the dose for the level of renal function (at times assessed by measuring creatinine clearance rather than relying on serum creatinine levels alone), and monitoring the serum levels of the antimicrobial agents all are useful measures to limit nephrotoxicity and prevent the development of ARF in the patient with burns.

BURN WOUND MANAGEMENT

Topical antimicrobial agents to limit bacterial proliferation and fungal colonization, better nursing care of patients and of burn wounds, early and aggressive burn wounds excision, and adequate use of systemic antibiotics have successfully resulted in a decrease in the mortality rate due to sepsis.[18–20, 49, 50]

NUTRITIONAL SUPPORT

The postburn catabolic state is usually associated with depletion of protein, vitamin, and mineral stores, together with impaired immunity. All of these factors can delay wound healing and increase incidence of sepsis as well as mortality.[51] Early nutritional support has been decisive in improving survival of burn patients.[51, 52] Current recommendations include using the enteral route for nutrition. This method releases intestinal hormones and growth factors that are useful in maintaining trophism of the gastrointestinal tract.[52] The use of recombinant growth hormone may improve nitrogen balance and increase muscle mass in hypercatabolic burn patients.[53]

Although carbohydrate supplements can act as a source for energy, protein supplements can replete the protein stores and aid in the wound-healing process. Several amino acids have been shown to be more efficacious than others are in managing postburn patients. Glutamine, which is decreased in plasma of patients following severe burns, has been shown to improve the function of the immune system, in addition to supplying energy to the intestinal mucosal cells. On the other hand, arginine, a precursor for nitric oxide, and a secretagogue for several hormones, has been shown to improve nitrogen balance, wound healing, and immune function.[51, 52]

The inclusion of ω-3 fatty acids in the diet was shown to decrease wound infections and length of hospital stays of burned patients by enhancing immune response.[54] Dietary ω-3 fatty acid can modulate cytokine production by decreasing the production of PGE_2 and leukotriene B_4.[17] These effects elicited by ω-3 fatty acids have also been shown in experimental animal models. Hayashi and coworkers[55] fed ω-3 fatty acid to burned rats. They demonstrated that dietary ω-3 fatty acids reduced proinflammatory cytokines such as interleukin-8 and interleukin-10 and prevented immunosuppression in these rats.

Specific Measures in the Management of Acute Renal Failure

If the patient has prerenal azotemia secondary to hypovolemia, intravenous resuscitation with normal saline is often adequate to resolve RBF and correct the azotemia. Forced diuresis, alkalinization of the urine using sodium bicarbonate and use of mannitol infusion are often helpful in the setting of rhabdomyolysis and myoglobinuria to prevent oliguric ARF.

In patients with extensive burn injury with ensuing hemolysis, releases of hemoglobin in excess of haptoglobin-binding capability result in increased free serum hemoglobin and hemoglobinuria. In these patients, administration of haptoglobin has been used successfully to prevent ARF.[56, 57] Yoshioka and colleagues[56] studied 10 extensively burned patients with overt hemoglobinuria. Five patients received haptoglobin, whereas the other five acted as controls and received only fluid resuscitation. Although one patient in the control group died due to ARF, none of the haptoglobin-treated group developed ARF. The investigators also noted that the time required to clear macroscopic hemoglobinuria was much less in the haptoglobin-treated group than in the control group.

ARF developing after the first week following burn injury is associated with multiple complications, including hypotension, sepsis, and use of nephrotoxic drugs. Measures including early excision of the wound along with adequate systemic antibiotic coverage should be applied promptly. Antimicrobial agents with the potential for nephrotoxicity should be used with care in the patient with burns and infection. Monitoring renal function with timed urine collection and measuring the creatinine clearance are more useful than relying on serum creatinine levels or measuring urine output alone. Nonoliguric ARF is also common in the patient with burn and sepsis. Serum creatinine level may be only minimally elevated despite considerable reduction in the creatinine clearance. This is because the patient with burns may have considerable increase in tissue catabolism and decline in muscle mass quite rapidly. When possible, measuring the serum level of the antimicrobial agent is useful in determining the dose and frequency of administration of the drug.

It is our recommendation, and also that of others, that early initiation of dialysis is preferable in the patient with burns and multiple complications including ARF.[36, 40] The clinician today has several options available in the management of the patient's azotemia and fluid excess. These include peritoneal dialysis (PD), intermittent hemodialysis, and continuous renal replacement therapy (CRRT) including hemofiltration/dialysis. The choice of the modality used varies widely and depends on the availability of these techniques, the clinician's preference, and the hemodynamic status of the patient (Table 18–2).[19, 36, 40, 41, 58]

Peritoneal dialysis (PD) has been used successfully in patients with burns and ARF.[58] Although PD is widely available and has potential benefits for better fluid balance and the lack of need for anticoagulants, it does have several restrictions. PD is quite effective in children but may be less effective in the management of the adult patient with increased catabolism and significant azotemia. Patients with extensive burn injuries affecting the abdominal wall or those with prior abdominal surgery may not be suitable candidates for PD. In addition, healthy abdominal skin might be needed as a future donor site and may make PD difficult. The risk of peritonitis with worsening sepsis could further limit the use of PD.

Hemodialysis has been the major procedure used in the management of ARF in association with massive burns for almost 3 decades.[59] Hemodialysis using dialyzers with biocompatible membranes is effective in the fluid removal and correction of azotemia and electrolyte disturbances in the patient with burns and ARF. Vascular access for hemodialysis is readily established with double-lumen femoral or internal jugular catheters. Heparin is the standard anticoagulant used during the procedure, but at times if the patient has bleeding complications, only minimal or even no heparin may be used during the hemodialysis procedure. The massive amount of intravenous fluids required to stabilize burned patients, in addition to the parenteral nutrition needs and significant azotemia due to increased catabolism, may require daily hemodialysis. Another limitation of the use of intermittent hemodialysis is that patients suffering from severe burn injuries and sepsis are often hemodynamically unstable and unable to tolerate this modality.

CRRT including continuous hemofiltration/dialysis offers the advantage of slow, continuous clearance of waste products and easier fluid removal in the hemodynamically unstable patient. The technique for continuous hemofiltration/dialysis has improved significantly recently. The improvement in technology and the availability of simpler machines have made the procedure more widely accepted. Vascular access may be established using a double-lumen venous catheter. This technique is labeled *venovenous* and requires a pump to drive the blood through the hemofilter. In some centers an arterial catheter is used for blood flow into the dialyzer. This technique is called *arteriovenous* and does not require a blood pump. The hemofilter may be used simply to ultrafiltrate fluid from the patient without the use of dialysis fluid or replacement fluid.

TABLE 18–2. Dialysis Options for Patients With Burns and Acute Renal Failure

MODALITY	ADVANTAGE	LIMITATIONS
Continuous therapies including venovenous or arteriovenous hemofiltration/dialysis	Better fluid and electrolyte management Needs less expertise Allows massive fluid infusion and nutrition support	Inefficient; requires several days for correction of azotemia Need for anticoagulant may lead to bleeding problems
Continuous peritoneal dialysis (either manual or with automated delivery systems)	Adequate fluid and electrolyte management Allows nutritional support No need for anticoagulation	Cannot do if abdominal injury Might need abdominal skin as future donor site Low clearance Prior abdominal surgery
Intermittent hemodialysis	Adequate clearance	Cannot be used if patient unstable Ultrafiltration of massive fluid is limited

This procedure called *slow continuous ultrafiltration* may be suitable for the patient with considerable fluid excess but modest renal impairment and minimal azotemia. The use of replacement fluid (hemofiltration) and/or dialysate (hemodialysis) greatly enhances the removal of waste products and correction of electrolyte disturbances. These continuous procedures may be varied and tailored to meet the individual needs of the patient. Heparin is necessary as an anticoagulant in all CRRT systems. This can be a limiting factor in the patient with burns and ARF who may require repeated surgical procedures in the care of the burned skin and have an increased risk of bleeding. Recently, citrate has been used as an effective anticoagulant for CRRT. Citrate may be particularly useful in the patient in whom heparin cannot be used due to immune thrombocytopenia.[21, 60]

The use of dialysis in the critically ill patient with burns who may also have other organ dysfunction has been helpful in saving several lives. We recently presented our experience with dialysis in patients with burns and ARF.[40] Since then, we have cared for several additional patients with burns and renal failure. During the past 20 years at our institution, a total of 23 patients have required dialysis for ARF developing as a complication after burns. The overall survival of this group of patients has been 35%. These patients were critically ill and would have died without dialysis. Only one of four patients requiring dialysis in the first week after burn injury survived. Several patients required dialysis for prolonged periods (up to 105 days) before recovering renal function. Two patients did not recover renal function and required maintenance hemodialysis and/or renal transplantation.

CONCLUSION

ARF complicating the postburn period is associated with higher morbidity and mortality rates. ARF may be prevented by aggressive fluid resuscitation in the immediate postburn period. The early diagnosis of rhabdomyolysis, possible use of haptoglobin, and cautious use of antibiotics are useful to prevent renal injury. New strategies to prevent and manage sepsis adequately are being developed. The advances in topical and systemic antibiotic regimens, along with new surgical techniques including cadaveric and cultured skin grafts, have been great aids in the fight against sepsis. Management of ARF developing later in the postburn course has shown promising results but still poses a great challenge to the clinician. Early and aggressive use of dialysis and/or CRRT may save some critically ill burned patients. In the patient with ARF after burns, dialysis may be necessary for prolonged periods. In the occasional patient, renal function may not recover, necessitating maintenance dialysis or renal transplantation.

ACKNOWLEDGMENTS

I would like to thank Dr. W. K. Bolton and Dr. A. Khidr for their help in reviewing this manuscript.

REFERENCES

1. Hanumadass ML, Voora SB, Kagan RJ, et al: Acute electrical burns: a 10-year clinical experience. Burns 1986; 12:427–431.
2. Herruzo-Cabrera R, Fernandez-Arjona M, Garcia-Torres V, et al: Mortality evolution study of burn patients in a critical burn unit between 1971 and 1991. Burns 1995; 21:106–109.
3. Haberal MA: An eleven-year survey of electrical burn injuries. J Burn Care Rehabil 1995; 16:43–48.
4. Haberal MA, Ucar N, Bilgin N: Epidemiological survey of burns treated in Ankara, Turkey, and desirable burn prevention strategies. Burns 1995; 21:601–606.
5. Munster AM: The 1996 Presidential Address: Burns of the World. J Burn Care Rehabil 1996; 17:477–484.
6. Muguti GI, Mazabane BN: An analysis of the factors contributing to mortality rates in burns patients treated at Mpilo Central Hospital, Zimbabwe. J R Coll Surg Edinb 1997; 42:259–261.
7. De-Souza DA, Marchesan WG, Greene LJ: Epidemiological data and mortality rate of patients hospitalized with burns in Brazil. Burns 1998; 24:433–438.
8. El-Badawy A, Mabrouk AR: Epidemiology of childhood burns in the burn unit of Ain Shams University in Cairo, Egypt. Burns 1998; 24:728–732.
9. Forjuoh SN: The mechanisms, intensity of treatment, and outcomes of hospitalized burns: issues for prevention. J Burn Care Rehabil 1998; 19:456–460.
10. Wilkinson E: The epidemiology of burns in secondary care, in a population of 2.6 million people. Burns 1998; 24:139–143.
11. Ryan CM, Schoenfeld DA, Thorpe WP, et al: Objective estimates of the probability of death from burn injuries. N Engl J Med 1998; 338:362–366.
12. Ferreiro I, Meléndez J, Regalado J, et al: Factors influencing the sequelae of high-tension electrical injuries. Burns 1998; 24:649–653.
13. Mann R, Heimbach D: Prognosis and treatment of burns. West J Med 1996; 165:215–220.
14. Keswani MH: The 1996 Everett Idris Evans Memorial Lecture: The Cost of Burns and the Relevance of Prevention. J Burn Care Rehabil 1996; 17:485–490.
15. Brigham PA, McLoughlin E: Burn incidence and medical care use in the United States: estimates, trends, and data sources. J Burn Care Rehabil 1996; 17:95–107.
16. Monafo WW: Initial management of burns. N Engl J Med 1996; 335:1581–1586.
17. Blok WL, Katan MB, Van der Meer JW: Modulation of inflammation and cytokine production by dietary (n-3) fatty acid. J Nutr 1996; 126:1515–1533.
18. Nguyen TT, Gilpin DA, Meyer NA, et al: Current treatment of severely burned patients. Ann Surg 1996; 223:14–25.
19. Rose JK, Herndon DN: Advances in the treatment of burn patients. Burns 1997; 23:S19–S26.
20. Rose JK, Barrow RE, Desai MH, et al: Advances in burn care. Adv Surg 1997; 30:71–95.
21. Hubsher J, Olshan AR, Schwartz AB, et al: Continuous arteriovenous hemofiltration for the treatment of anasarca and acute renal failure in severely burned patients. Trans ASAIO 1986; 32:401–404.
22. Lee RC: Injury by electrical forces: pathophysiology, manifestations, and therapy. Curr Probl Surg 1997; 34:677–764.
23. Sheridan RL, Ryan CM, Yin LM, et al: Death in the burn unit: sterile multiple-organ failure. Burns 1998; 24:307–311.
24. Sevitt S: Renal function after burning. J Clin Pathol 1965; 18:572–578.
25. Graber IG, Sevitt S: Renal function in burned patients and its relationship to morphological changes. J Clin Pathol 1959; 12:25–44.
26. Sosa JL, Ward CG, Hammond JS: The relationship of burn wound fluid to serum creatinine and creatinine clearance. J Burn Care Rehabil 1992; 13:437–442.
27. Goodwin CW, Aulick LH, Becker RA, et al: Increased renal perfusion and kidney size in convalescent burn patients. JAMA 1980; 244:1588–1590.
28. Lindquist J, Drueck C, Simon NM, et al: Proximal renal tubular dysfunction in severe burn. Am J Kidney Dis 1984; 4:44–47.
29. Klein GL, Nicolai M, Langman CB, et al: Dysregulation of cal-

cium homeostasis after severe burn injury in children: possible role of magnesium depletion. J Pediatr 1997; 131:246–251.

30. Berger MM, Rothen C, Cavadini C, et al: Exudative mineral losses after serious burns: a clue to the alterations of magnesium and phosphate metabolism. Am J Clin Nutr 1997; 65:1473–1481.

31. Tweddell JS, Waymack JP, Warden GD, et al: Hematuria in the burned child. J Pediatr Surg 1987; 22:899–903.

32. Emil S, Rockstad R, Vannix D: Hemolytic-uremic syndrome in a child with burn injuries. J Burn Care Rehabil 1998; 19:135–137.

33. Wilkins RG, Faragher EB: Acute renal failure in an intensive care unit: incidence, prediction, and outcome. Anaesthesia 1983; 38:628–634.

34. Davies MP, Evans J, McGonigle RJS: The dialysis debate: acute renal failure in burns patients. Burns 1994; 20:71–73.

35. Cameron JS, Miller-Jones CMH: Renal function and renal failure in badly burned children. Br J Surg 1967; 54:132–141.

36. Sawada Y, Momma S, Takamizawa A, et al: Survival from acute renal failure after severe burns. Burns 1984; 11:143–147.

37. Jeschke MG, Barrow RE, Wolf SE, et al: Mortality in burned children with acute renal failure. Arch Surg 1998; 133:752–756.

38. Chrysopoulo MT, Jeschke MG, Dziewulski P, et al: Acute renal dysfunction in severely burned adults. J Trauma 1999; 46:141–144.

39. Schiavon M, Di Landro D, Baldo M, et al: A study of renal damage in seriously burned patients. Burns 1988; 14:107–114.

40. Abdel-Rahman EM, Moorthy AV, Helgerson RB, et al: ARF requiring dialysis in patients with burns: 16 years' experience in one center (abstract). J Am Soc Nephrol 1997; 8:121A.

41. LeBlanc M, Thibeault Y, Quérin S: Continuous haemofiltration and haemodiafiltration for acute renal failure in severely burned patients. Burns 1997; 23:160–165.

42. Gupta M, Bansal M, Gupta A, et al: An unusual case of acute renal failure in burns. Burns 1995; 21:469–470.

43. Sevitt S: A review of the complications of burns, their origin, and importance for illness and death. J Trauma 1979; 19:353–369.

44. Aikawa N, Wakabayashi G, Ueda M, et al: Regulation of renal function in thermal injury. J Trauma 1990; 30:S174–S178.

45. Lazarus D, Hudson DA: Fatal rhabdomyolysis in a flame burn patient. Burns 1997; 23:446–450.

46. Guechot J, Cynober L, Lioret N, et al: Rhabdomyolysis and ARF in a patient with thermal injury. Intensive Care Med 1986; 12:159–160.

47. Huribal M, Cunningham ME, D'aiuto ML, et al: Endothelin-1 and prostaglandin E_2 levels increase in patients with burns. J Am Coll Surg 1995; 180:318–322.

48. Jonsson CE, Ericsson F: Impairment of renal function after treatment of a burn patient with diclofenac, a nonsteroidal anti-inflammatory drug. Burns 1995; 21:471–473.

49. Dacso CC, Luterman A, Curreri RW: Systemic antibiotic treatment in burned patients. Surg Clin North Am 1987; 67:57–68.

50. Monafo WW, West MA: Current treatment recommendations for typical burn therapy. Drugs 1990; 40:364–373.

51. Mayes T: Enteral nutrition for the burn patient. Nutr Clin Pract 1997; 12:S43–S45.

52. De-Souza DA, Greene LJ: Pharmacological nutrition after burn injury. J Nutr 1998; 128:797–803.

53. Herndon DN, Pierre EJ, Stokes KN, et al: Growth hormone treatment for burned children. Horm Res 1996; 45(Suppl 1):29–31.

54. Gottschlich MM, Jenkins M, Warden GD, et al: Differential effects of three enteral dietary regimens on selected outcome variables in burn patients. JPEN J Parenter Enteral Nutr 1990; 14:225–236.

55. Hayashi N, Tashiro T, Yamamori H, et al: Effects of intravenous omega-3 and omega-6 fat emulsion on cytokine production and delayed type hypersensitivity in burned rats receiving total parenteral nutrition. JPEN J Parenter Enteral Nutr 1998; 22:363–367.

56. Yoshioka T, Sugimoto T, Ukai T, et al: Haptoglobin therapy for possible prevention of renal failure following thermal injury: a clinical study. Trauma 1985; 25:281–287.

57. Imaizumi H, Tsunoda K, Ichimiya N, et al: Repeated large-dose haptoglobin therapy in an extensively burned patient: case report. J Emerg Med 1994; 12:33–37.

58. Pomeranz A, Reichenberg Y, Schurr D, et al: Acute renal failure in a burn patient: the advantages of continuous peritoneal dialysis. Burns 1985; 11:367–370.

59. Bartlett RH, Gentle DE, Allyn PA, et al: Hemodialysis in the management of massive burns. Trans ASAIO 1973; 19:269–276.

60. Paradiso C: Hemofiltration: an alternative to dialysis. Heart Lung 1989; 18:282–290.

CHAPTER 19

Acute Renal Failure With Cardiovascular Disease

Juan Fort

It is well recognized that various cardiovascular diseases can cause deterioration of renal function, both in acute forms, such as renal artery embolism and atheroembolic disease, and in chronic forms, such as atherosclerotic disease of the renal artery, also known as *ischemic nephropathy*.[1] The incidence of patients with terminal renal insufficiency secondary to ischemic nephropathy is unknown, but it seems to be increasing. The most common cause of ischemic renal disease in adults is bilateral renal atheromatous disease or unilateral stenosis in the case of a single kidney.

There are now functional tests, as well as invasive and noninvasive radiologic studies, to detect and diagnose renal atheromatous disease in patients with suspected ischemic pathology. Treatment options, including medical intervention, surgical revascularization, or transluminal angioplasty, must be evaluated in individual patients according to multiple factors in an attempt to offer the ideal treatment for the particular situation.

Renal and systemic ischemia due to atheroembolism usually occurs in patients with erosive, diffuse atherosclerosis, mainly after instrumentation of the aorta during arteriography, angioplasty, or surgery.[2] Ischemia can also occur spontaneously or after treatment with anticoagulants or thrombolytic agents. Since there is no specific treatment for atheroembolic disease, it is extremely important to recognize patients at high risk to avoid the procedures that can favor the development of this pathology.

Renal artery embolism is a relatively infrequent cause of renal insufficiency in patients with valvular cardiopathy or aortic atheromatosis.[3] Diagnosis of renal artery embolism is difficult, and its real incidence is probably underestimated. The embolism can be bilateral or affect a patient with a single functioning kidney. Although it is nonspecific, determination of serum lactate dehydrogenase (LDH) can facilitate the diagnosis in patients with consistent clinical symptoms and history. Several authors have suggested the importance of rapid revascularization in renal artery embolism,[4] but successful late revascularization has also been described. Treatment is controversial, and surgery and administration of fibrinolytic agents are the present treatments of choice.

This chapter deals with the spectrum of processes associated with cardiovascular disease that can cause acute renal insufficiency and renal ischemia. Special emphasis is placed on early diagnosis, since these pathologies often remain undetected but in many cases can be treated. In addition, a review is provided of renal dysfunction in patients suffering from heart failure and acute renal failure (ARF) in patients treated with open heart surgery.

ATHEROEMBOLIC DISEASE

Systemic and renal ischemia attributable to thrombolytic disease was first described in 1862 by Panum.[4] In 1945, Flory reported the presence of atheroembolism in 3.5% of necropsy studies performed in patients with atherosclerotic vascular disease.[5] Since that time, numerous cases of cholesterol embolism have been documented antemortem,[6] suggesting a higher incidence of this entity than has been previously recognized.

It is important to detect patients at risk of developing atheroembolic disease and to be familiar with the pathogenesis, clinical manifestations, and treatment options for this pathology. There are two forms of atheromatous embolism: (1) those that originate with dislodgment of a large atheromatous plaque, producing occlusion of a major systemic vessel (eg, coronary or cerebral artery) with consequent dysfunction of the affected organ[7]; and (2) a more common form consisting of occlusion of several small vessels by cholesterol microcrystals. In the latter case, the sequelae are usually subclinical, but when vascular occlusion is extensive, the clinical manifestations can mimic those of chronic multiorgan disease.[8]

Predisposing Factors

Renal cholesterol embolization occurs most frequently in hypertensive men older than 60 years of age with severe atherosclerosis of the abdominal aorta.[9] Although it can develop spontaneously, most patients have antecedents of aortic surgery, angiography of the large vessels, or treatment with anticoagulants or fibrinolytics.[10] Several investigators have found a strong correlation between the degree of atherosclerosis and renal cholesterol embolization.[11] This renal pathology has never been found in patients free from atherosclerotic aortic disease.[12] Triggering factors have been reported in 31% to 90% of cases.[13]

Development of the clinical process of cholesterol embolism can occur within 24 hours after an angiographic procedure or be delayed for several weeks.[14] Presumably, embolism by cholesterol crystals originates when rigid angiographic catheters traumatize vessel walls and cause lesions to the atheromatous plaque. The current use of more flexible catheters is associated with a lower risk of embolism.

Several authors have described a clear correlation between atheroembolic disease and systemic anticoagulant[15] or fibrinolytic[16] treatments. Although the precise mechanism by which these agents favor the devel-

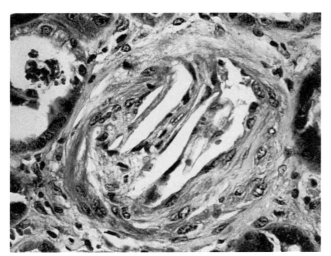

FIGURE 19–1 ■ Biconcave cholesterol clefts occluding an interlobular artery (H&E ×400).

opment of atheroembolic disease is unknown, some authors have hypothesized that anticoagulant and fibrinolytic drugs could precipitate cholesterol embolization by dissolving preformed thrombi that cover the atheromatous plaques, permitting access of the cholesterol matrix to systemic circulation.

Pathology

The lesions produced by renal cholesterol embolism are well defined. On gross examination, the kidneys show significant atrophy with depressed, wedge-shaped cortical areas of scarring that are sharply defined.[6] This patchy atrophy and scarring results in a characteristic nodular coarse surface of the kidney. Typical lesions that affect the arcuate and interlobular arteries, showing biconvex clefts that remain after fixation, are seen on histologic study (Figs. 19–1 and 19–2). In fresh tissue, the cholesterol crystals can be found alone or

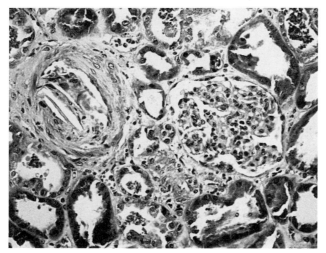

FIGURE 19–2 ■ Cholesterol clefts occluding an interlobular artery close to a glomerulus (H&E ×250).

in parallel groups and are identified by their characteristic birefringence to polarized light.

Clinical Presentation

The extrarenal manifestations of cholesterol embolization are often multisystemic and can be clinically evident or silent. Although embolization of the kidney is the most frequent, necropsy studies[5, 13, 17] have evidenced cholesterol emboli in areas such as the spleen, pancreas, stomach, liver, adrenal glands, thyroids, skin, and retinal vessels. Cutaneous involvement, demonstrated by biopsy or necropsy study, is the most frequent extrarenal manifestation (30% to 35%). Livedo reticularis, a lacy, bluish discoloration, typically affecting the lower extremities and the trunk, is the most common cutaneous sign. Onset is usually abrupt, but the appearance may wax and wane. Because of the strong association between livedo reticularis and cholesterol embolization, it has been suggested that the disease should be suspected in all patients who present this clinical manifestation.[18] The peripheral pulses are usually normal; however, in patients with arteriosclerotic disease involving the large vessels, pulses can be decreased or absent. Other potential manifestations of systemic embolization include visual deficits secondary to embolization of the retinal arterioles and abdominal pain attributable to pancreatic or mesenteric ischemia.[19]

Renal involvement occurs in 50% of cases[13] and renal symptoms range from moderate renal insufficiency to rapidly progressive insufficiency with uremia. Patients can present fluctuations in renal function associated with recurrent episodes of embolization.[20] Renal atheroembolism after surgery or angiography should be differentiated from postischemic tubular necrosis or necrosis due to iodinated contrast agent administration. The association of extrarenal embolism favors the diagnosis of atheroembolism. Likewise, the distinction between a clinical course of ARF with progressive recovery of renal function, as seen in acute tubular necrosis, and the persistence of renal insufficiency, as occurs in atheroembolism, is also helpful in diagnosing these two entities.[21] Arterial hypertension is frequent in cholesterol embolization. Its pathogenesis has not been completely defined, although it seems to be the result of an increase in the secretion of renin, angiotensin, and aldosterone.[22]

Laboratory

Some laboratory data are useful in the diagnosis of atheroembolism. The degree of azotemia tends to be proportional to the degree of renal parenchymal involvement. In episodes of fulminant atheroembolism, renal insufficiency appears abruptly and can progress rapidly to severe renal failure. In other cases renal function deteriorates more slowly and renal insufficiency is moderate.[14] The erythrocyte sedimentation rate (ESR) is frequently elevated; there is thrombocytopenia in some cases and, more commonly, leukocytosis.[13, 15] Eosinophilia, defined as an eosinophil count higher than 300/mL or more than 3% of the total of leukocytes, is a characteristic finding.[23] The presence of eosinophilia, seen in 39% to 80% of cases of atheroembolic renal disease,[15, 23] helps differentiate this pathology from other causes of renal failure. Eosinophilia generally appears between 1 and 3 weeks after the embolic episode and is transitory, persisting only for a few days.[24]

Hypocomplementemia, reflecting an enhancement of the inflammatory response, is also frequent and may contribute to the pathogenesis of vascular injury associated with cholesterol embolism. Urinalysis can show proteinuria (always in small quantities) and microscopic hematuria in some patients. Various authors have highlighted the presence of eosinophiluria,[25] whereas others cite it as little prevalent[23]; thus, the use of this parameter for diagnosing cholesterol embolization is controversial.

Differential Diagnosis

The symptoms and signs associated with atheroembolic disease are not specific and can mimic an underlying systemic disease, such as polyarteritis nodosa, subacute bacterial endocarditis, and atrial myxoma. The form of presentation of atheroembolic disease and certain vasculitides, such as polyarteritis nodosa, shows many similarities. Several symptoms, such as weight loss, anorexia, renal insufficiency, inflammatory markers, leukocytosis, elevated ESR, and eosinophilia, are seen in both disorders.[10] However, the presence of inciting factors, such as aortic manipulation, arteriography, and disseminated atherosclerotic vascular disease, can help to differentiate atheroembolic disease from polyarteritis.

Definite diagnosis can be established by identifying the characteristic lesions of intravascular cholesterol crystals in the affected organs, mainly the skin. Some authors suggest that even in the absence of cutaneous lesions, skin or muscle biopsies should be performed when atheroembolic disease is suspected.[13, 26] The sensitivity of biopsies is 75% for a single sample and 94% when two samples of the same tissue are obtained.[10] Biopsy of the skin lesions, when present, is the first step toward diagnosis. In patients with renal dysfunction who lack cutaneous involvement, kidney biopsy is recommended.

Prognosis

Patients with renal atheroembolism have a dismal prognosis for recovery of renal function and survival. However, recent publications have shown improvements in survival and some amelioration in renal function[11, 27] because of early detection of the disease, withdrawal of anticoagulants, and application of supportive measures, such as dialysis. Despite this progress, atheroembolic disease should be considered as a pathology with poor prognosis, particularly in patients who develop the disease spontaneously without the intervention of triggering factors. Overall mortality ranges from 72% to 100% and is usually the result of multiorgan involvement or secondary to severe generalized atherosclerosis.[13, 28]

Treatment

Prevention is the best form of treatment for atheroembolic disease. Arteriographic studies and prolonged systemic anticoagulation therapy should be avoided whenever possible in patients with diffuse aortic atheromatosis.[11, 28] The risk of atheroembolism can also be decreased by limiting the number of angiographic instrumentations during the same procedure and using catheters that are more flexible. There is no effective treatment for this illness and therapy is usually supportive. When anticoagulation treatment has been demonstrated to be a precipitating factor, it should be discontinued. In some cases this measure has resulted in prompt cessation of symptoms and improvement of renal function.[29] The use of oral anticoagulants is not recommended. In cases in which anticoagulation must be maintained, intermittent parenteral anticoagulation should be used to minimize the development of atheroemboli.[30]

THROMBOEMBOLIC RENAL INFARCTION AND RENAL ARTERY EMBOLISM

Acute ischemia of the kidney is a relatively infrequent presentation of renovascular pathology. It is generally due to thrombotic or embolic occlusion of the renal arteries. Acute kidney ischemia can be of iatrogenic origin, secondary to aortic dissection or traumatism, or secondary to embolism in patients affected with cardiovascular pathology. In contrast with other manifestations of renovascular pathology, ischemia is acute and, therefore, early diagnosis and treatment are important to preserve renal function.

Renal Artery Thrombosis

The most frequent causes of renal artery thrombosis are (1) traumatism in a polytraumatized patient who presents laceration or dissection of the renal artery; (2) advanced progression of critical stenosis of the renal artery; and (3) iatrogenic causes in the context of transluminal angioplasty.

Renal Artery Embolism

Renal artery embolism is an infrequent but significant cause of renal function loss in patients suffering from valvular cardiopathy (Fig. 19–3) or arrhythmias.[2] The first bibliographic reference to kidney embolism

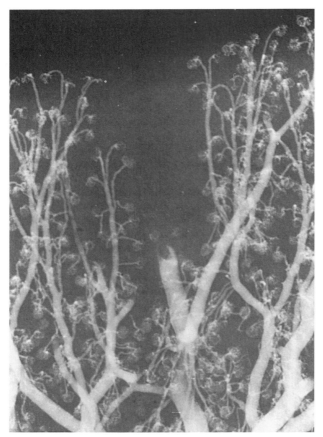

FIGURE 19–3 ■ Embolic arterial infarct shown with microangiography. High-power (×30) view of a small area of infarction demonstrates the embolus of subacute bacterial endocarditis within an interlobular artery. Note the total abrupt cortical destruction, without evidence of collateral flow. (From Bookstein JJ, Clark RL, eds: Renal Microvascular Disease: Angiographic-Microangiographic Correlates. Boston: Little, Brown; 1980; with permission.)

dates back to 1856.[31] Since clinical diagnosis is quite difficult, the real incidence of the disease is probably underestimated, as was suggested by Hoxie and Coggin in 1940.[32] In their interesting article including a series of more than 14,000 postmortem studies, these authors found 205 cases of renal artery embolism; however, correct antemortem diagnosis had been made in only 2 of these 205 cases. More recently, other authors[33] have reported that correct diagnosis at admission was made in only 4 of 17 patients diagnosed with renal artery embolism.

It is known that diagnosis of unilateral embolism is often delayed and that the process can even remain undetected. Laboratory analyses can reveal renal insufficiency only in patients suffering from bilateral renal embolism or in those with unilateral renal embolism in which the contralateral kidney is nonfunctional or has been removed.

CLINICAL PRESENTATION

In cases of polytraumatism with suspected renal artery thrombosis, the patient refers to lumbar pain, pain on palpation of the lumbar fossa, and macroscopic hematuria. Complete obstruction of the renal artery as a result of progression of a critical stenosis is subclinical in most cases and should be suspected in all elderly patients with progressive renal insufficiency, arterial hypertension, and peripheral vascular pathology.[1]

In most patients, renal artery embolism has a cardiac origin. In 30% of cases both kidneys are affected, and in 5% extrarenal embolization is produced.[34] Renal artery embolism should be suspected when there are features of acute renal ischemia in the presence of atrial fibrillation, myocardial infarction, heart failure, myocardiopathy, and prosthetic heart valves. Patients present with sharp, prolonged lumbar pain of acute onset resembling nephric colic pain, nausea, vomiting,[33, 34] and sometimes hematuria. Anuria is present only when renal embolism is bilateral or unilateral in a patient with one functional kidney. If the physician responsible for examining the patient in the emergency department is not aware of the possibility of embolism, an erroneous diagnosis of nephric colic can be made.

DIAGNOSIS: LABORATORY AND COMPLEMENTARY PROCEDURES

Elevated LDH (I and II fractions) has been considered a good biochemical parameter for screening patients suffering from renal embolism,[35, 36] even though it is nonspecific and can occur in many other conditions. Serum LDH levels remain elevated for some time after renal artery embolism occurs.[37] Slight elevations of serum glutamic-oxaloacetic transaminase, glutamic-pyruvic transaminase, and alkaline phosphatase values have been described, but they are less reliable indicators.

Microscopic or chemical hematuria is the most common finding on urinalysis. Serum creatinine can be abnormal in cases of bilateral embolism or unilateral embolism in the one functional kidney. Our group[38] has recently designed an algorithm for diagnosis of renal embolism, based on LDH determination at the hospital emergency department in all patients in whom renal artery embolism is suspected (Fig. 19–4).

Although transfemoral arteriography performed early on seems to offer the best diagnostic sensitivity,[33] renal power Doppler, scintigraphy, and computed tomography have also been found useful.[3, 39]

According to several authors,[40, 41] the duration of ischemia is an important factor for recovering renal function; however, successful late revascularization has also been reported.[40, 42] Preserved vascularization, either by incomplete obstruction or by collateral circulation, enables the ischemic kidney to restore its renal output when renal flow is re-established and tubular lesions have healed.

TREATMENT

Prompt treatment is stressed by all authors. Partial or segmental renal artery occlusion and the finding of

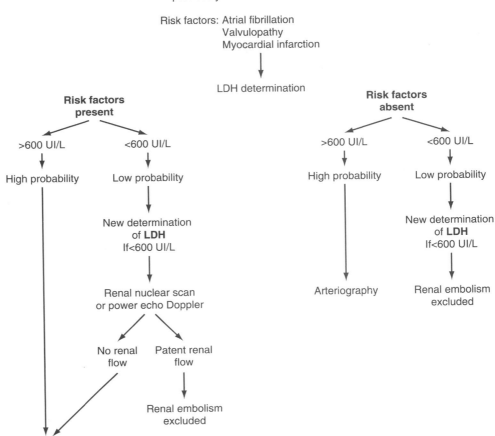

Suspected Renal Artery Embolism
1. Clinical symptoms:
   Atypical lumbar pain
   resembling colic nephric pain
2. A rise in serum creatinine in patient with
   previously normal renal function

Risk factors: Atrial fibrillation
              Valvulopathy
              Myocardial infarction

LDH determination

Risk factors present
>600 UI/L → High probability
<600 UI/L → Low probability → New determination of **LDH** If<600 UI/L → Renal nuclear scan or power echo Doppler → No renal flow / Patent renal flow
No renal flow → Arteriography
Patent renal flow → Renal embolism excluded
High probability → Arteriography

Risk factors absent
>600 UI/L → High probability → Arteriography
<600 UI/L → Low probability → New determination of **LDH** If<600 UI/L → Renal embolism excluded

FIGURE 19–4 ■ Algorithm for the diagnosis of renal artery embolism (RAE). *LDH,* lactate dehydrogenase.

good collateral circulation are associated with favorable outcome for both surgical and thrombolytic treatments.[43–45] The choice of treatment is still controversial.[46] Several authors[45, 47, 48] are in favor of surgical embolectomy when renal artery embolism is bilateral or unilateral with a solitary functioning kidney, the embolus occurring in the main renal artery. Both conditions are frequent in a considerable number of elderly patients with only one kidney contributing to glomerular filtration. Other authors[49] suggest that surgical embolectomy should be reserved for patients with total parenchymal embolization whose conditions have failed to respond to less invasive models of therapy (Figs. 19–5 and 19–6).

Since the successful introduction of fibrinolytic treatment by Halpern,[50] a number of reports have been published using intra-arterial fibrinolytics as the therapy of choice, particularly when the embolism is located in the intrarenal arteries (Figs. 19–6 and 19–7). Intra-arterial perfusions of streptokinase,[51, 52] urokinase[43, 53, 54] and, later on, tissue-type plasminogen activator (t-PA)[55, 56] all have been successfully administered.

Fibrinolytic therapy has several theoretical advantages over the more traditional methods, such as anticoagulation, thrombectomy, and embolectomy. Anticoagulation only limits the extension of the thrombosis, facilitating fibrinolysis through the endogenous plasminogen activators. Embolectomy, performed in centers with extensive experience, is the most effective technique for treating recent embolism in normal arteries; however, embolectomy is not useful for intrarenal embolism.

Urokinase, originally obtained from human urine[57] in 1947 and presently from human kidney cells,[58] is the most commonly used fibrinolytic.[59, 60] It is a trypsin-like serine protease capable of direct activation of fibrinolysis with no antigenicity and low pyrogenicity. t-PA is a clot-specific serine protease. First identified in 1947, its DNA structure was sequenced and cloned in 1983.[61] This agent has a high affinity for thrombus-bound plasminogen in the absence of fibrin. Thus, it exerts a powerful local effect on the thrombus with minimum systemic activation. Although it is considered to be an ideal fibrinolytic,[62] the relatively high

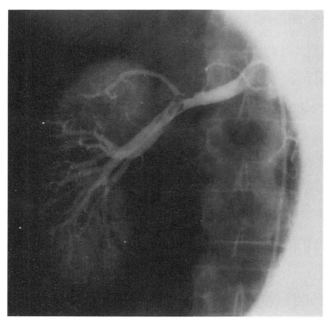

FIGURE 19–5 ▪ Selective arteriography of the right renal artery showing partial emboli occlusion at bifurcation of the main renal artery.

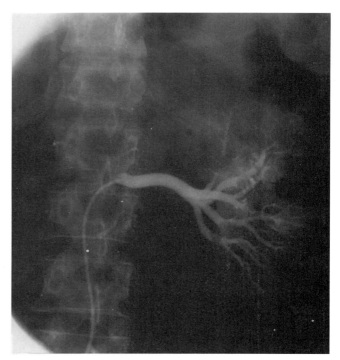

FIGURE 19–7 ▪ Left selective renal arteriography showing multiple segmentary intrarenal emboli.

cost of t-PA remains a problem. To achieve the best results, treatment should be managed by a team of specialists in nephrology, vascular surgery, and interventional radiology.

Urokinase is currently given immediately after arteriography, via a catheter in the main renal artery at an initial dose of 4000 IU/min until re-establishment of circulation and then at a reduced dose of 1000 IU/

min until total thrombi lysis is achieved[63–65] (see Figs. 19–5 and 19–6). Bolus administration of 250,000 IU over 30 minutes followed by 100,000 IU/h for 8 to 24 hours has also been described (Figs. 19–7 and 19–8). Radiologic control is used to monitor the embolus. If it persists, urokinase perfusion is prolonged; if revascularization is achieved, the catheter is removed and

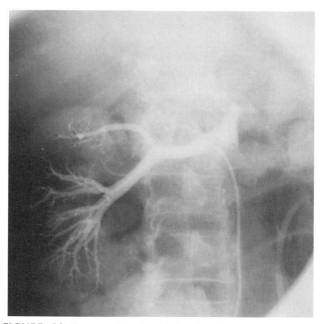

FIGURE 19–6 ▪ Total emboli lysis after 24 hours of systemic fibrinolytic treatment.

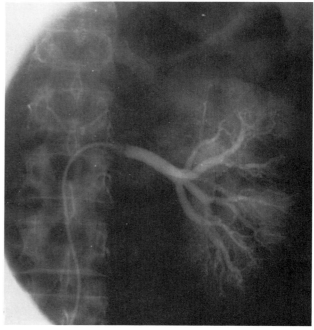

FIGURE 19–8 ▪ Emboli lysis after fibrinolytic treatment with partial recuperation of perfusion of the parenchyma.

sodium heparin perfusion is administered to keep the activated partial thromboplastin time ratio at 1.5 to 2. A long time lapse after the embolism occurs should not be considered a contraindication for revascularization when arteriography shows signs of viability.[31, 66]

It is important that emergency department physicians include renal artery embolism in the differential diagnosis of elderly patients with atrial fibrillation or cardiovascular background who complain of abrupt lumbar pain and present with anuria or renal insufficiency. When renal artery embolism occurs, prompt diagnosis is essential to restore renal function and avoid end-stage renal disease and chronic dialysis, which is badly tolerated in these patients and implies high morbidity and social cost.

Traumatic renal artery occlusion is treated surgically when indicated, although the results have not been encouraging.[67]

CONTRAINDICATIONS TO FIBRINOLYTIC THERAPY

The exclusion criteria for fibrinolytic therapy were described in 1980 in the "Consensus Development Conference."[68]

- Absolute contraindication: active hemorrhage, recent cerebrovascular accident, active intracranial process
- Major relative contraindication: major surgery, peripartum, puncture biopsy of an organ, recent gastrointestinal hemorrhage, severe arterial hypertension
- Minor relative contraindication: recent cardiopulmonary resuscitation maneuvers, presence of left heart thrombi, bacterial endocarditis, age older than 75 years, hemorrhagic retinopathy

The presence of intracardiac thrombi should be evaluated by ultrasound. Although this factor is only a relative contraindication, the possibility that microemboli can be produced from the major thrombus during fibrinolytic treatment must be considered in the choice of therapy.

COMPLICATIONS

Hemorrhage is the most frequent complication of fibrinolytic therapy,[69] followed by local hematomas at the puncture site. The incidence of hemorrhage varies in the different series and ranges from 4% to 25%, although with correct selection of patients associated with careful clinical and analytic control, the frequency of hemorrhage can be reduced considerably. Other potential complications, such as fragmentation of the embolus and migration to the peripheral renal branches, have not been regarded as relevant in the literature. Allergic reactions have been described with streptokinase, but urokinase and t-PA have been used with virtually no such adverse reactions.

CONSIDERATIONS

Although fibrinolysis is an attractive and less invasive option than surgery in the severely ill patient with cardiovascular compromise, it must be borne in mind that its use still carries a certain risk. Only when there is bilateral occlusion of the renal arteries or when a solitary functioning kidney is affected is surgery necessary to salvage renal function. If one of two functioning kidneys has a vascular occlusion in a high-risk patient, it may be safer to accept the loss of the kidney and to avoid aggressive treatment.

ATHEROSCLEROTIC ISCHEMIC RENAL DISEASE

Atherosclerotic renovascular disease has been recognized as a cause of occlusion of the renal artery leading to ARF since the first publications describing improved renal function after revascularization.[70, 71] After analyzing large series of patients with ARF, Kalra and colleagues[72] found that renovascular atherosclerotic disease was the cause of deterioration of renal function in 16% of cases. The term *ischemic nephropathy* refers to reduced glomerular filtration caused by hemodynamically significant obstruction of the renal artery.[73] The most frequent cause of ischemic renal illness in adults is bilateral atheromatous renal disease or unilateral stenosis in patients with a single kidney.

In this chapter, we do not go into the diagnosis or treatment of this pathology, which are more related to the study of vascular nephropathy and renovascular hypertension. But it is important to mention the role that the angiotensin-converting enzyme (ACE) inhibitors have in the exacerbation of renal failure in patients with critical renal stenosis.[74, 75] The use of ACEs is becoming increasingly frequent in elderly patients with cardiac failure, diabetic nephropathy, or arterial hypertension who present with atheromatous renal pathology. Administration of these agents requires careful monitoring of renal function, especially in situations of sodium depletion, when the glomerular filtration rate is particularly dependent on angiotensin II.[76]

ACUTE RENAL FAILURE IN HEART FAILURE

The heart, the kidney, and the blood vessels are the essential limbs of the cardiovascular perfusion system whose functions are regulated in an organized manner. Cardiac failure compromises the compensatory mechanisms that the kidney presents in normal conditions. Patients with cardiac failure have reduced cardiac output (reduced ejection fraction), sometimes associated with enlargement of the atrial and ventricular chambers and accompanied by structural changes in the myocardium and cardiac muscle and vessels ("ventricular remodeling"). Cardiac failure is associated with increased pressure and engorgement of central veins and with their physiologic sequela, peripheral edema. The kidney responds to the perturbations of cardiac failure by more avid salt and water retention than occurs in physiologic circumstances.[77]

ACUTE RENAL FAILURE AFTER OPEN HEART SURGERY

Although the incidence of dialysis-dependent ARF after cardiac surgery is low,[78, 79] the morbidity and mortality associated with this condition are high.[80, 81] Moreover, ARF in these circumstances lengthens the patient's stay in the intensive care unit, with the consequent increases in health care cost.[82] Discrete alterations of renal function that do not require dialysis are more frequent and correlate with lower morbidity as compared with patients experiencing severe renal failure. In the preoperative period, patients who present various risk factors can be exposed to renal insults, such as ischemia and nephrotoxicity. It is of utmost importance to identify a patient at risk and avoid possible renal insults during and after cardiopulmonary bypass (CPB) and open heart surgery.[82] The intraoperative period exposes the kidney to the obligatory nonphysiologic state of CPB; however the role that CPB plays in ARF is controversial.[83] The impact of the post-bypass period is intensified by the devastating effect of low cardiac output on renal function after cardiac surgery. Once renal failure becomes established, the therapeutic capacity to restore renal function is limited.

Risk Factors

Preoperative risk factors, such as previous renal dysfunction, advanced age, diabetes, chronic cardiac failure, as well as ischemic insult and nephrotoxicity, play an important role in the development of ARF in cardiac surgery. The most important predictor of postoperative ARF identified in the literature is previous renal dysfunction.[84] During cardiac surgery the kidney can be damaged by the type of surgery and the number of nephrotoxins administered. The type of cardiac surgery is an important factor affecting the development of ARF. Schmitt and coworkers[81] have reported a rate of renal failure of 0.9% in coronary bypass surgery and 4.5% in combined coronary and valve replacement surgery. Repeated cardiac surgery was found to be an independent risk factor for the development of renal failure in a multivariate analysis,[84] taking into account that patients who had to be reoperated had a multitude of additional medical and surgical problems. Heart transplant surgery carries a high risk of producing alterations in renal function[85] because of the greater complexity and duration of the surgery and the need to administer nephrotoxic agents, such as cyclosporine. Slogoff and associates[86] identified emergency reintervention as the type of surgery most often associated with renal dysfunction.

Cardiopulmonary bypass is a highly nonphysiologic situation for various organs, including the kidney. The effects of hemodilution, low blood pressure/flow, hypothermia, nonpulsatility, acid-base alterations, microemboli and macroemboli, and the generalized inflammatory responses to CPB contribute greatly to the morbidity and mortality of cardiac surgery. Since 1980 cardiac surgery without CPB has been carried out in selected patients.[87] However, a larger number of patients from several centers are required to evaluate the effect of these techniques on renal function.

Apart from cyclosporine, other drugs, such as aminoglycosides, have been cited as responsible for perioperative impairment of renal function. In cardiac patients, aminoglycosides are generally used as prophylactic therapy or in combination with other drugs when bacterial endocarditis is present. Aprotinin, used to inhibit fibrinolysis, blunts the inflammatory response to CPB and reduces bleeding and the need for transfusion. The participation of aprotinin in renal dysfunction[88] has been attributed to renal tubular dysfunction and microvascular thrombosis.

Prophylaxis for Renal Failure

Prophylaxis for renal failure consists of avoiding the controllable risk factors and applying active techniques to prevent renal dysfunction. Prevention of renal dysfunction begins with careful preparation of the patients, which includes postponing the intervention if creatinine levels are over 1.9 mg/dL and correcting reversible factors, ie, limiting the amount of contrast agent, performing previous hydration, avoiding nephrotoxic agents, and administering calcium antagonists.[89] Abundant preoperative hydration instead of fluid restriction is important for decreasing the risk of renal failure. Placement of a catheter in the pulmonary artery to measure pulmonary capillary wedge pressure is essential for intraoperative and postoperative hemodynamic management. The most effective way to avoid renal ischemia is to maintain correct renal plasmatic flow with adequate cardiac output. The urine flow rate is not predictive of renal function evolution, since 50% to 70% of ARF is nonoliguric.[90]

The renal protective role of dopamine is controversial.[91] Although the majority of studies have demonstrated its diuretic action,[92] few have proven its effectiveness in increasing renal plasmatic flow and, therefore, providing renal protection.

Although mannitol has been used extensively in attempts to attenuate perioperative renal dysfunction in cardiac surgery patients, there is considerable debate about its usefulness.[93] Mannitol may even have some detrimental effects on the cardiac patient after CPB. Its use during CPB washes out the hypertonic renal medulla and renders the kidney incapable of concentrating urine.

Other drugs, such as ACE inhibitor captopril,[94] atrial natriuretic peptide,[95] urodilatin,[96] prostaglandins,[97] pentoxifylline,[98] and the calcium entry blocker felodipine all have been studied with the aim of decreasing the incidence of renal failure associated with cardiac surgery. Patients who need dialysis are now usually provided supportive treatment with continuous venovenous hemofiltration.

REFERENCES

1. Jacobson H: Ischemic renal disease. Kidney Int 1988; 34:729.
2. Gleen JF, Boyce WH, Kaufman JJ, Salvat S (eds): In: *Textbook of Cirugía Urológica*. Barcelona; 1986:297.

3. Höbarth K, Kratzik CH, Schurawitzki H: Diagnosis of renal artery occlusion by duplex sonography and successful lysis therapy. Urol Int 1991; 46:136.

4. Panum PL: Experimentalle Beitrage zur Lehre Von Der Emboli. Virchows Archiv Pathol Anat Physiol Klin Med 1863; 25:308.

5. Flory CM: Arterial occlusions produced by emboli from eroded aortic atheromatous plaques. Am J Pathol 1945; 21:549.

6. Moldveen-Geronimus M, Merriam JC: Cholesterol embolization: from pathological curiosity to clinical entity. Circulation 1967; 35:946.

7. Tunick PA, Culliford AT, Lamparello PI, et al: Atheromatosis of the aortic arch as an occult source of multiple systemic emboli. Ann Intern Med 1991; 114:391.

8. Eliot RS, Kanjuh VI, Edwards JE: Atheromatous embolism. Circulation 1964; 30:611.

9. Handler FP: Clinical and pathologic significance of atheromatous embolization with emphasis on an etiology of renal hypertension. Am J Med 1956; 20:366.

10. Case records of the Massachusetts General Hospital: Weekly clinicopathological exercises. Case 2-1991. A 60-year-old woman with hypertension, seizures, and mild renal failure. N Engl J Med 1991; 325:563.

11. Smith MC, Ghose MK, Henry AR: The clinical spectrum of renal cholesterol embolization. Am J Med 1981; 71:174.

12. Thurlbeck WM, Castleman B: Atheromatous emboli to the kidneys after aortic surgery. N Engl J Med 1957; 257:442.

13. Fine MJ, Kapoor W, Falanga W: Cholesterol crystal embolization: a review of 221 cases in the English literature. Angiology 1987; 38:769.

14. Case records of the Massachusetts General Hospital: Weekly clinicopathological exercises. Case 34-1991. A 51-year-old man with severe hypertension and rapidly progressive renal failure. N Engl J Med 1991; 324:113.

15. Dahlberg PJ, Frecentese DF, Cogbill TH: Cholesterol embolism: experience with 22 histologically proven cases. Surgery 1989; 105:737.

16. Mendia R, Cavaliere G, Sparacio F, et al: Does thrombolysis produce cholesterol embolisation? Lancet 1992; 339:562.

17. Freund NS: Cholesterol emboli syndrome following cardiac catheterization. Postgrad Med 1990; 87:55.

18. Falanga V, Fine MJ, Kapoor WN: The cutaneous manifestations of cholesterol crystal embolization. Arch Dermatol 1936; 122:1194.

19. Fisher ER, Hellstrom HR, Myers JD: Disseminated atheromatous emboli. Am J Med 1960; 29:176.

20. Gore I, Collins DP: Spontaneous atheromatous embolization: review of the literature and a report of 16 additional cases. Am J Clin Pathol 1960; 33:416.

21. Alexander RD, Berkes SL, Abuelo G: Contrast media–induced oliguric renal failure. Arch Intern Med 1978; 138:381.

22. Dalakos TG, Streeten DHP, Jones D, et al: Malignant hypertension resulting from atheromatous embolization predominantly of one kidney. Am J Med 1974; 57:135.

23. Kasinath BS, Corwin HL, Bidani AK, et al: Eosinophilia in the diagnosis of atheroembolic renal disease. Am J Nephrol 1987; 7:173.

24. Kasinath BS, Lewis EJ: Eosinophilia as a clue to the diagnosis of atheroembolic renal disease. Arch Intern Med 1987; 147:1384.

25. Wilson DM, Salazer TL, Farkouh ME: Eosinophiluria in atheroembolic renal disease. Am J Med 1991; 91:186.

26. Carbajal JA, Anderson WR, Weiss L, et al: Atheroembolism: an etiologic factor in renal insufficiency, gastrointestinal hemorrhages, and peripheral vascular diseases. Arch Intern Med 1967; 119:593.

27. Schipper H, Gordon M, Berris B: Atheromatous embolic disease. Can Med Assoc J 1975; 113:640.

28. Glassock RJ: Renal arterial thrombosis and embolism. In: Massry SG, Glassock RJ, eds: Textbook of Nephrology. Baltimore: Williams & Wilkins; 1989:916.

29. McGowan JA, Greenberg A: Cholesterol atheroembolic renal disease: report of three cases with emphasis on diagnosis by skin biopsy and extended survival. Am J Nephrol 1986; 6:135.

30. Acker CG: Cholesterol microembolization and stable renal function with continued anticoagulation. South Med J 1992; 85:210.

31. Traube L: Uber den Zusammenhang vo Herz und Nierenkrankheit. Berlin; 1856:77.

32. Hoxie HJ, Coggin CB: Renal infarction: statistical study of two hundred and five cases and detailed report of an unusual case. Arch Intern Med 1940; 65:587.

33. Lessman RK, Johnson SF, Coburn JW, et al: Renal artery embolism: clinical features and long-term follow-up of 17 cases. Ann Intern Med 1978; 89:477.

34. Gasparini M, Hofmann R, Stoller M: Renal artery embolism: clinical features and therapeutic options. J Urol 1992; 147:567.

35. Winzelberg CG, Hull JP, Agar JW, et al: Elevation of serum lactate dehydrogenase levels in renal infarction. JAMA 1979; 247:268.

36. Fort J, Camps J, Ruíz P, et al: Renal artery embolism successfully revascularized by surgery after 5 days' anuria: is it never too late? Nephrol Dial Transplant 1996; 11:1843.

37. Gault MH, Steiner G: Serum and urinary enzyme activity after renal infarction. Arch Intern Med 1972; 129:958.

38. Fort J, Segarra A, Camps J, et al: Diagnostico precoz del embolismo de arteria renal mediante determinación de lacto deshidrogenasa en urgencias de un gran hospital. Nefrologia 1998; 18(Suppl 3):26.

39. Hansen KJ, Tribble RW, Reavis SW, et al: Renal duplex sonography: evaluation of clinical utility. J Vasc Surg 1990; 12:227.

40. Perkins RP, Jacobsen DS, Feder FP, et al: Return of renal function after late embolectomy: report of a case. N Engl J Med 1967; 276:1194.

41. Ouriel K, Andrus CH, Ricotta, et al: Acute renal artery occlusion: when is revascularization justified? J Vasc Surg 1987; 5:348.

42. Fort J: Renal artery embolism [Editorial]. Ren Fail 1997; 19:vii–viii.

43. Blum V, Billman P, Krause T: Effect of local low-dose thrombolysis on clinical outcome in acute embolic renal artery occlusion. Radiology 1993; 189:549.

44. Salam TA, Lumsden AB, Martin LG: Local infusion of fibrinolytic agents for acute renal artery thromboembolism: report of ten cases. Ann Vasc Surg 1993; 7:21.

45. Bouttier S, Valverde JP, Lacombe M: Renal artery emboli: the role of surgical treatment. Ann Vasc Surg 1988; 2:161.

46. Lacombe M: Surgical versus medical treatment of renal artery emboli. J Cardiovasc Surg 1977; 18:281.

47. Moyer JD, Rao CN, Widrich C, et al: Conservative management of renal artery embolus. J Urol 1973; 109:138.

48. Scharamek A, Hashmonal M, Chaimovitz C, et al: Survival following late renal embolectomy in a patient with a single functional kidney. J Urol 1973; 108:342.

49. Nicholas GG, DeMuth WE Jr: Treatment of renal artery embolism. Arch Surg 1984; 119:278.

50. Halpern M: Acute renal artery embolus: a concept of diagnosis and treatment. J Urol 1967; 98:552.

51. Pilmore HL, Walker RJ, Salomon C, et al: Acute bilateral renal artery occlusion: successful revascularization with streptokinase. Am J Nephrol 1995; 15:90.

52. Wilms G, Vermylen J, Baert A: Intra-arterial low-dose streptokinase infusion in the treatment of acute renal thromboembolism. Eur J Radiol 1987; 7:72.

53. Fischer C, Konnak J, Chop KJ, et al: Renal artery embolism: therapy with intra-arterial thrombolytic therapy. J Urol 1981; 78:402.

54. Kennedy JS, Gerety BM, Silverman R: Simultaneous renal artery and venous thrombosis associated with idiopathic nephrotic syndrome: treatment with intra-arterial urokinase. Am J Med 1991: 90:124.

55. Mügge A, Gulba DC, Frei U, et al: Renal artery embolism thrombolysis with recombinant tissue-type plasminogen activator. J Intern Med 1990; 228:279.

56. Risius B, Graor RA, Geisinger MA, et al: Recombinant human tissue-type plasminogen activator for thrombolysis in peripheral arteries and bypass grafts. Radiology 1986; 160:183.

57. McFarlane RG, Pilling J: Fibrinolytic activity of normal urine. Nature 1947; 159:779.

58. McFarlane RG, Pilling J: Observations on fibrinolysis, plasminogen, plasmin, and antiplasmin content of human blood. Lancet 1965; 2:562.

59. Van Breda A, Katzen BJ, Deutsch AS: Urokinase versus streptokinase in local thrombolysis. Radiology 1987; 165:109–111.

60. Belkin M, Belkin B, Bucknam CA, et al: Intra-arterial fibrinolytic

therapy: efficacy of streptokinase versus urokinase. Arch Surg 1986; 121:769–773.

61. Pennica D, Holmes WE, Kohr WJ, et al: Cloning and expression of human tissue-type plasminogen activator cDNA in *E. coli.* Nature 1983; 301:214.

62. Berridge DC, Gregson RH, Hopkinson BR, et al: Intra-arterial thrombolysis using recombinant tissue plasminogen activator (r-tPA): the optimal agent, at the optimal dose? Eur J Vasc Surg 1989; 3:327.

63. McNamara TO, Fischer JR: Thrombolysis of peripheral arterial and graft occlusions: improved results using high-dose urokinase. Am J Radiol 1985; 144:769.

64. McNamara T: Technique and results of "higher dose" infusion. Cardiovasc Intervent Radiol 1988; 11:S48.

65. Segarra A, Rius JM, Moreiras M, et al: Tratamiento no quirúrgico de la embolia de arteria renal. In: Vaquero F, Uriach J (eds): *Isquemias Agudas,* 3rd ed. Barcelona; 1994:349.

66. Ramsay AG, Olagati V, Dietz PA: Renal function recovery 47 days after renal artery occlusion. Am J Nephrol 1983; 3:325.

67. Clark DE, Georgitis JE, Ray FS: Renal arterial injuries caused by trauma. Surgery 1981; 90:87.

68. Consensus Development Conference. Biol Clin Hematol 1980; 2:257.

69. Berridge DC, Makin GS, Hopkinson BR: Local low-dose intra-arterial thrombolytic therapy: the risk of stroke or major haemorrhage. Br J Surg 1989; 76:1230.

70. Sheil AGR, May J, Stokes GS, et al: Reversal of renal failure by revascularization of kidneys with thrombosed renal arteries. Lancet 1973; 2:865.

71. Bengtsson U, Bergentz SE, Norback B: Surgical treatment of renal artery stenosis with impending uremia. Clin Nephrol 1974; 2:222.

72. Kalra PS, Mamtora H, Holmes AM, et al: Renovascular disease and renal complications of angiotensin-converting enzyme inhibitor therapy. Q J Med 1990; 282:1013.

73. Jacobson H: Ischemic renal disease. Kidney Int 1988; 34:1572.

74. Hricik DE, Browning PJ, Kopelman R, et al: Captopril-induced functional renal insufficiency in patients with bilateral renal artery stenoses or renal artery stenosis in a solitary kidney. N Engl J Med 1983; 308:373.

75. Hannedouche T, Godin M, Fries D, et al: Acute renal thrombosis induced by angiotensin-converting enzyme inhibitors in patients with renovascular hypertension. Nephron 1991; 57:230.

76. Hall JE, Guyton AC, Jackson TE, et al: Control of glomerular filtration rate by the renin-angiotensin system. Am J Physiol 1977; 233:F366.

77. Colin JN: The management of chronic heart failure. N Engl J Med 1996; 335:490.

78. Gailiunas P, Chawla R, Lazarus JM, et al: Acute renal failure following cardiac operations. J Thorac Cardiovasc Surg 1980; 79:241.

79. Hilberman M, Myers BD, Carrie BJ, et al: Acute renal failure following cardiac surgery. J Thorac Cardiovasc Surg 1979; 77:880.

80. Zanardo G, Michielon P, Paccagnella A, et al: Acute renal failure in the patient undergoing cardiac operation. J Thorac Cardiovasc Surg 1994; 107:1489.

81. Schmitt H, Riehl J, Boseila A, et al: Acute renal failure following cardiac surgery: pre- and perioperative clinical features. Contrib Nephrol 1991; 93:98.

82. Endre Z: Post–cardiac surgery acute renal failure in the 1990s. Aust N Z J Med 1995; 25:28.

83. Krian A: Incidence, prevention, and treatment of acute renal failure following cardiopulmonary bypass. Int Anaesthiol Clin 1976; 1:87.

84. Mora Mangano C, Diamondstone L, Ramsav J, et al: Perioperative renal dysfunction in coronary revascularization patients: risk factors, morbid outcomes, and hospital resource utilization. Anesth Analg 1996; 82:SCA4B.

85. Sehgal V, Radhakrishnan J, Appel G, et al: Progressive renal insufficiency following cardiac transplantation: cyclosporine, lipids, and hypertension. Am J Kid Dis 1995; 26:193.

86. Slogoff S, Raul GJ, Keats AS, et al: Role of perfusion pressure and flow in major organ dysfunctions after cardiopulmonary bypass. Ann Thorac Surg 1990; 50:911.

87. Calafiore A, Giammarco G, Teodori G, et al: Left anterior descending coronary artery grafting via left anterior small thoracotomy without cardiopulmonary bypass. Ann Thorac Surg 1996; 61:1658.

88. Sundt TM, Kouchoukos NT, Saffitz JE, et al: Renal dysfunction and intravascular coagulation with aprotinin and hypothermic circulatory arrest. Ann Thorac Surg 1993; 55:1418.

89. Neumayer H, Junge W, Kufner A: Prevention of radiocontrast media–induced nephrotoxicity by the calcium channel blocker nitrendipine: a prospective randomised clinical trial. Nephrol Dial Transplant 1989; 4:1030.

90. Moran S, Myers B: Pathophysiology of protracted acute renal failure in man. J Clin Invest 1985; 76:1440.

91. Hines R: Pro: dopamine and renal preservation. J Cardiovasc Thorac Anesth 1995; 3:333.

92. Hilberman M, Maseda J, Stinson EB, et al: The diuretic properties of dopamine in patients after open heart operation. Anesthesiology 1984; 61:489.

93. Gelman S: Does mannitol save the kidney? Anesth Analg 1996; 82:889.

94. Colson P, Ribstein J, Mimran A, et al: Effect of angiotensin-converting enzyme inhibition on blood pressure and renal function during open heart surgery. Anesthesiology 1990; 72:23.

95. Shannon R, Libby E, Elahi D: Impact of acute reduction in chronically elevated left atrial pressure on sodium and water excretion. Ann Thorac Surg 1988; 46:430.

96. Hummel M, Kuhn M, Dub A: Urodilatin: a new peptide with beneficial effects in the postoperative care of cardiac transplant patients. J Clin Invest 1992; 70:674.

97. Hashimoto K, Miyamoto H, Suzuki K, et al: Evidence of organ damage after cardiopulmonary bypass: the role of elastase and vasoactive mediators. J Thorac Cardiovasc Surg 1992; 104:666.

98. White J Jr, Rockwood T, Wilson D, et al: The effects of pentoxifylline on the prevention of cyclosporine-induced nephrotoxicity in cardiac transplant patients. Clin Ther 1994; 16:673.

CHAPTER **20**

Acute Renal Failure in Liver Disease

Murray Epstein

The interrelationship of liver disease and simultaneous kidney dysfunction has been recognized for thousands of years. Basically, three major categories of disease states subtend such interrelationships: (1) disorders involving the liver and kidney directly, (2) primary disorders of the kidney with secondary hepatic involvement, and (3) primary disorders of the liver with secondary renal dysfunction. This chapter does not cover the entire spectrum of diseases that simultaneously involve the liver and kidney. Rather, consideration is given only to the syndromes of acute azotemia that secondarily complicate primary disorders of the liver. Because the hepatorenal syndrome (HRS) constitutes a prominent disorder among this category, this syndrome is emphasized.

The hepatorenal syndrome is a unique form of acute renal failure (ARF) occurring in patients with liver disease for which a specific cause cannot be elucidated. Despite the intense clinical and investigative interest that this syndrome has stimulated, until recently, relatively little progress had been made in the understanding and management of this syndrome. The past several years, however, have witnessed newer insights in both the pathophysiology and therapeutics of this syndrome. The role of a number of pathogenic mechanisms has been more rigorously delineated. The characterization of endothelin (ET) and the nitric oxide (NO)-arginine pathway and their roles in biology and medicine has provided additional new insights with regard to the pathogenesis of HRS. Finally, recently initiated therapeutic approaches including the maturation of orthotopic liver transplantation (OLTX) and transjugular intrahepatic portosystemic shunt (TIPS) lend a note of optimism to the future management of a syndrome that is so often incompatible with recovery.

Progressive oliguric renal failure commonly complicates the course of advanced hepatic disease.[1-4] Although this condition has been designated by many names—including *functional renal failure, hemodynamic renal failure, hepatic nephropathy,* the *renal failure of cirrhosis,* and others—the more appealing, albeit less specific, term *HRS* is the most commonly used. For the purpose of this discussion, HRS is defined as unexplained renal failure occurring in patients with liver disease in the absence of clinical, laboratory, or anatomic evidence of other known causes of renal failure.

When confronted with a patient who has concomitant renal and hepatic disease, the clinician should consider not only HRS but a number of potentially treatable disorders that simultaneously involve the liver and the kidney.[3, 4] These disorders, termed *pseudo-HRSs,* include toxic, hematologic, neoplastic, genetic, hemodynamic, and infectious processes. The importance of recognizing these disorders lies in the fact that they may be reversible if detected early and treated appropriately.

CLINICAL FEATURES

The clinical features of HRS have been detailed in several recent reviews[1-4] and are summarized in Table 20-1. In brief, HRS usually occurs in cirrhotic patients who are alcoholic, although cirrhosis is not a sine qua non for the development of HRS. Numerous reports have emphasized the development of renal failure after events that reduce effective blood volume, including abdominal paracentesis, vigorous diuretic therapy, and gastrointestinal bleeding, although renal failure can occur in the absence of an apparent precipitating event. In this context, several careful observers have noted that HRS patients seldom arrive in the hospital with preexisting renal failure; rather, HRS seems to develop in the hospital, indicating that iatrogenic events in the hospital might precipitate this syndrome.[1, 4]

The majority of patients die within 3 weeks of the onset of azotemia.[1, 4, 5] Despite the bleak prognosis, it is difficult to attribute the poor outcome directly to renal failure in patients in whom azotemia is moderate. Such observations suggest that the renal failure may be more of a reflection of a broader lethal event and

TABLE 20–1. Major Clinical Features of Hepatorenal Syndrome

Usually occurs in patients after they have been admitted to the hospital
No apparent precipitating factor
Renal failure usually occurs in patients with moderate to tense ascites
No consistent relationship to jaundice
Some degree of hepatic encephalopathy present in most patients
Blood pressure often lower than usual for that specific patient
Marked oliguria, almost complete absence of sodium, and usually hyponatremia
Urinary indices similar to those of prerenal azotemia and contrast with those seen in acute tubular necrosis
Spontaneous recovery unusual

Adapted from Epstein M: The Kidney in Liver Disease. 4th ed. Philadelphia: Hanley & Belfus; 1996; with permission.

Portions of this review, including Tables 20–1 and 20–2, have been reproduced and adapted with permission from an earlier review by the author: Epstein M: The Hepatorenal Syndrome. In: Epstein M, ed: *The Kidney in Liver Disease.* 4th ed. Philadelphia: Hanley & Belfus; 1996:75–108.

that, in most instances, it is not in itself the major determinant of survival. A truly uremic death is a rarity.

PATHOGENESIS

A substantial body of evidence lends strong support to the concept that the renal failure in HRS is functional in nature. Despite the severe derangement of renal function, pathologic abnormalities are minimal and inconsistent.[1, 4, 6] Furthermore, tubular functional integrity is maintained during the renal failure, as manifested by a relatively unimpaired sodium reabsorptive capacity and concentrating ability. Finally, more direct evidence is derived (1) from the demonstration that kidneys transplanted from patients with HRS are capable of resuming normal function in the recipient[7] and (2) by the return of renal function when the patient with HRS successfully receives a liver transplant.[8]

Despite extensive study, the precise pathogenesis of HRS has not been delineated. Many studies using diverse hemodynamic techniques have documented a significant reduction in renal perfusion.[9–11] Because a similar decrement of renal perfusion is compatible with urine volumes exceeding 1 L in many patients with chronic renal failure, it is unlikely that a decrease in mean blood flow per se is responsible for the encountered oliguria.[12]

Our laboratory applied the ^{133}Xe washout technique and selective renal arteriography to the study of HRS and demonstrated a significant reduction in calculated mean blood flow as well as a preferential reduction in cortical perfusion.[10] In addition, cirrhotic patients manifested marked vasomotor instability that was characterized not only by variability between serial xenon washout studies but also by instability within a single curve.[10] This phenomenon has not been encountered in renal failure of other etiologies. In addition, Epstein and coworkers[10] performed simultaneous renal arteriography to delineate further the nature of the hemodynamic abnormalities. Selective renal arteriograms disclosed marked beading and tortuosity of the interlobar and proximal arcuate arteries and an absence of distinct cortical nephrograms and vascular filling of the cortical vessels (Fig. 20–1A). Postmortem angiography performed on the kidneys of five patients studied during life disclosed a striking normalization of the vascular abnormalities with a reversal of all of the vascular abnormalities in the kidneys (Fig. 20–1B). These findings provide additional evidence for the functional basis of the renal failure, operating through active renal vasoconstriction.[10] This is further illustrated by a

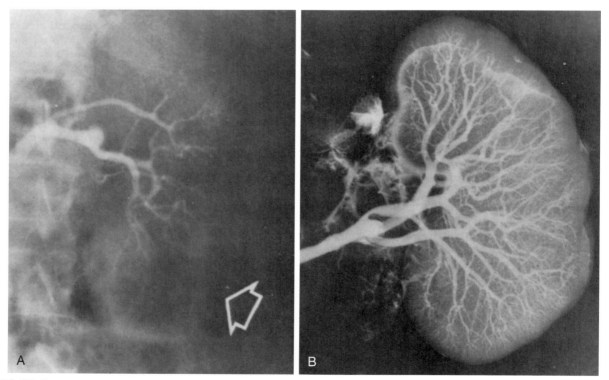

FIGURE 20–1 ■ *A,* A selective renal arteriogram carried out in a patient with oliguric renal failure and cirrhosis. Note the extreme abnormality of the intrarenal vessels, including the primary branches off the main renal artery and the interlobar arteries. The arcuate and cortical arterial system is not recognizable, nor is a distinct cortical nephrogram present. The *arrow* indicates the edge of the kidney. *B,* Angiogram of the same kidney carried out postmortem with the intra-arterial injection of Micropaque in gelatin as the contrast agent. Note filling of the renal arterial system throughout the vascular bed to the periphery of the cortex. The peripheral arterial tree that did not opacify in vivo now fills completely. The vascular attenuation and tortuosity are no longer present. The vessels were also histologically normal. (From Epstein M, Berk DP, Hollenberg NK, et al: Renal failure in the patient with cirrhosis: the role of active vasoconstriction. Am J Med 1970; 49:175–185; with permission.)

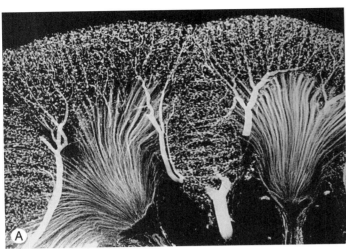

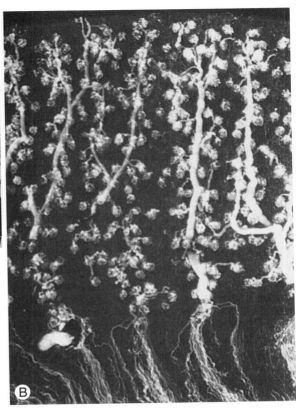

FIGURE 20–2 ■ *A,* Normal cortex, 3-mm section. Typical microangiographic appearance through two adjacent renal lobes and an intervening cortical septum of Bertin. Note the striking difference between the microvascular pattern of the cortex containing interlobular arteries and glomeruli and the medulla containing the bundles of vasa recta. Note also the slight residual fetal lobation at the outer cortical margin opposite the septum of Bertin. The relationship of the two renal papillae to their corresponding calices can also be seen. *B,* Normal cortex, 1-mm section. Higher power view (×20). Note the interlobular arteries and their corresponding glomeruli. Several corticomedullary glomeruli can be seen to supply efferent arterioles, which will divide into bundles of medullary vasa recta. (From Bookstein JJ, Clark RL, eds: *Renal Microvascular Disease: Angiographic-Microangiographic Correlates.* Boston: Little, Brown; 1980; with permission.)

comparison of the appearance of normal renal microangiograms (Fig. 20–2) with those obtained from patients with ARF occurring in association with the HRS (Fig. 20–3).

Although renal hypoperfusion with preferential renal cortical ischemia has been shown to underlie the renal failure of HRS,[10, 13] the factors responsible for sustaining reduction in cortical perfusion and suppression of filtration in HRS have not been elucidated. In a recent comprehensive review,[3] the author has considered the afferent events that participate in the pathogenesis of the HRS. Specifically this review focused on the role of the extracellular fluid translocations or sequestration into serous spaces or interstitial fluid compartments that characterize advanced liver disease. The present review focuses on efferent events, encompassing a survey of the hormonal and neural mechanisms proposed or implicated in the pathogenesis of the renal failure. Emphasis is placed on recent studies characterizing the sympathetic nervous system, the NO-arginine pathway, and the possible contribution of ET.

EFFERENT EVENTS

The effectors that promote renal ischemia and a decrease in glomerular filtration rate (GFR) remain incompletely defined. Several major hypotheses have been implicated or suggested, including the following: (1) alterations of the renin-angiotensin system; (2) an increase in sympathetic nervous system activity; (3) alterations in renal eicosanoids, including a relative decrease in renal vasodilatory prostaglandins and an increase in vasoconstrictor thromboxanes; (4) enhanced NO production with peripheral vasodilation; (5) elevated plasma ET levels; (6) a relative impairment of renal kallikrein production; and (7) endotoxemia (Table 20–2).

Renin-Angiotensin System

Several lines of evidence suggest a role for the renin-angiotensin axis in sustaining the vasoconstriction in HRS. Patients with decompensated cirrhosis frequently manifest marked elevations of plasma renin levels.[4, 14–17] An examination of the relationship between renal function and plasma renin levels has disclosed that cirrhotic patients with impaired renal function manifested the most profound elevations in plasma renin levels. Although the elevation of plasma renin is attributable in part to the decreased hepatic inactivation of renin, it is evident that the major determinant is increased renin secretion by the kidney. It is noteworthy that the elevation of plasma renin often occurs despite diminished hepatic synthesis of the α_2-globulin, renin substrate.[18]

The activation of the renin-angiotensin system has profound implications for renal function. In light of compelling experimental evidence that angiotensin plays an important role in the control of the renal

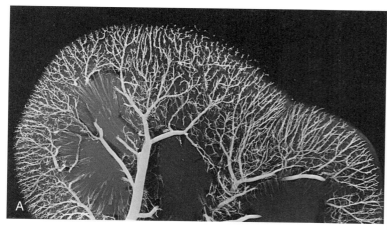

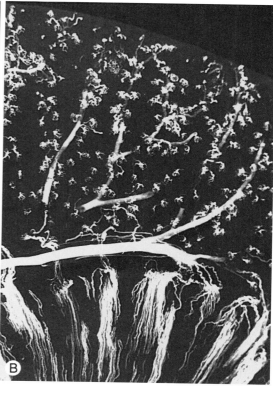

FIGURE 20–3 ■ Human acute renal failure due to hepatorenal syndrome. *A,* Note the "naked interlobular arteries" due to very poor glomerular perfusion, apparently due to preglomerular constriction. *B,* Note the absence of postglomerular capillary filling with prominent filling of the bundles of medullary vasa recta from a different patient under higher (×10) magnification. Both are autopsy specimens. (From Bookstein JJ, Clark RL, eds: *Renal Microvascular Disease: Angiographic-Microangiographic Correlates.* Boston: Little, Brown; 1980; with permission.)

circulation,[19, 20] it is tempting to speculate that enhanced angiotensin levels contribute to the renal vasoconstriction and the reduction in filtration rate seen in the renal failure in cirrhosis. Observations by Cade and associates[21] have underscored the role of angiotensin II in mediating the reduction in renal perfusion and GFR in patients with HRS. The infusion of angiotensin II caused a marked reduction of renal plasma flow in GFR, with a marked increase in filtration fraction.

TABLE 20–2. Known and Postulated Mechanisms That May Contribute to the Renal Failure of Liver Disease

Hormonal

Activation of the renin-angiotensin system
Alterations in renal eicosanoids
   Diminished vasodilatory prostaglandins
   Increased vasoconstrictor thromboxanes
Enhanced nitric oxide production
Elevated plasma endothelin levels
Endotoxemia
Relative impairment of renal kallikrein production
Diminished atrial natriuretic peptides
Vasoactive intestinal peptide
Glomerulopressin deficiency

Neural and Hemodynamic

Increase in sympathetic nervous system activity
Alterations in intrarenal blood flow distribution

Adapted from Epstein M: The Kidney in Liver Disease. 4th ed. Philadelphia: Hanley & Belfus; 1996; with permission.

Role of Renal Prostaglandins

Alterations of renal prostaglandins also participate in mediating the renal failure of cirrhosis.[22] Several investigators have demonstrated that the administration of inhibitors of prostaglandin synthetase (both indomethacin and ibuprofen) resulted in significant decrements in GFR and effective renal plasma flow in patients with alcoholic liver disease and ascites.[23, 24] Of interest, the decrement in renal hemodynamics varied directly with the degree of sodium retention, ie, the patients with the most avid sodium retention manifested the largest decrements in GFR.[24–26]

Because the earlier cited studies have examined the effect of inhibiting the endogenous production of renal prostaglandins, we were interested in assessing an opposite experimental manipulation, ie, investigating the effects of the augmentation of endogenous prostaglandins on renal function. Epstein and associates[27] have used water immersion to the neck, an experimental maneuver that redistributes blood volume with concomitant central hypervolemia and enhances prostaglandin E (PGE) excretion in normal humans. They demonstrated that decompensated cirrhotic patients manifested an increase in mean PGE excretion that was threefold greater than that observed in normal subjects studied under identical conditions.[28] This was attended by a marked natriuresis and an increase in creatinine clearance. When interpreted in concert with the earlier studies using prostaglandin synthetase inhibitors, these findings suggest that derangements in renal PGE production contribute to the renal dysfunction of cirrhosis. Specifically, it is tempting to postulate that, in the setting of cirrhosis of the liver, the ability to enhance prostaglandin synthesis constitutes a compensatory or adaptive response to incipient renal ischemia. The corollary of this formulation is that the administration of agents that impair such an adaptation can induce a clinically important deterioration of renal function.

These findings are not isolated observations. As I have noted,[26] one may conceive of renal prostaglandins as constituting critical modulators of renal function during conditions or disease states involving volume contraction. The demonstration that synthetase inhibition affected renal function only in decompensated (presence of ascites and/or edema) and not in compensated cirrhotic subjects and that the effects of synthetase inhibition vary as a function of the degree of renal sodium avidity is consistent with this formulation.[25, 26]

Increase in Sympathetic Nervous System Activity

An increase in sympathetic nervous system activity also contributes to the renal failure of cirrhosis.[29] It is now well established that alterations in the input of cardiopulmonary receptors induce changes in renal sympathetic activity.[30-33] Thus, a decrease in effective blood volume is sensed as a decrease in left atrial pressure (the sensor of the low-pressure vascular system). This "unloads" the left atrial mechanoreceptors, which in turn discharge into afferent vagal fibers that have appropriate central nervous system representation. As a consequence, efferent renal sympathetic nerve activity is augmented.[31, 32] Such an increase in sympathetic tone would tend to produce renal vasoconstriction and decrease GFR.

Although these theoretical considerations suggest a role for the sympathetic nervous system in the renal vasoconstriction and sodium retention of cirrhosis, only recently have studies been conducted to test this possibility. Earlier studies to assess the activity of the sympathetic nervous system in cirrhotic humans have measured plasma catecholamine levels during basal conditions and after postural manipulations.[32, 34-38] Most observers agree that mean peripheral norepinephrine levels are elevated in cirrhotic patients.[35-38]

As detailed in several comprehensive reviews,[39-41] however, the plasma concentration of norepinephrine is an inadequate guide to either total or regional sympathetic activity. Global measures of sympathetic activity, such as plasma norepinephrine measurements, fail to identify sources of norepinephrine release and cannot delineate regional patterns of sympathetic nervous activation. Esler and coworkers[41] conducted a physiologic and neurochemical evaluation of patients with cirrhosis, applying tracer kinetic techniques using radiolabeled norepinephrine, thereby allowing a more precise description of the regional pattern of the sympathetic nervous derangement in cirrhosis. They demonstrated that the elevated plasma norepinephrine concentration in patients with cirrhosis is attributable to higher overall rates of spillover of the neurotransmitter to plasma and not to reduced plasma clearance caused by liver disease. The administration of clonidine reduced previously elevated norepinephrine overflow rates for the whole body, kidneys, and hepatomesenteric circulation. This sympathetic inhibition was accompanied by several potentially clinically beneficial effects: the lowering of renal vascular resistance, an augmentation of GFR, and the reduction of portal venous pressure.[41]

In summary, the available data indicate that the sympathetic nervous system is activated in cirrhosis, both in the kidney and in other regional vascular beds, consequently contributing substantively to the renal vasoconstriction and renal dysfunction of cirrhosis.

Nitric Oxide

A more recent approach to the investigation of the pathogenesis of the HRS has focused on the florid systemic hemodynamic disturbances that invariably accompany the syndrome. These include a hyperdynamic circulation, increased heart rate and cardiac output, and decreased blood pressure and systemic vascular resistance.[3, 4, 42-45] These observations have suggested the likelihood of excess production of a vasodilator.[46]

Recently, attention has focused on the role of NO as a mediator of both the hyperdynamic circulation and renal failure.[47] NO, a vasodilator synthesized from L-arginine, accounts for the biologic activity of endothelium-derived relaxing factor.[48-50] Vallance and Moncada[47] have postulated that endotoxemia induces an NO synthase in peripheral blood vessels and that this increased NO synthesis and release accounts for the associated hyperdynamic circulation. This formulation does not posit that renal vasoconstriction is directly related to NO but rather suggests that the renal hypoperfusion and renal insufficiency are secondary to a diversion of blood away from the kidney.

If this hypothesis is correct, the inhibition of NO synthesis should restore sensitivity to vasoconstrictors and reverse these hemodynamic abnormalities. Specific inhibitors of either the constitutive or the inducible NO synthase theoretically should facilitate a more precise manipulation of NO synthesis and help establish the pathophysiologic importance of NO in endotoxemia and cirrhosis.

Since Vallance and Moncada presented their hypotheses, several studies have appeared supporting this formulation. Niederberger and associates[51, 52] have provided compelling evidence to support the hypothesis that NO overproduction mediates the hyperdynamic circulation. First, these investigators demonstrated that cyclic guanosine monophosphate levels in arterial tissues of rats with carbon tetrachloride–induced cirrhosis were elevated in an N(G)-nitro-L-arginine methyl ester (L-NAME)-suppressible fashion.[51] Next, these investigators showed that the inhibition of NO synthase with L-NAME resulted in normalization of arterial blood pressure, cardiac index, and systemic vascular resistance, as well as decreases in plasma renin activity and vasopressin concentration in cirrhotic rats.[51]

Cirrhotic patients manifest increased plasma levels of endotoxin.[53, 54] Vallance and Moncada[47] proposed that endotoxemia would enhance the expression of inducible NO synthase in peripheral blood vessels with a resultant increased release of NO. NO is an unstable molecule and is rapidly converted in vivo and in vitro to nitrite and nitrate.[55, 56] Consequently, serum NO_2^- and NO_3^- have been used in vitro[57] and in vivo[58] as indices of NO generation.

Recently, Guarner and colleagues[59] tested the hypothesis of NO overproduction by measuring levels of NO_2^- and NO_3^- in serum of cirrhotic patients and evaluated their relationship with plasma endotoxin levels measured simultaneously with a sensitive assay. Cirrhotic patients manifested significant increases in serum nitrite/nitrate and plasma endotoxin compared with controls. Values were particularly increased in patients with decompensated cirrhosis, as manifested by ascites. The investigators reported that serum nitrite/nitrate levels were highest in their group 4 patients with functional renal failure (ie, HRS). Consideration of Figure 1 in their paper, however, discloses great overlap among the three groups of cirrhotic patients, and it is not readily evident that HRS patients as a group had the highest levels. Of interest, elevated serum nitrite/nitrate levels were associated with activation of vasoactive hormones, including high plasma renin activity, high aldosterone and antidiuretic hormone levels, and low urinary excretion of sodium, findings that are in accord with the hypothesis of Vallance and Moncada.[47] In addition, serum nitrite/nitrate levels correlated significantly with endotoxemia.

To further examine the possibility that the enhanced endotoxemia was causally related to the increased NO production, Guarner and colleagues[59] demonstrated that oral administration of colistin, a nonabsorbable antibiotic with antiendotoxin activity, to cirrhotic patients reduced plasma endotoxin levels. Consequently serum nitrite/nitrate levels declined. The authors interpreted their data as supporting the postulate that endotoxin promotes induction of NO synthase. In patients with alcoholic cirrhosis, Criado-Jimenez and coworkers[60] detected elevated nitrite production by monocytes obtained from cirrhotic patients, but not from noncirrhotic alcoholics. Additional studies are required to substantiate this hypothesis.

In concert these observations suggest that NO overproduction is in part responsible for the hyperdynamic circulation of portal hypertension and liver cirrhosis.

Endothelin

In the past 15 years, ETs have emerged as an important new peptide family in the hormonal regulation of body fluid and cardiovascular homeostasis.[61, 62] ETs are the most potent vasoconstrictors known to date. They release Ca^{2+} and also potentiate Ca^{2+} release stimulated by other vasoconstrictors, including argi-

nine vasopressin and angiotensin II. There is increasing evidence that ET plays a role in the pathogenesis of diverse disorders, contributing to hypertension and mediating renal injury via its vascular effects, ie, in ARF due to cyclosporine, contrast media, or endotoxemia as well as in chronic forms of renal impairment.[63, 64]

Although it is tempting to speculate that ET may be important in the pathogenesis of the HRS, as yet there is no firm evidence to support this postulate. Most studies have demonstrated elevated circulating plasma levels of ET-1.[65]

Moore and associates[66] have suggested the possibility that alterations in ET may play a pathogenetic role in the renal failure of the HRS. They reported that patients with HRS had markedly elevated plasma ET-1 and ET-3 concentrations compared with normal subjects, patients having acute or chronic renal failure, and patients with liver disease without renal dysfunction. These investigators interpreted their results to support the hypothesis that these substances play a role in the pathogenesis of the HRS.

In summary, despite documentation of elevated ET-1 levels, there are difficulties in attributing the renal failure of HRS to ET.[65] As we have noted in a recent review,[65] there are no published data regarding the local production of ET-1 by the liver or kidney in this setting, nor are data available regarding the status of hepatic and/or renal ET receptors in this syndrome.

Finally, cause and effect have not been established. As I have noted in an editorial, it is possible if not probable that the elevated ET-1 levels and the renal failure merely represent pari passu events.[67] The recent availability of several chemically diverse ET antagonists, including agents that block the generation of ET and those that antagonize its binding to cellular receptors, provides an opportunity for using such pharmacologic probes in delineating the pathogenetic role of ET.

TREATMENT

General Considerations

Because knowledge about the pathogenesis of HRS is inferential and incomplete, therapy to the present time has been supportive. As the author has noted in a review article,[3] because iatrogenic events often precipitate this syndrome and because therapy is difficult once the syndrome is established, prevention constitutes the linchpin of management. In addition to the usual support and measures of stabilizing circulatory hemodynamics and careful restriction of sodium and fluid intake, only three specific therapeutic measures stand out as offering promise for the future: dialysis, OLTX, and TIPS.

Dialysis

Dialysis was previously reported to be ineffective in the management of HRS.[68, 69] Our own recent experience, however, suggests that such a sweeping condemnation should be qualified.[70] Although most of the published literature indeed suggests a dismal prognosis for patients who are dialyzed, such early reports have dealt with patients with chronic end-stage liver disease. In a few instances, we have undertaken dialysis in HRS patients with acute hepatic disease and have been gratified by the ultimate favorable outcome. Our experience suggests that in selected patients, ie, those with acute hepatic dysfunction in whom there is reason to believe that the renal failure may reverse coincident with the resolution of the acute hepatic insult, dialytic therapy is indicated.

The most important event to have impacted dialysis is the success of liver transplantation. With the recent maturation and refinement of OLTX and its acceptance as the treatment of choice for end-stage liver disease, dialysis has assumed an important ancillary role. Dialysis is now widely used as a supportive measure in the management of many patients awaiting liver transplantation.

In addition to stabilizing renal function, it is often necessary to remove fluid, either to prevent life-threatening emergencies such as acute pulmonary edema or to permit the administration of requisite fluids such as bicarbonate solutions and hyperalimentation. Although hemodialysis often constitutes the therapeutic modality of choice for this purpose, it is not feasible in many patients with severe liver disease who have associated hemodynamic instability. Unfortunately, patients with decompensated cirrhosis frequently become hypotensive in response to the institution of hemodialysis. To circumvent this problem, we have used continuous arteriovenous hemofiltration as an alternative maneuver in a few patients with HRS and have been successful in mobilizing fluid without concomitant hemodynamic instability.[71, 72] Additional experience is required to clarify the role of this approach in managing patients with HRS.

Molecular Adsorbent Recirculating System (MARS)

To extend the applicability of dialysis to the treatment of these patients, a new dialysis procedure has been employed.[73] The so-called molecular adsorbent recirculating system (MARS) is a modified dialysis method using an albumin-containing dialysate that is recirculated and perfused online through charcoal and anion-exchanger columns. MARS enables the selective removal of albumin-bound substances like unconjugated bilirubin or free fatty acids from plasma and blood. In a prospective controlled trial designed to determine the effect of MARS treatment on 30-day survival, 13 patients with cirrhosis with HRS were studied. Eight patients were treated with the MARS method in addition to hemodiafiltration (HDF) and standard medical therapy, and five patients were in the control group (HDF and standard medical treatment alone). None of these patients underwent liver transplantation or received a transjugular intrahepatic por-

tosystemic shunt or vasopressin analogues during the observation period. A significant decrease in bilirubin and creatinine levels and an increase in serum sodium level and prothrombin activity were observed in the MARS group. Mortality rates were 100% in the control group at day 7 and 62.5% in the MARS group at day 7 and 75% at day 30, respectively.[74]

Orthotopic Liver Transplantation

OLTX has recently become the accepted treatment for end-stage liver disease.[75, 76] Of interest, many of these patients are admitted with varying degrees of concomitant renal dysfunction, including HRS. Of major importance, OLTX has been reported to reverse HRS acutely.[8, 77, 78] Gonwa and colleagues[75] reviewed the extensive experience of the Baylor University transplant group and reported a good long-term survival with return of acceptable renal function for prolonged periods. They retrospectively reviewed the first 308 patients undergoing OLTX. The incidence of HRS was 10.5%. HRS patients manifested an increase in GFR from a baseline of 20 ± 4 mL/min to a mean of 33 ± 3 mL/min at 6 weeks, with a further increase to 46 ± 6 mL/min at 1 year. GFR remained stable at 2 years postoperatively (38 ± 6 mL/min). There was no difference in perioperative (90-day) mortality between HRS and non-HRS patients, despite a worse preoperative status and a more unstable postoperative course. The actuarial 1- and 2-year survival rate for the HRS patients was 77%, not different from that of non-HRS patients. These investigators concluded that with aggressive pretransplant and posttransplant management, one can anticipate excellent results after OLTX in patients with the HRS. Gonwa and Wilkinson have now updated the extensive Baylor experience and have confirmed their earlier experience.[76] The major "take home" message is that concomitant renal dysfunction should not preclude consideration for OLTX.

It is notable that as many as 38% of combined liver-kidney transplant (LKTX) procedures performed nationally may be done for the renal diagnosis of HRS. Jeyarajah and coworkers[79] performed a study designed to determine if combined LKTX provides any benefit over isolated OLTX to HRS patients. They reported a five-year patient survival of 48.1% for LKTX patients, 67.1% for HRS patients receiving isolated OLTX, and 70.1% for other patients with an S_{Cr} level of > 2.0 mg/dL receiving isolated OLTX. They concluded that HRS patients can be successfully managed with isolated OLTX. Nonetheless, others have pointed out that cirrhotic patients with renal dysfunction experience an overall poorer surgical outcome following liver transplantation than their counterparts with normal renal function. Indeed, a multifactorial regression analysis has demonstrated that of all pretransplant factors analyzed, elevation in the S_{Cr} level was the strongest predictor of both ARF requiring dialysis and of death. However, the presence or absence of HRS syndrome did not influence the results.[80] The fact remains that when HRS occurs, all the proposed treatments have been shown to only moderately or temporarily improve renal function, thus leaving liver transplantation as the only choice of treatment for these patients.[81]

Transjugular Intrahepatic Portosystemic Shunt (TIPS)

Recently, a few anecdotal reports have appeared describing improvement in renal function in HRS patients following insertion of a TIPS.[82–84] The rationale for this procedure is similar to that for the establishment of a side-to-side portacaval shunt, thereby creating a portal-to-systemic vascular pathway that serves to decompress the portacaval system.[85] Although TIPS obviates the need for performing major vascular surgery, it is not nearly so simple and innocuous a procedure as some of its adherents would propose. It is operator dependent, requiring skilled and experienced interventional radiologists for its successful insertion. In addition, the reported experience is quite preliminary, and the available data consist in great part of a few preliminary and anecdotal reports. Somberg and associates' recent review[86] consists of an in-depth review of the rationale and experience with TIPS, as well as considerations regarding its potential future niche in the therapeutic armamentarium.

While the initial enthusiasm for TIPS in the management of patients with the HRS has been somewhat tempered,[87] this procedure may in fact be accompanied by a degree of renal functional improvement in the majority of nontransplantable cirrhotic patients with HRS.[88] In particular, clinical and hemodynamic results after TIPS have demonstrated it to be an effective bridge to liver transplantation.[89]

Systemic Vasoconstrictors

The most interesting of the new treatments that have been proposed to reverse HRS in cirrhosis is one that employs the simultaneous administration of plasma volume expansion and vasoconstrictors. That is, it has been reported that the long-term administration (1 to 3 weeks) of analogs of vasopressin (ornipressin or terlipressin) or other vasoconstrictors together with plasma volume expansion with albumin is associated with a dramatic improvement in circulatory function and normalization of S_{Cr} level in patients with severe HRS.[90] Although this program may be successful in reversing HRS, it carries with it the risk of significant ischemic complications.[91]

In some patients, ornipressin plus dopamine has been used as a bridge to liver transplantation.[92] In others, low-dose vasopressin alone may be useful in critical patients with renal shutdown while awaiting liver transplantation.[93] Also, the long-term administration of midodrine (a postsynaptic α-adrenergic receptor agonist) and octreotide (a long-acting octapeptide with pharmacologic properties mimicking those of the natural hormone somatostatin) seems to be an effective and safe treatment in some patients with HRS.[94]

CONCLUSION

In summary, despite considerable progress in the past 3 decades, we still lack a comprehensive understanding of the pathogenetic cascade that produces HRS. Much progress in the delineation of the intrarenal hemodynamic alterations that underlie the HRS has been witnessed in the past 3 decades. The characterization of ET and NO-arginine pathways and their roles in biology and medicine has provided additional new insights with regard to the pathogenesis of HRS. The numerous attempts at treating HRS empirically with vasodilators have not resulted in important therapeutic innovations. The failure of many HRS patients to survive despite partial correction of their renal hemodynamic abnormality is a reflection of the precarious state of the patient with liver failure. Hemorrhage, infection, and hepatic coma are the usual causes of death in these patients.

It is apparent that any future breakthroughs in providing definitive treatment of HRS must be predicated on a greater clarification of the mechanisms and a delineation of the mediators. The role of hemodialysis has recently undergone reappraisal, and it is apparent that dialysis clearly has a role in supporting patients awaiting hepatic transplantation. Dialysis also may be warranted as a supportive measure in some patients with apparently reversible hepatic dysfunction. Hepatic transplantation has evolved over the past decade to the point where it constitutes definitive therapy for patients with hepatic dysfunction and concomitant renal failure. Finally, preliminary reports describing an improvement in renal function in HRS patients following insertion of a TIPS suggest that this modality may be useful in the management of selected patients. It is hoped that future clinical trials will establish the precise contribution of each of these treatment modalities and its respective role in the therapeutic armamentarium.

ACKNOWLEDGMENTS

I thank Elsa V. Reina for her expert secretarial help.

REFERENCES

1. Papper S: Hepatorenal syndrome. In: Epstein M, ed: *The Kidney in Liver Disease.* 2nd ed. New York: Elsevier Biomedical; 1983:87–106.
2. Epstein M: Functional renal abnormalities in cirrhosis: pathophysiology and management. In: Zakim D, Boyer TD, eds: *Hepatology: A Textbook of Liver Disease.* 2nd ed. Philadelphia: WB Saunders; 1990:493–512.
3. Epstein M: Hepatorenal syndrome. In: Epstein M, ed: *The Kidney in Liver Disease.* 4th ed. Philadelphia: Hanley & Belfus; 1996:75–108.
4. Epstein M: The hepatorenal syndrome: emerging perspective of pathophysiology and therapy. J Am Soc Nephrol 1994; 4:1735–1753.
5. Goldstein H, Boyle JD: Spontaneous recovery from the hepatorenal syndrome: report of four cases. N Engl J Med 1965; 272:895–898.

6. Shear L, Kleinerman J, Gabuzda GJ: Renal failure in patients with cirrhosis of the liver: I. Clinical and pathologic characteristics. Am J Med 1965; 39:184–198.

7. Koppel MH, Coburn JW, Mims MM, et al: Transplantation of cadaveric kidneys from patients with hepatorenal syndrome: evidence for the functional nature of renal failure in advanced liver disease. N Engl J Med 1969; 280:1367–1371.

8. Iwatsuki S, Popovtzer MM, Corman JL, et al: Recovery from hepatorenal syndrome after orthotopic liver transplantation. N Engl J Med 1973; 289:1155–1159.

9. Schroeder ET, Shear L, Sanceta SM, Gabuzda GJ: Renal failure in patients with cirrhosis of the liver: III. Evaluation of intrarenal blood flow by para amino-hippurate extraction and response to angiotensin. Am J Med 1967; 43:887–896.

10. Epstein M, Berk DP, Hollenberg NK, et al: Renal failure in the patient with cirrhosis: the role of active vasoconstriction. Am J Med 1970; 49:175–185.

11. Epstein M, Schneider N, Befeler B: Relationship of systemic and intrarenal hemodynamics in cirrhosis. J Lab Clin Med 1977; 89:1175–1187.

12. Hollenberg NK, Epstein M, Basch RI, et al: Acute oliguric renal failure in man: evidence for preferential renal cortical ischemia. Medicine (Baltimore) 1968; 47:455–474.

13. Kew MC, Varma RR, Williams HS, et al: Renal and intrarenal blood flow in cirrhosis of the liver. Lancet 1971; 2:504–510.

14. Schroeder ET, Eich RH, Smulyan H, et al: Plasma renin level in hepatic cirrhosis. Am J Med 1970; 49:186–191.

15. Epstein M, Levinson R, Sancho J, et al: Characterization of the renin-aldosterone system in decompensated cirrhosis. Circ Res 1977; 41:818–829.

16. Barnardo DE, Summerskill WHJ, Strong CB, Baldus WP: Renal function, renin activity, and endogenous vasoactive substances in cirrhosis. Am J Dig Dis 1970; 15:419–425.

17. Barnardo DE, Baldus WP, Maher FT: Effects of dopamine on renal function in patients with cirrhosis. Gastroenterology 1970; 58:524–531.

18. Ayers CR: Plasma renin activity and renin-substrate concentration in patients with liver disease. Circ Res 1967; 20:594–598.

19. Levens NR, Peach MJ, Carey RM: Role of the intrarenal renin-angiotensin system in the control of the renal function. Circ Res 1981; 48:157–167.

20. Mitchell KD, Navar LG: Intrarenal actions of angiotensin II in the pathogenesis of experimental hypertension. In: Laragh JH, Brenner BM, eds: Hypertension: Pathophysiology, Diagnosis, and Management. 2nd ed. New York: Raven; 1995:1437–1450.

21. Cade R, Wagemaker H, Vogel S, et al: Hepatorenal syndrome: studies of the effect of vascular volume and intraperitoneal pressure on renal and hepatic function. Am J Med 1987; 82:427–438.

22. Laffi G, La Villa G, Pinzani M, Gentilini P: Lipid-derived autocoids and renal function in liver cirrhosis. In: Epstein M, ed: The Kidney in Liver Disease. 4th ed. Philadelphia: Hanley & Belfus; 1996:307–337.

23. Boyer TD, Zia P, Reynolds TB: Effect of indomethacin and prostaglandin A₁ on renal function and plasma renin activity in alcoholic liver disease. Gastroenterology 1979; 77:215–222.

24. Zipser RD, Hoefs JC, Speckart PF, et al: Prostaglandins: modulators of renal function and pressor resistance in chronic liver disease. J Clin Endocrinol Metab 1979; 48:895–900.

25. Epstein M, Lifschitz MD: Volume status as a determinant of the influence of renal PGE on renal function. Nephron 1980; 25:157–159.

26. Epstein M: Renal prostaglandins and the control of renal function in liver disease. Am J Med 1986; 80(Suppl 1A):46–55.

27. Epstein M, Lifschitz M, Hoffman DS, Stein JH: Relationship between renal prostaglandin E and renal sodium handling during water immersion in normal man. Circ Res 1979; 45:71–80.

28. Epstein M, Lifschitz M, Ramachandran M, Rappaport K: Characterization of renal PGE responsiveness in decompensated cirrhosis: implications for renal sodium handling. Clin Sci 1982; 63:555–563.

29. Zambraski EJ, DiBona G: Renal sympathetic nervous system in hepatic cirrhosis. In: Epstein M, ed: The Kidney in Liver Disease. 4th ed. Philadelphia: Hanley & Belfus; 1996:405–421.

30. Thames MD: Neural control of renal function: Contribution of cardiopulmonary baroreceptors to the control of the kidney. Fed Proc 1977; 37:1209–1213.

31. DiBona GF: The functions of the renal nerves. Rev Physiol Biochem Pharmacol 1982; 94:75–181.

32. DiBona GF: Renal neural activity in hepatorenal syndrome. Kidney Int 1984; 25:841–853.

33. Epstein M: Renal effects of head-out water immersion in humans: a 15-year update. Physiol Rev 1992; 72:563–621.

34. Bichet DG, VanPutten VJ, Schrier RW: Potential role of increased sympathetic activity in impaired sodium and water excretion in cirrhosis. N Engl J Med 1982; 307:1552–1557.

35. Ring-Larsen H, Hesse B, Henriksen JH, Christensen NJ: Sympathetic nervous activity and renal and systemic hemodynamics in cirrhosis: plasma norepinephrine concentration, hepatic extraction, and renal release. Hepatology 1982; 2:304–310.

36. Henriksen JH, Ring-Larsen H, Christensen NJ: Sympathetic nervous activity in cirrhosis: a survey of plasma catecholamine studies. J Hepatol 1984; 1:55–65.

37. Epstein M, Larios O, Johnson G: Effects of water immersion on plasma catecholamines in decompensated cirrhosis: implications for deranged sodium and water homeostasis. Miner Electrolyte Metab 1985; 11:25–34.

38. Bichet DG, Groves BM, Schrier RW: Mechanisms of improvement of water and sodium excretion by immersion in decompensated cirrhotic patients. Kidney Int 1983; 24:788–794.

39. Kopp UC, Dibona GF: The neural control of renal function. In: Seldin DW, Giebisch G, eds: The Kidney: Physiology and Pathophysiology. 2nd ed. New York: Raven; 1992:1157–1204.

40. Folkow B, DiBona G, Hjemdahl P, et al: Measurements of plasma norepinephrine concentration in human primary hypertension—a word of caution concerning their applicability for assessing neurogenic contribution. Hypertension 1983; 5:399–403.

41. Esler M, Dudley F, Jennings G, et al: Increased sympathetic nervous activity and the effects of its inhibition with clonidine in alcoholic cirrhosis. Ann Intern Med 1992; 116: 446–455.

42. Cohn JN: Renal hemodynamic alterations in liver disease. In: Suki WN, Eknoyan G, eds: The Kidney in Systemic Disease. 2nd ed. New York: John Wiley; 1981:509–519.

43. Schrier RW, Arroyo V, Bernardi M, Epstein M, et al: Peripheral arterial vasodilation hypothesis: a proposal for the initiation of renal sodium and water retention in cirrhosis. Hepatology 1988; 8:1151–1157.

44. Schrier RW, Niederberger M, Weigert A, Gines P: Peripheral arterial vasodilation: determinant of functional spectrum of cirrhosis. Semin Liver Dis 1994; 14:14–22.

45. Levy M: Pathogenesis of sodium retention in early cirrhosis of the liver: evidence for vascular overfilling. Semin Liver Dis 1994; 14:4–13.

46. Bosch J, Ginés P, Arroyo V, et al: Hepatic and systemic hemodynamics and the neurohumoral systems in cirrhosis. In: Epstein M, ed: The Kidney in Liver Disease. 3rd ed. Baltimore: Williams & Wilkins; 1988:286–305.

47. Vallance P, Moncada S: Hyperdynamic circulation in cirrhosis: a role for nitric oxide? Lancet 1991; 337:776–778.

48. Umans JG, Levi R: The nitric oxide system in circulatory homeostasis and its possible role in hypertensive disorder. In: Laragh JH, Brenner BM, eds: Hypertension: Pathophysiology, Diagnosis, and Management. 2nd ed. New York: Raven; 1995:1083–1096.

49. Palmer RMJ, Ferrige AG, Moncada S: Nitric oxide release accounts for the biological activity of endothelium-derived relaxing factor. Nature 1987; 327:524–526.

50. Palmer RMJ, Ashton DS, Moncada S: Vascular endothelial cells synthesize nitric oxide from L-arginine. Nature 1988; 333: 664–666.

51. Niederberger M, Gines P, Tsai P, et al: Increased aortic cyclic GMP concentration in experimental cirrhosis in rats: evidence for a role of nitric oxide in the pathogenesis of arterial vasodilation in cirrhosis. Hepatology 1995; 21: 1625–31.

52. Niederberger M, Martin PY, Gines P, et al: Normalization of nitric oxide production corrects arterial vasodilation and hyperdynamic circulation in cirrhotic rats. Gastroenterology 1995; 109:1624–30.

53. Lumsden A, Henderson J, Kutner M: Endotoxin levels measured by a chromogenic assay in portal, hepatic, and peripheral venous blood in patients with cirrhosis. Hepatology 1988; 8: 232–236.

54. Bourgoignie JJ, Valle GA: Endotoxin and renal dysfunction in liver disease. In: Epstein M, ed: *The Kidney in Liver Disease*. 3rd ed. Baltimore: Williams & Wilkins; 1988:486–507.

55. Stuehr DJ, Marletta MA: Mammalian nitrate biosynthesis: mouse macrophages produce nitrite and nitrate in response to *Escherichia coli* lipopolysaccharide. Proc Natl Acad Sci U S A 1985; 82: 7738–7742.

56. Marletta MA, Poksyn SY, Iyengar R, et al: Macrophage oxidation of L-arginine to nitrite and nitrate: nitric oxide is an intermediate. Biochemistry 1988; 27: 8706–8711.

57. Hunt NCA, Goldin RD: Nitric oxide production by monocytes in alcoholic liver disease. J Hepatol 1992; 14:146–50.

58. Langrehr JM, Murase N, Markus PM, et al: Nitric oxide production in host-versus-graft and graft-versus-host reactions in the rat. J Clin Invest 1992; 90:679–683.

59. Guarner C, Soriano G, Tomas A, et al: Increased serum nitrite and nitrate levels in patients with cirrhosis: relationship to endotoxemia. Hepatology 1993; 18:1139–1143.

60. Criado-Jimenez M, Rivas-Cabanero L, Martin-Oterino J, et al: Nitric oxide production by mononuclear leukocytes in alcoholic cirrhosis. J Mol Med 1995; 73:31–33.

61. King AJ: Endothelins: Multifunctional peptides with potent vasoactive properties. In: Laragh JH, Brenner BM, eds: *Hypertension: Pathophysiology, Diagnosis, and Management*. 2nd ed. New York: Raven; 1995:631–672.

62. Rubanyi GM: Endothelin in cardiovascular homeostasis. In: Laragh JH, Brenner BM, eds: *Hypertension: Pathophysiology, Diagnosis, and Management*. 2nd ed. New York: Raven; 1995:1109–1124.

63. Tomita K, Ujiie K, Nakanishi T, et al: Plasma endothelin levels in patients with acute renal failure. N Engl J Med 1989; 321:1127.

64. Deray G, Carayon A, Maistre G, et al: Endothelin in chronic renal failure. Nephrol Dial Transplant 1992; 7:300–305.

65. Epstein M, Goligorsky MS: Endothelin and nitric oxide in hepatorenal syndrome: a balance reset. J Nephrol 1997; 10:85–92.

66. Moore K, Wendon J, Frazer M, et al: Plasma endothelin immunoreactivity in liver disease and the hepatorenal syndrome. N Engl J Med 1992; 327:1774–1778.

67. Epstein M: The hepatorenal syndrome: newer perspectives [Editorial]. N Engl J Med 1992; 327:1810–1811.

68. Pérez GO, Oster JR: A critical review of the role of dialysis in the treatment of liver disease. In: Epstein M, ed: *The Kidney in Liver Disease*. New York: Elsevier; 1978:325–336.

69. Wilkinson SP, Weston MJ, Parsons V, Williams R: Dialysis in the treatment of renal failure in 1993: patients with liver disease. Clin Nephrol 1977; 8:287–292.

70. Perez GO, Golper TA, Epstein M, Oster JR: Dialysis, hemofiltration, and other extracorporeal techniques in the treatment of the renal complications of liver disease. In: Epstein M, ed: *The Kidney in Liver Disease*. 4th ed. Philadelphia: Hanley & Belfus; 1996:517–528.

71. Epstein M, Pérez GO: Continuous arterio-venous ultrafiltration in the management of the renal complications of liver disease. Int J Artif Organs 1986; 9:217–218.

72. Epstein M, Pérez GO, Bedoya LA, Molina R: Continuous arteriovenous ultrafiltration in cirrhotic patients with ascites or renal failure. Int J Artif Organs 1986; 9:253–256.

73. Stange J, Mitzner S, Ramlow W, et al: A new procedure for the removal of protein bound drugs and toxins. ASAIO J 1993; 39:M621–M625.

74. Mitzner SR, Stange J, Klammt S, et al: Improvement of hepatorenal syndrome with extracorporeal albumin dialysis MARS: results of a prospective, randomized, controlled clinical trial. Liver Transplantation 2000; 6:277–286.

75. Gonwa TA, Morris CA, Goldstein RM, et al: Long-term survival and renal function following liver transplantation in patients with and without hepatorenal syndrome—experience in 300 patients. Transplantation 1991; 51:428–430.

76. Gonwa TA, Wilkinson AH: Liver transplantation and renal function: results in patients with and without hepatorenal syndrome. In: Epstein M, ed: *The Kidney in Liver Disease*. 4th ed. Philadelphia: Hanley & Belfus; 1996:529–542.

77. Wood RP, Ellis D, Starzl TE: The reversal of the hepatorenal syndrome in four pediatric patients following successful orthotopic liver transplantation. Ann Surg 1987; 205:415–419.

78. Gunning TC, Brown MR, Swygert TH, et al: Perioperative renal function in patients undergoing orthotopic liver transplantation. Transplantation 1991; 51:422–427.

79. Jeyarajah DR, Gonwa TA, McBride M, et al: Hepatorenal syndrome: combined liver kidney transplants versus isolated liver transplant. Transplantation 1997; 64:1760–1765.

80. Lafayette RA, Pare G, Schmid CH, et al: Pretransplant renal dysfunction predicts poorer outcome in liver transplantation. Clin Nephrol 1997; 48:159–164.

81. Gentilini P, La Villa G, Casini-Raggi V, Romanelli RG: Hepatorenal syndrome and its treatment today. Eur J Gastroenterol Hepatol 1999; 11:1061–1065.

82. Conn H: Transjugular intrahepatic portal-systemic shunts: the state of the art. Hepatology 1993; 17:148–158.

83. Somberg K, Lake J, Tomlanovich S, et al: Transjugular intrahepatic portosystemic shunt for refractory ascites: assessment of clinical and humoral response and renal function [Abstract]. Gastroenterology 1994; 104:A998.

84. Lake J, Ring E, LaBerge J, et al: Transjugular intrahepatic portacaval stent shunt in patients with renal insufficiency. Transplant Proc 1992; 25:1766–1767.

85. Orloff MJ: Effect of side-to side portacaval shunt in intractable ascites, sodium excretion, and aldosterone metabolism in man. Am J Surg 1996; 112:287–298.

86. Somberg KA: Transjugular intrahepatic portosystemic shunt in the treatment of refractory ascites and hepatorenal syndrome. In: Epstein M, ed: *The Kidney in Liver Disease*. 4th ed. Philadelphia: Hanley & Belfus; 1996:507–516.

87. Stanley AJ, Redhead DN, Hayes PC: Review article: update on the role of transjugular intrahepatic portosystemic stent-shunt (TIPSS) in the management of complications of portal hypertension. Aliment Pharmacol Ther 1997; 11:261–272.

88. Brensing KA, Textor J, Perz J, et al: Long-term outcome after transjugular intrahepatic portosystemic stent-shunt in nontransplant cirrhotics with hepatorenal syndrome: a phase II study. Gut 2000; 47:288–295.

89. Brown RS Jr., Lake JR: Transjugular intrahepatic portosystemic shunt as a form of treatment for portal hypertension: indications and contraindications. Adv Intern Med 1997; 42:485–504.

90. Arroyo V, Jimenez W: Complications of cirrhosis. II. Renal and circulatory dysfunction. Lights and shadows in an important clinical problem. J Hepatol 2000; 32(Suppl 1):157–170.

91. Guevara M, Gines P, Fernandez-Esparrach G, et al: Reversibility of hepatorenal syndrome by prolonged administration of ornipressin and plasma volume expansion. Hepatology 1998; 27:35–41.

92. Gulberg V, Bilzer M, Gerbes AL: Long-term therapy and retreatment of hepatorenal syndrome type 1 with ornipressin and dopamine. Hepatology 1999; 30:870–875.

93. Eisenman A, Armali Z, Enat R, et al: Low-dose vasopressin restores diuresis both in patients with hepatorenal syndrome and in anuric patients with end-stage heart failure. J Intern Med 1999; 246:183–190.

94. Angeli P, Volpin R, Gerunda G, et al: Reversal of type 1 hepatorenal syndrome with the administration of midodrine and octreotide. Hepatology 1999; 29:1690–1697.

CHAPTER 21

Acute Renal Failure in Vasculitis

Patrick H. Nachman

Several vasculitic diseases can affect the kidney and lead to a syndrome of acute renal failure (ARF). Although these account for only a small minority of cases of ARF (about 5%), they can be associated with severe morbidity and sometimes death. Most often, the clinical presentation is that of a rapidly progressive glomerulonephritis (RPGN) with or without signs and symptoms of extrarenal manifestation. The notable exception to this general rule pertains to thrombotic microangiopathies that may present in the absence of the glomerular hematuria and proteinuria that characterize the other nephritic syndromes.

The approach to the diagnosis of ARF in the setting of glomerulonephritis or vasculitis can be based on the salient features of the patient's clinical presentation (eg, nephrotic, nephritic, renal-pulmonary, and renal-dermal syndromes). Clues as to the specific diagnosis are obtained from a careful history, review of systems, and physical examination, looking for evidence of extrarenal manifestations of disease. A careful urinalysis is crucial in distinguishing glomerulonephritides from other causes of ARF such as acute tubular necrosis, interstitial nephritis, and obstruction. The presence of dysmorphic red blood cells, red blood cell casts, or proteinuria that exceeds 500 mg per day is strong indication of glomerular injury. Laboratory studies, including serologic findings, and assessment of complement cascade activation may increase or decrease the likelihood of certain diseases.[1] Ultimately, the definitive diagnosis is attained by examination of the renal histology. In fulminant cases where the clinical syndrome is highly indicative of a specific disease, it may be necessary to initiate appropriate therapy prior to obtaining the definitive results of a renal biopsy or serologic work-up, because a delay in therapy may adversely affect the patient's outcome.

An alternative working classification of the glomerular and vasculitic syndromes associated with ARF is based on their pathogenetic mechanisms, namely (1) immune complex–mediated vasculitis, (2) direct anti-body attack–mediated disease, (3) pauci-immune necrotizing vasculitis, and (4) thrombotic microangiopathies.

This latter approach is followed in this chapter to discuss the major vasculitic syndromes associated with ARF (Tables 21–1 and 21–2).

IMMUNE COMPLEX–MEDIATED DISEASE

Systemic Lupus Erythematosus

CLINICOPATHOLOGIC SYNDROMES OF RENAL DISEASE

The diagnosis of a patient with systemic lupus erythematosus (SLE) is based on combined clinical, pathologic, and laboratory findings. The classification of patients with lupus is based on criteria established by the American Rheumatism Association.[2] To establish a diagnosis of SLE, patients must exhibit at least 4 of 11 signs or symptoms. The clinical diagnosis of lupus nephritis is most likely made following a diagnostic renal biopsy in the presence of positive serology and characteristic extrarenal manifestations of disease.

Lupus nephritis is the prototypic immune complex glomerulonephritis. Most patients with SLE have deposition of immunoglobulin and complement, even in the absence of clinically significant renal dysfunction. The location and quantity of immune reactants, and the host response to these immune reactants, result in a spectrum of renal lesions categorized by the World Health Organization (WHO) into different classes of lupus nephritis.

WHO class I is the mildest pathologic expression of lupus nephritis and is associated with normal renal histology. Class II is characterized by immune complex deposition confined to the mesangium, with (class IIB) or without (class IIA) varying degrees of focal to diffuse mesangial hypercellularity. Class II lupus nephritis

TABLE 21–1. Major Categories of Glomerulonephritis and Systemic Vasculitis Associated With Acute Renal Failure

IMMUNE COMPLEX MEDIATED	DIRECT ANTIBODY ATTACK	PAUCI-IMMUNE VASCULITIS	THROMBOTIC MICROANGIOPATHIES
Systemic lupus erythematosus	Anti-GBM disease	Microscopic polyangiitis	Thrombotic thrombocytopenic purpura
Cryoglobulinemic vasculitis	Goodpasture's syndrome	Wegener's granulomatosis	Hemolytic-uremic syndrome
Henoch-Schönlein purpura		Churg-Strauss syndrome	Systemic sclerosis renal crisis
			Malignant hypertension
			Preeclampsia

GBM, glomerular basement membrane.

TABLE 21–2. Names and Definitions of Small Vessel Vasculitis Adopted by the Chapel Hill Consensus Conference on the Nomenclature of Systemic Vasculitis

NAME	DEFINITION
Wegener's granulomatosis	Granulomatous inflammation involving the respiratory tract, and necrotizing vasculitis affecting small- to medium-sized vessels (capillaries, venules, arterioles, and arteries)
Churg-Strauss syndrome	Eosinophil-rich and granulomatous inflammation involving the respiratory tract and necrotizing vasculitis affecting small- to medium-sized vessels, and associated with asthma and blood eosinophilia
Microscopic polyangiitis (microscopic polyarteritis)	Necrotizing vasculitis with few or no immune deposits affecting small vessels (capillaries, venules, or arterioles); necrotizing arteritis involving small- and medium-sized arteries may be present
Henoch-Schönlein purpura	Vasculitis with IgA-dominant immune deposits affecting small vessels (capillaries, venules, or arterioles)
Essential cryoglobulinemic vasculitis	Isolated cutaneous leukocytoclastic angiitis without systemic vasculitis or glomerulonephritis

Adapted from Jennette JC, Falk RJ, Andrassy K, et al: Nomenclature of systemic vasculitides: the proposal of an international consensus conference. Arthritis Rheum 1994; 37:187–192; with permission.

usually causes only a mild nephritic picture with asymptomatic hematuria and proteinuria.

Focal proliferative (class III) or diffuse proliferative (class IV) lupus nephritis is characterized by endocapillary hypercellularity caused not only by mesangial and endothelial proliferation but also by leukocyte infiltration. The most active lesions are complicated by necrosis and crescent formation.

Class V lupus nephritis is characterized by the localization of immune complexes predominantly in the subepithelial zone. Similar to idiopathic membranous nephropathy, class V lupus nephritis usually causes a nephrotic rather than nephritic syndrome, unless substantial proliferative changes are also present. Class V lupus nephritis is further categorized as class Va when membranous changes are found exclusively, Vb when there is concurrent mesangial hypercellularity, Vc when there are focal endocapillary proliferative changes, and Vd in the presence of diffuse proliferative changes. Clinically, patients with class Vc and Vd nephritis follow a clinical course resembling that of focal or diffuse proliferative lupus glomerulonephritis (class III and IV),[3] whereas patients with class Va and Vb have a more predominantly nephrotic course similar to that of idiopathic membranous nephropathy.[4] Therefore, our approach is to treat patients with combined membranous and proliferative lesions (class Vc and Vd) as if they had class III or IV lupus nephritis.

Of the various classes of lupus nephritis, classes III, IV, and Vc and Vd are the most likely to present as a syndrome of RPGN and ARF and are the focus of discussion in this chapter. Classes I, II, and Va and Vb usually present as asymptomatic proteinuria and hematuria or as a nephrotic syndrome without renal failure.

Some patients with lupus develop a thrombotic microangiopathy that may be associated with antiphospholipid antibodies or with an overlap syndrome with systemic sclerosis. This complication is characterized by subendothelial expansion in glomerular capillaries, fibrinoid necrosis of arterioles, and edematous intimal expansion in arteries. The resultant narrowing of lumina, as well as superimposed thrombosis, may cause severe and rapid renal failure and microangiopathic hemolytic anemia.

Because of the typically relapsing and remitting nature of SLE, the nephritis eventually results in glomerular sclerosis, adhesions, fibrous crescents, interstitial fibrosis, and arteriosclerosis. The relative histologic markers of active inflammation and chronic injury can be expressed as activity and chronicity indices, the prognostic importance of which is a subject of controversy.[5]

One difficulty in managing patients with lupus nephritis lies in the fact that the pathologic lesion may change from one form of glomerular injury to another. It is common for a class III lupus nephritis to progress to a class IV lupus nephritis. Both class III and class IV lesions can transform into membranous (class V) lupus nephritis, either spontaneously or with immunosuppressive therapy. It is less common, but possible, for membranous lesions to transform into more proliferative lesions. Even repetitive clinical evaluations may not be sufficiently insightful in detecting these changes, and repeated renal biopsies are sometimes needed.

THE ROLE OF RENAL BIOPSY

The role of a renal biopsy in the evaluation of patients with SLE and nephritis has been the subject of debate fueled by the inability to reliably correlate the pathologic changes with long-term outcome.[6] Nonetheless, because of the substantial overlap in the clinical presentation of patients with the pathologic findings on biopsy, we use the renal biopsy to aid in the management of our patients. In our opinion, the renal biopsy helps clarify the clinicopathologic syndrome, as well as the relative degrees of active inflammation and chronic scarring. The finding of extensive glomerular sclerosis but no active inflammation, for example, may deter from further immunosuppressive therapy. The biopsy may also identify unsuspected causes for an acute worsening in renal function such as the development of a thrombotic microangiopathy or tubulointerstitial nephritis caused by the use of antimicrobial or anti-inflammatory drugs.

LABORATORY FINDINGS

Antinuclear antibodies (ANAs) are more than 90% sensitive but only 70% specific for SLE because they are also found with other rheumatic diseases, with infections, and in older age groups (Table 21–3). In contrast, up to 10% of patients who fulfill diagnostic criteria for lupus do not have a positive ANA. Tests for antibodies to nuclear or cytosolic antigens other than DNA are more specific for SLE. For example, antibodies to the Sm antigen are very specific for lupus but are found in only 25% of patients. Patients with anti-Sm antibodies have a higher risk of severe lupus, renal disease, CNS disease, cutaneous vasculitis, and death.[7, 8]

The total hemolytic complement (CH_{50}), C4, and C3 are typically low during active disease. Because decreased synthesis of complement components also results in depressed complement levels, a low complement concentration does not always indicate active disease. Longitudinally repeated measurements of these factors may be more helpful in determining the relative state of complement activation and disease activity of a patient.

TREATMENT

Therapeutic decisions for individual patients with lupus nephritis should be based on consideration of their clinical presentation, laboratory features, and histologic findings on biopsy. Patients with lupus focal proliferative or diffuse proliferative glomerulonephritis (WHO class III and IV, respectively) are at risk of progressive loss of renal function and end-stage renal disease and warrant consideration of aggressive immunosuppressive therapy. Patients with more "benign" lesions may also undergo a transformation to proliferative lesions associated with the development of nephritic sediment and increasing proteinuria.[9] In patients with proliferative lesions, the use of cytotoxic drugs cyclophosphamide or azathioprine in addition to corticosteroids leads to improved renal survival over treatment with corticosteroids alone[10, 11] and fewer scle-

TABLE 21–3. Serologic Findings in Patients With Systemic Vasculitis and/or Rapidly Progressive Glomerulonephritis

SYSTEMIC ILLNESS	SEROLOGIC FINDINGS
Systemic lupus erythematosus	ANA/anti–double-stranded DNA
Small vessel vasculitis	ANCA
Wegener's granulomatosis	PR3-ANCA > MPO-ANCA
Microscopic polyangiitis	MPO-ANCA > PR3-ANCA
Churg-Strauss syndrome	MPO-ANCA
Cryoglobulemic vasculitis	Mixed cryoglobulins
	Anti-hepatitis C antibodies
Anti-GMB disease and Goodpasture's disease	Anti-GBM antibodies
Thrombotic microangiopathy	von Willebrand factor cleaving protease inhibitor*
	Anticardiolipin antibodies†
Systemic sclerosis	Anti-DNA topoisomerase, anti-RNA polymerase III

*Test not currently clinically available.
†Found in patients with underlying systemic lupus erythematosus.
ANA, antinuclear antibody; *ANCA,* antineutrophil cytoplasmic autoantibodies; *GBM,* glomerular basement membrane; *PR3,* proteinase-3; *MPO,* myeloperoxidase.

rotic or atrophic lesions on repeat renal biopsy.[12] Delay of therapy is associated with an increase in renal scarring that is poorly responsive to immunosuppressive therapy.[13]

Cyclophosphamide. Although early studies suggested only a decrease in the long-term frequency of relapse[14, 15] with the use of cyclophosphamide in addition to corticosteroids, the role for intermittent intravenous cyclophosphamide therapy was established by two prospective, controlled clinical trials performed at the National Institutes of Health (NIH).[16, 17] These trials demonstrated greater long-term renal but not overall survival with the use of cyclophosphamide as compared with corticosteroids alone. Continuing quarterly pulse cyclophosphamide for at least 1 year after renal remission decreases the frequency of nephritic relapses and the risk of renal function deterioration.[17–19] The application of these results to the general population of patients with SLE requires caution because these studies included patients with various histologic lesions and excluded patients with severely impaired renal function.

Azathioprine. The role of azathioprine in the treatment of proliferative lupus nephritis is less well established than that of cyclophosphamide. Early studies suggested improved outcomes with the use of azathioprine in combination with corticosteroids over corticosteroids alone,[20, 21] whereas in the NIH randomized, controlled trial azathioprine was no more effective than prednisone alone in reducing renal failure.[16] However, azathioprine has fewer side effects than cyclophosphamide and may be considered for patients at low risk of ESRD, typically with focal proliferative (WHO class III) nephritis. Based on the results of a small study,[22] the role of azathioprine is currently being investigated in a prospective, randomized trial comparing the NIH regimen of long-course, intermittent intravenous cyclophosphamide with oral prednisone versus intravenous pulse methylprednisolone and azathioprine.[23]

Pulse Methylprednisolone. In two controlled trials for the treatment of proliferative lupus nephritis, the combination of cyclophosphamide and pulse methylprednisolone afforded a more rapid response and greater probability of renal remission.[24, 25]

Plasmapheresis. Plasmapheresis has been employed in the treatment of lupus nephritis to eliminate pathogenic antibodies and circulating immune complexes. However, a large-scale, prospective, controlled clinical trial showed no additional benefit of plasmapheresis compared with corticosteroids and short-course oral cyclophosphamide therapy alone.[26, 27] There is, therefore, no current support for the routine use of plasmapheresis in the treatment of lupus nephritis, although it may have a role in the treatment of patients with overwhelming disease in whom standard therapy is failing.

Cyclosporine. Most reports on treatment of lupus with cyclosporine have evaluated the effects of the drug on extrarenal manifestations of lupus with few patients with active nephritis treated. Cyclosporine has been shown to be effective in reducing clinical and histologic activity in proliferative lupus nephritis.[28] Autoantibody formation and hypocomplementemia did not uniformly improve and the frequent occurrence of hypertension and nephrotoxicity limits the usefulness of this therapy.[29]

In summary, patients with class IV or severe class III lupus nephritis are treated with pulse methylprednisolone [AU1](7 mg/kg daily for 3 days) followed by cyclophosphamide and prednisone. Prednisone is started at a dose of 1 mg/kg per day for the first month, followed by a gradual taper over the following 3 months. Frequently, extrarenal manifestations of the disease require the continued use of daily oral prednisone at doses between 5 and 10 mg/day. Intravenous cyclophosphamide is given according to the NIH protocol, once a month for 6 consecutive months. The dosage is titrated upward during the first 6 months, starting at a dose of 0.5 g/m² body surface area and increasing by 0.25 g/m² on successive treatments (not to exceed 1 g/m²), provided that the 2-week leukocyte count remains above 3000 cell/mm³. After the first 6 months, pulse cyclophosphamide is given every 3 months for a total of 24 months. Patients with significant renal impairment may need a reduction in the first dose of parenteral cyclophosphamide.

It is unclear whether high-dose prednisone, cyclophosphamide, or azathioprine is indicated for patients with mild to moderate focal proliferative glomerulonephritis (class III). Most patients are treated with corticosteroids for their extrarenal manifestations of disease. However, when there is necrosis or crescent formation in addition to the focal proliferative disease, the long-term outcome is probably similar to that of diffuse proliferative glomerulonephritis (class IV) and should be treated in the same fashion.

The best approach to therapy relies on an assessment of several factors. The clinician should assess disease activity, disease severity, the patient's previous history of disease activity, and the patient's own response to corticosteroid and immunosuppressive drugs.

There are several markers of disease activity. The clinical history is usually most helpful for assessing overall symptomatology. Renal disease activity may be indicated by the presence of numerous red blood cells and red blood cell casts in the urine. The presence of proteinuria may relate to previous renal damage rather than to an acute process, except in cases of membranous nephropathy and its attendant nephrotic syndrome. Overall, lupus activity may be further assessed by the use of serologic markers as adjunctive tests. Rises in the anti–double-stranded DNA titer, or declines in complement levels, especially CH₅₀, are particularly helpful.

PROGNOSIS

There is a general assertion that the long-term survival of patients with SLE has improved over last 50 years. Some of this progress is a consequence of the broadened appreciation of the picture of SLE, and some may be attributed to the judicious use of cortico-

steroids and the introduction and refinement of the use of cyclophosphamide and azathioprine. Overall, lupus mortality is still more likely to be a consequence of cerebritis or myocarditis than a loss of renal function, largely owing to the availability of dialysis and transplantation. The other major cause of death is attributable to overwhelming infection as a consequence of immunosuppressive therapy.

Certain prognostic factors affect the long-term outcome of renal disease. In a recent study of patients with diffuse proliferative glomerulonephritis treated with cyclophosphamide, poor long-term outcome was more likely for African American patients and for those whose biopsies revealed interstitial fibrosis.[30, 31] The increased risk for end-stage renal disease among African Americans may be due to genetic factors[32–34] as well as racial differences in socioeconomic factors.[35, 36]

In other studies, the entry serum creatinine level[6] and the biopsy findings have been suggested as predictors of eventual renal failure. Although no specific numerical cutoff on the chronicity index scale is associated with certainty to long-term outcome, substantial interstitial fibrosis, glomerulosclerosis, and tubular atrophy are likely predictors of progress to end-stage renal disease over the course of years.

Henoch-Schönlein Purpura

Henoch-Schönlein purpura affects primarily children and, less frequently, adults. This syndrome is characterized by leukocytoclastic vasculitis of the skin, abdominal pain sometimes associated with gastrointestinal hemorrhage, arthralgias, arthritis, and glomerulonephritis. The lesions of the skin are similar to those of other renal-dermal vasculitic syndromes. Although there are typically crops of macular and palpable purpuric rashes on the lower extremities, buttocks, and flanks, there may be urticarial lesions as well.

The frequency of clinically significant renal disease varies. When renal disease occurs, it is typically noted within days to weeks after the onset of symptoms. Most patients present with microscopic or, at times, macroscopic hematuria with red blood cell casts. Proteinuria is typically mild, although some patients may have nephrotic syndrome.

PATHOLOGY

The glomerular picture of Henoch-Schönlein purpura is identical to that of IgA nephropathy, with a spectrum of lesions ranging from mild mesangial proliferation to diffuse endocapillary proliferation, with or without crescent formation. Immunofluorescence microscopy reveals a mesangial deposition of IgA as well as complement components such as C3. By electron microscopy, electron-dense deposits are found predominantly in the mesangium, but capillary wall deposits can be found in patients with severe glomerulonephritis.

Skin biopsy typically reveals a leukocytoclastic vasculitis that involves postcapillary venules. This skin vasculitis can be differentiated from that of other vasculitic syndromes by the presence of IgA deposition in vessels. There are no specific laboratory tests that are either sensitive or specific markers of Henoch-Schönlein purpura.

CLINICAL COURSE AND TREATMENT RECOMMENDATIONS

In most children, Henoch-Schönlein purpura remains a self-limited disorder that usually resolves spontaneously. This is especially true of the dermal and joint complaints. The gastrointestinal symptoms may be severe and may prompt numerous diagnostic studies and even exploratory laparoscopy. Corticosteroids clearly improve the extrarenal manifestations of the disease, including abdominal pain. In general, the disease process follows a relapsing and remitting course.

Treatment recommendations for the nephritis vary according to the renal lesion. In individuals with mild mesangial hypercellularity, it is unlikely that any anti-inflammatory or immunosuppressive therapy is needed. A large number of patients undergo spontaneous remission and a generally favorable course. However, among patients who have acute nephritis or RPGN, a substantial proportion (up to 44%) have persisting hypertension or a decline in glomerular filtration rate.[37] In this latter group of patients, institution of high-dose corticosteroids and sometimes cyclophosphamide is indicated. This may be especially true for adult patients with Henoch-Schönlein purpura who have more frequent and more severe renal involvement than children. Despite the more severe glomerulonephritis, the institution of immunosuppressive and/or cytotoxic treatment affords adults as good a prognosis as that of children.[38] Treating nephrologists tend to follow regimens similar to those used in other forms of crescentic glomerulonephritis.

Cryoglobulinemic Vasculitis

Cryoglobulins are composed of different types of immunoglobulins, which makes possible their separation into three categories. Whereas type I cryoglobulins are characterized by the presence of monoclonal antibodies, usually IgM, types II and III are mixtures of monoclonal and polyclonal, or polyclonal with polyclonal immunoglobulins, respectively. In type II mixed cryoglobulins, the monoclonal component is usually an IgM and the polyclonal component is usually an IgG.[39]

The association of type II cryoglobulins with hepatitis C virus (HCV) infection is now well established.[40-42] This association is based on a high prevalence of HCV infection in patients with type II cryoglobulinemia, as well as the demonstration of anti-HCV antibodies and HCV RNA in the cryoglobulin precipitate.[43, 44]

Cryoglobulins are detectable in up to 30% of patients with HCV, but the clinical syndrome of mixed cryoglobulinemia occurs only in 1% to 2% of patients with HCV infection.

The mechanism by which HCV infection might lead to the development of type II cryoglobulinemia is unclear. The recent finding that peripheral blood leukocytes, especially B cells, can be the site of extrahepatic viral replication of HCV has led to the postulation that in a subgroup of patients with chronic infection, direct active viral replication in B cells triggers their activation to overproduce polyclonal IgM rheumatoid factors. An additional, as yet uncharacterized event might induce the abnormal proliferation of a single clone leading to the production of a monoclonal IgM rheumatoid factor and, consequently, type II mixed cryoglobulinemia.

PATHOLOGY

The most common renal lesion in patients with type II mixed cryoglobulinemia is type I membranoproliferative glomerulonephritis. Pathologic characteristics include endocapillary hypercellularity due to the proliferation of mesangial and endothelial cells and infiltration of monocytes and T lymphocytes. There are typically large amorphous eosinophilic, periodic acid–Schiff positive, Congo red negative deposits that may fill the capillary lumina ("hyaline thrombi"). The basement membrane is typically thickened with a "double-contour" appearance. A few patients have fibrinoid necrosis of the walls of arterioles and venules. Electron microscopy may reveal subendothelial electron-dense deposits consisting of a microtubular structure of hollow fibers, 100 to 1000 nm long. By immunofluorescence microscopy, there is granular to bandlike staining of the vessel walls for IgM, IgG, and complement C3. Some patients exhibit intense staining of large deposits that fill the capillary lumen.

CLINICAL MANIFESTATIONS

Type II mixed cryoglobulinemia is most often diagnosed in the fifth and sixth decades of life, often many years after the first symptoms appear. Cryoglobulinemic vasculitis is characterized clinically by weakness, purpura, arthralgias, arthritic vasculitis, neuropathy, and proliferative glomerulonephritis. Renal involvement occurs in 8% to 58% of patients and is more common in women with mixed cryoglobulinemia. Manifestations of renal involvement typically appear many years after the first symptoms of cryoglobulinemic vasculitis develop. The renal disease may appear concomitantly with the extrarenal manifestations on occasion, but rarely before. The most frequent renal syndrome is that of isolated proteinuria and microscopic hematuria with moderate chronic renal insufficiency. ARF and a picture of RPGN occurs only in 20% to 30% of patients and presents with severe proteinuria, hematuria, and hypertension. Twenty percent of patients may present with nephrotic syndrome.

CLINICAL COURSE AND PROGNOSIS

The clinical course of MPGN type I associated with HCV may vary. Ten percent to 15% of patients attain complete remission, even when presenting with acute nephritis. Thirty percent of patients follow an indolent course that does not progress to end-stage renal disease despite the persistence of abnormal urinary sediment and chronic renal insufficiency. Twenty percent of patients may have recurrent episodes of acute nephritis that may go into remission either spontaneously or in response to high-dose corticosteroids and/or plasmapheresis. This course usually leads eventually to chronic renal insufficiency. Only about 15% of patients progress to end-stage renal disease over a mean period of 10 years.[45] Cryoglobulinemic vasculitis, however, is associated with a high mortality rate secondary to the extrarenal disease. The 10-year probability of survival without end-stage renal disease is about 50%.[46] The major causes of death are cardiovascular disease, infection, liver failure, and neoplasia. The main risk factors for a poor outcome are age older than 50 years, vascular purpura, splenomegaly, cryocrit level greater than 10%, and C3 plasma levels less than 54 mg/dL. As with other glomerulonephritides, an abnormal serum creatinine is an important risk factor for chronic renal failure or death.

TREATMENT

The recognition of an association between HCV infection and type I MGPN has led to great interest in the treatment of this glomerular disease with antiviral agents. Although a large body of data has accumulated over the last several years concerning the treatment of HCV infection, most knowledge is derived from the treatment of HCV-related hepatic disease. An early study of the treatment of HCV-related mixed cryoglobulinemia with interferon-α[47] resulted in improvement in cutaneous vasculitis, cryocrit, serum creatinine, and a decrease in HCV RNA. However, the viremia and cryoglobulinemia recurred in all patients after discontinuation of interferon-α. Treatment of HCV-related hepatic disease with[48] interferon-α2b alone for 6 months resulted in a disappointing 8% rate of sustained response.

The mediocre results achieved with interferon-α alone led to the evaluation of combination therapy including interferon-α and the nucleoside analog ribavirin.[49] Ribavirin in standard doses combined with interferon-α in doses of 3 million units, three times weekly for 6 months, was found to significantly improve the sustained biochemical and virologic response rates compared with interferon-α alone. No study has yet been reported as to the use of this combination therapy in the treatment of HCV-related mixed cryoglobulinemia or MPGN.

Two nonrandomized case series on the use of plasmapheresis with and without small doses of corticosteroids in the treatment of acute exacerbation of cryoglobulinemic membranoproliferative glomerulonephritis[50, 51] report a beneficial effect of plasmapheresis. Patients with acute deterioration of renal function seem to benefit the most with such treatment, whereas patients with chronic stable renal insufficiency have a less marked benefit from the treatment. In some

patients,[50] plasma exchange can lead to a sustained remission without clinical relapse after the frequency of plasmapheresis is reduced or discontinued.

DIRECT ANTIBODY–MEDIATED DISEASE

Antiglomerular Basement Membrane Glomerulonephritis and Goodpasture's Disease

Depending on the series examined, anti–glomerular basement membrane (anti-GBM) disease accounts for about 10% to 20% of crescentic glomerulonephritides.[52] This disease is characterized by the presence of circulating antibodies to the GBM[53] and, on renal biopsy, the deposition of IgG or rarely IgA along the glomerular and tubular basement membrane.[54]

EPIDEMIOLOGY

The incidence of anti-GBM disease follows two peaks with respect to age. The first peak, in the third decade of life, consists predominantly of men who present with pulmonary hemorrhage (Goodpasture's disease). The second peak, between ages 50 and 70 years, has a predominance of women affected with anti-GBM glomerulonephritis without pulmonary hemorrhage. Overall, the male-to-female ratio approaches 1.3:1.

Genetic susceptibility to anti-GBM disease has been described to be associated with HLA DRw2 specificity of the DRB1 alleles, DRB1*1501 and DQB*0602.[55, 56]

PATHOLOGY

The hallmark findings of anti-GBM disease consist of crescent formation and focal glomerular fibrinoid necrosis.[57] Crescents can be found affecting 5% to 90% of glomeruli. The necrotizing lesions can also lead to disruption of Bowman's capsule, which is then associated with a conspicuous periglomerular inflammation. By light microscopy, these changes are similar to those seen in patients with antineutrophil cytoplasmic autoantibody (ANCA)—small vessel vasculitis and glomerulonephritis and may be distinguished from immune complex–mediated crescentic lesions by the normal thickness of the capillary loops and a lesser degree of proliferative changes. The characteristic changes of anti-GBM disease are seen on immunofluorescence microscopy and consist of a diffuse, global linear staining of the glomerular and sometimes the tubular basement membranes with IgG and, to a lesser degree, C3.[58] By electron microscopy, no electron-dense deposits are seen, a finding shared with pauci-immune glomerulonephritis.

PATHOGENESIS

The target antigen of anti-GBM antibodies is in the collagenase-resistant part of type IV collagen, the "noncollagenous domain," or "NC1 domain."[59, 60] The antigenic epitope is in an encrypted form because there is little antibody binding to the native hexameric structure of the NC1 domain, but it increases 15-fold when the hexameric NC1 domain is denatured and dissociates into dimers and monomers.[60] The majority of patients express antibodies to a restricted epitope on the α_3 chain of type IV collagen.[61, 62] Some patients with anti-GBM disease who do not have antibodies to the classic epitope on the α_3 chain have antibodies to entactin,[63] and a small percentage of patients may additionally have antibodies to the NC1 domains of the α_1 or α_4 chains of type IV collagen. In addition, 10% to 38% of patients with anti-GBM disease also have circulating ANCA.[64-66] When both autoantibodies coexist, anti-GBM antibodies are associated with anti-myeloperoxidase (anti-MPO) antibodies in about 70% of cases and with anti-proteinase-3 (anti-PR3) antibodies in about 30% of cases. The co-occurrence of ANCA and anti-GBM antibodies may be associated with more severe vasculitis, especially in capillary beds other than for the lung and the kidney.[65, 67]

The role of the T cell in the pathogenesis of anti-GBM disease is suggested by the increased susceptibility to the disease in the presence of the HLA DRw2 antigens[55] and from studies of T-cell proliferation in response to monomeric components of the GBM and synthetic oligopeptides.[68] Furthermore, when mice of eight different strains were immunized with purified bovine α_3 (IV) NC1 dimers, this led to the production of anti-α_3 (IV) NC1 antibodies in all strains of mice. However, only the mouse strains capable of mounting a Th1 type response developed nephritis and pulmonary hemorrhage.[69] In this model, the passive transfer of lymphocytes or antibodies from nephritogenic strains to syngeneic recipients led to the development of nephritis, whereas the passive transfer of antibodies to T-cell receptor–deficient mice failed to do so, bringing further evidence for a role of T cells in the pathogenesis of this disease.

CLINICAL FEATURES

The onset of disease is typically an abrupt, acute glomerulonephritis with severe oliguria or anuria. Rarely, patients present with a more insidious onset that remains essentially asymptomatic until the development of uremic symptoms and fluid retention.[53, 70] The onset of disease may be associated with arthralgias, fever, myalgias, and abdominal pain; however, gastrointestinal complaints or neurologic disturbances are rare.

Goodpasture's disease is distinguished from anti-GBM disease by the presence of pulmonary hemorrhage. The usual presentation is marked by severe and even life-threatening pulmonary hemorrhage, although it may present with mild pulmonary symptoms and a small infiltrate only. The occurrence of pulmonary hemorrhage is far more common in smokers than nonsmokers and with environmental exposures to hydrocarbons,[71] use of cocaine, or upper respiratory tract infection.[72] Occupational exposure to petroleum-based mineral oils is a risk factor for the development of anti-GBM antibodies per se. The association of pulmonary hemorrhage with environmental exposures and infection raises the theoretical possibility of exposure of the cryptic antigenic epitope in the alveolar basement membrane to circulating anti-GBM antibodies.

LABORATORY FINDINGS

Anti-GBM disease typically presents as part of acute nephritic syndrome associated with hematuria, including dysmorphic erythrocyturia and red blood cells casts. Although nephrotic-range proteinuria and even massive proteinuria may rarely occur, full nephrotic syndrome is rarely seen.[53, 70]

The characteristic laboratory finding in anti-GBM disease is that of circulating antibodies to the GBM. These antibodies may be detected by radioimmunoassay in more than 95% of patients. The anti-GBM antibodies are most often of the IgG1 subclass but may also be of IgG4 subclass, the latter being more often seen in women.[73]

TREATMENT

The standard of therapy for the treatment of anti-GBM disease and Goodpasture's syndrome includes intensive plasmapheresis combined with corticosteroids and cyclophosphamide or azathioprine.[74, 75] Plasmapheresis is performed daily until circulating antibody levels become undetectable and pulmonary hemorrhage ceases. Patients with pulmonary hemorrhage should receive replacement of clotting factors with fresh frozen plasma at the end of each treatment. Prednisone is started at a dose of 1 mg/kg of body weight for at least the first month and then tapered in an organized manner to alternate-day therapy during the second and third months of treatment. Although the administration of pulse methylprednisolone has not been systematically analyzed in Goodpasture's syndrome, the urgent nature of the clinical process typically prompts its use as part of induction therapy in this form of crescentic glomerulonephritis.[76, 77] Cyclophosphamide is administered either orally (at a dose of 2 mg/kg per day), or monthly intravenous cyclophosphamide is used at a starting dose of 0.5 g/m² of body surface area. The dose of cyclophosphamide must be adjusted with consideration of the degree of impairment of renal function and the white blood cell count. Cytotoxic therapy is usually continued for 6 to 12 months, with the possibility of switching cyclophosphamide to azathioprine after 3 to 4 months in selected patients.

The use of aggressive plasmapheresis with corticosteroids and cyclophosphamide has improved patient and renal survival to approximately 85% and 60%, respectively (where patient survival was less than 50% and 10% prior to the introduction of plasmapheresis).[78, 79] The major prognostic marker for the progression to end-stage renal disease is the serum creatinine level at the time treatment is initiated. Patients with a serum creatinine level above 7 mg/dL are unlikely to recover sufficient renal function to discontinue renal replacement therapy.[80] Whereas aggressive immunosuppression and plasmapheresis are warranted in patients with pulmonary hemorrhage (Goodpasture's disease), such therapy should be withheld in patients with renal-limited disease who present with widespread glomerular and interstitial scarring on renal biopsy and a serum creatinine level greater than 7 mg/dL. In such patients, the risks of therapy outweigh the potential benefits. For those patients with an elevated serum creatinine level, yet have active crescentic glomerulonephritis on biopsy, aggressive treatment should continue for at least 4 weeks and discontinue in the absence of recovery of renal function by 8 weeks.

In patients who have both circulating anti-GBM and ANCA, the chance of recovery of renal function is better when compared with that of patients with anti-GBM disease alone. In these patients, immunosuppressive therapy should not be withheld, even with serum creatinine levels above 7 mg/dL, because the concomitant presence of ANCA may be associated with a more favorable renal outcome.[81]

Once remission of anti-GBM disease is achieved with immunosuppressive therapy, recurrent disease occurs only rarely.[82, 83] Similarly, the recurrence of anti-GBM disease after renal transplantation is also rare, especially when transplantation is delayed until after disappearance or substantial diminution of anti-GBM antibody titers.[84]

Pauci-Immune Small Vessel Vasculitis

Pauci-immune forms of small vessel vasculitis are microscopic polyangiitis, Wegener's granulomatosis, or Churg-Strauss syndrome.[85] Some patients present with necrotizing and crescentic glomerulonephritis only without any signs of extrarenal vasculitis. These syndromes share several similarities, not only on the basis of the blood vessels that they involve (predominantly capillaries, venules, arterioles, and small arteries), but also with respect to the clinical phenotype of the diseases and their association with ANCA.

PATHOLOGY

The characteristic feature of the glomerular lesion in pauci-immune small vessel vasculitis is focal necrotizing glomerulonephritis associated with cellular or fibrocellular crescents that usually involve more than 50% of glomeruli. The glomerulonephritides associated with ANCA–small vessel vasculitis and anti-GBM disease are characterized predominantly by necrosis rather than hypercellularity. The reverse is true for immune complex glomerulonephritis, which tends to have prominent proliferative changes. Identification of vasculitis in vessels other than glomerular capillaries is seen in only approximately 10% of renal biopsies from patients with ANCA–small vessel vasculitis. Interstitial necrotizing granulomatous inflammation is rarely observed in renal biopsies from patients with Wegener's granulomatosis.

Most patients with ANCA-associated glomerulonephritis and small vessel vasculitis have little or no glomerular staining for immunoglobulin by immunofluorescence microscopy. Electron microscopy typically reveals no electron-dense deposits or only a few scattered deposits within the mesangium. However, some patients have a necrotizing ANCA–associated glomerulonephritis concurrent with anti-GBM disease or immune complex disease, in which case a well-defined background linear or granular staining for immunoglobulins can be seen.

CLINICAL MANIFESTATIONS

The clinical manifestations of ANCA–small vessel vasculitis are protean. These can be limited to the kidney alone (pauci-immune necrotizing and crescentic glomerulonephritis) or may involve a number of other organs in various combinations. Most patients present with constitutional findings such as fever, myalgias, and migratory arthralgias and describe a flulike prodrome.[86]

The renal manifestations of necrotizing glomerulonephritis are hematuria, with dysmorphic erythrocyturia and red blood cell casts, and proteinuria that can be mild to moderate or of nephrotic range.[87, 88] A common presentation of the necrotizing glomerulonephritis is that of a RPGN that may progress to end-stage renal disease if not treated emergently. Alternatively, some patients follow a more indolent, remitting, and relapsing course of episodes of focal necrosis and hematuria, which leads to substantial glomerulosclerosis. These individuals usually do not respond well to immunosuppressive therapy and eventually require dialytic support.

Prominent among the extrarenal manifestations of pauci-immune small vessel vasculitis are those of the respiratory tract and skin. Pulmonary disease is found in 50% of patients and varies from focal infiltrates to fulminant hemorrhagic alveolar capillaritis resulting in life-threatening hemorrhage. Patients with granulomatous disease (Wegener's granulomatosis or Churg-Strauss syndrome) may have more nodular and occasionally cavitating lesions. In Churg-Strauss syndrome, pulmonary involvement is the most predominant form of the disease and is associated with asthma and eosinophilia.

The upper respiratory tract disease associated with ANCA–small vessel vasculitis may take the form of nasal erosions, ulcers, and necrosis of the nasal septum. Sinusitis, found in one third of patients, typically involves more than one sinus cavity, and patients with Wegener's granulomatosis may have bony erosion into surrounding areas, including the orbit. Vasculitic inflammation in the nasal cavity and sinuses is sometimes difficult to differentiate from infection, especially in patients receiving immunosuppressive therapy. Patients with Wegener's granulomatosis may also have tracheal inflammation, especially in the subglottic region, resulting in stridor and sometimes critical airway narrowing that requires emergency tracheostomy. Upper airway disease may manifest itself as otitis media sometimes associated with entrapment of the seventh nerve and facial paralysis.

Some patients present with a renal-dermal vasculitic syndrome. The most common lesion consists of leukocytoclastic angiitis with purpuric lesions in the lower extremities. However, several other cutaneous lesions have been observed, including ecchymoses; erythematous, tender nodules; focal necrosis; ulceration; urticaria; and livedo reticularis.

Other organ system involvement with ANCA–small vessel vasculitis includes the gastrointestinal tract with abdominal complaints, nonhealing ulcers, and, rarely, transmural ischemic ulcers and bowel perforation. Nervous system disease primarily takes the form of a mononeuritis multiplex, whereas CNS vasculitis with seizures is less frequent. Cardiac involvement occurs uncommonly, taking the form of pericarditis or coronary artery vasculitis that results in either subendocardial or transmural myocardial infarctions. Ocular involvement may occur in the form of iritis or uveitis.

LABORATORY FINDINGS

Approximately 90% of patients with ANCA–small vessel vasculitis have autoantibodies either to MPO (MPO-ANCA) or to PR3 (PR3-ANCA).[89] MPO-ANCAs are predominant in patients with microscopic polyangiitis and Churg-Strauss syndrome, or with necrotizing and crescentic glomerulonephritis without extrarenal manifestations of disease, whereas PR3-ANCAs predominate in patients with Wegener's granulomatosis. Nonetheless, 20% to 30% of patients with Wegener's granulomatosis have MPO-ANCA, and approximately 20% to 30% of patients with necrotizing glomerulonephritis with no obvious extrarenal manifestations have a positive PR3-ANCA. Most patients have normal complement levels, and approximately 10% of patients have a positive ANA.

PROGNOSIS

The two main prognostic markers of the long-term outcome of patients with ANCA–small vessel vasculitis are the presence of pulmonary hemorrhage and entry serum creatinine. Pulmonary hemorrhage accounts for at least half of all deaths in the fulminant phase of disease. The long-term renal prognosis is largely associated with the entry serum creatinine.[90] The higher the serum creatinine level, the higher the risk of developing end-stage renal disease. Unlike in anti-GBM disease, no cutoff creatinine concentration could be identified above which the recovery of renal function was so unlikely as to withhold immunosuppressive therapy.

TREATMENT

The treatment of ANCA–small vessel vasculitis and glomerulonephritis rests primarily on the use of induc-tion methylprednisolone, high-dose corticosteroids, and cyclophosphamide in a regimen similar to that described for anti-GBM disease. Considering the importance of the serum creatinine concentration at the time treatment is initiated as a determinant of long-term renal outcome, pulse methylprednisolone (7 mg/kg per day for 3 days) is used to curb the active inflammation as soon as possible. This is followed by instituting daily prednisone at a dose of 1 mg/kg for the first month of therapy. Corticosteroids are then tapered over the second month to an alternate-day dosing and eventually discontinued by the end of the fourth to fifth month.

The beneficial role of cyclophosphamide in the treatment of acute ANCA–small vessel vasculitis is evidenced by the substantial improvement in the rate of re-emission (from 56% to 85%) and a threefold decrease in the risk of relapse associated with the use of this drug.[91] Cyclophosphamide may be administered either as monthly intravenous pulses or as a daily oral regimen. When the intravenous route is used, it is usually started at a dose of 0.5 g/m^2, which is subsequently increased to a maximal dose of 1 g/m^2. This dose is adjusted to maintain the 2-week leukocyte nadir above 3000 to 4000 cell/mm^3. The alternative approach is to use daily oral cyclophosphamide, given at a dose of 1.5 to 2 mg/kg per day.[92] To prevent severe leukopenia, careful attention to the leukocyte count must be maintained throughout this therapy. Cyclophosphamide is usually continued for a total of 6 to 12 months depending on the patient's response to treatment. Whether one form of cyclophosphamide therapy is superior to the other is a subject of continued investigation. Whereas a regimen of daily oral cyclophosphamide may be associated with a decreased risk of relapse (when compared with a regimen of monthly intravenous pulses),[93] this approach subjects the patients to three times the cumulative dose of cyclophosphamide and a higher rate of short- and long-term toxicities.

Patients presenting with pulmonary hemorrhage also benefit from the institution of plasmapheresis in a regimen similar to that used for anti-GBM disease. In our experience, early and aggressive institution of plasmapheresis has substantially diminished the mortality associated with massive pulmonary hemorrhage. Recent data suggest that plasmapheresis may also improve the renal outcome of patients who present with severe renal failure requiring dialysis. Plasmapheresis is typically performed daily until the pulmonary hemorrhage ceases and then every other day for a total of 7 to 10 treatments.

Once remission is attained, an alternative maintenance regimen consists of switching cyclophosphamide to oral azathioprine at the end of 3 months.[94] Azathioprine is then continued for a total of 12 to 24 months.

With the use of an alkylating agent, the rate of remission is of the order of 70% to 85%. Patients who require dialysis at the onset of their disease have a decreased probability of recovering sufficient renal function to discontinue dialysis (about 50%). Patients who do recover sufficient renal function do so within the first 3 months of treatment. For that reason, and in the absence of active extrarenal vasculitis, immunosuppression may be stopped after 3 months if no signs of renal recovery have occurred.

Relapse of ANCA–small vessel vasculitis occurs in about 30% of patients.[91] In our experience, 80% of relapses occur in the first 18 months after immunosuppressive therapy is discontinued. Recurrent disease may clinically resemble the initial presentation but is sometimes associated with new organ involvement. Whether ANCA titers are predictive of a relapse is a matter of controversy. To determine the occurrence of a relapse, serial measurements of ANCA titers should be interpreted only in the context of the clinical history and physical and laboratory examinations of the patient. Recurrent glomerulonephritis is usually indicated by the recurrence or worsening of hematuria with an increase in serum creatinine level. An increase in proteinuria alone or the gradual increase in the serum creatinine level without hematuria may be the result of progressive chronic scarring rather than recurrent active inflammation. Repeat renal biopsy is sometimes indicated to best differentiate between recurrent disease and progressive scarring, and avoid unnecessary immunosuppression in the latter case.

Relapsing ANCA–small vessel vasculitis responds to immunosuppression with corticosteroids and cytotoxic agents with a similar response rate as the initial disease. The decision regarding the repeat use of pulse methylprednisolone can be based on the total amount of corticosteroid that has been administered to the patient over the course of the disease, as well as the severity of the relapse. Patients with a history of relapsing disease may require the use of long-term "maintenance" immunosuppressive therapy with either low-dose prednisone or azathioprine.

ALTERNATIVE TREATMENT STRATEGIES

There has been substantial interest in the use of trimethoprim-sulfamethoxazole or co-trimoxazole in the treatment or the prevention of relapses in Wegener's granulomatosis.[95, 96] The beneficial effect of these antimicrobial agents appears to be limited to the management of nasal and upper respiratory tract vasculitis, whereas no benefit is seen with regard to disease affecting the kidneys or other organ systems.

Methotrexate has been evaluated in the treatment of ANCA–small vessel vasculitis as well, but its use is contraindicated in patients with a creatinine clearance below 60 mL/min.[97]

THERAPEUTIC CONSIDERATION COMMON TO ALL VASCULITIC SYNDROMES

Corticosteroids and intermittent intravenous cyclophosphamide therapy remain the mainstay of therapy of severe proliferative lupus nephritis, anti-GBM disease, and ANCA–small vessel vasculitis. This therapy is, however, associated with short- and long-term complications. The most prominent side effects of this form

of therapy are infection, ovarian failure (especially with a prolonged course of cyclophosphamide), bone disease, and cataract formation. Studies of long-term oral cyclophosphamide treatment for patients with Wegener's granulomatosis suggest that 15% of patients will develop transitional cell carcinoma of the bladder over the course of 5 to 10 years.[98] Whether the use of monthly pulse intravenous cyclophosphamide (which is associated with a smaller cumulative dose and a lower incidence of hemorrhagic cystitis) can reduce the rate of bladder cancer is not yet ascertained.

The institution of attentive supportive care is crucial in containing the short- and long-term side effects to a minimum level. Compulsive attention must be paid to the early detection and aggressive treatment of infections, especially in patients treated with pulse methylprednisolone, corticosteroids, and cyclophosphamide. Infectious complications of immunosuppression account for no less than 22% of deaths among patients with SLE.[99]

Whenever corticosteroids are used, measures must be taken to minimize the development of osteoporosis.[100] Specific recommendations include calcium (1.2 g of calcium daily) and vitamin D supplementation, and in selected patients with established osteoporosis, calcitonin nasal spray or alendronate for patients in whom the drug is not contraindicated (eg, azotemia or esophagitis). The role of estrogen replacement in patients with SLE is currently under investigation.

Rigorous control of blood pressure with sodium restriction and antihypertensive therapy is essential to minimize the additive effect of hypertension in loss of renal function following active nephritis. Current research directions include the preservation of gonadal function by hormonal manipulation during cytotoxic therapy. In a small study, the use of testosterone during cyclophosphamide treatment appeared to prevent azoospermia.[101] We are currently evaluating the use of the gonadotropin-releasing hormone agonist leuprolide for the prevention of cyclophosphamide-induced ovarian failure.

EXPERIMENTAL THERAPIES FOR ACUTE RPGN AND SYSTEMIC VASCULITIS

Some patients with proliferative lupus nephritis or ANCA–small vessel vasculitis and glomerulonephritis suffer from repeatedly relapsing disease. These patients are especially subject to the cumulative toxic effects of cytotoxic agents and corticosteroids, resulting in increased risk for long-term complications. It is in an effort to search for alternative—hopefully less toxic—therapies that a number of immunomodulatory drugs and antibodies are being evaluated. The efficacy of such agents is currently not established, and they should not be considered as first-line therapies, except as part of experimental protocols. Anecdotal reports and small pilot studies[102] suggest that mycophenolate mofetil may have a role in the treatment of lupus nephritis and ANCA–small vessel vasculitis. This role is currently under investigation in a randomized, multicenter trial for the treatment of lupus nephritis.

Other immunomodulatory molecules targeted to block specific inflammatory or lymphocyte costimulatory pathways are currently at various stages of evaluation in the treatment of SLE and ANCA–small vessel vasculitis.

THROMBOTIC MICROANGIOPATHIES

Thrombotic microangiopathies encompass a number of syndromes that are characterized by the presence of microangiopathic hemolytic anemia, thrombocytopenia associated with platelet aggregation in the microcirculation, and similar histologic findings of microvascular occlusion due in part to endothelial cell swelling, enlargement of the subendothelial space, and various degrees of thrombosis. They all may present with a syndrome of ARF, frequently associated with anuria, azotemia, and severe hypertension. The various syndromes include hemolytic-uremic syndrome (HUS), thrombotic thrombocytopenic purpura (TTP), scleroderma renal crisis, preeclampsia, and the thrombotic microangiopathy associated with malignant hypertension. The last diagnosis is usually one of exclusion in the absence of evidence supporting one of the other syndromes. The thrombotic microangiopathies may occur sporadically without an obvious precipitant, or they may be associated with an underlying infection (eg, diarrheal HUS or human immunodeficiency virus syndrome); rheumatologic disease (eg, SLE, progressive systemic sclerosis); malignancies; transplantation (especially bone marrow transplantation)[103]; the use of certain drugs (eg, cyclosporine, tacrolimus, mitomycin C,[104] ticlopidine,[105] and quinine[106]); coronary artery bypass surgery[107]; or pregnancy. This chapter focuses on TTP, HUS, and scleroderma renal crisis.

In part because of the similarities in clinical presentation, and because of our incomplete understanding of the pathogenetic mechanisms of the two syndromes, TTP and HUS are frequently lumped together and the two terms are sometimes used interchangeably. Clinically, the term *HUS* is usually ascribed to a syndrome more commonly seen in children, frequently associated with a diarrheal illness and marked by uremia, whereas TTP is usually ascribed to a syndrome more commonly seen in adults and marked by the prominence of neurologic symptoms. The clinical overlap of the two syndromes is such that a distinction between these two "diagnoses" is frequently difficult. Recent advances in the understanding of the pathogenetic mechanisms of disease may lead to a clearer classification of these diseases (Table 21–4).

Thrombotic Thrombocytopenic Purpura

TTP is classically defined as the pentad of microangiopathic hemolytic anemia, thrombocytopenia, renal failure, neurologic signs and symptoms, and fever. However, the full pentad of findings is often incomplete and may not be necessary to establish the diagnosis of TTP. Indeed, recent reviews suggest a decrease

TABLE 21–4. Major Features Differentiating "Typical" Hemolytic-Uremic Syndrome and Thrombotic Thrombocytopenic Purpura

HEMOLYTIC-UREMIC SYNDROME	THROMBOTIC THROMBOCYTOPENIC PURPURA
Predominantly in children	Predominantly in adults
Associated with diarrheal illness and verotoxin-producing *Escherichia coli*	No diarrheal illness, no pathogen
Predominance of uremic signs and symptoms	Predominance of neurologic signs and symptoms
Primary event is verotoxin-induced endothelial damage	Primary event is defect in von Willebrand factor (vWf) cleaving protease or vWf cleaving protease inhibitor

in the frequency of renal failure, neurologic symptoms, and fever over the last decades.[108] Clinically, the presentation of TTP differs from that of nondiarrheal HUS by its age group distribution and the prominence of neurologic signs and symptoms. However, the clinical overlap between the two diseases is such that they have been considered as the variable expression of a single disease entity.[109] In addition to idiopathic TTP, and the syndrome associated with the underlying diseases or treatments mentioned earlier, TTP may be a familial syndrome that follows an autosomal recessive inheritance, with a chronic, remitting and relapsing course.[110]

PATHOGENESIS

The pathogenesis of TTP is currently related to the production and release of unusually large multimers of von Willebrand factor (vWf) from endothelial cells. These unusually large multimers are more effective than the vWf multimers normally in plasma in binding to platelet receptors and stimulating their aggregation.[111] Normally these unusually large vWf multimers are reduced in size and stabilized by the action of a vWf cleaving protease.[112, 113] Recent studies of plasma from patients with chronic, relapsing TTP revealed a decrease or absence of vWf cleaving protease activity.[114] In patients with nonfamilial TTP, protease activity levels are severely or moderately depressed during the acute episode of TTP but normal at the time of remission.[115] In these patients the decrease in vWf cleaving protease activity was linked to the presence of an IgG inhibitor.[115, 116] In contrast, patients with nonfamilial HUS have either normal or near-normal levels of vWf cleaving protease.[115] In summary, it is proposed that patients with nonfamilial TTP have an autoimmune disease due to an acquired inhibitor of vWf cleaving protease, whereas patients with familial TTP have an underlying deficiency of this protease in the absence of an inhibitor.

TREATMENT

The cornerstone of treatment of TTP is therapeutic plasma exchange. Indeed, it is suggested that, in the absence of an alternative clinically apparent etiology, thrombocytopenia and microangiopathic hemolytic anemia are sufficient to establish a presumptive diagnosis of TTP and initiate plasma exchange. The current practices consist of daily plasma exchange (of 1 or 2 plasma volumes) until the platelet count exceeds 150,000/μL for 2 consecutive days[117] or until the lactate dehydrogenase level is near normal and the platelet count is above 100,000/μL and continues to rise after cessation of plasma exchange. There is center-to-center variation in the exact regimen followed and the choice of replacement fluid (fresh frozen plasma, cryoprecipitate poor plasma, or a combination of 5% albumin solution followed by fresh frozen plasma or cryoprecipitate poor plasma).[118] With plasma exchange, the median time to response is 8 days, but responses may take as long as 3 to 4 weeks to occur. Other therapies have included high-dose corticosteroids, antiplatelet agents, vincristine, intravenous gamma globulin, and splenectomy. Whether these agents have a beneficial effect beyond that of plasma exchange alone is not well established, and their use may be considered as adjunctive therapy for patients not responding to plasma exchange alone.

OUTCOME

The mortality rate of TTP remains about 10% to 20% even with the institution of therapeutic plasmapheresis,[119] and the relapse rate after plasma exchange is discontinued approaches 40%. The majority of deaths occur within the first 48 hours following presentation, underscoring the importance of a prompt diagnosis and immediate initiation of therapy.[118]

Hemolytic-Uremic Syndrome

HUS has traditionally been divided into categories called *typical* or *diarrhea-associated HUS* (D+HUS) and *atypical* or *nondiarrhea-associated HUS* (D-HUS). The epidemic syndrome typically associated with a diarrheal illness is mediated by a *Shigella*-like toxin, referred to as *shigatoxin* or *verotoxin*, and in North America is due to an infection with *Escherichia coli* O157:H7. A few patients present with the syndrome of HUS after urinary tract rather than gastrointestinal infection with the same organisms—which has prompted the use of the term *verotoxin* or *shigatoxin-associated HUS*.[120] This chapter addresses the pathogenesis and management of verotoxin-associated HUS.

CLINICAL PRESENTATION

Verotoxin-associated HUS is characterized by the sudden onset of microangiopathic hemolytic anemia with peripheral schistocytes, thrombocytopenia, and ARF typically following an episode of gastroenteritis and diarrhea. The diarrhea, which may be bloody, usually precedes the syndrome of HUS by 2 to 14 days. Unlike TTP, neurologic signs and symptoms are less prominent than those attributable to the ARF. HUS may vary in severity from a syndrome without anuria, need for dialysis, severe hypertension, and only rare seizures to one characterized by prolonged anuria requiring dialysis, severe hypertension, and seizures.[121]

Verotoxin-associated HUS may occur sporadically or may be part of an epidemic. The infections with verotoxin-producing *E. coli* (VTEC) are usually related to the consumption of poorly cooked meat products; however, person-to-person transmission is an important factor in the spread of epidemic HUS. This syndrome is more common in children than adults.

PATHOGENESIS

The pathogenesis of verotoxin-associated HUS is based on endothelial cell injury mediated by the verotoxin. After VTEC adhere to the colonic mucosal villi, they release the exotoxins. These exotoxins are made up of two subunits: The A subunit is enzymatically active, whereas the B subunit mediates binding to a glycolipid receptor Gb3.[120] Gb3 has been identified on renal epithelial, endothelial, and glomerular mesangial cells, as well as on erythrocytes, and germinal center B lymphocytes. After internalization of the verotoxin, endothelial cell injury ensues, as a result of cellular inhibition of protein synthesis by the A subunit.[122] Endothelial damage is further contributed by inflammatory mediators (tumor necrosis factor-α, interleukins), increased neutrophil adhesion and activation,[123, 124] and increased release of nitric oxide.[125] As a consequence of the endothelial cell damage, unusually large vWF multimers are released, resulting in sustained platelet activation and microvascular thrombosis.[126]

TREATMENT

The mainstay of treatment for verotoxin-associated HUS is supportive care, with particular attention to the management of fluid and electrolytes. Judicious volume replacement at the time of presentation is important in correcting the dehydration from diarrhea while avoiding volume overload or the development of hyponatremia.[127] Indications for hemodialysis are those of severe acidosis, volume overload, and hyperkalemia in an anuric patient. Azotemia alone, in the absence of oliguria, may not require the institution of renal replacement therapy.[128]

Neither fresh frozen plasma[129] nor plamapheresis[130] appears to be of benefit in the treatment of patients with verotoxin-associated HUS.

OUTCOME

The introduction of dialytic support has reduced the mortality rate associated with HUS from 30% of children to about 5%. Prolonged anuria is a predictor of poor short-term renal outcome and is a risk factor for chronic renal failure and eventually end-stage renal disease in patients who do recover renal function after the initial insult.[131, 132]

Progressive Systemic Sclerosis Renal Crisis

CLINICAL SYNDROME

As many as 75% of all patients with progressive systemic sclerosis have evidence of renal damage, and 50% have clinically evident renal disease. Some patients have mild proteinuria (typically <3 g/day) and varying degrees of mild renal insufficiency and hypertension. However, scleroderma renal crisis occurs in 10% to 15% of patients with progressive systemic sclerosis. It is defined as the new onset of accelerated arterial hypertension and/or acute onset of renal disease in a patient with either no or minimal prior evidence of renal injury.[133] The major risk factor for scleroderma renal crisis is the presence of diffuse systemic sclerosis because 20% to 25% of patients with diffuse disease suffer a renal crisis as opposed to only 1% of patients with limited disease.[134] Similarly, 75% to 80% of patients with renal crisis have obvious diffuse systemic sclerosis, and another 15% to 25% of patients are "destined" to develop diffuse disease.[135] Systemic sclerosis with diffuse scleroderma is characterized by (1) widespread skin involvement within months of disease onset affecting the trunk and proximal extremities and (2) the early visceral involvement of the gastrointestinal tract, heart, and kidneys. Serologically, diffuse systemic sclerosis is associated with the presence of antitopoisomerase I (anti-Scl-70) and anti-RNA polymerase III antibodies, the latter being more sensitive and specific.[136]

The estimated incidence of progressive systemic sclerosis is 100 to 200 per million, with a peak age of onset in the fourth to fifth decade and a female-to-male ratio of 4:1. It is more common in African Americans than whites. Scleroderma renal crisis occurs in about 10% of entire scleroderma population. Its incidence decreased from 22% of the population (at 5 years) between the years 1972 and 1979, to 9% at 5 years between 1980 and 1987. The decrease in incidence is probably due to the widespread use of D-penicillamine (shown in retrospective studies to decrease occurrence of scleroderma renal crisis), calcium channel blockers (for Raynaud's phenomenon), and angiotensin-converting enzyme (ACE) inhibitors (although there are no data demonstrating the ability of ACE inhibitors to prevent scleroderma renal crisis).

The symptoms associated with scleroderma renal crisis are related to the marked increase in blood pressure and consist of headache, blurred vision, encephalopathy, and sometimes seizures. The urinalysis may reveal a bland sediment, although some patients have microscopic hematuria, subnephrotic proteinuria, and granular casts. Red blood cell casts are rarely seen.

PATHOLOGY

The histologic findings in the acute renal crisis of progressive systemic sclerosis are those of a thrombotic microangiopathy. There is glomerular consolidation caused by subendothelial expansion and capillary thrombosis, fibrinoid necrosis of arterioles, and edematous intimal expansion in arteries. The chronic changes of progressive systemic sclerosis resemble chronic hypertensive injury and include fibrotic intimal thickening in arteries and glomerular sclerosis. As a consequence of the vascular changes, there may be signs of chronic tubulointerstitial disease, including interstitial fibrosis, tubular atrophy, and glomerular obsolescence. Some of the tubulointerstitial and glomerular disease may be a consequence of the thrombotic microangiopathy, whereas others are a consequence of hypertension.

PATHOGENESIS

The pathogenesis of scleroderma renal crisis is attributed to a decrease in renal plasma flow. This has been documented by a decrease in renal cortical perfusion in patients without renal failure and a loss of cortical flow in patients with scleroderma renal crisis. A phenomenon of acute decrease in renal blood flow with exposure to cold (renal Raynaud's) has also been described. The severe, persistent vasospasm is associated with a marked increase in renin levels during a renal crisis, whereas these levels are normal prior to the crisis. The activation of the renin-angiotensin system likely contributes to the perpetuation of the severe vasoconstriction and provides the basis for the treatment recommendations.

Precipitating factors of scleroderma renal crisis relate to situations in which renal blood flow is further compromised, such as cardiac dysfunction (effusions, arrhythmias, or congestive heart failure), hypotension (dehydration, sepsis, or antihypertensive medications), and nonsteroidal anti-inflammatory drugs (no convincing evidence). The use of corticosteroids at high doses (>40 mg) has been associated with the development of renal crisis.[137] It is, however, unclear as to whether corticosteroids precipitate renal crisis or whether they are most likely to be prescribed to patients with early aggressive, diffuse systemic sclerosis who are at high risk for scleroderma renal crisis.

The major risk factor for the development of scleroderma renal crisis is the presence of diffuse scleroderma.[138] African Americans are at a higher risk of developing scleroderma renal crisis than whites. Although antitopoisomerase antibodies are a marker of diffuse systemic sclerosis, they do not predict renal crisis among patients with diffuse disease. Anti-RNA polymerase III antibodies are almost exclusively seen in diffuse systemic sclerosis, and 24% of patients with these antibodies develop scleroderma renal crisis.

TREATMENT

Prior to the use of ACE inhibitors, less than 10% of patients with scleroderma renal crisis survived more than 3 months. This bleak prognosis even pushed treating physicians in late 1970s to resort to bilateral nephrectomy to aid in the management of hypertension and congestive heart failure.

The first report on the successful use of ACE inhibitor in the management of scleroderma renal crisis dates to 1979[139]; the findings were subsequently confirmed by other studies. Unfortunately, not all patients respond to ACE inhibitors in that these agents fail to control blood pressure alone or prevent renal failure in all patients. The major predictor of reversal of renal failure is the serum creatinine level, whereby renal failure is more likely to reverse if serum creatinine is less than 4 mg/dL. Despite the improved survival afforded by the use of ACE inhibitors, the mortality rate associated with scleroderma renal crisis remains as high as 44%. Predictors of death are age older than 55 years, male gender, initial serum creatinine level higher than 3 mg/dL, uncontrolled hypertension, and congestive heart failure. By multivariate analysis, only age and congestive heart failure remained predictors of death.[140]

On the other hand, renal failure resulting from scleroderma renal crisis (and other thrombotic microangiopathies) may recover several months after the institution of dialysis. In that respect, it is important to note that the continuation of ACE inhibitors after dialysis is started is associated with an increased chance of recovery of renal function, sometimes as late as after 18 months of dialysis.

A few patients may have scleroderma renal crisis without hypertension (*normotensive renal crisis*).[141] These patients may have a substantial increase in blood pressure (>20 mm Hg) above their baseline, even if the absolute measurement does not reach "hypertensive" levels (eg, an increase from 100/60 to 140/90 mm Hg). In these cases, the presence of an RPGN, microangiopathic hemolytic anemia, and/or thrombocytopenia must be documented. In their presence ACE inhibitors should be instituted to the maximum tolerated dose. Pulmonary hemorrhage is a life-threatening complication in patients with thrombocytopenia. Steroids and plasmapheresis have not been helpful in treating patients with normotensive renal crisis.

CONCLUSION

The acute glomerulonephritides and vasculitic syndromes account only for a small minority of ARF. They represent a varied group of diseases with protean clinical presentations and disparate etiologies and pathogenetic mechanisms. However, they share a common propensity to lead to a rapid deterioration of renal function and, left untreated, may be fatal. With a few exceptions, the short- and long-term outcomes of the patient rest on the early diagnosis and immediate institution of immunosuppressive treatment or plasmapheresis of exchange. Conversely, and despite the potential complications associated with these interventions, their astute institution has substantially decreased the mortality from these syndromes and often has led to dramatic clinical improvement.

REFERENCES

1. Hebert LA, Cosio FG, Neff JC: Diagnostic significance of hypocomplementemia. Kidney Int 1991; 39:811.
2. Tan EM, Cohen AS, Fries JF: The 1982 revised criteria for the classification of systemic lupus erythematosus. Arthritis Rheum 1982; 25:1271.
3. Sloan RP, Shwartz MM, Korbet SM, et al: Long-term outcome in systemic lupus erythematosus membranous glomerulonephritis. Lupus Nephritis Collaborative Study Group. J Am Soc Nephrol 1996; 7:299.
4. Pasquali S, Banfi G, Zucchelli A, et al: Lupus membranous nephropathy: long-term outcome. Clin Nephrol 1993; 39:175.
5. Appel GB, Cohen DJ, Pirani CL, et al: Long-term follow-up of lupus nephritis: a study based on the WHO classification. Am J Med 1987; 83:877.
6. Austin HA III, Muenz LR, Joyce KM, et al: Diffuse proliferative lupus nephritis: identification of specific pathologic features affecting renal outcome. Kidney Int 1984; 25:689.
7. Barada FA Jr, Andrews BS, Davis JS 4th, et al: Antibodies to Sm in patients with systemic lupus erythematosus: correlation of Sm antibody titers with disease activity and other laboratory parameters. Arthritis Rheum 1981; 24:1235.
8. Beaufils M, Kouki F, Mignan F, et al: Clinical significance of anti-SM antibodies in systemic lupus erythematosus. Am J Med 1983; 74:201.
9. Silva FG: The nephropathies of systemic lupus erythematosus. In: Rosen S, ed: *Pathology of Glomerular Diseases.* New York: Churchill Livingstone; 1983:79–124.
10. Felson DT, Anderson J: Evidence for the superiority of immunosuppressive drugs and prednisone over prednisone alone in lupus nephritis. N Engl J Med 1984; 311:1528.
11. Cameron JS: What is the role of long-term cytotoxic agents in the treatment of lupus nephritis? J Nephrol 1993; 6:172.
12. Balow JE, Austin HA, Muenz LR, et al: Effect of treatment on the evolution of renal abnormalities in lupus nephritis. N Engl J Med 1984; 311:491.
13. Esdaile JM, Joseph L, Mackenzie T, et al: The benefit of early treatment with immunosuppressive agents in lupus nephritis. J Rheumatol 1994; 21:2046.
14. Donadio JV, Holley KE, Ferguson RH, et al: Progressive lupus glomerulonephritis: treatment with prednisone and combined prednisone and cyclophosphamide. Mayo Clin Proc 1976; 51:484.
15. Donadio JV, Holley KE, Ferguson RH, et al: Treatment of diffuse proliferative lupus nephritis with prednisone and combined prednisone and cyclophosphamide. N Engl J Med 1978; 299:1151.
16. Austin HA, Klippel JH, Balow JE, et al: Therapy of lupus nephritis: controlled trial of prednisone and cytotoxic drugs. N Engl J Med 1986; 314:614.
17. Boumpas DT, Austin HA, Vaughn EM, et al: Controlled trial of pulse methylprednisolone versus two regimens of pulse cyclophosphamide in severe lupus nephritis. Lancet 1992; 340:741.
18. Balow JE, Boumpas DT, Fessler BJ, et al: Management of lupus nephritis. Kidney Int 1996; 53(Suppl):S-88.
19. Moroni G, Quaglini S, Maccario M, et al: "Nephritic flares" are predictors of bad long-term renal outcome in lupus nephritis. Kidney Int 1996; 50:2047.
20. Donadio JV, Holley KE, Wagoner RD, et al: Treatment of patients with lupus nephritis with prednisone and combined prednisone-azathioprine. Ann Intern Med 1972; 77:829.
21. Cade R, Spooner G, Schlein E, et al: Comparison of azathioprine, prednisone, and heparin alone or combined in treating lupus nephritis. Nephron 1973; 10:37.
22. Glas-Vos JW, Krediet RT, Weening JJ, et al: Treatment of proliferative lupus nephritis with methylprednisolone pulse therapy and oral azathioprine. Neth J Med 1995; 46:4.
23. Van Den Wall Bake AWL, Berden JHM, Derksen RHWM, et al: Therapy of proliferative lupus glomerulonephritis: a prospective trial in the Netherlands. Neth J Med 1994; 45:280.
24. Liebling MR, McLaughlin K, Boonsue S, et al: Monthly pulses of methylprednisolone in SLE nephritis. J Rheumatol 1982; 9:543.
25. Gourley MF, Austin HA III, Scott D, et al: Methylprednisolone and cyclophosphamide, alone or in combination, in patients with lupus nephritis: a randomized, controlled trial. Ann Internal Med 1996; 125:549.
26. Derksen RH, Hene RJ, Kallenberg CG, et al: Prospective multi-

centre trial on the short-term effects of plasma exchange versus cytotoxic drugs in steroid-resistant lupus nephritis. Neth J Med 1988; 33:168.

27. Lewis EJ, Hunsicker LG, Lan SP, et al: A controlled trial of plasmapheresis therapy in severe lupus nephritis. The Lupus Nephritis Collaborative Study Group. N Engl J Med 1992; 326:1373.

28. Favre H, Miescher PA, Huang YP, et al: Cyclosporin in the treatment of lupus nephritis. Am J Nephrol 1989; 9(Suppl 1):57.

29. Fu LW, Yang LY, Chen WP, Lin CY: Clinical efficacy of cyclosporin a neoral in the treatment of paediatric lupus nephritis with heavy proteinuria. Br J Rheumatol 1998; 37:217.

30. Dooley MA, Hogan S, Jennette CJ, et al: Cyclophosphamide therapy for lupus nephritis: poor renal survival in black Americans. Kidney Int 1997; 51:1188.

31. Austin HA, Boumpas DT, Vaughn EM, et al: High-risk features of lupus nephritis: importance of race and clinical and histological factors in 166 patients. Nephrol Dial Transplant 1995; 10:1620.

32. Freedman BI, Wilson CH, Spray BJ, et al: Familial clustering of end-stage renal disease in blacks with lupus nephritis. Am J Kidney Dis 1997; 29:729.

33. Howard PF, Hochberg MC, Bias WB, et al: Relationship between C4 null alleles, HLA-D region antigens, and genetic susceptibility to systemic lupus erythematosus in Caucasians and black Americans. Am J Med 1986; 81:187.

34. Salmon JE, Millard S, Schachter LA, et al: FcγRIIA alleles are heritable risk factors for lupus nephritis in African Americans. J Clin Invest 1996; 97:1348.

35. Petri M, Perez-Gutthann S, Longenecker C, et al: Morbidity of systemic lupus erythematosus: role of race and socioeconomic status. Am J Med 1991; 91:345.

36. Reveille JD, Bartolucci A, Alarcon GS: Prognosis in systemic lupus erythematosus: negative impact of increasing age at onset, Black race, and thrombocytopenia, as well as causes of death. Arthritis Rheum 1990; 33:37.

37. Goldstein AR, White RHR, Akuser R, et al: Long-term follow-up of childhood Henoch-Schönlein nephritis. Lancet 1992; 339:280.

38. Blanco R, Martiniz-Taboada VM, Rodriguez-Valverde V, et al: Henoch-Schönlein purpura in adulthood and childhood: two different expressions of the same syndrome. Arthritis Rheum 1997; 40:859.

39. Agnello V: The etiology and pathophysiology of mixed cryoglobulinemia secondary to hepatitis C virus infection. Springer Semin Immunopathol 1997; 19:111.

40. Pascual M, Perrin L, Giostra E, et al: Hepatitis C virus in patients with cryoglobulinemia type II. J Infect Dis 1990; 162:569.

41. Durand JM, Lefevre P, Harle JR, et al: Cutaneous vasculitis and cryoglobulinemia type II associated with hepatitis C virus infection. Lancet 1991; 337:599.

42. Burstein DM, Rodby RA: Membranous glomerulonephritis associated with hepatitis C virus infection. J Am Soc Nephrol 1993; 4:1288.

43. Misiani R, Bellavita P, Fenili D, et al: Hepatitis C virus infection in patients with essential mixed cryoglobulinemia. Ann Intern Med 1992; 117:573.

44. Agnello V, Chunt RT, Kaplan LM: A role for hepatitis C virus infection in type II cryoglobulinemia. N Engl J Med 1992; 327:1490.

45. D'Amico G, Fornasieri A: Cryoglobulinemic glomerulonephritis: a membranoproliferative glomerulonephritis induced by hepatitis C virus. Am J Kidney Dis 1995; 25:361.

46. Tarantino A, Campise M, Banfi G, et al: Long-term predictors of survival in essential mixed cryoglobulinemic glomerulonephritis. Kidney Int 1995; 47:618.

47. Misiani R, Bellavita P, Fenili D, et al: Interferon alpha-2a therapy in cryoglobulinemia associated with hepatitis C virus. N Engl J Med 1994; 330:751.

48. Carithers RL Jr, Emerson SS: Therapy of hepatitis C: meta-analysis of interferon alfa-2b trials. Hepatology 1997; 26 (Suppl 1):83S.

49. Reichard O, Schvarcz R, Weiland O: Therapy of hepatitis C: alpha interferon and ribavirin. Hepatology 1997; 26(Suppl 1):108S.

50. Ferri C, Moriconi L, Gremignai G, et al: Treatment of the renal involvement in mixed cryoglobulinemia with prolonged plasma exchange. Nephron 1986; 43:246–253.

51. Bombardieri S, Ferri C, Paleologo G, et al: Prolonged plasma exchange in the treatment of renal involvement in essential mixed cryoglobulinemia. Int J Art Organs 1983; 6(Suppl 1):47.

52. Jennette JC, Falk RJ: The pathology of vasculitis involving the kidney. Am J Kidney Dis 1994; 24:130.

53. Kelly PT, Haponik EF: Goodpasture syndrome: molecular and clinical advances. Medicine 1994; 73:171.

54. Border WA, Baehler RW, Bhathena D, et al: IgA antibasement membrane nephritis with pulmonary hemorrhage. Ann Intern Med 1979; 91:21.

55. Rees AJ, Peters DK: Strong association between HLA-DRw2 and antibody-mediated Goodpasture's syndrome. Lancet 1978; 1:966.

56. Fisher M, Pusey CD, Vaughan RW, et al: Susceptibility to antiglomerular basement membrane disease is strongly associated with HLA-DRB1 genes. Kidney Int 1997; 51:222.

57. McPhaul JJ Jr, Mullins JD: Glomerulonephritis mediated by antibody to glomerular basement membrane: immunological, clinical, and histopathological characteristics. J Clin Invest 1976; 57:351.

58. Poskitt TR: Immunologic and electron microscopic studies in Goodpasture's syndrome. Am J Med 1970; 49:250.

59. Wieslander J, Barr JF, Butkowski RJ, et al: Goodpasture antigen of the glomerular basement membrane: localization to noncollagenous regions of type IV collagen. Proc Natl Acad Sci U S A 1984; 81:3828.

60. Hellmark T, Segelmark M, Wieslander J: Anti-GBM antibodies in Goodpasture syndrome: anatomy of an epitope. Nephrol Dial Transplant 1997; 12:646.

61. Hellmark T, Johansson C, Wieslander J: Characterization of anti-GBM antibodies involved in Goodpasture's syndrome. Kidney Int 1994; 46:823.

62. Kalluri R, Sun MJ, Hudson BG, et al: The Goodpasture autoantigen: structural delineation of two immunologically privileged epitopes on alpha3(IV) chain of type IV collagen. J Biol Chem 1996; 271:9062.

63. Saxena R, Bygren P, Butkowski R, et al: Entactin: a possible auto-antigen in the pathogenesis of non-Goodpasture anti-GBM nephritis. Kidney Int 1990; 38:263.

64. Kalluri R, Meyers K, Mogyorosi A, et al: Goodpasture syndrome involving overlap with Wegener's granulomatosis and anti-glomerular basement membrane disease. J Am Soc Nephrol 1997; 8:1795.

65. Short AK, Esnault VL, Lockwood CM: Anti-neutrophil cytoplasm antibodies and anti-glomerular basement membrane antibodies: two coexisting distinct autoreactivities detectable in patients with rapidly progressive glomerulonephritis. Am J Kidney Dis 1995; 26:439.

66. Hellmark T, Niles JL, Collins AB, et al: Comparison of anti-GBM antibodies in sera with or without ANCA. J Am Soc Nephrol 1997; 8:376.

67. Heeringa P, Brouwer E, Klok PA, et al: Autoantibodies to myeloperoxidase aggravate mild anti-glomerular basement membrane–mediated glomerular injury in the rat. Am J Pathol 1996; 149:1695.

68. Merkel F, Kalluri R, Marx M, et al: Autoreactive T-cells in Goodpasture's syndrome recognize the N-terminal NC1 domain on α_3 type IV collagen. Kidney Int 1996; 49:1127.

69. Kalluri R, Danoff TM, Okada H, et al: Susceptibility to antiglomerular basement membrane disease and Goodpasture syndrome is linked to MHC class II genes and the emergence of T cell–mediated immunity in mice. J Clin Invest 1997; 100:2263.

70. Walker RG, Scheinkestel C, Becker GJ, et al: Clinical and morphological aspects of the management of crescentic antiglomerular basement membrane antibody (anti-GBM) nephritis/Goodpasture's syndrome. Q J Med 1985; 54:75.

71. Zimmerman SW, Groehler K, Beirne GJ: Hydrocarbon exposure and chronic glomerulonephritis. Lancet 1975; 2:199.

72. Rees AJ, Lockwood CM, Peters DK: Enhanced allergic tissue injury in Goodpasture's syndrome by intercurrent bacterial infection. BMJ 1977; 2:723.

73. Segelmark M, Butkowski R, Wieslander J: Antigen restriction and IgG subclasses among anti-GBM autoantibodies. Nephrol Dial Transplant 1990; 5:991.

74. Lang CH, Brown DC, Staley N, et al: Goodpasture syndrome treated with immunosuppression and plasma exchange. Arch Intern Med 1977; 137:1076.

75. Johnson JP, Whitman W, Briggs WA, et al: Plasmapheresis and immunosuppressive agents in antibasement membrane antibody-induced Goodpasture's syndrome. Am J Med 1978; 64:354.

76. Glassock RJ: The role of high-dose steroids in nephritic syndromes: the case for a conservative approach. In: Narins R, ed: *Controversies in Nephrology and Hypertension*. New York: Churchill Livingstone; 1984:421.

77. Bolton WK: The role of high-dose steroids in nephritic syndromes: the case for aggressive use. In: Narins R, ed: *Controversies in Nephrology and Hypertension*. New York: Churchill Livingstone; 1984:421.

78. Peters DK, Rees AJ, Lockwood CM, et al: Treatment and prognosis in antibasement membrane antibody-mediated nephritis. Tran Proc 1982; 14:513.

79. Madore F, Lazarus JM, Brady HR: Therapeutic plasma exchange in renal diseases. J Am Soc Nephrol 1996; 7:367.

80. Merkel F, Pullig O, Marx M, et al: Course and prognosis of anti-basement membrane antibody (anti-BM-Ab)-mediated disease: report of 35 cases. Nephrol Dial Transplant 1994; 9:372.

81. Jayne DR, Marshall PD, Jones SJ, et al: Autoantibodies to GBM and neutrophil cytoplasm in rapidly progressive glomerulonephritis. Kidney Int 1990; 37:965.

82. Dahlberg PJ, Kurtz SB, Donadio JV, et al: Recurrent Goodpasture's syndrome. Mayo Clin Proc 1978; 53:533.

83. Wu MJ, Moorthy AV, Beirne GJ: Relapse in anti-glomerular basement membrane antibody-mediated crescentic glomerulonephritis. Clin Nephrol 1980; 13:97.

84. Almkuist RD, Buckalew VM Jr, Hirszel P, et al: Recurrence of anti-glomerular basement membrane antibody-mediated glomerulonephritis in an isograft. Clin Immunol Immunopathol 1981; 18:54.

85. Jennette JC, Falk RJ, Andrassy K, et al: Nomenclature of systemic vasculitides: proposal of an International Consensus Conference. Arthritis Rheum 1994; 37:187.

86. Falk RJ, Hogan S, Carey TS, et al: Clinical course of antineutrophil cytoplasmic autoantibody-associated glomerulonephritis and systemic vasculitis. The Glomerular Disease Collaborative Network. Ann Intern Med 1990; 113:656.

87. Savage COS, Winearls CG, Evans DJ, et al: Microscopic polyarteritis: presentation, pathology, and prognosis. Q J Med 1985; 220:467.

88. Savage COS, Harper L, Adu D: Primary systemic vasculitis. Lancet 1997; 349:553.

89. Hagan EC, Ballieux BE, van Es LA, et al: Antineutrophil cytoplasmic autoantibodies: a review of the antigens involved, the assays, and the clinical and possible pathogenetic consequences. Blood 1993; 91:1996.

90. Hogan SL, Nachman PH, Wilkman AS, et al: Prognostic markers in patients with antineutrophil cytoplasmic autoantibody-associated microscopic polyangiitis and glomerulonephritis. J Am Soc Nephrol 1996; 7:23.

91. Nachman PH, Hogan SL, Jennette JC, et al: Treatment response and relapse in antineutrophil cytoplasmic autoantibody-associated microscopic polyangiitis and glomerulonephritis. J Am Soc Nephrol 1996; 7:33.

92. Hoffman GS, Kerr GS, Leavitt RY, et al: Wegener's granulomatosis: an analysis of 158 patients. Ann Intern Med 1992; 116:488.

93. Guillevin L, Cordier JF, Lhote F, et al: A prospective, multicenter, randomized trial comparing steroids and pulse cyclophosphamide versus steroids and oral cyclophosphamide in the treatment of generalized Wegener's granulomatosis. Arthritis Rheum 1997; 40:2187.

94. Pusey CD, Rees AJ, Evans DJ, et al: Plasma exchange in focal necrotizing glomerulonephritis without anti-GBM antibodies. Kidney Int 1991; 40:757.

95. DeRemee RA, McDonald TJ, Weiland LH: Wegener's granulomatosis: observations on treatment with antimicrobial agents. Mayo Clin Proc 1985; 60:27.

96. Stegeman CA, Cohen Tervaert JW, de Jong PE, et al: Trimethoprim-sulfamethoxazole (co-trimoxazole) for the prevention of relapses of Wegener's granulomatosis. Dutch Co-Trimoxazole Wegener Study Group. N Engl J Med 1996; 335:16.

97. Sneller MC, Hoffman GS, Talar-Williams C, et al: An analysis of forty-two Wegener's granulomatosis patients treated with methotrexate and prednisone. Arthritis Rheum 1995; 38:608.

98. Tarlar-Williams C, Hijazi YU, Walther MM, et al: Cyclophosphamide-induced cystitis and bladder cancer in patients with Wegener's granulomatosis. Ann Intern Med 1996; 124:477.

99. Ward MM, Pyun E, Studenski S: Causes of death in systemic lupus erythematosus: long-term follow up of an inception cohort. Arthritis Rheum 1995; 38:1492.

100. 1996 American College of Rheumatology Guidelines for the Prevention and Treatment of Glucocorticoid-Induced Osteoporosis. Arthritis Rheum 1996; 39:1791.

101. Masala A, Faedda R, Alagna S, et al: Use of testosterone to prevent cyclophosphamide-induced azoospermia. Ann Intern Med 1997; 126:292.

102. Dooley MA, Cosio FG, Nachman PH, et al: Mycophenolate mofetil therapy in lupus nephritis: clinical observations. J Am Soc Nephrol 1999; 10:833.

103. Verburgh CA, Vermeij CG, Zijlmans JM, et al: Haemolytic-uraemic syndrome following bone marrow transplantation: case report and review of the literature. Nephrol Dial Transplant 1996; 11:1332.

104. Moake JL, Byrnes JJ: Thrombotic microangiopathies associated with drugs and bone marrow transplantation. Hematol Oncol Clin North Am 1996; 10:485.

105. Bennett CL, Weinberg PD, Rozenberg-Ben-Dror K, et al: Thrombotic thrombocytopenic purpura associated with ticlopidine: a review of 60 cases. Ann Intern Med 1998; 128:541.

106. Gottschall JL, Neahring B, McFarland JG, et al: Quinine-induced immune thrombocytopenia with hemolytic-uremic syndrome: clinical and serological findings in nine patients and review of literature. Am J Hematol 1994; 47:283.

107. Pavlovsky M, Weinstein R: Thrombotic thrombocytopenic purpura following coronary artery bypass graft surgery: prospective observations of an emerging syndrome. J Clin Apheresis 1997; 12:159.

108. George JN, Gilcher RO, Smith JW, et al: Thrombotic thrombocytopenic purpura-hemolytic-uremic syndrome: diagnosis and management. J Clin Apheresis 1998; 13:120.

109. Remuzzi G: HUS and TTP: variable expression of a single entity. Kidney Int 1987; 32:292.

110. Berns JS, Kaplan BS, Mackow RC, et al: Inherited hemolytic-uremic syndrome in adults. Am J Kidney Dis 1992; 19:331.

111. Moake JL, Turner NA, Stathopoulos NA, et al: Shear-induced platelet aggregation can be mediated by vWF released from platelets, as well as by exogenous large or unusually large vWF multimers, requires adenosine diphosphate, and is resistant to aspirin. Blood 1988; 71:1366.

112. Moake JL, Chow TW: Increased von Willebrand factor (vWf) binding to platelets associated with impaired vWf breakdown in thrombotic thrombocytopenic purpura. J Clin Apheresis 1998; 13:126.

113. Furlan M, Robles R, Lamie B: Partial purification and characterization of a protease from human plasma cleaving von Willebrand factor to fragments produced by in vivo proteolysis. Blood 1996; 87:4223.

114. Furlan M, Robles R, Solenthaler M, et al: Deficient activity of von Willebrand factor cleaving protease in chronic relapsing thrombotic thrombocytopenic purpura. Blood 1997; 89:3097.

115. Furlan M, Robles R, Galbusera M, et al: von Willebrand factor cleaving protease in thrombotic thrombocytopenic purpura and the hemolytic-uremic syndrome. N Engl J Med 1998; 339:1578.

116. Tsai HM, Lian EC: Antibodies to von Willebrand factor cleaving protease in acute thrombotic thrombocytopenic purpura. N Engl J Med 1998; 339:1585.

117. Guidelines for therapeutic hemapheresis: American Association of Blood Banks, 1992–1993. Bethesda, MD: AABB Extracorporeal Therapy Committee; 1992.

118. Bandarenko N, Brecher ME: United States Thrombotic Thrombocytopenic Purpura Apheresis Study Group (US TTP ASG):

multicenter survey and retrospective analysis of current efficacy of therapeutic plasma exchange. J Clin Apheresis 1998; 13:133.

119. Bell WR, Braine HG, Ness PM, et al: Improved survival in thrombotic thrombocytopenic purpura–hemolytic-uremic syndrome: clinical experience in 108 patients. N Engl J Med 1991; 325:398.

120. Arbus GS: Association of verotoxin-producing E. coli and verotoxin with hemolytic-uremic syndrome. Kidney Int 1997; 58(Suppl):S91.

121. Kaplan BS, Katz J, Krawitz S, et al: An analysis of the results of therapy in 67 cases of the hemolytic-uremic syndrome. J Pediatr 1971; 78:420.

122. Remuzzi G, Ruggenenti P: The hemolytic-uremic syndrome. Kidney Int 1995; 48:2.

123. Forsyth KD, Simpson AC, Fitzpatrick MM, et al: Neutrophil-mediated endothelial injury in haemolytic-uraemic syndrome. Lancet 1989; 2:411.

124. Fitzpatrick MM, Shah V, Trompeter RS, et al: Interleukin-8 and polymorphoneutrophil leucocyte activation in hemolytic-uremic syndrome of childhood. Kidney Int 1992; 42:951.

125. Noris M, Ruggenenti P, Todeschini M, et al: Increased nitric oxide formation in recurrent thrombotic microangiopathies: a possible mediator of microvascular injury. Am J Kidney Dis 1996; 27:790.

126. Ruggenenti P, Lutz J, Remuzzi G: Pathogenesis and treatment of thrombotic microangiopathy. Kidney Int 1997; 58(Suppl): S97.

127. Kaplan BS, Meyers KE, Schulman SL: The pathogenesis and treatment of hemolytic-uremic syndrome. J Am Soc Nephrol 1998; 9:1126.

128. Schulman SL, Kaplan BS: Management of patients with hemolytic-uremic syndrome demonstrating severe azotemia but not anuria. Pediatr Nephrol 1996; 10:671.

129. Rizzoni G, Claris-Appiani A, Edefonti A, et al: Plasma infusion for hemolytic-uremic syndrome in children: results of a multicenter controlled trial. J Pediatr 1988; 112:284.

130. Gianviti A, Perna A, Caringella A, et al: Plasma exchange in children with hemolytic-uremic syndrome at risk of poor outcome. Am J Kidney Dis 1993; 22:264.

131. Schieppati A, Ruggenenti P, Cornejo RP, et al: Renal function at hospital admission as a prognostic factor in adult hemolytic-uremic syndrome. The Italian Registry of Haemolytic-Uremic Syndrome. J Am Soc Nephrol 1992; 2:1640.

132. Repetto HA: Epidemic hemolytic-uremic syndrome in children. Kidney Int 1997; 52:1708.

133. Steen VD: Scleroderma renal crisis. Rheum Dis Clin North Am 1996; 22:861.

134. Black CM: Scleroderma. In: Oxford Textbook of Clinical Nephrology. Oxford, England: Oxford University Press; 1992.

135. Steen VD, Medsger TA Jr: The palpable tendon friction rub: an important physical examination finding in patients with systemic sclerosis. Arthritis Rheum 1997; 40:1146.

136. Okano Y, Steen VD, Medsger TA Jr: Autoantibody reactive with RNA polymerase III in systemic sclerosis. Ann Intern Med 1993; 119:1005.

137. Steen VD, Medsger TA Jr: Case control study of corticosteroids and other drugs that either precipitate or protect from the development of scleroderma renal crisis. Arthritis Rheum 1998; 41:1613.

138. Steen VD, Medsger TA, Osial TA, et al: Factors predicting development of renal involvement in progressive systemic sclerosis. Am J Med 1984; 76:779.

139. Lopez-Overjero JA, Sall SD, D'Angelo WA, et al: Reversal of vascular and renal crises of scleroderma by oral angiotensin-converting enzyme blockade. N Engl J Med 1979; 300:1417.

140. Steen VD, Medsger TA Jr: Epidemiology and natural history of systemic sclerosis. Rheum Dis Clin North Am 1990; 16:1.

141. Helfrich DJ, Banner B, Steen VD, et al: Normotensive renal failure in systemic sclerosis. Arthritis Rheum 1989; 32:1128.

CHAPTER 22

Acute Renal Failure as a Result of Infectious Diseases

Luis Yu ▪ Emmanuel A. Burdmann

There is a close relationship between renal impairment and infectious diseases. Infections may cause several renal disorders such as acute renal failure (ARF), interstitial nephritis, glomerulonephritis, and hemolytic-uremic syndrome (HUS) (Table 22–1). Indeed, the risk of developing ARF is greater in infected patients than in noninfected patients. Additionally, infectious agents may complicate the course of ARF, affecting adversely patients' outcome.[1–4]

Infection-induced ARF is more frequent in hospitalized patients, especially in critically ill patients, than in community patients.[5–8] On the other hand, drug-induced nephrotoxicity and infection-related causes were the most common etiologies in community-acquired ARF as reported by Kaufman and associates.[9] In hospitalized patients, infections are more frequent in intensive care unit (ICU) patients as compared with non-ICU patients. The incidence of sepsis in ARF patients from renal units varies from 22% to 41%[5, 7, 10] compared with 57% to 75% in medical and surgical ICUs.[11–14] In a multicenter study performed in Madrid, the incidence of sepsis in ICU patients was 35.4% compared with 26.9% in non-ICU patients.[15] In a French multicenter study,[16] the incidence of sepsis in severe critically ill ARF patients was 48%. Infections are frequent in the ICU: The Centers for Disease Control and Prevention found a median overall infection rate of 9.2 infections per 100 patients with a strong positive correlation with average length of ICU stay.[17] Additionally, sepsis has been increasingly reported as a cause of ARF over the last decades, becoming one of the main causes of ARF. Turney and colleagues[8] analyzed the evolution of ARF from 1956 to 1988 and observed that the incidence of sepsis rose from 13.3% in late 1960s to 23.9% in the period between 1980 to 1988. Biesenbach and coworkers[3] reported that in 710 cases of ARF treated over a 15-year period, sepsis was a major cause of ARF, and the incidence increased in trauma patients from 7% in the period of 1975 to 1979 to 28% during the period of 1985 to 1989. In our tertiary university hospital, sepsis was present in 9% of ARF patients during the period between 1957 and

TABLE 22–1. Renal Disorders in Infectious Diseases

Acute renal failure and acute tubular necrosis
Postinfectious glomerulonephritis
Interstitial nephritis
Hemolytic-uremic syndrome
Disseminated intravascular coagulation

TABLE 22–2. Infectious Agents Associated With Acute Renal Disorders

TYPE	AGENTS OR INFECTION
Bacteria	*Staphylococcus, Streptococcus, Pseudomonas aeruginosa, Salmonella, Shigella, Legionella, Leptospira, Listeria, Pasteurella, Bacillus cereus, Clostridium perfringens*
Viruses	HIV, Hantaviruses, hepatitis A and B, echovirus, Epstein-Barr virus, influenza virus, Coxsackie A and B, cytomegalovirus, adenovirus, varicella, measles, mumps
Mycoplasms and rickettsia	
Fungi	*Candida,* mucormycosis
Parasites	Malaria

HIV, human immunodeficiency virus.

1966, increasing afterward to 15% during 1980 to 1982, and finally reaching an incidence of 35% in 1993.[18]

Several infectious agents may cause or complicate ARF patients (Table 22–2). There is little information regarding infection-related cause in community ARF patients, mostly consisting of episodic reports of specific infections causing ARF. In hospitals, especially in the ICU, several pathogens may cause infections associated to ARF. Jarvis[19] reported in a 10-year epidemiologic investigation of nosocomial outbreaks that 62% were caused by bacterial pathogens, 9% by fungi, 8% by viruses, 4% by mycobacteria, and 18% by toxins or other organisms. The European Prevalence of Infection in Intensive Care (EPIC) study in Europe,[20] which evaluated the prevalence of nosocomial infection in the ICU, found that 44.8% of patients were infected, with 20.6% of these patients with ICU-acquired infections. The most frequent types of ICU infections were pneumonia, lower respiratory tract infection, urinary tract infection, and blood stream infection. The most frequent microorganisms were Enterobacteriaceae (34.4%), *Staphylococcus aureus* (30.1%), *Pseudomonas aeruginosa* (28.7%), coagulase-negative staphylococci (19.1%), and fungi (17.1%).

RENAL DISORDERS IN INFECTIOUS DISEASES

Infections, especially bacterial infections, may cause multiple renal dysfunctions such as sepsis-induced ARF, which is one of the main causes of ARF currently.

In addition, ARF may occur in viral diseases, especially human immunodeficiency virus (HIV)–infected patients and in parasitic infections. Renal involvement in infectious diseases may occur in other forms, such as postinfectious glomerulonephritis, acute interstitial nephritis (AIN), and HUS. Although these latter renal disorders are less frequent, renal insufficiency in these circumstances may be as severe as ARF in multiorgan dysfunction syndrome (MODS).

Postinfectious Glomerulonephritis

Acute poststreptococcal glomerulonephritis is the most common form of postinfectious glomerulonephritis, accounting for 10% to 20% of the ARF due to glomerular disease. It is more frequent in children than in adults in whom idiopathic forms of rapidly progressive glomerulonephritis occur more often.[21, 22] A similar renal disorder may occur following several other types of infections, such as bacterial, rickettsial, viral, mycoplasmal, fungal, protozoal, helminthic, and spirochetal.[23] In most cases, nonstreptococcal agents cause a similar glomerulonephritis, usually milder, that resolves with infection eradication. However, severe cases of acute proliferative glomerulonephritis have been described in septic patients, primarily related to chronic localized infection such as visceral abscesses,[24] subacute bacterial endocarditis,[25, 26] and infected ventriculoatrial shunts.[27] In these situations, eradication of abscesses or localized infections is also the treatment for glomerulonephritis. Furthermore, infections are frequently implicated in initiating or causing relapses of vasculitis diseases, such as in Wegener's granulomatosis, microscopic polyarteritis, and Henoch-Schönlein purpura. Usually, renal involvement is manifested by focal necrotizing glomerulonephritis, often with glomerular epithelial crescents that may lead to a rapidly progressive outcome.[28] Because these vasculitis disorders, particularly Wegener's granulomatosis, often occur in the presence of active infection, prophylactic use of antibiotics has been postulated to prevent relapses of the disease.[29]

Acute Interstitial Nephritis

Acute interstitial nephritis was reported associated with bacteria, viruses, and other organisms such as *Mycoplasma* and *Rickettsia*,[30, 31] *Chlamydia*,[32] *Yersinia*,[33] *Candida*,[34] and *Leptospira*.[35, 36] It is a common renal complication of viral infections such as cytomegalovirus[37] and Epstein-Barr virus.[38, 39] Molecules from the infectious agents may be present in the renal parenchyma that could lead to a crossing inflammatory reaction with tubulointerstitial structures.[40] Usually, patients with infectious AIN are simultaneously using analgesics, anti-inflammatory drugs, and/or antibiotics that also could cause interstitial nephritis. Clinical and laboratory manifestations of infection and drug-induced AIN, including fever, skin rash, eosinophilia, and eosinophiluria, are similar except for the skin rash

that is more frequent in allergic AIN, especially when caused by β-lactam antibiotics.[39, 41] However, the absence of these manifestations does not exclude the diagnosis of AIN. The classic AIN triad—rash, fever, eosinophilia—was seen in less than 30% of the patients in some series.[42] The interstitial infiltrate in drug-induced AIN usually presents lymphocytes, monocytes/macrophages, plasmocytes, and eosinophils, whereas in infectious-induced AIN, neutrophils predominate, with few eosinophils.[43, 44] Treatment of AIN is mostly supportive, in which potentially offending drugs should be discontinued and infections treated. In patients whose renal function does not improve after infection treatment and/or drug withdrawal, a renal biopsy should be considered to confirm an AIN diagnosis and to evaluate the degree of interstitial fibrosis. In those patients with histology showing acute inflammation and minimal interstitial fibrosis, immunosuppressive drugs such as corticosteroids may be considered. There are a few small, uncontrolled studies demonstrating a beneficial effect of steroids on the course of AIN.[40, 45, 46] However, there is no prospective, randomized clinical trial assessing the efficacy of such a regimen.[47]

Hemolytic-Uremic Syndrome

Hemolytic-uremic syndrome is characterized by a nonimmune hemolytic anemia, thrombocytopenia, platelet thrombi in kidney microcirculation, and renal failure.[48] The overall incidence rate is estimated to be 2.1 cases/100,000 persons/year, with a peak incidence in children younger than 5 years old.[49] Most cases are associated with bloody diarrheal prodrome caused by *Escherichia coli*, which produces Shiga-like toxins (verotoxins 1 and 2), and the most common *E. coli* serotype is 0157:H7.[50, 51] There is only one another significant agent associated with HUS, the *Shigella dysenteriae* I (shigellosis), which produces Shiga toxin.[52, 53] It is estimated that following exposure to this *E. coli* serotype, 38% to 61% of the contaminants will develop hemorrhagic colitis, with 2% to 7% of these patients developing complete HUS.[48] In Argentina, free verotoxin was demonstrated in 48% of children, whereas *E. coli* infection was present in only 2%, suggesting that other verotoxin-producing agents may cause HUS.[54] The incidence of HUS is higher in Argentina compared with other countries. In addition, the incidence of Shiga toxin causing gastroenteritides is around 23% in Argentina compared with 0.6% to 2.4% in other countries.[55] Reports have noted an association of HUS with HIV infection as well as with other viruses such as Coxsackie,[56] influenza, and hepatitis A.[48, 57] The main feature in HUS is the endothelial injury with activation and adherence of platelets to the site of damage, causing thrombotic microangiopathy. Although knowledge of the pathophysiology has greatly expanded, the exact pathogenic mechanism remains to be elucidated. Therapeutic management includes supportive therapy, aiming at prompt correction of hypovolemia due to diarrhea and vomiting and control of hypertension, which usually is renin mediated and, therefore, angiotensin-converting enzyme (ACE) inhibitors are preferred for the treatment. If ARF supervenes, clinical and dialysis treatment should be initiated. Antibiotics are not effective except in some forms of *S. dysenteriae*. Actually, antibiotics such as trimethoprim-sulfamethoxazole may increase verotoxin production by *E. coli* 0157:H7, thereby increasing the risk of developing HUS.[48] Specific therapeutic measurements may be used to limit vascular injury. These strategies include fresh frozen plasma infusion. A loading dose of 30 to 40 mL/kg and then a daily dose of 15 to 20 mL/kg has been recommended until the platelet count normalizes or hemolysis ceases. In addition, plasma exchange is usually advocated, especially in cases of HUS with neurologic involvement, yet it remains to be proved as effective therapy in HUS. Several other treatments such as steroids, antiplatelets, anticoagulants, and immunoglobulins have been tried, but all were found to be ineffective.[53, 57]

Acute Renal Failure in Sepsis

Sepsis is the systemic response to infection. It is characterized by systemic inflammatory response syndrome (SIRS) together with definitive evidence of infection. Systemic inflammatory response syndrome is characterized by a widespread inflammatory response to a variety of severe clinical insults, according to the Society of Critical Care Consensus.[58] This syndrome is clinically recognized by the presence of two or more of the following signs:

- Temperature > 38°C or < 36°C
- Heart rate > 90 beats/min
- Respiratory rate > 20 breaths/min or $PaCO_2$ < 32 mm Hg
- White blood cell count > 12,000 cells/mm³, < 4000 cells/mm³, or > 10% immature forms

Sepsis is considered severe when it is associated with organ dysfunction, hypoperfusion, or hypotension. The exact incidence of sepsis is not known. Current estimates in the United States suggest an incidence of more than 500,000 cases/year with more than 100,000 deaths as a consequence of severe sepsis and septic shock.[59, 60] Sepsis is traditionally attributed to a gram-negative bacteremia but it can also be a consequence of gram-positive organisms, as well as fungi, viruses, and parasites. In the last few years, there has been an increase of reported frequency of gram-positive bacteremia and sepsis. Bone reported an incidence of 30% to 40% of gram-positive sepsis in United States.[61] In Europe, in a one-day point prevalence study,[62] it was found that 44.8% of patients in ICUs were infected. The most frequently reported microorganisms were Enterobacteriaceae (34.4%), *S. aureus* (30.1%), and *P. aeruginosa* (28,7%). Furthermore, sepsis is more frequently observed in middle-aged and elderly patients, in which comorbidities are frequently causes of further health impairment.[29, 63–65]

Sepsis and especially septic shock are important risk factors for the development of ARF. Prevalences ranging from 9% to 40% of ARF in sepsis have been reported.[66] Liano and associates[67] reported in a multicenter trial that sepsis caused acute tubular necrosis (ATN) in 35.4% of ICU patients and 26.9% of non-ICU patients. In a French multicenter study,[68] ARF was related to sepsis in 48% of the patients who presented a higher significant mortality rate compared with nonseptic patients (73% vs. 45%). Furthermore, in a recent prospective study including 2527 patients who met the criteria for SIRS, the evolution to sepsis and septic shock was studied. The incidence of ARF was 19% in sepsis, 23% in severe sepsis, and 51% in septic shock.[69] Abbs and Cameron, in a multidisciplinary ICU analysis of 544 patients admitted from 1982 to 1996, reported that sepsis and ARF following cardiothoracic surgery were the predominant causes of ARF.[10] Several reports[70] have addressed the issue of identifying risk or predictive factors for development of ARF in community, hospitalized, or ICU patients. Although comparisons among these studies are difficult to perform because of different populations, definitions, and methodologies, sepsis is invariably identified among the important variables either for development of or mortality in ARF.

The sepsis syndrome is a dynamic process, with severity ranging from mild infection evolving to sepsis and/or septic shock and, ultimately, to MODS. Several complex events take place during this process. Initiating factors related to infection, such as endotoxin and bacterial products (eg, lipopolysaccharide of gram-negative bacteria), induce a host defense with recruitment of various cell types including macrophages, endothelial cells, and polymorphonuclear cells. Activation of these cells triggers an inflammatory response with release of several inflammatory mediators such as TNF-α, interleukin-1 (IL-1), IL-6, IL-8, and interferon-γ and other mediators such as coagulation factors, complement system, proteases, eicosanoids, platelet-activating factor, and nitric oxide (NO). This inflammatory response aims to localize the area of tissue injury through vasodilation, formation of microthrombi, and changes in endothelial cell function resulting in blood flow alterations, increased vascular permeability, and edema. If the septic process persists, a more generalized response (SIRS) may develop affecting otherwise normal tissue that could ultimately lead to circulatory failure (septic shock) and widespread tissue injury (MODS).

The hemodynamic responses to sepsis syndrome have been characterized as especially due to endotoxin released by gram-negative bacteremia. Peripheral vascular resistance initially decreases, causing a reduction in mean arterial pressure and a secondary increase in cardiac output.[71] The altered renal hemodynamics in septicemia is usually attributed to renal hypoperfusion. However, a wide range of renal blood flows (RBFs) has been reported, probably related to differences in models, techniques, and severity of shock.[72] An increased RBF and a decreased renal vascular resistance may be observed during the initial stage of sepsis as a consequence of a decreased peripheral vascular resistance.[73] This renal vasodilation may be mediated by prostaglandins, NO, and/or the kallikrein system.[72, 74, 75] However, the characteristic renal consequences of the septic altered hemodynamics are an increase in renal vascular resistance with a subsequent reduction in RBF and glomerular filtration rate (GFR).[76–78] These renal alterations may occur even with preserved RBF and without mean arterial pressure reduction.[79, 80] In these circumstances, an intrarenal redistribution of blood flow may occur as a consequence of a shift of flow away from the cortex to the juxtaglomerular and medullary areas. This blood flow redistribution was exacerbated by nitrous oxide inhibition.[81–83] Additionally, endotoxin infusion has minor effects on renal perfusion in isolated perfused kidneys, suggesting that endotoxin systemic response rather than a direct renal effect is responsible for renal hemodynamic changes.[84]

Although renal ischemia due to a sepsis-induced decrease in RBF is not a uniform finding, the most significant renal alteration in sepsis is a decrease in GFR. In many cases, GFR reduction is determined by a fall in renal plasma flow (RPF) and glomerular perfusion pressure in the presence of systemic hypotension. Moreover, a reduction in GFR may be the result of a decrease in the filtration fraction, ie, the ratio of glomerular filtration to RBF.[85, 86] The main determinants of filtration fraction are the afferent and efferent arteriolar resistances and the total surface area. Thus, constriction of the afferent arteriole and/or dilation of the efferent arteriole reduce filtration fraction as shown by Lugon and colleagues in endotoxemic rats.[77] In this situation, several vasoactive mediators, such as leukotrienes, adenosine, thromboxane A$_2$, angiotensin II, and endothelin may affect filtration fraction, also by reducing filtration area through mesangial cell contraction.[86–89] However, wide variations in filtration fraction have also been reported during septic shock in humans, indicating that GFR can be affected by sepsis and endotoxemia independently of renal perfusion.[80]

In addition to renal hemodynamic alterations during sepsis, glomerular capillaries may be affected by acute endothelial injury.[76] Endotoxin may activate coagulation and fibrinolysis cascades, releasing a tissue factor with deposition of platelets and fibrin within capillaries.[72, 86] In fact, there is evidence of the occurrence of microthrombi in glomerular and peritubular capillaries in sepsis-induced ARF.[90] Moreover, leukocytes may be activated by endotoxin-enhancing endothelium alterations with changes in the release of vascular mediators such as NO and endothelin-1 and release of oxidants that further enhances renal injury.[91, 92] NO released by activated neutrophils and locally released is an important mediator of RBF regulation and participates in renal ischemic injury.[93, 94] Excessive NO generation has been implicated in septic shock.[95] In experimental septic models, inhibition of NO impaired blood flow, further increasing afferent and efferent arteriolar constriction. Thus, NO is an important vascular regulatory mediator, maintaining microvascular flow under basal conditions and probably counteracting vasoconstrictors during sepsis.[96] Fur-

thermore, NO also inhibits leukocyte interactions with endothelial cells and platelet aggregation.[97] In fact, it was demonstrated that inhibition of NO in an experimental endotoxin model caused glomerular thrombosis and contributed to GFR decline.[98]

Besides the hemodynamic and glomerular alterations in sepsis-induced ARF, tubular dysfunction may also occur. In early stages of ARF, a pure hemodynamic form of ARF may occur in which RBF is reduced sufficiently to cause GRF decline without tubular damage. In these circumstances, fractional excretion of sodium (FENa) is low as demonstrated in endotoxemic experimental models. With progression of ARF, there is an increase in sodium wasting with high FENa,[76, 99] probably reflecting the onset of tubular injury that may result in ATN. Patients with established ARF caused by sepsis are generally regarded as presenting ATN.[86] Therefore, preventive measures to restore renal perfusion and optimize oxygen delivery are important in preventing and limiting ischemic damage to the kidneys. In addition to RBF, optimal arterial oxygenation and hemoglobin concentration are important determinants of renal oxygen delivery, especially because renal oxygen requirement may be high and renal oxygen extraction may be impaired in sepsis.[100–102] Furthermore, reperfusion injury may supervene after temporary hypoperfusion especially in the setting of endotoxemia.[103] In fact, there is evidence that mild ischemia activates primed neutrophils to cause ARF through oxidant or protease-mediated mechanisms.[92, 104] In addition, several other factors may also participate in the reperfusion injury, such as reactive oxygen species, NO, calcium accumulation, and activation of phospholipases and proteases. Therefore, several different mediators may interact to further cause cell injury when restoration of blood flow occurs after a period of hypoperfusion.[93, 94, 105–108]

Finally, although ischemic ATN seems to occur in most patients with established sepsis-induced ARF, experimental models have demonstrated that it is relatively difficult to induce severe tubular injury from ischemia alone; usually 1 hour of complete cessation of RBF is necessary. The author and his associates demonstrated that indeed kidneys are quite resistant to hypoperfusion. They observed that awake rats subjected to hemorrhagic shock for 3 hours presented a very mild renal impairment 24 hours after correction of hypotension with blood reinfusion.[109] Moreover, endotoxin alone did not cause significant tubular injury with inconsistent effects on isolated perfused kidney.[84] It is likely that in patients with sepsis-induced ARF, multiple insults are involved in the pathogenesis of ARF. Several endogenous and exogenous factors may interact to cause ARF in sepsis. For example, endotoxemia enhanced postischemic tubular necrosis and reduced GRF without interfering with RBF.[110] Body temperature may have an impact on the severity of ischemic and nephrotoxic insults to the kidneys. Zager and others have demonstrated that hyperthermia profoundly enhanced renal ischemia as well as gentamicin nephrotoxicity.[111–113] Additionally, modest renal hypoperfusion and aminoglycosides may have a synergistic effect causing tubular injury.[114, 115] Endotoxemia and aminoglycosides may also interact, each causing renal vasoconstriction and having a synergistic effect on renal filtration reduction.[112, 116] Therefore, multiple factors are present in the setting of sepsis, each of them potentially interacting to cause an early functional hemodynamic renal disturbance until a severe ATN occurs, which often is part of a complicated event such as MODS.

The initial assessment of a patient with ARF in the presence of sepsis is to differentiate among prerenal, postrenal, and renal failure as a usual procedure in any case of ARF. The prerenal and postrenal ARF are considered functional disturbances and therefore immediate correction of the causative mechanism should restore renal function. Obstruction of the urinary tract is easily diagnosed with ultrasound and radiology methods. Differentiation between prerenal and ATN may be more complicated, especially as described earlier, a reduction in RBF and GFR with sodium retention may occur in spite of normal blood pressure and an absence of significant tubular damage in early stages of sepsis. The differential diagnosis may include laboratory tests, which are described in a previous chapter.

Treatment of a patient with ARF of sepsis origin is usually managed in an ICU environment where monitoring of fluids, electrolytes, and acid-base disorders can be continuously performed. In addition, in certain circumstances hemodynamic and tissue oxygenation monitoring may be required for an adequate patient management. An early recognition of septic shock increases the chances of successful therapy. The presence of signals of sepsis such as fever or hypothermia, hyperventilation, tachycardia, or changes in mental status should prompt acquisition of blood cultures and possible initiation of therapy. Blood pressure may be normal or slightly reduced with adequate extremities' perfusion early in the course of sepsis. If sepsis is not adequately controlled it will progress, resulting in hypotension and inadequate tissue perfusion. The cardiovascular changes of septic shock are characterized by a spectrum beginning with decreased systemic vascular resistance and increased cardiac output (warm shock), then progressing to decreased cardiac output and increased systemic vascular resistance (cold shock).

Treatment of ARF in sepsis includes standard therapy for ARF together with prompt treatment of sepsis. Treatment strategy should include antibiotics, fluids, oxygen, and cardiotropic agents such as dopamine and dobutamine. Surgical search of septic foci and widespectrum antibiotics are fundamental in sepsis management. Selection of an appropriate antibiotic treatment must take into account the site of infection and presumptive pathogens. Initial empiric therapy should be broad enough to include gram-negative as well as gram-positive microorganisms because of the reported increasing incidence of sepsis caused by the latter pathogens.[20, 117] Antibiotics should also be adjusted according to patient's hepatic and renal functions to avoid iatrogenic or synergic effects of these antibiotics

and endotoxemia as described before. Further complications of infectious therapy on renal function are discussed in the next section. Controversial therapies of septic shock include use of steroids, heparin, opiate antagonists (naloxone), cyclooxygenase inhibitors (nonsteroidal anti-inflammatory drugs [NSAIDs]), and experimental therapies such as passive immunization (human antisera) and monoclonal antibodies directed to endotoxin.[118–120] Intermittent or continuous dialysis therapies may be required for correction of electrolyte and acid-base disturbances, uremia, and/or for an adequate fluid and nutritional balance. Continuous renal replacement therapy has been used with increasing frequency in the management of critically ill patients even in the absence of ARF or specifically for therapy of sepsis.[121–123] However, there is no convincing evidence demonstrating superiority of continuous therapy (eg, hemodiafiltration) over intermittent modalities (conventional hemodialysis) for the treatment of sepsis-induced ARF.[124–126] Most of the reported studies were retrospective, and a randomized, controlled study in sepsis is lacking.

ACUTE RENAL FAILURE IN VIRAL DISEASES

Viral diseases are distributed worldwide and represent the majority of human infectious diseases. Some of these viruses (Table 22–3) may cause renal diseases in humans.[127] Despite the high frequency of viral infections, renal involvement is surprisingly low in such patients, indicating that other factors such as host response and virus immunogenicity are determinant of renal injury. Most of the evidence of acute renal function impairment has been documented as isolated case reports in viral diseases such as hepatitis A, influenza A, measles, and Epstein-Barr virus.[128–134] However, renal involvement has been increasingly reported in HIV infection and hemorrhagic fever with renal syndrome (HFRS) caused by Hantaviruses in parallel with the increased incidence of these infectious diseases worldwide.

Renal Disorders in HIV Infection

Several renal disorders have been reported in HIV-infected patients since the first publications describing a nephropathy associated with this disease, now termed *HIV-associated nephropathy* (HIVAN).[135–137] These disorders include ARF, diverse fluid and electrolyte abnor-

TABLE 22–3. Viruses Causing Renal Diseases

Adenovirus	Hepatitis A, B, C
Coxsackie	HIV
Cytomegalovirus	Influenza
Echo	Measles
Epstein-Barr	Mumps
Hantaan	Varicella

HIV, human immunodeficiency virus.

TABLE 22–4. Renal Disorders Associated With HIV Infection

DISORDERS	MANIFESTATION
HIV-associated nephropathy	Focal segmental glomerulosclerosis
	Other forms of glomerulonephritis
Acute renal failure	Acute tubular necrosis
	Acute interstitial nephritis
	Hemolytic-uremic syndrome
	Postinfectious glomerulonephritis
Electrolyte and acid-base disorders	Hyponatremia
	Disturbances of potassium, uric acid, calcium, magnesium, and ADH secretion
	Renal tubular acidosis
	Lactic acidosis
Infiltrative and malignant disorders	Lymphoma
	Kaposi sarcoma
	Renal cell carcinoma
Renal infections	
Obstructive nephropathy	Drugs
	Extrinsic obstruction

HIV human immunodeficiency virus; *ADH,* antidiuretic hormone.

malities, renal infections, infiltrative and malignant disorders, and obstructive uropathy (Table 22–4).[138]

HIV-ASSOCIATED NEPHROPATHY

Human immunodeficiency virus–associated nephropathy usually presents clinically as massive proteinuria, often with a full picture of nephrotic syndrome that rapidly progress to chronic renal insufficiency in a matter of weeks to months. Kidneys are usually enlarged at presentation, remaining large during the progression of renal insufficiency.[139–142] The predominant glomerular lesion is a collapsing form of focal and segmental glomerulosclerosis, frequently associated with severe acute tubular and interstitial involvement. Acute tubular necrosis, interstitial edema, and lymphocytic infiltration are also observed. Ultrastructural changes include tubuloreticular structures widespread in endothelial cells and leukocytes and the presence of nuclear bodies in tubular and interstitial cells.[143–145] Treatment of HIVAN is based on reported benefits of antiviral therapy, immunosuppressive drugs (eg, corticosteroids), and nonspecific medications to reduce proteinuria such as ACE inhibitors. However, there has been no randomized trial assessing the efficacy of any form of therapy.[146–151]

ACUTE RENAL FAILURE IN HIV INFECTION

ARF is a common complication in HIV-infected patients that may result from the HIV infection and/or as consequence of diagnostic and therapeutic procedures.[138, 152] Acute renal failure in HIV patients is diverse in nature, with many causes similar to that in non-HIV patients. However, HIV patients are usually younger and sicker. The most common syndrome, as in non-HIV patients, is ATN due to ischemia (dehydration, hypovolemia, hypotension, sepsis) and nephrotoxicity (pentamidine, aminoglycosides, trimethoprim-

sulfamethoxazole, NSAIDs).[153, 154] Other causes of ARF in HIV-patients include hypoalbuminemia due to malnutrition or cachexia; rhabdomyolysis and myoglobinuria; interstitial nephritis; HUS; and postinfectious glomerulonephritis. There is a recent report that retrospectively analyzed 92 HIV-infected patients with ARF; 60 of them underwent renal biopsy. The main cause of acute or rapidly progressing renal failure was HUS followed by ATN (ischemic/toxic or rhabdomyolysis), obstructive renal failure, and HIVAN.[155]

The choice of dialysis method for ARF treatment in HIV patients remains arbitrary. All the available methods—peritoneal dialysis, hemodialysis, and continuous renal replacement therapy—have been used for the treatment of ARF in HIV patients, depending mostly on the medical status and institutional resources. Decisions concerning whether to suspend or withhold dialysis therapy are usually difficult, considering ethical and medical aspects.

In the early series, ARF was usually considered as a preterminal event. However, mortality rates of ARF in HIV patients have been recently reported to be similar to non-HIV infected patients.[153] Rao and Friedman[154] compared the course of severe ARF in 146 HIV-infected patients with 306 contemporaneous non-HIV infected subjects. Despite an increased incidence of sepsis and worse medical condition in the former group, the mortality rate was similar (60% vs. 56%). A recent French study[155] reported that the overall mortality in 92 HIV-patients with ARF was 20%, whereas in ischemic ATN in this series, the mortality rate was 44%. Thus, many forms of ARF in HIV patients are treatable or reversible rather than a preterminal event. Nevertheless, ARF in the setting of an HIV infection or full-blown acquired immunodeficiency syndrome certainly increases morbidity and mortality, frequently presenting clinical and ethical dilemmas that require the assistance of a multidisciplinary medical group together with patient and family participation.

Hemorrhagic Fever With Renal Syndrome

Hemorrhagic fever with renal syndrome is a group of illnesses caused by viruses from the genus *Hantavirus* of the family Bunyaviridiae.[156] This name was recommended by a World Health Organization Working Group[157] to unify similar clinical diseases occurring mainly in Europe and Asia. It is an acute febrile nephropathy caused by zoonotic viruses spread to humans from persistently infected rodents and small mammals. There are about 180 Hantavirus isolates from 23 species of animals.[158] The first Hantavirus, identified by Lee, was the Hantaan virus,[159] which is the causative agent of the Korean hemorrhagic fever. Three other Hantaviruses were identified: Seoul, Puumala, and Prospect Hill.[156, 160, 161] Seoul virus is implicated in urban cases and laboratory-acquired cases of HFRS in Korea. It is transmitted to humans from domestic and laboratory rats.[162, 163] Puumala virus was identified as the agent of a mild form of HFRS prevailing in Europe, also designated *nephropathia epidem-*

ica.[164, 165] Prospect Hill virus does not appear to cause disease in humans.[161] Recently, an emerging infectious disease caused by Hantavirus named *Hantavirus pulmonary syndrome* has been described after an outbreak in southwestern United States.[166–168] This syndrome is characterized by a febrile prodrome progressing to severe noncardiogenic pulmonary edema, usually without renal involvement. It is caused by newly described Hantaviruses: (1) Sin Nombre virus; (2) Four Corners virus, identified in Louisiana; and (3) Black Creek Canal virus.[169–172] HFRS is primarily an Eurasian disease, whereas this pulmonary syndrome appears to be confined to the Americas; this geographic distinction appears to correlate with the phylogenies of the rodent hosts and the viruses that coevolved with them.[173]

Hantavirus infections are transmitted to humans mainly through aerosols originated from secretions of infected animals. Staff of animal rooms and rodent breeders have an increased risk of infection. Hemorrhagic fever with renal syndrome is characterized by the presence of febrile, gastrointestinal, cardiovascular, hemorrhagic, renal, and neurologic manifestations. The major symptoms are fever, chills, headache, weakness, dizziness, myalgia, back pain, nausea, vomiting, abdominal pain, and blurred vision. Respiratory and cardiac signs may also be present. Physical signs include facial flushing, puffy face, bleeding signs, hypotension followed by hypertension, and bradycardia. The clinical course is divided into five subsequent phases: (1) febrile, (2) hypotensive, (3) oliguric, (4) diuretic and polyuric, and (5) convalescent, lasting about 4 to 8 weeks. Clinical manifestations vary from subclinical and mild to severe. In mild cases, the hypotensive and oliguric phases may not appear and serologic tests are usually necessary for the diagnosis. Although the clinical pattern is similar in Europe and Asia, HFRS is usually much milder in Scandinavia and Western Europe as well as the HFRS caused by the Seoul virus in Korea. Laboratory features include thrombocytopenia, leukocytosis, and liver enzyme elevation. Renal function abnormalities are universal, including proteinuria and microhematuria. HFRS is considered an immune-mediated disease. Circulating immune complexes and complement consumption were described. Specific antibodies (IgM, IgG, and IGE) can be detected at or close to the onset of symptoms. Virus may also be detectable in plasma and mononuclear cells, in which it persists for a longer period.[161, 163]

Renal function in HFRS is initially preserved with normal RPF and GFR during the febrile phase. During the next hypotensive and oliguric phases, both RPF and GFR decline, with a more pronounced effect on GFR, resulting in decreased filtration fraction. Renal plasma flow and GFR begin to improve during the diuretic phase; polyuria and reversal of azotemia are rapidly established. Most patients will fully recover renal function, but re-establishment of normal tubular function may take months. Irreversible renal lesions may occur in a limited number of patients, irrespective of severity of the acute illness, leading to chronic renal failure.

Kidney histology of patients dying of HFRS demonstrates intense congestion and dilation of medullary vessels, accompanied by interstitial edema filled with red blood cells. Tubular changes include compression and distortion, necrosis and degeneration of tubular cells, and presence of tubular casts.[161] In two series of renal biopsies in Finland, where a mild form of HFRS (Puumala virus) is one of the most frequent causes of ARF,[174] Collan and coworkers[165] collected 80 biopsies from 65 patients, demonstrating the presence of slight tubular dilation and interstitial edema with diffuse and sparse inflammatory infiltrate. Occasional necrotic cells or mitosis were observed. Medullary interstitial hemorrhages were seen in 60% of samples. Immunofluorescence was positive for IgG or IgM and C3 in tubular basement membrane. Mustonen and associates[175] performed renal biopsies in 86 of 126 adult HFRS patients in Finland. They found that severity of renal failure correlated slightly with blood inflammatory parameters and the degree of hematuria rather than the proteinuria. The most common histopathologic lesion was acute tubulointerstitial nephritis. The histologic lesions were mild and not specific, except for the presence of hemorrhage in the outer medulla. Similar renal pathologic changes were described in Slovenia, where 20 of 33 patients were infected with Hantaan virus and the remainder with Puumala virus.[176]

Treatment of HFRS is mainly supportive, aiming at correction of hypovolemia and electrolyte and acid-base disturbances. Treatment of complications and platelet transfusions are often necessary. Renal impairment may be severe enough to require hemodialysis or peritoneal dialysis, especially during the oliguric phase. Therapy with the antiviral drug ribavirin at the onset of disease may be beneficial. Immune therapy with α-interferon and vaccination are currently under investigation, and their efficacy has not yet been determined.[158, 171, 177] Mortality in HFRS caused by the Hantaan virus infection varies from 2% to 7%, whereas in Seoul viral infection it is less than 1%.[163] Prognosis of the mild form of HFRS in Europe is fairly good, with a mortality rate below 0.5%.[165, 178]

ACUTE RENAL FAILURE CAUSED BY MISCELLANEOUS AGENTS

Acute Renal Failure in Malaria

Malaria is a parasitic disease prevalent in the tropics. However, because of the great air travel expansion, cases of Malaria have been reported worldwide.[179] Malarial infection is caused by the protozoan of the genus *Plasmodium*. Four species affect humans: *P. vivax, P. malariae, P. ovale,* and *P. falciparum*. The disease is characterized by periodic fever with chills, headache, prostration, anemia, and splenomegaly. Renal disorders may complicate infections of *P. malariae* and *P. falciparum*. Renal involvement with the former agent is associated with glomerulonephritis that may progress to chronic renal failure, whereas falciparum malaria can cause acute water and electrolyte disturbances as well as ARF.[180] Furthermore, malaria has been recently recognized as a complication of renal transplantation either as a new infection or reactivation of the disease in an immunosuppressed patient.[181]

Plasmodium parasites (sporozoites) are injected into the blood stream by the mosquito's bite, finding their way to the patient's liver, where they mature into tissue schizonts, releasing merozoites that will infect red blood cells. In infected erythrocytes, merozoites progress to trophozoites and finally to schizonts, which release new generations of merozoites that will infect other red blood cells, establishing the clinically cyclic nature of malaria. The relationship between red blood cell parasitization and the host's monocyte activation determines the clinical expressions of malaria.[181]

Fluid and electrolyte disturbances in falciparum malaria include hypovolemia or hypervolemia, hyponatremia, hyperkalemia, hypocalcemia, hypophosphatemia, hyperuricemia, and hypoglicemia.[182] Renal complications are ATN, AIN, and glomerulonephritis. ARF is the main renal complication, usually caused by ATN. It occurs in 1% to 4% of falciparum malaria patients, but it may reach 60% in malignant malaria.[180, 183] ARF is usually oliguric and hypercatabolic, often associated with vasodilation, hemolysis, rhabdomyolysis, and disseminated intravascular coagulation. Hyperbilirubinemia, as consequence of hemolysis and intrahepatic cholestasis, is frequently associated with ARF in falciparum malaria. Peripheral pooling is a common manifestation leading to reduced blood flow and diminished tissue perfusion.[184]

Prognosis of malarial ARF depends on the severity of the illness, the presence of extrarenal complications, and especially the response to antiparasitic treatment (chloroquine, quinine, primaquine, and artemisinin derivatives), exchange blood transfusion, and availability of dialysis therapy.[182, 185] Reported mortality ranges from 10% to 44%.[179, 183, 185–187]

Acute Renal Failure in Leptospirosis

Leptospirosis is a disease caused by several serotypes of a spirochetal bacteria, *Leptospira interrogans*. This disease is a common zoonosis in domestic and wild animals. It is unusual in Western countries, but it is an important cause of ARF in certain tropical countries.[188, 189]

Patients with leptospirosis present clinically with sudden onset of fever, chills, generalized muscle pain (especially in the lower limbs), and variable degrees of jaundice. Leptospirosis diagnosis can be done by serologic or saliva tests[190, 191] and identification or culture of the agent in blood or tissue sample. Pulmonary and cardiovascular complications may occur, usually manifesting as hypoxemia, pulmonary hemorrhage, and cardiac arrythmias.[192, 193] Renal involvement occurs almost invariably in leptospirosis, and the reported incidence of ARF varies from 15% to 69%.[189, 194] ARF in leptospirosis is more prevalent in young men. It is characterized as a nonoliguric ARF with normokalemia

or hypokalemia, seldom with hyperkalemia. Oliguric patients on admission may present with dehydration that usually responds to volume expansion. Moreover, most ARF patients present with jaundice and rhabdomyolysis that may cause or complicate ARF.[35, 194–197] The absence of hyperkalemia in leptospirosis is attributed to urinary losses due to increased distal potassium secretion as a consequence of increased distal sodium delivery.[196, 198] Furthermore, high levels of aldosterone and cortisol were detected in leptospirosis ARF patients that could contribute for renal potassium excretion.[195] Pathologic examinations disclosed that the primary lesion was tubulointerstitial nephritis with local or diffuse mononuclear cell infiltration in association with proximal and distal tubular cell degeneration.[199] Mortality in leptospirosis is reported varying from 2% in children to 14.7% in adult populations living in endemic areas. The main cause of death appears to be pulmonary hemorrhage.[188, 197, 200–202]

Prevention and treatment of leptospirosis include better hygienic and sanitary conditions, eradication of natural hosts (rodents), and antibiotic prophylaxis or treatment. Doxycycline has been successfully used as a prophylactic measure.[200, 203] Penicillin and doxycycline treatment, especially administered early in the course of the disease, have proved effective.[204, 205]

REFERENCES

1. Spiegel DM, Ullian ME, Zerbe GO, Berl T: Determinants of survival and recovery in acute renal failure patients dialyzed in intensive care units. Am J Nephrol 1991; 11:44–47.
2. Turney JH: Why is mortality persistently high in acute renal failure [letter]? Lancet 1990; 335:971.
3. Biesenbach G, Zazgornik J, Kaiser W, et al: Improvement in prognosis of patients with acute renal failure over a period of 15 years: an analysis of 710 cases in a dialysis center. Am J Nephrol 1992; 12:319–325.
4. Wiecek A, Zeier M, Ritz E: Role of infection in the genesis of acute renal failure. Nephrol Dial Transplant 1994; 9(Suppl 4):40–44.
5. Abreo K, Moorthy AV, Osborne M: Changing patterns and outcome of acute renal failure requiring hemodialysis. Arch Intern Med 1986; 146:1338–1441.
6. Corwin HL, Teplick RS, Schreiber MJ, et al: Prediction of outcome in acute renal failure. Am J Nephrol 1987; 7:8–12.
7. Beaman M, Turney JH, Rodger RS, et al: Changing pattern of acute renal failure. Q J Med 1987; 62:15–23.
8. Turney JH, Marshall DH, Brownjohn AM, et al: The evolution of acute renal failure, 1956–1988. Q J Med 1990; 74:83–104.
9. Kaufman J, Dhakal M, Patel B, Hamburger R: Community-acquired acute renal failure. Am J Kidney Dis 1991; 17:191–198.
10. Abbs IC, Cameron JS: Epidemiology of Acute Renal Failure in the Intensive Care Unit. In: Ronco C, Bellomo R, eds: *Critical Care Nephrology*. Netherlands: Kluwer; 1997:133–142.
11. Jochimsen F, Schafer JH, Maurer A, Distler A: Impairment of renal function in medical intensive care: predictability of acute renal failure. Crit Care Med 1990; 18:480–485.
12. Groeneveld AB, Tran DD, van der Meulen J, et al: Acute renal failure in the medical intensive care unit: predisposing, complicating factors, and outcome. Nephron 1991; 59:602–610.
13. Schaefer JH, Jochimsen F, Keller F, et al: Outcome prediction of acute renal failure in medical intensive care. Intensive Care Med 1991; 17:19–24.
14. Neveu H, Kleinknecht D, Brivet F, et al: Prognostic factors in acute renal failure due to sepsis: results of a prospective multicentre study. The French Study Group on Acute Renal Failure. Nephrol Dial Transplant 1996; 11:293–299.

15. Liano F, Pascual J: Epidemiology of acute renal failure: a prospective, multicenter, community-based study. Madrid Acute Renal Failure Study Group. Kidney Int 1996; 50:811–818.

16. Brivet FG, Kleinknecht DJ, Loirat P, Landais PJ: Acute renal failure in intensive care units: causes, outcome, and prognostic factors of hospital mortality—a prospective, multicenter study. French Study Group on Acute Renal Failure [see comments]. Crit Care Med 1996; 24:192–198.

17. Jarvis WR, Edwards JR, Culver DH, et al: Nosocomial infection rates in adult and pediatric intensive care units in the United States. National Nosocomial Infections Surveillance System. Am J Med 1991; 91:185S–191S.

18. Burdmann EA, Oliveira MB, Ferraboli R, et al: Epidemiologia. In: Schor N, Boim MA, Santos OFP, eds: Insuficiência Renal Aguda: Fisiopatologia, Clínica, e Tratamento. Sao Paulo: Sarvier; 1997:1–8.

19. Jarvis WR: Nosocomial outbreaks: the Centers for Disease Control's Hospital Infections Program experience, 1980–1990. Epidemiology Branch, Hospital Infections Program. Am J Med 1991; 91:101S–106S.

20. Vincent JL, Bihari DJ, Suter PM, et al: The prevalence of nosocomial infection in intensive care units in Europe: results of the European Prevalence of Infection in Intensive Care (EPIC) Study. EPIC International Advisory Committee (see comments). JAMA 1995; 274:639–644.

21. Lieberman E: Management of acute renal failure in infants and children. Nephron 1973; 11:193–208.

22. Stilmant MN, Bolton WK, Sturgill BC, et al: Crescentic glomerulonephritis without immune deposits: clinicopathologic features. Kidney Int 1979; 15:184–195.

23. Levine JS, Lieberthal W, Bernard DB, Salant DJ: Acute Renal Failure Associated With Renal Vascular Disease, Vasculitis, Glomerulonephritis, and Nephrotic Syndrome. In: Lazarus JM, Brenner BM, eds: Acute Renal Failure. New York: Churchill Livingstone; 1993:247–356.

24. Beaufils M, Morel-Maroger L, Sraer JD, et al: Acute renal failure of glomerular origin during visceral abscesses. N Engl J Med 1976; 295:185–189.

25. Neugarten J, Baldwin DS: Glomerulonephritis in bacterial endocarditis. Am J Med 1984; 77:297–304.

26. Conlon PJ, Jefferies F, Krigman HR, et al: Predictors of prognosis and risk of acute renal failure in bacterial endocarditis. Clin Nephrol 1998; 49:96–101.

27. Arze RS, Rashid H, Ward MK, et al: Shunt nephritis: report of two cases and review of the literature. Clin Nephrol 1983; 19:48–53.

28. Zappacosta AR, Ashby BL: Gram-negative sepsis with acute renal failure: occurrence from acute glomerulonephritis. JAMA 1977; 238:1389–1390.

29. Ziegler EJ, Fisher CJJ, Sprung CL, et al: Treatment of gram-negative bacteremia and septic shock with HA-1A human monoclonal antibody against endotoxin: a randomized, double-blind, placebo-controlled trial. The HA-1A Sepsis Study Group (see comments). N Engl J Med 1991; 324:429–436.

30. Andrews PA, Lloyd CM, Webb MC, Sacks SH: Acute interstitial nephritis associated with Mycoplasma pneumoniae infection. Nephrol Dial Transplant 1994; 9:564–566.

31. Conlon PJ, Procop GW, Fowler V, et al: Predictors of prognosis and risk of acute renal failure in patients with Rocky Mountain spotted fever. Am J Med 1996; 101:621–626.

32. Branley P, Speed B: Acute interstitial nephritis due to Chlamydia psittaci. Aust N Z J Med 1999; 25:365.

33. Iijima K, Yoshikawa N, Sato K, Matsuo T: Acute interstitial nephritis associated with Yersinia pseudotuberculosis infection. Am J Nephrol 1989; 9:236–240.

34. Ramsay AG, Olesnicky L, Pirani CL: Acute tubulointerstitial nephritis from Candida albicans with oliguric renal failure. Clin Nephrol 1985; 24:310–314.

35. Sitprija V, Pipatanagul V, Mertowidjojo K, et al: Pathogenesis of renal disease in leptospirosis: clinical and experimental studies. Kidney Int 1980; 17:827–836.

36. Lai KN, Aarons I, Woodroffe AJ, Clarkson AR: Renal lesions in leptospirosis. Aust N Z J Med 1982; 12:276–279.

37. Platt JL, Sibley RK, Michael AF: Interstitial nephritis associated with cytomegalovirus infection. Kidney Int 1985; 28:550–552.

38. Kopolovic J, Pinkus G, Rosen S: Interstitial nephritis in infectious mononucleosis. Am J Kidney Dis 1988; 12:76–77.

39. Buysen JG, Houthoff HJ, Krediet RT, Arisz L: Acute interstitial nephritis: a clinical and morphological study in 27 patients. Nephrol Dial Transplant 1990; 5:94–99.

40. Neilson EG: Pathogenesis and therapy of interstitial nephritis. Kidney Int 1989; 35:1257–1270.

41. Murray KM, Keane WR: Review of drug-induced acute interstitial nephritis. Pharmacotherapy 1992; 12:462–467.

42. Eapen SS, Hall PM: Acute tubulointerstitial nephritis. Cleve Clin J Med 1992; 59:27–32.

43. Joh K, Aizawa S, Yamaguchi Y, et al: Drug-induced hypersensitivity nephritis: lymphocyte stimulation testing and renal biopsy in 10 cases. Am J Nephrol 1990; 10:222–230.

44. Grunfeld JP, Kleinknecht D, Droz D: Acute Interstitial Nephritis. In: Schrier RW, Gottschalk CW, eds: Diseases of the Kidney. Boston: Little, Brown; 1992:1331–1354.

45. Galpin JE, Shinaberger JH, Stanley TM, et al: Acute interstitial nephritis due to methicillin. Am J Med 1978; 65:756–765.

46. Pusey CD, Saltissi D, Bloodworth L, et al: Drug-associated acute interstitial nephritis: clinical and pathological features and the response to high-dose steroid therapy. Q J Med 1983; 52:194–211.

47. Michel DM, Kelly CJ: Acute interstitial nephritis. J Am Soc Nephrol 1998; 9:506–515.

48. Remuzzi G, Ruggenenti P: The hemolytic-uremic syndrome. Kidney Int 1995; 48:2–19.

49. Su C, Brandt LJ: Escherichia coli 0157:H7 infection in humans. Ann Intern Med 1995; 123:698–714.

50. Chart H, vd Kar N, Monnens LA: Serological identification of Escherichia coli 0157 as cause of haemolytic-uraemic syndrome in Netherlands. Lancet 1991; 337:437.

51. Chart H, Smith HR, Scotland SM, et al: Serological identification of Escherichia coli 0157:H7 infection in haemolytic-uraemic syndrome. Lancet 1991; 337:138–140.

52. Boyce TG, Swerdlow DL, Griffin PM: Escherichia coli 0157:H7 and the hemolytic-uremic syndrome. N Engl J Med 1995; 333:364–368.

53. Neild GH: Hemolytic-uremic syndrome/thrombotic thrombocytopenic purpura: pathophysiology and treatment. Kidney Int Suppl 1998; 64:S45–S49.

54. Lopez EL, Diaz M, Grinstein S, et al: Hemolytic-uremic syndrome and diarrhea in Argentine children: the role of Shiga-like toxins. J Infect Dis 1989; 160:469–475.

55. Repetto HA: Haemolytic-uraemic syndrome—the experience in Argentina [editorial]. Nephrol Dial Transplant 1999; 14:548–550.

56. Austin TW, Ray CG: Coxsackie virus group B infections and the hemolytic-uremic syndrome. J Infect Dis 1973; 127:698–701.

57. Remuzzi G, Ruggenenti P: The hemolytic-uremic syndrome. Kidney Int Suppl 1998; 66:S54–S57.

58. American College of Chest Physicians/Society of Critical Care Medicine Consensus Conference: definitions for sepsis and organ failure and guidelines for the use of innovative therapies in sepsis [see comments]. Crit Care Med 1992; 20:864–874.

59. Centers for Disease Control and Prevention: Increase in National hospital discharge survey rates in septicemia—United States, 1979–1987. MMWR Morb Mort Wkly Rep 1990; 39:31.

60. Centers for Disease Control and Prevention, National Center for Health Statistics: Mortality Patterns—United States, 1990. Monthly Vital Stat Rep 1990; 41:5.

61. Bone RC: Gram-positive organisms and sepsis. Arch Intern Med 1994; 154:26–34.

62. Vincent JL, Bihari DJ, Suter PM, et al: The prevalence of nosocomial infection in intensive care units in Europe: results of the European Prevalence of Infection in Intensive Care (EPIC) Study. EPIC International Advisory Committee [see comments]. JAMA 1995; 274:639–644.

63. Sands KE, Bates DW, Lanken PN, et al: Epidemiology of sepsis syndrome in eight academic medical centers. Academic Medical Center Consortium Sepsis Project Working Group. JAMA 1997; 278:234–240.

64. Bone RC, Fisher CJJ, Clemmer TP, et al: A controlled clinical trial of high-dose methylprednisolone in the treatment of severe sepsis and septic shock. N Engl J Med 1987; 317:653–658.

65. Dhainaut JF, Vincent JL, Richard C, et al: CDP571, a humanized antibody to human tumor necrosis factor-alpha: safety, pharmacokinetics, immune response, and influence of the antibody on cytokine concentrations in patients with septic shock. CPD571 Sepsis Study Group. Crit Care Med 1995; 23:1461–1469.

66. Thijs A, Thijs LG: Pathogenesis of renal failure in sepsis. Kidney Int Suppl 1998; 66:S34–S37.

67. Liano F, Junco E, Pascual J, Madero R, Verde E: The spectrum of acute renal failure in the intensive care unit compared with that seen in other settings. The Madrid Acute Renal Failure Study Group. Kidney Int Suppl 1998; 66:S16–S24.

68. Brivet FG, Kleinknecht DJ, Loirat P, Landais PJ: Acute renal failure in intensive care units—causes, outcome, and prognostic factors of hospital mortality—a prospective, multicenter study. French Study Group on Acute Renal Failure [see comments]. Crit Care Med 1996; 24:192–198.

69. Rangel-Frausto MS, Pittet D, Costigan M, et al: The natural history of the systemic inflammatory response syndrome (SIRS): a prospective study [see comments]. JAMA 1995; 273:117–123.

70. Kleinknecht D: Risk Factors for Acute Renal Failure in Critically Ill Patients. In: Ronco C, Bellomo R, eds: Critical Care Nephrology. Netherlands: Kluwer; 1998:143–152.

71. Danner RL, Elin RJ, Hosseini JM, et al: Endotoxemia in human septic shock. Chest 1991; 99:169–175.

72. Khan RZ, Badr KF: Endotoxin and renal function: perspectives to the understanding of septic acute renal failure and toxic shock [editorial]. Nephrol Dial Transplant 1999; 14:814–818.

73. Lucas CE, Rector FE, Werner M, Rosenberg IK: Altered renal homeostasis with acute sepsis: clinical significance. Arch Surg 1973; 106:444–449.

74. Badr KF, Kelley VE, Rennke HG: Roles for thromboxane A_2 and leukotrienes in endotoxin-induced acute renal failure. Kidney Int 1986; 30:474–480.

75. Tolins JP, Palmer RM, Moncada S, Raij L: Role of endothelium-derived relaxing factor in regulation of renal hemodynamic responses. Am J Physiol 1990; 258:H655–H662.

76. Kikeri D, Pennel JP, Hwang KH, et al: Endotoxemic acute renal failure in awake rats. Am J Physiol 1986; 250:F1098–F1106.

77. Lugon JR, Boim MA, Ramos OL, et al: Renal function and glomerular hemodynamics in male endotoxemic rats. Kidney Int 1989; 36:570–575.

78. Zager RA: Sepsis-associated acute renal failure: some potential pathogenetic and therapeutic insights. Nephrol Dial Transplant 1994; 9(Suppl 4):164–167.

79. Zager RA, Prior RB: Gentamicin and gram-negative bacteremia: a synergism for the development of experimental nephrotoxic acute renal failure. J Clin Invest 1986; 78:196–204.

80. Brenner M, Schaer GL, Mallory DL, et al: Detection of renal blood flow abnormalities in septic and critically ill patients using a newly designed indwelling thermodilution renal vein catheter. Chest 1990; 98:170–179.

81. Cronenwett JL, Lindenauer SM: Distribution of intrarenal blood flow during bacterial sepsis. J Surg Res 1978; 24:132–141.

82. van Lambalgen AA, van Kraats AA, van den Bos GC, et al: Renal function and metabolism during endotoxemia in rats: role of hypoperfusion. Circ Shock 1991; 35:164–173.

83. Garrison RN, Wilson MA, Matheson PJ, Spain DA: Nitric oxide mediates redistribution of intrarenal blood flow during bacteremia. J Trauma 1995; 39:90–96.

84. Cohen JJ, Black AJ, Wertheim SJ: Direct effects of endotoxin on the function of the isolated perfused rat kidney. Kidney Int 1990; 37:1219–1226.

85. Groeneveld AB: Pathogenesis of acute renal failure during sepsis. Nephrol Dial Transplant 1994; 9(Suppl 4):47–51.

86. Goddard J, Cumming AD: Renal Alterations in the Septic Patient. In: Ronco C, Bellomo R, eds: Critical Care Nephrology. Netherlands: Kluwer; 1997:517–526.

87. Mene P, Dunn MJ: Contractile effects of TxA_2 and endoperoxide analogues on cultured rat glomerular mesangial cells. Am J Physiol 1986; 251:F1029–F1035.

88. Cumming AD, McDonald JW, Lindsay RM, et al: The protective effect of thromboxane synthetase inhibition on renal function in systemic sepsis. Am J Kidney Dis 1989; 13:114–119.

89. Voerman HJ, Stehouwer CD, van Kamp DJ, et al: Plasma endothelin levels are increased during septic shock. Crit Care Med 1992; 20:1097.

90. Anderson BO, Bensard DD, Harken AH: The role of platelet-activating factor and its antagonists in shock, sepsis, and multiple organ failure. Surg Gynecol Obstet 1991; 172:415–424.

91. Weitzberg E, Lundberg JM, Rudehill A: Elevated plasma levels of endothelin in patients with sepsis syndrome. Circ Shock 1991; 33:222–227.

92. Linas SL, Whittenburg D, Repine JE: Role of neutrophil-derived oxidants and elastase in lipopolysaccharide-mediated renal injury. Kidney Int 1991; 39:618–623.

93. Yu L, Gengaro PE, Niederberger M, et al: Nitric oxide: a mediator in rat tubular hypoxia/reoxygenation injury. Proc Natl Acad Sci U S A 1994; 91:1691–1695.

94. Tome LA, Yu L, de Castro, I, Campos SB, Seguro AC: Beneficial and harmful effects of L-arginine on renal ischaemia. Nephrol Dial Transplant 1999; 14:1139–1145.

95. Millar CGM, Thiemermann C: NO in Septic Shock. In: Goligorsky MS, Gross SS, eds: Nitric Oxide and the Kidney: Physiology and Pathophysiology. New York: Chapman & Hall; 1997:271–306.

96. Spain DA, Wilson MA, Garrison RN: Nitric oxide synthase inhibition exacerbates sepsis-induced renal hypoperfusion. Surgery 1994; 116:322–330.

97. Moncada S, Palmer RM, Higgs EA: Nitric oxide: physiology, pathophysiology, and pharmacology. Pharmacol Rev 1991; 43:109–142.

98. Shultz PJ, Raij L: Endogenously synthesized nitric oxide prevents endotoxin-induced glomerular thrombosis. J Clin Invest 1992; 90:1718–1725.

99. Churchill PC, Bidani AK, Schwartz MM: Renal effects of endotoxin in the male rat. Am J Physiol 1987; 253:F244–F250.

100. Hussain SN, Roussos C: Distribution of respiratory muscle and organ blood flow during endotoxic shock in dogs. J Appl Physiol 1985; 59:1802–1808.

101. Hussain SN, Rutledge F, Graham R, et al: Effects of norepinephrine and fluid administration on diaphragmatic O_2 consumption in septic shock. J Appl Physiol 1987; 62:1368–1376.

102. Gullichsen E, Nelimarkka O, Halkola L, Niinikoski J: Renal glucose and lactate metabolism in endotoxin shock in dogs. Acta Chir Scand 1989; 155:561–565.

103. Groeneveld AB: Pathogenesis of acute renal failure during sepsis. Nephrol Dial Transplant 1994; 9(Suppl 4):47–51.

104. Linas SL, Whittenburg D, Parsons PE, Repine JE: Mild renal ischemia activates primed neutrophils to cause acute renal failure. Kidney Int 1992; 42:610–616.

105. Greene EL, Paller MS: Oxygen free radicals in acute renal failure. Miner Electrolyte Metab 1991; 17:124–132.

106. Paller MS, Weber K, Patten M: Nitric oxide–mediated renal epithelial cell injury during hypoxia and reoxygenation. Ren Fail 1998; 20:459–469.

107. Thadhani R, Pascual M, Bonventre JV: Acute renal failure [see comments]. N Engl J Med 1996; 334:1448–1460.

108. Kribben A, Wieder ED, Wetzels JF, et al: Evidence for role of cytosolic free calcium in hypoxia-induced proximal tubule injury. J Clin Invest 1994; 93:1922–1929.

109. Yu L, Seguro AC, Rocha AS: Acute renal failure following hemorrhagic shock: protective and aggravating factors. Ren Fail 1992; 14:49–55.

110. Zager RA: Escherichia coli endotoxin injections potentiate experimental ischemic renal injury. Am J Physiol 1986; 251:F988–F994.

111. Zager RA, Altschuld R: Body temperature: an important determinant of severity of ischemic renal injury. Am J Physiol 1986; 251:F87–F93.

112. Zager RA, Prior RB: Gentamicin and gram-negative bacteremia: a synergism for the development of experimental nephrotoxic acute renal failure. J Clin Invest 1986; 78:196–204.

113. Zager RA: Hyperthermia: effects on renal ischemic/reperfusion injury in the rat. Lab Invest 1990; 63:360–369.

114. Zager RA: Endotoxemia, renal hypoperfusion, and fever: interactive risk factors for aminoglycoside and sepsis-associated acute renal failure. Am J Kidney Dis 1992; 20:223–230.

115. Spiegel DM, Shanley PF, Molitoris BA: Mild ischemia predisposes the S3 segment to gentamicin toxicity. Kidney Int 1990; 38:459–464.

116. Schor N, Ichikawa I, Rennke HG, et al: Pathophysiology of altered glomerular function in aminoglycoside-treated rats. Kidney Int 1981; 19:288–296.

117. Schaberg DR, Culver DH, Gaynes RP: Major trends in the microbial etiology of nosocomial infection. Am J Med 1991; 91:72S–75S.

118. Abraham E, Wunderink R, Silverman H, et al: Efficacy and safety of monoclonal antibody to human tumor necrosis factor alpha in patients with sepsis syndrome: a randomized, controlled, double-blind, multicenter clinical trial. TNF-Alpha MAb Sepsis Study Group. JAMA 1995; 273:934–941.

119. Bone RC: Sepsis and SIRS. Nephrol Dial Transplant 1994; 9(Suppl 4):99–103.

120. Cambi V, David S: Basic therapeutic requirements in the treatment of sepsis in acute renal failure. Nephrol Dial Transplant 1994; 9(Suppl 4):183–186.

121. van Bommel EF: Should continuous renal replacement therapy be used for "non-renal" indications in critically ill patients with shock? Resuscitation 1997; 33:257–270.

122. Schetz MR: Classical and alternative indications for continuous renal replacement therapy. Kidney Int Suppl 1998; 66:S129–S132.

123. Bellomo R, Baldwin I, Cole L, Ronco C: Preliminary experience with high-volume hemofiltration in human septic shock. Kidney Int Suppl 1998; 66:S182–S185.

124. van Bommel EF: Are continuous therapies superior to intermittent haemodialysis for acute renal failure on the intensive care unit [editorial]? Nephrol Dial Transplant 1995; 10:311–314.

125. Bellomo R, Ronco C: Continuous versus intermittent renal replacement therapy in the intensive care unit. Kidney Int Suppl 1998; 66:S125–S128.

126. De Vriese AS, Vanholder RC, De Sutter JH, et al: Continuous renal replacement therapies in sepsis: where are the data [editorial]? Nephrol Dial Transplant 1998; 13:1362–1364.

127. Siamopoulos KC: Virus-related acute renal failure: the clinical course and outcome of haemorrhagic fever with renal syndrome. Nephrol Dial Transplant 1994; 9(Suppl 4):111–115.

128. Geltner D, Naot Y, Zimhoni O, et al: Acute oliguric renal failure complicating type A nonfulminant viral hepatitis: a case presentation and review of the literature. J Clin Gastroenterol 1992; 14:160–162.

129. Phillips AO, Thomas DM, Coles GA: Acute renal failure associated with non-fulminant hepatitis A. Clin Nephrol 1999; 39:156–157.

130. Malbrain ML, De Meester X, Wilmer AP, et al: Another case of acute renal failure (ARF) due to acute tubular necrosis (ATN), proven by renal biopsy in non-fulminant hepatitis A virus (HAV) infection [letter; comment]. Nephrol Dial Transplant 1997; 12:1543–1544.

131. Berry L, Braude S: Influenza A infection with rhabdomyolysis and acute renal failure—a potentially fatal complication. Postgrad Med J 1991; 67:389–390.

132. Dell KM, Schulman SL: Rhabdomyolysis and acute renal failure in a child with influenza A infection [see comments]. Pediatr Nephrol 1997; 11:363–365.

133. Goebel J, Harter HR, Boineau FG, el-Dahr SS: Acute renal failure from rhabdomyolysis following influenza A in a child. Clin Pediatr (Phila) 1997; 36:479–481.

134. Seibold S, Merkel F, Weber M, Marx M: Rhabdomyolysis and acute renal failure in an adult with measles virus infection. Nephrol Dial Transplant 1998; 13:1829–1831.

135. Rao TK, Filippone EJ, Nicastri AD, et al: Associated focal and segmental glomerulosclerosis in the acquired immunodeficiency syndrome. N Engl J Med 1984; 310:669–673.

136. Gardenswartz MH, Lerner CW, Seligson GR, et al: Renal disease in patients with AIDS: a clinicopathologic study. Clin Nephrol 1984; 21:197–204.

137. Pardo V, Aldana M, Colton RM, et al: Glomerular lesions in the acquired immunodeficiency syndrome. Ann Intern Med 1984; 101:429–434.

138. Rao TKS, Berns AS: Acute Renal Failure in Patients with HIV Infection. In: Kimmel PL, Berns JS, eds: *Renal and Urologic Aspects of HIV Infection.* New York: Churchill Livingstone; 1995:41–58.

139. Rao TK, Friedman EA, Nicastri AD: The types of renal disease in the acquired immunodeficiency syndrome. N Engl J Med 1987; 316:1062–1068.

140. Bourgoignie JJ: Renal complications of human immunodeficiency virus type 1 [clinical conference]. Kidney Int 1990; 37:1571–1584.

141. Glassock RJ, Cohen AH, Danovitch G, Parsa KP: Human immunodeficiency virus (HIV) infection and the kidney. Ann Intern Med 1990; 112:35–49. [erratum: Ann Intern Med 1990; 112:476.]

142. Frassetto L, Schoenfeld PY, Humphreys MH: Increasing incidence of human immunodeficiency virus–associated nephropathy at San Francisco General Hospital. Am J Kidney Dis 1991; 18:655–659.

143. Chander P, Soni A, Bhagwat R, et al: Renal ultrastructural markers in AIDS-associated nephropathy. Am J Pathol 1987; 126:513–526.

144. D'Agati V, Appel GB: HIV infection and the kidney. J Am Soc Nephrol 1997; 8:138–152.

145. D'Agati V, Appel GB: Renal pathology of human immunodeficiency virus infection. Semin Nephrol 1998; 18:406–421.

146. Briggs WA, Tanawattanacharoen S, Choi MJ, et al: Clinicopathologic correlates of prednisone treatment of human immunodeficiency virus–associated nephropathy. Am J Kidney Dis 1996; 28:618–621.

147. Burns GC, Paul SK, Toth IR, Sivak SL: Effect of angiotensin-converting enzyme inhibition in HIV-associated nephropathy. J Am Soc Nephrol 1997; 8:1140–1146.

148. Ifudu O, Rao TK, Tan CC, et al: Zidovudine is beneficial in human immunodeficiency virus–associated nephropathy. Am J Nephrol 1995; 15:217–221.

149. Kimmel PL, Mishkin GJ, Umana WO: Captopril and renal survival in patients with human immunodeficiency virus nephropathy. Am J Kidney Dis 1996; 28:202–208.

150. Michel C, Dosquet P, Ronco P, et al: Nephropathy associated with infection by human immunodeficiency virus: a report on 11 cases, including 6 treated with zidovudine. Nephron 1992; 62:434–440.

151. Smith MC, Pawar R, Carey JT, et al: Effect of corticosteroid therapy on human immunodeficiency virus–associated nephropathy. Am J Med 1994; 97:145–151.

152. Rao TK: Acute renal failure syndromes in human immunodeficiency virus infection. Semin Nephrol 1998; 18:378–395.

153. Valeri A, Neusy AJ: Acute and chronic renal disease in hospitalized AIDS patients [see comments]. Clin Nephrol 1991; 35:110–118.

154. Rao TK, Friedman EA: Outcome of severe acute renal failure in patients with acquired immunodeficiency syndrome. Am J Kidney Dis 1995; 25:390–398.

155. Peraldi MN, Maslo C, Akposso K, et al: Acute renal failure in the course of HIV infection: a single-institution retrospective study of ninety-two patients and sixty renal biopsies. Nephrol Dial Transplant 1999; 14:1578–1585.

156. Schmaljohn CS, Hasty SE, Dalrymple JM, et al: Antigenic and genetic properties of viruses linked to hemorrhagic fever with renal syndrome. Science 1985; 227:1041–1044.

157. WHO Working Group: WHO. Bull WHO 1983; 61:269–275.

158. Tkachenko EA, Lee HW: Etiology and epidemiology of hemorrhagic fever with renal syndrome. Kidney Int Suppl 1991; 35:S54–S61.

159. Lee HW, Lee PW, Johnson KM: Isolation of the etiologic agent of Korean hemorrhagic fever. J Infect Dis 1978; 137:298–308.

160. Lee HW, van der Groen G: Hemorrhagic fever with renal syndrome. Prog Med Virol 1989; 36:62–102.

161. Cosgriff TM, Lewis RM: Mechanisms of disease in hemorrhagic fever with renal syndrome. Kidney Int Suppl 1991; 35:S72–S79.

162. Lee HW, Johnson KM: Laboratory-acquired infections with Hantaan virus, the etiologic agent of Korean hemorrhagic fever. J Infect Dis 1982; 146:645–651.

163. Lee JS: Clinical features of hemorrhagic fever with renal syndrome in Korea. Kidney Int Suppl 1991; 35:S88–S93.

164. Settergren B, Juto P, Wadell G, et al: Incidence and geographic distribution of serologically verified cases of nephropathia epidemica in Sweden. Am J Epidemiol 1988; 127:801–807.

165. Collan Y, Mihatsch MJ, Lahdevirta J, et al: Nephropathia epidemica: mild variant of hemorrhagic fever with renal syndrome. Kidney Int Suppl 1991; 35:S62–S71.

166. Centers for Disease Control and Prevention: Hantavirus pulmonary syndrome—United States, 1993. MMWR CDC Surveill Summ 1994; 43:45–48.
167. Nichol ST, Spiropoulou CF, Morzunov S, et al: Genetic identification of a hantavirus associated with an outbreak of acute respiratory illness [see comments]. Science 1993; 262:914–917.
168. Duchin JS, Koster FT, Peters CJ, et al: Hantavirus pulmonary syndrome: a clinical description of 17 patients with a newly recognized disease. The Hantavirus Study Group [see comments]. N Engl J Med 1994; 330:949–955.
169. Childs JE, Ksiazek TG, Spiropoulou CF, et al: Serologic and genetic identification of *Peromyscus maniculatus* as the primary rodent reservoir for a new hantavirus in the southwestern United States. J Infect Dis 1994; 169:1271–1280.
170. Rollin PE, Ksiazek TG, Elliott LH, et al: Isolation of Black Creek Canal virus, a new hantavirus from *Sigmodon hispidus* in Florida. J Med Virol 1995; 46:35–39.
171. Morrison YY, Rathbun RC: Hantavirus pulmonary syndrome: the Four Corners disease. Ann Pharmacother 1995; 29:57–65.
172. Khan AS, Gaviria M, Rollin PE, et al: Hantavirus pulmonary syndrome in Florida: association with the newly identified Black Creek Canal virus. Am J Med 1996; 100:46–48.
173. Peters CJ, Simpson GL, Levy H: Spectrum of Hantavirus infection: hemorrhagic fever with renal syndrome and Hantavirus pulmonary syndrome. Annu Rev Med 1999; 50:531–545.
174. Zeier M, Andrassy K, Zoller L, Ritz E: Hantavirus infection presenting as acute renal failure [letter] [see comments]. Lancet 1990; 336:1441–1442.
175. Mustonen J, Helin H, Pietila K, et al: Renal biopsy findings and clinicopathologic correlations in nephropathia epidemica. Clin Nephrol 1994; 41:121–126.
176. Bren AF, Pavlovcic SK, Koselj M, et al: Acute renal failure due to hemorrhagic fever with renal syndrome. Ren Fail 1996; 18:635–638.
177. Lu Q, Zhu Z, Weng J: Immune responses to inactivated vaccine in people naturally infected with Hantaviruses. J Med Virol 1996; 49:333–335.
178. Siamopoulos KC: Virus-related acute renal failure: the clinical course and outcome of haemorrhagic fever with renal syndrome. Nephrol Dial Transplant 1994; 9(Suppl 4):111–115.
179. Barsoum RS: Malarial nephropathies. Nephrol Dial Transplant 1998; 13:1588–1597.
180. Sitprija V: Nephropathy in falciparum malaria (clinical conference). Kidney Int 1988; 34:867–877.
181. Turkmen A, Sever MS, Ecder T, et al: Posttransplant malaria. Transplantation 1996; 62:1521–1523.
182. Eiam-Ong S, Sitprija V: Falciparum malaria and the kidney: a model of inflammation. Am J Kidney Dis 1998; 32:361–375.
183. Prakash J, Gupta A, Kumar O, et al: Acute renal failure in falciparum malaria—increasing prevalence in some areas of India—a need for awareness (news) [see comments]. Nephrol Dial Transplant 1996; 11:2414–2416.
184. Taylor WR, Prosser DI: Acute renal failure, acute rhabdomyolysis, and falciparum malaria. Trans R Soc Trop Med Hyg 1992; 86:361.
185. Wilairatana P, Westerlund EK, Aursudkij B, et al: Treatment of malarial acute renal failure by hemodialysis. Am J Trop Med Hyg 1999; 60:233–237.
186. Naqvi R, Ahmad E, Akhtar F, et al: Predictors of outcome in malarial renal failure. Ren Fail 1996; 18:685–688.
187. Sheiban AK: Prognosis of malaria-associated severe acute renal failure in children. Ren Fail 1999; 21:63–66.
188. Sitprija V: Renal involvement in human leptospirosis. BMJ 1968; 2:656–658.
189. Abdulkader RC: Acute renal failure in leptospirosis. Ren Fail 1997; 19:191–198.
190. da Silva MV, Nakamura PM, Camargo ED, et al: Immunodiagnosis of human leptospirosis by dot-ELISA for the detection of IgM, IgG, and IgA antibodies. Am J Trop Med Hyg 1997; 56:650–655.
191. da Silva MV, Dias CE, Vaz AJ, Batista L: Immunodiagnosis of human leptospirosis using saliva. Trans R Soc Trop Med Hyg 1992; 86:560–561.
192. de Brito T, Morais CF, Yasuda PH, et al: Cardiovascular involvement in human and experimental leptospirosis: pathologic findings and immunohistochemical detection of leptospiral antigen. Ann Trop Med Parasitol 1987; 81:207–214.
193. O'Neil KM, Rickman LS, Lazarus AA: Pulmonary manifestations of leptospirosis. Rev Infect Dis 1991; 13:705–709.
194. Martinelli R, Luna MA, Rocha H: Is rhabdomyolysis an additional factor in the pathogenesis of acute renal failure in leptospirosis? Rev Inst Med Trop Sao Paulo 1994; 36:111–114.
195. Abdulkader RC, Seguro AC, Malheiro PS, et al: Peculiar electrolytic and hormonal abnormalities in acute renal failure due to leptospirosis. Am J Trop Med Hyg 1996; 54:1–6.
196. Seguro AC, Lomar AV, Rocha AS: Acute renal failure of leptospirosis: nonoliguric and hypokalemic forms. Nephron 1990; 55:146–151.
197. Park SK, Lee SH, Rhee YK, et al: Leptospirosis in Chonbuk Province of Korea in 1987: a study of 93 patients. Am J Trop Med Hyg 1989; 41:345–351.
198. Magaldi AJ, Yasuda PN, Kudo LH, et al: Renal involvement in leptospirosis: a pathophysiologic study. Nephron 1992; 62:332–339.
199. Davila de Arriaga AJ, Rocha AS, Yasuda PH, de Brito T: Morpho-functional patterns of kidney injury in the experimental leptospirosis of the guinea-pig (*L. icterohaemorrhagiae*). J Pathol 1982; 138:145–161.
200. Everard CO, Edwards CN, Everard JD, Carrington DG: A twelve-year study of leptospirosis on Barbados. Eur J Epidemiol 1995; 11:311–320.
201. Sasaki DM, Pang L, Minette HP, et al: Active surveillance and risk factors for leptospirosis in Hawaii. Am J Trop Med Hyg 1993; 48:35–43.
202. Sitprija V, Pipatanagul V, Mertowidjojo K, et al: Pathogenesis of renal disease in leptospirosis: clinical and experimental studies. Kidney Int 1980; 17:827–836.
203. Takafuji ET, Kirkpatrick JW, Miller RN, et al: An efficacy trial of doxycycline chemoprophylaxis against leptospirosis. N Engl J Med 1984; 310:497–500.
204. Watt G, Padre LP, Tuazon ML, et al: Placebo-controlled trial of intravenous penicillin for severe and late leptospirosis. Lancet 1988; 1:433–435.
205. Marotto PC, Marotto MS, Santos DL, et al: Outcome of leptospirosis in children. Am J Trop Med Hyg 1997; 56:307–310.

CHAPTER 23

Acute Renal Failure in Pregnancy

Dipti Shah ▪ Susan Hou

Acute renal failure (ARF) in pregnancy usually results from obstetric complications and not intrinsic renal disease. The frequency of pregnancy-associated ARF is a reflection of the overall quality and availability of obstetric care and the availability of safe pregnancy termination.

EPIDEMIOLOGY

Historically, ARF in pregnancy once represented 20% to 40% of all cases of ARF and was responsible for 50% of cases in women.[1] In 1958, the estimated incidence of ARF in pregnancy was as high as 1 in 1400. Today, in industrialized countries, the incidence is approximately 1 in 20,000.[2] In pregnancy, ARF occurs with a bimodal distribution. A peak in early pregnancy is associated with septic abortion, whereas a third trimester peak is associated with late obstetric complications such as preeclampsia, abruptio placentae, postpartum hemorrhage, amniotic fluid embolism, and retained dead fetus.[1, 3]

The relationship between the decrease in obstetric renal failure and the legalization of abortion is inescapable. In Western Europe, there has been almost complete elimination of the first peak.[4] The legalization of abortion in France was followed by a decrease in the percentage of cases of ARF attributable to obstetric causes from 40% in 1966 to 4.5% in 1978.[2] When abortion was made illegal in Romania in 1966, complications of illegal abortion became a major cause of ARF. In a report of 653 patients dialyzed for ARF between 1966 and 1989, in 131 (20%) ARF resulted from complications of illegal abortion.[5] Between 1990 and 1992, obstetric ARF accounted for only 1.52% of the total ARF.

In developing countries, obstetric ARF remains a serious problem. Randeree and colleagues described the changing picture of obstetric ARF as the health care system in South Africa improved.[6] Between 1978 and 1991 the frequency of ARF in a hospital serving a poor community declined from 1 in 450 pregnancies to 1 in 900 pregnancies. With improvement in prenatal care, the percentage of obstetric ARF secondary to septic abortion decreased from 65% in 1978 to 19% in 1991, whereas the percentage of obstetric ARF from preeclampsia increased from 10% to 48%. With further improvement in obstetric care and early recognition of preeclampsia, the frequency of ARF from this cause would be expected to decrease.

ACUTE RENAL FAILURE ASSOCIATED WITH INFECTION

Postabortion Sepsis

There are many contributing factors to ARF failure following abortion, including hypotension, hemorrhage, sepsis, and disseminated intravascular coagulation. Spontaneous abortion rarely leads to infection.[7] Deliberate interference with pregnancy without sterile operating conditions is the major cause of postabortion ARF. Because these conditions are most common when abortion is illegal, patients often present after a delay and show features of septicemia and shock.

A variety of organisms are cultured from these patients, including *Escherichia coli*, a variety of *Clostridium* species, enterococci, *Pseudomonas aeruginosa*, β-hemolytic streptococci, *Staphylococcus aureus*, and *Klebsiella*.[8] Although ARF can occur with sepsis from any of these organisms, it is most common and severe during infections with *Clostridium* species because of their production of a toxin causing hemolysis.[9] The organism is difficult to culture and may be present in normal vaginal flora, but the infection is usually accompanied by severe abdominal pain. Gas in the uterine wall on plain abdominal film or on computed tomographic (CT) scan of the abdomen is characteristic and rare in infections with other organisms, but the presence of *Clostridium* should be suspected and the organism covered even in the absence of gas in the uterus.

Management of *Clostridium* infection involves supportive care, intravenous antibiotics, and fluid resuscitation. Since infections following septic abortion often involve multiple organisms, broad-spectrum coverage including gram-negative types and anaerobes should be the initial therapy. Dialysis may be required for correction of metabolic disturbances and fluid overload. Because of hemolysis, patients with *Clostridium* sepsis and renal failure are at particular risk for hyperkalemia. There are reports on the successful use of exchange transfusion to remove the toxin and free hemoglobin.[10, 11] The need for surgical intervention has been debated. At one time, infection with *Clostridium* was considered an automatic indication for hysterectomy.[11] Firmat and colleagues recommended hysterectomy only in the presence of gangrene or documented uterine perforation.[12] Hawkins and colleagues reported that 17 of 19 patients treated with intensive antibiotic therapy, dialysis, and a minimum of surgical intervention survived, and preserved fertility was documented in 9.[13]

Pyelonephritis

Urinary tract infection is one of the most common medical complications of pregnancy and can be associated with preterm labor and prematurity.[14–16] A number of the normal physiologic changes that take place during pregnancy predispose to urinary tract infection. There is dilation of the upper collecting system that leads to stasis of up to 300 mL of urine in the collecting system. Hormonal factors lead to relaxation of the smooth muscle of the ureter and bladder. These changes are more pronounced on the right side. The enlarged uterus may cause partial obstruction of the ureters.[17, 18]

Urinary tract infection in pregnancy can present as asymptomatic bacteriuria (ASB), cystitis, or pyelonephritis. ASB, defined as persistent, asymptomatic bacterial colonization of the urinary tract, occurs in 5% to 10% of women. Pregnancy itself does not cause ASB. The prevalence is similar in pregnant and nonpregnant patients; however, 30% of ASB in pregnant women will progress to pyelonephritis.[19] All women should be screened with a urine culture at the first prenatal visit. Other methods of screening for ASB, such as measurement of urinary leukocyte esterase or nitrates, are not adequately sensitive. The growth of >100,000 colony-forming units of a single uropathogen indicates the presence of ASB, and women with positive cultures should be treated for 7 to 10 days with an antibiotic, based on sensitivity testing and safety of the drug during pregnancy. Repeat urine cultures should be performed 1 week after completing a course of antibiotics and then monthly for the remainder of the pregnancy. A second positive urine culture warrants a 14-day course with a different antibiotic followed by suppressive therapy. Patients with persistent or recurrent infection should undergo a urologic evaluation 3 to 6 months after delivery, when normal pregnancy-related urinary tract changes resolve.[17, 18]

Cystitis refers to inflammation of the bladder in the presence of bacteriuria and in association with symptoms of dysuria, frequency, or suprapubic discomfort. The incidence of cystitis in pregnant women is 0.3% to 2%, which is slightly higher than in nonpregnant, sexually active women.[20] Patients with cystitis should be treated and followed in the same way as patients with ASB.

Pyelonephritis occurs in 1% to 2% of all pregnancies. With the advent of screening programs, the incidence has been reduced over the last 20 years from 4% to 0.8%. Although ARF rarely occurs from pyelonephritis, 25% of patients develop a transient decline in glomerular filtration rate (GFR).[21] Of these patients, most demonstrate a return to normal renal function 3 to 8 weeks after successful treatment of the acute infection. Pyelonephritis in pregnancy is frequently complicated by other serious medical problems with bacteremia in 10% of cases and respiratory failure in 2% of cases. Thus, these patients should be treated aggressively with intravenous antibiotics followed by oral antibiotics to complete a 2-week course of therapy. After successful treatment, suppressive therapy should be continued for the rest of the pregnancy. Women who fail to improve within 72 hours of treatment should be evaluated for obstructive uropathy.

Obstruction

Despite the changes in the urinary tract, obstructive uropathy is an uncommon cause of renal failure in pregnancy. Renal stones form no more frequently in pregnant women than in the general population. Changes in factors that influence stone formation occur in pregnancy but tend to cancel each other out. Urinary stasis in the dilated collecting system is accompanied by hypercalciuria; increased supersaturation of calcium, oxalate, and phosphate; and an alkaline urine. However, there is an increased excretion of magnesium citrate as well as the glycoprotein nephrocalcin, which inhibits stone formation.[22] Nephrolithiasis may be a cause of pain and infection in pregnancy, but bilateral obstruction is required for ARF from obstruction.

There are rare instances of renal failure caused directly by obstruction of the ureter(s) by the pregnant uterus.[23, 24] This is most common in the setting of a single kidney with polyhydramnios during the third trimester. Obstruction should be considered in the appropriate clinical setting when there is nothing to suggest renal failure from other causes.

The interpretation of ultrasound, the usual screening test for obstruction, may be difficult in pregnancy. Hydronephrosis is progressive throughout the course of pregnancy, but the average degree of dilation cannot determine whether a given degree of dilation is too great for the stage of gestation in an individual patient.[25] In the setting of ARF, the need for diagnosis justifies the radiation exposure associated with spiral CT scan.

When polyhydramnios causes ARF, renal function may improve with amniocentesis and recurrence prevented by treatment of the polyhydramnios with nonsteroidal anti-inflammatory agents. The approach depends on the demands of the obstetric problem causing polyhydramnios. Ureteral stents can be placed during pregnancy but require considerable technical skill on the part of the urologist. Percutaneous nephrostomy tubes can also be used. These may not be necessary if the obstetric problem requires delivery of the fetus.

ACUTE RENAL FAILURE IN THE THIRD TRIMESTER

Bilateral Cortical Necrosis

In a majority of instances, ARF secondary to preeclampsia or peripartum hemorrhage follows a course typical of acute tubular necrosis with recovery of renal function. In obstetric ARF, a substantial minority of patients develops bilateral cortical necrosis in which renal function may fail to recover or recovery may be partial with later progression to end-stage renal disease. Bilateral cortical necrosis may occur in any type of ischemic ARF, but a disproportionate number of cases occur in obstetric patients. In a report of 38 instances of cortical necrosis that occurred at Necker Hospital between 1953 and 1972, obstetric patients accounted for 26 (68%).[26] The incidence of cortical necrosis was 2% in the nonpregnant adult with ARF and 21% of obstetric patients with ARF. There may be a vulnerability of the renal vasculature that is peculiar to pregnancy. It is notable that the Schwartzman reaction can be induced in postpartum animals after one exposure to endotoxin, whereas nonpregnant animals develop it only after a second exposure.[27] Cortical necrosis can be diagnosed by CT scan or angiography.[28] The diagnosis is made primarily for prognostic purposes.

Acute Renal Failure in Preeclampsia

Decreased GFR and renal blood flow and decreased sodium excretion are characteristic of preeclampsia, but frank renal failure is unusual. Acute renal failure in preeclamptic women occurs most often when another obstetric complication such as abruptio placentae is present or when preeclampsia has progressed to the HELLP (hemolysis, elevated liver enzymes, low platelet count) syndrome.[29–31] In the largest series of patients with HELLP, 7.7% suffered ARF. In one report of 17 preeclamptic women with ARF, 80% of women who developed cortical necrosis had abruptio placentae compared with one third of those who recovered renal function.[30] When ARF follows preeclampsia, there is substantial risk of maternal mortality (9.6% in one series).[29] Pulmonary edema occurs in more than 50% of women with ARF, emphasizing the need for judicious fluid administration in women with preeclampsia. Women with who survive ARF in the setting of preeclampsia without essential hypertension or underlying renal disease have normal renal function at long-term follow-up. When ARF occurs in women with underlying chronic renal disease and renal insufficiency, as many as 80% are dialysis dependent at follow-up.[29] In these women it is frequently difficult to distinguish between ARF secondary to preeclampsia and the poorly understood acceleration of renal failure in women with preexisting renal insufficiency, particularly because these women are frequently hypertensive when they lose renal function.

Acute Fatty Liver of Pregnancy

Acute fatty liver of pregnancy is an obstetric emergency that, if untreated, may progress to fulminant hepatic failure, which is life threatening for both the mother and fetus. The disease most often presents in the third trimester with complaints of headache, fatigue, malaise, nausea, and abdominal pain. Late signs include jaundice, bleeding, seizures, and hepatic encephalopathy, which may progress to frank coma. Liver biopsy shows microvesicular fatty infiltration of hepatocytes in a centrilobular distribution.[32] The maternal mortality rate for the disease has improved from 80% to 85% in the 1970s to less than 20% in recent series, with the lowest mortality rate reported being 6.6%.[33–35] The improvement in outcome can be attributed to earlier recognition and treatment, the recognition of milder cases, and better supportive care of fulminant hepatic failure. Acute fatty liver is frequently accompanied by preeclampsia, and there may be a link between the two syndromes. The etiology of the syndrome is unknown, but recent investigations have found a familial metabolic defect in fatty acid metabolism.[36–38]

Some degree of ARF occurs in up to 90% of women with acute fatty liver of pregnancy.[33, 35] Renal biopsy findings in acute fatty liver of pregnancy include acute tubular necrosis, fatty vacuolization of tubular cells, and occlusion of capillary lumens by fibrin-like material. Clinically, the ARF in this syndrome may resemble hepatorenal syndrome with low fractional excretion of sodium and benign sediment. Treatment includes delivery of the baby and supportive care. ARF usually resolves post partum, as does the liver failure. The availability of orthotopic liver transplant offers a lifesaving treatment to women who do not recover post partum. The timing of liver transplant is difficult since waiting may result in deterioration of the patient to the point where liver transplant carries a high mortality and performing a transplant prematurely may commit a woman who might have had a complete recovery to life-long immunosuppression.

Postpartum Hemolytic-Uremic Syndrome

Initially described in children with antecedent diarrheal illness and in association with verotoxin, hemolytic-uremic syndrome (HUS) is characterized by a microangiopathic hemolytic anemia, thrombocytopenia, and renal failure. It is also recognized in adults in association with diarrheal illnesses, certain forms of adenocarcinoma, medications, and pregnancy. Early reports of postpartum HUS refer to the syndrome as *postpartum renal failure*, but although it usually occurs between 1 day and 3 months' postpartum, HUS may occur prior to delivery as well.[39, 40] Thrombotic thrombocytopenic purpura (TTP), considered to be related to HUS along a continuum, occurs during and less often following pregnancy. It combines the features of HUS and TTP. Renal failure in both HUS and TTP is often severe enough to require temporary dialysis, and patients may suffer residual renal damage, some severe enough to require chronic dialysis or transplant.[41]

In a review of 68 adults with HUS/TTP of various etiologies diagnosed between 1980 and 1982, Conlon and associates found a normal urinalysis at presentation in only 3%.[42] Eighty-six percent had microscopic hematuria, and 89% had proteinuria. In one series of 11 women with pregnancy-associated HUS, 81% had impaired renal function at presentation. Cases of HUS/TTP have been reported in sisters.[43, 44]

The mainstay of treatment for HUS/TTP is plasma

TABLE 23–1. Clinical Characteristics of HELLP Syndrome, Lupus, and Hemolytic-Uremic Syndrome

CHARACTERISTICS	HELLP	LUPUS	HUS
Timing	>20 wk	Any time	Postpartum, rarely during
Blood pressure	↑	↑/normal	↑/normal
Edema	Present	Sometimes present	Sometimes present
Urine sediment	Benign	RBC casts, active	RBCs
Hemoglobin	↓	↓/normal	↓
Complement	Normal/↑	↓/normal	Normal
Platelet count	↓	↓/normal	↓
LDH	↑	Normal/↑	↑
Transaminases	↑↑	Normal	Normal

HELLP, hemolysis, elevated liver enzymes, low platelet count; *HUS,* hemolytic-uremic syndrome; *RBC,* red blood cell; *LDH,* lactate dehydrogenase.

exchange. Prior to the advent of plasmapheresis, the maternal mortality rate was 90%. With this treatment, maternal survival has increased to 70% to 80%. Plasma exchange during pregnancy has not shown adverse effects on the fetus.[45, 46] Plasma exchange is thought to work by removing factors that promote platelet aggregation and replacing inhibitory factors that may be lacking in the serum of patients with HUS/TTP. The number of treatments necessary varies among patients, ranging from 5 to 47 days in one series of 67 women.[47] The duration of treatment is determined by monitoring hematologic, neurologic, and renal parameters. Other treatments used have included prednisone, aspirin, dipyridamole, heparin, immunoglobulin, vincristine, and splenectomy. These should be considered only as adjuncts to plasma exchange.

Recurrence of HUS has been described both in subsequent pregnancies and in response to other inciting factors, including oral contraceptives, infections, and drugs such as cyclosporine.

There is sometimes difficulty in distinguishing HUS/TTP from severe preeclampsia accompanied by the HELLP syndrome (Table 23–1). Thrombocyto-penia, microangiopathic hemolytic anemia, renal insufficiency, proteinuria, and hypertension may occur in both. Some distinguishing features include isolated elevation of lactate dehydrogenase in HUS/TTP as opposed to elevation of transaminases in preeclampsia/HELLP. Elevations of prothrombin and partial thromboplastin times are unusual in HUS/TTP and suggest preeclampsia. Preeclampsia generally improves following delivery, although there may be transient worsening for 48 hours. Thrombotic thrombocytopenia purpura/HUS is not improved by termination of pregnancy. The distinction is important since preeclampsia resolves with supportive care following delivery, and HUS/TTP is generally irreversible without plasma exchange.

Biopsy findings in HUS/TTP include glomerular capillary endothelial swelling and subendothelial deposition of fibrinoid material that may cause occlusion of capillaries[48] (Fig. 23–1). Thrombi composed of fibrin and platelets are found within capillaries and arterioles.

The pathophysiology of microthrombus formation in HUS/TTP is thought to involve endothelial injury

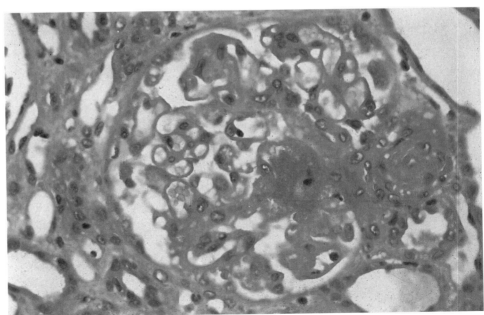

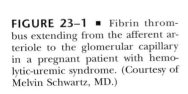

FIGURE 23–1 ■ Fibrin thrombus extending from the afferent arteriole to the glomerular capillary in a pregnant patient with hemolytic-uremic syndrome. (Courtesy of Melvin Schwartz, MD.)

along with other factors contributing to enhancement of platelet aggregation or a decrease in inhibitors to platelet aggregation. Among those factors, abnormally large multimers of von Willebrand factor have been observed in TTP, and these can cause aggregation of activated platelets. Calpain, a cysteine protease capable of causing aggregation of normal platelets and of enhancing platelet binding by von Willebrand factor, has been found in some patients with active TTP. Decreased fibrinolysis may play a role. Plasminogen activator inhibitor-1, the major inhibitor of plasminogen activator, has been found to be increased in some cases of postdiarrheal HUS. Decreased synthesis and increased degradation of prostacyclin have been suggested on the basis of studies using plasma from individuals with TTP. There may also be some genetic predisposition to HUS/TTP. There are known familial occurrences, and pregnancy-associated HUS has been reported in sisters.[49, 50]

Even though advances in treatment have dramatically increased patient survival in obstetric HUS/TTP, it still poses a significant threat to both mother and child, particularly if not diagnosed and treated promptly. Patients with pregnancy-associated HUS/TTP should be aware of the possibility of recurrence in future pregnancies and with estrogen-containing oral contraceptives, although at present there is no method to identify those who will be affected a second time.

ACUTE RENAL FAILURE SECONDARY TO NONOBSTETRIC RENAL DISEASE

Differentiating Nonobstetric Renal Disease From Preeclampsia

Primary renal disease may be a cause of ARF in pregnancy. Acute glomerulonephritis is the major nonobstetric renal disease that may be difficult to differentiate from preeclampsia (see Table 23–1). With interstitial nephritis, the history of a drug exposure is usually given. For ischemic or toxic ARF, the precipitating event or exposure can usually be identified. Acute renal failure secondary to cocaine and other illicit drugs may be difficult to obtain. In the case of cocaine-induced renal failure, evidence of rhabdomyolysis is usually present.

Glomerulonephritis may present with ARF accompanied by proteinuria and hypertension. If symptoms occur before 20 weeks' gestation, causes of renal failure other than preeclampsia must be sought. Beyond 20 weeks' gestation, ARF would be expected only in severe preeclampsia. It is common to see red blood cells and white blood cells in the urine sediment of pregnant women,[51] but red blood cell casts indicate the presence of glomerulonephritis.[52] Serum complement levels can be helpful. Pregnancy is usually associated with increased levels of complement. Hypocomplementemia strongly suggests intrinsic glomerular disease.

Lupus nephritis has its highest incidence in women

of childbearing age. Like preeclampsia, it can be a multisystem disease. Thrombocytopenia and hemolytic anemia can be seen in both lupus and preeclampsia. Pulmonary edema in a woman with preeclampsia may resemble pulmonary hemorrhage seen in lupus. Seizures may be either eclampsia or lupus cerebritis. The hemolytic anemia of preeclampsia is accompanied by microangiopathic changes on peripheral smear, not a characteristic finding in lupus. Elevated transaminase levels are uncommon in lupus. Arthralgias and skin rash are not usually seen in preeclampsia. Urine sediment and serologic determinations are helpful in distinguishing the two. Pregnancy may precipitate a flare of preexisting lupus nephritis or the development of lupus nephritis in a woman with extrarenal lupus.[53] Women with preexisting lupus should be followed with monthly measurements of serum complement since there may be a drop within the normal range because of the high complements in normal pregnancy.

If the cause of ARF is not clear, renal biopsy can be done. Late in pregnancy, it can be done in the sitting or lateral position. In the hands of experienced operators, biopsy during pregnancy does not carry a higher risk than in the nonpregnant state.[54] Biopsy is indicated in new-onset lupus during pregnancy. This is because the histology frequently shows a diffuse proliferative glomerulonephritis that requires aggressive treatment.

Occasionally proteinuria and an elevated serum creatinine level from preexisting renal disease are noted for the first time during pregnancy. Decreased renal size and findings of hyperparathyroidism on hand films are indicative of long-standing renal disease. Women with even mild degrees of renal insufficiency who become pregnant are usually severely anemic, out of proportion to iron deficiency, because they are unable to increase red blood cell production as needed for normal pregnancy. With chronic renal disease there may be proteinuria and hypertension together with ARF. The sediment may be bland and the serologies normal. Early prenatal care allows for the recognition of preexisting renal disease early enough that it is not confused with preeclampsia. It is usually reasonable to follow a woman over a period of days to a week to determine whether renal function is changing, if the woman is otherwise stable. Women with preexisting renal insufficiency (serum creatinine > 1.4 mg/dL) have a 35% to 50% chance that their renal function will deteriorate during pregnancy, sometimes to the point of needing dialysis.[55]

Acute renal failure in renal transplant recipients has the same differential diagnosis as when the patient is not pregnant. There are a few considerations specific to pregnancy. Acute rejection may occur because of changing cyclosporine levels in the absence of a change in dose. Occasionally, a poorly educated transplant recipient will stop her immunosuppressive medication in a misguided attempt to protect the baby from their effects. Cyclosporine toxicity may occur as a result of drug interaction. In particular, erythromycin is commonly prescribed to pregnant women for respiratory illnesses because of its safety for the fetus. Forty percent of pregnant transplant recipients develop urinary tract infections with the risks noted earlier.[56] Obstruction of a solitary kidney should always be considered. Many of these pitfalls can be avoided by appropriate education about pregnancy from the time the patient first considers transplant for end-stage renal disease.

Treatment of Intrinsic Renal Disease

Acute renal failure from glomerulonephritis, particularly lupus nephritis, requires aggressive treatment with immunosuppressive drugs. In the patient with diffuse proliferative lupus nephritis, cyclophosphamide may offer the only chance of recovering renal function. The drug is teratogenic in the first trimester.[57] Experience with cyclophosphamide in the second and third trimesters is limited, and it is frequently used as part of a multidrug chemotherapeutic regimen for treatment of cancer.[58] It is associated with fetal neutropenia, and infants exposed to cyclophosphamide in utero should be monitored for the development of cancer during childhood. A woman who is treated with cyclophosphamide during the second and third trimesters need not be encouraged to terminate the pregnancy because of the effects of the drug on the fetus.

High-dose steroids have been used for many conditions in pregnant women.[59] In low doses, the fetal exposure may be small, but in large doses, the baby is at risk for adrenal insufficiency. Betamethasone and dexamethasone cross the placenta more readily than does prednisone.[60]

Other immunosuppressive drugs have been widely used in pregnancy. Azathioprine may also be associated with fetal neutropenia.[61] Cyclosporine does not appear to be teratogenic but is associated with small-for-gestational-age babies.[62] Both these drugs have been used extensively during pregnancy in organ transplant recipients, and the risk associated with them may be acceptable. However, these drugs are usually inadequate for treatment of ARF. They may be used following completion of a 2-month course of oral cyclophosphamide.

Some women with lupus and ARF might have ARF from another cause. A woman with mild mesangial lupus may have acute tubular necrosis. A renal biopsy should be done before terminating a pregnancy or exposing a fetus to cyclophosphamide. A frozen section of the biopsy can be done, or the woman can be treated with high-dose steroids until the need for cyclophosphamide is confirmed.

Acute Renal Failure in Pregnant Renal Transplant Recipients

Management of ARF in pregnant transplant recipients includes the diagnosis and treatment of ARF in nonpregnant transplant recipients, which are covered in Chapter 25. There are a few considerations specific to pregnancy. Transplant recipients are generally advised to wait 1.5 to 2 years after transplant to become

pregnant, and acute rejection is uncommon if this recommendation is followed. However, acute rejection may occur as a result of changes in drug levels. Serum levels of cyclosporine may change during pregnancy in unpredictable ways, and these should be measured weekly during the early stages of pregnancy until a stable therapeutic dose is established. Rarely, a previously conscientious patient may discontinue medication in a misguided attempt to protect the fetus from the effects of immunosuppression. The latter mistake can be avoided by beginning education about pregnancy as soon as a woman of childbearing age begins to consider transplant. Because pregnant women have several physicians involved in their care, there is a risk that erythromycin, which is safe in pregnancy, may be prescribed for treatment of a respiratory infection. The drug interaction may lead to worsening renal function as a result of cyclosporine toxicity.

Like women with other renal diseases, transplant recipients are at increased risk for preeclampsia, and it is occasionally necessary to perform a renal biopsy to differentiate preeclampsia from acute rejection.

Obstruction of the transplant ureter by the pregnant uterus is uncommon despite the pelvic location of the renal allograft.

Dialysis of Pregnant Women

Dialysis can be initiated during pregnancy if ARF is not secondary to preeclampsia and the patient is remote from term (< 34 weeks' gestation). Seventy to 80% of women who start dialysis during pregnancy because of chronic renal failure have surviving infants.[63] The experience with ARF is more limited, but there are numerous case reports of successful pregnancy in women with ARF.

Either hemodialysis or peritoneal dialysis can be done. An experienced surgeon can place a peritoneal catheter even during the third trimester. During pregnancy, there is some risk of laceration of a uterine vein by the peritoneal catheter, and bloody peritoneal fluid requires admission to hospital for observation and evaluation for bleeding from the surface of the uterus and for impending placental separation.

When recovery is expected, hemodialysis can be done through a temporary catheter. Heparin does not cross the placenta and heparin-free dialysis need not be done unless there is active bleeding.

There are no firm guidelines for the amount of dialysis done in pregnant women, but there is some suggestion that in women with complete renal shutdown, women receiving more than 20 hours of dialysis per week have a better outcome. This recommendation is based on experience in women with chronic renal failure and may not prove to be applicable in ARF.

Six-times-weekly dialysis allows for improved blood pressure control and eliminates the need for removal of large volumes of fluid with each dialysis treatment. With daily dialysis, a 2.5 mEq/L dialysis bath should be used. The normal bicarbonate for pregnancy is 18 to 20 mEq/L and a low-bicarbonate bath is required.[64] Hemodiafiltration can be used to control severe alkalosis. Pregnant women require higher doses of supplementary water-soluble vitamins than either normal pregnant women or nonpregnant dialysis patients.

Preterm labor and preeclampsia are common in women with renal failure. A woman with residual renal function may develop hyperkalemia and increased dialysis requirements if preterm labor is treated with indomethacin. The use of magnesium for either preterm labor or preeclampsia carries the risk of magnesium toxicity and respiratory arrest. The patient can be given an initial loading dose of magnesium. Magnesium can be supplemented after each hemodialysis treatment, and it can be put in the peritoneal dialysate to maintain serum levels. Continuous infusions of magnesium should not be used.

In summary, ARF is uncommon in pregnancy where good prenatal care is available and illegal abortion is unnecessary. ARF still occurs occasionally in the setting of third-trimester obstetric complications or in the event that intrinsic renal disease presents during pregnancy. Several of the causes of ARF in pregnancy require specific treatment, and prompt diagnosis is essential. Administration of medication and of dialysis must take into account the effect on both the mother and the fetus. ARF is often part of a life-threatening disease, but with appropriate treatment, the woman and, frequently, the baby should survive, and a majority of women should have a return of renal function.

REFERENCES

1. Ober WE, Reid DE, Romney SL, Merrill JP: Renal lesions and acute renal failure in pregnancy. Am J Med; 20:781–810.
2. Grünfeld JP, Ganavel D, Bournérias F: Acute renal failure in pregnancy. Kidney Int 1980; 18:179–191.
3. Harkins JL, Wilson DR, Muggah HF: Acute renal failure in obstetrics. Am J Obstet Gynecol 1974; 118:331–336.
4. Krane NK: Acute renal failure in pregnancy. Arch Intern Med 1988; 148:2347–2357.
5. Vladintia DS, Spanu C, Patio IM, et al: Abortion prohibition and acute renal failure: the tragic Romanian experience. Ren Fail 1995; 17:605–609.
6. Randeree IGH, Czarnocki A, Moodley J, et al: Acute renal failure in pregnancy in South Africa. Ren Fail 1995; 17:147–153.
7. Isaac V, Hemlatha H: Abortion and renal failure. J Obstet Gynecol India 1976; 26:657–661.
8. Utian WH: The cause of death following abortion: an analysis of 28 consecutive cases at Groote Schuur Hospital: I. Obstet Gynecol Br Commonwealth 1968; 75:705–712.
9. Hou S, Peano C: Acute renal failure in pregnancy. Saudi J Kidney Dis Transplant 1998; 9:261–266.
10. Smith LP, McLean APH, Maughan GB: *Clostridium welchii* septicotoxemia. Am J Obstet Gynecol 1971; 110:135–149.
11. Strum W, Cade JR, Shires DL: Postabortal septicemia due to *Clostridium welchii.* Arch Intern Med 1968; 122:73–74.
12. Firmat J, Zucchini A, Martin R, Aguirre C: A study of 500 cases of acute renal failure. Ren Fail 1994; 16:91–99.
13. Hawkins DF, Sevitt LH, Fairbrother PF, Tothill U: Management of septic chemical abortion with renal failure. N Engl J Med 1975; 292:722–725.
14. Kinningham RB: Asymptomatic bacteriuria in pregnancy. Am Fam Physician 1993; 47: 1232–1238.
15. Naeye RL: Causes of excess rates of perinatal mortality and prematurity in pregnancies complicated by maternal urinary tract infections. N Engl J Med 1979; 300:819–823.
16. Patterson TF, Andriole VT: Detection, significance, and therapy of bacteriuria in pregnancy. Infect Dis Clin North Am 1997; 11:593–608.
17. Millar LK, Cox SM: Urinary tract infections complicating pregnancy. Infect Dis Clin North Am 1997; 11:13–26.
18. Bint AJ, Hill D: Bacteriuria in pregnancy—an update on significance, diagnosis, and management. J Antimicrob Chemother 1994; 33(Suppl A):93–97.
19. Hodgeman DE: Management of urinary tract infection in pregnancy. J Perinatol Neonatol 1994; 8:1–11.
20. Harris RE, Gilstrap LC: Prevention of recurrent pyelonephritis during pregnancy. Obstet Gynecol 1974; 44:637–641.
21. Whalley PJ, Cunningham FG, Martin FG: Transient renal dysfunction associated with acute pyelonephritis of pregnancy. Obstet Gynecol 1975; 46:174–177.
22. Maikrantz P, Coe F, Parks J, Lindheimer MD: Nephrolithiasis in pregnancy. Am J Kidney Dis 1987; 9:354–358.
23. Homans DC, Blake GD, Harrington JT, Cetrulo CL: Acute renal failure caused by ureteral obstruction by a gravid uterus. JAMA 1981; 246:1230–1231.
24. D'Elia FL, Brennan RE, Brownstein PK: Acute renal failure secondary to ureteral obstruction by a gravid uterus. J Urol 1982; 128:803–804.
25. Faúndes A, Brícola-Filho M, Luiz J: Dilatation of the urinary tract during pregnancy: proposal of a curve of maximal calyceal diameter by gestational age. Am J Obstet Gynecol 1998; 178:1082–1086.
26. Kleinknect D, Grünfeld JP, Gomez PC, et al: Diagnostic procedures and long-term prognosis in bilateral renal cortical necrosis. Kidney Int 1973; 4:390–400.
27. Conger JD, Falk SA, Guggenheim SJ: Glomerular dynamics and morphologic changes in the generalized Schwartzman reaction in postpartum rats. J Clin Invest 1975; 67:1334–1346.
28. Salloni DF, Yaqoob M, White E, Finn R: Case report: the value of contrast-enhanced computed tomography in acute bilateral renal cortical necrosis. Clin Radiol 1955; 50:126–127.
29. Sibai BM, Ramadan MK: Acute renal failure in pregnancies complicated by hemolysis, elevated liver enzymes, and low platelets. Am J Obstet Gynecol 1993; 168:1682–1690.
30. Stratta P, Canavese C, Colla L, et al: Acute renal failure in preeclampsia-eclampsia. Gynecol Obstet Invest 1987; 24:225–231.
31. Barton JR, Sibai BM: Acute life-threatening emergencies in preeclampsia-eclampsia. Clin Obstet Gynecol 1992; 35:402–413.
32. Bernan JP, Degott C, Novel O, et al: Non-fatal acute fatty liver of pregnancy. Gut 1983; 24:340–344.
33. Usta M, Barton JR, Avrem EA, et al: Acute fatty liver of pregnancy: an experience with the diagnosis and management of 14 cases. Am J Obstet Gynecol 1994; 171:1342–1347.
34. Reyes H, Sandoval S, Weinstein A, et al: Acute fatty liver of pregnancy: a clinical study of 12 episodes in 11 patients. Gut 1994; 35:101–106.
35. Pockros PJ, Peters RL, Reynolds TB: Idiopathic fatty liver of pregnancy: findings in ten cases. Medicine 1984; 63:1–11.
36. Treem WR, Rinaldo P, Hqale DE, et al: Acute fatty liver of pregnancy and long-chain 3-hydroxyacyl-coenzyme A dehydrogenase deficiency. Hepatology 1994; 19:339–345.
37. Dani R, Mendez SG, Medeiros J d'L, et al: Study of liver changes occurring in preeclampsia and their possible pathogenetic connection with acute fatty liver of pregnancy. Am J Gastroenterol 1996; 91:292–294.
38. Sims HF, Brackett JC, Powell CK, et al: The molecular basis of pediatric long-chain 3-hydroxyacyl-CoA dehydrogenase deficiency associated with maternal acute fatty liver of pregnancy. Proc Natl Acad Sci U S A 1995; 92:841–845.
39. Remuzzi G, Ruggerenenti P: The hemolytic-uremic syndrome. Kidney Int 1995; 47:2–19.
40. Martinez Roman S, Gratacócos E, Tomé A, et al: Successful pregnancy in a woman with hemolytic-uremic syndrome during the second trimester of pregnancy. J Reprod Med 1996; 41:211–214.
41. Egerman RS, Witlin AG, Friedman SA, Sibai BM: Thrombotic thrombocytopenic purpura and the hemolytic-uremic syndrome in pregnancy: review of 11 cases. Am J Obstet Gynecol 1996; 175:950–956.

42. Conlon PJ, Howell DN, Macik G, et al: The renal manifestations and outcome of thrombotic thrombocytopenic purpura/hemolytic-uremic syndrome in adults. Nephrol Dial Transplant 1995; 10:1189–1193.
43. Fuch WE, George JN, Dotin LN, Sears DA: Thrombotic thrombocytopenic purpura occurrence two years apart during late pregnancy in two sisters. JAMA 1976; 19:235.
44. Wiznitzer A, Mazor M, Leiberman JR, et al: Familial occurrence of thrombotic thrombocytopenic purpura. Am J Obstet Gynecol 1992; 166:20–21.
45. Ezra Y, Rose M, Eldor A: Therapy and prevention of thrombotic thrombocytopenic purpura and hemolytic uremic syndrome: a clinical study of 16 pregnancies. Am J Hematol 1996; 15:1–6.
46. Rose M, Rowe JM, Elder A: The changing course of thrombotic thrombocytopenic purpura and modern therapy. Blood Rev 1993; 7:95–103.
47. Hayward CPM, Sutters DMC, Carter WH, et al: Treatment outcomes in patients with adult thrombotic thrombocytopenic purpura/hemolytic-uremic syndrome. Arch Intern Med 1994; 154:982–988.
48. McCrae KR, Cines DB: Thrombotic microangiopathy during pregnancy. Semin Hematol 1997; 34:148–158.
49. Fuch WE, George JN, Dotin LN, Sears DA: Thrombotic thrombocytopenic purpura occurrence two years apart during late pregnancy in two sisters. JAMA 1976; 19:235.
50. Berns JS, Kaplan BS, Mackow RC, Hefter LG: Inherited hemolytic-uremic syndrome in adults. Am J Kidney Dis 1992; 19:331–334.
51. Gallery ED, Ross M, Gyory AZ: Urinary red blood cells and cast excretion in normal and hypertensive pregnancy. Am J Obstet Gynecol 1993; 168:67–70.
52. Hou S, Schwartz M: Hypertension, proteinuria, and hypocomplementemia in a multigravida. Am J Kidney Dis 1996; 27:292–298.
53. Hou S: Pregnancy in Women with Lupus Nephritis. In: Lewis EJ, Schwartz MM, Korbet SM, eds: Lupus Nephritis. Oxford: Oxford University Press; 1999:262–283.
54. Packham D, Fairly K: Renal biopsy: indications and complications in pregnancy. Br J Obstet Gynaecol 1987; 94:935–939.
55. Jones DC, Hayslett JP: Outcome of pregnancy in women with moderate or severe renal insufficiency. N Engl J Med 1996; 335:226–232.
56. Davison JM: Pregnancy in renal allograft recipients: prognosis and management. Clin Obstet Gynaecol (Baillière's) 1994; 8:501–525.
57. Kirshon B, Wasserstrum N, Willis R, et al: Teratogenic effects of first trimester cyclophosphamide therapy. Obstet Gynecol 1988; 72:462–464.
58. Doll DC, Ringenberg QS, Yarbro JW: Antineoplastic agents and pregnancy. Semin Oncol 1989; 16:337–346.
59. Beitins IZ, Baird F, Aces IG, et al: The transplacental passage of prednisone and prednisolone in pregnancy near term. J Pediatr 1975; 5:936–945.
60. Bradford AT, Murphy BEP: In vitro metabolism of prednisolone, betamethasone, and cortisol by the human placenta. Am J Obstet Gynecol 1997; 127:264–267.
61. Davison JM, Dellagrammatikas H, Parkin JM: Maternal azathioprine therapy and depressed haematopoiesis in the babies of renal allograft patients. Br J Obstet Gynecol 1985; 92:233–239.
62. Armenti VT, Ahlswede KM, Ahlswede BA, et al: Variables affecting 197 pregnancies in cyclosporine-treated renal transplant recipients. Transplantation 1995; 59:476–479.
63. Okundaye IB, Abrinko P, Hou S: A registry for pregnancy in dialysis patients. Am J Kidney Dis 1998; 31:766–773.
64. Hou S: Pregnancy in chronic renal insufficiency and end-stage renal disease. Am J Kidney Dis 1999; 33:235–252.

CHAPTER 24

Acute Renal Failure as a Result of Malignancy

J. Carlos T. da Silva, Jr. ▪ Douglas E. Mesler

The approach to acute renal failure (ARF) in the setting of malignancy is no different from that to renal failure in general, except that underlying neoplasia always raises suspicion of obstruction.[1-3] However, once postrenal processes are ruled out, important prerenal and parenchymal causes of renal failure remain (Table 24–1).

OBSTRUCTIVE UROPATHY

The symptoms, signs, and implications of urinary tract obstruction depend its location and completeness and the acuity with which it develops. Although acute obstruction (such as that with a stone) is characterized by sudden, severe, and colicky pain, subacute or incomplete obstruction, particularly when unilateral, develops slowly over time and may be relatively free of symptoms. When symptomatic, upper ureteral lesions radiate pain to the flanks, lower ureteral distention radiates to the groin, and bladder outlet obstruction is associated primarily with suprapubic symptoms.

Bladder Outlet Obstruction and Urinary Retention

Lower urinary tract obstruction results from neurologic or mechanical processes that impair the normal bladder emptying mechanism. More commonly seen in older men, it should also be suspected in the postoperative period when pain, opiate analgesia, and recum-

TABLE 24–1. Cancer-Associated Acute Renal Failure

POSTRENAL CAUSES

    Bladder outlet obstruction
    Upper tract obstruction

PRERENAL CAUSES

    Dehydration
    Bleeding, hypotension, sepsis
    CHF, hepatorenal syndrome, superior vena cava obstruction
    Hypercalcemia

RENAL CAUSES

    Established ischemic ATN
    Nephrotoxic ATN
    Acute interstitial nephritis
    Myeloma kidney
    Lymphomatous infiltration
    Hemolytic-uremic syndrome
    Rapidly progressive glomerulonephritis
    Intratubular obstruction (tumor-lysis syndrome)

CHF, congestive heart failure; *ATN,* acute tubular necrosis.

bence lead to functional obstruction or can exacerbate previously asymptomatic benign prostatic hyperplasia or urethral strictures.[4]

Bladder outlet obstruction due to direct tumor involvement, although typically slowly progressive over a period of weeks or months, can present acutely when provoked pharmacologically or mechanically by an acute retention crisis or when associated with acute neurologic compromise. Rarely, constipation has resulted in acute urinary retention.[5] Obstructive symptoms may also be provoked by forced hydration and the anticholinergic effects of antiemetic agents during the administration of chemotherapy. Local injury to the sacral plexus may arise from retroperitoneal invasion from prostatic, colorectal, or cervical carcinomas. CNS processes such as tumors arising in or metastatic to the brain or spinal cord may interfere with central control of micturition and neuromuscular coordination of bladder emptying.[3] For example, herpes simplex viral meningitis has been reported to cause acute urinary retention.[6]

Upper Urinary Tract Obstruction

Ureteral obstruction may be bilateral or unilateral. Complete bilateral ureteral compression (or luminal obstruction of the collecting system of a single functioning kidney) usually results in anuric renal insufficiency. Obstruction that develops slowly over time, however, can be painless and asymptomatic until azotemia finally ensues. Partial obstruction can also result in renal insufficiency, particularly in the setting of preexisting renal dysfunction and progressive worsening of the obstructive component. In this situation, urine output can be preserved but variable, with an acquired renal concentrating defect occasionally leading to polyuria.[7]

Obstruction of the upper collecting system may be caused by extraureteral compression by primary tumor or associated lymph nodes, or by direct tumor or metastatic invasion of the ureter itself. Seventy percent of malignant ureteral obstructions are due to pelvic cancers (cervical, bladder, or prostate). The balance is usually the result of retroperitoneal lymphadenopathy due to either lymphoma or metastatic solid malignancies of the abdomen such as gastric, colorectal, pancreatic cancer, or to metastatic breast cancer.[3] Rarely ureteral obstruction is a consequence of candidal fungus ball in patients with repeated instrumentation of the urinary tract, prolonged course of broad-spectrum antibiotics, and compromised immune response.[8]

Although uncommon, retroperitoneal fibrosis may

be the presentation of a new malignancy such as lymphoma, or more frequently, a complication of surgery or pelvic irradiation. For some long-term cancer survivors, the cumulative risk of retroperitoneal fibrosis may become substantial.[3] Retroperitoneal fibrosis also deserves special mention because of its tendency (along with circumferential tumor encasement of the ureter [Fig. 24–1]) to obstruct with minimal or no dilation of the urinary tract on imaging studies (Fig. 24–2A and B).[9–14]

Diagnosis of Urinary Tract Obstruction

Urinary tract obstruction can be diagnosed by intravenous urography, antegrade or retrograde pyelography, or renal ultrasound.[15] However, abdominal computed tomography (CT) (or magnetic resonance imaging) uniquely identifies the nature and magnitude of any extrarenal involvement in addition to the location of obstruction.[3] Nondilated obstruction can be seen in recent onset of obstruction (< 48 hours), retroperitoneal fibrosis, ureteral encasement by tumor (see Fig. 24–1), and obstruction with concurrent sepsis or hypotension. Retrograde pyelography may be particularly useful when the probability of obstruction is high (such as in the setting of a known pelvic malignancy), but hydronephrosis is not detected by ultrasound.

Management of Urinary Tract Obstruction

Acute urinary retention is usually associated with suprapubic pain and a palpably distended bladder,

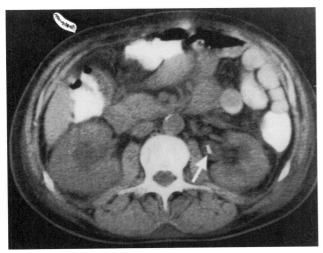

FIGURE 24–1 ■ Abdominal CT scan showing mild bilateral hydronephrosis and slight dilation of the left ureter (*arrow*). A left ureteral stent is in place. This 53-year-old man presented with urinary tract obstruction, respiratory distress, cerebral infarcts and blindness, and acute renal failure in the setting of widespread metastatic gastric carcinoma. (From Weekly clinicopathological exercises (Case 10-1999): A 53-year-old man with acute renal failure, cortical blindness, and respiratory distress. N Engl J Med 1999; 340:1099; with permission. Copyright 1999, Massachusetts Medical Society. All rights reserved.)

both of which can be relieved by successful placement of a Foley catheter. Caution should always be taken with Foley catheter insertion, particularly so in the setting of suspected or known malignancy. The experienced provider avoids forcing the catheter, which might result in urethral laceration, false passage formation, bleeding, and occasionally catastrophic infection. In men, it is imperative that the catheter be inserted until its hub and urine return is observed to avoid inflating the catheter in the urethra. If a transurethral catheter cannot be placed by experienced personnel, a percutaneous suprapubic nephrostomy tube may be required to decompress the bladder until more permanent arrangements can be made. Successful insertion of a Foley catheter does not rule out obstruction in patients with known prostatic, bladder, or cervical cancer, because vesicoureteral junction involvement of the ureters will not resolve with bladder drainage.

Once inserted, the timing of catheter removal must be addressed. The infectious complications of prolonged bladder catheterization are well known, with a cumulative frequency of urinary tract infection of 5% to 10% a day.[16] Also, many patients with acute urinary retention will void if given another chance after being decompressed.[17] However, in patients with malignancy, enthusiasm for a voiding trial is tempered by the need to await passing of the postoperative period, to manage malignancy-associated or postoperative pain with or without opiates, and to cope with the increased urinary flow needs of chemotherapy. The intermittent clamping of a Foley catheter to "retrain" the bladder has no scientific support and should no longer be practiced.[3] However, if persistent bladder neck obstruction does not allow spontaneous micturition, clean, intermittent self-catheterization has proven to be useful. Many patients with functional outlet obstruction regain the ability to empty their bladder within 8 to 10 weeks without the need for surgical intervention.[4]

Once mechanical bladder outlet obstruction is bypassed to re-establish urine flow, consideration should be given to intervention that is more definitive. Transurethral resection of the prostate remains the treatment of choice for patients with benign prostatic hypertrophy or obstructing prostatic malignancy. However, urethral stenting is an option for locally advanced or hormonally unresponsive prostate cancer,[18, 19] and aggressive hormonal therapy without stenting may be effective in treatment-naive patients.

Once an assessment of the need for intervention in ureteral obstruction is made, surgical or endourologic intervention is typically required. Thinning of the renal cortex usually reflects long-standing obstruction and little chance of functional recovery, and in cases of bilateral ureteral obstruction, the organ with best-preserved cortex should be salvaged (see Fig. 24–3A and B). Closed-space infection is an indication for drainage, regardless of the level of renal function. Treatment with cystoscopy and retrograde urography is usually the first approach, unless visualization and catheterization of the ureteral orifices through the bladder are not feasible, in which case a percutaneous nephrostomy with antegrade urography should be per-

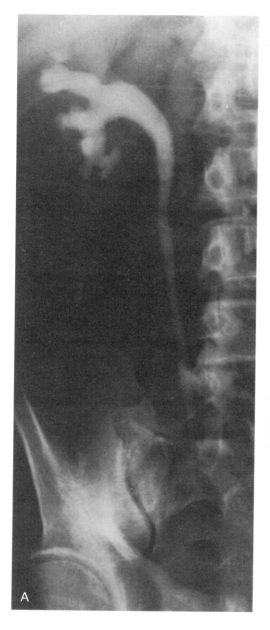

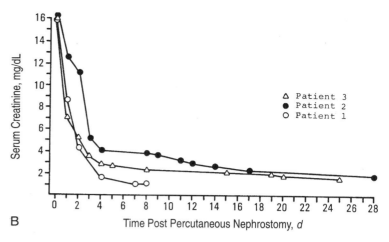

FIGURE 24–2 ■ *A*, Antegrade urogram showing minimally dilated collecting system and total obstruction at the level of pelvic inlet. *B*, Serum creatinine level as a function of time following percutaneous nephrostomy performed in the patient depicted in *A* (*open triangles*) and two other patients with similar presentation of minimally dilated severe obstructive nephropathy. (*A* and *B*, From Curry N, Gobien RP, Schabel SI: Minimal dilation obstructive nephropathy. Radiology 1982; 143:533: with permission.)

formed to confirm the diagnosis. The retrograde approach also allows for correction of uretero-enteric stenoses in ileal conduits. Both retrograde and percutaneous approaches allow for therapeutic interventions like insertion of double-J polyurethane stents, transluminal ureteroplasty, and insertion of self-expandable metallic stents. The antegrade approach allows ultrasound- or CT scan–guided placement of a percutaneous nephrostomy tube. Complications of endourologic techniques include infection, encrustation and obstruction, migration of double-J stents, and rarely hemorrhage or accidental injury to the kidneys or collecting system.

A special case is retroperitoneal fibrosis, where reports of successful medical management have been published.[20, 21] Although a surgical therapeutic approach is often necessary, there is anecdotal evidence of remission of retroperitoneal fibrosis with the use of mycophenolate mofetil and prednisone[20] or tamoxifen.[21]

Once lower or bilateral upper urinary tract obstruction is relieved, polyuria (that may reach several liters a day) may supervene. On rare occasions this represents a true concentrating defect due to nephrogenic diabetes insipidus presumably related to down-regulation of water channels.[22] However, more often than not the initial polyuria represents an appropriate response to prior volume and solute retention during the period of complete obstruction.[7] In this setting, overzealous intravenous volume replacement perpetuates the excessive urinary output. Prudent management involves close hemodynamic monitoring, initial volume replacement with 1/2 normal saline to replace salt lost to renal wasting, usually at a rate no higher

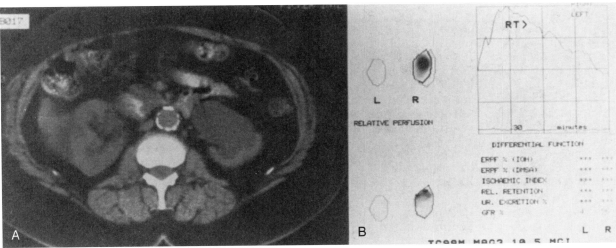

FIGURE 24–3 ■ *A*, CT of the abdomen demonstrates left hydronephrosis with cortical atrophy secondary to pelvic recurrence of cervical cancer in a 58-year-old woman. *B*, Radionuclide renogram (dimercaptosuccinic acid [DMSA]) demonstrates no function in the left kidney and normal function of the right one. Because of documented lack of function in the left kidney, decompression was not recommended. (*A* and *B*, From Russo P: Oncologic emergencies. In: DeVita VT, Hellman S, Rosenberg S, eds: *Cancer: Principles and Practice of Oncology.* 5th ed. Philadelphia: Lippincott-Raven; 1997:2514; with permission.)

than 75 mL/min, and correction of significant electrolyte losses.

Prognosis of Urinary Tract Obstruction

The information about morbidity, technique, and patient survival after use of newer endourologic maneuvers of ureteral decompression is still evolving in the medical literature. However, it appears that major determinants are the stage and severity of the underlying malignancy. In this respect, the outcome for urologic malignancies appears to differ from that for nonurologic malignancies, with the latter generally conferring a poorer prognosis. Even locally advanced prostatic carcinoma may be manageable with radical prostatectomy, particularly in patients with well or moderately differentiated tumors.[23-25]

For nonurologic malignancies, the need for intervention needs to be weighed against the frequent incidence of treatment complications and the limited survival benefit achieved in these patients. Donat and Russo[26] from Memorial Sloan-Kettering Cancer Center in New York published their experience with 78 patients with advanced or metastatic nonurologic tumors causing ureteral obstruction: 68% underwent successful transurethral decompression and 32% required percutaneous nephrostomy. Half of the patients had at least one complication (eg, obstruction, infection, or migration); the median number of hospitalizations per patient related to the decompression procedure was eight. Median patient survival was 6.8 months; actuarial survival was 55% at 1 year and 30% at 3 years. Patients with gastric and pancreatic cancer fared worse, with median survival of only 1.4 months. Lugmayr and Pauer reported the results of ureteral decompression using metallic self-expandable permanent endoluminal stents to treat 40 patients, and 54 with malignant

ureteral stenosis.[27] The mean follow-up time was 10.5 months; about half of the ureters needed reintervention to re-establish patency; and three ureters were eventually abandoned. The estimated primary patency rate was 31% at 1 year. However, patient survival was unrelated to stent placement in this study where the most common malignancies were colon, ovarian, uterine, and breast carcinoma.

PRERENAL AZOTEMIA

Given the vulnerable condition of the cancer patient, the high prevalence of comorbid conditions, and the need to defend the internal milieu against a multiplicity of interventions, it is not surprising that prerenal azotemia is common. Potentially reversible decreased renal perfusion can be consequent to mucositis-related gastrointestinal losses, hemorrhage due to marrow suppression or surgical procedures, or third spacing because of serositis secondary to peritoneal carcinomatosis. Low albumin levels due to malnutrition and/or accelerated catabolism may also contribute to third spacing. Finally, hepatorenal syndrome due to liver metastases and portal hypertension may result in renal hypoperfusion.

Even in the presence of adequate intravascular volume, ineffective circulation can result in prerenal azotemia. Superior vena cava syndrome, pericardial effusion with tamponade physiology, or depressed myocardial function due to effects of chemotherapy (eg, doxorubicin) all can contribute to reduced cardiac output and potentially reversible hemodynamic insult. Sepsis may impair renal perfusion through several mechanisms: maldistribution of cardiac output and decreased left ventricular ejection fraction through cytokine-induced vasodilation and myocardial depression, and alteration of the relation between total peripheral resistance and renal vascular resistance.

Cancer patients often experience pain and discomfort, and the use of nonsteroidal anti-inflammatory drugs (NSAIDs) in the setting of poor oral intake or ongoing extrarenal volume losses serves to further compromise the renal function. It is worth emphasizing the importance of considering lymphoproliferative disease or plasma cell dyscrasia as a parenchymal cause for renal insufficiency in the clinical scenario of an elderly patient with back pain and anemia initially diagnosed with NSAID-induced azotemia.

HYPERCALCEMIA OF MALIGNANCY

Hypercalcemia is a common complication of neoplastic disorders,[28, 29] most often associated with squamous cell carcinoma of the lung, head, and neck; renal cell carcinoma; metastatic breast carcinoma; multiple myeloma; and lymphomas. Several mechanisms contribute to increased bone resorption: local actions of resorptive cytokines in lytic tumors,[30] tumor release of 1,25-dihydroxyvitamin D3,[31] and local[32] or distant effects of tumor release of parathyroid hormone (PTH)-related peptide (PTHrP).[29, 33, 34] Parathyroid hormone–related peptide has 70% homology to the first 13 amino acids of the amino-terminal portion of PTH, binds to PTH/PTHrP receptors, and shares similar biologic activity to PTH.[35] Parathyroid hormone–related peptide, like PTH, increases bone reabsorption and enhances renal calcium reabsorption and phosphorus excretion, resulting in increased calcium levels due to both bone reabsorption and decreased calcium clearance by the kidney.[36, 37]

Malignancy-associated hypercalcemia causes acute arteriolar vasoconstriction, defective urinary concentration leading to volume depletion, and tubulointerstitial calcium deposition and injury (nephrocalcinosis).[38, 39] Treatment for malignancy-associated hypercalcemia focuses on reversal of these processes, replacing intravascular volume, reducing tubular calcium reabsorption with a saline-forced diuresis (in patients with intact renal function), and inhibiting bone reabsorption with calcitonin (4 IU/kg) subcutaneously and bisphosphonates (eg, pamidronate 60 to 90 mg intravenously over 4 hours). The former acts quickly, with reductions in serum calcium levels seen within 3 hours, whereas the latter achieves a response after 24 hours that peaks at 4 to 5 days.[40–42]

PARENCHYMAL RENAL FAILURE

Common parenchymal causes of acute renal insufficiency in patients with cancer result from sustained prerenal injury leading to acute tubular necrosis or the noxious tubular effect of nephrotoxins. Typical offending agents include aminoglycosides, radiologic contrast agents, platinum-based chemotherapy, amphotericin B, or antiviral therapy (eg, foscarnet, acyclovir). Acute interstitial nephritis can also be seen, as in the general hospitalized population, associated with the use of antibiotics such as nafcillin, ciprofloxa-

cin, use of NSAIDs, or viral infections (eg, Epstein-Barr virus, cytomegalovirus). There are, however, several causes of parenchymal renal failure unique to malignancy.

Multiple Myeloma

Multiple myeloma is a plasma cell dyscrasia resulting from the uncontrolled proliferation of a single plasma cell clone. The disease produces myriad clinical symptoms ranging from focal plasma cell proliferation with skeletal destruction to systemic manifestations of immunoglobulin excess. It is predominantly a disease of the elderly, with peak incidence in the seventh decade, and presentation before 40 years of age occurring less than 2% of the time.[43, 44] Multiple myeloma causes only 1% of all malignancies but is disproportionately associated with renal disease, contributing 47% of end-stage renal disease cases resulting from malignancy in the United States.[45, 46]

Renal failure frequently accompanies the diagnosis of multiple myeloma, with 20% to 50% having residual renal insufficiency after volume replacement at initial presentation.[47, 48] Regardless of its cause, renal failure at the time of myeloma diagnosis carries grave prognostic significance, with probability of 1-year survival for patients with an initial creatinine level greater than 2.3 mg/dL being 37% less than the group with creatinine levels under 1.5 mg/dL, and a strong link between survival and response of renal disease to therapy.[49, 50]

CAUSES OF ACUTE RENAL FAILURE IN MYELOMA

Light-chain nephropathy and amyloidosis are typically associated with chronic, as opposed to acute, renal failure. However, myeloma cast nephropathy ("myeloma kidney") and, less commonly, hypercalcemia and cryoglobulinemia are known causes of ARF in this population. Myeloma patients also are at uniquely increased risk for ARF associated with radiocontrast administration,[51] use of NSAIDs,[52] and angiotensin-converting enzyme (ACE) inhibitors.[53] The mechanism for hypercalcemic ARF in multiple myeloma is identical to that described previously for other malignancies, with the additional risk of potentiation of tubular light-chain toxicity.[54] Cryoglobulinemia occurs in multiple myeloma and has been reported in amyloidosis, although its implication for therapy in the latter remains unclear.[55, 56]

PATHOGENESIS OF MYELOMA KIDNEY

Immunoglobulin light chains usually do not appear in the urine in any great quantity, being freely filtered by the glomerulus and reabsorbed by proximal tubular cells. However, when produced in substantial excess, and/or in the setting of tubular dysfunction, the threshold for tubular reabsorption can be exceeded. In

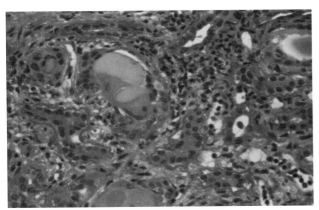

FIGURE 24–4 ▪ Intraluminal cast formation in myeloma kidney. Note reactive inflammation and giant cell formation in surrounding tubule. (Periodic acid–Schiff × 350). (Courtesy of Helmut Rennke, MD, Brigham and Women's Hospital, Boston, MA.)

this setting Bence Jones proteinuria can be substantial; however, since light chains are not dipstick reactive, it will be missed on routine urinalysis unless specifically examined for. Sulfasalicylic acid reactivity (turbidity) in the absence of dipstick albuminuria suggests the presence of nonalbumin protein, usually excess light chains.

The most common histologic finding in myeloma kidney is intratubular cast formation.[57] Casts form in the distal and collecting tubule, forming dense, obstructing lesions that may be associated with a local inflammatory giant cell reaction (Fig. 24–4).[58] Casts also contain other proteins, most notably Tamm-Horsfall protein (THP), and it may be the strength of the association with THP that determines light chains' pathogenic potential.[59]

Not all light chains are equally nephrotoxic, because some patients excrete large amounts of light-chain protein without significant renal complications. Indeed, studies suggest that unique physicochemical characteristics of light chains determine nephrotoxicity, with infusion of light chains from diseased patients recapitulating the original disease in experimental animals.[59, 60]

ROLE OF PRECIPITANTS IN MYELOMA KIDNEY

Radiocontrast media exposure has been long suspected to provoke ARF in patients with myeloma. Although recent reports suggest that the risk of ARF in myeloma patients exposed to radiocontrast media may have been overestimated, and indeed may be less than 1.5%,[51] contrast media has been demonstrated to promote light-chain toxicity in vitro and in experimental animals.[61, 62] Nonsteroidal anti-inflammatory drugs and ACE inhibitors have been associated with both reversible and irreversible renal failure in patients with myeloma.[52, 53, 63, 64] Hypercalcemia is a common finding in myeloma patients with ARF.[65] Although a direct effect of calcium on light-chain characteristics is indeed possible and has been demonstrated,[54] it is likely that the urinary concentration of light chains, either through

reduction in glomerular filtration rate or volume depletion is the major factor.

THERAPY FOR MYELOMA KIDNEY

The urgency to treat myeloma kidney derives from a prognosis that is strongly associated with worsening renal insufficiency[49] and the potential for reversibility. Treatment consists of specific steps to interrupt cast formation, chemotherapy for the underlying myeloma to reduce Bence Jones proteinuria, and control of the complications of ARF. Of these, prophylaxis and treatment of intraluminal cast formation should receive the highest priorities, because reversibility of the ARF is common with removal of precipitants, restoration of intravascular volume, and forced alkaline diuresis (in patients with adequate circulating volume and preserved cardiac and renal function).[65]

Chemotherapy is the mainstay of reducing the quantity of circulating light chains. Melphalan and prednisone are most commonly used, although vincristine, doxorubicin, and dexamethasone (VAD) have a more rapid onset of action and a primarily hepatic metabolism that offers theoretical advantages in patients with renal failure.[66] Plasmapheresis more rapidly reduces plasma monoclonal protein levels and the few small, controlled trials suggest improved renal survival; however, the magnitude of this advantage and its application to clinical practice remain controversial.[65, 67–69] Dialysis itself removes light chains (although at a rate nearly one tenth that of plasmapheresis), and recovery of patients after weeks and months of dialysis has been documented.[70] In dialysis-dependent patients, or in those with more gradual onset of renal failure, renal biopsy may be necessary to ensure proper diagnosis and guide intervention.[71] In addition to ruling out other causes of renal failure, documentation of significant interstitial fibrosis may suggest a lower likelihood of reversibility.[57, 65]

The association between development and degree of renal insufficiency in myeloma and survival has been scrutinized recently. In particular, the assumption that renal insufficiency itself portends a poor prognosis has been questioned.[72] Although tumor mass and initial degree of renal insufficiency are related, response to therapy appears to be independent of level of renal insufficiency.[48] Furthermore, survival of patients whose renal failure is dialysis dependent appears to be the same as for those with milder renal insufficiency, and irreversibility of renal insufficiency may not portend a worse prognosis.[72, 73] Survival in myeloma depends most strongly on the disappearance of the monoclonal protein after treatment,[74] and some have even advocated renal transplantation for long-term survivors.[75]

Renal failure has rarely been associated with light-chain excretion in malignant lymphoma, in which case clinical behavior appears indistinguishable from that in myeloma.[76] Animal models and case reports suggest that even polyclonal light chains with appropriate characteristics when present in excess are potentially toxic to the kidney.[77, 78]

Lymphomatous Kidney Infiltration

Infiltration of the kidney is not rare in lymphoma autopsy series, ranging from 6% to 60%[79–81] and averaging 34% in the largest series.[82] Presentation would be typical of lymphoma, with a subacute course of fevers, weight loss, with elevated serum lactate dehydrogenase and uric acid levels, with the additional findings of microscopic hematuria and occasionally flank pain or a renal mass. However, acute renal insufficiency is considerably less frequent, with an estimated incidence of only 0.5%. Even more remote is the chance of renal infiltration as the first manifestation of lymphoma. Therefore, even with the demonstration of massively enlarged kidneys (Fig. 24–5A) and histologic proof of infiltration (Fig. 24–5B), other causes of acute renal insufficiency should be ruled out, and improvement of renal function after successful chemotherapy or radiation treatment should be documented to ascribe acute renal insufficiency to the lymphomatous infiltration.[79]

Glomerular Diseases

Although the association between glomerular diseases and malignancy is well established in the literature, these syndromes do not typically present with acute renal insufficiency. Nephrotic syndrome with little or no renal insufficiency may be seen in Hodgkin's lymphoma (minimal change disease), solid tumors of the colon and lung (membranous nephropathy), and renal cell carcinoma (secondary amyloidosis). Renal insufficiency may be seen with minimal-change disease, particularly in the setting of diuretic-induced volume depletion.

Nephritic presentations have been seen in malignancy, although the strength of the association is less clear. Membranoproliferative glomerulonephritis, crescentic glomerulonephritis, and anti-glomerular basement membrane glomerulonephritis all have been seen, and in some cases improvement of renal function and proteinuria with tumor resection or successful chemotherapy lends credence to a causal relationship.[83–85] The association may be most robust for membranoproliferative glomerulonephritis and chronic lymphocytic leukemia, although monotypic IgG deposits in a fibrillary configuration have been seen as well.[86] Rapidly progressive glomerulonephritis has been seen in malignancy, although again the strength of the association is not certain.[83]

Mixed cryoglobulinemia is most commonly related to hepatitis C infection; however, it is also seen in association with lymphoid malignancies. Clinical presentation often includes hematuria, subacute renal insufficiency (sometimes with waxing and waning course), hypocomplementemia, and occasionally arthralgias, fevers, and skin ulcers. The histologic picture is of proliferative and exudative glomerulonephritis seen on light microscopy, subendothelial deposits with "thumbprint" crystalline ultrastructure seen on electron microscopy, and occasionally intraluminal thrombi positive for IgM and IgG on immunofluorescence.[87]

An uncommon and unique situation is the develop-

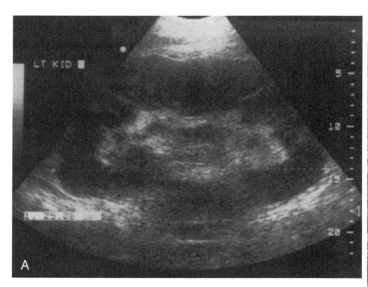

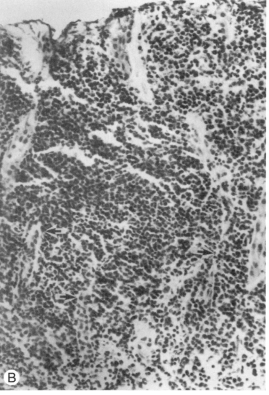

FIGURE 24–5 ■ *A,* Renal ultrasound study showing massive enlargement of the left kidney of a 47-year-old man who presented with painful gross hematuria, hesitancy, and acute renal insufficiency. The right kidney had a similar ultrasonographic appearance. *B,* Histology of the kidney shown in *A.* Diffuse lymphocytic infiltration; *arrows* point to compressed renal tubules. (Periodic acid–Schiff ×350). (*A* and *B,* From Obrador GT, Price B, O'Meara Y, Salant DJ: Acute renal failure due to lymphomatous infiltration of the kidneys. J Am Soc Nephrol 1997; 8:1348.)

ment of ARF in the setting of Waldenstrom macroglobulinemia due hyperviscosity and intraglomerular occlusive thrombi consisting of IgM protein. Clinical improvement with intensive plasmapheresis and alkylating agents has been reported.[88]

THROMBOTIC MICROANGIOPATHY AND HEMOLYTIC-UREMIC SYNDROME

Thrombotic angiopathy can be seen in the setting of malignancy, most often in the form of disseminated intravascular coagulation related to sepsis, but occasionally in the form of hemolytic-uremic syndrome (HUS) related to either the underlying tumor or chemotherapy. Mucin-producing tumors such as gastric, pancreatic, or prostatic adenocarcinomas are most often associated with HUS, but presentations more consistent with thrombotic thrombocytopenic purpura (TTP) have been reported as well.[89, 90] HUS is most frequently encountered as a consequence of combination chemotherapy or radiation plus high-dose cyclophosphamide in preparation for bone marrow transplantation (see section on ARF associated with cancer chemotherapy). The recognition of this syndrome is important, given reports of improved outcome of patients promptly treated with plasmapheresis, immunoadsorption, and fresh frozen plasma infusion.[91-93]

SPONTANEOUS TUMOR LYSIS SYNDROME

Tumor lysis syndrome is most often seen after institution of chemotherapy; however, it can occur prior to any cancer treatment. Frequency appears rare, but some series have documented from 10% to 25% of all cases arising spontaneously.[94, 95] Spontaneous tumor lysis should be suspected in patients with massive tumor burden with rapid turnover, such as with high-grade lymphomas. Hallmark findings are a markedly elevated uric acid level, usually above 16 mg/dL, associated with oligoanuric ARF. In contrast with that occurring after chemotherapy, hyperphosphatemia may not be prominent.[94] Treatment prior to anuria consists of allopurinol, saline, and loop diuretics to flush out uric acid crystals. Once oliguric renal failure has occurred, intermittent dialysis or continuous therapies can be effective in reducing uric acid levels, with renal function usually returning promptly after uric acid levels fall back into the normal range.

REFERENCES

1. Garnick MB, Mayer RJ: Acute renal failure associated with neoplastic disease and its treatment. Semin Oncol 1978; 5:155.
2. Mindell JA, Chertow GM: A practical approach to acute renal failure. Med Clin North Am 1997; 81:731.
3. Russo P: Oncologic Emergencies. In: DeVita VT Jr, Hellman S, Rosenberg S, eds: Cancer: Principles and Practice of Oncology. 5th ed. Philadelphia: Lippincott-Raven; 1997:2514.
4. Anderson JB, Grant JB: Postoperative retention of urine: a prospective urodynamic study. BMJ 1991; 302:894.
5. Murray K, Massey A, Freneley RCL: Acute urinary retention—a urodynamic assessment. Br J Urol 1984; 56:468–473.
6. Steinberg J, Rukstalis DB, Vickers MA: Acute urinary retention secondary to herpes simplex meningitis. J Urol 1991; 145:359–360.
7. Klahr S: Nephrology Forum: Pathophysiology of obstructive nephropathy. Kidney Int 1983; 23:414–426.
8. Scerpella EG, Alhalel R: An unusual cause of acute renal failure: bilateral ureteral obstruction due to Candida tropicalis fungus balls. Clin Infect Dis 1994; 18:440.
9. Weekly clinicopathological exercises (Case 10–1999): A 53-year-old man with acute renal failure, cortical blindness, and respiratory distress. N Engl J Med 1999; 340:1099.
10. Kocurek JN, Orihuela E, Saltzstein DR: Nondilated obstructive uropathy and renal failure as a result of carcinoma of the intrapelvic area. Surg Gynecol Obstet 1991; 173:470.
11. Lalli AF: Retroperitoneal fibrosis and inapparent obstructive uropathy. Radiology 1977; 122:339.
12. Tabenkin H, Schwarzman P, Steinmatz D, et al: Acute renal failure in a patient with prostatic carcinoma: a case of benign uropathy. Postgrad Med 1992; 91:155.
13. Tripodi SA, Mattei FM, Giovannelli V, et al: Idiopathic retroperitoneal fibrosis simulating renal malignancy. J Urol 1998; 160:2145.
14. Rascoff JH, Golden RA, Spinowitz BS, et al: Nondilated obstructive nephropathy. Arch Intern Med 1983; 143:696.
15. Kaye AD, Pollack HM: Diagnostic imaging approach to the patient with obstructive uropathy. Semin Nephrol 1982; 2:55.
16. Stamm WE: Nosocomial infections: etiologic changes, therapeutic challenges. Hosp Pract 1981; 16:75–88.
17. Taube M, Gajraj H: Trial without catheter following acute retention of urine. Br J Urol 1989; 63:180–182.
18. Anson KM, Barnes DG, Briggs TP, et al: Temporary prostatic stenting and androgen suppression: a new minimally invasive approach to malignant prostatic retention. J R Soc Med 1993; 86:634–636.
19. Thomas DJ, Balaji VJ, Copcoat MJ, Abercrombie GF: Acute urinary retention secondary to carcinoma of the prostate: is initial channel TURP beneficial? J R Soc Med 1992; 85:318–319.
20. Grotz W, von Zedtwitz I, Andre M, et al: Treatment of retroperitoneal fibrosis by mycophenolate mofetil and corticosteroids. Lancet 1998; 352:1195.
21. al-Musawi D, Mitchenere P, Al-Akraa M: Idiopathic retroperitoneal fibrosis treated with tamoxifen only. Br J Urol 1998; 82:442.
22. Marples JJ, Knepper MA, Nielsen S: Bilateral ureteral obstruction downregulates expression of vasopressin-sensitive AQP-2 water channel in rat kidney. Am J Physiol 1996; 270:F657.
23. Cheng L, Sebo TJ, Slezac J, et al: Predictors of survival for prostate carcinoma patients treated with salvage radical prostatectomy after radiation therapy. Cancer 1998; 83:2164–2171.
24. Krongrad A, Lai H, Lai S: Survival after radical prostatectomy. JAMA 1997; 278:44–46.
25. Van Den Ouden D, Hop WC, Schroder FH: Progression in and survival of patients with locally advanced prostate cancer (T3) treated with radical prostatectomy as monotherapy. J Urol 1998; 160:1392–1397.
26. Donat SM, Russo P: Ureteral decompression in advanced nonurologic malignancies. Ann Surg Oncol 1996; 3:393.
27. Lugmayr HF, Pauer W: Wallstents for the treatment of extrinsic malignant ureteral obstruction: midterm results. Radiology 1996; 198:105.
28. Jones CH, Warren CW: Acute renal failure secondary to hypercalcemia reversible after resection of a benign ovarian teratoma. Nephrol Dial Transplant 1996; 11:1860.
29. Mundy GR, Guise TA: Hypercalcemia of malignancy. Am J Med 1997; 103:134.
30. Garrett IR, Durie BG, Nedwin GE, et al: Production of lymphotoxin, a bone-resorbing cytokine, by cultured human myeloma cells. N Engl J Med 1987; 317:526–532.
31. Seymour JF, Gagel RF: Calcitriol: the major humoral mediator of hypercalcemia in Hodgkin's disease and non-Hodgkin's lymphomas. Blood 1993; 82:1383–1394.
32. Guise TA, Yin JJ, Taylor SD, et al: Evidence for a causal role of parathyroid hormone–related protein in the pathogenesis of human breast cancer-mediated osteolysis. J Clin Invest 1996; 98:1544–1549.

33. Rosol T, Capen C: Mechanisms of cancer-induced hypercalcemia. Lab Invest 1992; 67:680–702.

34. Rankin W, Gritt V, Martin TJ: Parathyroid hormone–related protein and hypercalcemia. Cancer 1997; 80:1564.

35. Horiuchi N, Caulfield MP, Fisher JE, et al: Similarity of synthetic peptide from human tumor to parathyroid hormone in vivo and in vitro. Science 1987; 238:1566–1568.

36. Rizzoli R, Ferrari SL, Pizurki L, et al: Actions of parathyroid hormone and parathyroid hormone–related protein. J Endocrinol Invest 1992; 15:51–56.

37. Fraher LJ, Hodsman AB, Jonas K, et al: A comparison of the in vivo biochemical responses to exogenous parathyroid hormone-(1–34) (PTH-(1–34) and PTH-related peptide-(1–34) in man. J Endocrinol Metab 1992; 75:417–423.

38. Lins LE: Reversible renal failure caused by hypercalcemia: a retrospective study. Acta Med Scand 1978; 203:309.

39. Levi M, Ellis MA, Berl T: Control of renal hemodynamics and glomerular filtration rate in chronic hypercalcemia: role of prostaglandins, renin-angiotensin system, and calcium. J Clin Invest 1983; 71:1624.

40. Binstock ML, Mundy GR: Effect of calcitonin and glucocorticoids in combination on the hypercalcemia of malignancy. Ann Intern Med 1980; 93:269–272.

41. Berenson JR, Rosen L, Vescio R, et al: Pharmacokinetics of pamidronate disodium in patients with cancer with normal or impaired renal function. J Clin Pharmacol 1997; 37:285.

42. Machado CE, Flombaum CD: Safety of pamidronate in patients with renal failure and hypercalcemia. Clin Nephrol 1996; 45:175.

43. Blade J, Kyle RA, Greipp PR: Presenting features and prognosis in 72 patients with multiple myeloma who were younger than 40 years. Br J Haematol 1996; 93:345–351.

44. Kyle RA: Multiple myeloma: review of 869 cases. Mayo Clin Proc 1975; 50:29–40.

45. US Renal Data System (USRDS) 1999 Annual Data Report. Bethesda, MD: National Institutes of Health, National Institute of Diabetes and Digestive and Kidney Diseases, 1999.

46. Kyle RA, Beard CM, O'Fallon WM, et al: Incidence of multiple myeloma in Olmsted County, Minnesota, 1978 through 1990, with a review of the trend since 1945. J Clin Oncol 1994; 12:1577.

47. MacLennan I, Drayson M, Dunn J: Multiple myeloma. BMJ 1994; 308:1033–1036.

48. Alexanian R, Barlogie B, Dixon D: Renal failure in multiple myeloma: pathogenesis and prognostic implications. Arch Intern Med 1990; 150:1693.

49. MacLennan IC, Cooper EH, Chapman CE, et al: Renal failure in myelomatosis. Eur J Haematol 1989; 43:60–65.

50. Blade J, Fernandez-Llama P, Bosch F, et al: Renal failure in multiple myeloma: presenting features and predictors of outcome in 94 patients from a single institution. Arch Intern Med 1998; 158:1889–1893.

51. McCarthy CS, Becker JA: Multiple myeloma and contrast media. Radiology 1992; 183:519–521.

52. Irish AB, Winearls CG, Littlewood T: Presentation and survival of patients with severe renal failure and myeloma. Q J Med 1997; 90:773–780.

53. Rabb H, Gunasekaran H, Gunasekaran S, Saba SR: Acute renal failure from multiple myeloma precipitated by ACE inhibitors. Am J Kidney Dis 1999; 33:E5.

54. Smolens P, Barnes JL, Kreisberg R: Hypercalcemia can potentiate the nephrotoxicity of Bence Jones proteins. J Lab Clin Med 1987; 110:460–465.

55. Brouet JC, Clavel JP, Danon F, et al: Biologic and clinical significance of cryoglobulins: a report of 86 cases. Am J Med 1974; 57:775–788.

56. Moroni G, Banfi G, Maccario M, et al: Extracapillary glomerulonephritis and renal amyloidosis. Am J Kidney Dis 1996; 28:695–699.

57. Pasquali S, Zucchelli P, Casanova S, et al: Renal histological lesions and clinical syndromes in multiple myeloma. Renal Immunopathology Group. Clin Nephrol 1987; 27:222–228.

58. Pirani CL, Silva F, D'Agati V, et al: Renal lesions in plasma cell dyscrasias: ultrastructural observations. Am J Kidney Dis 1987; 10:208–221.

59. Sanders PW, Booker BB: Pathobiology of cast nephropathy from human Bence Jones proteins. J Clin Invest 1992; 89:630–639.

60. Solomon A, Weiss DT, Kattine AA: Nephrotoxic potential of Bence Jones proteins. N Engl J Med 1991; 324:1845–1851.

61. Schwartz RH, Berdon WE, Wagner HE, et al: Tamm-Horsfall urinary muroprotein predipitation by urographic contrast agents. Am J Rheumatol 1970; 108:698–701.

62. Holland MD, Galla HH, Sanders PW, Luke RG: Effect of urinary pH and diatrizoate on Bence Jones protein nephrotoxicity in the rat. Kidney Int 1985; 27:46–50.

63. Yussim E, Schwartz E, Sidi Y, Ehrehfeld M: Acute renal failure precipitated by non-steroidal anti-inflammatory drugs (NSAIDs) in multiple myeloma. Am J Hematol 1998; 58:142–144.

64. Rota S, Mougenot B, Baudouin B, et al: Multiple myeloma and severe renal failure: a clinicopathologic study of outcome and prognosis in 34 patients. Medicine 1987; 66:126–137.

65. Winearls CG: Acute myeloma kidney. Kidney Int 1995; 48:1347–1361.

66. Alexanian R, Dimopoulos M: Drug therapy: the treatment of multiple myeloma. N Engl J Med 1994; 330:484–489.

67. Moist L, Nesrallah G, Kortas C, et al: Plasma exchange in rapidly progressive renal failure due to multiple myeloma: a retrospective case series. Am J Nephrol 1999; 19:45–50.

68. Johnson WJ, Kyle RA, Pineda AA, et al: Treatment of renal failure associated with multiple myeloma: plasmapheresis, hemodialysis, and chemotherapy. Arch Intern Med 1990; 150:863.

69. Zuchelli P, Pasquali S, Cagnoli L, Ferrari G: Controlled plasma exchange trial in acute renal failure due to multiple myeloma. Kidney Int 1988; 33:1175–1180.

70. Pichette V, Querin S, Desmeules M, et al: Renal function recovery in end-stage renal disease. Am J Kidney Dis 1993; 22:398–402.

71. Montseny JJ, Kleinknecht D, Meyrier A, et al: Long-term outcome according to renal histological lesions in 118 patients with monoclonal gammopathies. Nephrol Dial Transplant 1998; 13:1438–1445.

72. Sharland A, Snowdon L, Joshua DE, et al: Hemodialysis: an appropriate therapy in myeloma-induced renal failure. Am J Kidney Dis 1997; 30:786–792.

73. Torra R, Blade J, Cases A, et al: Patients with multiple myeloma requiring long-term dialysis: presenting features, response to therapy, and outcome in a series of 20 cases. Br J Haematol 1995; 91:854–859.

74. Clark AD, Shetty A, Soutar R: Renal failure and multiple myeloma: pathogenesis and treatment of renal failure and management of underlying myeloma. Blood Rev 1999; 13:79–90.

75. Walker F, Bear RA: Renal transplantation in light-chain multiple myeloma. Am J Nephrol 1983; 3:34–37.

76. Burke JR, Flis R, Lasker N, Simenhoff M. Malignant lymphoma with "myeloma kidney" acute renal failure. Am J Med 1976; 60:1055–1060.

77. Soffer O, Nassar VH, Campbell WG, Bourke E: Light-chain cast nephropathy and acute renal failure associated with rifampin therapy: renal disease akin to myeloma kidney. Am J Med 1987; 82:1052–1056.

78. Fattori E, Cocca CD, Costa P, et al: Development of progressive kidney damage and myeloma kidney in interleukin-6 transgenic mice. Blood 1994; 83:2570–2579.

79. Obrador GT, Price B, O'Meara Y, Salant DJ: Acute renal failure due to lymphomatous infiltration of the kidneys. J Am Soc Nephrol 1997; 8:1348.

80. Coggins CH: Renal failure in lymphoma. Kidney Int 1980; 17:847.

81. Ferry JA, Harris NL, Papanicolaou N, et al: Lymphoma of the kidney: a report of 11 cases. Am J Surg Pathol 1995; 19:134.

82. Richmond J, Sherman RS, Diamond HD, et al: Renal lesions associated with malignant lymphomas. Am J Med 1962; 32:184.

83. Alpers CE, Cotran RS: Neoplasia and glomerular injury. Kidney Int 1986; 30:465.

84. Ahmed M, Solangi K, Abbi R, et al: Nephrotic syndrome, renal failure, and renal malignancy: an unusual tumor-associated glomerulonephritis. J Am Soc Nephrol 1997; 8:848.

85. Maes B, Vanwalleghem J, Kuypers D, et al: IgA antiglomerular basement membrane disease associated with bronchial carcinoma and monoclonal gammopathy. Am J Kidney Dis 1999; 33:E3.

86. Moulin B, Ronco PM, Mougenot B, et al: Glomerulonephritis in chronic lymphocytic leukemia and related B-cell lymphomas. Kidney Int 1992; 42:127.

87. Feiner H, Gallo G: Ultrastructure in glomerulonephritis associated with cryoglobulinemia. Am J Pathol 1977; 88:145.

88. Morel-Maroger L, Basch A, Danon F, et al: Pathology of the kidney in Waldestrom's macroglobulinemia. N Engl J Med 1970; 283:123.

89. VanderMerwe WM, Collins JF: The haemolytic-uremic syndrome and prostatic carcinoma. N Z Med J 1987; 100:483.

90. Ortega-Marcos O, Miguel JL: Hemolytic-uremic syndrome in a patient with gastric adenocarcinoma: partial recovery of renal function after gastrectomy. Clin Nephrol 1985; 24:265.

91. Lesesne JB, Rothschild N, Erickson B, et al: Cancer-associated hemolytic-uremic syndrome: analysis of 85 cases from a national registry. J Clin Oncol 1989; 7:781–789.

92. Ruggenenti P, Remuzzi G: The pathophysiology and management of thrombotic thrombocytopenic purpura. Eur J Haematol 1996; 56:191.

93. Gordon LI, Kwaan HC: Cancer- and drug-associated thrombotic thrombocytopenic purpura and hemolytic-uremic syndrome. Semin Hematol 1997; 34:140.

94. Kjellstrand CM, Campbell CC, Hartitzch BV, Buselmeier TJ: Hyperuricemic acute renal failure. Arch Intern Med 1974; 133:349–359.

95. Tsokos GC, Balow JE, Spiegel RJ, McGrath IT: Renal and metabolic complications of undifferentiated and lymphoblastic lymphomas. Medicine 1981; 60:218–229.

CHAPTER 25

Acute Renal Failure in Solid-Organ Transplantation

Colm C. Magee ■ Joseph J. Walshe

INTRODUCTION

This chapter focuses firstly on acute renal failure (ARF) occurring after renal transplantation. Acute renal failure in the setting of liver, heart, or pancreas transplantation is then discussed. There is significant overlap in the causes and management of ARF in patients with different solid-organ transplants.

ACUTE RENAL FAILURE IN THE SETTING OF RENAL ALLOGRAFT TRANSPLANTATION

Acute renal allograft failure remains one of the most common complications of renal transplantation. Acute failure of the transplanted kidney may occur at any point in time after transplantation but is most common during the early postoperative period. The causes of ARF depend on the time period after transplantation, which allows a rational diagnostic and therapeutic approach in most cases. The time periods considered here are immediately after transplantation, early (1–12 weeks) after transplantation, and late (more than 3–6 months) after transplantation, but there is obviously overlap between these periods.

Delayed Graft Function During the Immediate Post-Transplantation Period

Delayed graft function (DGF) is usually defined as failure of the renal allograft to function immediately after transplant, with the need for one or more dialysis sessions within a specified period, usually 1 week. Thus, DGF is a clinical diagnosis. By using the requirement for dialysis as the sole criterion for diagnosis, some patients with residual native kidney function are excluded, however. The reported rates for DGF from recent series in patients receiving cadaveric kidney transplants are between 9% and 25%.[1, 2] Table 25–1 lists the causes of DGF, considered as prerenal, intrarenal, and postrenal insults. Frequently there is an overlap of causes, in particular between ischemia and rejection. Ischemic acute tubular necrosis (ATN) is by far the most common cause of DGF; in fact, the two terms are often used interchangeably, although they are *not* equivalent.

The risk factors for DGF include advanced donor age (over 50 years old),[3] prolonged cold or warm ischemia times, intraoperative or postoperative hypovolemia-hypotension, probably initial high cyclosporin A

(CsA) dosage, and sensitized or previously transplanted recipients.[4] Many of these factors obviously act by increasing the risk of ischemic damage and therefore ATN, but the last factor indicates an underlying immunologic etiology in some cases.

The diagnosis of the underlying cause of DGF is based on clinical, radiologic, and sometimes histologic findings. Figure 25–1 illustrates an algorithm for the diagnosis and management of transplant-kidney nonfunction and oliguria immediately after surgery. Careful review of the donor history and of the harvesting and transplantation process may provide clues to the etiology of DGF. Note that interpretation of the urine output requires knowledge of the pretransplant native kidney output. Prerenal and postrenal causes (including simple problems such as urinary catheter malposition or obstruction) must always be considered. A response to a fluid challenge implicates prerenal factors. If administration of fluids and diuretics fails to improve urine output, further investigation is warranted. The urgency with which further investigations are undertaken depends on the individual case. Persistent oliguria in the setting of a living donor kidney despite adequate hydration and administration of high-dose loop diuretics requires immediate radiologic evaluation of renal blood flow (by Doppler flow study or radionuclide scan) or immediate surgical re-exploration, because the cause of impaired function is more likely to be a major surgical complication than ATN. In contrast, a cadaveric kidney at high risk for ATN (eg, elderly donor, prolonged ischemia time) would generally be less urgently investigated.

Radiologic evaluation of the graft is undertaken to assess perfusion and to rule out urinary obstruction or leakage. Standard ultrasonography is useful, because it is inexpensive, noninvasive, and effective in excluding

TABLE 25–1. Causes of Delayed Graft Function in Renal Transplantation

Prerenal
    Severe hypovolemia-hypotension
    Renal vessel thrombosis
Intrarenal
    Ischemic ATN
    Hyperacute rejection
    Accelerated or acute rejection superimposed on ATN
    Acute CsA-tacrolimus nephrotoxicity (± ATN)
Postrenal
    Urinary tract obstruction/leakage

ATN, acute tubular necrosis; *CsA,* cyclosporin A.

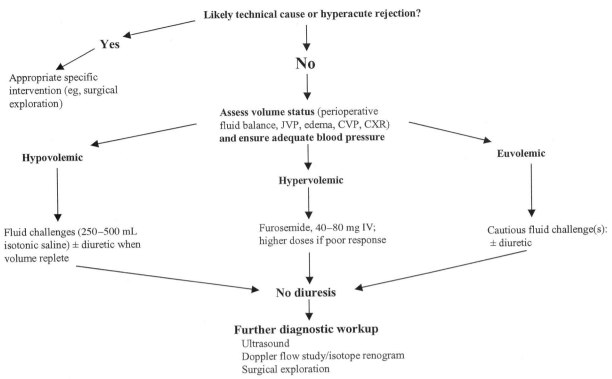

FIGURE 25–1 ■ Management of renal allograft nonfunction and oliguria immediately post transplant. (Adapted from McKay DB, et al: Clinical Aspects of Renal Transplantation. In: Brenner BM, ed: *The Kidney.* 5th ed. Philadelphia: WB Saunders; 1996:2602–2652; with permission.)

postrenal causes of renal failure. Doppler flow studies are helpful in assessing renal arterial and venous blood flow but cannot reliably distinguish intrarenal causes based on changes in intrarenal vascular resistance.[5] Nuclear medicine imaging may provide additional information regarding renal perfusion and function. Absent renal blood flow suggested by Doppler studies is best confirmed by isotope renography. In rare cases, the presence of a urine leak or urinary tract obstruction is detectable by isotope renography but not by initial ultrasonography. Although changes are seen on the radionuclide scan with intrarenal insults such as ATN or rejection, reliably distinguishing these is again not possible.

In many cases of DGF, prerenal and postrenal causes can be excluded and the clinical and radiologic findings are consistent with an intrarenal insult. Definitive diagnosis of the underlying cause requires allograft biopsy, but biopsy is generally avoided until at least 5 days after transplant. The decision to biopsy depends mainly on the duration of DGF and the likelihood of the underlying cause being ATN as opposed to a more graft-threatening cause such as rejection. An algorithm for diagnostic biopsy and treatment of persistent DGF is shown in Figure 25–2. Specific treatment of DGF depends on the underlying cause and is discussed later in this chapter.

ISCHEMIC ACUTE TUBULAR NECROSIS

Ischemic ATN is the most common cause of DGF in cadaveric kidney transplant recipients. The etiology of ATN in transplanted kidneys is presumed to be similar to that in native kidneys. At multiple steps during the surgical transplantation procedure the cadaveric graft is at risk for ischemic damage (Table 25–2). Reperfusion injury via mechanisms such as direct endothelial trauma, oxygen free-radical damage, and neutrophil activation also contributes to the development of this condition.[6, 7] Interactions between the graft endothelium and host neutrophils via ligands such as platelet-activating factor (PAF) and adhesion molecules play an important role in local neutrophil activation.

There are no clinical or radiologic features unique to transplant ATN. As is the case with ARF in native kidneys, transplant ATN should be a diagnosis of exclusion. Several of the risk factors identified in Table 25–2 may be present. Radiologic studies confirm intact graft perfusion, and the findings are consistent with an intrarenal insult. Histology, if available, shows tubular cell damage and necrosis (Fig. 25–3) similar to that found in native kidneys with ATN, although Solez and coworkers[8] have noted that transplant tubular necrosis is much more overt. Patchy interstitial lymphocytic infiltrates, but not tubulitis, may be present. The natural history of uncomplicated ATN is one of spontaneous resolution. Usually, improvements in urine output begin from 5 to 10 days after transplant, but ATN may persist for weeks.

The management of the patient during this period is essentially supportive: avoidance of fluid overload; nutritional support and dialysis as needed. Intravenous calcium gluconate and glucose plus insulin may be

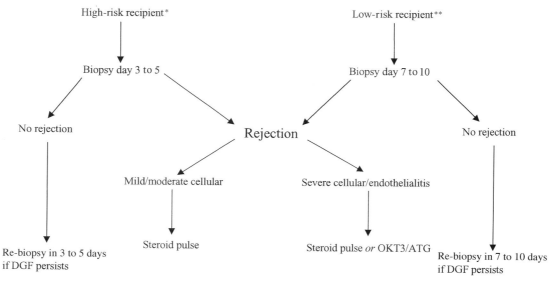

High-risk recipient*

Biopsy day 3 to 5

No rejection

Rejection

Low-risk recipient**

Biopsy day 7 to 10

No rejection

Mild/moderate cellular

Severe cellular/endothelialitis

Re-biopsy in 3 to 5 days
if DGF persists

Steroid pulse

Steroid pulse *or* OKT3/ATG

Re-biopsy in 7 to 10 days
if DGF persists

*eg, Sensitized/previous transplant

**More likely to be ischemic ATN

FIGURE 25–2 ■ Algorithm for diagnostic biopsy and treatment of persistent delayed graft function (DGF). (Adapted from McKay DB, et al: Clinical Aspects of Renal Transplantation. In: Brenner BM, ed: *The Kidney.* 5th ed. Philadelphia: WB Saunders; 1996:2602–2652; with permission.)

useful in controlling hyperkalemia and thus postponing the requirement for dialysis. Kayexalate should be avoided in the early postoperative period, because of the risk of colonic dilation and perforation.[9] To reduce the risk of postsurgical bleeding, low-dose anticoagulation should be used during hemodialysis. Care must be taken to avoid intradialytic hypotension, which carries the risk of worsening graft damage. Although there is little direct evidence for the superiority of biocompatible over bioincompatible hemodialysis membranes in the setting of post-transplant ATN,[10] many centers routinely use biocompatible membranes. In general, peritoneal dialysis is best avoided in the first week after transplant, because of the risk of peritonitis or leakage of dialysis fluid into the wound area.

A major concern in the management of the patient with post-transplant ATN is that the diagnosis of new-onset surgical or medical complications involving the graft is difficult. Rejection, for example, may easily be missed. In fact, acute rejection occurs more frequently in grafts with delayed, as opposed to immediate, function.[11] The postulated mechanism is that ischemic and reperfusion injury increases the immunogenicity of the graft and thereby predisposes to acute rejection. Experimental animal models have demonstrated that ischemic ATN is associated with increased expression and production within the renal parenchyma of class I and II major histocompatibility (MHC) molecules, co-stimulatory molecules, proinflammatory cytokines, and adhesion molecules.[12, 13] Such an altered local mi-

TABLE 25–2. Causes of Ischemic Damage to the Cadaveric Renal Allograft

Preharvest donor state
  Shock syndrome
  Endogenous and exogenous catecholamines
  Nephrotoxic drugs
Organ procurement surgery
  Hypotension
  Trauma to renal vessels
  Inadequate flushing
Organ transport and storage
  Prolonged storage (cold ischemia time)
  Pulsatile perfusion injury
Transplantation of recipient
  Prolonged second warm-ischemia time
  Trauma to renal vessels
  Hypovolemia-hypotension
Postoperative period
  CsA-tacrolimus
  Acute heart failure

CsA, cyclosporin A.

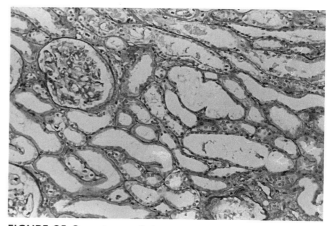

FIGURE 25–3 ■ Acute tubular necrosis. Biopsy of renal allograft with delayed function demonstrates flattening and disruption of the tubular cell lining. There is no significant mononuclear cell infiltrate, and the glomeruli appear normal (PAS ×160). (Courtesy of Dr. Eileen Campbell, Beaumont Hospital, Dublin, Ireland.)

lieu would amplify alloimmune responses. Further evidence of the importance of these mechanisms in human transplantation is that poorer human leukocyte antigen (HLA) matching accentuates the detrimental effect of DGF on allograft survival.[14] A high degree of suspicion for additional complications related to the allograft must therefore be maintained. Radiologic evaluation of the graft should be repeated regularly to detect new urinary or vascular complications. In some centers, core kidney biopsies are repeated in patients with prolonged ATN (see Fig. 25–2).

In the case of DGF secondary to ischemic ATN, an initial induction immunosuppression regimen with antithymocyte globulin (ATG) or OKT3 substituted for full-dose CsA has been advocated.[15] This has the potential benefit of preventing CsA nephrotoxicity while reducing the chances of occult rejection in the nonfunctioning graft. The use of induction therapy is expensive and increases the risk of serious infection, particularly with cytomegalovirus (CMV). Recent analysis of the United Network of Organ Sharing (UNOS) Scientific Renal Transplant Registry showed that the use of antibody induction protocols significantly reduced the incidence of early acute rejection in recipients with DGF; no improvement in 1- or 3-year graft survival or graft half-life was seen, however.[16] Daclizumab and basiliximab, the interleukin (IL)-2–receptor blockers, have not yet been formally tested in this setting.

HYPERACUTE REJECTION

Hyperacute rejection is now a rare cause of immediate renal allograft nonfunction. In addition to ABO blood group incompatibility, hyperacute rejection is caused by preformed recipient anti-HLA class I antibodies cross-reacting with antigens on the endothelial surface of the allograft and hence activating the complement and coagulation cascades. These anti-HLA class I antibodies are formed in response to previous transplantation, blood transfusion, or pregnancy. Rarer causes are mediated by anti-HLA class II antibodies (associated with a positive B-cell cross-match) or anti-donor endothelial-monocyte antibodies. Macroscopic changes may be seen minutes after vascular anastomosis is established. Clinically there is cyanosis and mottling of the kidney, anuria, and sometimes disseminated intravascular coagulation. Radiologic studies confirm absent or minimal renal perfusion, in contrast to what occurs in ATN, in which blood supply is relatively well maintained. Histology shows widespread small vessel endothelial damage and thrombosis, usually with neutrophil polymorphonuclear leukocytes incorporated into the thrombus. There is no effective treatment, and transplant nephrectomy is indicated. Screening for recipient-donor ABO or class I MHC incompatibility (the presence of the latter is often referred to as a "positive T-cell cross-match") has ensured that hyperacute rejection is now uncommon. Rare cases occur because of clerical errors or because of the presence of the other preformed antibodies described previously that are not detected by routine screening methods. Anti-donor endothelial-monocyte antibodies may cause a delayed-onset hyperacute rejection syndrome in HLA-identical grafts.

Several centers have described small series in which anti-donor HLA antibodies have been removed by immunoadsorption prior to transplantation.[17–19] Although this technique may allow transplantation of highly sensitized patients, rates of rejection and graft loss remain relatively high.

ACCELERATED REJECTION SUPERIMPOSED ON ACUTE TUBULAR NECROSIS

Accelerated acute rejection refers to rejection episodes occurring roughly between days 2 and 5 post transplant. The cause of rejection is thought to be pre-transplant sensitization of the recipient to donor alloantigens. This arises from previous transplantation or, less commonly, from blood transfusion. Accelerated acute rejection may be superimposed on ischemic ATN, in which case there may be no signs of rejection, or it may occur in an initially functioning allograft. Diagnosis is by renal biopsy, which usually shows predominantly antibody, rather than cell-mediated, immune damage.[20] The classic finding is necrotizing arteritis, ie, "fibrinoid" necrosis and inflammation of the arterial wall. Immunofluorescence shows that the fibrinoid material contains immunoglobulin, complement, and fibrin. Patients with presumed ischemic ATN who are at high risk for developing this form of rejection (eg, sensitized by previous transplantation) should undergo biopsy 3 to 5 days after transplantation. First-line treatment of accelerated acute rejection is either high-dose steroids or OKT3. Overall, the prognosis for recovery of good allograft function is guarded. Plasma exchange has been used for clearance of donor-specific alloantibody in antibody-mediated rejection, but definitive evidence of a benefit from this treatment is lacking.[21] Small series suggest this procedure is particularly effective when combined with tacrolimus and mycophenolate mofetil.

ACUTE CsA OR TACROLIMUS NEPHROTOXICITY SUPERIMPOSED ON ACUTE TUBULAR NECROSIS

CsA or tacrolimus, especially in high doses, causes an acute reversible decrease in glomerular filtration rate (GFR) by renal vasoconstriction, particularly of the afferent glomerular arteriole.[22] This is discussed in more detail later in this chapter. Delayed graft function may occur in severe cases, particularly if underlying ischemic ATN is present.

VASCULAR AND UROLOGIC COMPLICATIONS OF SURGERY

Renal vessel thrombosis, urinary leaks, and obstruction are rarer but important causes of DGF. These complications may also cause allograft dysfunction in the early postoperative period and are discussed later in this chapter.

OUTCOME AND SIGNIFICANCE OF DELAYED GRAFT FUNCTION

Patients with DGF require longer hospitalization and more interventional studies and are at higher risk for occult rejection or other insults to the graft. Postoperative fluid and electrolyte management is more difficult. In most cases, recovery of renal function is sufficient to become independent of dialysis. In fewer than 5% of cases, allografts with delayed function do not recover function: these are said to have primary nonfunction. However, although the majority of patients become independent of dialysis, most recent studies have demonstrated that recipients with DGF have poorer long-term graft outcome compared with those without DGF.[2, 23] Whether this effect is mediated by immune mechanisms (the increased risk of rejection) or nonimmune mechanisms, or both, is disputed. However, a recent analysis of primary cadaveric renal transplants in the US Renal Data System (USRDS) showed that DGF was an *independent predictor* of 5-year graft loss (relative risk = 1.53). The additional presence of acute rejection had an additive adverse effect with a 5-year graft survival of only 35%.[11] The importance of ischemic injury is further emphasized by the impressive graft survival outcomes in living nonrelated donor transplantation in which ischemic times are very short.[24]

Measures for limiting the incidence and duration of DGF are therefore very worthwhile. Obvious strategies include optimization of the hemodynamic status of the donor and recipient. Invasive vascular monitoring is useful for titrating fluid administration—in most cases a central venous pressure line is sufficient. Intraoperative mean arterial blood pressure should be maintained at more than 70 mm Hg. Intraoperative administration of mannitol is recommended by some clinicians, but high doses should be avoided.[2, 25] Meticulous surgical technique, rapid transport of harvested grafts, and the use of optimal preservation solutions are also of obvious extreme importance. The use of University of Wisconsin preservation solution during the cold ischemia period reduces the incidence of DGF,[3] and its use is now standard practice in most centers. Whether machine perfusion of cadaveric renal allografts is more effective than simple cold storage in preventing DGF remains controversial. It is certainly more expensive and complex. Prospective controlled trials in which one kidney from each donor is allocated to machine perfusion and the other to cold storage (thus controlling for donor factors) have yielded conflicting results.[26, 27] There is evidence that machine perfusion of grafts from non–heart-beating donors lowers the incidence of DGF.[28] If kidneys from marginal ("expanded criteria") donors are being used, transplantation of both kidneys into one recipient might be expected to lower the risk of DGF (see discussion later in this chapter); preliminary results are encouraging.[29]

The benefits and risks of induction therapy with OKT3 or ATG in the setting of ATN have been discussed briefly previously. Calcium channel blockers have been shown in experimental models to prevent ischemic injury and ameliorate CsA-mediated vasoconstriction.[30] These properties suggested that administration of calcium channel blockers to cadaveric-kidney transplant recipients in the perioperative period or to the donor before organ harvesting might reduce the incidence or duration of ischemic ATN. Unfortunately, studies have not provided definitive answers.[31, 32] Perioperative administration of dopamine to the recipient is of no benefit.[33] Atrial natriuretic peptide has been of limited benefit in the setting of nontransplant ARF[34] and is therefore unlikely to find use in the transplant situation. Strategies based on preventing neutrophil-mediated reperfusion injury by blocking PAF-PAF receptor or adhesion molecule interactions are under investigation. BN 52021, a PAF antagonist, significantly reduced the incidence of DGF in a pilot study in human cadaveric renal allograft recipients.[35] Anti–LFA-1 antibody but not anti–ICAM-1 antibody has shown promise in human trials.[36, 37] Delayed graft function from ATN is likely to remain a significant problem in cadaveric kidney transplantation as the use of "marginal" donors continues to increase.

Early Post-Transplantation Period

Table 25–3 shows the causes of allograft dysfunction during the early (1 to 12 weeks) post-transplant period. There is obviously some overlap in the causes of delayed and early allograft dysfunction. Despite its known limitations, the primary measure of early and late transplant kidney function remains the serum creatinine (S_{Cr}). Large elevations in S_{Cr} (more than 25% over baseline) usually represent a significant, potentially graft-endangering event. Again, prerenal and postrenal failure should be systematically excluded.

The role of fractional sodium excretion (FE_{Na}) and urinalysis and urine microscopy in distinguishing the various syndromes of ARF is less well established than in native kidney disease.[38, 39] Lymphocyturia and collecting duct exfoliation into the urine are sensitive markers of rejection but are not specific.[40]

TABLE 25–3. Causes of Renal Allograft Dysfunction in the Early Postoperative Period

Prerenal
 Hypovolemia-hypotension
 Renal vessel thrombosis
 Drugs: ACE inhibitors–NSAIDs
 Transplant renal artery stenosis
Intrarenal
 Acute rejection (most common)
 Acute CsA-tacrolimus nephrotoxicity
 CsA-tacrolimus–induced thrombotic microangiopathy
 Recurrence of primary disease
 Acute pyelonephritis
 Acute interstitial nephritis
Postrenal
 Urinary tract obstruction–leakage

ACE, Angiotensin-converting enzyme; *CsA*, cyclosporin A; *NSAIDs*, nonsteroidal anti-inflammatory drugs.

PRERENAL DYSFUNCTION

Hypovolemia may develop secondary to high-volume diuresis from the transplanted kidney or from "third space" losses. Patients, accustomed to rigid fluid restriction on dialysis, may have difficulty in "keeping up" with fluid losses. Angiotensin-converting enzyme (ACE) inhibitors and nonsteroidal anti-inflammatory drugs (NSAIDs) should generally be avoided in the early post-transplant period, because of the risk of functional prerenal failure with the often-fluctuating volume status; this risk is enhanced by the renal vasoconstrictive effects of CsA. In cases of acute prerenal failure associated with hypotension and falling hematocrit values, graft-related bleeding must be considered.

Renal Vessel Thrombosis

Transplantation-induced renal artery or renal vein thrombosis usually occurs in the first 72 hours but may be delayed for up to 10 weeks post transplant. Acute vascular thrombosis is the most common cause of graft loss in the first post-transplant week.[41] Patients with renal artery thrombosis present with abrupt onset of anuria (unless there is a native urine output) and rapidly rising S_{Cr} but often little localized graft pain or discomfort. Doppler flow studies show absent arterial and venous blood flow. Scintiscans show absent perfusion and absent visualization of the transplanted kidney. Removal of the infarcted kidney is indicated.

Renal vein thrombosis also presents with anuria and rapidly increasing creatinine. Pain, tenderness, swelling in the graft, and hematuria are usually much more pronounced than in renal artery thrombosis. Life-threatening complications, such as embolization or graft rupture and hemorrhage, may occur. Doppler flow studies show absent renal venous blood flow and characteristic highly abnormal renal arterial signals. Again, transplant nephrectomy is indicated. If the venous thrombosis extends beyond the renal vein, anticoagulation is necessary to reduce the risk of embolization.[42] There are case reports of salvaging renal function after early diagnosis of renal vessel thrombosis and intervention with thrombolysis[43, 44] or thrombectomy.[45] In almost all cases, however, infarction occurs too quickly to make this treatment worthwhile. Furthermore, thrombolysis is a high-risk strategy so soon after transplantation, because of the high risk of graft-related bleeding.

Meticulous surgical technique and avoidance of hypovolemia minimize the incidence of this devastating complication. Use of the low-molecular-weight heparin, enoxaparin, significantly reduced the incidence of graft thrombosis in one study of pediatric recipients.[46] The risk of postoperative bleeding in the enoxaparin group was high, however, and few centers routinely use anticoagulation.

INTRARENAL DYSFUNCTION

Acute Rejection

Acute rejection is defined as an acute deterioration in renal allograft function associated with specific pathologic changes in the graft. Most cases of acute rejection occur in the first 6 months post transplant, but this complication may occur at any time. With continued improvement in immunosuppressive regimens and overall patient management, the incidence of acute rejection continues to decrease: the 6-month acute rejection rate in recipients of a first cadaveric kidney transplant is now less than 25%.[47]

Acute rejection is presumed to be secondary to both cellular- and humoral-mediated immune responses, but evidence of cell-mediated responses predominates on most biopsies. In addition to an increasing S_{Cr}, common clinical signs are oliguria, hematuria, and increasing proteinuria. Fever and symptoms localized to the graft are usually not marked in CsA-treated patients. The presence of fever requires that underlying infection be ruled out. Note that a raised S_{Cr} is a relatively late marker of pathologic changes occurring within the graft—hence the interest in developing markers of early immune system activation and rejection. Renal scintiscan, ultrasound, and Doppler flow studies are usually abnormal in acute rejection, but the changes are not specific enough to exclude other causes. Definitive diagnosis requires biopsy, but where there is a high likelihood of uncomplicated acute rejection, empirical treatment is often instituted.

The Banff classification (Table 25–4) is a widely used schema for grading histologic signs of renal allograft rejection and is useful in comparing the effects of different treatments for acute rejection.[48] The classic histologic findings in acute cell-mediated rejection are (1) edema and mononuclear cell infiltration of the interstitium, mainly with CD4$^+$ and CD8$^+$ T lymphocytes but also with some macrophages and plasma cells

TABLE 25–4. Banff Classification of Acute Rejection

Normal
Hyperacute rejection
Borderline changes ("very mild acute rejection"): No intimal arteritis, only mild or moderate focal mononuclear cell infiltration with foci of mild tubulitis (1 to 4 mononuclear cells/tubular cross-section).
Acute rejection
  Grade I: Mild acute rejection (cases with significant interstitial infiltration [> 25% of parenchyma affected] and foci of moderate tubulitis [> 4 mononuclear cells/tubular cross-section or group of 10 tubular cells]).
  Grade II: Moderate acute rejection (cases with A: significant interstitial infiltration and foci of severe tubulitis [> 10% mononuclear cells/tubular cross-section] and/or B: mild or moderate intimal arteritis).
  Grade III: Severe acute rejection (cases with severe intimal arteritis and/or transmural arteritis with fibrinoid change and necrosis of medial smooth muscle cells); or, recent focal infarction and interstitial hemorrhage without obvious cause.
Chronic allograft nephropathy: Graded as mild, moderate, or severe (I, II, III) chronic transplant nephropathy, interstitial fibrosis, and tubular atrophy.
Other (changes not considered to be due to rejection).

Adapted from Solez K, Axelsen RA, Benediktsson H: International standardization of criteria for the histologic diagnosis of renal allograft rejection: the Banff working classification of kidney transplant pathology. Kidney Int 1993; 44:411–412.

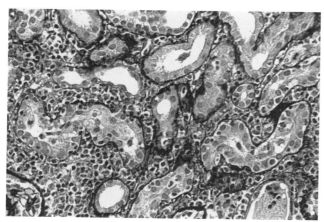

FIGURE 25–4 ■ Acute cellular rejection. Marked infiltration of the interstitium and tubular epithelium with mononuclear cells (PASM and H&E counterstain ×800). (Courtesy of Dr. Eileen Campbell, Beaumont Hospital, Dublin, Ireland.)

and (2) tubulitis (infiltration of tubular epithelium by lymphocytes). A typical example is shown in Figure 25–4. Glomerular involvement is rare, but vascular involvement is common if sought carefully.[20] The latter reflects more severe rejection and is termed "endotheliolitis" or "arteritis." Here, mononuclear cells undermine endothelium (but rarely extend into the muscularis), and the endothelial cells are swollen and detached (Fig. 25–5). Endotheliolitis is frequently a focal process and may therefore be easily missed on biopsy. The term "vascular rejection" is best avoided, because it fails to distinguish between cell-mediated vascular damage (endotheliolitis) and humoral-mediated vascular damage (necrotizing arteritis). The former is much more responsive to antirejection treatment than is the latter. It is important to note that focal infiltrates of mononuclear cells without endotheliolitis or tubulitis may occur in the presence of stable allograft function. Neutrophil infiltration is unusual and should suggest the alternative diagnosis of infec-

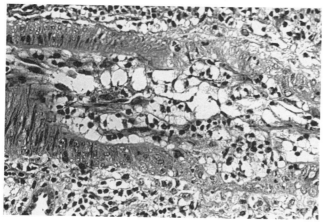

FIGURE 25–5 ■ Severe acute rejection with endothelialitis. Marked disruption of the endothelium of a small artery is seen. Mononuclear cells undermine the endothelium and extend into the media (H&E ×800). (Courtesy of Dr. Eileen Campbell, Beaumont Hospital, Dublin, Ireland.)

tion. The presence of eosinophils in the cellular infiltrate suggests severe rejection,[49] but allergic interstitial nephritis should also be considered.

Uncomplicated acute cellular rejection is generally treated with a short course of high-dose steroids—so-called "pulse" treatment. Urinary tract infection should first be excluded. OKT3 or thymoglobulin and ATG are highly effective in treating first episodes of rejection, reversing them in more than 80% of cases.[50, 51] Because of cost and toxicity, these agents are usually reserved for steroid-resistant cases or when there is severe rejection on the initial biopsy. Typically, 500 to 1000 mg/day of methylprednisolone are given intravenously for 3 to 5 days. There is approximately a 70% response rate to this regimen. The main complication of such high-dose steroid therapy is an increased risk of infection. After completion of pulse therapy, the maintenance oral steroid dose can be resumed immediately, although some centers prefer to taper back to the maintenance dose. The CsA-tacrolimus dosage should be increased if blood levels are "low."

Steroid-resistant acute rejection cases, defined somewhat arbitrarily as failure of improvement in urine output or S_{Cr} elevation within 5 days of starting pulse treatment, are usually treated with OKT3 or ATG. If steroid treatment was based on an empirical rather than a histologic diagnosis of acute rejection, a biopsy is recommended to confirm this diagnosis before instituting anti–T-cell antibody treatment. The response rate to OKT3 in these situations is 80% to 90%.[52] Approximately similar results are obtained with the polyclonal preparations.

If severe rejection with endotheliolitis is found on the initial biopsy, OKT3 is often used as the first-line treatment, because it is thought to be the most effective agent. Of note, treatment with OKT3 in this setting may be associated with an increase in creatinine, 3 to 4 days into the course of OKT3. This transient nephrotoxic effect is presumed to be mediated by increased circulatory levels of cytokines such as tumor necrosis factor-alpha (TNF-α).[53] OKT3 should be continued, because this effect is transient and does not herald a poorer response to the drug. The most important adverse effects of monoclonal or polyclonal antibody treatment, namely, the increased risk of life-threatening infections and lymphoproliferative disease, are well known and should prompt careful analysis of the risks and benefits associated with its use in the treatment of aggressive rejection.[54] Rebound rejection may occur after OKT3 treatment, but this is usually mild and reversible with pulse steroids.

Refractory Acute Rejection. Refractory acute rejection is generally defined as persistent rejection resistant to a course of OKT3. Therapeutic options include a repeat course of OKT3, switching from CsA to tacrolimus or switching from azathioprine to mycophenolate mofetil (MMF).[55] Changing to treatment with tacrolimus is probably the best strategy: there are no head-to-head comparisons of these interventions, however. Uncontrolled studies of tacrolimus rescue therapy have demonstrated improved renal function in more than 70% of such cases.[56, 57] If repeat courses of OKT3 are used, the dosage may need to be increased in patients who produce neutralizing anti-mouse antibodies. Patients undergoing such aggressive immunosuppression should be continued on anti-PCP prophylaxis with sulfamethoxazole-trimethoprim (SMX-TMP) and must be monitored carefully for opportunistic infection.

Significance of Acute Rejection. Although acute rejection is frequently reversed (at least as assessed by S_{Cr}), retrospective studies show that it remains a major predictor of the development of chronic rejection and is associated with poorer allograft survival.[47] Poorer outcome also correlates with the severity of rejection, the number of rejection episodes, and resistance to steroid therapy. Whatever the outcome in terms of graft function, treatment involves exposing the patient to supplemental potentially life-threatening immunosuppression.

Reducing the incidence of acute rejection remains a major goal in transplantation. Fortunately, the incidence is decreasing over the last 20 years, mainly because of improvements in immunosuppression. CsA has been a major factor in this regard. Prophylactic use of OKT3/ATG is effective in decreasing the incidence of *early acute rejection* but is expensive, and later rejections may occur more frequently.[16] A major advantage of the recently introduced IL-2–receptor blocker (induction) therapy is the very low incidence of side effects. When it is used with CsA and steroids, acute rejection rates are reduced by approximately one third.[58, 59] In three recent randomized multicenter trials, MMF has been shown to reduce the incidence of early acute rejection after renal transplantation by almost 50%,[60] and many centers now use this drug routinely in place of azathioprine. Tacrolimus was more effective than CsA in preventing acute renal allograft rejection in two recent multicenter trials.[61, 62]

Acute Calcineurin Inhibitor Nephrotoxicity

The calcineurin inhibitor CsA, especially in high doses, causes an acute, reversible decrease in GFR by renal vasoconstriction, particularly of the afferent glomerular arteriole.[63] Tacrolimus causes a similar syndrome of vasomotor acute renal dysfunction. This is manifested clinically as dose-dependent and blood-level–dependent acute reversible increases in S_{Cr} level. As acute CsA-tacrolimus nephrotoxicity is mainly vasomotor-prerenal, it is not surprising that the histologic changes in this setting may be unimpressive. With very high drug levels, direct proximal tubular damage and dysfunction may occur. This has not been seen as commonly in the last 10 years, because of the lower doses of CsA employed.[8] In such cases, histology shows tubular dilation, tubular cell flattening, and scattered individual tubular cell necrosis. Giant mitochondria and isometric vacuolization in tubular cells reflect more severe damage (Fig. 25–6). Hyaline thickening of arterioles is thought to be a more specific finding.[8] Acute calcineurin inhibitor nephrotoxicity responds to dosage reduction.

Distinguishing Between Acute CsA-Tacrolimus Nephrotoxicity and Acute Rejection

Unfortunately, even with the aid of measurement of blood drug levels, distinguishing between acute cal-

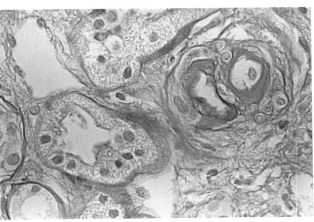

FIGURE 25–6 ▪ Severe acute CsA toxicity. There is isometric vacuolization of tubular cells. Hyaline thickening of the arteriolar wall is also seen (PAS ×800). (Courtesy of Dr. Eileen Campbell, Beaumont Hospital, Dublin, Ireland.)

cineurin inhibitor nephrotoxicity and acute rejection clinically can be difficult. Low and high blood drug levels in the presence of deteriorating renal function suggest, but do not imply, rejection and drug nephrotoxicity, respectively. Both syndromes may coexist. Indicators of acute CsA-tacrolimus nephrotoxicity are signs of extrarenal toxicity, such as severe tremor, a "moderate" increase in the S_{Cr} level (<50% over baseline), and high CsA (eg, >350 ng/mL in whole blood) or tacrolimus levels (>20 ng/mL in whole blood). Indicators of acute rejection are fever, allograft pain and tenderness, rapid, nonplateauing increases in S_{Cr} levels, and low drug levels (eg, CsA <150 ng/mL in whole blood). Oliguria is more pronounced in severe acute rejection than in calcineurin inhibitor toxicity. Sodium retention and edema may occur with either condition. Fever and symptoms localized to the allograft do not occur in calcineurin inhibitor toxicity, but by no means do they imply rejection: infections such as acute pyelonephritis must be considered.

The criteria for deciding on biopsy in order to more firmly establish the diagnosis of rejection vary among centers. An algorithm for approaching this common clinical problem is shown in Figure 25–7. One common strategy is to institute a "trial of therapy" and, if the clinical response to this is unsatisfactory, to proceed to biopsy within 48 to 96 hours. For example, if acute CsA nephrotoxicity were suspected, the CsA dose would be reduced, which should lead to improvement in renal function within 24 to 48 hours, if this diagnosis were correct. A presumptive diagnosis of acute rejection would mean empirical treatment with a steroid pulse. Lack of response after several days of antirejection treatment because of resistant rejection, CsA nephrotoxicity, or another cause would be diagnosed by biopsy. The threshold for biopsy is lower in "high-risk" patients: those who are highly sensitized, have previously rejected a graft, or are at high risk of early recurrent primary renal disease, especially focal segmental glomerulosclerosis (FSGS) or hemolytic-uremic syndrome (HUS). Biopsy results alone should not dic-

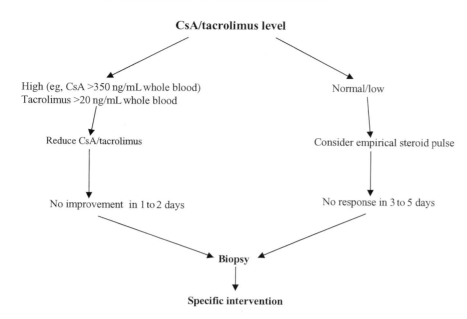

CsA/tacrolimus level

High (eg, CsA >350 ng/mL whole blood)
Tacrolimus >20 ng/mL whole blood

Reduce CsA/tacrolimus

No improvement in 1 to 2 days

Normal/low

Consider empirical steroid pulse

No response in 3 to 5 days

Biopsy

Specific intervention

FIGURE 25–7 ■ Algorithm for management of allograft dysfunction in the early post-transplant period (prerenal and postrenal causes excluded). (Adapted from McKay DB, et al: Clinical Aspects of Renal Transplantation. In: Brenner BM, ed: *The Kidney.* 5th ed. Philadelphia: WB Saunders; 1996: 2602–2652; with permission.)

tate management; rather, the constellation of clinical and histologic findings should be used to shape a treatment plan.[64] In some cases, histologic findings of CsA-tacrolimus–induced damage and acute rejection may coexist.

It has been suggested that measuring the levels of serum or urinary cytokines,[65] IL-2 receptor, adhesion molecules,[66] or other inflammatory markers such as complement and acute-phase proteins[67] may be useful in diagnosing acute allograft rejection. A serum or urine marker with high positive and negative predictive values might obviate biopsy or aid the follow-up of treated rejection. These markers await validation in large-scale multicenter human studies, however. Another concern is that infections, including those caused by CMV, could mimic acute rejection by elevating the levels of inflammatory and immunologic markers. Core kidney biopsy with appropriate histologic examination therefore remains the gold standard for diagnosing intrarenal causes of allograft dysfunction. Quantitative determination by reverse transcription–polymerase chain reaction of certain gene transcripts within renal biopsy tissue has been shown to be a sensitive and specific marker of acute rejection.[68] Combined analysis of Fas ligand, perforin, and granzyme B gene expression yielded the most accurate results. Interestingly, preliminary data from the same group suggest that expression of certain genes in peripheral blood leukocytes also correlates with acute rejection of the renal allograft.[69] Such specialized techniques, when proved to be highly reproducible, may assume a useful role in clinical practice.

Thrombotic Microangiopathy

Thrombotic microangiopathy (TMA) after renal transplantation is a rare but serious complication. CsA and tacrolimus, as well as other factors, have been associated with the development of this syndrome, which is presumed to be initiated by direct endothelial

cell damage. Onset is usually in the early post-transplant period. The classic laboratory findings are increasing S_{Cr} and lactate dehydrogenase levels, thrombocytopenia, falling hematocrit, and the presence of schistocytes on the blood film. The hematologic features of thrombotic microangiopathy may easily be missed, however. Renal biopsy shows platelet and fibrin thrombi in the lumina of arterioles and glomerular capillaries (Fig. 25–8). Similar histologic changes occur in cases of malignant hypertension, recurrent HUS, pulsatile perfusion injury, and hyperacute rejection. Early diagnosis of TMA is essential in order to salvage worthwhile renal function. Treatment involves cessation or reduction of calcineurin inhibitor therapy, control of any hypertension present, and plasmapheresis. Prognosis for the allograft is poor, although in one retrospective series of 13 cases, a regimen of aspirin, isradipine, and pentoxifylline combined with tempo-

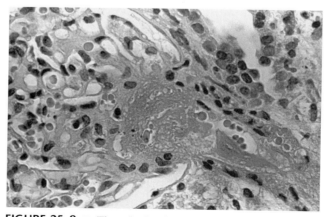

FIGURE 25–8 ■ Thrombotic microangiopathy. Transplant kidney biopsy performed 2 weeks post transplant in a patient on tacrolimus and with hematologic evidence of thrombotic microangiopathy. Fibrin thrombus is seen in the glomerular capillaries and arteriole (H&E ×800). (Courtesy of Dr. Eileen Campbell, Beaumont Hospital, Dublin, Ireland.)

rary discontinuation of CsA-tacrolimus gave an initial response rate of 69%.[70] Long-term graft function (creatinine clearance) remained inferior to nonaffected control subjects. Absence of recurrence after initial treatment has been reported with both reintroduction of CsA and switching from CsA to tacrolimus.[70, 71] There is evidence that TMA in some cases may be related to the presence of anticardiolipin antibodies in hepatitis C–positive recipients.[72]

Acute Pyelonephritis

Urinary tract infections (UTIs) may occur at any time period but most frequently occur shortly after transplantation, because of catheterization, stenting, and aggressive immunosuppression. Other risk factors for UTI are anatomic abnormalities and neurogenic bladder. In general, UTIs occurring in the first few months post transplant are more severe and complicated and require more aggressive therapy than those occurring later.[73] There is evidence that acute pyelonephritis in the early post-transplant period predisposes to acute rejection. Fortunately, acute pyelonephritis and urosepsis are much less common since the widespread use of prophylactic SMX-TMP. Fever, allograft pain and tenderness, and raised peripheral white blood cell count are usually more pronounced in acute pyelonephritis than in acute rejection. Diagnosis requires urine culture, but empirical antibiotic treatment is started immediately. The most commonly implicated microorganisms are gram-negative bacilli, coagulase-negative staphylococci, and enterococci, organisms similarly found in nontransplant patients.[74] Renal function usually returns to baseline quickly with antimicrobial therapy and volume expansion. Recurrent cases of pyelonephritis require investigation to rule out underlying urologic abnormalities.

Acute Allergic Interstitial Nephritis

Distinguishing acute allergic interstitial nephritis and acute rejection is difficult. Mononuclear cell and eosinophil infiltration of the transplanted kidney may occur with either condition. Both conditions usually respond to steroids. Colvin[20] has suggested that invasion of multiple tubules by eosinophils is strong evidence of drug-induced acute allergic interstitial nephritis. Sulfamethoxazole-trimethoprim is the drug most probably implicated in renal transplant patients. Nonsteroidal anti-inflammatory drugs have also been reported as causes of this syndrome (see later discussion).

De Novo Glomerulonephritis

De novo anti–glomerular basement membrane (GBM) disease may arise in the early post-transplant period in grafts transplanted into recipients with Alport's syndrome. Here, the recipient with abnormal type IV collagen α chains produces antibodies against the previously "unseen" normal α chain in the basement membrane of the transplanted kidney. Patients with graft dysfunction should be treated with plasma exchange and cyclophosphamide.[75] Graft failure due to anti-GBM disease in the transplanted kidney is more common in re-transplants.

Recurrence of Primary Disease

Several renal diseases may recur in the early post-transplant period and cause acute allograft dysfunction. It is difficult to draw firm conclusions regarding the recurrence rate of primary kidney disease post transplant for several reasons: the original cause of end-stage renal disease (ESRD) is often unknown, and most relevant studies are small and retrospective with variable follow-up periods. Randomized prospective trials of treatment regimens for recurrent disease do not exist. The conditions associated with recurrence in transplanted kidneys may be classified into 3 groups: (1) glomerulonephritis, (2) metabolic diseases such as primary oxalosis, and (3) systemic diseases such as hemolytic-uremic syndrome–thrombotic thrombocytopenic purpura (HUS–TTP).[76] Table 25–5 summarizes the conditions that recur during different time periods after transplantation. Focal segmental glomerulosclerosis is considered in more detail in the paragraph that follows, because of its relatively high frequency of recurrence and its propensity to cause severe graft injury.

Focal Segmental Glomerulosclerosis. Focal segmental glomerulosclerosis (FSGS) has a reported recurrence rate of 20% to 40% and causes graft loss in approximately 50% of recurrent cases.[77, 78] Risk factors for recurrence include early onset (<15 years of age), rapidly progressive FSGS in the recipient's native kidneys, and mesangial proliferation on the original biopsies. Recurrence of disease in a previous allograft puts the patient at very high risk for subsequent recurrence. Most cases present hours to weeks post transplant. This rapidity of recurrence suggests the presence of a pathogenic circulating plasma factor—there is now some experimental evidence for this.[79] Proteinuria, which may be massive, is the main clinical feature. Early biopsy (Fig. 25–9) is indicated in those at risk who develop proteinuria. Treatment strategies include plasma exchange, immunoadsorption, high-dose CsA, cyclophosphamide, or ACE inhibitors, but controlled

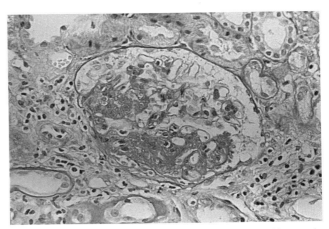

FIGURE 25–9 ■ Recurrent FSGS post transplant. Glomerulus shows an area of segmental sclerosis at the vascular pole. The patient had developed proteinuria and renal impairment in the early post-transplant period. (Courtesy of Dr. Eileen Campbell, Beaumont Hospital, Dublin, Ireland.)

TABLE 25–5. Recurrent Disease After Renal Transplantation

DISEASE	CLINICAL RECURRENCE, %	TIME TO RECURRENCE AFTER TRANSPLANTATION	TREATMENT OF RECURRENCE	LIVING RELATED DONORS	COMMENTS
Metabolic					
Primary oxalosis	Was high; now much improved	Immediately and continuing	Prevention is achievable goal	Yes, but cadaveric liver + kidney transplantation better	Early combined liver + kidney transplantation and intensive perioperative treatment to protect graft are best options
Systemic diseases					
Wegener's granulomatosis	40	From 1st week	Cyclophosphamide	Yes	Avoid transplant if disease active, ?role of monitoring ANCA
HUS/TTP	50	Up to 5 y	Plasma exchange/ infusion	Yes, if not familial HUS	Hold transplant until >3 mo after acute disease
Glomerulonephritis					
FSGS	40–50	Hours to weeks	Plasma exchange, NSAIDs, steroids, ACE-I	No, if high risk of recurrence	Increased risk in children, those with rapid progression to ESRD or mesangial proliferation on biopsy
IgA GN	1–10	2 mo and continuing	With crescents: plasma exchange, cytotoxics	Yes	Overall, graft survival is increased compared with other renal diseases
Henoch-Schönlein purpura	Rare	Immediately and continuing	?Steroids	Avoid	Avoid transplant if relapsing purpura
Anti-GBM disease	25	Immediately	Plasma exchange, cyclophospha-mide	Yes	Hold transplant until clinical remission and negative antibodies for 6–12 mo

ACE-I, angiotensin-converting enzyme inhibitor; *ANCA,* antineutrophil cytoplasmic antibody; *ESRD,* end-stage renal disease; *FSGS,* focal segmental glomerulo-sclerosis; *GBM,* glomerular basement membrane; *GN,* glomerulonephritis; *HUS,* hemolytic-uremic syndrome; *NSAIDs,* nonsteroidal inflammatory drugs; *TTP,* thrombocytopenic purpura.

Adapted from Michielsen P: Recurrence of the original disease: does this influence renal graft failure? Kidney Int Suppl 1995; 52:S79–S84.

studies proving efficacy are lacking.[75] Those at high risk for recurrence should be offered cadaveric, rather than living related, kidneys.

POSTRENAL DYSFUNCTION

The incidence of serious urologic complications and associated morbidity in transplant recipients has decreased significantly over the last 20 years to less than 10%.[80] Graft loss from urologic complications is now rare. Nevertheless, postrenal causes must always be considered in the differential diagnosis of ARF post transplant. Most urologic complications are secondary to technical factors at the time of transplant and manifest themselves in the early postoperative period, but immunologic factors may play a role in some cases.

Urine Leaks

Urine leaks usually occur in the first few weeks after transplantation. Leaks may occur at the level of the renal calyx, the ureter, or the bladder. The causes include infarction of the (distal) ureter, resulting from perioperative disruption of its blood supply, and break-

down of the ureterovesical anastomosis. Severe obstruction may also result in rupture of the urinary tract with leakage. The clinical features include abdominal pain and swelling; the plasma urea and creatinine levels increase secondary to reabsorption across the peritoneal membrane. If a perirenal drain is being used, however, a urine leak may occur with high-volume drainage of fluid. Ultrasound may demonstrate a fluid collection (urinoma). Aspiration of fluid from the fluid collection by sterile technique allows comparison of the fluid creatinine with the S_{Cr}. In cases in which ultrasound diagnosis is difficult, renal scintigraphy may be useful in demonstrating extravasation of tracer from the urinary system, provided there is adequate renal function. Rough localization of the site of the leak is sometimes possible with this technique (Fig. 25–10). Antegrade pyelography allows precise diagnosis and localization of proximal urinary leaks. Cystography is the best test for demonstrating a bladder leak.

It is important to note that the clinical features may mimic those of acute rejection. An incorrect diagnosis of acute rejection and administration of supplemental immunosuppression in this context may have serious

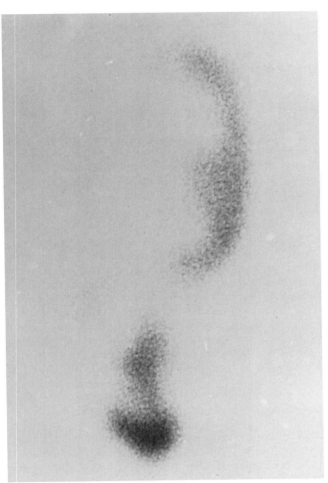

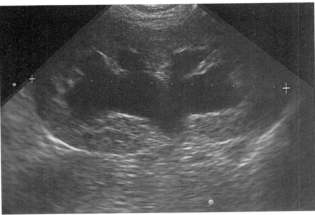

FIGURE 25–11 ■ Ultrasound showing marked hydronephrosis of transplant kidney. (Courtesy of Dr. F. Keeling, Beaumont Hospital, Dublin, Ireland.)

the transplant's urinary collecting system is often seen in the early postoperative period, serial scans showing worsening hydronephrosis may be needed to confirm the diagnosis. Renal scintiscan with diuretic washout is useful in equivocal cases.[83] Percutaneous antegrade pyelography is the best radiologic technique for determining the site of obstruction (Fig. 25–12) and can be combined with interventional endourologic techniques. In expert hands, endourologic techniques (eg, balloon dilatation, stenting) may be effective in treating ureteric stenosis or stricture. More complicated cases require open surgical repair. Extrinsic compression requires specific intervention, such as draining of the lymphocele.

FIGURE 25–10 ■ Isotope renogram demonstrates leakage of urine into abdominal cavity. (Courtesy of Dr. F. Keeling, Beaumont Hospital, Dublin, Ireland.)

Late Acute Allograft Dysfunction

The causes and evaluation of *late* (more than 12 weeks post transplant) *acute renal allograft* dysfunction are broadly similar to those of early acute dysfunction.

consequences. Whenever urine leakage is suspected, a bladder catheter should be immediately inserted to decompress the urinary tract. Selected patients may do well with endourologic treatment.[81] Most cases, however, require urgent surgical exploration and repair. The type of repair depends on the level of the leak and the viability of involved tissues.

Urinary Tract Obstruction

Urinary tract obstruction can cause allograft dysfunction at any time after transplantation but is most commonly manifested during the early postoperative period. The main intrinsic causes are poor reimplantation of the ureter into the bladder, intraluminal blood clots or slough material, and fibrosis of the ureter caused by ischemia or rejection. Extrinsic compression (eg, by a lymphocele) can occur but is less common. Calculi are less common causes of urinary tract obstruction and renal dysfunction.[82]

A typical clinical feature of urinary tract obstruction is a rising S_{Cr} level without localizing symptoms. In severe cases, high pressure within the urinary tract may result in rupture. Ultrasound usually demonstrates hydronephrosis (Fig. 25–11). Because some dilation of

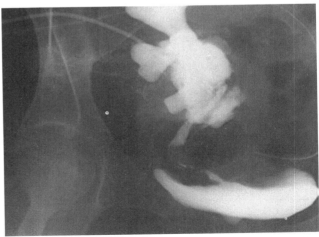

FIGURE 25–12 ■ Antegrade pyelogram demonstrates hydronephrosis and stenosis of transplant ureter. (Courtesy of Dr. F. Keeling, Beaumont Hospital, Dublin, Ireland.)

Acute prerenal failure may occur at any time. The causes are similar to those seen with native kidneys—such as shock syndromes and ACE inhibitor–NSAID hemodynamic effects. Urinary tract obstruction must also be considered in the differential diagnosis of ARF in the late post-transplant period. The causes are similar to those associated with native kidney obstruction, eg, stones, bladder outlet obstruction, and obstruction by neoplasm. Several causes of late acute allograft dysfunction are reviewed in more detail in this chapter.

ACUTE REJECTION

With adequate immunosuppression, acute rejection is uncommon after the first 6 months. Late acute rejection should alert the physician to prescription of inadequate immunosuppression or, more commonly, patient noncompliance.[84] The risk factors for noncompliance include younger patient age, more immunosuppressant side effects, lower socioeconomic status, and psychological stress or illness.[85–87]

The cessation of steroids is well known to increase the risk of deterioration of graft function over the long term. Acute rejection may also occur when steroids are stopped.[88] Hence, patients must be carefully monitored for elevations in creatinine when maintenance steroids are stopped. African-American patients appear to be at high risk for late acute rejection and graft loss.[89] Late acute rejection is usually treated with pulse steroids. Antilymphocyte antibody preparations are less effective in reversing acute rejection that occurs more than 3 to 6 months after transplantation. The aggressiveness of antirejection therapy depends on the clinical situation and biopsy findings. Importantly, late acute rejection has a particularly deleterious effect on long-term graft outcome.[90]

ACUTE CsA-TACROLIMUS NEPHROTOXICITY

Acute CsA-tacrolimus nephrotoxicity is less common in the late post-transplant period. This reflects the lower dosage of these drugs needed to prevent rejection. Inadvertent prescription of medications that impair metabolism of CsA-tacrolimus (Table 25–6) may induce acute deterioration in renal function, but this should be reversible with appropriate drug adjustment.

TRANSPLANT RENAL ARTERY STENOSIS

Transplant renal artery stenosis is usually a late complication of transplantation. The incidence is undetermined; retrospective studies report functionally significant stenosis in approximately 8% of transplant patients.[91] Luminal narrowing of 70% to 80% is probably required to make a stenosis functionally significant. The stenosis may occur in the donor artery or the recipient artery or at the anastomotic site. The causes include operative trauma or hemodynamic stress to these vessels, atheroma of the recipient vessels, or faulty suture technique. Immunologic factors have been postulated to play a role, because case control studies have found an association with the number of acute rejection episodes.[92] Signs suggestive of functionally significant stenosis are resistant hypertension; fluctuating renal function, especially with hypovolemia or ACE inhibition; edema; new bruits over the kidney; and polycythemia.

Color Doppler flow imaging, but not scintigraphy, is a useful screening test,[93] but definitive diagnosis

TABLE 25–6. Commonly Used Drugs That May Induce Acute Renal Failure in Patients With Kidney or Other Solid-Organ Transplants

DRUGS	PATHOPHYSIOLOGY	COMMENT
NSAIDs	Functional prerenal failure, particularly if hypovolemia or renal artery stenosis present; interstitial nephritis	Avoid in renal transplant patients; use with caution in nonrenal transplants
Acyclovir, foscarnet (high-dose)	Crystal deposition in tubules, causing obstruction and damage; also ATN	Hydration prevents crystal deposition
ACE inhibitors	Functional prerenal failure, particularly if hypovolemia or renal artery stenosis present	Monitor renal function carefully after starting ACE-I; avoid in early post-transplant period
SMX-TMP	Proximal and distal tubular secretion of creatinine (no effect on GFR); interstitial nephritis	In general, drug is well tolerated in transplant recipients
Amphotericin	Proximal and distal tubular damage; cumulative dose effect	Lysosomal preparation is less nephrotoxic but very expensive
Interferon alpha	Immune-stimulating effects promote acute rejection; other nephrotoxic effects reported	Risk-benefit ratio of using interferon alpha must be determined for individual patient
Erythromycin, verapamil, diltiazem, ketoconazole	Inhibit metabolism of CsA-tacrolimus	Monitor CsA-tacrolimus levels carefully
HMG-CoA reductase inhibitors, eg, simvastatin	Levels increased with concomitant CsA therapy, increasing risk of rhabdomyolysis	Use lowest dose initially; monitor S_{CR}, CK, etc.
Radiocontrast	Unclear; ?hemodynamic effects	Hydration and use of nonionic contrast medium reduce risk of contrast nephropathy. Acetylcysteine may also be of benefit.

ACE-I, Angiotensin-converting enzyme inhibitor; *ATN,* acute tubular necrosis; *CsA,* cyclosporin A; *GFR,* glomerular filtration rate; *HMG-CoA,* 3-hydroxy-3-methylglutaryl coenzyme A; *NSAIDs,* nonsteroidal anti-inflammatory drugs; *SMX-TMP,* sulfamethoxazole-trimethoprim.

requires renal angiography (Fig. 25–13). The initial treatment of choice is usually percutaneous transluminal stenting, although conservative medical management may suffice in less severe cases.[94] The clinical response rate to angioplasty is approximately 40% to 75%. Restenosis is a problem and may require repeat angioplasty or surgical repair. Surgical repair is performed when angioplasty has failed or is not possible. This is generally considered difficult and associated with a high frequency of graft loss, but good results have been reported from specialist centers.[95]

INFECTIONS

Human Polyomavirus Infection

The polyomaviruses are DNA viruses, the best known of which are the BK virus, the JC virus, and the SV40 virus. Sixty to eighty percent of adults have serologic evidence of past (usually subclinical) exposure. The clinical features associated with infection of renal transplant patients include asymptomatic infection (most common), acute graft dysfunction, and hemorrhagic cystitis. The acute graft dysfunction usually occurs secondary to interstitial nephritis, although

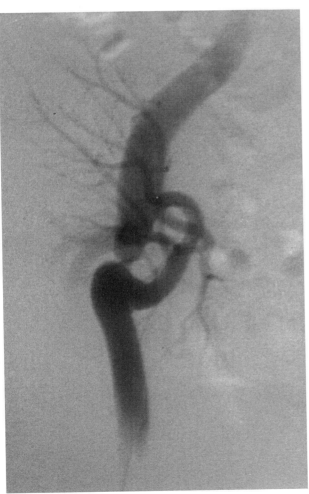

FIGURE 25–13 ▪ Angiogram demonstrates tight stenosis of external iliac artery at level of anastomosis with transplant renal artery. (Courtesy of Dr. F. Keeling, Beaumont Hospital, Dublin, Ireland.)

ureteric stenosis has also been described. Diagnosis of infection (either primary infection or reactivation) is by urine cytology or culture, serology, or demonstration of viral particles within the graft. Viral particles are seen as inclusions within the nucleus of tubular cells. In cases of interstitial nephritis, the histologic findings may overlap with those of acute rejection, which complicates management.[96] Judicious reduction in immunosuppression may result in clearance of the virus, but the long-term outlook for graft survival appears to be compromised.[96]

Hepatitis C and Interferon Alpha

Hepatitis C virus (HCV) infection of the recipient may complicate all forms of solid-organ transplantation but is of particular importance in hepatic and renal transplantation. Infection of the recipient usually occurs before transplantation but may also arise from transplantation of HCV-infected organs. Among renal transplant recipients, the prevalence of anti-HCV antibodies before transplantation is 11% to 49%[97]; there is wide geographic variation in these figures. Predictably, immunosuppression accelerates the progression of this systemic disease. The clinical presentation usually includes proteinuria and nephrotic syndrome, rather than renal failure. Membranoproliferative glomerulonephritis (MPGN) is the most common renal pathology, although membranous nephropathy has also been described.[98] The MPGN form may be associated with cryoglobulinemia, although systemic vasculitis is rare.[99]

The management of progressive hepatitis C disease in renal transplant recipients remains unsatisfactory. Treatment with interferon-alfa (IFN-α) may induce temporary remission, but the rate of relapse is high. Furthermore, up-regulation of the immune response by IFN-α results in a high rate of acute rejection (>40%) and even graft loss.[97] Acute renal transplant failure associated with interstitial edema on biopsy has also been reported.[100] Interestingly, there is speculation that the direct nephrotoxic effects of IFN-α may depend to some extent on the preparation used and its purity.[100]

An association of TMA with anticardiolipin antibodies in hepatitis C–positive patients has also been reported.[72] Hepatitis C–associated glomerular disease may occur in liver transplant recipients. Again, the renal response to IFN-α was disappointing.[101]

Cytomegalovirus

One group has described a series of 21 patients with asymptomatic CMV infection and late acute allograft dysfunction who did not respond to conventional antirejection therapy.[91] Treatment with ganciclovir resulted in stable improved renal function in 80% of cases. This syndrome requires further confirmation. Foscarnet therapy for CMV in transplant patients has been associated with ARF[102]; this is not a problem with ganciclovir.

DRUG- AND RADIOCONTRAST-INDUCED ACUTE RENAL FAILURE IN SOLID-ORGAN TRANSPLANTATION

In the setting of solid-organ transplantation, a variety of drugs can cause acute deterioration in renal function. In many cases, the offending agent (eg, an aminoglycoside or amphotericin) is a well-recognized cause of ARF in native kidneys. However, a number of drug-related nephrotoxic effects are more common in the setting of organ transplantation (see Table 25–6). Many of these are due to interaction with CsA or tacrolimus. Diltiazem, verapamil, ketoconazole, and the macrolide antibiotics impair CsA-tacrolimus metabolism and may lead to acute CsA-tacrolimus nephrotoxicity unless there is a concomitant dose reduction of the calcineurin inhibitor.[103] There are recent case reports implicating the newer antidepressants in this regard.[104, 105] Readers are directed to recent reviews for more information on this important topic of drug interactions with the calcineurin inhibitors.[106, 107] Sulfamethoxazole-trimethoprim therapy may cause an acute increase in S_{Cr} either secondary to inhibition of tubular secretion of creatinine (in this case GFR per se is not compromised, and S_{Cr} decreases within 5 days of stopping SMX-TMP) or resulting from allergic interstitial nephritis.[108] The latter complication is rare and is treated with pulse steroid therapy and cessation of the drug.

Not surprisingly, ACE inhibitors or angiotensin II antagonists have been implicated in precipitating ARF in the presence of transplant renal artery stenosis.[109, 110] Overall, if carefully prescribed, these agents are well tolerated. The use of ACE inhibitors or angiotensin II antagonists in the immediate post-transplant period, when volume status and CsA-tacrolimus levels are fluctuating, is not recommended.

Drugs with known nephrotoxic effects, such as aminoglycosides or amphotericin, may have enhanced toxicity when used concomitantly with a calcineurin inhibitor.[107] Nevertheless, they are sometimes required in transplant recipients. Use of the lysosomal preparation of amphotericin is preferred, because it is less nephrotoxic than the standard preparation.[111]

Nonsteroidal anti-inflammatory drugs have been implicated in several cases of acute interstitial nephritis in renal transplant recipients.[112] Of more concern is their use when renal prostaglandins play a critical role in maintaining renal blood flow and GFR. This occurs in the setting of hypovolemia, low output heart failure, and probably with CsA-tacrolimus therapy. Administration of NSAIDs may block production of prostaglandins, resulting in functional ARF.[113] This is reversible with cessation of the offending drug. Nevertheless, the usage of NSAIDs in patients with a renal transplant or who are on CsA or both should be minimized.

Lipid-lowering agents are increasingly being prescribed for solid organ transplant recipients. The most commonly used class of drugs includes the 3-hydroxy-3-methylglutaryl coenzyme A (HMG CoA)–reductase inhibitors. These drugs are generally well tolerated. However, there is a well-described increased risk of rhabdomyolysis and ARF when they are used with CsA-tacrolimus. This is discussed in more detail later.

The risk of developing ARF after administration of radiocontrast material to organ transplant recipients has not been well described. Presumably, risk factors for postcontrast ARF are similar to those seen in non-transplant patients. Thus, the same preventive measures should be used.

Acute Renal Failure in Simultaneous Pancreas-Kidney Transplantation

Simultaneous pancreas-kidney (SPK) transplantation is the preferred form of pancreas transplantation for patients with diabetes mellitus and ESRD. The causes of ARF in pancreas-kidney transplant recipients are generally similar to those seen in diabetic kidney transplant recipients. There are several noteworthy differences, however. Rates of delayed graft function have been lower, probably reflecting donor and recipient selection factors.[114] In contrast, rates of acute renal rejection have generally been higher. The latter finding may reflect the greater antigen "load" of two transplanted organs and a lower threshold for diagnosing acute rejection (renal dysfunction is often used as a surrogate marker of pancreas rejection). Acute rejection rates are decreasing with newer, more potent oral immunosuppression regimens.[115] With improvements in surgical techniques and immunosuppression, the incidence of septic complications after SPK transplantation has also greatly decreased. Nevertheless, these patients remain at higher risk of ATN secondary to sepsis syndrome and nephrotoxic antimicrobial therapy. Acute torsion and infarction of the transplanted kidney in the setting of combined pancreas-kidney transplantation has also been described.[116]

Features Common to Cardiac, Liver, or Lung Transplant Recipients

Many patients undergoing nonrenal organ transplantation have some impairment of renal function, although this may not be apparent by assessment of the S_{Cr} level. For example, severe heart failure may be associated with prerenal failure, or severe liver failure may cause the hepatorenal syndrome (HRS; see later). Not surprisingly, with restoration of normal organ function after successful transplantation, there is a tendency for renal function to improve in such cases. Opposing this tendency in most patients is the use of nephrotoxic doses of CsA from the time of engraftment. CsA has significantly improved the outcome of nonrenal solid-organ transplantation but at the expense of an increased risk of both acute and chronic nephrotoxicity. There is no evidence that tacrolimus is less nephrotoxic. Note that in most patients lean body mass increases in the weeks to months after successful organ transplantation; this may cause a small increase in S_{Cr} level. This increase may be accentuated by the use of prophylactic SMX-TMP. Thus, accurate determination of renal function before and after solid-organ transplantation requires sophisticated testing, such as iothalamate clearance; these tests are not commonly employed, however.

When ARF occurs in solid-organ recipients, it is usually in the early postoperative period and is usually related to predictable insults, such as volume depletion, hypotension, sepsis, or CsA-tacrolimus nephrotoxicity. Careful review of perioperative events and fluid balance usually yields the diagnosis. Urine biochemistry and microscopy are useful: low FE_{Na} and inactive urine sediment indicate prerenal causes, including acute CsA-tacrolimus toxicity, whereas high FE_{Na} and multiple granular casts suggest ATN. In contrast to renal transplantation, renal biopsy is very rarely performed. CsA-tacrolimus nephrotoxicity can occur when drug levels are not "high": perhaps because preoperative renal disease and intact sympathetic nerve innervation of native kidneys enhance the nephrotoxic effects of these drugs (renal allografts have no sympathetic nerve innervation, at least in the early postoperative period). Meticulous surgical and medical care, as well as judicious dosing of CsA, are vital in limiting the incidence of ARF after transplantation. In patients at high risk for ARF, intravenous administration of CsA should be avoided, if possible. Delayed introduction of CsA (eg, when $S_{Cr} < 3.0$ mg/dL) is sometimes used in such patients; the use of antilymphocyte preparations allows this to be done without an increased risk of graft rejection. The perioperative use of radiocontrast material should be minimized.

The approach to management of ARF is similar to that of the nontransplant postoperative patient except that some degree of CsA-tacrolimus toxicity is present. When renal replacement therapy is required, hemodialysis or continuous renal replacement therapy (CRRT) is usually employed.

THROMBOTIC MICROANGIOPATHY

Thrombotic microangiopathy (TMA) can occur after all forms of solid-organ transplantation.[117, 118] The pathology and clinical features of this condition were discussed previously. Both CsA and tacrolimus have been implicated. Management is similar to that for TMA that occurs in the renal transplant recipient.

Acute Renal Failure in Cardiac Transplantation

Acute renal failure continues to be an important complication of cardiac transplantation. The incidence is higher than that seen in nontransplant heart surgery. Various series (with different definitions of ARF) have reported incidences ranging from 0% to 30%.[119-122] These studies used doses of CsA higher than those typical of current practice. In one series, dialysis was required in 5% of cases overall.[119] The risk factors for ARF after cardiac transplantation include usage of calcineurin inhibitors, hospitalization before transplantation (reflecting more severe illness), pretransplant impairment of renal function, and perioperative cardiovascular complications.[119, 120]

The typical clinical features of ARF in this setting are shown in Table 25–7. Onset is usually in the first few days after transplantation. Oliguria, rising S_{Cr} level,

TABLE 25–7. Typical Clinical Features of Acute Renal Failure After Cardiac Transplantation

Onset within 5 days of transplant
Oliguria
Inactive urine sediment
Rising plasma BUN, creatinine
Disproportionately elevated plasma K^+
Low urinary sodium excretion
Recovery with reduction in dose of calcineurin inhibitor

BUN, blood urea nitrogen.

inactive urine sediment, and low FE_{Na} (<1%) are characteristic.[123, 124] As cardiac function is improved postoperatively and volume depletion is rare, the picture is thus one of functional prerenal failure. This acute nephrotoxic effect of CsA and tacrolimus has been described in detail earlier in this chapter. The treatment of ARF in this setting is supportive: maintenance of renal perfusion, reduction in dosage of CsA-tacrolimus if appropriate, and dialysis when necessary. Most cases improve within 2 weeks of transplant unless additional complications such as sepsis arise.

Reduction in the dosage of calcineurin inhibitors administered in the perioperative period should lessen the risk of ARF; this must be balanced against the increased risk of acute rejection. Induction therapy with ATG or OKT3 allows safe use of lower doses of calcineurin inhibitors,[120, 125] but this strategy entails the risk of excessive immunosuppression. Data on the use of IL-2 receptor blockers in this setting are not yet available. Urodilatin is a peptide derived from human urine that exerts atrial natriuretic peptide–like effects in vivo. Early work suggesting that urodilatin might reduce the requirement for dialysis after cardiac or liver transplantation has not been confirmed in phase II studies.[126, 127] There is no solid evidence that calcium channel blockers or dopamine prevents ARF after cardiac transplantation.

It should be emphasized that chronic renal failure–ESRD remains an important complication of long-term calcineurin inhibitor therapy. There is little evidence, however, that perioperative ARF per se predisposes to chronic CsA nephrotoxicity. The mortality associated with ARF after cardiac transplantation is lower than that seen with ARF in nontransplant cardiac surgery.[123] Presumably, this reflects the different etiologies of ARF and incidence of multiorgan failure between these two groups.

HMG-CoA–REDUCTASE INHIBITORS

Rhabdomyolysis and acute myoglobinuric renal failure have been reported with the combined use of HMG-CoA–reductase inhibitors and CsA in cardiac transplant recipients. In fact, cardiac transplant patients are the transplant group most likely to be taking these lipid-lowering drugs. Rhabdomyolysis was first reported with lovastatin in cardiac transplantation[128, 129]; other drugs in this class have been implicated.[130] The enhanced toxicity of HMG-CoA–

reductase inhibitors with concomitant CsA usage is not fully understood, but it is thought that CsA decreases biliary excretion of these agents and impairs their metabolism (through the cytochrome P-450 system), thereby significantly increasing blood levels. The additional use of fibrates such as gemfibrozil heightens the risk of myositis. Treatment of established cases involves cessation of HMG-CoA–reductase inhibitor therapy, reduction in CsA dosage if levels are high, and supportive measures, including hydration. With the use of lower doses of HMG-CoA–reductase inhibitors, the incidence of rhabdomyolysis in the transplant population appears to have decreased. In addition, newer HMG-CoA–reductase inhibitors, such as fluvastatin, are probably safer.[131] Nevertheless, initial doses of these agents should be low, plasma creatine kinase levels should be monitored, and patients advised to seek medical attention if muscle symptoms occur.

Acute Renal Failure in Lung Transplantation

Renal function may be impaired before transplantation in patients with severe respiratory failure, particularly those with primary pulmonary hypertension.[132] This is thought to reflect the renal effects of low cardiac output, hypoxia, and polycythemia. Moderate acute renal impairment is common after lung transplantation. CsA is the principal cause in this setting; less commonly NSAIDs or aminoglycosides have been implicated.[132, 133] Reduction in the dosage of the CsA may improve renal function; unfortunately, progression to ESRD may still occur.[133] Interestingly, in the series of Navis and coworkers,[132] the patients with primary pulmonary hypertension before diagnosis had *improved* renal function after transplantation—this presumably reflects the beneficial effects of the new organ on cardiovascular function, hematocrit level, and so on.[132, 134] Rhabdomyolysis and ARF have been reported in a lung-transplant recipient ingesting the combination of simvastatin, CsA, and itraconazole.[135] There is at least one report of CsA-associated TMA and irreversible renal failure after lung transplantation.[136]

Acute Renal Failure in Heart-Lung Transplantation

It has been suggested that heart-lung transplantation would carry a risk of renal complications greater than that of heart transplantation alone because of the more frequent use of nephrotoxic antimicrobial drugs such as amphotericin. However, in the largest reported single-center series to date, the risks of acute and chronic renal impairment were the same with either transplant procedure.[137] The biphasic decrease in renal function typical of CsA nephrotoxicity was found: a rapid fall in GFR over the first 6 months and then a slower decrease.

Acute Renal Failure in Liver Transplantation

Orthotopic liver transplantation is now the treatment of choice for end-stage liver disease (ESLD). Because many patients undergoing liver transplantation have some degree of acute or chronic renal impairment,[138] the immediate pretransplant period is considered here also. It should be noted that high plasma bilirubin levels may affect certain assays of S_{Cr}, resulting in falsely lower levels. Distant and Gonwa[139] have emphasized the poor correlation between S_{Cr} and GFR in liver disease patients, because of their frequently poor nutritional status and have recommended preoperative and postoperative monitoring of renal function using iothalamate clearance studies.

The principal causes of renal impairment in patients undergoing liver transplantation are prerenal failure, ATN, and HRS (Table 25–8). Glomerular lesions, particularly IgA glomerulonephritis, may also be present, but these rarely cause severe acute renal impairment. Fulminant acute hepatic failure (requiring transplantation) and ARF may also occur secondary to the direct hepatotoxic and nephrotoxic effects of acetaminophen, carbon tetrachloride, or other toxins. Renal failure associated with liver disease, in particular HRS, is discussed in Chapter 20. To summarize, HRS may be defined as unexplained renal failure occurring in patients with liver disease in the absence of clinical or laboratory evidence of other known causes of renal failure.[140]

An important issue confronting nephrologists caring for the pre–liver transplant patient is determining the *reversibility* of the renal failure. Diagnosis of its underlying cause is the first step but may be difficult. Supportive measures, such as volume expansion and treatment of sepsis, may improve renal function in the pretransplant period and aid in the diagnosis of conditions such as prerenal failure and ATN. The hepatorenal syndrome, as noted previously, is a diagnosis of exclusion. This syndrome usually reverses in the first few days to weeks after liver transplantation.[139, 141] Thus, dual liver-kidney transplant is rarely indicated in ESLD patients with renal failure. In a small number of cases,

TABLE 25–8. Etiology of ARF in Patients With ESLD Undergoing Liver Transplantation

FACTOR	ARF PRETRANSPLANT, %	ARF POSTTRANSPLANT, %
ATN, ischemic	54	52
ATN, nephrotoxic	21	18
CsA-tacrolimus toxicity	0	40
Hepatorenal syndrome	43	8
Contrast nephropathy	8	7
Sepsis	11	2
Rhabdomyolysis	4	1

Note that one patient may have multiple etiologies.
Adapted from Fraley DS, Burr R, Bernardini J, et al: Impact of acute renal failure on mortality in end-stage liver disease with or without transplantation. Kidney Int 1998; 54:518–524; with permission.
ATN, acute tubular necrosis; *CsA*, cyclosporin A.

there may be irreversible structural renal damage, eg, cortical necrosis secondary to prolonged severe renal ischemia. If this is suspected, renal biopsy should be performed. Biopsy results allow diagnosis of irreversible renal disease; dual liver-kidney transplantation may then be appropriate.[141] Even if liver transplantation alone is planned, biopsy of the kidneys during the transplant procedure can provide useful information regarding the prognosis for renal function.

In a significant number of patients with severe liver disease and ARF, dialysis is required as a bridge to transplantation, with the expectation that renal function will improve after successful transplantation. Cardiovascular system stability, changes in intracranial pressure, and requirements for anticoagulation are important issues to consider when one chooses the dialysis modality for the perioperative period. Peritoneal dialysis is not commonly utilized. Conventional hemodialysis allows efficient removal of fluid and solutes with minimal anticoagulation. However, hemodialysis may precipitate episodes of hypotension and also increase the risk of cerebral edema and increased intracranial pressure.[142] The latter syndrome is an important cause of mortality in patients with liver failure. A major advantage of CRRT is that it induces less fluctuation in cardiovascular stability and intracranial pressure.[142] One drawback of CRRT is that the standard regimen for the prevention of clotting in the extracorporeal circuit involves continuous systemic anticoagulation with heparin. If necessary, this problem can be circumvented by a number of measures: no anticoagulation (which shortens filter life and efficiency), regional heparin or citrate anticoagulation, or use of prostacyclin.[143] Citrate use may be problematic because citrate requires metabolism by the liver. There is some evidence that "biocompatible" membranes are preferable to "bioincompatible" membranes in these patients.[144] Finally, bicarbonate-based replacement solutions are preferable to lactate-based solutions because of the risk of impaired metabolism of lactate.

Research is ongoing to identify effective mechanisms for reversing the ARF of HRS.[141] Terlipressin is a vasopressin analogue that induces splanchnic and peripheral vasoconstriction and decreases renin-angiotensin-aldosterone activity. There is preliminary evidence that terlipressin reverses the renal failure of HRS and thus can act as a bridge to liver transplantation.[145] Some success has been reported with octreotide and the orally active vasoconstrictor, midodrine. However, the efficacy of these drugs has not yet been assessed in randomized controlled trials. Placement of a transjugular intrahepatic portosystemic shunt (TIPS) has also shown encouraging preliminary results.[146] Studies to date do not support a role for urodilatin in protection of renal function during liver transplantation.[127]

Rates of ARF after liver transplantation in recent series have been between 17% and 90% (reflecting different definitions of ARF) with dialysis required in 9% to 20%.[147–150] With improved surgical and supportive care, the incidence of ARF appears to be decreasing. By multivariate analysis, risk factors for postoperative ARF include a preoperative S_{Cr} level greater than 1.5 mg/dL, ascites, intraoperative blood transfusion requirements, and liver graft dysfunction.[147, 150–152] The principal causes of ARF in the early post-transplant period are ATN and CsA-tacrolimus toxicity[153] (see Table 25–8). The ATN occurs secondary to ischemia, sepsis, or nephrotoxic drugs. Many studies have shown that severe perioperative ARF (particularly the need for dialysis) correlates with poorer survival.[148, 150, 152–155] The excess morbidity and mortality associated with ARF occurs mainly in those with HRS.[154] This mortality effect is manifested mainly in the early postoperative period. To what extent ARF is an *independent* cause of poorer outcome (as opposed to being a marker of severe liver dysfunction, circulatory collapse, or shock) is difficult to determine. Most of the "effect" of ARF on poor prognosis probably reflects comorbid illness, particularly sepsis.[153] Thus, survival is poorest in ARF patients requiring CRRT as opposed to conventional hemodialysis or no dialysis, mainly because the requirement for CRRT defines a subgroup with more severe hemodynamic compromise. Undoubtedly, severe renal failure per se significantly complicates management. Patients with HRS spend longer periods of time in the intensive care setting after the transplant procedure and require more dialysis than do their non-HRS counterparts. It should be emphasized, however, that with improvements in the surgical procedure itself and in supportive care, the impact of HRS on overall outcomes is modest. Five-year survival in the large series of Gonwa and coworkers[154] was 60% in those with HRS vs. 68% in those without HRS. Thus, the presence of HRS is not a contraindication to liver transplantation. The situation is less clear when ARF occurs in the setting of fulminant hepatic failure, eg, drug-induced hepatic and renal failure.[155]

Management of ARF after transplantion involves supportive therapy, hemodialysis and CRRT, and reduction in the dosage of calcineurin inhibitor if appropriate. Recovery of renal function is the normal outcome. Unfortunately, chronic CsA-tacrolimus nephrotoxicity remains a problem in liver transplantation.

PREVENTIVE MEASURES

Careful analysis of GFR by inulin clearance has shown marked intraoperative impairment of renal function, particularly during the anhepatic phase when renal blood flow is reduced because of blockage of splanchnic and inferior vena cava venous return to the heart.[147] Intraoperative venovenous bypass is used in some centers to improve cardiovascular stability during the anhepatic phase of liver transplantation. Uncontrolled studies suggested that venovenous bypass ameliorated the adverse hemodynamic effects of obstructed inferior vena caval return on renal blood flow during the anhepatic phase of surgery. However, in the one randomized, controlled trial of venovenous bypass reported to date, no significant reduction in the need for dialysis was found with bypass intervention.[147]

The evidence to support the renal protective effects of calcium channel blockers in CsA-tacrolimus–treated liver transplant patients is inconclusive.[156, 157] The use of intravenous CsA-tacrolimus should be avoided in patients at high risk for ARF. Prophylactic use of OKT3 for the first 10 to 14 days after transplantation allows delayed introduction of CsA and better early preservation of renal function.[158, 159] This form of induction therapy probably has little benefit on renal function or rejection rates over the long-term, however.[159, 160] In addition, the cost and toxicity of OKT3 precludes its routine use. One retrospective study[161] suggested that perioperative administration of dopamine had renal protective effects, but this finding was not confirmed in a randomized, controlled trial.[162]

CONCLUSION

Acute renal failure remains an important complication of solid-organ, particularly heart and liver, transplantation. Hypovolemia and hypotension, sepsis, and CsA-tacrolimus nephrotoxicity are the most common causes of ARF in nonrenal transplantation. Severe ARF complicates post-transplant management and is associated with a poorer prognosis. This inferior outcome is mainly a reflection of more severe comorbid illness rather than a detrimental effect of ARF per se. Meticulous surgical, anesthetic, and medical management techniques are required to minimize the risk and complications of ARF in the peritransplant period. It is hoped that newer induction immunosuppressive regimens (eg, using IL-2 receptor blockers, which have an excellent profile) will allow the safe use of lower—and less nephrotoxic—doses of CsA-tacrolimus in patients at high risk for ARF following solid-organ transplantation.

REFERENCES

1. Shackleton CR, Keown PA, McLoughlin MG, et al: Cadaver kidney transplantation with minimal delayed function: experience with perioperative strategies to enhance initial renal allograft function. Transplant Proc 1995; 27:1075–1077.
2. Koning OH, Ploeg RJ, van Bockel JH, et al: Risk factors for delayed graft function in cadaveric kidney transplantation: a prospective study of renal function and graft survival after preservation with University of Wisconsin solution in multiorgan donors. European Multicentre Study Group. Transplantation 1997; 63:1620–1628.
3. Ploeg RJ, van Bockel JH, Langendijk PT, et al: Effect of preservation solution on results of cadaveric kidney transplantation. The European Multicentre Study Group. Lancet 1992; 340:129–137.
4. Scornik JC, Cecka JM: Immune Responsiveness and Renal Transplantation. In: Cecka JM, Terasaki PI, eds. Clinical Transplants 1996. Los Angeles: UCLA Tissue Typing Laboratory; 1997:373–379.
5. Phillips AO, Deane C, O'Donnell P, et al: Evaluation of Doppler ultrasound in primary nonfunction of renal transplants. Clin Transplant 1994; 8:83–86.
6. Shoskes DA, Halloran PF: Delayed graft function in renal transplantation: etiology, management, and long-term significance. J Urol 1996; 155:1831–1840.
7. Grinyo JM: Reperfusion injury. Transplant Proc 1997; 29:59–62.
8. Solez K, Racusen LC, Marcussen N, et al: Morphology of ischemic acute renal failure, normal function, and cyclosporine

9. Pirenne J, Lledo-Garcia E, Benedetti E, et al: Colon perforation after renal transplantation: a single-institution review. Clin Transplant 1997; 11:88–93.
10. Valeri A, Radhakrishnan J, Ryan R, Powell D: Biocompatible dialysis membranes and acute renal failure: a study in postoperative acute tubular necrosis in cadaveric renal transplant recipients. Clin Nephrol 1996; 46:402–409.
11. Ojo AO, Wolfe RA, Held PJ, et al: Delayed graft function: risk factors and implications for renal allograft survival. Transplantation 1997; 63:968–974.
12. Takada M, Chandraker A, Nadeau KC, et al: The role of the B7 costimulatory pathway in experimental cold ischemia-reperfusion injury. J Clin Invest 1997; 100:1199–1203.
13. Halloran PF, Homik J, Goes N, et al: The "injury response": a concept linking nonspecific injury, acute rejection, and long-term transplant outcomes. Transplant Proc 1997; 29:79–81.
14. Shoskes DA, Hodge EE, Goormastic M, et al: HLA matching determines susceptibility to harmful effects of delayed graft function in renal transplant recipients. Transplant Proc 1995; 27:1068–1069.
15. Benvenisty AI, Cohen D, Stegall MD, Hardy MA: Improved results using OKT3 as induction immunosuppression in renal allograft recipients with delayed graft function. Transplantation 1990; 49:321–327.
16. Katznelson S, Cecka JM: Immunosuppressive Regimens and Their Effects on Renal Allograft Outcome. In: Cecka JM, Terasaki PI, eds. Clinical Transplants 1996. Los Angeles: UCLA Tissue Typing Laboratory; 1997:361–371.
17. Higgins RM, Bevan DJ, Carey BS, et al: Prevention of hyperacute rejection by removal of antibodies to HLA immediately before renal transplantation. Lancet 1996; 348:1208–1211.
18. Hiesse C, Kriaa F, Rousseau P, et al: Immunoadsorption of anti-HLA antibodies for highly sensitized patients awaiting renal transplantation. Nephrol Dial Transplant 1992; 7:944–951.
19. Reisaeter AV, Leivestad T, Albrechtsen D, et al: Pretransplant plasma exchange or immunoadsorption facilitates renal transplantation in immunized patients. Transplantation 1995; 60:242–248.
20. Colvin RB: The renal allograft biopsy. Kidney Int 1996; 50:1069–1082.
21. Madore F, Lazarus JM, Brady HR: Therapeutic plasma exchange in renal diseases [editorial]. J Am Soc Nephrol 1996; 7:367–386.
22. Kopp JB, Klotman PE: Cellular and molecular mechanisms of cyclosporin nephrotoxicity. J Am Soc Nephrol 1990; 1:162–179.
23. Shoskes DA, Cecka JM: Effect of Delayed Graft Function on Short- and Long-Term Kidney Graft Survival. In: Cecka JM, Terasaki PI, eds: Clinical Transplants 1997. Los Angeles: UCLA Tissue Typing Laboratory; 1998:297–303.
24. Cecka JM, Terasaki PI: Living donor kidney transplants: superior success rates despite histoincompatibilities. Transplant Proc 1997; 29:203.
25. van Valenberg PL, Hoitsma AJ, Tiggeler RG, et al: Mannitol as an indispensable constituent of an intraoperative hydration protocol for the prevention of acute renal failure after renal cadaveric transplantation. Transplantation 1987; 44:784–788.
26. Alijani MR, Cutler JA, DelValle CJ, et al: Single-donor cold storage versus machine perfusion in cadaver kidney preservation. Transplantation 1985; 40:659–661.
27. Merion RM, Oh HK, Port FK, et al: A prospective controlled trial of cold-storage versus machine-perfusion preservation in cadaveric renal transplantation. Transplantation 1990; 50:230–233.
28. Daemen JH, de Wit RJ, Bronkhorst MW, et al: Short-term outcome of kidney transplants from non–heart-beating donors after preservation by machine perfusion. Transpl Int 1996; 9:S76–S80.
29. Alfrey EJ, Lee CM, Scandling JD, et al: When should expanded criteria donor kidneys be used for single versus dual kidney transplants? Transplantation 1997; 64:1142–1146.
30. Bia MJ, Tyler K: Evidence that calcium channel blockade prevents cyclosporine-induced exacerbation of renal ischemic injury. Transplantation 1991; 51:293–295.

8. (continued) toxicity in cyclosporine-treated renal allograft recipients. Kidney Int 1993; 43:1058–1067.

31. Ladefoged SD, Pedersen E, Hammer M, et al: Influence of diltiazem on renal function and rejection in renal allograft recipients receiving triple-drug immunosuppression: a randomized, double-blind, placebo-controlled study. Nephrol Dial Transplant 1994; 9:543–547.

32. Neumayer HH, Wagner K: Prevention of delayed graft function in cadaver kidney transplants by diltiazem: outcome of two prospective, randomized clinical trials. J Cardiovasc Pharmacol 1987; 10:S170–S177.

33. Denton MD, Chertow GM, Brady HR: "Renal-dose" dopamine for the treatment of acute renal failure: scientific rationale, experimental studies and clinical trials. Kidney Int 1996; 50:4–14.

34. Allgren RL, Marbury TC, Rahman SN, et al: Anaritide in acute tubular necrosis. Auriculin Anaritide Acute Renal Failure Study Group. N Engl J Med 1997; 336:828–834.

35. Grino JM: BN 52021: a platelet activating factor antagonist for preventing post-transplant renal failure. A double-blind, randomized study. The BN 52021 Study Group in Renal Transplantation. Ann Intern Med 1994; 121:345–347.

36. Hourmant M, Bedrossian J, Durand D, et al: A randomized multicenter trial comparing leukocyte function-associated antigen-1 monoclonal antibody with rabbit antithymocyte globulin as induction treatment in first kidney transplantations. Transplantation 1996; 62:1565–1570.

37. Salmela K, Wramner L, Ekberg H, et al: A randomized multicenter trial of the anti-ICAM-1 monoclonal antibody (enlimomab) for the prevention of acute rejection and delayed onset of graft function in cadaveric renal transplantation: a report of the European Anti-ICAM-1 Renal Transplant Study Group. Transplantation 1999; 67:729–736.

38. Hong CD, Kapoor BS, First MR, et al: Fractional excretion of sodium after renal transplantation. Kidney Int 1979; 16:167–178.

39. Morales JM, Andres A, Prieto C, et al: Fractional excretion of sodium represents an index of cyclosporine nephrotoxicity in the early post-transplant period. Transplant Proc 1987; 19:4005–4007.

40. Eggensperger D, Schweitzer S, Ferriol E, et al: The utility of cytodiagnostic urinalysis for monitoring renal allograft injury. A clinicopathological analysis of 87 patients and over 1000 urine specimens. Am J Nephrol 1988; 8:27–34.

41. Parrott NR: Early graft loss: the Cinderella of transplantation. Nephrol Dial Transplant 1995; 10:32–35.

42. Vachharajani TJ, Asari AJ, Tucker B, Baker LR: Ipsilateral deep venous thrombosis in renal transplant recipients: the need for prolonged anticoagulation [letter]. Nephrol Dial Transplant 1997; 12:627–628.

43. Schwieger J, Reiss R, Cohen JL, et al: Acute renal allograft dysfunction in the setting of deep venous thrombosis: a case of successful urokinase thrombolysis and a review of the literature. Am J Kidney Dis 1993; 22:345–350.

44. Chiu AS, Landsberg DN: Successful treatment of acute transplant renal vein thrombosis with selective streptokinase infusion. Transplant Proc 1991; 23:2297–2300.

45. Clarke SD, Kennedy JA, Hewitt JC, et al: Successful removal of thrombus from renal vein after renal transplantation. BMJ 1970; 1:154–155.

46. Broyer M, Gagnadoux MF, Sierro A, et al: Prevention of vascular thromboses after renal transplantation using low molecular weight heparin. Ann Pediatr (Paris) 1991; 38:397–399.

47. Cecka JM: The UNOS Scientific Renal Transplant Registry: Ten Years of Kidney Transplants. In: Cecka JM, Terasaki PI, eds. Clinical Transplants 1997. Los Angeles: UCLA Tissue Typing Laboratory; 1998:1–14.

48. Solez K, Axelsen RA, Benediktsson H, et al: International standardization of criteria for the histologic diagnosis of renal allograft rejection: the Banff working classification of kidney transplant pathology. Kidney Int 1993; 44:411–422.

49. Weir MR, Hall-Craggs M, Shen SY, et al: The prognostic value of the eosinophil in acute renal allograft rejection. Transplantation 1986; 41:709–712.

50. Gaber AO, First MR, Tesi RJ, et al: Results of the double-blind, randomized, multicenter, phase III clinical trial of Thymoglobulin versus Atgam in the treatment of acute graft rejection

episodes after renal transplantation. Transplantation 1998; 66:29–37.

51. Kamath S, Dean D, Peddi VR, et al: Efficacy of OKT3 as primary therapy for histologically confirmed acute renal allograft rejection. Transplantation 1997; 64:1428–1432.

52. Thistlethwaite JR, Jr, Gaber AO, Haag BW, et al: OKT3 treatment of steroid-resistant renal allograft rejection. Transplantation 1987; 43:176–184.

53. Simpson MA, Madras PN, Cornaby AJ, et al: Sequential determinations of urinary cytology and plasma and urinary lymphokines in the management of renal allograft recipients. Transplantation 1989; 47:218–223.

54. Conlon PJ, Jr, Carmody M, Donohoe J, et al: Cytomegalovirus infection as a complication of OKT3 therapy in kidney transplant recipients. Ir J Med Sci 1992; 161:630–632.

55. TMMRRRS Group: Mycophenolate mofetil for the treatment of refractory, acute, cellular renal transplant rejection. The Mycophenolate Mofetil Renal Refractory Rejection Study Group. Transplantation 1996; 61:722–729.

56. Jordan ML, Naraghi R, Shapiro R, et al: Tacrolimus rescue therapy for renal allograft rejection: five-year experience. Transplantation 1997; 63:223–228.

57. Woodle ES, Thistlethwaite JR, Gordon JH, et al: A multicenter trial of FK506 (tacrolimus) therapy in refractory acute renal allograft rejection: a report of the Tacrolimus Kidney Transplantation Rescue Study Group. Transplantation 1996; 62:594–599.

58. Vincenti F, Kirkman R, Light S, et al: Interleukin-2-receptor blockade with daclizumab to prevent acute rejection in renal transplantation: Daclizumab Triple Therapy Study Group. N Engl J Med 1998; 338:161–165.

59. Nashan B, Moore R, Amlot P, et al: Randomised trial of basiliximab versus placebo for control of acute cellular rejection in renal allograft recipients. CHIB 201 International Study Group (published erratum appears in Lancet 1997; 350:1484). Lancet 1997; 350:1193–1198.

60. Vanrenterghem Y: The use of mycophenolate mofetil (Cellcept) in renal transplantation (clinical conference). Nephron 1997; 76:392–399.

61. Pirsch JD, Miller J, Deierhoi MH, et al: A comparison of tacrolimus (FK506) and cyclosporine for immunosuppression after cadaveric renal transplantation. FK506 Kidney Transplant Study Group. Transplantation 1997; 63:977–983.

62. Mayer AD, Dmitrewski J, Squifflet JP, et al: Multicenter randomized trial comparing tacrolimus (FK506) and cyclosporine in the prevention of renal allograft rejection: a report of the European Tacrolimus Multicenter Renal Study Group. Transplantation 1997; 64:436–443.

63. Remuzzi G, Perico N: Cyclosporine-induced renal dysfunction in experimental animals and humans. Kidney Int Suppl 1995; 52:S70–S74.

64. Curtis JJ, Julian BA, Sanders CE, et al: Dilemmas in renal transplantation: when the clinical course and histological findings differ. Am J Kidney Dis 1996; 27:435–440.

65. Corey HE: Urine cytology: an underused method to diagnose acute renal allograft rejection. Pediatr Nephrol 1997; 11:226–230.

66. Bechtel U, Scheuer R, Landgraf R, et al: Assessment of soluble adhesion molecules (sICAM-1, sVCAM-1, sELAM-1) and complement cleavage products (sC4d, sC5b-9) in urine: clinical monitoring of renal allograft recipients. Transplantation 1994; 58:905–911.

67. Hartmann A, Eide TC, Fauchald P, et al: Serum amyloid A protein is a clinically useful indicator of acute renal allograft rejection. Nephrol Dial Transplant 1997; 12:161–166.

68. Strehlau J, Pavlakis M, Lipman M, et al: Quantitative detection of immune activation transcripts as a diagnostic tool in kidney transplantation. Proc Natl Acad Sci USA 1997; 94:695–700.

69. Vasconcellos LM, Schachter AD, Zheng XX, et al: Cytotoxic lymphocyte gene expression in peripheral blood leukocytes correlates with rejecting renal allografts (published erratum appears in Transplantation 1998; 66:1264). Transplantation 1998; 66:562–566.

70. Young BA, Marsh CL, Alpers CE, Davis CL: Cyclosporine-associated thrombotic microangiopathy-hemolytic uremic syndrome

following kidney and kidney-pancreas transplantation. Am J Kidney Dis 1996; 28:561–571.

71. Zent R, Katz A, Quaggin S, et al: Thrombotic microangiopathy in renal transplant recipients treated with cyclosporin A. Clin Nephrol 1997; 47:181–186.

72. Baid S, Pascual M, Williams WW, Jr, et al: Renal thrombotic microangiopathy associated with anticardiolipin antibodies in hepatitis C-positive renal allograft recipients. J Am Soc Nephrol 1999; 10:146–153.

73. Rubin RH: Infectious disease complications of renal transplantation (clinical conference). Kidney Int 1993; 44:221–236.

74. Fox BC, Sollinger HW, Belzer FO, Maki DG: A prospective, randomized, double-blind study of trimethoprim-sulfamethoxazole for prophylaxis of infection in renal transplantation: clinical efficacy, absorption of trimethoprim-sulfamethoxazole, effects on the microflora, and the cost-benefit of prophylaxis. Am J Med 1990; 89:255–274.

75. Kotanko P, Pusey CD, Levy JB: Recurrent glomerulonephritis following renal transplantation. Transplantation 1997; 63:1045–1052.

76. Michielsen P: Recurrence of the original disease: does this influence renal graft failure? Kidney Int Suppl 1995; 52:S79–S84.

77. Artero M, Biava C, Amend W, et al: Recurrent focal glomerulosclerosis: natural history and response to therapy. Am J Med 1992; 92:375–383.

78. Tejani A, Stablein DH: Recurrence of focal segmental glomerulosclerosis posttransplantation: a special report of the North American Pediatric Renal Transplant Cooperative Study. J Am Soc Nephrol 1992; 2(suppl 12):S258–S263.

79. Savin VJ, Sharma R, Sharma M, et al: Circulating factor associated with increased glomerular permeability to albumin in recurrent focal segmental glomerulosclerosis. N Engl J Med 1996; 334:878–883.

80. Waltzer WC: Urological aspects of renal transplantation. J Urol 1995; 153:619.

81. Rosenthal JT. Urological complications of renal transplantation. J Urol 1993; 150:1121–1122.

82. Rhee BK, Bretan PN, Jr, Stoller ML: Urolithiasis in renal and combined pancreas-renal transplant recipients. J Urol 1999; 161:1458–1462.

83. Khauli RB: Surgical aspects of renal transplantation: new approaches. Urol Clin North Am 1994; 21:321–341.

84. De Geest S, Borgermans L, Gemoets H, et al: Incidence, determinants, and consequences of subclinical noncompliance with immunosuppressive therapy in renal transplant recipients. Transplantation 1995; 59:340–347.

85. Frazier PA, Davis-Ali SH, Dahl KE: Correlates of noncompliance among renal transplant recipients. Clin Transplant 1994; 8:550–557.

86. Butkus DE, Meydrech EF, Raju SS: Racial differences in the survival of cadaveric renal allografts. Overriding effects of HLA matching and socioeconomic factors. N Engl J Med 1992; 327:840–845.

87. Meyers KE, Thomson PD, Weiland H: Noncompliance in children and adolescents after renal transplantation. Transplantation 1996; 62:186–189.

88. Tarantino A, Montagnino G, Ponticelli C: Corticosteroids in kidney transplant recipients. Safety issues and timing of discontinuation. Drug Saf 1995; 13:145–156.

89. Sanders CE, Curtis JJ, Julian BA, et al: Tapering or discontinuing cyclosporine for financial reasons—a single-center experience. Am J Kidney Dis 1993; 21:9–15.

90. Leggat JE, Jr, Ojo AO, Leichtman AB, et al: Long-term renal allograft survival: prognostic implication of the timing of acute rejection episodes. Transplantation 1997; 63:1268–1272.

91. Reinke P, Fietze E, Ode-Hakim S, et al: Late-acute renal allograft rejection and symptomless cytomegalovirus infection. Lancet 1994; 344:1737–1738.

92. Wong WS, Rahwan RG, Stephens RL, Jr: Examination of the potential antiulcer activity of the calcium antagonist propyl-methylenedioxyindene. III. Lack of effect on cysteamine-induced duodenal ulcers in rats. Pharmacology 1990; 41:215–223.

93. Baxter GM, Ireland H, Moss JG, et al: Colour Doppler ultrasound in renal transplant artery stenosis: which Doppler index? Clin Radiol 1995; 50:618–622.

94. Sankari BR, Geisinger M, Zelch M, et al: Post-transplant renal artery stenosis: impact of therapy on long-term kidney function and blood pressure control. J Urol 1996; 155:1860–1864.

95. Roberts JP, Ascher NL, Fryd DS, et al: Transplant renal artery stenosis. Transplantation 1989; 48:580–583.

96. Randhawa PS, Finkelstein S, Scantlebury V, et al: Human polyoma virus-associated interstitial nephritis in the allograft kidney. Transplantation 1999; 67:103–109.

97. Pereira BJ, Levey AS: Hepatitis C virus infection in dialysis and renal transplantation. Kidney Int 1997; 51:981–999.

98. Morales JM, Campistol JM, Andres A, Rodicio JL: Glomerular diseases in patients with hepatitis C virus infection after renal transplantation. Curr Opin Nephrol Hypertens 1997; 6:511–515.

99. Cruzado JM, Gil-Vernet S, Ercilla G, et al: Hepatitis C virus-associated membranoproliferative glomerulonephritis in renal allografts. J Am Soc Nephrol 1996; 7:2469–2475.

100. Rostaing L, Modesto A, Baron E, et al: Acute renal failure in kidney transplant patients treated with interferon alpha 2b for chronic hepatitis C. Nephron 1996; 74(3):512–516.

101. Davis CL, Gretch DR, Perkins JD, et al: Hepatitis C–associated glomerular disease in liver transplant recipients. Liver Transpl Surg 1995; 1:166–175.

102. Zanetta G, Maurice-Estepa L, Mousson C, et al: Foscarnet-induced crystalline glomerulonephritis with nephrotic syndrome and acute renal failure after kidney transplantation. Transplantation 1999; 67:1376–1378.

103. Spicer ST, Liddle C, Chapman JR, et al: The mechanism of cyclosporine toxicity induced by clarithromycin. Br J Clin Pharmacol 1997; 43:194–196.

104. Olyaei AJ, deMattos AM, Norman DJ, Bennett WM: Interaction between tacrolimus and nefazodone in a stable renal transplant recipient. Pharmacotherapy 1998; 18:1356–1359.

105. Vella JP, Sayegh MH: Interactions between cyclosporine and newer antidepressant medications. Am J Kidney Dis 1998; 31:320–323.

106. Mignat C: Clinically significant drug interactions with new immunosuppressive agents. Drug Saf 1997; 16:267–278.

107. Campana C, Regazzi MB, Buggia I, Molinaro M: Clinically significant drug interactions with cyclosporin: an update. Clin Pharmacokinet 1996; 30:141–179.

108. Smith EJ, Light JA, Filo RS, Yum MN: Interstitial nephritis caused by trimethoprim-sulfamethoxazole in renal transplant recipients. JAMA 1980; 244:360–361.

109. van Son WJ, van der Woude FJ, Tegzess AM, et al: Captopril-induced deterioration of graft function in patients with a transplant renal artery stenosis. Proc Eur Dial Transplant Assoc 1983; 20:325–330.

110. Ostermann M, Goldsmith DJ, Doyle T, et al: Reversible acute renal failure induced by losartan in a renal transplant recipient. Postgrad Med J 1997; 73:105–107.

111. Hay RJ: Liposomal amphotericin B, AmBisome. J Infect 1994; 28(suppl 1):35–43.

112. Stoves J, Rosenberg K, Harnden P, Turney JH: Acute interstitial nephritis due to over-the-counter ibuprofen in a renal transplant recipient [letter]. Nephrol Dial Transplant 1998; 13:227–228.

113. Stahl RA: Nonsteroidal anti-inflammatory agents in patients with a renal transplant. Nephrol Dial Transplant 1998; 13:1119–1121.

114. Hrick DE, Phinney MS, Weigel KA, et al: Long-term renal function in type I diabetics after kidney or kidney-pancreas transplantation: influence of number, timing, and treatment of acute rejection episodes. Transplantation 1997; 64:1283–1288.

115. Odorico JS, Becker YT, Van der Werf W, et al: Advances in Pancreas Transplantation: The University of Wisconsin Experience. In: Cecka JM, Terasaki PI, eds: Clinical Transplants 1997. Los Angeles: UCLA Tissue Typing Laboratory; 1998:157–165.

116. Roza AM, Johnson CP, Adams M: Acute torsion of the renal transplant after combined kidney-pancreas transplant. Transplantation 1999; 67:486–488.

117. Trimarchi HM, Truong LD, Brennan S, et al: FK506-associated thrombotic microangiopathy: report of two cases and review of the literature. Transplantation 1999; 67:539–544.

118. Singh N, Gayowski T, Marino IR: Hemolytic uremic syndrome in solid-organ transplant recipients. Transpl Int 1996; 9:68–75.

119. Greenberg A, Egel JW, Thompson ME, et al: Early and late forms of cyclosporine nephrotoxicity: studies in cardiac transplant recipients. Am J Kidney Dis 1987; 9:12–22.

120. Deeb GM, Kolff J, McClurken JB, et al: Antithymocyte gamma globulin, low-dosage cyclosporine, and tapering steroids as an immunosuppressive regimen to avoid early kidney failure in heart transplantation. J Heart Transplant 1987; 6:79–83.

121. Macris MP, Ford EG, Van Buren CT, Frazier OH: Predictors of severe renal dysfunction after heart transplantation and intravenous cyclosporine therapy. J Heart Transplant 1989; 8:444–448.

122. Merli M, Milazzo F, Visigalli MM, Civati G: Renal function, early postoperatively, in patients undergoing heart transplantation: experience with 61 patients. J Cardiothorac Anesth 1989; 3(suppl 1):62.

123. Cruz DN, Perazella MA: Acute renal failure after cardiac transplantation: a case report and review of the literature. Yale J Biol Med 1996; 69:461–468.

124. Greenberg A: Renal failure in cardiac transplantation. Cardiovasc Clin 1990; 20:189–198.

125. Keith FM, Magilligan DJ, Jr, Lakier JB, Drost CJ: Prevention of early postoperative renal dysfunction in cardiac transplantation. Transplant Proc 1988; 20(suppl 3):323–326.

126. Brenner P, Meyer M, Reichenspurner H, et al: Significance of prophylactic urodilatin (INN: ularitide) infusion for the prevention of acute renal failure in patients after heart transplantation. Eur J Med Res 1995; 1:137–143.

127. Langrehr JM, Kahl A, Meyer M, et al: Prophylactic use of low-dose urodilatin for prevention of renal impairment following liver transplantation: a randomized placebo-controlled study. Clin Transplant 1997; 11:593–598.

128. Corpier CL, Jones PH, Suki WN, et al: Rhabdomyolysis and renal injury with lovastatin use: report of two cases in cardiac transplant recipients. JAMA 1988; 260:239–241.

129. Norman DJ, Illingworth DR, Munson J, Hosenpud J: Myolysis and acute renal failure in a heart-transplant recipient receiving lovastatin [letter]. N Engl J Med 1988; 318:46–47.

130. Wombolt DG, Jackson A, Punn R, et al: Case report: rhabdomyolysis induced by mibefradil in a patient treated with cyclosporine and simvastatin. J Clin Pharmacol 1999; 39:310–312.

131. Goldberg R, Roth D: Evaluation of fluvastatin in the treatment of hypercholesterolemia in renal transplant recipients taking cyclosporine. Transplantation 1996; 62:1559–1564.

132. Navis G, Broekroelofs J, Mannes GP, et al: Renal hemodynamics after lung transplantation: a prospective study. Transplantation 1996; 61:1600–1605.

133. Zaltzman JS, Pei Y, Maurer J, et al: Cyclosporine nephrotoxicity in lung transplant recipients. Transplantation 1992; 54:875–878.

134. Broekroelofs J, Navis G, Stegeman CA, et al: Lung transplantation. Lancet 1998; 351:1064.

135. Malouf MA, Bicknell M, Glanville AR: Rhabdomyolysis after lung transplantation. Aust N Z J Med 1997; 27:186.

136. Butkus DE, Herrera GA, Raju SS: Successful renal transplantation after cyclosporine-associated hemolytic-uremic syndrome following bilateral lung transplantation. Transplantation 1992; 54:159–162.

137. Pattison JM, Petersen J, Kuo P, et al: The incidence of renal failure in one hundred consecutive heart-lung transplant recipients. Am J Kidney Dis 1995; 26:643–648.

138. Eckardt KU: Renal failure in liver disease. Intensive Care Med 1999; 25:5–14.

139. Distant DA, Gonwa TA: The kidney in liver transplantation. J Am Soc Nephrol 1993; 4:129–136.

140. Epstein M: Hepatorenal syndrome: emerging perspectives. Semin Nephrol 1997; 17:563–575.

141. Le Moine O: Hepatorenal syndrome: outcome after liver transplantation. Nephrol Dial Transplant 1998; 13:20–22.

142. Davenport A: The management of renal failure in patients at risk of cerebral edema-hypoxia. New Horiz 1995; 3:717–724.

143. Davenport A, Will EJ, Davison AM: Comparison of the use of standard heparin and prostacyclin anticoagulation in spontaneous and pump-driven extracorporeal circuits in patients with combined acute renal and hepatic failure. Nephron 1994; 66:431–437.

144. Davenport A, Davison AM, Will EJ: Membrane biocompatibility: effects on cardiovascular stability in patients on hemofiltration. Kidney Int Suppl 1993; 41:S230–S234.

145. Le Moine O, el Nawar A, Jagodzinski R, et al: Treatment with terlipressin as a bridge to liver transplantation in a patient with hepatorenal syndrome. Acta Gastroenterol Belg 1998; 61:268–270.

146. Brensing KA, Textor J, Strunk H, et al: Transjugular intrahepatic portosystemic stent–shunt for hepatorenal syndrome. Lancet 1997; 349:697–698.

147. Grande L, Rimola A, Cugat E, et al: Effect of venovenous bypass on perioperative renal function in liver transplantation: results of a randomized, controlled trial. Hepatology 1996; 23:1418–1428.

148. McCauley J, Van Thiel DH, Starzl TE, Puschett JB: Acute and chronic renal failure in liver transplantation. Nephron 1990; 55:121–128.

149. Andres A, Morales JM, Farias J, et al: Acute renal failure after liver transplantation in patients treated with cyclosporine. Transplant Proc 1992; 24:126–127.

150. Nuno J, Cuervas-Mons V, Vicente E, et al: Renal failure after liver transplantation: analysis of risk factors in 139 liver transplant recipients. Transplant Proc 1995; 27:2319–2320.

151. Bilbao I, Charco R, Balsells J, et al: Risk factors for acute renal failure requiring dialysis after liver transplantation. Clin Transplant 1998; 12:123–129.

152. Lafayette RA, Pare G, Schmid CH, et al: Pretransplant renal dysfunction predicts poorer outcome in liver transplantation. Clin Nephrol 1997; 48:159–164.

153. Fraley DS, Burr R, Bernardini J, et al: Impact of acute renal failure on mortality in end-stage liver disease with or without transplantation. Kidney Int 1998; 54:518–524.

154. Gonwa TA, Klintmalm GB, Levy M, et al: Impact of pretransplant renal function on survival after liver transplantation. Transplantation 1995; 59:361–365.

155. Mendoza A, Fernandez F, Mutimer DJ: Liver transplantation for fulminant hepatic failure: importance of renal failure. Transpl Int 1997; 10:55–60.

156. Chan C, Maurer J, Cardella C, et al: A randomized controlled trial of verapamil on cyclosporine nephrotoxicity in heart and lung transplant recipients. Transplantation 1997; 63:1435–1440.

157. Gunning TC, Brown MR, Swygert TH, et al: Perioperative renal function in patients undergoing orthotopic liver transplantation: a randomized trial of the effects of verapamil. Transplantation 1991; 51:422–427.

158. Millis JM, McDiarmid SV, Hiatt JR, et al: Randomized prospective trial of OKT3 for early prophylaxis of rejection after liver transplantation. Transplantation 1989; 47:82–88.

159. Farges O, Ericzon BG, Bresson-Hadni S, et al: A randomized trial of OKT3-based versus cyclosporine-based immunoprophylaxis after liver transplantation: long-term results of a European and Australian multicenter study. Transplantation 1994; 58:891–898.

160. McDiarmid SV, Busuttil RW, Levy P, et al: The long-term outcome of OKT3 compared with cyclosporine prophylaxis after liver transplantation. Transplantation 1991; 52:91–97.

161. Polson RJ, Park GR, Lindop MJ, et al: The prevention of renal impairment in patients undergoing orthotopic liver grafting by infusion of low dose dopamine. Anaesthesia 1987; 42:15–19.

162. Swygert TH, Roberts LC, Valek TR, et al: Effect of intraoperative low-dose dopamine on renal function in liver transplant recipients. Anesthesiology 1991; 75:571–576.

CHAPTER 26

Acute Renal Failure After Bone Marrow Transplantation

Eric P. Cohen

DEFINITION

Renal failure may occur early after bone marrow transplant (BMT), or it may begin months or years later. This chapter focuses on the acute renal failure (ARF) that occurs in the early post-BMT period, generally up to 30 days after BMT, and in patients with no prior kidney disease.

OCCURRENCE

Acute renal failure after BMT is most often an early complication of BMT. Although it may occur many months after BMT, that is, in subjects whose marrow transplant has engrafted, ARF after BMT generally occurs just after the time of marrow ablation, which is the first 3 weeks after BMT.

The timing of ARF after BMT varies somewhat according to the precise cause of the ARF but generally clusters in the first month after BMT.[1–4] A large study of ARF at the Seattle BMT unit showed an average doubling of the serum creatinine level by 14 days after BMT.[1] At the Medical College of Wisconsin unit, and in 21 cases of ARF seen over the past 2 years, the median time to maximum plasma creatinine (P_{Cr}) level was 15 days after BMT.

EPIDEMIOLOGY

An adequate understanding of ARF after BMT requires some knowledge of the BMT itself. Bone marrow transplantation, either autologous or allogeneic, is most commonly undertaken for treatment of cancer. More than 15,000 BMTs are done per year in the United States, of which about one third are allogeneic, ie, from a donor other than self, and the remainder are autologous, ie, from self. Use of BMT was experimental and thus uncommon until the mid-1980s. Thus, complications of BMT were even more uncommon and of only minor importance. The progressive rise in use of BMT in the past decade has been accompanied by larger numbers of early and late survivors of BMT, as well as increasing numbers of subjects having complications of BMT. Quantitative data on BMT may be viewed on the Internet, at http://www.ibmtr.org

A subject undergoing BMT may have had previous surgery, radiation therapy, and/or chemotherapy. In the week preceding a BMT, a subject undergoes systemic chemotherapy ± total-body irradiation (TBI) to ablate both residual malignant cells and to ablate the subject's own bone marrow. The BMT that follows thus "rescues" the subject from what would otherwise have been a rapidly lethal dose of chemoirradiation. In the case of allogeneic BMT, the pre-BMT chemoirradiation is generally more intense and more often includes TBI. This is to ensure complete ablation of the host marrow and eradication of the host immune system, but it carries with it a higher systemic toxicity. To this pre-BMT toxicity must be added the use of cyclosporin A (CsA), used in allogeneic BMT for 6 months or longer, to prevent or treat graft-versus-host-disease, which is not an issue in autologous BMT. Toxicities due to the BMT are generally more severe in allogeneic compared with autologous BMT.[5] Accordingly, ARF after BMT is more common after allogeneic BMT as compared with autologous BMT. Lane and associates reported ARF requiring dialysis in 4 of 241 autologous BMT compared with 26 of 408 allogeneic BMT, all in children.[2] In a series of 275 adults, Gruss and colleagues reported ARF in 6 of 92 autologous BMT as compared with 66 of 193 allogeneic BMT.[3] In the author's recent series of 168 adult BMT (1996 to 1998), there were 3 cases of ARF in 108 autologous BMT and 18 cases of ARF in 60 allogeneic BMT. Combining these three series yields a 3% rate of ARF after autologous BMT and a 16% rate of ARF after allogeneic BMT.

This difference in rates may relate to the somewhat more rapid engraftment of autologous compared with allogeneic marrow, with less prolonged neutropenia, less risk of sepsis, and less use of nephrotoxic antibiotics. Also, lack of use of CsA in autologous transplants lessens the risk of nephrotoxicity. These considerations might suggest that autologous BMT is preferable to allogeneic BMT; however, risk of disease relapse is higher in autologous BMT.[6]

PATHOGENESIS

The timing of ARF after BMT corresponds to the period of post-BMT neutropenia and is often accompanied by fevers, sepsis, and use of nephrotoxic antibiotics. Not surprisingly, the first large review of ARF after BMT implicated the use of amphotericin in the development of ARF with the need for dialysis.[1] This had been reported previously, with emphasis on possible additive toxicity from CsA.[7] Hypotension and sepsis, which are obvious factors for ARF in any patient, have also been implicated in post-BMT ARF.

Jaundice may be present in patients with ARF after BMT, and a liver biopsy in such patients may show veno-occlusive disease (VOD). Correlations have been made between VOD or jaundice and ARF after BMT.[1-3] Indeed, Zager and coworkers[1] have made a strong case for a hepatorenal-like syndrome in such patients. This is based on the timing of liver disease before renal disease, the low urine sodium concentration (U_{Na}), and relative lack of histologic renal injury at postmortem in their series.[8] This author and colleagues' recent experience has not been as uniform. In their recent series of 21 cases of ARF after BMT, 9 had autopsies, and only 1 had VOD of the liver. Moreover, U_{Na} values ranged from 11 to 92 mEq/L (mean, 40 mEq/L), which does not suggest a sodium-avid state as would exist in hepatorenal syndrome.

The most common form of ARF after BMT, however, does not occur as a straightforward entity with one or two causes. Not only may sepsis and hypotension be present but also the patient may simultaneously be exposed to well-known nephrotoxins such as amphotericin and CsA. It is difficult, in an individual case, to assign a specific cause. This is made more difficult by absence of severe histologic injury to kidneys at postmortem in such cases.[8] That has been the author's experience as well, with the additional comment that the kidneys are often edematous and swollen. None of the author's recent cases showed classic acute tubular necrosis (ATN) at postmortem. Typical charges of ATN could have been missed because they were starting to heal or because of autolysis.

Other causes of ARF after BMT have a different pathogenesis. The tumor lysis syndrome can occur, even though it is quite rare. At the author's center, only one case of tumor lysis syndrome with ARF has occurred in 12 years, out of 800 BMTs over that same period. Tumor lysis syndrome is the result of rapid and abundant cancer cell death. Its most well-known occurrence is in rapidly growing cancers such as Burkitt's lymphoma. Cells killed by cancer chemotherapy undergo lysis, which may cause hyperuricemia, hyperphosphatemia, and even hyperkalemia.[9] This may be complicated by acute hyperuricemic nephropathy. Adequate hydration and use of allopurinol usually blunt this phenomenon, thus avoiding the syndrome.

As noted, CsA is a factor associated with early ARF after BMT. This drug is used in allogeneic BMT to prevent the development of graft-versus-host disease. In three well-documented cases reported in 1981, renal failure occurred within a month after allogeneic BMT, accompanied by hemolysis and, at postmortem, glomerular capillary thrombosis.[10] In each case, 12.5 mg/kg per day of CsA was given from the time of BMT, a dose that is higher than doses of CsA used currently.[11] Similar CsA nephrotoxicity in BMT has been documented by others.[12] At present, the doses of CsA have been decreased to avoid this risk. By way of example, at the author's BMT unit, the starting daily dose of CsA is 3 mg/kg per day, given intravenously in divided doses. With this lesser dose, florid CsA toxicity is less evident, although the kidney function in the first month after BMT may still fluctuate according to the blood concentrations of CsA. The pathogenesis of CsA nephrotoxicity after BMT is similar to its toxicity with other use. The early CsA toxicities are probably cased by vasoconstriction, and the longer-term toxicities are associated with arterial intimal fibrosis and tubular atrophy.[13] Recognition of these toxicities has led to a reduction in the doses of CsA used in BMT over the past decade. CsA appears to have a toxic effect on the endothelium, causing reduction in anticoagulant function of that tissue.[14] When endotoxin was given parenterally to rabbits, it potentiated the endothelial injury caused by CsA, resulting in kidney damage similar to that seen clinically when CsA causes microangiopathic toxicity.[15] Conceivably, in neutropenic BMT patients, there is circulating endotoxin that may potentiate the effects of even "normal" blood levels of CsA.

The role of TBI has clearly been shown for the later development of chronic renal failure after BMT.[16] That syndrome, termed *BMT nephropathy*, presents clinically at 6 or more months after BMT, with azotemia, hypertension, and disproportionately severe anemia. It is histologically distinctive, with emphasis on mesangiolysis and glomerular subendothelial expansion. For the doses of TBI that are used in BMT, such effects many months after BMT are not completely unexpected. Usually, there is a latent interval of weeks or months between irradiation and renal injury.[17] Nonetheless, in analysis of postmortem kidney tissue obtained in patients dying with ARF after BMT, we have, from time to time, encountered histologic changes reminiscent of radiation nephropathy. It is therefore possible that radiation is a contributor to ARF after BMT. This would be consistent with the greater frequency of ARF after allogeneic compared with autologous BMT. The univariate analysis of Gruss and associates also showed that use of TBI was a risk factor for ARF after BMT.[3]

At the time of marrow infusion, hemolyzed red blood cells have been associated with nephrotoxicity.[18] The preservation procedure of the marrow may cause hemolysis of any red blood cells that are present, and the hemolysate may then cause hemoglobinuria on infusion into the patient. Hemoglobin is probably directly toxic to renal tubular epithelium, and hemoglobinuria may be followed by ARF. This marrow infusion problem is avoided in current BMT practice by leukapheresis during the marrow preparation, so that the final product is mostly devoid of red blood cells.

Iron has been amply studied as a factor in oxidative injuries, and its actions are discussed elsewhere. One clinical study has shown twofold elevation in serum iron level during BMT, which could clearly potentiate cellular injury acutely.[19] Experimental data suggest that iron may potentiate renal injury, and its depletion may alleviate it. In particular, experimental ischemic ARF is exacerbated by prior iron loading.[20] This finding may be relevant in that patients who undergo BMT may well have had prior blood transfusions and thus have a surfeit of bodily iron. However, no such link has thus far been established.

The pathogenetic factors discussed earlier—iron, tumor lysis, irradiation, hypotension, sepsis, amphotericin, CsA, and liver disease—are positive ones (Table 26–1). That is, they appear to cause ARF by their presence. There are three negative factors that deserve attention. These are the possible nephroprotective effect of cilastatin, the lack of protection by use of pentoxifylline, and the fact that ARF after BMT often occurs in neutropenic subjects.

Cilastatin is a component of the antibiotic imipenem (Primaxin). The cilastatin component inhibits a renal tubular brush border peptidase, which would otherwise hydrolyze the β-lactam ring of the antibiotic imipenem. A retrospective analysis of 104 allogeneic BMT performed between 1991 and 1995 suggested that the use of imipenem/cilastatin in the early post-BMT period was associated with a lesser occurrence of ARF as compared with no use of imipenem/cilastatin (20% vs. 48% occurrence of ARF, respectively).[21] In heart transplant patients receiving CsA-based immunosuppression, a randomized masked study showed that use of the imipenem/cilastatin preparation during the first week after transplant was associated with significantly less ARF than was the use of placebo.[22] The mechanism of this protective effect remains unclear. In a single case of ARF after autologous BMT, therapeutic use of imipenem/cilastatin was associated with recovery and survival despite ARF requiring dialysis, but this observation must be considered anecdotal.[23]

Tumor necrosis factor-alpha (TNF-α) is known to be elevated within the first day after clinical BMT.[24] Pentoxifylline has inhibitory effects on TNF-α synthesis, and a preliminary trial suggested that it was beneficial in limiting toxicity after BMT, but subsequent comparative evaluation showed no such benefit.[25]

Neutrophils have been proposed as an important cellular factor in ischemic-reperfusion injury. Recent experimental studies have supported this idea.[26] Indeed, there is a recent report of ARF after BMT in five patients in which ARF coincided with engraftment of the marrow, ie, increasing WBC.[26a] Yet the ARF that occurs after BMT often occurs in patients with very low white blood cell counts, and in them as in most forms of ATN, neutrophils are not a prominent histologic feature.[27]

PREVENTION

The frequency of ARF after BMT is compounded by its association with greater mortality in those affected.

TABLE 26–1. Acute Renal Failure After Bone Marrow Transplantation (BMT)

Risk factors
    Allogeneic vs. autologous BMT
    Use of total-body irradiation
    Use of cyclosporine
    Use of amphotericin
    Jaundice
Preventive factors
    Use of cilastatin
    Use of liposomal rather than standard amphotericin

Without ARF, mortality in the early BMT period is 20%, whereas in BMT patients who develop ARF requiring dialysis treatment, mortality rises to 80% or higher.[1, 3] Preventive measures need to be considered.

As in any population at risk for ARF, volume depletion requires early intervention. Adequate intravenous fluids need to be provided, especially during periods when early post-BMT patients cannot take in fluids by mouth. At the author's BMT unit, in such patients, at least 2 L per day of intravenous crystalloid is usual.

Tumor lysis syndrome is a rare occurrence in modern BMT practice. This is probably due in part to policies ensuring adequate volume repletion as well as use of allopurinol in any patient at risk for this syndrome.

Aminoglycoside antibiotics have clear-cut nephrotoxicity and should be avoided, if possible, yet they may be required in certain situations. Many centers have pharmacokinetic drug monitoring protocols, in an effort to avoid toxic aminoglycoside drug levels. A recent comparative study was not able to show benefit of pharmacist-assisted drug monitoring when compared with aminoglycoside dosing without pharmacist assistance.[28] Obtaining drug levels is probably still useful, however.

The toxicity of amphotericin B has clearly been associated with ARF after BMT. Within the last few years, the development of a lipid-based formulation of this drug has been closely watched for its potential of lesser toxicity, including nephrotoxicity. This has been borne out, as published in two recent studies.[29, 30] A randomized double-masked study of 700 subjects showed equal efficacy but lesser toxicity of the liposomal amphotericin compared with conventional amphotericin. Half of the subjects in this trial were BMT patients. Increased use of liposomal amphotericin may result in significantly less ARF after BMT in the future.

DETECTION

The detection of ARF is usually straightforward—a drop in urine output, along with a rising blood urea nitrogen (BUN) level and P_{Cr} occurring over several days is a usual scenario. In a BMT patient, this may also occur, yet some features may be atypical. Urine output may not fall, because of ongoing intravenous fluids and a volume-expanded state. The P_{Cr} may not rise rapidly or even rise much more than 1 or 2 mg/dL, perhaps because of volume expansion but also because of decreased muscle mass and activity in the often-weakened patient with cancer and BMT. In the study of ARF after BMT, Gruss and associates[3] found that patients required hemodialysis at an average P_{Cr} of only 4.6 mg/dL, and in the study by Zager and colleagues,[1] the average P_{Cr} was only 3.2 mg/dL before the first dialysis. The average BUN level in the latter study, however, was 98 mg/dL. This lack of great rise in the P_{Cr} is not dissimilar to what occurs in general intensive care units (ICUs). For example, Liano and coworkers found that the maximal P_{Cr} was only 5.2 mg/dL in 253 cases of ARF in an ICU setting.[31] Twelve or 24-hour urine collections may be useful to calculate the urea and creatinine clearances, the average of which closely approximates the glomerular filtration rate.[32] A urinalysis may be helpful, and in most cases of clear-cut ARF, will show typical muddy brown granular casts. In a single case of ARF after BMT seen at the author's center last year, the urinalysis showed acyclovir crystals, which pointed to that drug as contributing to ARF.

TREATMENT

Acute renal failure after BMT requires the same attention to volume status and nephrotoxins that ARF does in any setting. Tachycardia and/or hypotension may indicate volume depletion, although there can be myocardial depression after a BMT,[33] and too vigorous volume repletion may lead to volume overload. Avoidance of potential nephrotoxins requires assiduous care. In these often catabolic patients, who are also on parenteral glucocorticoids, the BUN level may rise to well over 150 mg/dL. This may in turn necessitate reduction in nitrogen intake, specifically in parenteral hyperalimentation solutions. Sufficient caloric intake is probably as important in these patients as it is in any critically ill patient with ARF. Thirty-five kcal/kg per day of total calories is recommended.[34]

Specific forms of ARF require specific attention. Aside from cases of nephrotoxic renal failure, such as that from aminoglycosides or amphotericin, the case of the early hemolytic-uremic syndrome/thrombotic thrombocytopenic purpura-like syndrome may occur. This syndrome, as described by Shulman and others,[10] may improve by withdrawal of CsA. Plasmapheresis has been advocated for such patients. Even though it may improve the hematologic picture, plasmapheresis does not improve the renal failure and should not be used solely for that purpose.[35, 36]

There are no firmly established criteria for starting dialysis in patients with ARF after BMT. This is the reflection of a similar uncertainty in all critically ill patients with ARF.[37] Intractable and significant volume overload or major electrolyte disturbances are obvious classic indications. More difficult is the nonoliguric BMT patient whose BUN level is near 100 mg/dL and whose P_{Cr} is 3 mg/dL. A trial of intravenous crystalloid may be useful, but if there are signs of uremia such as lethargy and asterixis, dialysis will be needed. This almost always is hemodialysis, peritoneal being probably not efficient enough for these hypercatabolic patients. A separate hemodialysis access is needed, because indwelling Hickman-type catheters do not have the capacity to support high blood flow, and because of the need for separate intravenous access for medication and nutrition.

The intensity of dialysis for ARF or the level of azotemia that is desirable to achieve is not well defined. Recent data on ARF in critically ill patients suggest that better dialysis (urea removal of 60% or more per dialysis session) is associated with better outcomes as compared with less intensive dialysis.[38] At the

TABLE 26–2. Unanswered Questions in Acute Renal Failure (ARF) After Bone Marrow Transplantation (BMT)

Do previous transfusions and iron overload enhance the risk of ARF after BMT?
What is the effect of dialysis dose on outcome?
Can outcome be predicted using scoring systems?

same time, continuous filtration/dialysis in critically ill patients with ARF does not appear to improve outcome over intermittent dialysis. There are no published data on these questions in patients with ARF after BMT. With regard to prognosis, although the Liano scoring system for ARF has now been tested fairly well, there are no published reports of its use in BMT patients with ARF. It is possible that its judicious application may provide clearer guidelines on continuing intensive treatments for BMT patients in ARF with poor prognosis.

FUTURE DEVELOPMENTS

Although it is likely that 5% to 15% of future BMT patients will continue to develop ARF much as they do now, improved treatments for cancer may diminish the need for BMT. Novel cancer chemotherapies or even biologic therapies may render BMT obsolete, but that prospect is in the distant future. At present, then, efforts to better understand and treat ARF after BMT are thus worthy and practical. Table 26–2 lists some of the questions pertaining to this issue, which may hopefully be answered in the near future.

ACKNOWLEDGMENTS

Supported in part by NIH Grant CA24652.
Data on BMT at the Medical College of Wisconsin have been provided and verified by Claudia Kabler-Babbit, Clinical Study Coordinator.

REFERENCES

1. Zager RA, O'Quigley J, Zager BK, et al: Acute renal failure following bone marrow transplantation: a retrospective study of 272 patients. Am J Kidney Dis 1989; 13:210–216.
2. Lane PH, Mauer SM, Blazar BR, et al: Outcome of dialysis for acute renal failure in pediatric bone marrow transplantation. Bone Marrow Transplant 1994; 13:613–617.
3. Gruss E, Bernis C, Tomas JF, et al: Acute renal failure in patients following bone marrow transplantation: prevalence, risk factors, and outcome. Am J Nephrol 1995; 15:473–479.
4. Kone BC, Whelton A, Santos G, et al: Hypertension and renal dysfunction in bone marrow transplant recipients. Q J Med 1988; 69:985–995.
5. Bearman SI, Applebaum FR, Buckner CD, et al: Regimen-related toxicity in patients undergoing bone marrow transplantation. J Clin Oncol 1988; 6:1562–1568.
6. Armitage JO: Bone marrow transplantation. N Engl J Med 1994; 330:827–838.
7. Kennedy MS, Deeg JH, Siegel M, et al: Acute renal toxicity with

combined use of amphotericin B and cyclosporine after marrow transplantation. Transplantation 1983; 35:211–215.

8. Zager RA: Acute renal failure in the setting of bone marrow transplantation. Kidney Int 1994; 46:1443–1458.

9. Tsokos GC, Balow JE, Spiegel RJ, MacGrath IT: Renal and metabolic complications of undifferentiated and lymphoblastic lymphomas. Medicine 1981; 60:218–229.

10. Shulman H, Striker G, Deeg HJ, et al: Nephrotoxicity of cyclosporine A after allogeneic bone marrow transplantation. N Engl J Med 1981; 305:1392–1395.

11. Ash RC, Casper JT, Chitambar CR, et al: Successful allogeneic transplantation of T-cell depleted bone marrow from closely HLA-matched unrelated donors. N Engl J Med 1990; 322:485–494.

12. Atkinson K, Biggs JC, Hayes J, et al: Cyclosporine A–associated nephrotoxicity in the first 100 days after allogeneic bone marrow transplantation: three distinct syndromes. Br J Haematol 1983; 54:59–67.

13. Nizze H, Mihatsch MJ, Zollinger HU, et al: Cyclosporine-associated nephropathy in patients with heart and bone marrow transplants. Clin Nephrol 1988; 30:248–260.

14. Neild OH, Rocchi G, Imberti L, et al: Effects of cyclosporine A on prostacycline synthesis by vascular tissue. Thromb Res 1983; 32:373–379.

15. Faraco PR, Hewitson TD, Kincaid-Smith P: An animal model for the study of the microangiopathic form of cyclosporine nephrotoxicity. Transplantation 1991; 51:1129–1131.

16. Cohen EP, Lawton CA, Moulder JE, et al: Bone marrow transplant nephropathy: radiation nephritis revisited. Nephron 1995; 70: 217–222.

17. Robbins MEC, Bonsib SM: Radiation nephropathy: a review. Scanning Microsc 1995; 9:535–560.

18. Smith DM, Weisenburger DD, Bierman P, et al: Acute renal failure associated with autologous bone marrow transplantation. Bone Marrow Transplant 1987; 2:195–201.

19. Gordon LI, Brown SG, Tallman MS, et al: Sequential changes in serum iron and ferritin in patients undergoing high-dose chemotherapy and radiation with autologous bone marrow transplantation: possible implications for treatment-related toxicity. Free Radic Biol Med 1995; 18:383–389.

20. Wu ZL, Paller MS: Iron loading enhances susceptibility to renal ischemia in rats. Ren Fail 1994; 16:471–480.

21. Gruss B, Tomas JF, Bernis C, et al: Nephroprotective effect of cilastatin in allogeneic bone marrow transplantation: results from a retrospective analysis. Bone Marrow Transplant 1996; 18:761–765.

22. Markewitz A, Hammer C, Pfeiffer M, et al: Reduction of cyclosporine-induced nephrotoxicity by cilastatin following clinical heart transplantation. Transplantation 1994; 57:865–870.

23. Wagner A, Mayer G, Roggla G, Linkesch W: Successful treatment of acute renal failure related to bone marrow transplantation. Nephrol Dial Transplant 1995; 10:1255–1256.

24. Girinsky TA, Pallardy M, Comoy B, et al: Peripheral blood corti-cotrophin-releasing factor, adrenocorticotropic hormone, and cytokine (interleukin-β, interleukin-γ, tumor necrosis factor-α) levels after high- and low-dose total body irradiation in humans. Radiat Res 1994; 139:360–363.

25. Clift RA, Bianco JA, Appelbaum FR, et al: A randomized, controlled trial of pentoxifylline for the prevention of regimen-related toxicities in patients undergoing allogeneic bone marrow transplantation. Blood 1993; 82:2025–2030.

26. Kelly KJ, Williams WW, Colvin RB, et al: Intercellular adhesion molecule-1–deficient mice are protected against ischemic renal injury. J Clin Invest 1996; 97:1056–1063.

26a. Bhatt UY, Plott DT, Fu J, et al: Bone marrow engraftment and acute renal failure. J Am Soc Nephrol 2000; 11:126a.

27. Solez K, Morel-Maroger L, Sraer JD: The morphology of "acute tubular necrosis" in man: analysis of 57 renal biopsies and a comparison with the glycerol model. Medicine 1979; 58:362–376.

28. Leehey DJ, Braun BI, Tholl DA, et al: Can pharmacokinetic dosing decrease nephrotoxicity associated with aminoglycoside therapy? J Am Soc Nephrol 1993; 4:81–90.

29. Luke RG, Boyle JA: Renal effects of amphotericin B lipid complex. Am J Kidney Dis 1998; 31:780–785.

30. Walsh TJ, Finberg RW, Arndt C, et al: Liposomal amphotericin B for empirical therapy in patients with persistent fever and neutropenia. National Institute of Allergy and Infectious Diseases Mycoses Study Group. N Engl J Med 1999; 340:764–771.

31. Liano F, Junco E, Madero R, et al: The spectrum of acute renal failure in the intensive care unit compared with that seen in other settings. Kidney 1998; 53:(Suppl 66):S16–S24.

32. Lubowitz H, Statopolsky E, Shankel S, et al: Glomerular filtration rate: determination in patients with chronic renal disease. JAMA 1967; 199:100–104.

33. Braverman AC, Antin JH, Plappert MT, et al: Cyclophosphamide cardiotoxicity in bone marrow transplantation: a prospective evaluation of new dosing regimens. J Clin Oncol 1991; 9:1215–1223.

34. Hirschberg R, Maroni B: Protein and energy metabolism in acute renal failure. Semin Dial 1997; 10:74–82.

35. Silva VA, Frei-Lahr D, Brown RA, Herzig GP: Plasma exchange and vincristine in the treatment of hemolytic-uremic syndrome/thrombotic thrombocytopenic purpura associated with bone marrow transplantation. J Clin Apheresis 1991; 6:16–20.

36. Sarode R, McFarland JG, Flomenberg N, et al: Therapeutic plasma exchange does not appear to be effective in the management of thrombotic thrombocytopenic purpura/hemolytic uremic syndrome following bone marrow transplantation. Bone Marrow Transplant 1995; 16:271–275.

37. Bellomo R, Ronco C: Indications and criteria for initiating renal replacement therapy in the intensive care unit. Kidney Int 1998; 53(Suppl 66):S106–S109.

38. Paganini EP, Tapolyai M, Goormastic M, et al: Establishing a dialysis therapy/patient outcome link in intensive care unit acute dialysis for patients with acute renal failure. Am J Kidney Dis 1996; 28(Suppl 3):S81–89.

CHAPTER 27

Nephrotoxicity From Antibacterial, Antifungal, and Antiviral Drugs

John J. Dillon

INTRODUCTION

The antibiotics were one of the last century's greatest achievements. The antibiotic dream, however, of developing substances toxic to microorganisms without adverse effects on humans has never been realized completely. The kidneys, as concentrators of many antibiotics, are uniquely vulnerable to the toxicity that does occur. Acute renal failure (ARF) from the early sulfonamides was one of the first antibiotic side effects to be noted.[1]

The most common types of antibiotic nephrotoxicity are acute tubular necrosis (ATN), tubular dysfunction without necrosis (electrolyte disorders, renal tubular acidosis, water-handling defects or Fanconi's syndrome), acute interstitial nephritis (AIN), and obstruction (intratubular or ureteral) from drug precipitation. Less frequently, the antibiotics may cause glomerulonephritis or vasculitis. In addition to these direct toxic effects, antibiotics may cause indirect nephrotoxicity by interfering with the metabolism of other nephrotoxic drugs, such as cyclosporine, or by damaging nonrenal tissues whose breakdown products cause renal failure, as would occur with drug-induced hemolytic anemias or drug-induced rhabdomyolysis.

This chapter is divided into three sections: antibacterial toxicity, antifungal nephrotoxicity, and antiviral toxicity. Each section contains a summary table of the drugs that cause toxicity as well as detailed descriptions of their effects.

NEPHROTOXICITY FROM ANTIBACTERIAL DRUGS

The antibacterial drugs, in use for more than six decades, have become safer, as more-harmful compounds have been replaced by less-harmful ones and as the experience with these drugs has grown. Counter to this trend has been a tendency for patients to survive with increasingly serious illnesses, predisposing to both antibiotic use and renal complications. The nephrotoxicities of the antibacterial drugs are summarized in Table 27–1.

Aminoglycosides

The aminoglycosides are potent tubular toxins. In use since streptomycin was isolated in 1944,[2] they are bactericidal antibiotics that kill by binding to bacterial ribosomes, inhibiting protein synthesis. They are effective against aerobic gram-negative organisms and are particularly useful for bacterial species resistant to other antibiotics, such as *Pseudomonas aeruginosa* . The aminoglycosides are also effective against *Listeria monocytogenes* and against methicillin-sensitive staphylococci. Acute tubular necrosis is the most severe and best-appreciated form of nephrotoxicity. Tubular dysfunction resulting in hypomagnesemia, hypocalcemia, or hypokalemia is also common.

MECHANISM OF TOXICITY

The kidneys are targets for toxicity because the renal tubular epithelial cells concentrate aminoglycosides. Renal cortical concentrations may be 10 to 100 times those of plasma.[3, 4] Once present, the drug may persist for several weeks; the half-life of gentamicin in the renal cortex of the rat exceeds 100 hours.[3, 5]

Structurally, the aminoglycosides contain two or more amino sugars attached to an aminocyclitol ring. They are freely filtered by the glomeruli.[6, 7] The nephrotoxic sequence begins in the tubular lumens when the positively charged amino groups bind to anionic, acidic phospholipids present on the brush border membranes of the proximal tubular epithelial cells.[8] Brush border membrane binding increases with an increasing number of ionizable amino groups: six for neomycin; five for gentamicin, tobramycin, netilmicin, and sisomicin; four for amikacin and kanamycin; and three for streptomycin.[9]

Once bound, aminoglycosides enter the cells by pinocytosis and are sequestered in the lysosomes.[10, 11] There, they inhibit phospholipases and sphingomyelinase,[12] causing phospholipid accumulation. An increase in the number and size of proximal tubular lysosomes and lysosomal myeloid bodies, lamellar structures consisting of concentrically arranged phospholipid, are early manifestations of aminoglycoside nephrotoxicity.[13–15] Cytoplasmic vacuolization, dilation of the cisternae of the rough endoplasmic reticulum, and a decrease in the height and density of the brush border microvilli follow. As injury progresses, the mitochondria swell, and necrosis and desquamation of the tubular epithelial cells occur. The tubules clog with cellular debris, intratubular pressures increase, and glomerular filtration decreases. The S1 and S2 segments of the proximal tubules are most severely affected. Tubular epithelial regeneration coexists with necrosis.[13] Curiously, animals with aminoglycoside nephrotoxicity become insensitive to the nephrotox

TABLE 27–1. Nephrotoxicity From Antibacterial Drugs

DRUG	ATN	TUBULAR DYSFUNCTION	INTERSTITIAL NEPHRITIS	INTRATUBULAR OBSTRUCTION OR CALCULI	OTHER
Aminoglycosides	+ + +	+ + +	+	−	−
Vancomycin	+	−	+	−	−
Penicillins	−	−	+ +	−	−
Cephalosporins	?	−	+	−	−
Carbapenems	−	−	−	−	−
Monobactams	−	−	−	−	−
Sulfonamides	?	−	+ +	+	+
Trimethoprim	−	+	−	−	−
Fluoroquinolones	?	−	+	?	+
Macrolides	−	−	+	−	+
Tetracyclines	−	+	+	−	+
Rifampin	+	−	+	−	+
Polypeptides	+ + +	−	?	−	−
Nitrofurantoin	−	−	+	−	−
Metronidazole	−	−	−	−	?
Spectinomycin	−	−	−	−	−
Chloramphenicol	−	−	−	−	−
Clindamycin	−	−	−	−	−
Lincomycin	−	−	−	−	−

− = none; ? = possible or reported but etiology uncertain; + = very uncommon; + + = uncommon; + + + = common.

effects of aminoglycosides and recover even if drug administration continues.[16, 17] One component of this insensitivity is probably selective inhibition of aminoglycoside uptake across the apical membranes of the proximal tubular cells.[18]

CLINICAL TOXICITY

Acute tubular necrosis occurs in 5% to 20% of aminoglycoside-treated individuals, even with careful attention to dosing using sophisticated drug level–monitoring programs.[19–23] Renal failure of severity sufficient to require dialysis is much less frequent. Many cases develop after courses of therapy have been completed.[23]

Aminoglycoside-induced ATN is usually nonoliguric. Virtually all patients without severe, pre-existing renal insufficiency recover renal function.[23] Indeed, end-stage renal failure attributable solely to aminoglycoside therapy may not occur.[24, 25]

Urinary magnesium wasting causing hypomagnesemia, with secondary hypocalcemia and hypokalemia, is common.[26–34] This may occur with or without associated renal insufficiency. Fanconi syndrome is a less common complication of aminoglycoside therapy.[35–37]

Acute interstitial nephritis has been described with aminoglycoside therapy.[38–40] However, this complication must be rare.

RISK FACTORS

Table 27–2 lists conditions predisposing to ATN among aminoglycoside-treated patients.[23, 41–54] The duration of therapy is probably the most important factor under physician control.[23, 41–44] In one study, nephrotoxicity developed in 43% of patients treated for 14 or more days versus 15% in those treated for 11 or fewer

days.[23] In another, nephrotoxicity developed in 50% of those treated for more than 14 days versus 4% of those treated for 7 or fewer days.[42]

The relative toxicities of the different aminoglycosides in human beings remain poorly defined, despite many published studies. Neomycin, with the most amino groups, is clearly more nephrotoxic than the other aminoglycosides, and streptomycin, with the fewest amino groups, is clearly less nephrotoxic. Neomycin is no longer used parenterally, and streptomycin use is limited by widespread bacterial resistance. Among almost 10,000 individuals participating in prospective clinical trials of the other aminoglycosides between 1975 and 1982,[55] nephrotoxicity occurred with the following frequencies: gentamicin 14.0%; tobramycin 12.9%; amikacin 9.4%; and netilmicin 8.7%. Amikacin was more ototoxic and netilmicin was less ototoxic than gentamicin or tobramycin.

Other nephrotoxic drugs, such as cisplatin or amphotericin, or other insults, such as shock, probably

TABLE 27–2. Risk Factors for Nephrotoxicity With Aminoglycoside Therapy

PHYSICIAN-PRESCRIBED FACTORS	PATIENT FACTORS
Longer duration of therapy	Serious illness requiring ICU admission
Greater total dose	Shock
Recent aminoglycoside therapy	Advanced age
Type of aminoglycoside used	Liver disease
Vancomycin	Renal insufficiency
Furosemide (or volume depletion)	Hypoalbuminemia
Cephalothin	Hypokalemia*
Contrast medium or other nephrotoxic drugs	Metabolic acidosis*
	Nonrenal tissue necrosis*

*Demonstrated in experimental animals only.

have additive effects. Cephalothin plus an aminoglycoside was more nephrotoxic than a penicillin plus an aminoglycoside in three prospective, randomized trials.[52-54] Cephalothin is no longer available in the United States, and its nephrotoxicity has not been reported with the other cephalosporins. Sodium depletion enhances aminoglycoside nephrotoxicity in the rat.[56] Potassium depletion enhances aminoglycoside nephrotoxicity in the rat and in the dog.[57-60] Sodium depletion is the probable mechanism by which furosemide increases aminoglycoside nephrotoxicity; potassium depletion may also contribute. Alternatively, the interaction between furosemide and the aminoglycosides may be artifactual, based either on prerenal azotemia, not ATN, among patients receiving furosemide, or on a tendency for clinicians to prescribe furosemide for patients developing, or at risk for, ARF.

PREVENTION

Limiting the duration of therapy and limiting the total dose are the most effective ways of minimizing aminoglycoside nephrotoxicity. Aminoglycosides, initiated empirically while awaiting culture results, should be stopped if bacterial sensitivities indicate that the infection can be treated with less toxic antibiotics. Stopping empirical aminoglycoside therapy should be considered seriously if the culture results are negative. If full-course aminoglycosides are required, the risk increases substantially when the duration exceeds 10 days.

In theory, once-daily aminoglycoside dosing is attractive. This approach exploits three aminoglycoside properties: they kill bacteria best when peak levels are high, they have a substantial postantibiotic effect, and their renal cortical uptake is saturable within the usual dosing range. A postantibiotic effect means that the bactericidal effect of an antibiotic persists after the antibiotic has been removed or has declined to less-than-bactericidal levels. The first two properties allow the administration of large, infrequent doses without diminishing efficacy. A consequence of the second property, saturable uptake, is that cortical accumulation is minimized by administering large, infrequent doses and is maximized by administering the same quantity of drug by continuous infusion or as small, frequent doses. The extent to which cortical uptake is saturable differs for the different aminoglycosides. Uptake is most saturable for gentamicin, less saturable for netilmicin and amikacin, and not saturable (ie, linear) for tobramycin.[61-65] Therefore, the advantage of once-daily dosing should be greatest for gentamicin, less for netilmicin and amikacin, and absent for tobramycin. This approach has been subjected to numerous clinical trials and 10 meta-analyses.[19, 66-74] The aggregate results indicate that extending the dosing interval conferred a modest nephrotoxicity risk reduction, that is, 20% to 33% for gentamicin.[19] Extending the dosing interval did not affect nephrotoxicity for netilmicin or amikacin and has not been well studied for tobramycin. Antibacterial efficacy and ototoxicity were equivalent. Although this approach has no medical

advantages for aminoglycosides other than gentamicin, it is less costly and more convenient.

Dosing to obtain trough serum concentrations below 2 μg/mL for gentamicin and tobramycin, 4 μg/mL for netilmicin, and 10 μg/mL for amikacin, although practiced widely, has little experimental basis. In general, elevated trough levels are consequences of, rather than predictors of, nephrotoxicity. Elevated first-trough concentrations usually reflect pre-existing renal insufficiency.[41]

Sodium chloride depletion should be avoided among aminoglycoside-treated patients. Polyaspartic acid,[75-81] potassium,[57] calcium,[82] methimazole,[83] fish oil,[83] and the combination of sodium bicarbonate, potassium bicarbonate, and acetazolamide[84] have reduced aminoglycoside nephrotoxicity in experimental animals. These approaches have not been evaluated in humans.

Aminoglycoside therapy increases the urinary excretion of a variety of proteins, including β_2-microglobulin, lysozyme, retinol-binding protein and N-acetyl-beta-D-glucosaminidase (NAG). The first three do not signal toxicity and are probably excreted because the aminoglycosides inhibit their uptake by the proximal tubular cells.[85] N-acetyl-beta-D-glucosaminidase excretion increases several days before the serum creatinine increases and may be useful as a marker of impending toxicity.[85, 86] However, whether toxicity can be prevented by stopping aminoglycosides in response to rising urinary NAG levels has not been established.

Vancomycin

Vancomycin is a tricyclic glycopeptide active against gram-positive bacteria. Bacterial resistance to vancomycin has been slow to develop but is present now among both enterococci[87, 88] and *Staphylococcus aureus*.[89-91] Vancomycin is excreted by glomerular filtration, but probably enters the tubular epithelial cells across the basolateral membranes.[92]

Whether vancomycin is significantly nephrotoxic is uncertain. Vancomycin was considered highly nephrotoxic after it was introduced in the late 1950s. Impurities in early preparations may have been responsible.[93] In animals, extremely high doses are required to produce ATN.[94-96] Human studies have been confounded by other causes of ATN, such as septicemia and aminoglycoside therapy. Among patients treated with vancomycin, but not an aminoglycoside, in eight studies, nephrotoxicity developed in 8%.[46, 97-103] Nephrotoxicity, in these studies, was most often defined as a 0.5 mg/dL increase in the serum creatinine concentration. The fraction of this 8% attributable to vancomycin, rather than to other causes, is uncertain. A meta-analysis demonstrated that the incidence of nephrotoxicity was 4% greater among patients treated with vancomycin plus an aminoglycoside than among patients treated with an aminoglycoside alone.[101] This figure may have been confounded, however, by more serious illnesses among the patients receiving combination therapy.

Greater total doses,[101] longer durations of therapy,[44, 46, 101] elevated peak levels,[44] and elevated trough levels[44, 46, 98, 101, 104, 105] have correlated with nephrotoxicity. As with the aminoglycosides, determining whether higher levels cause nephrotoxicity or result from nephrotoxicity is difficult.

Overall, the evidence suggests that vancomycin does cause ATN. However, this complication, from vancomycin alone, is probably very rare when drug levels are maintained within the therapeutic range.

Acute interstitial necrosis is rare with vancomycin. Only five cases have been described over the four decades that the drug has been in use.[106–110]

Beta-Lactams (Penicillins, Cephalosporins, Carbapenems, and Monobactams)

The penicillins, cephalosporins, carbapenems, and monobactams all contain a beta-lactam ring. They are bactericidal antibiotics that target bacterial cell-wall formation. Most of these drugs are concentrated and eliminated by the kidneys. However, although renal exposure is high, renal toxicity is low. Renal toxicity usually results from hypersensitivity reactions, most commonly acute interstitial necrosis.

The beta-lactams are too small to be directly immunogenic. Hypersensitivity occurs when they or their metabolites bind to larger molecules, acting as haptens. Although many penicillins and cephalosporins may cause AIN,[40, 111–120] this is best described and probably most common with methicillin.

The clinical characteristics of methicillin-induced AIN are shown in Table 27–3.[121, 122] Proteinuria is usually, but not always, less than 3.5 g/day. Hematuria may occur and is occasionally gross. Histologically, methicillin-induced interstitial nephritis is characterized by a patchy interstitial infiltrate composed mainly of lymphocytes, plasma cells, and eosinophils. The lymphocytes often invade the tubular basement membranes and the spaces between the tubular epithelial cells. The tubular lumens may contain a mixture of sloughed, degenerated epithelial and inflammatory cells. Tubular necrosis may be present. Immunofluorescence is usually negative, but staining of the tubular basement membranes for IgG, C3, and a methicillin

TABLE 27–3. Clinical Characteristics of Methicillin-Induced Acute Interstitial Nephritis

CHARACTERISTIC	PATIENTS AFFECTED, %
Signs and symptoms	
Fever	87–100
Rash	22–29
Oliguria	18–29
Arthralgias	0–7
Laboratory findings	
Pyuria	93–100
Eosinophiluria	≤100
Eosinophilia	79–100
Azotemia	46–100
Proteinuria	36–94

antigen, possibly dimethoxyphenylpenicilloyl, has been reported.[123] A renal biopsy is required for a definitive diagnosis but is not always necessary in the clinical setting. Renal gallium uptake, a nonspecific marker for inflammation, is usually present with AIN.[116, 117]

As many as 90% of individuals with methicillin-induced AIN recover completely.[121] Recovery is more certain if the offending drug is withdrawn promptly. Recovery occurs rapidly in nonazotemic patients after drug withdrawal but may require weeks or months (ranging up to 1 year) in those with azotemia. Glucocorticoid therapy is controversial because a large, randomized study has not been performed. In one small, nonrandomized study,[122] steroid-treated patients recovered more quickly (the average recovery time was 9 days among steroid-treated patients vs. 54 days among untreated patients) and more completely (75% of steroid-treated patients versus 35% of untreated patients recovered completely). These individuals had severe renal involvement; the median serum creatinine concentration was 6.5 mg/dL and was similar in the treated and untreated patients. The average steroid dose was 60 mg of oral prednisone daily for 10 days. Similar results were obtained in another nonrandomized study.[124]

Other forms of nephrotoxicity are extremely uncommon with the beta-lactam antibiotics. The cephalosporins are transported into the proximal tubular epithelial cells by the organic anion transport system and are secreted across the luminal membranes.[125] Acute tubular necrosis may occur if high concentrations accumulate in the tubular cells. This is best seen with cephaloridine. Cephaloridine is transported into the cells as just described. Unlike the other cephalosporins, it is not readily secreted across the luminal membrane, and high concentrations accumulate within the cells. Acute tubular necrosis was common with this drug,[126, 127] and it is no longer marketed. The other cephalosporins have limited potential to cause ATN. Very large doses have caused ATN in experimental animals,[125] and cephalothin plus an aminoglycoside caused more nephrotoxicity than a penicillin plus an aminoglycoside in three randomized clinical trials.[52–54] Monotherapy with the current cephalosporins at the recommended doses probably does not cause ATN. One case of cortical necrosis has been reported with cefuroxime, but the mechanism was probably a hypersensitivity reaction.[128]

Imipenem is metabolized rapidly by dehydropeptidase-1, an enzyme located in the proximal tubular brush border. The metabolites are potentially nephrotoxic, and high doses of imipenem, alone, have caused ATN in rabbits.[129] Cilastatin blocks dehydropeptidase-1, permitting adequate urinary concentrations and preventing toxicity. Nephrotoxicity has not been observed with the imipenem-cilastatin combination. Nephrotoxicity has not been reported with meropenem or with the monobactam aztreonam.

Sulfonamides and Trimethoprim

The antibiotic era began with sulfanilamide in the 1930s.[130] The early sulfonamides, and their acetylated metabolites, were poorly soluble, especially at acid pH, and precipitated in the renal tubules or in the collecting system, causing an intrarenal obstructive uropathy or renal calculi.[1] This was much less true of sulfanilamide than of its successors, sulfapyridine, sulfathiazole, and sulfadiazine. Renal calculi developed in 2% to 3% of individuals treated with the latter drugs,[1, 131] and renal failure, sometimes fatal, was not uncommon. Hydrating (to maintain a high urine flow rate) and alkalinizing the urine minimized this complication.

The solubility problem was attacked in two ways. One approach was to create sulfonamide mixtures, taking advantage of the fact that the compounds of which such mixtures are composed have additive antibacterial effects but independent solubilities. Trisulfapyrimidines (sulfadiazine, sulfamerazine, and sulfamethazine), also called triple sulfa, used this approach. This strategy was only partially successful. The second approach was to create more soluble sulfonamides. Complications from crystalluria are uncommon, but not unknown, with the newer compounds (sulfamethizole, sulfisoxazole, sulfadoxine, and sulfamethoxazole). Sulfamethoxazole and sulfisoxazole are acetylated to poorly soluble metabolites, and stones or renal failure may result from precipitation of these derivatives.[132–134] Individuals receiving these drugs should remain adequately hydrated, especially if high doses are employed or if pre-existing renal insufficiency is present.

Interstitial nephritis is the other common form of sulfonamide nephrotoxicity and may be the more frequent form of nephrotoxicity with today's more soluble agents.[40, 135–137] Stopping the drug in a timely fashion is important. The data on steroid therapy for sulfonamide-induced interstitial nephritis are limited. These data,[40] and the data for methicillin-induced interstitial nephritis, suggest that glucocorticoids may be beneficial, especially for severely affected patients.[122, 124]

The sulfonamides may produce hemolysis, with resulting renal injury. Acute tubular necrosis has also been reported.[138–140] Whether this resulted from direct tubular toxicity, from intratubular precipitation that had resolved by the time of biopsy, from hemolysis, or as a complication of infection, is uncertain.

Trimethoprim, a nonsulfonamide, inhibits bacterial and protozoal dihydrofolate reductases, blocking tetrahydrofolic acid synthesis. Trimethoprim has an amiloride-like effect on the distal nephron that may produce hyperkalemia[141–143] and metabolic acidosis.[144, 145] In addition, trimethoprim blocks tubular creatinine secretion, raising the serum creatinine concentration without changing the glomerular filtration rate.[146]

Fluoroquinolones

The fluoroquinolones inhibit bacterial DNA gyrase. Their primary renal toxicity is interstitial nephritis.[147–156] Most, but not all,[149] cases occurred with ciprofloxacin. Interstitial nephritis may by accompanied, occasionally, by a necrotizing vasculitis.[155] Data from a small number of patients indicate that individuals with interstitial nephritis have autoantibodies to a 65-kDa protein expressed by renal microsomes.[156] Hepatic microsomes express the same protein, and similar autoantibodies have been observed in individuals developing hepatitis with quinolone therapy.[156]

The fluoroquinolones are not very soluble at alkaline pH, and high doses have produced crystalluria and azotemia in experimental animals.[157] Human beings are less susceptible, because human urine tends to be more acidic. Norfloxacin crystals have been observed in human urine after single doses of 1200 mg,[158] suggesting that humans could be at risk for intratubular obstruction if doses are high, patients are dehydrated, or urine is alkaline.

Some patients treated with temafloxacin developed severe hemolytic anemia; this was accompanied by renal failure in a majority of cases.[159–161] Temafloxacin was withdrawn from the market in 1992. A single case of biopsy-proven ATN has been reported in a patient treated with ciprofloxacin.[162]

Macrolides

The macrolide antibiotics erythromycin, clarithromycin, azithromycin, and dirithromycin bind to the 50S subunit of bacterial ribosomes, preventing protein-chain elongation. They have little direct nephrotoxicity. Two cases of interstitial nephritis have developed with erythromycin therapy,[163, 164] and two cases of systemic vasculitis, causing hematuria but not renal failure, have been reported with clarithromycin.[165, 166]

The macrolides are inhibitors of the cytochrome P-450 isoenzyme CYP 3A4 and may cause indirect nephrotoxicity by interfering with cyclosporine or tacrolimus metabolism.[167–174] This effect may be more pronounced with erythromycin and clarithromycin than with azithromycin or dirithromycin.[174] In addition, erythromycin potentiates the renal vasoconstrictive effect of cyclosporine, at least in the rat.[175]

Lovastatin is also metabolized by CYP 3A4. Rhabdomyolysis, with ensuing ARF, has occurred when erythromycin was added to lovastatin.[176]

Tetracyclines

The tetracyclines inhibit bacterial protein synthesis by binding to the 30S ribosomal subunit. Five nephrotoxic effects have been described with these drugs: AIN; nephrogenic diabetes insipidus from demeclocycline; ARF among patients with cirrhosis who were treated with demeclocycline; phosphaturia among individuals with the syndrome of inappropriate antidiuretic hormone secretion (SIADH); and Fanconi syndrome from old tetracycline. In addition, their inhibitory effect on protein synthesis occurs to a lesser extent, but is not absent, in mammals. Therefore, because amino acids not used for protein synthesis are converted primarily to urea, the tetracyclines may elevate the blood urea nitrogen concentration without changing the glomerular filtration rate.[177]

Interstitial nephritis is rare with the tetracyclines. Two[178, 179] or possibly three[180] biopsy-proven cases have been reported with minocycline, one[181] with tetracycline. All patients had severe renal failure. Three were treated with steroids.[179–181] One was not.[178] All patients recovered.

Demeclocycline interferes with antidiuretic hormone at a site distal to hormone binding, probably by impairing cyclic AMP generation and action.[182] Nephrogenic diabetes insipidus is universal and dose-related. This effect may be exploited to treat hyponatremia caused by SIADH[183] or congestive heart failure.[184] This approach is dangerous among individuals with hyponatremia due to cirrhosis, however. The drug induces a water diuresis, but most patients with demeclocycline-treated cirrhosis develop reversible renal failure.[185, 186] Urinary phosphate wasting has been reported when patients with SIADH received demeclocycline[187, 188] or doxycycline.[189]

The early 1960s witnessed the publication of several reports that described patients who developed Fanconi syndrome after ingesting outdated or degraded tetracycline.[190–192] Anhydro-4-epitetracycline, a degradation product that forms under the influence of moisture, heat, and low pH, may have been responsible.[191, 193] Expiration dates and tetracycline reformulation have eliminated this problem.

Rifampin

Rifampin is a large, lipid-soluble molecule that blocks bacterial RNA synthesis by binding to DNA-dependent RNA polymerase. It is a broad-spectrum antibacterial, effective against mycobacteria, anaerobes, most gram-positive aerobes, and some gram-negative aerobes. It causes four types of nephrotoxicity.[194] The most common type, occurring in about 1 in every 2000 treated patients,[195] is a syndrome of ARF developing with discontinuous treatments. Less common are three types of renal failure that may occur with continuous treatments: AIN; rapidly progressive glomerulonephritis; and light-chain cast nephropathy.

The discontinuous therapy syndrome was described best in a series of 60 patients who were treated at a single center in Romania.[195] Acute renal failure developed suddenly, with symptoms typically beginning within 1 day of the time that rifampin was reintroduced. The most common symptoms were nausea, vomiting, diarrhea, abdominal or flank pain, fever, and chills. Hemolysis was common, but not universal. Leukocytosis, thrombocytopenia, and abnormalities of liver function tests were also common. Affected individuals were almost always anuric. The mean duration of anuria was 11 days. Almost all patients recovered normal renal function within 90 days. Renal biopsies from patients with this syndrome have usually shown the presence of ATN or interstitial nephritis.[194, 195] Rifampin-dependent antibodies were present in the plasma of almost all patients.[194] These may be directed against the erythrocyte I antigen[194, 196] and, presumably, cause the syndrome. They are probably suppressed or cleared with continuous therapy. Most of the affected patients have not been treated with immunosuppression. Whether steroids hasten recovery is uncertain.

At least six cases of AIN have been described with continuous therapy.[197–202] In addition, some of these patients had glomerular immune complexes resulting in heavy proteinuria.[199] Rapidly progressive, crescentic glomerulonephritis has been described in four patients receiving continuous therapy.[203–206] Three of these developed within the first 2 months of treatment, the fourth[204] after a 10-month course was completed. At least one[206] had rifampin-dependent antibodies. Finally, at least five cases of reversible renal failure due to light-chain cast nephropathy have been described with continuous rifampin.[207–210] The light chains were polyclonal in each case.

Polypeptides (Polymyxins and Bacitracin)

The polymyxins polymyxin B and colistin (polymyxin E) are cyclic polypeptides active against aerobic gram-negative bacteria. They contain cationic amino groups that bind to bacterial cell-membrane phospholipids, disrupting the membranes. As with the aminoglycosides, these amino groups also bind to phospholipids present in the membranes of the renal tubular epithelium. Nephrotoxicity and neurotoxicity limit their systemic use. Parenteral polymyxin B is no longer available in the United States, and parenteral colistin is used primarily for treating *Pseudomonas* infections resistant to other antibiotics. Topical preparations are used widely.

Approximately 20% of individuals treated with parenteral colistin develop ARF.[211] Acute tubular necrosis is seen in some patients, but the renal pathology is normal in many. Renal function usually continues to decline after the drug has been withdrawn, reaching a nadir about 1 week after the drug has been stopped. Surviving patients usually recover completely.

A single case of AIN has been attributed to polymyxin B.[212] Its nephrotoxicity is otherwise similar to that of colistin.

Bacitracin, a cyclic polypeptide mixture, is active primarily against gram-positive bacteria. It was used widely between 1946 and 1960 against penicillin-resistant staphylococci. It is highly nephrotoxic, causing urinary abnormalities (hematuria, proteinuria, glycosuria, leukocyturia, or granular casts) in almost all patients, and ARF, probably ATN, in 31% of patients.[213] Only topical preparations remain available in the United States.

Nitrofurantoin

Nitrofurantoin is used to treat or to suppress urinary tract infections. Acute interstitial necrosis occurs occasionally.[214–218]

Metronidazole

Nephrotoxicity has not been reported with metronidazole. It inhibits the cytochrome P-450 isoenzyme

CYP 3A4, so the potential for nephrotoxicity resulting from elevated cyclosporine or tacrolimus levels exists.

NEPHROTOXICITY FROM ANTIFUNGAL DRUGS

Individuals requiring systemic antifungal therapy often have serious underlying illnesses that predispose them to both opportunistic infections and ARF. When ARF develops in such individuals, it has a high mortality. Unfortunately, the most potent antifungal drug, amphotericin B, is highly nephrotoxic. The nephrotoxicities of the antifungal drugs are summarized in Table 27–4.

Amphotericin B

Amphotericin B is the most effective drug available for severe fungal infections. Despite newer antifungal drugs, its use has increased as more complex therapies have increased the number of immunosuppressed or otherwise compromised patients developing such infections.[219] Nephrotoxicity is its dose-limiting side effect.

MECHANISM OF TOXICITY

Structurally, amphotericin B is a polyene antibiotic. It attacks fungi by binding to cell-membrane sterols, principally ergosterol, creating pores that increase membrane permeability.[220] Mammalian cell membranes lack ergosterol, and mammalian toxicity results from lower-affinity binding to cholesterol. As with fungi, cell damage results from increased membrane permeability. In the kidney, small doses increase tubular epithelial cell permeability to water and small solutes, reducing tubular function. With larger doses, the cell's ability to compensate for increased membrane permeability is overwhelmed, and tubular necrosis occurs.

CLINICAL TOXICITY

Glomerular filtration is reduced both by the direct toxic effect on the tubular epithelium, resulting in ATN,[221] and by renal vasoconstriction.[222] Almost all amphotericin B–treated individuals develop some renal dysfunction.[223-225] The serum creatinine concentration can be expected to double in about one third of individuals treated with doses of conventional amphotericin B consisting of an average of 0.6 mg/kg per day for 10 days.[226] Additional abnormalities of tubular function are common and may be present without reductions in the glomerular filtration rate. These include hypokalemia, hypomagnesemia, a concentrating defect, and a distal renal tubular acidosis.

Renal potassium wasting, resulting in hypokalemia,[227, 228] is common. Severe hypokalemia developed in 52% of amphotericin B–treated patients versus 23% of fluconazole-treated patients in one randomized trial.[229] Hypomagnesemia is also common[226, 230] and may exacerbate hypokalemia. A concentrating defect occurs in almost all patients.[223, 224] It is not reversed by vasopressin.[231] Hypokalemia may contribute to the concentrating defect but is probably not the sole cause.[219] The distal renal tubular acidosis is dose-related[232, 233] but does not require renal insufficiency.[227] Like other types of nephrotoxicity, the acidosis probably results from increased membrane permeability, in this case increased membrane permeability of the epithelium in the distal nephron to hydrogen ions.[234, 235]

Renal abnormalities generally resolve or improve after drug withdrawal,[236] but permanent deficits may occur, especially if total doses exceed 3 to 4 g. In one series, renal dysfunction persisted among 44% of individuals who received total doses exceeding 4 g vs. that among 17% of those who received less.[237] The incidence of permanent dysfunction has usually been assessed with the use of methods that have low sensitivity, serum creatinine concentrations, or creatinine clearance, so the incidence may by understated.

Histologically, most patients treated with amphotericin B develop intratubular calcium deposits involving the proximal and distal tubules.[221, 237] Acute degenerative changes, consisting of proximal and distal tubular epithelial necrosis, disintegration, and desquamation, with intratubular cast formation, are common.[221] Vacuolization of the media of the small arteries and arterioles has also been described.[238]

RISK FACTORS AND PREVENTION

Greater total doses, diuretic therapy, and pre-existing renal insufficiency all are risk factors for ARF

TABLE 27–4. Nephrotoxicity From Antifungal Drugs

DRUG	ATN	TUBULAR DYSFUNCTION	INTERSTITIAL NEPHRITIS	INTRATUBULAR OBSTRUCTION OR CALCULI	OTHER
Amphotericin B	+ + +	+ + +	−	−	+ + +
Ketoconazole	−	−	−	−	+
Fluconazole	−	−	−	−	+
Itraconazole	−	−	−	−	+
Griseofulvin	−	−	?	−	?
Flucytosine	−	−	−	−	−
Terbinafine	−	−	−	−	−

− = none; ? = possible or reported but etiology uncertain; + = very uncommon; + + = uncommon; + + + = common.

during amphotericin B therapy.[239] The risk is reduced if a fixed total dose is administered over a longer period.[239] The adverse effect of diuretics is dose-dependent and probably results from sodium chloride depletion. Individuals treated with amphotericin B frequently receive other nephrotoxic agents or have conditions, such as sepsis, known to cause ARF. These additional insults add to the risk; in clinical practice, the specific contribution of amphotericin B to azotemia is often uncertain.

Saline is the only therapy known to reduce the risk of ARF from amphotericin B in human beings.[240, 241] The optimal sodium dose has not been established. The single randomized, controlled human trial[241] administered 1 L of normal saline daily. Saline-treated patients required more potassium supplementation than did control patients in order to maintain serum potassium concentrations of 3 mEq/L: 90 mEq/day by the end of the treatment course for saline-treated patients vs. 20 mEq/d in control patients. Saline administration did not affect the plasma or tissue concentrations of amphotericin B.

In vitro, pH values of 5.6 to 6.0, similar to those found in the distal nephron, impeded the recovery of renal tubular epithelial cells from amphotericin B nephrotoxicity.[242] This suggests that bicarbonate therapy may be protective, at least in the distal nephron. This concept has not been tested clinically. Theophylline[222] and calcium channel blockers[243, 244] have blunted experimental amphotericin B toxicity but have not been evaluated in humans.

Incorporating a drug into lipid vesicles may allow the drug to be targeted to specific tissues or pathogens capable of taking up such vesicles, sparing other tissues. This approach has been particularly successful with amphotericin B, and three lipid-based formulations are now available in the United States. These include amphotericin B colloidal dispersion (ABCD), amphotericin B lipid complex (ABLC), and liposomal amphotericin B. Both the renal uptake[245] and the nephrotoxicity[226, 245, 246] of these formulations are considerably less than that of conventional amphotericin B. Indeed, renal function of patients who had developed nephrotoxicity with conventional amphotericin B improved as therapy continued with ABLC.[247]

The tissue dispositions, toxicities, and antifungal properties of the different lipid-based preparations depend on their chemical compositions and physical properties. In addition, their relative antifungal activities may depend on the specific fungal pathogen.[248] Generalizations should be made with great caution. To date, no comparative clinical trials of the different lipid-based preparations have been performed. Considerable work remains to be done to define the optimal preparation and dose for each clinical situation.

Azoles

Among the azoles, ketoconazole, an imidazole, and two triazoles, fluconazole and itraconazole, are available. All damaged fungal cell membranes interfere with ergosterol synthesis by inhibiting the cytochrome P-450 system. All, especially ketoconazole, have some affinity for the mammalian P-450 system. None of the azoles is directly nephrotoxic. All, especially ketoconazole, may cause indirect nephrotoxicity among cyclosporine or tacrolimus-treated patients by interfering with the metabolism of these drugs.[249–254]

Griseofulvin

One case of AIN has been reported with long-term griseofulvin therapy[255]; the diagnosis was not confirmed with a renal biopsy. Glomerular changes (mesangial cell proliferation and increased mesangial matrix) and tubular epithelial-cell changes (dilated mitochondria and smooth endoplasmic reticulum) have developed with high doses in mice.[256] Such changes have not been described in humans. Griseofulvin, in theory, may cause renal transplant rejection by inducing cyclosporine or tacrolimus metabolism.[257]

NEPHROTOXICITY FROM ANTIVIRAL DRUGS

Five antiviral drugs cause nephrotoxicity: foscarnet; indinavir; acyclovir (related drugs may have minor nephrotoxic effects); cidofovir, and interferon-α (IFN-α). The toxicities of the first three result chiefly from their poor solubilities, a mechanism that had become uncommon among antimicrobial agents after the early sulfonamides were replaced by more soluble drugs. The mechanism of cidofovir's nephrotoxicity is unknown, while that of IFN-α is immunologic. The nephrotoxicities of the antiviral drugs are summarized in Table 27–5.

Foscarnet

Foscarnet (trisodium phosphonoformate) is a pyrophosphate analogue that inhibits herpesvirus DNA polymerase and retrovirus reverse transcriptase. It is excreted by the kidneys. It has been used primarily for treating infections caused by cytomegalovirus. Nephrotoxicity is dose dependent[258] and common. Acute renal failure has developed in 13% to 66% of foscarnet-treated patients.[259–262] Intravenous saline, infused at a rate of 2.5 L/day, reduced the incidence of ARF substantially.[260]

Acute renal failure results from glomerulonephritis and ATN. The apparent mechanism of glomerulonephritis is peculiar: deposition of foscarnet sodium and calcium salts in the glomerular capillaries.[263–266] The glomerulonephritis may be crescentic. Similar crystals also form, to a lesser extent, in the tubules. Crystallization may be all or part of the mechanism by which foscarnet causes ATN. Foscarnet crystals disappear and renal function improves after foscarnet withdrawal, but residual fibrosis is probably common.[265, 266]

Foscarnet has more affinity for calcium than for

TABLE 27–5. Nephrotoxicity From Antiviral Drugs

DRUG	ATN	TUBULAR DYSFUNCTION	INTERSTITIAL NEPHRITIS	INTRATUBULAR OBSTRUCTION OR CALCULI	OTHER
Foscarnet	+ + +	+	+	+ + +	+ + +
Indinavir	?	–	+	+ + +	–
Acyclovir	+	–	+	+ + +	–
Valacyclovir	?	–	?	?	–
Ganciclovir	–	–	–	?	–
Famciclovir	–	–	–	–	–
Cidofovir	+ + +	+ + +	–	–	–
Interferon-α	–	–	+	–	+
Amantadine	–	–	–	–	–
Rimantadine	–	–	–	–	–
Ribavirin	–	–	–	–	–
Lamivudine	–	–	–	–	–
Zidovudine	–	–	–	–	–

– = none; ? = possible or reported but etiology uncertain; + = very uncommon; + + = uncommon; + + + = common.

sodium, and the calcium salt is less soluble. Replacement of sodium by calcium is required for foscarnet precipitation in vivo. In vitro, it precipitates in solutions containing more than 2.5 mmol/L of calcium chloride.[264] In humans, foscarnet infusions may cause hypocalcemia as plasma calcium binds to the drug in place of sodium.

Hypomagnesemia was more common with foscarnet than with ganciclovir in a large, randomized trial comparing these therapies.[262] Two cases of reversible nephrogenic diabetes insipidus have been attributed to foscarnet.[267] One of these individuals also had distal renal tubular acidosis. Interstitial nephritis among renal transplant patients was reported in one series[268]; the mechanism was uncertain but may have been tubular precipitation, rather than hypersensitivity.

Indinavir

Indinavir is a protease inhibitor active against the human immunodeficiency virus. It is metabolized primarily by the liver. However, as much as 10% of the intact drug and smaller amounts of indinavir metabolites are excreted in the urine.[269] The parent compound is poorly soluble in aqueous solutions, and intrarenal or urinary crystallization is common. Kopp and coworkers[270] described three syndromes, all associated with indinavir crystalluria, among a large group of indinavir-treated patients: 5% developed back or flank pain, with renal parenchymal filling defects usually, but not always, present on CT scans; 4% developed indinavir nephrolithiasis; and 3% developed dysuria and urinary urgency. Serum creatinine elevations occurred in a minority of the patients with parenchymal defects or stones. The parenchymal defects probably resulted from intratubular precipitation. Twenty percent of Kopp's patients had asymptomatic crystalluria.

Indinavir crystals are distinctive and consist of layered, roughly rectangular plates, sheaves of densely packed needles, and starbursts or rosettes.[270–272] Hydration, though not formally tested, is probably useful in

preventing toxicity. Indinavir is more soluble in acid than in alkaline solutions, but the acidity required may be beyond that achievable. In vitro, a pH of 4.5 is required to dissolve indinavir crystals in human urine.[270] In vivo urinary acidification has not been tested as a prophylactic or therapeutic measure.

As with the other poorly soluble antiviral drugs, interstitial nephritis has been attributed to indinavir.[273–276] The cause, although not definitely established, may have been tubular precipitation, rather than hypersensitivity, in some or all of these cases.

Deoxyguanosine Analogues (Acyclovir, Valacyclovir, Ganciclovir, and Famciclovir)

The deoxyguanosine analogues inhibit DNA polymerase and prevent viruses of the herpes family from replicating. They are eliminated by both glomerular filtration and tubular secretion. Valacyclovir and famciclovir are prodrugs and are converted rapidly to acyclovir and penciclovir, respectively.

Acyclovir is poorly soluble in tubular fluid and urine. Acute renal failure from intratubular precipitation is common when high doses are administered intravenously.[277–281] Crystalluria may be observed with polarized microscopy; the crystals are needle-shaped and may be engulfed by leukocytes.[281, 282] Infusing the drug slowly, over at least 1 hour, reducing the dose for individuals with renal impairment, and hydrating the patient to maintain high urine flow rates minimize the intratubular concentrations of acyclovir and diminish the risk.[278]

Acyclovir is absorbed slowly and incompletely from the gastrointestinal tract. Oral acyclovir is much less nephrotoxic than the intravenous form. Occasionally, ARF develops with oral acyclovir,[283–286] especially when high doses are administered, dehydration exists, or renal function is impaired.

Individuals developing ARF generally recover after drug withdrawal and hydration. Acyclovir is removed readily by hemodialysis. In theory, and in limited practice,[287] hemodialysis is useful for decreasing plasma drug concentrations after overdoses and among individuals with ARF and high plasma levels.

Acute interstitial necrosis[288] and ATN[289] have been reported after acyclovir administration. It is unknown whether these complications resulted from hypersensitivity, in the case of interstitial nephritis; from toxicity to the tubular epithelial cells, in the case of ATN; or from crystallization.

Valacyclovir, better absorbed from the gastrointestinal tract than acyclovir and converted rapidly to acyclovir after absorption, should be more nephrotoxic than oral acyclovir. In practice, nephrotoxicity has not occurred.[290, 291] In particular, renal transplant patients who were enrolled in a large randomized, placebo-controlled trial that used relatively high oral doses (8 g/d with reduced doses for glomerular filtration rates below 75 mL/min) experienced no nephrotoxicity.[292]

Ganciclovir probably causes little renal dysfunction in humans; only a few instances of relatively mild ARF have been reported.[293] High doses of ganciclovir have not caused ARF in rats.[294] Famciclovir is not known to be nephrotoxic.

Cidofovir

Cidofovir, a nucleoside analogue of cytosine, is active against herpesviruses. To date, it has been used primarily for cytomegalovirus retinitis in patients with the acquired immunodeficiency syndrome. Virtually all of the drug is eliminated unchanged by glomerular filtration and tubular secretion. Probenecid blocks its tubular secretion.[295, 296] Despite rapid elimination from plasma, it has a long intracellular duration of action[297] and may be dosed biweekly. Dose-dependent nephrotoxicity is its major side effect.

Cidofovir is a proximal tubular toxin[298] and causes proteinuria, Fanconi's syndrome, and ATN. The mechanism of toxicity is unknown. Toxicity may be reduced, but not eliminated, by concomitant administration of probenecid and saline.[299] Cidofovir is usually stopped if 2^+ proteinuria (quantitative methods, such as the urinary ratio of protein to creatinine have not been investigated) or serum creatinine concentrations of at least 2 mg/dL occur. In two trials employing these measures, proteinuria occurred in 45% and serum creatinine elevations occurred in 13% of patients receiving individual doses of 5 mg/kg.[300, 301] These problems improved after drug withdrawal but did not always resolve completely.

Interferon-α

The interferons are immunomodulatory glycoproteins with broad antiviral and antineoplastic activities. There are three types, designated alpha, beta, and gamma, and many subtypes. Their roles are under investigation. Currently, the most commonly used drug in this group is IFN-α for hepatitis C.

Interferon-α causes systemic side effects frequently, but renal side effects are uncommon. Those that occur seem to result from enhanced immunologic activity. Thrombotic microangiopathies,[302–305] focal segmental glomerulosclerosis,[306–308] and minimal change glomerulopathy[309–311] have been described most often. There have also been reports of AIN,[306, 310, 311] membranoproliferative glomerulonephritis,[302, 312] membranous glomerulopathy,[313] and one case of a unique glomerulonephritis.[314] That some of these renal diseases were caused by underlying illnesses, rather than interferon, is possible. However, one case of minimal change glomerulopathy and AIN recurred when the patient received a second course of IFN-α.[311]

Renal transplant patients treated with IFN-α have done poorly. In one series, ARF, not always reversible, developed in more than one third of patients.[315]

REFERENCES

1. Brown WH, Thornton WB, Wilson JS: An evaluation of the clinical toxicity of sulfanilamide and sulfapyridine. JAMA 1940; 114:1605–1611.
2. Waksman SA: Streptomycin: background, isolation, properties, and utilization. Science 1953; 118:259–266.
3. Luft FC, Kleit SA: Renal parenchymal accumulation of aminoglycoside antibiotics in rats. J Infect Dis 1974; 130:656–659.
4. Edwards CQ, Smith CR, Baughman KL, et al: Concentrations of gentamicin and amikacin in human kidneys. Antimicrob Agents Chemother 1976; 9:925–927.
5. Fabre J, Rudhardt M, Blanchard P, et al: Persistence of sisomicin and gentamicin in renal cortex and medulla compared with other organs and serum of rats. Kidney Int 1976; 10:444–449.
6. Senekjian HO, Knight TF, Weinman EJ: Micropuncture study of the handling of gentamicin by the rat kidney. Kidney Int 1981; 19:416–423.
7. Pastoriza-Munoz E, Timmerman D, Feldman S, et al: Ultrafiltration of gentamicin and netilmicin in vivo. J Pharmacol Exp Ther 1982; 220:604–608.
8. Sastrasinh M, Knauss TC, Weinberg JM, et al: Identification of the aminoglycoside receptor of renal brush border membranes. J Pharmacol Exp Ther 1982; 222:350–358.
9. Williams PD, Bennett DB, Gleason CR, et al: Correlation between renal membrane binding and nephrotoxicity of aminoglycosides. Antimicrob Agents Chemother 1987; 31:570–574.
10. Silverblatt FJ, Kuehn C: Autoradiography of gentamicin uptake by the rat proximal tubule cell. Kidney Int 1979; 15:335–345.
11. Wedeen RP, Batuman V, Cheeks C, et al: Transport of gentamicin in rat proximal tubule. Lab Invest 1983; 48:212–223.
12. Laurent G, Carlier MB, Rollman B, et al: Mechanism of aminoglycoside-induced lysosomal phospholipidosis: in vitro and in vivo studies with gentamicin and amikacin. Biochem Pharmacol 1982; 31:3861–3870.
13. Houghton DC, Harnett M, Campbell-Boswell MV, et al: A light and electron microscopic analysis of gentamicin nephrotoxicity in rats. Am J Pathol 1976; 255:589–599.
14. Houghton DC, Campbell-Boswell MV, Bennett WM, et al: Myeloid bodies in the renal tubules of humans: relationship to gentamicin therapy. Clin Nephrol 1978; 10:140–145.
15. De Broe ME, Paulus GJ, Verpooten GA, et al: Early effects of gentamicin, tobramycin, and amikacin on the human kidney. Kidney Int 1984; 25:643–652.
16. Elliott WC, Houghton DC, Gilbert DN, et al: Gentamicin nephrotoxicity. I. Degree and permanence of acquired insensitivity. J Lab Clin Med 1982; 100:501–512.
17. Elliott WC, Houghton DC, Gilbert DN, et al: Gentamicin nephrotoxicity. II. Definition of conditions necessary to induce acquired insensitivity. J Lab Clin Med 1982; 100:513–525.
18. Sundin DP, Meyer C, Dahl R, et al: Cellular mechanism of aminoglycoside tolerance in long-term gentamicin treatment. Am J Physiol 1997; 272:C1309–C1318.

19. Munckhof WJ, Grayson ML, Turnidge JD: A meta-analysis of studies on the safety and efficacy of aminoglycosides given either once daily or as divided doses. J Antimicrob Chemother 1996; 37:645–663.

20. Dillon KR, Dougherty SH, Casner P, et al: Individualized pharmacokinetic versus standard dosing of amikacin: comparison of therapeutic outcomes. J Antimicrob Chemother 1989; 24:581–589.

21. Burton ME, Ash CL, Hill DP Jr, et al: A controlled trial of the cost benefit of computerized bayesian aminoglycoside administration. Clin Pharmacol Ther 1991; 49:685–694.

22. Whipple JK, Ausman RK, Franson TR, et al: Effect of individualized pharmacokinetic dosing on patient outcome. Crit Care Med 1991; 19:1480–1485.

23. Leehey DJ, Braun BI, Tholl DA, et al: Can pharmacokinetic dosing decrease nephrotoxicity associated with aminoglycoside therapy. J Am Soc Nephrol 1993; 4:81–90.

24. Luft FC: Clinical significance of renal changes engendered by aminoglycosides in man. J Antimicrob Chemother 1984; 13 (Suppl A):23–30.

25. Kleinknecht D, Landais P, Goldfard B: Drug-Associated Acute Renal Failure. A Prospective Multicenter Report. In Davison AM, Guillou PJ, eds: Proceedings of the European Dialysis and Transplantation Association—European Renal Association. Vol. 22. London: Bailliere Tindall, 1985:1002–1007.

26. Landau D, Kher KK: Gentamicin-induced Bartter-like syndrome. Pediatr Nephrol 1997; 11:737–740.

27. Slayton W, Anstine D, Lakhdir F, et al: Tetany in a child with AIDS receiving intravenous tobramycin. South Med J 1996; 89:1108–1110.

28. Wu B, Atkinson SA, Halton JM, et al: Hypermagnesiuria and hypercalciuria in childhood leukemia: an effect of amikacin therapy. J Pediatr Hematol Oncol 1996; 18:86–89.

29. Zaloga GP, Chernow B, Pock A, et al: Hypomagnesemia is a common complication of aminoglycoside therapy. Surg Gynecol Obstet 1984; 158:561–565.

30. Kes P, Reiner Z: Symptomatic hypomagnesemia associated with gentamicin therapy. Magnes Trace Elements 1990; 9:54–60.

31. Nanji AA, Denegri JF: Hypomagnesemia associated with gentamicin therapy. Drug Intell Clin Pharm 1984; 18:596–598.

32. Patel R, Savage A: Symptomatic hypomagnesemia associated with gentamicin therapy. Nephron 1979; 23:50–52.

33. Keating MJ, Sethi MR, Bodey GP, et al: Hypocalcemia with hypoparathyroidism and renal tubular dysfunction associated with aminoglycoside therapy. Cancer 1977; 39:1410–1414.

34. Bar RS, Wilson HE, Mazzaferri EL: Hypomagnesemic hypocalcemia secondary to renal magnesium wasting. Ann Intern Med 1975; 82:646–649.

35. Gainza FJ, Minguela JI, Lampreabe I: Aminoglycoside-associated Fanconi's syndrome: an underrecognized entity. Nephron 1997; 77:205–211.

36. Melnick JZ, Baum M, Thompson JR: Aminoglycoside-induced Fanconi's syndrome. Am J Kidney Dis 1994; 23:118–122.

37. Schwartz JH, Schein P: Fanconi syndrome associated with cephalothin and gentamicin therapy. Cancer 1978; 41:769–772.

38. Chakurski I, Minkova V, Belovezhdov N: Acute interstitial nephritis following the use of gentamycin. Vutr Boles 1986; 25:125–126.

39. Viero RM, Cavallo T: Granulomatous interstitial nephritis. Hum Pathol 1995; 26:1347–1353.

40. Pusey CD, Saltissi D, Bloodworth L, et al: Drug associated acute interstitial nephritis: clinical and pathological features and the response to high dose steroid therapy. QJM 1983; 52:194–211.

41. Prins JM, Weverling GJ, de Blok K, et al: Validation and nephrotoxicity of a simplified once-daily aminoglycoside dosing schedule and guidelines for monitoring therapy. Antimicrob Agents Chemother 1996; 40:2494–2499.

42. Paterson DL, Robson JM, Wagener MM: Risk factors for toxicity in elderly patients given aminoglycosides once daily. J Gen Intern Med 1998; 13:735–739.

43. Bertino J Jr, Booker LA, Franck PA, et al: Incidence of and significant risk factors for aminoglycoside-associated nephrotoxicity in patients dosed by using individualized pharmacokinetic monitoring. J Infect Dis 1993; 167:173–179.

44. Pauly DJ, Musa DM, Lestico MR, et al: Risk of nephrotoxicity with combination vancomycin-aminoglycoside antibiotic therapy. Pharmacotherapy 1990; 10:378–382.

45. Moore RD, Smith CR, Lipsky JJ, et al: Risk factors for nephrotoxicity in patients treated with aminoglycosides. Ann Intern Med 1984; 100:352–357.

46. Rybak MJ, Albrecht LM, Boike SC, et al: Nephrotoxicity of vancomycin, alone and with an aminoglycoside. J Antimicrob Chemother 1990; 25:679–687.

47. Gamba G, Contreras AM, Cortes J, et al: Hypoalbuminemia as a risk factor for amikacin nephrotoxicity. Rev Invest Clin 1990; 42:204–209.

48. Cortes J, Gamba G, Contreras A, et al: Amikacin nephrotoxicity in patients with chronic liver disease. Rev Invest Clin 1990; 42:93–98.

49. Hsu CH, Kurtz TW, Easterling RE, et al: Potentiation of gentamicin nephrotoxicity by metabolic acidosis. Proc Soc Exp Biol Med 1974; 146:894–897.

50. Elliott WC, Parker RA, Houghton DC, et al: Effect of sodium bicarbonate and ammonium chloride ingestion in experimental nephrotoxicity in rats. Res Commun Chem Pathol Pharmacol 1980; 28:483–495.

51. Zager RA: A focus of tissue necrosis increases renal susceptibility to gentamicin administration. Kidney Int 1988; 33:84–90.

52. Klastersky J, Hensgens C, Debussscher L: Empiric therapy for cancer patients: comparative study of ticarcillin-tobramycin, ticarcillin-cephalothin, and cephalothin-tobramycin. Antimicrob Agents Chemother 1975; 7:640–645.

53. The EORTC International Antimicrobial Therapy Project Group: Three antibiotic regimens in the treatment of infection in febrile granulocytopenic patients with cancer. J Infect Dis 1978; 137:14–29.

54. Wade JC, Smith CR, Petty BG, et al: Cephalothin plus an aminoglycoside is more nephrotoxic than methicillin plus an aminoglycoside. Lancet 1978; 2:604–606.

55. Kahlmeter G, Dahlager JI: Aminoglycoside toxicity: a review of clinical studies published between 1975 and 1982. J Antimicrob Chemother 1984; 13:9–22.

56. Bennett WM, Hartnett MN, Gilbert D, et al: Effect of sodium intake on gentamicin nephrotoxicity in the rat. Proc Soc Exp Biol Med 1976; 151:736–738.

57. Thompson JR, Simonsen R, Spindler MA, et al: Protective effect of KCl loading in gentamicin nephrotoxicity. Am J Kidney Dis 1990; 15:583–591.

58. Brinker KR, Bulger RE, Dobyan DC, et al: Effect of potassium depletion on gentamicin nephrotoxicity. J Lab Clin Med 1981; 98:292–301.

59. Dobyan DC, Cronin RE, Bulger RE: Effect of potassium depletion on tubular morphology in gentamicin-induced acute renal failure in dogs. Lab Invest 1982; 47:586–594.

60. Klotman PE, Boatman JE, Volpp BD, et al: Captopril enhances aminoglycoside nephrotoxicity in potassium-depleted rats. Kidney Int 1985; 28:118–127.

61. Giuliano RA, Verpooten GA, De Broe ME: The effect of dosing strategy on kidney cortical accumulation of aminoglycosides in rats. Am J Kidney Dis 1986; 8:297–303.

62. Giuliano RA, Verpooten GA, Verbist L, et al: In vivo uptake kinetics of aminoglycosides in the kidney cortex of rats. J Pharmacol Exp Ther 1986; 236:470–475.

63. De Broe ME, Giuliano RA, Verpooten GA: Aminoglycoside nephrotoxicity: mechanism and prevention. Adv Exp Med Biol 1989; 252:233–245.

64. De Broe ME, Verbist L, Verpooten GA: Influence of dosage schedule on renal cortical accumulation of amikacin and tobramycin in man. J Antimicrob Chemother 1991; 27:41–47.

65. Verpooten GA, Giuliano RA, Verbist L, et al: Once-daily dosing decreases renal accumulation of gentamicin and netilmicin. Clin Pharmacol Ther 1989; 45:22–27.

66. Blaser J, Konig C: Once-daily dosing of aminoglycosides. Eur J Clin Microbiol Infect Dis 1995; 14:1029–1038.

67. Galloe AM, Graudal N, Christensen HR, et al: Aminoglycosides: single or multiple daily dosing? A meta-analysis on efficacy and safety. Eur J Clin Pharmacol 1995; 48:39–43.

68. Barza M, Ioannidis JP, Cappelleri JC, et al: Single or multiple daily doses of aminoglycosides: a meta-analysis. BMJ 1996; 312:338–345.

69. Ferriols-Lisart R, Alos-Alminana M: Effectiveness and safety of once-daily aminoglycosides: a meta-analysis. Am J Health Syst Pharm 1996; 53:1141–1150.
70. Hatala R, Dinh T, Cook DJ: Once-daily aminoglycoside dosing in immunocompetent adults: a meta-analysis. Ann Intern Med 1996; 124:717–725.
71. Freeman CD, Strayer AH: Mega-analysis of meta-analysis: an examination of meta-analysis with an emphasis on once-daily aminoglycoside comparative trials. Pharmacotherapy 1996; 16:1093–1102.
72. Ali MZ, Goetz MB: A meta-analysis of the relative efficacy and toxicity of single daily dosing versus multiple daily dosing of aminoglycosides. Clin Infect Dis 1997; 24:796–809.
73. Hatala R, Dinh TT, Cook DJ: Single daily dosing of aminoglycosides in immunocompromised adults: a systematic review. Clin Infect Dis 1997; 24:810–815.
74. Bailey TC, Little JR, Littenberg B, et al: A meta-analysis of extended-interval dosing versus multiple daily dosing of aminoglycosides. Clin Infect Dis 1997; 24:786–795.
75. Gilbert DN, Wood CA, Kohlhepp SJ, et al: Polyaspartic acid prevents experimental aminoglycoside nephrotoxicity. J Infect Dis 1989; 159:945–953.
76. Kishore BK, Kallay Z, Lambricht P, et al: Mechanism of protection afforded by polyaspartic acid against gentamicin-induced phospholipidosis. I. Polyaspartic acid binds gentamicin and displaces it from negatively charged phospholipid layers in vitro. J Pharmacol Exp Ther 1990; 255:867–874.
77. Kohlhepp SJ, McGregor DN, Cohen SJ, et al: Determinants of the in vitro interaction of polyaspartic acid and aminoglycoside antibiotics. J Pharmacol Exp Ther 1992; 263:1464–1470.
78. Ramsammy LS, Josepovitz C, Lane BP, et al: Polyaspartic acid protects against gentamicin nephrotoxicity in the rat. J Pharmacol Exp Ther 1989; 250:149–153.
79. Ramsammy L, Josepovitz C, Lane B, et al: Polyaspartic acid inhibits gentamicin-induced perturbations of phospholipid metabolism. Am J Physiol 1990; 258:C1141–C1149.
80. Swan SK, Gilbert DN, Kohlhepp SJ, et al: Duration of the protective effect of polyaspartic acid on experimental gentamicin nephrotoxicity. Antimicrob Agents Chemother 1992; 36:2556–2558.
81. Todd JH, Hottendorf GH: Renal brush border membrane vesicle aminoglycoside binding and nephrotoxicity. J Pharmacol Exp Ther 1995; 274:258–263.
82. Humes HD, Sastrasinh M, Weinberg JM: Calcium is a competitive inhibitor of gentamicin-renal membrane binding interactions and dietary calcium supplementation protects against gentamicin nephrotoxicity. J Clin Invest 1984; 73:134–147.
83. El Daly ES: Effect of methimazole and fish oil treatment on gentamicin nephrotoxicity in rats. J Pharm Belg 1997; 52:149–156.
84. Aynedjian HS, Nguyen D, Lee HY, et al: Effects of dietary electrolyte supplementation on gentamicin nephrotoxicity. Am J Med Sci 1988; 295:444–452.
85. Ylitalo P, Morsky P, Parviainen MT, et al: Nephrotoxicity of tobramycin. Value of examining various protein and enzyme markers. Methods Find Exp Clin Pharmacol 1991; 13:281–287.
86. Assadamongkol K, Tapaneya-Olarn W, Chatasingh S: Urinary N-acetyl-beta-D-glucosaminidase (NAG) in aminoglycoside nephrotoxicity. J Med Assoc Thai 1989; 1:42–46.
87. Goossens H: Spread of vancomycin-resistant enterococci: differences between the United States and Europe. Infect Control Hosp Epidemiol 1998; 19:546–551.
88. Martone WJ: Spread of vancomycin-resistant enterococci: why did it happen in the United States?. Infect Control Hosp Epidemiol 1998; 19:539–545.
89. Sieradzki K, Roberts RB, Haber SW, et al: The development of vancomycin resistance in a patient with methicillin-resistant Staphylococcus aureus infection. N Engl J Med 1999; 340:517–523.
90. Smith TL, Pearson ML, Wilcox KR, et al: Emergence of vancomycin resistance in glycopeptide-intermediate Staphylococcus, a Staphylococcus aureus ureus Working Group. N Engl J Med 1999; 340:493–501.
91. Waldvogel FA: New resistance in Staphylococcus aureus. N Engl J Med 1999; 340:556–557.
92. Sokol PP: Mechanism of vancomycin transport in the kidney:

studies in rabbit renal brush border and basolateral membrane vesicles. J Pharmacol Exp Ther 1991; 259:1283–1287.
93. Kirby WMM: Vancomycin therapy of staphylococcal infections. Antibiot Chemother 1963; 11:84–96.
94. Torel Ergur A, Onarlioglu B, Gunay Y, et al: Does vancomycin increase aminoglycoside nephrotoxicity? Acta Paediatr Jpn 1997; 39:422–427.
95. Wold JS, Turnipseed SA: Toxicology of vancomycin in laboratory animals. Rev Infect Dis 1981; 3:S224–S229.
96. Wood CA, Kohlhepp SJ, Kohnen PW, et al: Vancomycin enhancement of experimental tobramycin nephrotoxicity. Antimicrob Agents Chemother 1986; 30:20–24.
97. European Organization for Research and Treatment of Cancer (EORTC) International Antimicrobial Therapy Cooperative Group and the National Cancer Institute of Canada-Clinical Trials Group: Vancomycin added to empirical combination antibiotic therapy for fever in granulocytopenic cancer patients. J Infect Dis 1991; 163:951–958.
98. Cimino MA, Rotstein C, Slaughter RL, et al: Relationship of serum antibiotic concentrations to nephrotoxicity in cancer patients receiving concurrent aminoglycoside and vancomycin therapy. Am J Med 1987; 83:1091–1097.
99. Downs NJ, Neihart RE, Dolezal JM, et al: Mild nephrotoxicity associated with vancomycin use. Arch Intern Med 1989; 149:1777–1781.
100. Farber BF, Moellering R Jr: Retrospective study of the toxicity of preparations of vancomycin from 1974 to 1981. Antimicrob Agents Chemother 1983; 23:138–141.
101. Goetz MB, Sayers J: Nephrotoxicity of vancomycin and aminoglycoside therapy separately and in combination. J Antimicrob Chemother 1993; 32:325–334.
102. Mellor JA, Kingdom J, Cafferkey M, et al: Vancomycin toxicity: a prospective study. J Antimicrob Chemother 1985; 15:773–780.
103. Sorrell TC, Collignon PJ: A prospective study of adverse reactions associated with vancomycin therapy. J Antimicrob Chemother 1985; 16:235–241.
104. Kralovicova K, Spanik S, Halko J, et al: Do vancomycin serum levels predict failures of vancomycin therapy or nephrotoxicity in cancer patients? J Chemother 1997; 9:420–426.
105. Zimmermann AE, Katona BG, Plaisance KI: Association of vancomycin serum concentrations with outcomes in patients with gram-positive bacteremia. Pharmacotherapy 1995; 15:85–91.
106. Azar R, Bakhache E, Boldron A: Acute interstitial nephropathy induced by vancomycin. Nephrologie 1996; 17:327–328.
107. Bergman MM, Glew RH, Ebert TH: Acute interstitial nephritis associated with vancomycin therapy. Arch Intern Med 1988; 148:2139–2140.
108. Codding CE, Ramseyer L, Allon M, et al: Tubulointerstitial nephritis due to vancomycin. Am J Kidney Dis 1989; 14:512–515.
109. Michail S, Vaiopoulos G, Nakopoulou L, et al: Henoch-Schöenlein purpura and acute interstitial nephritis after intravenous vancomycin administration in a patient with a staphylococcal infection. Scand J Rheumatol 1998; 27:233–235.
110. Wai AO, Lo AM, Abdo A, et al: Vancomycin-induced acute interstitial nephritis. Ann Pharmacother 1998; 32:1160–1164.
111. Al Shohaib S, Satti MS, Abunijem Z: Acute interstitial nephritis due to cefotaxime. Nephron 1996; 73:725.
112. Baldwin DS, Levine BB, McCluskey RT, et al: Renal failure and interstitial nephritis due to penicillin and methicillin. N Engl J Med 1968; 279:1245–1252.
113. Grcevska L, Polenakovic M: Second attack of acute tubulointerstitionephritis induced by cefataxim and pregnancy. Nephron 1996; 72:354–355.
114. Ladagnous JF, Rousseau JM, Gaucher A, et al: Acute interstitial nephritis. Role of ceftazidime. Ann Fr Anesth Reanim 1996; 15:677–680.
115. Lewis JA, Rindone JP: Acute interstitial nephritis associated with cephapirin. Drug Intell Clin Pharm 1987; 21:380–381.
116. Linton AL, Clark WF, Driedger AA, et al: Acute interstitial nephritis due to drugs: review of the literature with a report of nine cases. Ann Intern Med 1980; 93:735–741.
117. Shibasaki T, Ishimoto F, Sakai O, et al: Clinical characterization of drug-induced allergic nephritis. Am J Nephrol 1991; 11:174–180.

118. Thieme RE, Caldwell SA, Lum GM: Acute interstitial nephritis associated with loracarbef therapy. J Pediatr 1995; 127:997–1000.

119. Walter L, Rosen S, Schur PH: Allergic interstitial nephritis: report of a case with activation of complement by the alternate pathway. Clin Nephrol 1975; 3:153–159.

120. Wiles CM, Assem ES, Cohen SL, et al: Cephradine-induced interstitial nephritis. Clin Exp Immunol 1979; 36:342–346.

121. Ditlove J, Weidmann P, Bernstein M, et al: Methicillin nephritis. Medicine 1977; 56:483–491.

122. Galpin JE, Shinaberger JH, Stanley TM, et al: Acute interstitial nephritis due to methicillin. Am J Med 1978; 65:756–765.

123. Border WA, Lehman DH, Egan JD, et al: Antitubular basement-membrane antibodies in methicillin-associated interstitial nephritis. N Engl J Med 1974; 291:381–384.

124. Laberke HG: Treatment of acute interstitial nephritis. Klin Wochenschr 1980; 58:531–532.

125. Tune BM: Relationship between the transport and toxicity of cephalosporins in the kidney. J Infect Dis 1975; 132:189–194.

126. Hinman AR, Wolinsky E: Nephrotoxicity associated with the use of cephaloridine. JAMA 1967; 200:724–726.

127. Tune BM, Fravert D: Mechanisms of cephalosporin nephrotoxicity: a comparison of cephaloridine and cephaloglycin. Kidney Int 1980; 18:591–600.

128. Manley HJ, Bailie GR, Eisele G: Bilateral renal cortical necrosis associated with cefuroxime axetil. Clin Nephrol 1998; 49:268–270.

129. Kahan FM, Kropp H, Sundelof JG, et al: Thienamycin: development of imipenem-cilastatin. J Antimicrob Chemother 1983; 12(suppl D):1–35.

130. Spink WE: The drama of sulfanilamide, penicillin and other antibiotics 1936–1972. Minn Med 1973; 56(6):551–556.

131. Dowling HF, Lepper MH: Toxic reactions following therapy with sulfapyridine, sulfathiazole and sulfadiazine. JAMA 1943; 121:1190–1194.

132. Albala DM, Prien E, Galal HA: Urolithiasis as a hazard of sulfonamide therapy. J Endourol 1994; 8:401–403.

133. Schwarz A, Perez-Canto A: Nephrotoxicity of antiinfective drugs. Int J Clin Pharmacol Ther 1998; 36:164–167.

134. Van der Ven AJ, Mantel MA, Vree TB, et al: Formation and elimination of sulphamethoxazole hydroxylamine after oral administration of sulphamethoxazole. Br J Clin Pharmacol 1994; 38:147–150.

135. Chandra M, Chandra P, McVicar M, et al: Rapid onset of co-trimoxazole induced interstitial nephritis. Int J Pediatr Nephrol 1985; 6:289–292.

136. Cryst C, Hammar SP: Acute granulomatous interstitial nephritis due to co-trimoxazole. Am J Nephrol 1988; 8:483–488.

137. Smith EJ, Light JA, Filo RS, et al: Interstitial nephritis caused by trimethoprim-sulfamethoxazole in renal transplant recipients. JAMA 1980; 244:360–361.

138. Prien EL: The mechanism of renal complications in sulfonamide therapy. N Engl J Med 1945; 232:63–68.

139. Kalowski S, Nanra RS, Mathew TH, et al: Deterioration in renal function in association with co-trimoxazole therapy. Lancet 1973; 1:394–397.

140. Rudra T, Webb DB, Evans AG: Acute tubular necrosis following co-trimoxazole therapy. Nephron 1989; 53:85–86.

141. Choi MJ, Fernandez PC, Patnaik A, et al: Brief report: trimethoprim-induced hyperkalemia in a patient with AIDS. N Engl J Med 1993; 328:703–706.

142. Eiam-Ong S, Kurtzman NA, Sabatini S: Studies on the mechanism of trimethoprim-induced hyperkalemia. Kidney Int 1996; 49:1372–1378.

143. Reiser IW, Chou SY, Brown MI, et al: Reversal of trimethoprim-induced antikaliuresis. Kidney Int 1996; 50:2063–2069.

144. Kaufman AM, Hellman G, Abramson RG: Renal salt wasting and metabolic acidosis with trimethoprim-sulfamethoxazole therapy. Mt Sinai J Med 1983; 50:238–239.

145. Porras MC, Lecumberri JN, Castrillon JL: Trimethoprim/sulfamethoxazole and metabolic acidosis in HIV-infected patients. Ann Pharmacother 1998; 32:185–189.

146. Berglund F, Killander J, Pompeius R: Effect of trimethoprim-sulfamethoxazole on the renal excretion of creatinine in man. J Urol 1975; 114:802–808.

147. Bailey JR, Trott SA, Philbrick JT: Ciprofloxacin-induced acute interstitial nephritis. Am J Nephrol 1992; 12:271–273.

148. Ball P: Ciprofloxacin: an overview of adverse experiences. J Antimicrob Chemother 1986; 18:187–193.

149. Hadimeri H, Almroth G, Cederbrant K, et al: Allergic nephropathy associated with norfloxacin and ciprofloxacin therapy: report of two cases and review of the literature. Scand J Urol Nephrol 1997; 31:481–485.

150. Helmink R, Benediktsson H: Ciprofloxacin-induced allergic interstitial nephritis. Nephron 1990; 55:432–433.

151. Lien YH, Hansen R, Kern WF, et al: Ciprofloxacin-induced granulomatous interstitial nephritis and localized elastolysis. Am J Kidney Dis 1993; 22:598–602.

152. Reece RJ, Nicholls AJ: Ciprofloxacin-induced acute interstitial nephritis. Nephrol Dial Transplant 1996; 11:393.

153. Rippelmeyer DJ, Synhavsky A: Ciprofloxacin and allergic interstitial nephritis. Ann Intern Med 1988; 109:170.

154. Rosado LJ, Siskind MS, Copeland JG: Acute interstitial nephritis in a cardiac transplant recipient receiving ciprofloxacin. J Thorac Cardiovasc Surg 1994; 107:1364–1366.

155. Shih DJ, Korbet SM, Rydel JJ, et al: Renal vasculitis associated with ciprofloxacin. Am J Kidney Dis 1995; 26:516–519.

156. Gauffre A, Mircheva J, Glotz D, et al: Autoantibodies against a kidney-liver protein associated with quinolone-induced acute interstitial nephritis or hepatitis. Nephrol Dial Transplant 1997; 12:1961–1962.

157. Patterson DR: Quinolone toxicity: methods of assessment. Am J Med 1991; 91:35S–37S.

158. Swanson BN, Boppana VK, Vlasses PH, et al: Norfloxacin deposition after sequentially increasing oral doses. Antimicrob Agents Chemother 1983; 23:284–288.

159. Blum MD, Graham DJ, McCloskey CA: Temafloxacin syndrome: review of 95 cases. Clin Infect Dis 1994; 18:946–950.

160. Deamer RL, Prichard JG, Koenker N, et al: Temafloxacin-induced hemolytic anemia and renal failure. Clin Pharm 1993; 12:380–382.

161. Maguire RB, Stroncek DF, Gale E, et al: Hemolytic anemia and acute renal failure associated with temafloxacin-dependent antibodies. Am J Hematol 1994; 46:363–366.

162. Wilmer WA, Dillon JJ, Bay WH, et al: Acute renal failure associated with oral quinolone therapy (abstract). J Am Soc Nephrol 1992; 3:323.

163. Ding SL, Bailey RR, Gardner J: Acute interstitial nephritis and acute renal failure following erythromycin treatment: case report. N Z Med J 1996; 109:322.

164. Rosenfeld J, Gura V, Boner G, et al: Interstitial nephritis with acute renal failure after erythromycin. BMJ Clin Res Ed 1983; 286:938–939.

165. Gavura SR, Nusinowitz S: Leukocytoclastic vasculitis associated with clarithromycin. Ann Pharmacother 1998; 32:543–545.

166. De Vega T, Blanco S, Lopez C, et al: Clarithromycin-induced leukocytoclastic vasculitis. Eur J Clin Microbiol Infect Dis 1993; 12:563.

167. Ben-Ari J, Eisenstein B, Davidovits M, et al: Effect of erythromycin on blood cyclosporine concentrations in kidney transplant patients. J Pediatr 1988; 112:992–993.

168. Ferrari SL, Goffin E, Mourad M, et al: The interaction between clarithromycin and cyclosporine in kidney transplant recipients. Transplantation 1994; 58:725–727.

169. Jensen CW, Flechner SM, Van Buren CT, et al: Exacerbation of cyclosporine toxicity by concomitant administration of erythromycin. Transplantation 1987; 43:263–270.

170. Kessler M, Louis J, Renoult E, et al: Interaction between cyclosporin and erythromycin in a kidney transplant patient. Eur J Clin Pharmacol 1986; 30:633–634.

171. Padhi ID, Long P, Basha M, et al: Interaction between tacrolimus and erythromycin. Ther Drug Monit 1997; 19:120–122.

172. Spicer ST, Liddle C, Chapman JR, et al: The mechanism of cyclosporine toxicity induced by clarithromycin. Br J Clin Pharmacol 1997; 43:194–196.

173. Wadhwa NK, Schroeder TJ, O'Flaherty E, et al: Interaction between erythromycin and cyclosporine in a kidney and pancreas allograft recipient. Ther Drug Monit 1987; 9:123–125.

174. Watkins VS, Polk RE, Stotka JL: Drug interactions of macrolides: emphasis on dirithromycin. Ann Pharmacother 1997; 31:349–356.

175. McCormack AJ, Snipes RG, Dillon JJ, et al: Primary renovascular effects of erythromycin in the rat: relationship to cyclosporine nephrotoxicity. Ren Fail 1990; 12:241–248.

176. Wong PW, Dillard TA, Kroenke K: Multiple organ toxicity from addition of erythromycin to long-term lovastatin therapy. South Med J 1998; 91:202–205.

177. Shils ME: Renal disease and the metabolic effect of tetracycline. Ann Intern Med 1963; 58:389–408.

178. Walker RG, Thomson NM, Dowling JP, et al: Minocycline-induced acute interstitial nephritis. BMJ 1979; 1:524.

179. Wilkinson SP, Stewart WK, Spiers EM, et al: Protracted systemic illness and interstitial nephritis due to minocycline. Postgrad Med J 1989; 65:53–56.

180. Fletcher S, Sellars L: Minocycline-induced chronic interstitial nephritis? Nephrol Dial Transplant 1996; 11:540–541.

181. Bihorac A, Ozener C, Akoglu E, et al: Tetracycline-induced acute interstitial nephritis as a cause of acute renal failure. Nephron 1999; 81:72–75.

182. Singer I, Rotenberg D: Demeclocycline-induced nephrogenic diabetes insipidus: in-vivo and in-vitro studies. Ann Intern Med 1973; 79:679–683.

183. De Troyer A: Demeclocycline. Treatment for syndrome of inappropriate antidiuretic hormone secretion. JAMA 1977; 237:2723–2726.

184. Zegers de Beyl D, Naeije R, de Troyer A: Demeclocycline treatment of water retention in congestive heart failure. BMJ 1978; 1:760.

185. Miller PD, Linas SL, Schrier RW: Plasma demeclocycline levels and nephrotoxicity: correlation in hyponatremic cirrhotic patients. JAMA 1980; 243:2513–2515.

186. Perez-Ayuso RM, Arroyo V, Camps J, et al: Effect of demeclocycline on renal function and urinary prostaglandin E_2 and kallikrein in hyponatremic cirrhotics. Nephron 1984; 36:30–37.

187. Taylor HC, Fallon MD, Velasco ME: Oncogenic osteomalacia and inappropriate antidiuretic hormone secretion due to oat-cell carcinoma. Ann Intern Med 1984; 101:786–788.

188. Decaux G, Soupart A, Unger J, et al: Demeclocyclin-induced phosphate diabetes in patients with inappropriate secretion of antidiuretic hormone. N Engl J Med 1985; 313:1480–1481.

189. Decaux G: Tetracycline-induced renal hypophosphatemia in a patient with a syndrome of inappropriate secretion of antidiuretic hormone. Nephron 1988; 48:40–42.

190. Gross JM: Fanconi syndrome (adult type) developing secondary to the ingestion of outdated tetracycline. Ann Intern Med 1963; 58:523–528.

191. Frimpter GW, Timpanelli AE, Eisenmenger WJ, et al: "Fanconi syndrome" caused by degraded tetracycline. JAMA 1963; 184:111–113.

192. Folup M, Drapkin A: Potassium-depletion syndrome secondary to nephropathy apparently caused by "outdated tetracycline." N Engl J Med 1965; 272:986–989.

193. Cox M: Tetracycline Nephrotoxicity. In Porter GA, ed: *Nephrotoxic Mechanisms of Drug and Environmental Toxins*. 1. New York: Plenum; 1982:65–77.

194. De Vriese AS, Robbrecht DL, Vanholder RC, et al: Rifampicin-associated acute renal failure: pathophysiologic, immunologic, and clinical features. Am J Kidney Dis 1998; 31:108–115.

195. Covic A, Goldsmith DJ, Segall L, et al: Rifampicin-induced acute renal failure: a series of 60 patients. Nephrol Dial Transplant 1998; 13:924–929.

196. Pereira A, Sanz C, Cervantes F, et al: Immune hemolytic anemia and renal failure associated with rifampicin-dependent antibodies with anti-I specificity. Ann Hematol 1991; 63:56–58.

197. Quinn BP, Wall BM: Nephrogenic diabetes insipidus and tubulointerstitial nephritis during continuous therapy with rifampin. Am J Kidney Dis 1989; 14:217–220.

198. Power DA, Russell G, Smith FW, et al: Acute renal failure due to continuous rifampicin. Clin Nephrol 1983; 20:155–159.

199. Neugarten J, Gallo GR, Baldwin DS: Rifampin-induced nephrotic syndrome and acute interstitial nephritis. Am J Nephrol 1983; 3:38–42.

200. Lai FM, Lai KN, Chong YW: Papillary necrosis associated with rifampicin therapy. Aust N Z J Med 1987; 17:68–70.

201. Bansal VK, Bennett D, Molnar Z: Prolonged renal failure after rifampin. Am Rev Resp Dis 1977; 116:137–140.

202. Lamy P, Cacoub P, Deray G, et al: Acute renal failure and nephrotic syndrome caused by rifampicin: polymorphism of the nephrotoxicity of rifampicin. Ann Med Interne Paris 1989; 140:323–325.

203. Hirsch DJ, Bia FJ, Kashgarian M, et al: Rapidly progressive glomerulonephritis during antituberculous therapy. Am J Nephrol 1983; 3:7–10.

204. Kohler LJ, Gohara AF, Hamilton RW, et al: Crescentic fibrillary glomerulonephritis associated with intermittent rifampin therapy for pulmonary tuberculosis. Clin Nephrol 1994; 42:263–265.

205. Murray AN, Cassidy MJ, Templecamp C: Rapidly progressive glomerulonephritis associated with rifampicin therapy for pulmonary tuberculosis. Nephron 1987; 46:373–376.

206. Ogata H, Kubo M, Tamaki K, et al: Crescentic glomerulonephritis due to rifampin treatment in a patient with pulmonary atypical mycobacteriosis. Nephron 1998; 78:319–322.

207. Kumar S, Mehta JA, Trivedi HL: Light-chain proteinuria and reversible renal failure in rifampin-treated patients with tuberculosis. Chest 1976; 70:564–565.

208. Soffer O, Nassar VH, Campbell W Jr, et al: Light chain cast nephropathy and acute renal failure associated with rifampin therapy: renal disease akin to myeloma kidney. Am J Med 1987; 82:1052–1056.

209. Warrington RJ, Hogg GR, Paraskevas F, et al: Insidious rifampin-associated renal failure with light-chain proteinuria. Arch Intern Med 1977; 137:927–930.

210. Winter RJ, Banks RA, Collins CM, et al: Rifampicin induced light chain proteinuria and renal failure. Thorax 1984; 39:952–953.

211. Koch-Weser J, Sidel VW, Federman EB, et al: Adverse effects of sodium colistimethate: manifestations and specific reaction rates during 317 courses of therapy. Ann Intern Med 1970; 72:857–868.

212. Bevine GJ, Hansing CE, Octaviano GN, et al: Acute renal failure caused by sensitivity to polymyxin B sulfate. JAMA 1967; 202:62–64.

213. Pulaski E, Connell JF: Bacitracin in surgical wound infections. Bull US Army Med Dept 1949; 9:141–147.

214. Kahn SR: Acute interstitial nephritis associated with nitrofurantoin. Lancet 1996; 348:1177–1178.

215. Korzets Z, Elis A, Bernheim J, et al: Acute granulomatous interstitial nephritis due to nitrofurantoin. Nephrol Dial Transplant 1994; 9:713–715.

216. Ondrus J: Acute tubulointerstitial nephritis as a manifestation of furantoin poisoning. Cesk Pediatr 1993; 48:24–25.

217. Simenhoff ML, Guild WR, Dammin GJ: Acute diffuse interstitial nephritis: review of the literature and case report. Am J Med 1968; 44:618–625.

218. Muehrcke RC, Pirani CL, Kark RM: Interstitial nephritis: a clinicopathological renal biopsy case. Ann Intern Med 1967; 66:1052.

219. Sawaya BP, Briggs JP, Schnermann J: Amphotericin B nephrotoxicity: the adverse consequences of altered membrane properties. J Am Soc Nephrol 1995; 6:154–164.

220. Andreoli TE: On the anatomy of amphotericin B-cholesterol pores in lipid bilayer membranes. Kidney Int 1973; 4:337–345.

221. Wertlake PT, Butter WT, Hill GJ, et al: Nephrotoxic tubular damage and calcium deposition following amphotericin B therapy. Am J Pathol 1963; 43:449–457.

222. Sawaya BP, Weihprecht H, Campbell WR, et al: Direct vasoconstriction as a possible cause for amphotericin B–induced nephrotoxicity in rats. J Clin Invest 1991; 87:2097–2107.

223. Bell NH, Andriole VT, Sabesin SM, et al: On the nephrotoxicity of amphotericin B in man. Am J Med 1962; 33:64–69.

224. Holeman CWJ, Einstein H: Toxic effects of amphotericin B in man. Calif Med 1963; 99:90–93.

225. Wilson R, Feldman S: Toxicity of amphotericin B in children with cancer. Am J Dis Child 1979; 133:731–734.

226. Walsh TJ, Finberg RW, Arndt C, et al: Liposomal amphotericin B for empirical therapy in patients with persistent fever and neutropenia. National Institute of Allergy and Infectious Diseases Mycoses Study Group. N Engl J Med 1999; 340:764–771.

227. Burgess JL, Birchall R: Nephrotoxicity of amphotericin B, with emphasis on changes in tubular function. Am J Med 1972; 53:77–84.

228. McChesney JA, Maraquardt JF: Hypokalemic paralysis induced by amphotericin B. JAMA 1964; 189:1029–1031.

229. Malik IA, Moid I, Aziz Z, et al: A randomized comparison of fluconazole with amphotericin B as empiric anti-fungal agents in cancer patients with prolonged fever and neutropenia. Am J Med 1998; 105:478–483.

230. Barton CH, Pahl M, Vaziri ND, et al: Renal magnesium wasting associated with amphotericin B therapy. Am J Med 1984; 77:471–474.

231. Barbour GL, Straub KD, O'Neal BL, et al: Vasopressin-resistant nephrogenic diabetes insipidus: a result of amphotericin B therapy. Arch Intern Med 1979; 139:86–88.

232. Douglas JB, Healy JK: Nephrotoxic effects of amphotericin B, including renal tubular acidosis. Am J Med 1969; 46:154–162.

233. McCurdy DK, Frederic M, Elkinton JR: Renal tubular acidosis due to amphotericin B. N Engl J Med 1968; 278:124–131.

234. Gil FZ, Malnic G: Effect of amphotericin B on renal tubular acidification in the rat. Pflugers Arch 1989; 413:280–286.

235. Steinmetz PR, Lawson LR: Defect in urinary acidification induced in vitro by amphotericin B. J Clin Invest 1970; 49:596–601.

236. Miller RP, Bates JH: Amphotericin B toxicity. A follow-up report of 53 patients. Ann Intern Med 1969; 71:1089–1095.

237. Butler WT, Bennett JE, Alling DW, et al: Nephrotoxicity of amphotericin B: early and late effects in 81 patients. Ann Intern Med 1964; 61:175–187.

238. Bullock WE, Lake RG, Nuttall CE, et al: Can mannitol reduce amphotericin B nephrotoxicity? Double-blind study and description of a new vascular lesion in kidneys. Antimicrob Agents Chemother 1976; 10:555–563.

239. Fisher MA, Talbot GH, Maislin G, et al: Risk factors for amphotericin B-associated nephrotoxicity. Am J Med 1989; 87:547–552.

240. Stein RS, Alexander JA: Sodium protects against nephrotoxicity in patients receiving amphotericin B. Am J Med Sci 1989; 298:299–304.

241. Llanos A, Cieza J, Bernardo J, et al: Effect of salt supplementation on amphotericin B nephrotoxicity. Kidney Int 1991; 40:302–308.

242. Walev I, Bhakdi S: Possible reason for preferential damage to renal tubular epithelial cells evoked by amphotericin B. Antimicrob Agents Chemother 1996; 40:1116–1120.

243. Tolins JP, Raij L: Adverse effect of amphotericin B administration on renal hemodynamics in the rat: neurohumoral mechanisms and influence of calcium channel blockade. J Pharmacol Exp Ther 1988; 245:594–599.

244. Tolins JP, Raij L: Chronic amphotericin B nephrotoxicity in the rat: protective effect of calcium channel blockade. J Am Soc Nephrol 1991; 2:98–102.

245. Wong-Beringer A, Jacobs RA, Guglielmo BJ: Lipid formulations of amphotericin B: clinical efficacy and toxicities. Clin Infect Dis 1998; 27:603–618.

246. Sharkey PK, Graybill JR, Johnson ES, et al: Amphotericin B lipid complex compared with amphotericin B in the treatment of cryptococcal meningitis in patients with AIDS. Clin Infect Dis 1996; 22:315–321.

247. Walsh TJ, Hiemenz JW, Seibel NL, et al: Amphotericin B lipid complex for invasive fungal infections: analysis of safety and efficacy in 556 cases. Clin Infect Dis 1998; 26:1383–1396.

248. Joly V, Bolard J, Saint-Julien L, et al: Influence of phospholipid/amphotericin B ratio and phospholipid type on in vitro renal cell toxicities and fungicidal activities of lipid-associated amphotericin B formulations. Antimicrob Agents Chemother 1992; 36:262–266.

249. Novakova I, Donnelly P, de Witte T, et al: Itraconazole and cyclosporin nephrotoxicity. Lancet 1987; 2:920–921.

250. Lopez-Gil JA: Fluconazole-cyclosporine interaction: a dose-dependent effect? Ann Pharmacother 1993; 27:427–430.

251. Garcia R, Marin C, Herrera J, et al: Usefulness of ketoconazole combined with cyclosporin in renal transplantation. Invest Clin 1991; 32:115–121.

252. Collignon P, Hurley B: Interaction between fluconazole and cyclosporin. Lancet 1989; 2:867–868.

253. Canafax DM, Graves NM, Hilligoss DM, et al: Interaction between cyclosporine and fluconazole in renal allograft recipients. Transplantation 1991; 51:1014–1018.

254. Assan R, Fredj G, Larger E, et al: FK 506/fluconazole interaction enhances FK 506 nephrotoxicity. Diabetes Metabol 1994; 20:49–52.

255. Haskell LP, Mennemyer RP, Greenman R, et al: Isolated erythroid hypoplasia and renal insufficiency induced by long-term griseofulvin therapy. South Med J 1990; 83:1327–1330.

256. Magno WB, Shapiro SH: Serial light and electron microscopic changes in renal glomeruli in mice fed griseofulvin. Ann Clin Lab Sci 1993; 23:189–195.

257. Anonymous: Drugs used for superficial infections of the skin and mucous membranes. In Bennett DR, ed: Drug Evaluations Annual 1994. Rockville, MD: American Medical Association, 1994:1579–1610.

258. Seidel EA, Koenig S, Polis MA: A dose escalation study to determine the toxicity and maximally tolerated dose of foscarnet. AIDS 1993; 7:941–945.

259. Jacobson MA, Crowe S, Levy J, et al: Effect of foscarnet therapy on infection with human immunodeficiency virus in patients with AIDS. J Infect Dis 1988; 158:862–865.

260. Deray G, Martinez F, Katlama C, et al: Foscarnet nephrotoxicity: mechanism, incidence and prevention. Am J Nephrol 1989; 9:316–321.

261. Palestine AG, Polis MA, De Smet MD, et al: A randomized, controlled trial of foscarnet in the treatment of cytomegalovirus retinitis in patients with AIDS. Ann Intern Med 1991; 115:665–673.

262. Anonymous: Morbidity and toxic effects associated with ganciclovir or foscarnet therapy in a randomized cytomegalovirus retinitis trial: studies of ocular complications of AIDS Research Group, in collaboration with the AIDS Clinical Trials Group. Arch Intern Med 1995; 155:65–74.

263. Trolliet P, Dijoud F, Cotte L, et al: Crescentic glomerulonephritis and crystals within glomerular capillaries in an AIDS patient treated with foscarnet. Am J Nephrol 1995; 15(3):256–259.

264. Maurice-Estepa L, Daudon M, Katlama C, et al: Identification of crystals in kidneys of AIDS patients treated with foscarnet. Am J Kidney Dis 1998; 32:392–400.

265. Justrabo E, Zanetta G, Martin L, et al: Irreversible glomerular lesions induced by crystal precipitation in a renal transplant after foscarnet therapy for cytomegalovirus infection. Histopathology 1999; 34:365–369.

266. Zanetta G, Maurice-Estepa L, Mousson C, et al: Foscarnet-induced crystalline glomerulonephritis with nephrotic syndrome and acute renal failure after kidney transplantation. Transplantation 1999; 67:1376–1378.

267. Navarro JF, Quereda C, Quereda C, et al: Nephrogenic diabetes insipidus and renal tubular acidosis secondary to foscarnet therapy. Am J Kidney Dis 1996; 27:431–434.

268. Nyberg G, Blohme I, Persson H, et al: Foscarnet-induced tubulointerstitial nephritis in renal transplant patients. Transplant Proc 1990; 22:241.

269. Balani SK, Arison BH, Mathai L, et al: Metabolites of L-735,524, a potent HIV-1 protease inhibitor, in human urine. Drug Metab Dispos 1995; 23:266–270.

270. Kopp JB, Miller KD, Mican AM, et al: Crystalluria and urinary abnormalities associated with indinavir. Ann Intern Med 1997; 127:119–125.

271. Gagnon RF, Tsoukas CM, Watters AK: Light microscopy of indinavir crystals. Ann Intern Med 1998; 128:321.

272. Tsao JW, Kogan SC: Indinavir crystalluria. N Engl J Med 1999; 340:1329.

273. Rutstein RM, Feingold A, Meislich D, et al: Protease inhibitor therapy in children with perinatally acquired HIV infection. AIDS 1997; 11:F107–F111.

274. Tashima KT, Horowitz JD, Rosen S: Indinavir nephropathy. N Engl J Med 1997; 336:138–140.

275. Sarcletti M, Petter A, Zangerle R: Indinavir and interstitial nephritis. Ann Intern Med 1998; 128:320–321.

276. Marroni M, Gaburri M, Mecozzi F, et al: Acute interstitial nephritis secondary to the administration of indinavir. Ann Pharmacother 1998; 32:843–844.

277. Bianchetti MG, Roduit C, Oetliker OH: Acyclovir-induced renal failure: course and risk factors. Pediatr Nephrol 1991; 5:238–239.

278. Brigden D, Rosling AE, Woods NC: Renal function after acyclovir intravenous injection. Am J Med 1982; 73:182–185.

279. Firat H, Brun P, Loirat C, et al: Kidney failure induced by administration of acyclovir: apropos of 2 cases. Arch Fr Pediatr 1992; 49:641–643.
280. Tucker W, Jr, Macklin AW, Szot RJ, et al: Preclinical toxicology studies with acyclovir: acute and subchronic tests. Fundam Appl Toxicol 1983; 3:573–578.
281. Sawyer MH, Webb DE, Balow JE, et al: Acyclovir-induced renal failure: clinical course and histology. Am J Med 1988; 84:1067–1071.
282. Perazella MA: Crystal-induced acute renal failure. Am J Med 1999; 106:459–465.
283. Ahmad T, Simmonds M, McIver AG, et al: Reversible renal failure in renal transplant patients receiving oral acyclovir prophylaxis. Pediatr Nephrol 1994; 8:489–491.
284. Eck P, Silver SM, Clark EC: Acute renal failure and coma after a high dose of oral acyclovir. N Engl J Med 1991; 325:1178–1179.
285. Hernandez E, Praga M, Moreno F, et al: Acute renal failure induced by oral acyclovir. Clin Nephrol 1991; 36:155–156.
286. Johnson GL, Limon L, Trikha G, et al: Acute renal failure and neurotoxicity following oral acyclovir. Ann Pharmacother 1994; 28:460–463.
287. Krieble BF, Rudy DW, Glick MR, et al: Case report: acyclovir neurotoxicity and nephrotoxicity: the role for hemodialysis. Am J Med Sci 1993; 305:36–39.
288. Rashed A, Azadeh B, Abu Romeh SH: Acyclovir-induced acute tubulo-interstitial nephritis. Nephron 1990; 56:436–438.
289. Becker BN, Fall P, Hall C, et al: Rapidly progressive acute renal failure due to acyclovir: case report and review of the literature. Am J Kidney Dis 1993; 22:611–615.
290. Jacobson MA, Gallant J, Wang LH, et al: Phase I trial of valaciclovir, the L-valyl ester of acyclovir, in patients with advanced human immunodeficiency virus disease. Antimicrob Agents Chemother 1994; 38:1534–1540.
291. Wang LH, Schultz M, Weller S, et al: Pharmacokinetics and safety of multiple-dose valaciclovir in geriatric volunteers with and without concomitant diuretic therapy. Antimicrob Agents Chemother 1996; 40:80–85.
292. Lowance D, Neumayer HH, Legendre CM, et al: Valacyclovir for the prevention of cytomegalovirus disease after renal transplantation. International Valacyclovir Cytomegalovirus Prophylaxis Transplantation Study Group. N Engl J Med 1999; 340:1462–1470.
293. Aguado JM, Gomez-Sanchez MA, Lumbreras C, et al: Prospective randomized trial of efficacy of anti-cytomegalovirus (CMV) immunoglobulin to prevent CMV disease in CMV-seropositive heart transplant recipients treated with OKT3. Antimicrob Agents Chemother 1995; 39:1643–1645.
294. Dos Santos MF, Dos Santos OF, Boim MA, et al: Nephrotoxicity of acyclovir and ganciclovir in rats: evaluation of glomerular hemodynamics. J Am Soc Nephrol 1997; 8:361–367.
295. Cundy KC, Petty BG, Flaherty J, et al: Clinical pharmacokinetics of cidofovir in human immunodeficiency virus–infected patients. Antimicrob Agents Chemother 1995; 39:1247–1252.
296. Lacy SA, Hitchcock MJ, Lee WA, et al: Effect of oral probenecid coadministration on the chronic toxicity and pharmacokinetics of intravenous cidofovir in cynomolgus monkeys. Toxicol Sci 1998; 44:97–106.
297. Ho HT, Woods KL, Bronson JJ, et al: Intracellular metabolism of the antiherpes agent (S)-1-[3-hydroxy-2-(phosphonylmethoxy)propyl] cytosine. Mol Pharmacol 1992; 41:197–202.
298. Bedard J, May S, Lis M, et al: Comparative study of the anti-human cytomegalovirus activities and toxicities of a tetrahydrofuran phosphonate analogue of guanosine and cidofovir. Antimicrob Agents Chemother 1999; 43:557–567.
299. Lalezari JP, Drew WL, Glutzer E, et al: (S)-1-[3-hydroxy-2-(phosphonylmethoxy)propyl] cytosine (cidofovir): results of a phase I/II study of a novel antiviral nucleotide analogue. J Infect Dis 1995; 171:788–796.
300. Studies of Ocular Complications of AIDS Research Group in Collaboration with the AIDS Clinical Trials Group: Parenteral cidofovir for cytomegalovirus retinitis in patients with AIDS: the HPMPC peripheral cytomegalovirus retinitis trial. A randomized, controlled trial. Ann Intern Med 1997; 126:264–274.
301. Lalezari JP, Stagg RJ, Kuppermann BD, et al: Intravenous cidofovir for peripheral cytomegalovirus retinitis in patients with AIDS. A randomized, controlled trial. Ann Intern Med 1997; 126:257–263.
302. Cardineau E, Le Goff C, Henri P, et al: Nephropathies caused by interferon alpha: apropos of 2 cases. Rev Med Interne 1995; 16:691–695.
303. Honda K, Ando A, Endo M, et al: Thrombotic microangiopathy associated with alpha-interferon therapy for chronic myelocytic leukemia. Am J Kidney Dis 1997; 30:123–130.
304. Kobayashi H, Utsunomiya Y, Miyazaki Y, et al: Case of chronic myelogenous leukemia with hemolytic-uremic syndrome–like kidney during long-term interferon-alpha therapy. Nippon Naika Gakkai Zasshi 1997; 86:1259–1261.
305. Ravandi-Kashani F, Cortes J, Talpaz M, et al: Thrombotic microangiopathy associated with interferon therapy for patients with chronic myelogenous leukemia: coincidence or true side effect? Cancer 1999; 85:2583–2588.
306. Coroneos E, Petrusevska G, Varghese F, et al: Focal segmental glomerulosclerosis with acute renal failure associated with alpha-interferon therapy. Am J Kidney Dis 1996; 28:888–892.
307. Nassar GM, Pedro P, Remmers RE, et al: Reversible renal failure in a patient with the hypereosinophilia syndrome during therapy with alpha interferon. Am J Kidney Dis 1998; 31:121–126.
308. Shah M, Jenis EH, Mookerjee BK, et al: Interferon-α–associated focal segmental glomerulosclerosis with massive proteinuria in patients with chronic myeloid leukemia following high dose chemotherapy. Cancer 1998; 83:1938–1946.
309. Dhib M, Bakhache E, Postec E, et al: Nephrotic syndrome complicating treatment with interferon alpha. Presse Med 1996; 25:1066–1068.
310. Tashiro M, Yokoyama K, Nakayama M, et al: A case of nephrotic syndrome developing during postoperative gamma interferon therapy for renal cell carcinoma. Nephron 1996; 73:685–688.
311. Averbuch SD, Austin HA, Sherwin SA, et al: Acute interstitial nephritis with the nephrotic syndrome following recombinant leukocyte alpha interferon therapy for mycosis fungoides. N Engl J Med 1984; 310:32–35.
312. Kimmel PL, Abraham AA, Phillips TM: Membranoproliferative glomerulonephritis in a patient treated with interferon-α for human immunodeficiency virus infection. Am J Kidney Dis 1994; 24:858–863.
313. Endo M, Ohi H, Fujita T, et al: Appearance of nephrotic syndrome following interferon-α therapy in a patient with hepatitis B virus and hepatitis C virus coinfection. Am J Nephrol 1998; 18:439–443.
314. Lederer E, Truong L: Unusual glomerular lesion in a patient receiving long-term interferon-α. Am J Kidney Dis 1992; 20:516–518.
315. Rostaing L, Modesto A, Baron E, et al: Acute renal insufficiency in renal transplants treated with interferon-α for chronic hepatitis C. Nephrologie 1996; 17:247–254.

CHAPTER 28

Acute Renal Failure Associated With Cancer Chemotherapy

Mahendra Agraharkar ▪ Susan C. Guba ▪ Robert L. Safirstein

Chemotherapy is used with increasing frequency for treating malignant disorders in combination with surgery and radiation therapy. A variety of neoplastic conditions tend to cause acute renal failure (ARF) and increase the kidney's vulnerability to the nephrotoxic effect of antineoplastic drugs. The antineoplastic agents can cause or contribute to the renal and electrolyte abnormalities that are commonly associated with neoplasia. They also can indirectly cause tubular toxicity from hemoglobinuria and myoglobinuria. Tubulointerstitial disease and renal failure due to obstructive uropathy are also observed with some of the chemotherapeutic agents. Whatever its cause, ARF worsens the prognosis of patients with cancer because it can interfere with the effective management of the tumor. This chapter focuses first on those factors that are known to augment the nephrotoxic potential of antineoplastic drugs and then describes what is thought to be their direct nephrotoxic effects. The general notion to be pursued is that an awareness of the special susceptibility of the cancer patient to the nephrotoxic potential of these agents will promote better preparation of the patient before exposure is considered.

FACTORS THAT AUGMENT THE NEPHROTOXIC POTENTIAL OF ANTINEOPLASTIC DRUGS

Factors That Reduce the Effective Circulating Blood Volume

Anorexia, nausea, and vomiting as a direct consequence of malignant tumors or its treatment may lead to loss of effective circulating blood volume. If the thirst mechanism is also deranged due to the underlying neoplasm, it further augments hypovolemia from reduced fluid intake. Diabetes insipidus and diarrhea can also lead to profound fluid loss. Third-space fluid sequestration as seen in bowel obstruction, pancreatitis, and malignant effusions can lead to reduction in effective circulating blood volume. Similarly, liver failure, cardiac failure, and hypoalbuminemic states can contribute to prerenal azotemia and hypovolemic renal failure. The presence of these factors enhances the nephrotoxicity of antineoplastic drugs. Most patients with tenuous fluid status should be prehydrated to minimize the risk of damage to the kidney. Patients with poor performance status, extremely poor nutrition, and cardiac failure may not be treated with chemotherapy, since the overall toxicity of chemotherapy, not just nephrotoxicity, outweighs any potential benefit in a fragile cancer patient. Patients who have third-space fluid may not receive methotrexate because methotrexate may enter third-space fluid and enhance unacceptable myelotoxicity and gastrointestinal toxicity.

Intrinsic Renal Disease

Solid tumors and hematologic malignancies such as Hodgkin's disease, multiple myeloma, and leukemia are known to cause glomerular lesions such as membranous glomerulonephritis and minimal-change glomerulonephritis. This can cause hypoalbuminemia and diminished serum oncotic pressure. Sometimes these glomerulopathies may even compromise renal function, alter excretion of drugs, and enhance the nephrotoxic effects of the antineoplastic drugs.

Chronic Renal Failure

Those who already have some impairment of renal function are especially prone to the nephrotoxic effects of antineoplastic agents. In addition to obvious effects on the plasma level of potentially nephrotoxic drugs that reduced excretion imposes, body mass estimates may be erroneous because of the cachexia, weight loss, and edema that are present. Thus, estimates of glomerular filtration from plasma creatinine levels and body weight may be erroneous and dosing of antineoplastic agents would be seriously flawed.

Tumor Invasion of the Kidneys

The kidneys can be directly involved with tumor due to primary renal cancer or secondary invasion of the renal parenchyma from adjacent organs involved in a neoplastic condition. This can result in a significant loss of functioning renal tissue and thus reduce the glomerular filtration rate (GFR).

Tubulointerstitial Disease

Cancer patients may have tubulointerstitial disease due either to infiltration of the kidney parenchyma by tumor cells or to several of the medications that are administered. These patients invariably require pain medications, which can make them prone to interstitial nephritis. Prior exposure to radiocontrast material, radiation, and antibiotics has been associated with renal damage that has not been fully appreciated. These patients are particularly susceptible to the nephrotoxic potential of antineoplastic drugs, as is highlighted later when the nephrotoxic potential of individual drugs is discussed.

Obstructive Uropathy

Obstruction to the urinary tract is quite common in cancer patients. It is usually due either to extrinsic compression by a mass or to direct invasion of the urinary tract. Obstruction to the bladder neck and bilateral ureteral obstruction may be encountered in gynecologic malignancies, prostate cancer, and bladder cancer. Lymphomas and sarcomas are not infrequently encountered, causing mechanical obstruction as well. The obstruction may not be due to tumor alone but can also be due to stones or blood clots established by obstruction and invasion of tumor. Retroperitoneal fibrosis, secondary to breast cancer, drugs, or radiation, may interfere with ureteric peristalsis and cause obstructive renal failure.

Obstruction to the Tubules

Malignancies such as multiple myeloma and certain lymphomas secrete paraproteins, which can be filtered by the glomerulus at a rate exceeding the tubular capacity for reabsorption, causing the formation of proteinaceous casts. This condition is also termed *cast nephropathy*. Other conditions causing similar paraprotein syndromes are disorders of the hematopoietic system such as macroglobulinemia and cryoglobulinemia. These disorders may also be associated with glomerulopathy.

Acute Renal Failure Related to Severe Electrolyte Disorders

Hypercalcemia is perhaps the most common metabolic complication of cancer. It is related either to local osteolysis or humoral factors that cause bone resorption. Hypercalcemia can reduce the GFR and also potentiate the nephrotoxicity of antineoplastic drugs. Other electrolyte abnormalities causing ARF are hypokalemia and hypophosphatemia. Although rare, both conditions can cause rhabdomyolysis-related ARF. Hyperuricemia/urate nephrology may also result in ARF. Tumor lysis syndrome (hyperuricemia, hyperkalemia, hyperphosphatemia, and hypocalcemia) is a serious oncologic problem seen most commonly in hematologic malignancies and small cell lung cancer. Tumor lysis toxicity can be minimized with adequate hydration of the patient, alkalinization of the urine, allopurinol, and correction of electrolyte abnormalities prior to administration of chemotherapy.

ANTINEOPLASTIC AGENTS THAT CAUSE ACUTE RENAL FAILURE

A survey of incidence of ARF occurring within hospitalized patients revealed that 20% of such cases are related to antineoplastic therapy.[1] Several antineoplastic agents and their metabolites have predictable nephrotoxicity. These agents include the alkylating agents such as cisplatin and streptozotocin, the antimetabolite methotrexate, the antitumor antibiotic mithramycin (plicamycin), and the cytokine interleukin-2 (IL-2). These agents cause a fall in GFR in a more or less predictable manner, and the fall in GFR is dose related. Other agents may cause renal failure only after repeated doses, especially in combination with other antineoplastic agents, as a single exposure rarely causes renal failure. Such drugs are the alkylating agents such as lomustine (CCNU) and semustine (methyl-CCNU) and the antibiotic mitomycin (Table 28–1).

Alkylating Agents

CISPLATIN

Cisplatin is perhaps the most commonly used alkylating agent to treat solid tumors and also is perhaps the most studied antineoplastic drug for nephrotoxicity, both in animal models and in humans. It is commonly used in the malignancies involving the genitourinary tract, tumors of the head and neck, and lung cancers.

Pharmacokinetics. Cisplatin is highly protein bound; within 2 hours after a bolus infusion of cisplatin, 90% is protein bound mainly to albumin, transferrin, and gamma globulin.[2] The maximum red blood cell concentration is reached within 90 to 150 minutes, and it declines in a biphasic manner with a terminal half-life of 36 to 47 days. The highest concentrations are seen in the liver, prostate, and kidneys.

After a 40- to 140-mg/m² bolus administration of cisplatin, only 10% to 40% is excreted by the kidneys in 24 hours. Over 5 days, 35% to 51% is excreted in the urine. The renal clearance of free platinum exceeds the GFR, suggesting active secretion of the drugs by the kidney. The renal clearance of free platinum is nonlinear and variable. It is dependent on the dose, urine flow rate, and tubular secretion. There is no evidence of tubular reabsorption, suggesting that the kidneys accumulate cisplatin by peritubular uptake.

Pathogenesis. The uptake of cisplatin by the kidneys is energy dependent and mediated, in part, by the organic base transport systems. The principal sites of cisplatin nephrotoxicity is the proximal straight tubules in the S3 segment of the outer medullary stripe (the S3 segment accumulates the highest content of cisplatin) and where the maximum necrosis is observed. Minor changes in the distal nephron also have

TABLE 28–1. Antineoplastic Agents With Nephrotoxic Potential

DRUGS	INDICATIONS	TOXICITY	PRECAUTIONS
Alkylating agents			
Nitrogen mustards			
Cyclophosphamide	Hematologic malignancies Solid tumors Vasculitides and immune- mediated disorders	↑ Secretion and ↑ response to Hemorrhagic cystitis and bladder	Hydration Mesna
Ifosfamide	Germ cell tumors Soft tissue sarcomas Osteosarcoma Ewing tumor	Tubular dysfunction Distal RTA SIADH Hemorrhagic cystitis ↓ GFR	Hydration Divided dosing instead of single boluses Mesna
Nitrosoureas			
Carmustine (BCNU)	Lymphomas Multiple myeloma	Acute renal failure	Keep cumulative dose ≤ 1000 mg/m²
Lomustine (CCNU) Semustine (methyl-CCNU)	Primary brain tumors Melanoma Gastrointestinal tumors	Acute renal failure Glomerular sclerosis Interstitial fibrosis Tubular atrophy	Not known Not known
Streptozotocin	Pancreatic carcinoma Carcinoid tumor	Fanconi syndrome	Use at cumulative dose < 4000 mg/m²
Chlorozotocin	Pancreatic carcinoma	Fanconi syndrome and renal failure	Use at cumulative dose < 1500 mg
Metal salts			
Cisplatin	Genitourinary cancers Head and neck tumors Lung cancer	Reduced GFR Nonoliguric renal failure Hypomagnesemia Hemolytic-uremic syndrome	Solute diuresis with saline amifostine infusion
Carboplatin	Ovarian cancer	Renal failure	Hydration
Antimetabolites			
Methotrexate	Choriocarcinoma Osteosarcoma Bone marrow transplant Wegener granulomatosis Dermatomyositis Rheumatoid arthritis Crohn disease	Intratubular precipitation Direct tubular toxicity Acute tubular necrosis Nonoliguric renal failure	Hydration Alkalization of urine Methotrexate level monitoring Folinic acid administration
Cytosine arabinoside (cytarabine or ara-C)	Acute leukemia Non-Hodgkin lymphoma	Renal failure	Not known Avoid other nephrotoxic drugs
5-Fluorouracil (5-FU)	Carcinoma of the breast Gastrointestinal cancer Carcinoma of ovary Cervical carcinoma	Renal failure	Avoid cisplatin combination
Antitumor antibiotics			
Mitomycin C	Carcinoma of colon Carcinoma of stomach Bladder carcinoma	Acute tubular necrosis Microangiopathic renal failure	Avoid other nephrotoxic drugs Avoid dose > 50 mg/m²
Mithramycin (plicamycin)	Testicular cancer Glioblastoma Hypercalcemia of malignancy	↓ GFR	Avoid repeated administration
Biologic agents			
Interferon-α	Hematologic malignancies Many other cancers	Minimal change GN Renal insufficiency	Not known
Interleukin-2	Solid tumors Melanoma Renal cell carcinoma Colorectal cancer	Hypotension-related renal failure ↓ GFR	? Hydration
Vitamin A derivative			
Tretinoin (all-trans-retinoic acid)	Acute promyelocytic leukemia	Retinoic acid syndrome	High-dose dexamethasone Withhold therapy Supportive therapy

GFR, glomerular filtration rate; GN, glomerulonephritis; RTA, renal tubular acidosis; SIADH, syndrome of inappropriate secretion of antidiuretic hormone.

been observed, such as mitochondrial swelling and nuclear pallor. Glomerular involvement, however, is not observed.[3]

The exact mechanism of damage to the kidney is not known and may be mediated through cisplatin's well-known effect on DNA. Although the excreted platinum is predominantly cisplatin, once it enters the cell it is converted to a different platinum compound as it undergoes aqueous reaction and loses its labile chloride ligands. This renders the compound highly reactive and generates a positively charged electrophilic product. It is currently thought that the principal target of cisplatin that causes cell death is the generation of adducts produced by the binding of cisplatin to purine bases in DNA. The resultant structural alteration to DNA inhibits the template function of DNA and inhibits replication. This lesion is not produced by the oxiliplatin (Transplatin) isomer, which is neither nephrotoxic nor antineoplastic. Cisplatin may also cause damage to cells by depleting critical sulfhydryl centers, including glutathione, and provoking oxidant stress.[4] Either mechanism or both can lead to cell death either by virtue of necrosis or apoptosis, both of which are seen following cisplatin nephrotoxicity.[4]

Genotoxic stress could play a critical role in the nephrotoxic potential of cisplatin, as indicated by the nature of the molecular response of the kidney following its administration. Among the earliest responses to cisplatin exposure, and before significant morphologic or functional evidence of renal injury is evident, is a typical immediate early gene response and the activation of the p21[WAF1/CIP1] gene.[5] These genes are activated by oxidants and DNA-binding agents, and p21[WAF1/CIP1], which binds to and inhibits the cyclin-dependent kinases, prevents the replication of damaged DNA. Cells undergoing such inhibition to DNA replication may die if the injury cannot be repaired or survive if it can be repaired. p21 knockout animals are more susceptible to cisplatin-induced renal injury, suggesting that the same mechanisms may be applied to kidney cells. It would appear that the particular vulnerability of the kidney to cisplatin is in part determined by the kidney's role in its transport, which elevates the intracellular concentration of cisplatin to a critical level, and the consequent generation of DNA adducts that cannot be repaired.[5]

Clinical Manifestation. Cisplatin lowers the GFR predictably in a dose-dependent manner even after a single drug exposure.[6] The onset of renal failure is gradual and evolves 3 to 5 days after the administration of the drug. Early mild proteinuria (<500 mg per day), glycosuria, and enzymuria are common, even in the mildest form of ARF. In some patients a severe form of sodium divalent cation and phosphate wasting is seen, but this presentation is uncommon and is associated with high-dose therapy. The most common presentation, however, is the gradual onset of nonoliguric renal failure, with water excretion in excess of solute.[7] As evidenced in the micropuncture experiments, the cause of the concentrating defect is due to altered water reabsorption in the otherwise normal-appearing collecting ducts. In animal models, the reduced GFR is due to afferent vasoconstriction and possibly an altered ultrafiltration coefficient, before evidence of tubular obstruction.[8]

In a large percentage of patients receiving cisplatin, hypomagnesemia is also observed. It is usually seen in those who are repeatedly exposed to cisplatin therapy over a long period but may also occur in the acute setting.[9] It is more common when additional drugs such as gentamicin and amphotericin, which are known to cause hypomagnesemia, are simultaneously administered.[10] It appears that at least in animal models dietary magnesium deficiency plays a significant role in causing clinical magnesium deficiency.[11] Although hypomagnesemia remits when cisplatin therapy is discontinued, in some cases it may persist even after the withdrawal of treatment.[12] Hypokalemia and hypocalcemia may be seen in relation to cisplatin-induced hypomagnesemia and is reverted with the correction of hypomagnesemia. Hyponatremia is also observed, which may clinically manifest itself with postural hypotension.

Several studies have established that cisplatin reduces the GFR chronically in a dose-dependent manner.[6, 13–15] One study showed that patients receiving up to 850 mg of cisplatin in multiple courses had only a 9% reduction in hippuran clearance, whereas those receiving more than 850 mg of cisplatin had a 40% reduction in GFR over a 5-year period. The same study also observed a significant potentiation of cisplatin nephrotoxicity in those patients who received cisplatin in combination with radiation therapy.[6]

Cisplatin is also known to cause hemolytic-uremic syndrome (HUS). Usually the HUS resulting from cisplatin is aggressive and severe. Plasmapheresis and immunoadsorption using a staphylococcal protein A column have been successfully used in sporadic cases. Most often, cisplatin-induced HUS has a fatal outcome.[16]

Protective Measures. The best known protective measure is to establish a solute diuresis. A commonly used protocol is to ensure adequate hydration by infusing normal saline 12 to 24 hours prior to cisplatin therapy. This is followed by administration of the dose in isotonic saline over a 3-hour period, followed by saline infusion for 24 hours. The cisplatin dose is given daily for 5 days until the maximum total dose of 120 mg/m^2 of body surface area is reached. Higher doses are associated with an unacceptably higher degree of ARF even with proper hydration and diuresis.

The exact mechanism of the protection is unclear. Although the urinary concentration of cisplatin with these measures is lowered, neither the tissue concentration nor the cytotoxicity is reduced. It was initially considered that the higher chloride concentration in the urine after saline diuresis might be responsible for the renoprotective effect by reducing speciation into a toxic metabolite. However, a similar renal protective effect was observed after mannitol diuresis, where the urinary chloride concentration was reduced, suggesting some other mechanism.[17]

Diethyldithiocarbamate and sodium thiosulfate are chelating agents that have been used to reduce cisplatin toxicity. Diethyldithiocarbamate, a metabolite of disulfiram, was shown to compete for platinum binding to DNA. It has shown promise in experimental models; however, in human trials it was less successful due to its toxic effects and its failure to reduce other organ toxicity, such as ototoxicity.[18] Bismuth, by inducing another binding protein, metallothionein, offers some protection against cisplatin toxicity. Ethyol (amifostine) is an organic thiophosphate that is dephosphorylated by alkaline phosphatase in vivo into a free, active thiol metabolite. This metabolite has been proven to offer some protection against cisplatin nephrotoxicity. At this stage only amifostine (Ethyol) is clinically used at a recommended starting dose of 910 mg/m² administered daily by an intravenous infusion over 15 minutes, 30 minutes before the administration of cisplatin. Nausea, vomiting, hypotension, and hypocalcemia are prominent side effects.

CARBOPLATIN

Carboplatin is a newer platinum compound with less nephrotoxicity than cisplatin. The aqueous reaction, which is thought to be responsible for the nephrotoxicity, occurs at a slower pace and without affecting its antineoplastic property. It is used mainly in ovarian cancer but is also used in many other tumors, including neoplasm of the lung, head and neck, and cervix. The mechanism of action appears to be cell-cycle nonspecific, and, like cisplatin, it acts by DNA cross-linkage that inhibits the template function of DNA and its subsequent replication. Despite the difference in the aqueous reaction rate, which is slower in carboplatin, both cisplatin and carboplatin induced equal numbers of drug-DNA cross-links, causing equivalent lesions and biologic defects. The nephrotoxicity, however, is mild and rare. Usually, renal dysfunction may be detected only by measuring urinary tubular enzymes. Serum creatinine or creatinine clearance is rarely affected.

Anecdotal reports of renal failure have been described, especially when administered in high dosage without proper hydration. Severe hematuria possibly due to the sloughing of the transitional epithelium, causing urinary obstruction and ARF, has been reported in a patient treated with higher doses of carboplatin without aggressive hydration for the treatment of ovarian malignancy. Myelosuppression, especially thrombocytopenia, remains the major limiting factor for its use.[19, 20]

Precautions. Aggressive hydration similar to that used with cisplatin therapy may be all that is required.

CYCLOPHOSPHAMIDE

Cyclophosphamide is an alkylating agent that acts mainly by cross-linking DNA and inhibiting DNA replication. The generation of reactive intermediates in the liver is necessary via the cytochrome P450 system because the drug itself is inactive. Unlike the platinum compound, whose cytotoxicity is linked to intrastrand DNA linkage, the cytotoxicity of this alkylating com-

pound correlates well with interstrand DNA cross-linkage. The metabolites may also covalently link DNA and proteins and thus disrupt its template function. It is used to treat many hematologic malignancies and several solid tumors. It is also used in a variety of non-neoplastic conditions, such as systemic lupus erythematosus and other immune-mediated disorders.

Carcinogenesis, myelosuppression, and impairment of fertility are the most prominent side effects. Cyclophosphamide, when given in high doses, can enhance the release of antidiuretic hormone and increase the cellular response to it.[21, 22] This causes excretion of concentrated urine. Metabolites that are toxic to the bladder mucosa, such as acrolein, are therefore concentrated in the urine, enhancing toxicity to the bladder mucosa and causing hemorrhagic cystitis. In the long term this may cause bladder fibrosis.

IFOSFAMIDE

Ifosfamide, a synthetic analogue of cyclophosphamide, is effective in the treatment of germ cell testicular tumor. It is also used in treating other pediatric soft tissue sarcomas, osteosarcoma, and Ewing sarcoma.[23] Its metabolic activation also requires liver P450 activation, and these metabolites appear to bind to DNA. The major urinary metabolites, 4-carboxyifosfamide, thiodiacetic acid, and acrolein, are probably responsible for hemorrhagic cystitis. Ifosfamide, unlike cyclophosphamide, is also known to cause tubular dysfunction. The dose-related nephrotoxicity can be significantly reduced by administering the total dose in four divided doses rather than a single bolus infusion.[23] A proximal tubular reabsorptive defect and a small decline in the GFR are consistently observed in patients receiving multiple courses of non–platinum-containing protocols with ifosfamide. Previous renal disease, as with the use of cisplatin, increases the risk of nephrotoxicity with ifosfamide. Distal renal tubular acidosis, diabetes insipidus, and the syndrome of inappropriate secretion of antidiuretic hormone have each been reported with ifosfamide.[24–27]

Precautions and Prevention. Aggressive hydration alone is adequate to reduce toxicity in most cases. However, if a high dose of cyclophosphamide or ifosfamide is used, a detoxifying agent (mesna) may be used. The active ingredient of mesna is a synthetic sulfhydryl compound. Once in the body, mesna is oxidized to mesna disulfide, which is reduced to a free thiol compound in the kidney. It reacts chemically with the urotoxic metabolites acrolein and 4-hydroxy ifosfamide, rendering them innocuous.

Nitrosoureas

CARMUSTINE, LOMUSTINE, AND SEMUSTINE

Carmustine (BCNU), lomustine (CCNU), and semustine (methyl-CCNU) are lipophilic and therefore easily cross the blood-brain barrier. Therefore, they are widely used in the treatment of brain tumors.[28, 29]

Carmustine usually is given intravenously at a dose of 150 to 200 mg/m² infused over 1 to 2 hours. Its half-life is 15 to 90 minutes, with rapid dissociation into the cerebrospinal fluid. About 30% to 80% of the drug appears in the urine within 24 hours.[30] It is also used in the treatment of Hodgkin disease, other lymphomas, and multiple myeloma. It causes pulmonary fibrosis, hepatic failure, and renal failure when used in doses greater than 1000 mg/m².[31, 32] Lomustine and semustine are analogues of carmustine and have the same spectrum of clinical activity, but they are rarely used.[32]

STREPTOZOTOCIN

Streptozotocin was originally discovered as an antibiotic. It is a methylnitrosourea (MNU) moiety, has a special affinity for β-cells of the islets of Langerhans, and causes diabetes mellitus in experimental animals. It is used in the treatment of metastatic carcinoma of the pancreas and carcinoid tumor. Nephrotoxicity remains the chief limiting side effect, occurring in 75% of patients who receive prolonged streptozotocin treatment.[33]

The kidney is the major excretory route of streptozotocin. Proximal tubules appear to be the principal site of damage, and prolonged administration of streptozotocin may induce tubular reabsorptive abnormalities similar to those of Fanconi syndrome. Although not firmly established, it appears that the cumulative dose that is nephrotoxic is 4 g/m² body surface area. However, proximal tubular dysfunction may be seen even after a single exposure.[34, 35] It is best avoided in the presence of preexisting renal insufficiency, and great caution should be exercised in using it with other nephrotoxic drugs.[36]

Antimetabolites

METHOTREXATE

Methotrexate is an analogue of folic acid and is usually used in combination with other antineoplastic drugs to reduce tumor burden. It was the first drug to produce a striking, although temporary, remission in leukemia and the first drug to cure a solid tumor malignancy. It is used in the treatment of choriocarcinoma, osteogenic sarcoma, bladder cancer, and breast cancer as well as in cytoreductive protocols for bone marrow transplant recipients. Methotrexate is also used in non-neoplastic conditions requiring potent inhibitors of cell-mediated immune response such as dermatomyositis, rheumatoid arthritis, Wegener granulomatosis, and Crohn disease.[37]

After a conventional intravenous dose, more than 90% of the drug appears unchanged in the urine. It is principally excreted via the kidney by glomerular filtration and tubular secretion. Nephrotoxicity is rarely a problem at low doses. In certain malignancies, such as osteogenic sarcoma, higher doses are needed and nephrotoxicity can occur unless proper precau-

tions are taken. In the presence of renal insufficiency, the bone marrow, gastrointestinal, and renal toxicity are more pronounced. The exact mechanism of nephrotoxicity is unclear, but intratubular precipitation of methotrexate in an acidic urine appears to be the most likely mechanism. Adequate hydration and alkalization of the urine seem to offer some protection against methotrexate-mediated nephrotoxicity. Proximal tubular necrosis without precipitation of methotrexate has also been noted, suggesting a direct nephrotoxic effect of methotrexate.[38–40]

Clinical Course. Typically, methotrexate-related renal failure is nonoliguric. Reduction of glomerular filtration further increases the serum methotrexate level, amplifying renal damage. Plasma levels exceeding 0.5 μM, 48 hours after methotrexate infusion, are associated with a 40% incidence of severe toxicity.

Preventive Measures. Adequate hydration and alkalization of the urine may be all that are necessary to prevent toxicity. Monitoring of methotrexate levels is helpful, especially in high-risk patients (see earlier). Neither peritoneal dialysis nor hemodialysis is useful for the removal of the drug. Plasma exchange is also ineffective in enhancing drug clearance.[40]

CYTOSINE ARABINOSIDE

Cytosine arabinoside, also known as *cytarabine* or *ara-C*, is a pyrimidine nucleoside that inhibits DNA synthesis when activated by the enzyme deoxycytidine kinase. Deamination of cytosine arabinoside yields uracil arabinoside, which is the principal metabolite that appears in the urine. Cytosine arabinoside is used in the treatment of acute leukemia and non-Hodgkin lymphoma in multidrug protocols. Renal failure develops in 50% of patients treated with a regimen using cytosine arabinoside, even if the other drugs used are not known to be nephrotoxic. The incidence of renal failure is especially high if used in combination with cisplatin and hydroxyurea. When used in patients with prior renal insufficiency, cytosine arabinoside causes a higher degree of nephrotoxicity and neurotoxicity. The exact mechanism of the injury, however, is unknown.[41, 42]

5-FLUOROURACIL

5-Fluorouracil, also known as *5-FU*, is a pyrimidine analogue that inhibits the methylation reaction of deoxyuridylic acid to thymidylic acid and thus interferes with the synthesis of both RNA and DNA. It is used in the treatment of metastatic carcinomas of the breast and gastrointestinal tract. It is also used as an adjuvant drug for the treatment of colorectal cancers. Beneficial effects have also been reported in treating hepatoma and carcinomas of the ovary, cervix, urinary bladder, prostate, pancreas, and oropharynx. When given with mitomycin-C, 5-fluorouracil provokes severe renal insufficiency in 10% of patients treated for carcinoma of the gastrointestinal tract and pancreas. In several reports, a clinical picture of microangiopathy is described and the histopathology reveals fibrin thrombi in the arterioles, with intimal hyperplasia. Interstitial fibrosis, tubular atrophy, and glomerular necrosis are observed in the chronic form. The combination of 5-fluorouracil and cisplatin used in the treatment of resistant advanced solid tumor of the head and neck and esophageal and invasive cervical cancer[43, 44] is especially nephrotoxic.

FIVE-AZACYTIDINE

Five-Azacytidine is a cytidine analogue, which, like 5-fluorouracil, interferes with RNA and DNA synthesis. It has negligible nephrotoxicity when used alone but does induce renal tubular acidosis, glycosuria, phosphaturia, and mild azotemia when used in combination with other chemotherapeutic agents.[45, 46]

Antitumor Antibiotics

MITOMYCIN-C

Mitomycin-C is an antibiotic isolated from *Streptomyces caespitosus* and participates in alkylation reactions with DNA, causing single-strand and chromosomal breaks. The drug inhibits DNA synthesis, causes single-strand breaks in DNA, and also causes chromosomal breaks. The drug undergoes external biologic conversion because less than 10% of the active drug is excreted in the urine or the bowel. It is primarily used to treat anal and sometimes gastric cancer.

Chemical Toxicity. Late-onset myelotoxicity with leukopenia and thrombocytopenia appears to be the major toxic effect. In preclinical studies, acute tubular necrosis was induced by a single intravenous dose, although only a small fraction of the drug is excreted by the kidneys. Animal studies show a direct tubulotoxic effect.[47–49] The mechanism of the nephrotoxicity is unknown. The nephrotoxicity is usually mild and most likely dose related. However, nephrotoxicity of mitomycin-C is more frequent and severe when used in combination with other nephrotoxic drugs. It manifests clinically as ARF associated with microangiopathy, especially at a dose that exceeds 50 mg/m², well above currently used dose regimens.

MITHRAMYCIN

Mithramycin inhibits RNA synthesis and has a limited role in treating testicular cancer and glioblastomas. Its antiosteoclastic function is secondary to its inhibition of messenger-RNA synthesis. It is therefore used in treating hypercalcemia associated with malignancy. At a usual single intravenous dose of 25 μg/kg of body weight, the serum calcium level is normalized in most cases and no nephrotoxicity is observed. However, repeated administration has been reported to cause nephrotoxicity in up to 40% of cases. The mechanism of this nephrotoxicity is not known.[50–53]

Biologic Agents

INTERFERONS

Interferons are glycoproteins that have antiviral, immunomodulatory, and antitumor activity. Interferon-α and interferon-β each cause evidence of renal damage.[54–56] Proteinuria is more common with interferon-α, and nephrotic syndrome with histopathologic changes of minimal change glomerulopathy has been reported.[57] The occurrence of renal failure is rare.[58] Interferon-γ, however, is associated with ARF and histologic evidence of acute tubular necrosis.[59] Interferons might also cause the development of autoantibodies that trigger interstitial nephritis and glomerular injury.

INTERLEUKIN-2

Interleukin-2 is a polypeptide cytokine that is not directly cytotoxic but enhances a T-cell response that is cytolytic for tumor cells. A control study infusing IL-2–activated cells, termed *lymphokine-activated-killer* (LAK) *cells,* concurrently with IL-2 is associated with regression of several solid tumors, including malignant melanoma, renal cell carcinoma, and colorectal cancer.[60] A reduction in blood pressure, GFR, and sodium excretion occurs during the period of drug infusion, which resolves when the infusion is stopped,[61] and a fall in GFR is documented in 90% of patients receiving IL-2.[62] Although the clinical picture is consistent with prerenal azotemia, with a fall in blood pressure, GFR, salt retention, and azotemia, massive fluid infusion does not abrogate the fall in GFR, suggesting a primary intrarenal hemodynamic effect of the drug.[63]

Gallium Nitrate

Although gallium nitrate was originally developed as an antineoplastic drug, it has little antitumor activity. Rather, it is used in cancer patients for its antibone resorption effect and to treat the hypercalcemia of malignancy. In preliminary studies, gallium nitrate infusions were associated with renal insufficiency that was thought to be caused by the precipitation of gallium-calcium-phosphate crystals in the tubules. However, subsequent experiments have shown that continuous infusion of gallium nitrate of as high a dose as 200 mg/m² for 5 days caused mild reduction in GFR and hypophosphatemia in a few cases.[64–66]

Retinoic Acid Derivatives

Tretinoin (all-*trans*-retinoic acid) is a vitamin A derivative that is known to induce cellular differentiation and apoptosis in blood precursors and particularly in the cells from patients with acute promyelocytic leukemia. Tretinoin enhances morphologic and functional maturation of leukemic promyelocytes and the appearance of normal hematopoietic cells, eventually reduces blood cell counts, and reduces the number of relapses.

Although tretinoin is well tolerated in most patients, a few cases of what has been termed *retinoic acid syndrome* have been reported. This syndrome is characterized by weight gain, respiratory distress, serous effusions, and sometimes cardiac and renal failure. It is associated with an increase in leukocyte count, suggesting the release of several cytokines as the cause. In the Acute Promyelocytic Leukemia 93 trial in which 61 patients developed retinoic acid syndrome, 41% also developed renal failure.[67–69]

Precautions and Treatment. High-dose dexamethasone intravenously is used soon after the detection of the first symptom of the syndrome. Other measures include transient discontinuation of tretinoin and supportive treatment, including mechanical ventilation and hemodialysis when required.

CHEMOTHERAPY, TUMOR LYSIS, AND ACUTE RENAL FAILURE

Tumors with high rates of growth can release potential nephrotoxic products, especially after response to chemotherapy. These "high-turnover tumors," after massive cytolysis, generate high levels of potassium, phosphate, uric acid, xanthine, and other substances that can cause ARF. It can also significantly worsen preexisting renal insufficiency. This syndrome is more commonly seen after the treatment of acute leukemia, malignant lymphoma, and bulky solid tumors.[70, 71]

Hyperuricemia

Acute hyperuricemia-induced renal failure is frequently seen with the therapy of leukemia and lymphomas and has been reported in disseminated carcinoma. It can also occur spontaneously. In one series the incidence of ARF after therapy for non-Hodgkin lymphoma was 6% of all patients but was significantly higher in those with high-grade malignancy and renal insufficiency. Preventive measures, including pretreatment with allopurinol and alkaline diuresis, have reduced the incidence of this complication greatly.[70–74]

Xanthine Nephropathy

Rarely, xanthine concentrations in the blood can increase to levels that cause intratubular precipitation during cytolysis, when allopurinol is used to prevent uric acid nephropathy. Those patients who have minor degrees of hypoxanthine-guanine-phosphoribosyl transferase deficiency are more likely to develop xanthine nephropathy. Xanthine, like uric acid, is poorly soluble in acid urine. Alkalization of the urine therefore may be helpful.[75, 76]

Hyperphosphatemic Nephropathy

Hyperphosphatemia can cause ARF. Although the exact mechanism of extreme hyperphosphatemia is not known, therapy directed toward reducing phosphate levels improves GFR, which may require hemodialysis.[77–79]

BONE MARROW TRANSPLANT–RELATED ACUTE RENAL FAILURE

The role of bone marrow transplant is rapidly expanding in the treatment of neoplastic and non-neoplastic conditions. The current indications for bone marrow transplantation include aplastic anemia, hematologic malignancies and solid tumors, some of the immunodeficiency states, a small number of hereditary enzyme deficiency states, and certain hemoglobinopathies. The incidence of renal failure in the patients treated with bone marrow transplant can be 40% or higher.[80–83]

The timing of the ARF in relation to the bone marrow transplant suggests its cause. During the first 10 days after the bone marrow transplant, less than 5% of patients develop renal failure, which is most likely due to either the tumor lysis syndrome or the infusion of bone marrow.[84, 85] Tumor lysis may be a consequence of the inductive chemotherapy regimen with or without total body irradiation to enhance engraftment. However, more commonly, the renal failure is secondary to the bone marrow infusate itself, most probably a result of the lysis of cells in the stored infusate. More than 75% of patients receiving bone marrow develop hemoglobinuria, and a portion of these patients develop ARF. ARF occurring within 10 to 21 days of the bone marrow infusion is usually associated with hepatorenal syndrome and veno-occlusive hepatic dysfunction. The mortality in these patients requiring dialysis may be as high as 80% to 90%.[86–91]

Twenty percent of patients who have survived the initial period of bone marrow transplant may develop delayed renal failure. Renal failure may appear without overt signs and may have subclinical renal dysfunction, especially those who received total body irradiation. Chronic cyclosporine toxicity may also be observed in those patients who received the drug for protection against graft-versus-host disease.

Bone Marrow Transplant Nephropathy

Bone marrow transplant nephropathy occurs several months after the bone marrow transplant and manifests as HUS with hypertension, anemia, thrombocytopenic purpura, proteinuria, microscopic hematuria, and renal failure. Four to 12 months after bone marrow transplant, thrombotic angiopathy–related ARF may appear, which could be related to either bone marrow transplant or chemotherapy. This HUS/thrombotic thrombocytopenic purpura–like syndrome may clinically and histopathologically mimic radiation nephritis with mesangiolysis, arterial fibrinoid necrosis, and ill-defined subendothelial deposits, along with glomerular capillary fibrin thrombi. The pathogenesis is unknown, but aggressive inductive therapy with cyclosporine is a risk factor. Angiotensin-converting enzyme inhibitors, angiotensin receptor blockers, and plasma exchange have been successfully used for the prevention of bone marrow transplant nephropathy.[92–95] Improvement in the peripheral smear may take several weeks after discontinuation of the drug.

CONCLUSION

Several factors potentiate the development of ARF in cancer patients. The treatment of the malignant conditions with nephrotoxic antineoplastic drugs increases the likelihood of inducing ARF. The mortality in this population is significantly higher with the development of renal failure, and the occurrence of renal failure in these patients reduces their survival. Identification of factors such as preexisting renal disease, renal insufficiency, and contracted intravascular volume may help in minimizing the nephrotoxic potential of these drugs by either correcting the underlying conditions or adjusting the dose of nephrotoxic antineoplastic agents for the level of renal dysfunction. The use of other nephrotoxic drugs, such as nonsteroidal anti-inflammatory drugs, aminoglycosides, and amphotericin, is best avoided when nephrotoxic antineoplastic drugs are included in the protocol. Optimum hydration and use of potent antiemetics for some time after treatment are probably the most important preventive measures available. More detailed knowledge of the mechanisms of ARF and repair undoubtedly will aid in the treatment of these disorders.

REFERENCES

1. Eliahou HE, Boichis H, Bott-Kanner G, et al: An epidemiologic study of renal failure: II. Acute renal failure. Am J Epidemiol 1975; 101:281.
2. Safirstein R, Miller P, Guttenplan JB: Uptake and metabolism of cisplatin by rat kidney. Kidney Int 1984; 25:753.
3. Gonzales-Vitale JC, Hayes DM, Cvitkovic E, et al: The renal pathology in clinical trials of cis-platinum (II) diaminodichloride. Cancer 1977; 39:1362.
4. Levi J, Jacobs C, Kalman SM, et al: Mechanism of cis-platinum nephrotoxicity: I. Effects on sulfhydryl groups in rat kidneys. Pharmacol Exp Ther 1980; 213:545.
5. Megyesi J, Safirstein RL, Price PM: Induction of p21[wafl/cip1/sdi1] in kidney tubule cells affects the course of cisplatin-induced acute renal failure. J Clin Invest 1998; 101:777–782.
6. Aass N, Fossa SD, Asa M, et al: Renal function related to different treatment modalities for malignant germ cell tumors. Br J Cancer 1990; 62:842.
7. Safirstein R, Miller P, Dikman S, et al: Cisplatin nephrotoxicity in rats: defect in papillary hypertonicity. Am J Physiol 1982; 241:F175.
8. Winston JA, Safirstein R: Reduced renal blood flow in early cisplatin-induced acute renal failure in the rat. Am J Physiol 1985; 249:F490.
9. Schilsky RL, Anderson T: Hypomagnesemia and renal magnesium wasting in patients receiving cisplatin. Ann Intern Med 1979; 90:929.
10. Buckley JE, Clark VL, Meyer TJ, et al: Hypomagnesemia after cisplatin combination chemotherapy. Arch Intern Med 1984; 144:2347.
11. Mavichak V, Wong NL, Quamme GA, et al: Studies on the pathogenesis of cisplatin-induced hypomagnesemia in rats. Kidney Int 1985; 28:914.
12. Daugaard G, Abildgaard U: Cisplatin nephrotoxicity. Cancer Chemother Pharmacol 1989; 25:1.
13. Meijer S, Sleijfer DT, Mulder NK, et al: Some effects of combination chemotherapy with cis-platinum on renal function in patients with nonseminomatous testicular carcinoma. Cancer 1983; 51:2035.
14. Fjeldborg P, Sorensen J, Helkjaer PE: The long-term effect of cisplatin on renal function. Cancer 1986; 58:2214.
15. Daugaard G, Rossing N, Rorth M: Effects of cisplatin on different measures of glomerular function in the human kidney with special emphasis on high dose. Cancer Chemother Pharmacol 1988; 21:163.
16. Palmisano J, Agraharkar M, Kaplan A: Successful treatment of cisplatin-induced hemolytic-uremic syndrome (HUS) using therapeutic plasma exchange (TPE). Am J Kidney Dis 1998; 32:314.
17. Bodenner DL, Dedon PC, Keng PC, et al: Effect of diethyldithiocarbamate on cis-diamminedichloroplatinum (II)–induced cytotoxicity, DNA cross-linking, and gamma-glutamyl transpeptidase inhibition. Cancer Res 1986; 46:2745.
18. Berry JM, Jacobs C, Sikic B, et al: Modification of cisplatin toxicity with diethyldithiocarbamate. J Clin Oncol 1990; 8:1585.
19. Egorin MJ, Van Echo DA, Tipping SJ, et al: Pharmacokinetics and dosage reduction of cis-diammine (1,1-cyclobutanedicarboxylate) platinum in patients with impaired renal function. Cancer Res 1984; 44:5432.
20. Agraharkar M, Palmisano J, Kaplan A: Carboplatin-induced hematuria and acute renal failure. Am J Kidney Dis 1998; 32:E5.
21. DeFronzo RA, Colvin OM, Braine H, et al: Proceedings: cyclophosphamide and the kidney. Cancer 1974; 33:483.
22. Bode U, Seif SM, Levine AS: Studies on the antidiuretic effect of cyclophosphamide: vasopressin release and sodium excretion. Med Pediatr Oncol 1980; 8:295.
23. Zalupski M, Baker LH: Ifosfamide. J Natl Cancer Inst 1988; 80:556.
24. Antman KH, Montella D, Rosenbaum KC, et al: Phase II trial of ifosfamide with mesna in previously treated metastatic sarcoma. Cancer Treat Rep 1985; 69:499.
25. Goren MP, Wright RK, Pratt CB, et al: Potentiation of ifosfamide neurotoxicity, hematotoxicity, and tubular nephrotoxicity by pri-cis-diamminedichloroplatinum (II) therapy. Cancer Res 1987; 4:1456.
26. Patterson WP, Khojasteh A: Ifosfamide-induced renal tubular defects. Cancer 1989; 63:649.
27. Rossi R, Godde A, Kleinebrand A, et al: Unilateral nephrectomy and cisplatin as risk factors for ifosfamide-induced nephrotoxicity: analysis of 120 patients. J Clin Oncol 1994; 12:159.
28. Carter SK, Wasserman TH: The nitrosoureas—thoughts for the future. Cancer Treat Rep 1976; 60:807.
29. Oliverio VT: Toxicology and pharmacology of the nitrosoureas: III. Cancer Chemother Rep 1973; 4:13.
30. Sponzo RW, DeVita VT, Oliverio VT: Physiologic disposition of 1-(2-chloroethyl)-3-(4-methylcyclohexyl)-1-nitrosourea (Me CCNU) in man. Cancer 1973; 31:1154.
31. Schacht RG, Feiner HD, Gallo GR, et al: Nephrotoxicity of nitrosoureas. Cancer 1981; 48:1328.
32. Micetich KC, Jensen-Akula M, Mandard JC, et al: Nephrotoxicity of semustine (methyl CCNU) in patients with malignant melanoma receiving adjuvant chemotherapy. Am J Med 1981; 71:967.
33. Weiss RB: Streptozocin: a review of its pharmacology, efficacy, and toxicity. Cancer Treat Rep 1982; 66:427.
34. Bhuyan BK, Kuentzel SL, Gray LG, et al: Tissue distribution of streptozotocin (NSC-85998). Cancer Chemother Rep 1974; 58:157.
35. Loftus L, Cuppage FE, Hoogstraten B: Clinical and pathological effects of streptozotocin. J Lab Clin Med 1974; 84:407.
36. Schein PS, O'Connell MJ, Blom J, et al: Clinical antitumor activity and toxicity of streptozotocin (NSC-85998). Cancer 1974; 34:993.
37. Bukowski RM, Tangen C, Lee R, et al: Phase II trial of chlorozo-

tocin and fluorouracil in islet cell carcinoma: a Southwest Oncology Group study. J Clin Oncol 1992; 10:1914.

38. Hande KR, Donehower RC, Chabner BA: Pharmacology and pharmacokinetics of high-dose methotrexate in man. In: Pindeo HM, ed: *Clinical Pharmacology of Antineoplastic Drugs*. North Holland: Elsevier; 1978:97–114.

39. Pitman SW, Parker LM, Tattersall MHN, et al: Clinical trial of high-dose methotrexate (NSC 740) with citrovorum factor (NSC 3590): toxicologic and therapeutic observations. Cancer Chemother Rep 1975; 6:43.

40. Stoller RG, Hande KR, Jacobs SA, et al: Use of plasma pharmacokinetics to predict and prevent methotrexate toxicity. N Engl J Med 1977; 297:630.

41. Thierry FX, Vernier I, Dueymes JM, et al: Acute renal failure after high-dose methotrexate therapy: role of hemodialysis and plasma exchange in methotrexate removal. Nephron 1989; 51:416.

42. Pitman SW, Frei E III: Weekly methotrexate–calcium leukovorin rescue: effect of alkalinization on nephrotoxicity—pharmacokinetics in the CNS and use in CNS non-Hodgkin's lymphoma. Cancer Treat Rep 1977; 61:695.

43. Hidemann W: Cytosine arabinoside in the treatment of acute myeloid leukemia: the role and place of high-dose regimens. Ann Hematol 1991; 62:119.

44. Capizzi RL, White JC, Powell BL, et al: Effect of dose on the pharmacokinetic and pharmacodynamic effects of cytarabine. Semin Hematol 1991; 28:54.

45. Jassem J, Gyergyay F, Kerpel-Fronius S, et al: Combination of daily 4-h infusion of 5-fluorouracil and cisplatin in the treatment of advanced head and neck squamous cell carcinoma: a Southeast European Oncology Group study. Cancer Chemother Pharmacol 1993; 31:489.

46. Park TK, Choi DH, Kim SN, et al: Role of induction chemotherapy in invasive cervical cancer. Gynecol Oncol 1991; 41:107.

47. Von Hoff DD, Penta JS, Helman LJ, et al: Incidence of drug-related deaths secondary to high-dose methotrexate and citrovorum factor administration. Cancer Treat Rep 1977; 61:745.

48. Peterson BA, Collins AJ, Vogelzang NJ, et al: 5-Azacytidine and renal tubular dysfunction. Blood 1981; 57:182.

49. Philips FS, Schwartz HS, Sternberg SS: Pharmacology of mitomycin-C: I. Toxicity and pathologic effects. Cancer Res 1960; 20:1354.

50. Ratanatharathorn V: Clinical and pathological study of mitomycin C nephrotoxicity. In: Carter SK, Crooke ST, eds: *Mitomycin C: Current Status and New Developments*. New York: Academic Press; 1979:219–230.

51. Price TM, Murgo AJ, Keveney JJ, et al: Renal failure and hemolytic anemia associated with mitomycin C. Cancer 1985; 55:51.

52. Kennedy BJ: Metabolic and toxic effects of mithramycin during tumor therapy. Am J Med 1970; 49:494.

53. Kennedy BJ, Brown JH, Yarbro JW: Mithramycin (NSC-24559) therapy for primary glioblastomas. Cancer Chemother Rep 1965; 48:59.

54. Cortes EP, Holland JF, Moskowitz R, et al: Effects of mithramycin on bone resorption in vitro. Cancer Res 1972; 34:74.

55. Hall TJ, Schaeublin M, Chambers TJ: The majority of osteoclasts require mRNA and protein synthesis for bone resorption in vitro. Biochem Biophys Res Commun 1993; 195:12245.

56. Bean B: Antiviral therapy: current concepts and practices. Clin Microbiol Rev 1992; 5:146.

57. Krown SE: Interferons and interferon inducers in cancer treatment. Semin Oncol 1986; 13:207.

58. Talpaz M, Kantarjian HM, Kurzrock R, et al: Therapy of chronic myelogenous leukemia: chemotherapy and interferons. Semin Hematol 1988; 25:62.

59. Selby P, Kohn J, Raymond J, et al: Nephrotic syndrome during treatment with interferon. BMJ 1985; 290:1180.

60. Sherwin SA, Knost JA, Fein S, et al: A multiple-dose phase I trial of recombinant leukocyte A interferon in cancer patients. JAMA 1982; 319:1397.

61. Ault BH, Stapleton FB, Gaber L, et al: Acute renal failure during therapy with recombinant human gamma interferon. N Engl J Med 1988; 296:1134.

62. Rosenberg SA: Immunotherapy of cancer by systemic administra-

tion of lymphoid cells plus interleukin-2. J Biol Response Mod 1984; 3:501.

63. Textor SC, Margolin K, Bloyney D, et al: Renal, volume, and hormonal changes during therapeutic administration of recombinant interleukin-2 in man. Am J Med 1987; 83:1055.

64. Belldegrun A, Webb DE, Austin HA III, et al: Effects of interleukin-2 on renal function in patients receiving immunotherapy for advanced cancer. Ann Intern Med 1987; 106:817.

65. Ponce P, Cruz J, Travassos J, et al: Renal toxicity mediated by continuous infusion of recombinant interleukin-2. Nephron 1993; 64:114.

66. Warrell RP Jr, Israel R, Frisone M, et al: Gallium nitrate for acute treatment of cancer-related hypercalcemia. Ann Intern Med 1988; 108:669–674.

67. Krakoff IH, Newman RA, Goldberg RSL: Clinical toxicologic and pharmacologic studies of gallium nitrate. Cancer 1979; 44:1722–1727.

68. Warrell RP Jr, Murphy WK, Schulman P, et al: A randomized, double-blind study of gallium nitrate compared with etidronate for acute control of cancer-related hypercalcemia. J Clin Oncol 1991; 9:1467–1475.

69. Fenaux P, Chastang C, Sanx M, et al: ATRA followed by chemotherapy versus ATRA plus chemotherapy and the role of maintenance therapy in newly diagnosed APL: first interim results of APL93 trial [abstract]. Blood 1997; 90(Suppl 1):122a.

70. Fenaux P, De Botton S: Retinoic acid syndrome: recognition, prevention, and management. Drug Safety 1998; 18:273–279.

71. Hatake K, Uwai M, Ohtsuki T, et al: Rare but important adverse effects of all-trans-retinoic acid in acute promyelocytic leukemia and their management. Int J Hematol 1997; 66:13–19.

72. Cohen L, Balow JE, Magrath IT, et al: Acute tumor lysis syndrome: a review of 37 patients with Burkitt's lymphoma. Am J Med 1980; 68:486.

73. Vogelzang NJ, Nelimark RA, Nath KA: Tumor lysis syndrome after induction chemotherapy of small cell bronchogenic carcinoma. JAMA 1983; 249:513.

74. O'Connor NT, Prentice HG, Hoffbrand AV: Prevention of urate nephropathy in the tumour lysis syndrome. Clin Lab Haematol 1989; 11:97.

75. Jasek AM, Day HJ: Acute spontaneous tumor lysis syndrome. Am J Hematol 1994; 47:29.

76. Hande KR, Yarrow GC: Acute tumor lysis syndrome in patients with high-grade non-Hodgkin's lymphoma. Am J Med 1993; 94:13.

77. Gomez GA, Stutzman L, Chu TM: Xanthine nephropathy during chemotherapy in deficiency of hypoxanthine-guanine phosphoribosyltransferase. Arch Intern Med 1978; 138:1017.

78. Aubert JD, Claeys M, Zwahlen A, et al: Hyperphosphatemia and transient renal insufficiency following chemotherapy of acute lymphoblastic leukemia. Schweiz Med Wochenschr 1988; 118:1953.

79. Kanfer A, Richet G, Roland J, et al: Extreme hyperphosphataemia causing acute anuric nephrocalcinosis in lymphosarcoma. BMJ 1979; 1:1320.

80. Boles JM, Dutel JL, Briere J, et al: Acute renal failure caused by extreme hyperphosphatemia after chemotherapy of an acute lymphoblastic leukemia. Cancer 1984; 53:2425.

81. Bortin MM, Horowitz MM, Rimm AA: Increasing utilization of allogeneic bone marrow transplantation. Ann Intern Med 1992; 116:505.

82. Zager RA, O'Quigley J, Zager BK, et al: Acute renal failure following bone marrow transplantation: a retrospective study of 272 patients. Am J Kidney Dis 1989; 13:210.

83. Beelen DW, Quabeck K, Kaiser B, et al: Six weeks of continuous intravenous cyclosporine and short-course methotrexate as prophylaxis for acute graft-versus-host disease after allogeneic bone marrow transplantation. Transplantation 1990; 50:421.

84. Tarbell NJ, Guinan EC, Chin L, et al: Renal insufficiency after total body irradiation for pediatric bone marrow transplantation. Radiother Oncol 1990; 18:139.

85. Zager RA: Acute renal failure in the setting of bone marrow transplantation [abstract]. Kidney Int 1994; 46:1443.

86. Davis JM, Rowley SD, Braine HG, et al: Clinical toxicity of cryopreserved bone marrow graft infusion. Blood 1990; 75:781.

87. Gruss E, Bernis C, Tomas JF, et al: Acute renal failure and bone marrow transplantation: Proceedings of the Third Satellite Symposium, Halkidiki, Greece, 1993.

88. McDonald GB, Sharma P, Matthews DE, et al: Venocclusive disease of the liver after bone marrow transplantation: diagnosis, incidence, and predisposing factors. Hepatology 1984; 4:116.

89. Jones RJ, Lee KS, Beschorner WE, et al: Veno-occlusive disease of the liver following bone marrow transplantation. Transplantation 1987; 44:778.

90. McDonald GB, Hinds MS, Fisher LD, et al: Veno-occlusive disease of the liver and multiorgan failure after bone marrow transplantation: a cohort study of 355 patients. Ann Intern Med 1993; 118:255.

91. Okamoto Y, Takaue Y, Saito S, et al: Toxicities associated with cryopreserved and thawed peripheral blood stem cell autografts in children with active cancer. Transfusion 1993; 33:578–581.

92. Kessinger A, Schmit-Pokorny D, Smith D, et al: Cryopreservation and infusion of autologous peripheral blood stem cells. Bone Marrow Transplant 1990; 5(Suppl 1):25–27.

93. Oyama Y, Komatsuda A, Imai H, et al: Late-onset bone marrow transplant nephropathy. Ann Intern Med 1996; 35:489–493.

94. Moulder JE, Fish BL, Cohen EP, Bonsib SM: Angiotensin II receptor antagonists in the prevention of radiation nephropathy. Radiat Res 1996; 146:106–110.

95. Moulder JE, Cohen EP, Fish BL, Hill P: Prophylaxis of bone marrow transplant nephropathy with captopril, an inhibitor of angiotensin-converting enzyme. Radiat Res 1993; 136:404–407.

Acute Renal Failure Associated With Radiocontrast Agents

Christiane M. Erley

The use of iodinated contrast media (CM) continues to be a common cause of hospital-acquired acute renal failure (ARF), and its development increases the in-hospital mortality significantly.[1] Contrast media–induced nephropathy (CMIN) is defined as an otherwise unexplained acute deterioration of renal function after intravascular administration of iodinated CM. Although the clinical features and the histopathologic findings of CMIN have been well described,[2-5] its pathogenesis, prevention, and best treatment modality still remain uncertain.

DEFINITION

Most authors define CMIN by an increase in the serum creatinine level of more than 1 mg/dL 2 to 3 days after CM exposure. Other reasons for an acute deterioration of renal function have to be excluded. Some investigators even believe that less of an increase in serum creatinine level (0.5 mg/dL 2 to 4 days after CM) also should be classified as CMIN. It would also be prudent to look for a decrease in the glomerular filtration rate (GFR), generally greater than 25% from baseline, with more sensitive methods (ie, inulin clearance).[6] Next to changes in the GFR or serum creatinine, an increase in urinary enzyme excretion seems also to be a sensitive marker of tubular damage after CM exposure.[6, 7] However, no conclusive relationship can be demonstrated between the detection of enzymes in urine and the decrease in GFR.[7-9]

CLINICAL FINDINGS AND HISTOPATHOLOGY

Usually, the increase in serum creatinine level starts 24 to 48 hours after CM exposure; the level then peaks after 3 to 5 days and returns to baseline 7 to 10 days thereafter. Except for patients with a higher degree of renal function impairment, CMIN presents as a nonoliguric form of ARF. Neither temporary nor continuous dialysis is required very often. Although most patients show only minor and transient effects on renal function after CM exposure, a recent study showed that even an increase of serum creatinine level without requirement of dialysis was related to a higher in-hospital mortality rate compared with patients without CMIN.[1]

Morphologic changes appear mainly as vacuolar changes in the proximal convoluted tubular cells.[5, 10, 11] These morphologic changes parallel the elevation in urinary enzyme excretion,[5, 12] but a strong relationship to renal function impairment after CM has not been demonstrated.[13]

Incidence

The incidence of CMIN in the literature ranges from less than 1% to more than 70%.[14-17] This discrepancy results from the lack of a single reliable definition, different methods of investigation, different types of radiologic procedures, use of high- or low-osmolar CM, and the presence or absence of risk factors. In patients without any risk factor, the incidence is less than 1% despite the use of volumes as much as 800 mL of CM.[18] An increasing number of cases of CMIN have been observed within the last years. This seems to be related to the wider use of diagnostic and therapeutic interventions in elderly and critically ill patients.[4, 19]

Risk Factors

A preexistent impairment of renal function is commonly regarded as the most important risk factor for CMIN.[2, 3, 15, 20, 21] Consistent with multivariate regression analyses, diabetes mellitus is frequently cited next to renal insufficiency as a self-standing risk factor for CMIN.[2, 3, 21, 22] However, in controlled studies it has not been shown that diabetic patients without renal functional impairment are at higher risk for developing CMIN.[23, 24] Because diabetic patients suffer from a number of vascular complications that contribute to renal damage, including abnormalities in endothelial function, this point still has to be clarified. After having developed renal insufficiency, diabetics are at significantly higher risk for CMIN compared with patients with other forms of renal failure.[25] In contrast with many other patients, they may develop an oliguric form of CMIN and subsequently need to be dialyzed more often. In contrast with findings in previous observations,[22, 26, 27] the volume of CM seems to be a risk factor in diabetic, azotemic patients only.[17, 28, 29] Because of a laboratory investigation on the intratubular precipitation of Bence-Jones protein after CM exposure, multiple myeloma has long been recognized as a self-standing risk factor. A recent retrospective analysis[30] demonstrated that patients with multiple myeloma seem not to have an increased risk for developing CMIN.

PATHOGENESIS

In general, CM exerts effects on renal hemodynamics and on the tubular system.[31] After injection of CM there is a transient increase, followed by a more prolonged decrease, in renal blood flow.[32-34] A variety of vasoactive substances may modulate the CM-induced vasoconstriction, including prostaglandins, atrial natriuretic peptide (ANP), adenosine, endothelin, vasopressin, noradrenaline, and angiotensin.[35] By measuring these substances after CM exposure and by using antagonists of these vasoactive substances (such as misoprostol, bosentan, angiotensin-converting enzyme [ACE] inhibitors, α-blockers),[34, 36-40] the degree of involvement in the process of developing CMIN has been investigated. So far only endothelin and adenosine seem to play a role as key factors in CMIN.[38, 39, 41]

CM induces intrarenal hypoxia, possibly related to the hemodynamic changes and/or an increased tubular energy expenditure due to osmotic stress.[31] It has been proposed that increased renal adenosine levels as a result of enhanced adenosine triphosphate hydrolysis may be a major factor in the development of ARF after CM application (Fig. 29-1). This is corroborated by the finding that application of CM increases urinary adenosine[42, 43] and the observation that dipyridamole, a nucleoside uptake blocker, enhances the renal hemodynamic effects of CM.[42, 43] Next to this there are some similarities between CM-induced nephrotoxicity and renal hemodynamic changes induced by adenosine. Sodium depletion is known to potentiate adenosine action in the kidney[44, 45] and also to augment the nephrotoxicity of CM.[33, 37] Blockade of the production of vasodilatory prostaglandins by indomethacin increases both the adenosine effect in the kidney[46] and the vasoconstriction induced by CM.[13, 47, 48] Ischemia prior to application of CM increases their toxicity[49] and renal ischemia enhances adenosine generation, leading to renal vasoconstriction.[44, 50, 51] CM and adenosine both

showed disparate effects regarding regional blood flow of the kidney with medullary vasodilation.[48, 52]

Experimental studies in different animal models of ARF revealed a nephroprotective effect of adenosine antagonism.[53-60] Theophylline, for instance, acts as an unspecific adenosine receptor antagonist. Studies in dogs and rats showed a nephroprotective effect of theophylline after application of CM.[42] Our own group showed that rats under chronic nitric oxide blockade are highly sensitive to CM damage, and adenosine antagonists (theophylline and 1, 3-dipropyl-8-cyclopentylxanthine [DPCPX]) showed favorable effects concerning the prevention of a decline in GFR and renal blood flow (Fig. 29-2) in this animal model of CMIN.[61]

PREVENTION AND TREATMENT

Choice of Contrast Media

Studies performed after the introduction of new low-osmolar (nonionic) CMs so far have failed to show that these substances reduce the incidence of CMIN in comparison with high-osmolar (ionic) CM.[3, 62-65] The largest trial involving a high number of azotemic patients (509 of 1196 patients), including 213 diabetics, also found a negligible incidence of CMIN with either low-osmolar or high-osmolar CM.[22] However, patients suffering from renal function impairment due to diabetic nephropathy have a twofold incidence of CMIN by using high-osmolar CM.[22] A recent published meta-analysis also showed that low-osmolar CM may be beneficial for patients with azotemia,[66] although the difference was small and the higher price of low-osmolar CM has to be taken into consideration. The definition of *low osmolar* still means substances with an osmolarity of around 600 mOsm/kg (compared with high-osmolar CM with an osmolarity of around 1400 mOsm/kg). Thus, the development of iso-osmolar CM (ie,

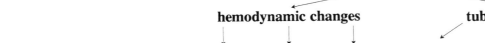
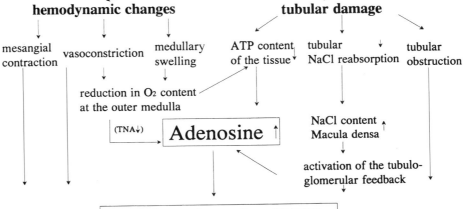

FIGURE 29-1 ■ Pathogenesis of contrast media–induced nephropathy. *ATP,* adenosine triphosphate; *GFR,* glomerular filtration rate.

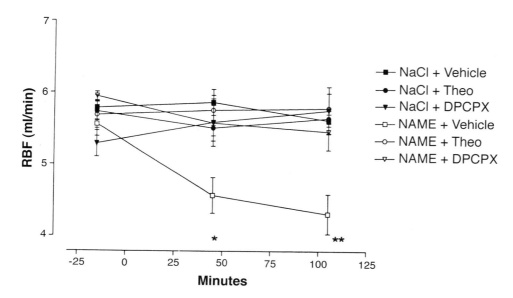

FIGURE 29-2 ■ Decline in renal blood flow (*RBF*) in rats with hypertension and renal vasoconstriction due to chronic nitric oxide inhibition by n(G)-nitro-L-arginine methyl ester (I-NAME) compared with controls after contrast medium application. Data obtained after the administration of adenosine antagonists (theophylline [*Theo*] and 1, 3-dipropyl-8-cyclopentylxanthine [*DPCPX*]) are also shown. (From Erley CM, Heyne N, Burgert K, et al: Prevention of radiocontrast-induced nephropathy by adenosine antagonists in rats with chronic nitric oxide deficiency. J Am Soc Nephrol 1997; 8:1125–1132; with permission.)

iodixanol) may bring another benefit regarding the development of CMIN.[35, 67, 68] An increasing number of studies use magnetic resonance imaging (MRI) CM as an alternative to prevent CMIN in azotemic patients for computed tomographic (CT) scanning or angiography.[69–71] However, the only proven benefit of these substances in conventional radiology (despite MRI) is the lack of iodine exposure in highly allergic patients. The disadvantages of the MRI CM are their high viscosity and osmolarity. This theoretically also limits their use for CMIN prevention (especially because the volume of contrast agents needed for a CT or angiography is much higher than for an MRI [100 mL vs. 15 mL]). Controlled studies in azotemic patients treated with either iso-osmolar CM or with MRI CM are not available. Another promising alternative to conventional radiographic CM seems to be the use of carbon dioxide, which provides a negative contrast. Studies performed so far showed less nephrotoxicity,[72, 73] although short-lasting ischemia of the perfused organs has been described. It cannot be used for investigation of cerebral vessels or for detecting smaller vessels. Although not proven yet, the development of alternative CM or alternative investigations might be an option in conventional investigations using iodinated CM in the future.

Hydration, Mannitol, and Diuretics

HYDRATION

Theoretically, prehydration of patients may have the following beneficial effects on the kidney:

- Decreased activity of the renin-angiotensin system
- Down-regulation of the tubuloglomerular feedback
- Augmentation of diuresis and sodium excretion
- Dilution of the CM and thus prevention of renal cortical vasoconstriction
- Reduced preconstriction of the vessels

- Avoidance of tubular obstruction
- Reduction of endothelin and other intrarenal vasoconstrictive mediators (eg, vasopressin)

MANNITOL

Most studies dealing with the issue of hydration in the prevention of CMIN have addressed the role of mannitol or the role of vasodilators such as dopamine, ANP, calcium antagonists, or ACE inhibitors with regard to the protection of the kidney from CM damage.[17, 25, 74–77] The authors have found that hydration alone was as effective as or even better than additional administration of hypertonic mannitol or the administration of one of the vasodilative agents. Other investigators have compared results in patients submitted to special hydration protocols with historical control groups[78, 79] or data reported in the literature.[80–82] Only hydration alone went along with a lowered incidence of ARF. So far, only one controlled, randomized study compared saline administration alone (0.45% saline over 24 hours, starting 12 hours before administration of radiocontrast dye) with mannitol (25 g of mannitol given 60 minutes before administration of radiocontrast dye) or furosemide (80 mg intravenously).[74] In this study administration of saline alone was the most successful strategy. In numerous studies dealing with the nephroprotective effect of nonionic CM, prehydration of the patients was included in the protocol,[22, 65] but patients with cardiac failure, liver cirrhosis, or edema mostly have been excluded from the studies to avoid overhydration.

USE OF DIURETICS

Which Fluid and When to Start. Most investigators administer 0.45% saline in combination with 5% dextrose intravenously in various amounts (around 1000 to 1500 mL, starting 12 hours before administration of radiocontrast agents). There is no controlled study that has assessed oral hydration in these patients. Until now, how long hydration should be continued has not been investigated. From a theoretical point of view the use of hyperosmolar fluids (such as 15% mannitol) in addition to the administration of the hyperosmolar CM may have adverse effects. Therefore, it is not surprising that most studies failed to observe a beneficial effect of mannitol in this setting.[25, 74, 78] In accordance with the experimental data, good results in humans have been obtained with hydration prior to and up to 12 hours after CM exposure.[74, 78, 81] Only a minor beneficial effect could be seen when fluid was administered during the procedure.[79, 82]

Effect of Diuretics. No conclusive evidence is available to support a protective role of loop-active diuretics with regard to the prevention of CMIN. It has been claimed that a reduction of the workload of the tubular cells by decreasing the rate of sodium reabsorption might be tubuloprotective. Additionally, there might be a dilution effect by an increment of diuresis after furosemide. Most investigators dealing with this point showed no or sometimes even worse results in the case of furosemide application.[74, 83, 84] The negative effect of furosemide could result from the reduction of cortical resistance inducing distribution of renal perfusion with reduced perfusion of the medulla. In combination with the CM-induced vasoconstriction the oxygen content could be reduced to a critical point and thereby deteriorate ischemia. Furosemide should be used with caution because there is always the fear of dehydration, which would enhance the nephrotoxicity of contrast agents.

Use of Vasoactive Substances as Prophylaxis

CALCIUM CHANNEL BLOCKERS

Owing to their vasodilating effect and the hope to prevent calcium overload in the tubular cells,[33] calcium channel blockers have been used in both experimental[55] and clinical studies.[42, 85, 86] Despite early promising results, large prospective trials have failed to observe a beneficial effect regarding the decline in GFR after CM exposure.[87–89] Taken together, a prophylactic value of calcium channel blockers (either short or long acting) has not been proven.

DOPAMINE

Dopamine given in the so-called "renal doses" of around 2 μg/kg per minute is widely used to prevent and treat ARF induced under various circumstances. So far, most prospective studies have failed to demonstrate any real benefit of dopamine in the setting of CMIN.[76, 90] An interesting point seems to be the observation that a prophylactic treatment with dopamine in 497 patients with ARF increased the mortality rate, which could be due to the proarrhythmic effect of this substance.[91]

ATRIAL NATRIURETIC PEPTIDE

Because of its natriuretic and vasodilative activity, next to its effect on the intracellular adenosine triphosphate concentration,[92] ANP seems to be a good candidate for the prevention of CMIN. Until now, no conclusive results have been obtained in clinical studies.[25, 75, 93] This may be due to the route of application (intravenous versus intra-arterial in experimental studies) and to intrarenal hemodynamic changes induced by ANP with induction of a steal phenomenon.

ADENOSINE ANTAGONISTS

In accordance with animal data, preliminary studies in humans indicated a nephroprotective effect of theophylline (an unspecific adenosine antagonist) concerning the reduction of GFR after application of CM.[43, 94] However, a large double-blind, placebo-controlled study performed in patients with chronic renal failure has failed to show a benefit of theophylline when given to otherwise stable and well-hydrated, mildly azotemic patients.[8] It can be argued that low tubular flow rates, as a result of dehydration and stimulation of the renin-angiotensin system, lead to prolonged tubular exposure to CM and that this combination is the main reason for a fall in GFR after CM. Adenosine seems to play a key role in developing CMIN only in cases of renal vasoconstriction.[41] Patients with heart failure or an inability to be sufficiently hydrated due to other conditions and a higher degree of renal insufficiency have been excluded from prospective trials that investigated the effects of theophylline. Clinical trials involving patients with contraindications for hydration should be carried out to clearly evaluate the value of theophylline in the prevention of CMIN. Preliminary results obtained through a retrospective study showed that theophylline administration on an intensive care unit showed good results regarding the incidence of CMIN in patients with cardiac insufficiency. (The incidence of ARF without theophylline was 15%; with theophylline, it was 7%.[95])

Antioxidant Agents

Reactive oxygen species may have a role in renal damage caused by contrast agents.[96, 97] In rats, contrast agents increased lipid peroxidation,[98] and superoxide dismutase, a scavenger of reactive oxygen species, preserved renal function.[99] Acetylcysteine, a thiol-containing antioxidant, has been used to treat a variety of pulmonary diseases and to treat acute acetaminophen poisoning. Recently, however, it has been used successfully to ameliorate the toxic effects of a variety of experimentally or clinically induced ischemia-reperfusion syndromes of the heart, kidney, lung, and liver.[100–102] In each of these syndromes, it is thought that the activity of acetylcysteine is related to its action as a free-radical scavenger, or as a reactive sulfhydryl compound that increases the reductive capacity of the cell. Tepel and coworkers[103] recently published the first clinical trial using acetylcysteine (1200 mg of acetylcysteine per day, given orally in divided doses on the day before and on the day of the administration of the radiocontrast agent) in order to prevent the decline in renal function in patients with moderate renal insufficiency, who were undergoing computed tomography. These preliminary data should be confirmed in a larger number of patients and in patients with even more seriously compromised renal function before acetylcysteine can be considered a potentially useful drug for prevention of CMIN, especially because, in the trial of Tepel and coworkers, the placebo group did not show a significant decline in renal function and significant differences resulted from the decline in creatinine levels in the acetylcysteine group compared with the stable creatinine levels in the placebo group.

Hemodialysis After Contrast Media Exposure

Many nephrologists use hemodialysis in azotemic patients to enhance the elimination rate of CM from the body. From a pathophysiologic point of view, hemodialysis normally initiated from 30 to 120 minutes after CM application cannot prevent the effects on the renal hemodynamic situation. The only prospective study done so far, by Lehnert and associates, showed no benefit regarding the development of ARF in dialyzed patients compared with controls.[104] In the author's own institute they performed another controlled study with azotemic patients. Fifteen patients with an impaired renal function (mean serum creatinine concentration 2.7 ± 0.2 mg/dL) were randomly assigned to receive either a hemodialysis procedure for 2 to 3 hours, started as early as possible after administration of CM (106 ± 25 minutes), or a conservative treatment. The course of absolute changes in serum creatinine level over the whole observation period was not different in both groups. The percentage of increase in serum creatinine level the day after CM application was higher in the group that underwent hemodialysis. The rate of CMIN (defined as serum creatinine level increase of ≥ 0.5 mg/dL within 48 hours after administration of CM) was significantly higher in the dialyzed group (43% in the hemodialysis group and 13% in the group with conservative treatment, respectively). The serum iodine concentration declined earlier in the dialyzed group. In summary, dialysis has no proven benefit in regard to prevention of CMIN in azotemic patients.

REFERENCES

1. Levy EM, Viscoli CM, Horwitz RI: The effect of acute renal failure on mortality: a cohort analysis. JAMA 1996; 275:1489–1494.
2. Berns AS: Nephrotoxicity of contrast media. Kidney Int 1989; 36:730–740.
3. Barrett BJ, Parfrey PS, Vavasour HM, et al: Contrast nephropathy in patients with impaired renal function: high versus low osmolar media. Kidney Int 1992; 41:1274–1279.
4. Rudnick MR, Berns JS, Cohen RM, Goldfarb S: Contrast media–associated nephrotoxicity. Curr Opin Nephrol Hypertens 1996; 5:127–133.
5. Moreau JF, Droz D, Sabto J, et al: Osmotic nephrosis induced by water-soluble triiodinated contrast media in man. Radiology 1975; 115:329–336.
6. Bettmann MA: The evaluation of contrast-related renal failure. AJR Am J Roentgenol 1991; 157:66–68.
7. Hunter JV, Kind PRN: Nonionic iodinated contrast media: potential renal damage assessed with enzymuria. Radiology 1992; 183:101–104.
8. Erley CM, Duda SH, Rehfuss D, et al: Prevention of radiocontrast-media–induced nephropathy in patients with preexisting renal insufficiency by hydration in combination with the adenosine antagonist theophylline. Nephrol Dial Transplant 1999; 14:1146–1149.
9. Donadio C, Tramonti G, Giordani R, et al: Glomerular and tubular effects of ionic and nonionic contrast media (diatrizoate and iopamidol). Contrib Nephrol 1988; 68:212–219.
10. Tervahartiala P, Kivisaari L, Kivisaari R, et al: Structural changes in the renal proximal tubular cells induced by iodinated contrast media. Nephron 1997; 76:96–102.
11. Dobrota M, Powell CJ, Holtz E, et al: Biochemical and morphological effects of contrast media on the kidney. Acta Radiol Suppl 1995; 399:196–203.
12. Battenfeld R, Khater AE, Drommer W, et al: Ioxaglate-induced light and electron microscopic alterations in the renal proximal tubular epithelium of rats. Invest Radiol 1991; 26:35–39.
13. Heyman SN, Brezis M, Reubinoff CA, et al: Acute renal failure with selective medullary injury in the rat. J Clin Invest 1988; 82:401–412.
14. Rich MW, Crecelius CA: Incidence, risk factors, and clinical course of acute renal insufficiency after cardiac catheterization in patients 70 years of age or older: a prospective study. Arch Intern Med 1990; 150:1237–1242.
15. Davidson CJ, Hlatky M, Morris KG, et al: Cardiovascular and renal toxicity of a nonionic radiographic contrast agent after cardiac catheterization: a prospective trial. Ann Intern Med 1989; 110:119–124.
16. D'elia JA, Gleason RE, Alday M, et al: Nephrotoxicity from angiographic contrast material: a prospective study. Am J Med 1982; 72:719–725.
17. Manske CL, Sprafka JM, Strony JT, Wang Y: Contrast nephropathy in azotemic diabetic patients undergoing coronary angiography. Am J Med 1990; 89:615–620.
18. Rosovsky MA, Rusinek H, Berenstein A, et al: High-dose administration of nonionic contrast media: a retrospective review. Radiology 1996; 200:119–122.
19. Tublin ME, Murphy ME, Tessler FN: Current concepts in contrast media-induced nephropathy. Am J Roentgenol 1998; 171:933–939.
20. Vanzee BE, Hoy WE, Talley TE, Jaenike JR: Renal injury associated with intravenous pyelography in nondiabetic and diabetic patients. Ann Intern Med 1978; 89:51–54.
21. Moore RD, Steinberg EP, Powe NR, et al: Nephrotoxicity of high-osmolality versus low-osmolality contrast media: randomized clinical trial. Radiology 1992; 182:649–655.
22. Rudnick MR, Goldfarb S, Wexler L, et al: Nephrotoxicity of ionic and nonionic contrast media in 1196 patients: a randomized trial. Kidney Int 1995; 47:254–261.
23. Parfrey PS, Griffiths SM, Barrett BJ, et al: Contrast material–induced renal failure in patients with diabetes mellitus, renal insufficiency, or both: a prospective controlled study. N Engl J Med 1989; 320:143–149.
24. Lautin EM, Freeman NJ, Schoenfeld AH, et al: Radiocontrast-associated renal dysfunction: incidence and risk factors. AJR Am J Roentgenol 1991; 157:49–58.
25. Weisberg LS, Kurnik PB, Kurnik BR: Risk of radiocontrast nephropathy in patients with and without diabetes mellitus. Kidney Int 1994; 45:259–265.
26. Gomes AS, Baker JD, Martin PV, et al: Acute renal dysfunction after major arteriography. AJR Am J Roentgenol 1985; 145:1249–1253.
27. Taliercio CP, McCallister SH, Holmes DR, et al: Nephrotoxicity of nonionic contrast media after cardiac angiography. Am J Cardiol 1989; 64:815–816.

28. Rudnick MR, Berns JS, Cohen RM, Goldfarb S: Contrast media–associated nephrotoxicity. Semin Nephrol 1997; 17:15–26.
29. Cigarroa RG, Lange RA, Williams RH, Hillis LD: Dosing of contrast material to prevent contrast nephropathy in patients with renal disease. Am J Med 1989; 86:649–652.
30. McCarthy CS, Becker JA: Multiple myeloma and contrast media. Radiology 1992; 183:519–521.
31. Heyman SN, Rosen S, Brezis M: Radiocontrast nephropathy: a paradigm for the synergism between toxic and hypoxic insults in the kidney. Exp Nephrol 1994; 2:153–157.
32. Katzberg RW, Morris TW, Burgener FA, et al: Renal renin and hemodynamic responses to selective renal artery catheterization and angiography. Invest Radiol 1977; 12:381–388.
33. Bakris GL, Burnett JCJ: A role for calcium in radiocontrast-induced reductions in renal hemodynamics. Kidney Int 1985; 27:465–468.
34. Caldicott WJ, Hollenberg NK, Abrams HL: Characteristics of response of renal vascular bed to contrast media: evidence for vasoconstriction induced by renin-angiotensin system. Invest Radiol 1970; 5:539–547.
35. Katzberg RW: Urography into the 21st century: new contrast media, renal handling, imaging characteristics, and nephrotoxicity. Radiology 1997; 204:297–312.
36. Workman RJ, Shaff MI, Jackson RV, et al: Relationship of renal hemodynamic and functional changes following intravascular contrast to the renin-angiotensin system and renal prostacyclin in the dog. Invest Radiol 1983; 18:160–166.
37. Larson TS, Hudson K, Mertz JI, et al: Renal vasoconstrictive response to contrast medium: the role of sodium balance and the renin-angiotensin system. J Lab Clin Med 1983; 101:385–391.
38. Heyman SN, Clark BA, Kaiser N, et al: Radiocontrast agents induce endothelin release in vivo and in vitro. J Am Soc Nephrol 1992; 3:58–65.
39. Oldroyd SD, Haylor JL, Morcos SK: Bosentan, an orally active endothelin antagonist: effect on the renal response to contrast media. Radiology 1995; 196:661–665.
40. Russo D, Minutolo R, Cianciaruso B, et al: Early effects of contrast media on renal hemodynamics and tubular function in chronic renal failure. J Am Soc Nephrol 1995; 6:1451–1458.
41. Erley CM, Osswald H: Prevention of contrast media–induced renal impairment by adenosine antagonists in humans. Drug Dev Res 1998; 45:172–175.
42. Arend LJ, Bakris GL, Burnett JCJ, et al: Role for intrarenal adenosine in the renal hemodynamic response to contrast media. J Lab Clin Med 1987; 110:406–411.
43. Katholi RE, Taylor GJ, McCann WP, et al: Nephrotoxicity from contrast media: attenuation with theophylline. Radiology 1995; 195:17–22.
44. Osswald H, Schmitz HJ, Heidenreich O: Adenosine response of the rat kidney after saline loading, sodium restriction, and hemorrhagia. Pflugers Arch 1975; 357:323–333.
45. Hall JE, Granger JP: Adenosine alters glomerular filtration control by angiotensin II. Am J Physiol 1986; 250:F917–F923.
46. Haas JA, Osswald H: Adenosine-induced fall in glomerular capillary pressure: effect of ureteral obstruction and aortic constriction in the Munich-Wistar rat kidney. Naunyn Schmiedebergs Arch Pharmacol 1981; 317:86–89.
47. Cantley LG, Spokes K, Clark B, et al: Role of endothelin and prostaglandins in radiocontrast-induced renal artery constriction. Kidney Int 1993; 44:1217–1223.
48. Heyman SN, Brezis M, Epstein FH, et al: Early renal medullary hypoxic injury from radiocontrast and indomethacin. Kidney Int 1991; 40:632–642.
49. Cederholm C, Almen T, Bergqvist D, et al: Acute renal failure in rats: interaction between contrast media and temporary renal arterial occlusion. Acta Radiol 1989; 30:321–326.
50. Deray G, Dubois M, Martinez F, et al: Renal effects of radiocontrast agents in rats: a new model of acute renal failure. Am J Nephrol 1990; 10:507–513.
51. Osswald H, Schmidt HJ, Kemper R: Tissue content of adenosine, inosine, and hypoxanthine in the rat kidney after ischemia and postischemic recirculation. Pflugers Arch 1977; 371:45–49.
52. Agmon Y, Peleg H, Greenfeld Z, et al: Nitric oxide and prostanoids protect the renal outer medulla from radiocontrast toxicity in the rat. J Clin Invest 1994; 94:1069–1075.
53. Osswald H, Helminger I, Jendralski A, Abrar B: Improvement of renal function by theophylline in the acute renal failure of the rat [abstract]. Naunyn Schmiedebergs Arch Pharmacol 1979; 307:R47.
54. Gouyon JB, Guignard JP: Theophylline prevents the hypoxemia-induced renal hemodynamic changes in rabbits. Kidney Int 1988; 33:1078–1083.
55. Deray G, Martinez F, Cacoub P, et al: A role for adenosine calcium and ischemia in radiocontrast-induced intrarenal vasoconstriction. Am J Nephrol 1990; 10:316–322.
56. Rossi N, Ellis V, Kontry T, et al: The role of adenosine in $HgCl_2$-induced acute renal failure in rats. Am J Physiol 1990; 258:F1554–F1560.
57. Lin JJ, Churchill PC, Bidani AK: Theophylline in rats during maintenance phase of postischemic acute renal failure. Kidney Int 1988; 33:24–28.
58. Lin JJ, Churchill PC, Bidani AK: Effect of theophylline on the initiation phase of postischemic acute renal failure in rats. J Lab Clin Med 1986; 108:150–154.
59. Bidani AK, Churchill PC: Aminophylline ameliorates glycerol-induced acute renal failure in rats. Can J Physiol Pharmacol 1983; 61:567–571.
60. Bidani AK, Churchill PC, Packer W: Theophylline-induced protection in myoglobinuric acute renal failure: further characterization. Can J Physiol Pharmacol 1987; 65:42–45.
61. Erley CM, Heyne N, Burgert K, et al: Prevention of radiocontrast-induced nephropathy by adenosine antagonists in rats with chronic nitric oxide deficiency. J Am Soc Nephrol 1997; 8:1125–1132.
62. Barrett BJ, Parfrey PS, McDonald JR, et al: Nonionic low-osmolality versus ionic high-osmolality contrast material for intravenous use in patients perceived to be at high risk: randomized trial. Radiology 1992; 183:105–110.
63. Deray G, Jacobs C: Radiocontrast nephrotoxicity: a review. Invest Radiol 1995; 30:221–225.
64. Katholi RE, Taylor GJ, Woods WT, et al: Nephrotoxicity of nonionic low-osmolality versus ionic high-osmolality contrast media: a prospective double-blind randomized comparison in human beings. Radiology 1993; 186:183–187.
65. Schwab SJ, Hlatky MA, Pieper KS, et al: Contrast nephrotoxicity: a randomized controlled trial of a nonionic and an ionic radiographic contrast agent. N Engl J Med 1989; 320:149–153.
66. Barrett BJ, Carlisle EJ: Meta-analysis of the relative nephrotoxicity of high- and low-osmolality iodinated contrast media. Radiology 1993; 188:171–178.
67. Jakobsen JA: Renal effects of iodixanol in healthy volunteers and patients with severe renal failure. Acta Radiol Suppl 1995; 399:191–195.
68. Jakobsen JA: Renal experience with Visipaque. Eur Radiol 1996; 6(Suppl 2):S16–S19.
69. Weissleder R: Can gadolinium be safely given in renal failure? AJR Am J Roentgenol 1996; 167:278–279.
70. Kaufman JA, Geller SC, Waltman AC: Renal insufficiency: gadopentetate dimeglumine as a radiographic contrast agent during peripheral vascular interventional procedures. Radiology 1996; 198:579–581.
71. Hatrick AG, Jarosz JM, Irvine AT: Gadopentetate dimeglumine as an alternative contrast agent for use in interventional procedures. Clin Radiol 1997; 52:948–952.
72. Seeger JM, Self S, Harward TR, et al: Carbon dioxide gas as an arterial contrast agent. Ann Surg 1993; 217:688–697.
73. Hawkins IF Jr, Wilcox CS, Kerns SR, Sabatelli FW: CO_2 digital angiography: a safer contrast agent for renal vascular imaging? Am J Kidney Dis 1994; 24:685–694.
74. Solomon R, Werner C, Mann D, et al: Effects of saline, mannitol, and furosemide on acute decreases in renal function induced by radiocontrast agents. N Engl J Med 1994; 331:1416–1420.
75. Kurnik BR, Weisberg LS, Cuttler IM, Kurnik PB: Effects of atrial natriuretic peptide versus mannitol on renal blood flow during radiocontrast infusion in chronic renal failure. J Lab Clin Med 1990; 116:27–36.
76. Weisberg LS, Kurnik PB, Kurnik BR: Dopamine and renal blood flow in radiocontrast-induced nephropathy in humans. Ren Fail 1993; 15:61–68.

77. Weisberg LS, Kurnik PB, Kurnik BR: Radiocontrast-induced nephropathy in humans: role of renal vasoconstriction. Kidney Int 1992; 41:1408–1415.
78. Anto HR, Chou SY, Porush JG, Shapiro WB: Infusion intravenous pyelography and renal function: effect of hypertonic mannitol in patients with chronic renal insufficiency. Arch Intern Med 1981; 141:1652–1656.
79. Eisenberg RL, Bank WO, Hedgock MW: Renal failure after major angiography can be avoided with hydration. Am J Radiol 1981; 136:859–861.
80. Carraro M, Stacul F, Collari P, et al: Contrast media nephrotoxicity: urinary protein and enzyme pattern in patients with or without saline infusion during digital subtracting angiography. Contrib Nephrol 1993; 101:251–254.
81. Kersrein MD, Puyau FA: Value of periangiography hydration. Surgery 1984; 96:919–922.
82. Louis BM, Hoch BS, Hernandez C, et al: Protection from the nephrotoxicity of contrast dye. Ren Fail 1996; 18:639–646.
83. Weinstein JM, Heyman S, Brezis M: Potential deleterious effect of furosemide in radiocontrast nephropathy. Nephron 1992; 62:413–415.
84. Golman K, Cederholm C: Contrast medium–induced acute renal failure: can it be prevented? Invest Radiol 1990; 25(Suppl 1):S127–S128.
85. Neumayer HH, Gellert J, Luft FC: Calcium antagonists and renal protection. Ren Fail 1993; 15:353–358.
86. Russo D, Testa A, Volpe LD, Sansone G: Randomised prospective study on renal effects of two different contrast media in humans: protective role of a calcium channel blocker. Nephron 1990; 55:254–257.
87. Carraro M, Mancini W, Aryero M, et al: Dose effect of nitrendipine on urinary enzymes and microproteins following non-ionic radiocontrast administration. Nephrol Dial Transplant 1996; 11:444–448.
88. Spengberg Viklund B, Berglund J, Nikonoff T, et al: Does prophylactic treatment with felodipine, a calcium antagonist, prevent low-osmolar contrast-induced renal dysfunction in hydrated diabetic and nondiabetic patients with normal or moderately reduced renal function? Scand J Urol Nephrol 1996; 30:63–68.
89. Khoury Z, Schlicht JR, Como J, et al: The effect of prophylactic nifedipine on renal function in patients administered contrast media. Pharmacotherapy 1995; 15:59–65.
90. Hall KA, Wong RW, Hunter GC, et al: Contrast-induced nephrotoxicity: the effects of vasodilator therapy. J Surg Res 1992; 53:317–320.
91. Chertow GM, Sayegh MH, Allgren RL, Lazarus JM: Is the administration of dopamine associated with adverse or favorable outcomes in acute renal failure? Auriculin Anaritide Acute Renal Failure Study Group. Am J Med 1996; 101:49–53.
92. Wambach G, Winkert T: Nierenfunktionsstörungen nach Röntgenkontrastmittelgabe: Prophylaxe durch das atriale natriuretische Peptid? Nieren und Hochdruckkrankheiten 1990; 19:312–317.
93. Kurnik BR, Allgren RL, Genter FC, et al: Prospective study of atrial natriuretic peptide for the prevention of radiocontrast-induced nephropathy. Am J Kidney Dis 1998; 31:674–680.
94. Erley CM, Duda SH, Schlepckow S, et al: Adenosine antagonist theophylline prevents the reduction of glomerular filtration rate after contrast media application. Kidney Int 1994; 45:1425–1431.
95. Erley CM: Prävention des kontrastmittelbedingten Nierenversagens. Intensivmed 1997; 34:769–777.
96. Yoshioka T, Fogo A, Beckman JK: Reduced activity of antioxidant enzymes underlies contrast media-induced renal injury in volume depletion. Kidney Int 1992; 41:1008–1015.
97. Baliga R, Ueda N, Walker PD, et al: Oxidant mechanisms in toxic acute renal failure. Am J Kidney Dis 1997; 29:465–477.
98. Parvez Z, Rahman MA, Moncada R: Contrast media-induced lipid peroxidation in the rat kidney. Invest Radiol 1989; 24:697–702.
99. Bakris GL, Lass N, Gaber AO, et al: Radiocontrast medium-induced declines in renal function: a role for oxygen free radicals. Am J Physiol 1990; 258:F115–F120.
100. Arstall MA, Yang J, Stafford I, et al: N-acetylcysteine in combination with nitroglycerin and streptokinase for the treatment of evolving acute myocardial infarction. Safety and biochemical effects. Circulation 1995; 92:2855–2862.
101. DiMari J, Megyesi J, Udvarhelyi N, et al: N-acetyl cysteine ameliorates ischemic renal failure. Am J Physiol 1997; 272:F292–F298.
102. Weinbroum AA, Rudick V, Ben-Abraham R, et al: N-acetyl-L-cysteine for preventing lung reperfusion injury after liver ischemia-reperfusion: a possible dual protective mechanism in a dose-response study. Transplantation 2000; 69: 853–859.
103. Tepel M, van-der-Giet M, Schwarzfeld C, et al: Prevention of radiographic contrast agent–induced reductions in renal function by acetylcysteine. N Engl J Med 2000; 343:180–184.
104. Lehnert T, Keller E, Gondolf K, et al: Effect of haemodialysis after contrast medium administration in patients with renal insufficiency. Nephrol Dial Transplant 1998; 13:358–362.

CHAPTER 30

Biological Nephrotoxins

Hai Yan Wang ▪ Mei Wang ▪ Taigen Cui ▪ Michelle Whittier

INTRODUCTION

Animals and plants produce a number of biological nephrotoxins (Table 30–1). Many toxins are known to cause significant kidney damage, and several have recently attracted considerable attention. This chapter discusses acute renal failure (ARF) associated with envenomation from snakes, spiders, bees, and wasps and describes the nephrotoxicity accompanying marine animals and certain medicinal herbs.

ACUTE RENAL FAILURE FROM ENVENOMATION

Snake Venoms

There are five families of venomous snakes worldwide (Table 30–2). Four of the families (Atractaspidae, Colubridae, Elapidae, and Viperidae) include venomous species dangerous to humans, and comprise a total of roughly 450 species or about 19% of all snake species. The global annual mortality from snakebite is around 40,000 people per year.[1] A particularly high incidence has been reported from Asia, Africa, and South America.[2, 3] Acute renal failure has been reported to occur in 5% to 30% of victims with severe envenomation. The two families responsible for the greatest morbidity and mortality are Elapidae (cobras, African mambas, and coral snakes) and Viperidae (vipers, adders, moccasins, and rattlesnakes).[4] The highly venomous snakes most commonly encountered are Russell's viper (subfamily Viperinae), snakes of the *Bothrops* species (subfamily Crotalinae), and rattle-

snakes. The incidence of ARF following Russell's viper bite has been estimated to be 13% to 32%,[5] and the prevalence of ARF following *Bothrops* snakebite ranges from 2% to 10%.[6–8] Snakebites occur most often during periods of stress, such as floods, earthquakes, and other environmental catastrophes as a consequence of the disruption of the snakes' natural habitat. Other bites are the result of inadvertent encounters.

VENOMS

Each species has unique venom, containing various amounts of toxic and nontoxic compounds. Venoms are at least 90% protein, and most of the proteins in venoms are enzymes. About 25 different enzymes have been isolated from snake venoms, 10 of which occur in the venoms of most snakes. Proteolytic enzymes, phospholipases, and hyaluronidases are the most common types of enzymes.[4, 9] Other enzymes include collagenases, ribonucleases, deoxyribonucleases, nucleotidases, amino acid oxidases, lactate dehydrogenases, and acidic and basic phosphatases. Not all of the toxic chemical compounds in snake venoms are enzymes. Polypeptide toxins, glycoproteins, and low-molecular-weight compounds may also be present.

In general, venoms are described as either neurotoxic or hematotoxic, although the venoms of many snakes contain both components. Neurotoxins act either presynaptically or postsynaptically and inhibit peripheral nerve impulses. Hemorrhagins affect vasculature permeability and cause both local and systemic bleeding. Potent procoagulants that activate the clotting cascade through Factor V and X have been described.[4, 9] Various proteolytic enzymes may cause local tissue necrosis. Other toxins, such as myocardial depressant factors and myotoxins, result in reduced car-

TABLE 30–1. Common Biological Nephrotoxins Produced by Animals and Plants

Snake
  Phospholipase A_2
  Myotoxins
  Procoagulant activating factors V and X
Spider
  Sphingomyelinase D *(Loxosceles)*
  Neurotoxins *(Latrodectus)*
Bee
  Melittin
  Phospholipase A_2
  Mast cell degranulating protein
Wasp
  Antigen 5
  Mastoparans
Carp
  Ichthyogalltoxin
  Cyprinol

TABLE 30–2. Classification of Venomous Snakes

Class Reptilia
  Subclass Lepidosauria
    Order Squamata
      Suborder Serpentes
        Infraorder Scolecophidia
        Infraorder Henophidia
        Infraorder Caenophidia
          Family Colubridae
          Family Elapidae
          Family Hydrophiidae
          Family Atractaspidae
          Family Viperidae
            Subfamily Azemiopinae
            Subfamily Viperinae
            Subfamily Crotalinae

diac output and substantial rhabdomyolysis, respectively. Lastly, a direct action of the venom may result in ARF, and there may be hypersensitivity reactions to either the venom or the antivenom protein itself.

CLINICAL EFFECTS

The clinical effects of these toxins include both local and systemic manifestations. The local toxicity occurs in minutes to hours and presents as pain, swelling, blistering, and tissue necrosis. The systemic effects consist of neurotoxicity, bleeding diatheses, shock, and ARF. The major manifestations of neurotoxic snakebite may include ptosis, impaired vision, slurred speech, difficulty in swallowing, hypersalivation, paresthesia, generalized muscle weakness, and respiratory insufficiency and arrest. In severe envenomation of a hemorrhagic snakebite, the major systemic manifestations may include hematemesis, melena, hemoptysis, and hematuria.[10]

Of the patients with ARF, 65% to 88% have been reported to be oliguric and some were hypercatabolic.[11-15] The risk of renal failure is increased with the age of the patient and by a delay in the interval between the time of the bite and the start of medical treatment.[12] The onset of symptoms can occur within minutes, but typically develop over a few hours. Renal abnormalities, such as anuria or oliguria, may also occur within a few hours, but may occur as late as 96 hours after the snakebite has occurred.[5, 16-18] This late manifestation of oliguria may contribute to the delay in seeking medical attention. Indeed, a wide spectrum of nephropathologic changes have been described.[19] In one series of 50 patients, critical oliguria (100%), local swelling (48%), and bleeding tendencies (50%) were the predominant clinical features. Disseminated intravascular coagulation was seen in 48% of the cases. Ninety percent of the patients required dialysis treatment.

The renal pathologic findings associated with snakebite include severe tubular and vascular lesions, increased apoptosis in the distal tubules, and the presence of eosinophils, mast cells, and hyperplastic fibroblasts in the interstitium.[20] The renal lesion most commonly described in envenomated patients is that of acute tubular necrosis (ATN).[21-22] Extracapillary glomerulonephritis,[23] acute interstitial nephritis,[24] and necrotizing arteritis of the interlobular arteries[25] also have been reported.[21, 26] Patchy or diffuse renal cortical necrosis occurs in the most serious cases. The patients with bilateral cortical necrosis may be those that develop chronic renal failure and become dependent on dialysis.[20, 22]

PATHOGENESIS

Several mechanisms have been proposed for the pathogenesis of ARF. First, circulatory shock develops as the result of hemorrhage, hemolysis, presynaptic neurotoxicity, vasodilation, release of endogenous autocoids, and interaction with monoamine receptors,[4] causing ischemic renal injury, and is probably the sequence of events most commonly thought to cause ARF.[18-20]

Second, some snake venoms are myotoxins, which cause rhabdomyolysis[27-29] and myoglobinuric ARF, resulting in abnormalities of the proximal convoluted tubule that range from loss of microvilli to frank epithelial cell necrosis.[30] The myoglobinemia and myoglobinuria are the result of both local tissue necrosis and circulating myotoxins. The latter is supported by the finding of foci of myonecrosis in areas remote from the site of the bite.[31]

Third, in animal studies, the intravenous injection of snake venom has led to an acute decrease in renal plasma flow and the glomerular filtration rate, with evidence of intravascular hemolysis and disseminated intravascular coagulation. Light and electron microscopy biopsy specimens have shown massive fibrin deposition in glomerular capillaries, proximal and distal tubular necrosis, and casts in renal tubules containing hemolyzed red blood cells.[32] In this instance, the renal histologic changes are consistent with renal ischemia caused by transient glomerular ischemia from fibrin deposition or by direct nephrotoxicity of the venom itself.[33]

Thus, it has been suggested that components of snake venom have nephrotoxic potential. For example, a study in rabbits injected with Russell's viper venom revealed proximal tubular abnormalities with intact basement membrane, suggesting a direct toxic effect.[34] In dog experiments, intravenous injection of Russell's viper venom also resulted in decreased renal blood flow and glomerular filtration rate and increased urinary N-acetyl-β-D-glucosaminidase.[35, 36] Pretreatment with indomethacin lessened the decrease in renal blood flow and prevented the change in the glomerular filtration rate.[35] In addition, it has been reported that in some cases, after envenomation, ARF occurred without evidence of neurotoxic envenomation, myoglobinuria, or disseminated intravascular coagulation and with only mild disturbance of coagulation.[37-39] These findings indicate that venom has renal vasoactive effects and direct tubular toxicity.

TREATMENT

The treatment of snakebites is primarily supportive. Immobilization of the affected limb, rapid transport to a medical facility, and identification of the snake species are helpful. Either specific or generalized antivenom should be given immediately[40] when there are symptoms or signs of envenomation. Antivenoms rarely offer cross-protection against snake species other than those used in their production unless the species are closely related. Since antivenom is derived from purified horse blood, it should be administered only in a medical facility under close supervision and after the patient has been tested for hypersensitivity to horse serum. Death is most often attributed to ARF, and early renal replacement therapy along with supportive treatment appears to be the mainstay of therapy.

Spider Venoms

Spider bite is a relatively uncommon cause of ARF, and the presentation can vary from species to species. Traditionally, disease states induced by the spider bite have been assigned specific names according to the genus of the spider. For example, a bite by the recluse spiders (genus *Loxosceles*) is known as *loxoscelism,* and the bite of widow spiders (genus *Latrodectus*) is termed *latrodectism.* While not all species in any given spider genus are venomous, this nomenclature is useful when one describes different types of spider envenomation.

RECLUSE SPIDERS

The recluse spiders (genus *Loxosceles*) belong to a unique family of arachnids known as the Sicariidae. This family consists of not only the recluse spiders but also the six-eyed crab spiders (genus *Sicarius*) of Central and South America, and of South Africa. At least 56 species of recluse spiders have been described across the world. Many of these species have only recently been recognized; thus, people are not familiar with them. In the United States, there are 11 indigenous species of recluse spiders and two others introduced from other countries. All recluse spiders, as well as the six-eyed crab spider, are considered venomous to humans.

Loxoscelism was first recognized in 1872 when Chilean physicians linked a peculiar skin lesion known as the "gangrenous spot of Chile" to the bite of the Chilean recluse spider, *Loxosceles laeta.* The brown recluse spider, *Loxosceles reclusa,* became the first spider in the United States to be associated with necrotic arachnidism in 1957 after a series of severe bites in the Midwest. Recluse spiders produce a toxic venom composed of sphingomyelinase D, which results in both local and systemic effects.[41] The bite of the recluse spider is unique, and signs and symptoms resulting from its venom include fever, chills, nausea, myalgias, and necrotic skin lesions. More serious systemic derangements include hemolysis, bleeding diatheses, and ARF. In a series of 267 cases of envenomation by *Loxosceles* species in Brazil, most patients experienced local pain, edema, and necrotic skin lesions. Acute renal failure was described in approximately 6% of cases. Almost all deaths occurred in young children.[42]

WIDOW SPIDERS

The widow spiders (genus *Latrodectus*) are among the most recognized species on earth. All species are venomous. Several widow spiders are found in the United States: the southern widow, the western black widow, the northern widow, the red widow, and the brown widow, which was introduced into Florida from tropical regions. In Europe, the malmignatte, or European black widow, is a significant health problem in various parts of its range. In Herzegovina (in the former Yugoslavia), this spider reportedly causes a large number of bites each autumn in fieldworkers who harvest grain by hand.

The bite of a widow spider is often initially painful. In contrast with the recluse spider, the local dermal reaction is minimal, with mild erythema that dissipates in a few hours. No tissue necrosis follows a widow spider bite. Widow spider venom contains a potent neurotoxin that induces the state of latrodectism. Latrodectism usually begins with severe cramping and spasms in the large muscles of the legs or abdomen. Some victims of widow spider bite may experience anxiety, profuse sweating, nausea, piloerection, and hypertension. Paralysis, stupor, and convulsions can also occur. Acute renal failure has been described secondary to the potent neurotoxin, causing neurogenic bladder with bilateral ureteral obstruction.[43] Death is unusual.

Bee and Wasp Venoms

Bee and wasp stings can cause several toxic effects when the envenomation is massive. Bees and wasps belong to the species *Hymenoptera,* with the majority of mass envenomations caused by two different families: Apidae, the honey and bumble bees, and Vespidae, including hornets, yellow jackets, and paper wasps. Mass envenomation is characterized by tens to hundreds of stings often in the head and neck region, occurring as the result of inadvertent disruption of the colony.[44]

The venom from bees and wasps results in injury either by direct toxicity on tissues or by inducing an immunologic response. Bee venom has many toxic mediators. Melittin is a polypeptide that induces pain, hemolysis, and smooth muscle contraction. Phospholipase A_2 works in conjunction with melittin to cause hemolysis by disruption of red blood cell membranes. Other mediators include apamin, hyaluronidase, and mast cell degranulating protein. Wasp venom differs from bee venom and consists of active amines, kinins, mastoparans, and antigen 5.[45, 46]

Massive envenomation can present with a spectrum of symptoms, depending on the amount of venom injected. Nausea, vomiting, diarrhea, and edema are often initially described, with severe reactions delayed for hours to days.[47] Acute renal failure is common and has been associated with hemolysis and rhabdomyolysis. Numerous case reports, however, have described ARF without associated hemoglobinuria or myoglobinuria. These cases may point to a direct toxic effect of the venom on tubules or tubular damage from ischemia. In these instances, renal biopsies reveal tubular damage and necrosis.[48] The treatment of ARF resulting from massive envenomation is largely supportive.

ICHTHYOGALLTOXIN

For years, there has been an association between the ingestion of raw bile taken from the gallbladder of carp fish species and ARF. It is believed in some rural areas in Asia that the ingestion of raw bile from carp can improve visual acuity and rheumatism, and promote overall good health.[49] Recently, there has been heightened awareness in North America of this association as the result of increased ethnic diversity, alternative medical therapies, food importation, and the introduction of the grass carp into regions in the Eastern United States. Five recognized species of *Cypriniformes* have been linked to ARF. The two most commonly cited species are *Ctenopharyngodon idella*, or grass carp, and *Cyprinus carpio*, or common carp.[50]

The pathogenesis of ARF following ingestion of carp gallbladder is poorly understood. Ichthyogalltoxin is found in the bile of all five carp species and is hypothesized to be a toxic mediator. Studies reveal that there is decreased cytochrome oxidase activity in the liver, kidney, and brain in animals given ichthyogalltoxin.[51] Alternatively, cyprinol, a C27 bile alcohol isolated from carp bile, has been shown to be toxic to mice.[52]

The severity of poisoning appears to be directly related to the amount of toxin ingested and the method of preparation of the fish. Carp that weigh less than 3 kg typically do not cause severe symptoms, but ingestion of raw, rather than boiled, gallbladder increases the severity of the intoxication.[53] Patients initially present with gastrointestinal symptoms, including nausea, vomiting, diarrhea, and abdominal pain. The onset of symptoms is usually within minutes to hours after exposure. Jaundice and hepatitis are common. Acute renal failure occurs in hours to days and varies from mild abnormalities in serum chemistries to oliguria, metabolic acidosis, and hyperkalemia. The urinary findings are significant for hematuria, mild proteinuria, and granular casts. Renal biopsies, if performed, frequently reveal tubular necrosis.[54] Treatment is largely supportive. Initial therapy should include gastric lavage, as animal experiments show that the bile can be detected in the gastrointestinal tract for up to 22 hours.[51] Other interventions should be directed toward patient symptomatology, specifically intravenous fluids, nutritional support, and renal replacement therapy. Death is rare.

ACUTE RENAL FAILURE FROM HERBAL REMEDIES

Products marked as "dietary supplements" include a diverse range of vitamins and minerals, high-potency free amino acids, botanicals (herbs), enzymes, animal extracts, and bioflavonoids. Herbal remedies include the processed or unprocessed plant parts (bark, leaves, flowers, fruits, and stems) as well as extracts and essential oils. Approximately one third of Americans use herbal products and spend more than $3 billion per year on these agents. It is estimated that 70% of patients who use complementary medicines, such as herbal products, do not tell their physician or pharmacist. Although it is believed that most herbal remedies of "natural" origin are harmless and without side effects, serious poisoning can occur when importers or retailers mistake one herb for another, owing to simi-

larity in appearance or confusion about the nomenclature.[55] In one series of 1701 patients admitted to two general medical wards, only in 0.2% of the cases was the admission attributed to the adverse effects of herbal remedies. In comparison, adverse reactions to "Western" drugs were responsible for 4.4% of the admissions.[56]

Factors Concerning Nephrotoxicity of Medicinal Herbs

The belief that herbal remedies are safe is a misconception. These herbs can be an insidious cause of ARF. The fundamental element in the nephrotoxicity of herbs is to determine the specific species of the herb. Confusion arises because there are certain medicinal herbs that belong to different species but are designated by similar names. For example, there are seven different species by the name "fangchi," a commonly prescribed Chinese herb.[57] It has been postulated that, in the cases described below, *Aristolochia fangchi* was mistaken for *Stephamia terandra*, as their names in Chinese differ by only one letter (Figs. 30–1A and B). Additionally, the preparation, amount of exposure, and route of administration are key elements that lead to toxicity.

ARISTOLOCHIA MANSHURIENSIS KOM

Aristolochia manshuriensis Kom (*AMK*) is a perennial vine of the Aristolochiaceae family endemic to North China. After being cut and dried, the stem of *AMK* is termed *Guanmutong*. This has long been used in Chinese traditional medicine, either alone or in combination with other herbs, for the treatment of renal stones or urinary tract infections, and to stimulate lactation. According to the Chinese pharmacopoeia, the total dose of *AMK* should be 3 to 6 g per day.[58] Doses higher than this can cause ARF,[59, 60] which may progress to chronic interstitial nephritis (Fig. 30–2). Prominent gastrointestinal symptoms develop immediately after ingestion, and oliguria develops within days.

OTHER PLANTS OF THE ARISTOLOCHIACEAE FAMILY

Aristolochia fangchi is another member of the Aristolochiaceae family grown in southern China. Aristolochic acid has been incriminated as the toxin in "Chinese herb nephropathy," but this is controversial. Belgian nephrologists have described Chinese herb nephropathy after a series of young women developed renal failure from a diet supplement that included *Aristolochia fangchi* powder. Intense renal interstitial fibrosis with relative sparing of the glomeruli was the pathologic feature.[61] A recent report on patients in Belgium who have end-stage renal disease as the consequence of *Aristolochia fangchi* exposure found that these individuals have an increased risk of developing urothelial carcinoma. As a result, it is recommended

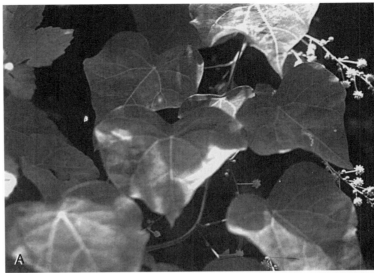
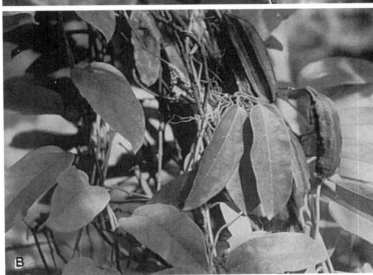

FIGURE 30–1 ■ *A, Aristolochia fangchi. B, Stephania tetrandra.*

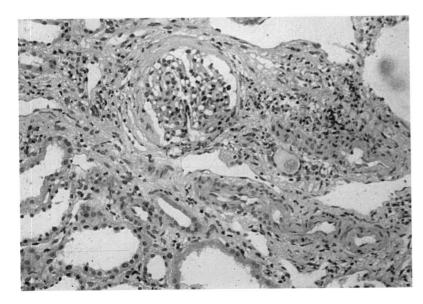

FIGURE 30–2 ■ Chronic tubulointerstitial nephritis caused by ingestion of *Aristolochia manshuriensis Kom.*

that these patients be followed closely with cystoscopy and possibly prophylactic removal of both native kidneys and ureters.[62] Alternatively, in studies conducted by Cosyns and coworkers,[63] rats were given either aristolochic acid or the other components in the dietary supplement for 3 months and no renal lesions were identified. In an additional study in China, Wistar rats were given *Aristolochia fangchi* powder for 4 months and no renal interstitial fibrosis was noted (unpublished data). Serotonin has also been implicated as the causative agent in Chinese herbal nephropathy after evidence revealed that serotonin could induce sustained preglomerular vasoconstriction, causing renal ischemia and fibrosis.[64] There is still much to be clarified concerning the possible mechanisms of ARF caused by medicinal herbs.

TRIPTERYGIUM WILFORDII HOOK F

Tripterygium wilfordii Hook f is a perennial twining vine of the Celastraceae family endemic to southern China. It has been used to treat rheumatoid arthritis, chronic nephritis, and skin disorders. All parts of the plant are toxic, particularly the root. Intoxication affects the gastrointestinal tract, heart, liver, and kidney. Acute renal failure is thought to be secondary to a direct toxic effect that causes tubular necrosis; however, acute interstitial nephritis has also been described.[65, 66]

OTHER HERBAL REMEDIES

Other less well-known herbal remedies can also cause ARF. *Taxus celebica* has been used in the treatment of diabetes mellitus. Tung Sheuh capsules have been shown to contain the nonlabeled adulterant mefenamic acid, which causes acute interstitial nephritis.[67]

REFERENCES

1. Chugh KS: Snakebite-induced acute renal failure in India. Kidney Int 1989; 35:891–907.
2. Chung KS, Sakhuja V: Renal failure from snake bites. Int J Artif Organs 1980; 3:319–321.
3. Pugh RNH, Theakston RDG: Incidence and mortality of snake bite in Savanna, Nigeria. Lancet 1980; 2:1181–1183.
4. Warrell DA: Venomous bites and stings in the tropical world. Med J Aust 1993; 159:773–779.
5. Chugh KS, Pal Y, Chakravarty RN, et al: Acute renal failure following poisonous snake bite. Am J Kidney Dis 1984; 4:30–38.
6. Kouyouumdjian JA, Polizelli C, Lobo SM, Guimarães SM: Acidentes ofidicos causados por *B. moojeni* na região de São José do Rio Preto-SP. Arq Bras Med 1990; 64:167–171.
7. Nishioka AS, Silveira PVP: A clinical and epidemiological study of 292 cases of lance-headed viper bite in a Brazilian teaching hospital. Am J Trop Med Hyg 1992; 47:805–810.
8. Queiroz LP, Moritz RD: Acidente botrópico em Florianópolis. Arq Catarinenses Med 1989; 18:163–166.
9. Shiffman S, Theodor I, Rapaport SI: Separation from Russell's viper venom of one fraction reacting with Factor X and another reacting with Factor V. Biochem J 1969; 8:1397–1404.
10. Chen J-B, Leung J, Hsu K-T: Acute renal failure after snakebite: a report of four cases. Chin Med J 1997; 59:65–69.
11. Ribeiro LA, Albuquerque MJ, de Campos VA, et al: Deaths caused by venomous snakes in the State of São Paulo: evaluation of 43 cases from 1988 to 1993. Rev Assoc Med Bras 1998; 44:312–318.
12. Silveira PV, Nishioka S: South American rattlesnake bite in a Brazilian teaching hospital: clinical and epidemiological study of 87 cases, with analysis of factors predictive of renal failure. Trans R Soc Trop Med Hyg 1992; 86:562–564.
13. Nishioka S de A, Silveira PV: A clinical and epidemiologic study of 292 cases of lance-headed viper in a Brazilian teaching hospital. Am J Trop Med Hyg 1992; 47:805–810.
14. Zou RL, Zhang-YM: Acute renal failure caused by viper: report of 48 cases. [Chinese]. Chin J Surg 1994; 32:119–120.
15. Wang YM, Zhu Z, Ye YX, et al: Acute renal failure caused by snake bite: report of 33 cases. [Chinese]. Chin J Nephrol 1998; 4:213–214.
16. Nelson BK: Snake envenomation, incidence, clinical presentation, and management. Med Toxicol Adverse Drug Exp 1989; 4:17–31.
17. Chugh KS, Alkat BK, Sharma BK, et al: Acute renal failure following snake bite. Am J Trop Med Hyg 1975; 24:692–697.
18. Dasilva OA, Lopez M, Godoy P: Intensive care unit treatment of acute renal failure following snake bite. Am J Trop Med Hyg 1979; 28:401–407.
19. Acharya VN, Khanna UB, Almeida AF, Merchant MR: Acute renal failure due to viperine snake bite as seen in tropical western India. Ren Fail 1989; 11:33–35.
20. Than-Than, Francis N, Tin-Nu-Swe, et al: Contribution of focal hemorrhage and microvascular fibrin deposition to fatal envenoming by Russell's viper (*Vipera russelli siamensis*) in Burma. Acta Trop 1989; 46:23–28.
21. Soe S, Win MM, Htwe TT, et al: Renal histopathology following Russell's viper (*Vipera russelli*) bite. Southeast Asian J Trop Med Public Health 1993; 24:193–197.
22. Milani JR, Jorge MT, de Campos FP, et al: Snake bites by the jararacucu (*Bothrops jararacussu*): clinicopathological studies of 29 proven cases in São Paulo State, Brazil. QJM 1997; 90:323–324.
23. Sitprija V, Boonpucknavig V: Extracapillary proliferative glomerulonephritis in Russell's viper bite. BMJ 1980; 2:1417.
24. Indraprasit S, Boonpucknavig V: Acute interstitial nephritis after a Russell's viper snake bite. Clin Nephrol 1986; 25:111.
25. Sitprija V, Benyajati C, Boonpucknavig PV: Further observations of renal insufficiency in snake bite. Nephron 1974; 13:396–403.
26. Ramachandran S: Acute Renal Failure in Sri Lanka. In: Chugh KH, ed: *Asian Nephrology.* Vol XI. Bombay: Oxford University Press; 1994:378.
27. Denis D, Lamireau T, Llanas B, et al: Rhabdomyolysis in European viper bite. Acta Pediatr 1998; 87:1013–1015.
28. Bush SP, Jansen PW: Severe rattlesnake envenomation with anaphylaxis and rhabdomyolysis. Am Emerg Med 1995; 25:845–848.
29. Cupo P, Azevedo-Marques MM, Hering SE: Clinical and laboratory features of South American rattlesnake (*Crotalus durissus terrificus*) envenomation in children. Trans R Soc Trop Med Hyg 1988; 82:924–929.
30. Ponraj D, Gopalakrishnakone P: Renal lesions in rhabdomyolysis caused by *Pseudechis stralis* snake myotoxin. Kidney Int 1997; 51:1956–1969.
31. Azevedo-Marques MM, Cupo P, Coimbra TM, et al: Myonecrosis, myoglobinuria and acute renal failure induced by South American rattlesnake (*Crotalus durissus terrificus*) envenomation in Brazil. Toxicon 1995; 23:631–636.
32. Burdmann EA, Woronik V, Prado EB, et al: Snakebite-induced acute renal failure: an experimental model. Am J Trop Med Hyg 1993; 48:82–88.
33. Burdmann EA, Antunes I, Saldanha LB, Abdulkader RC: Severe acute renal failure induced by the venom of *Lonomia* caterpillars. Clin Nephrol 1996; 46:337–339.
34. Soe-Soe, Than-Than, Khin-Ei-Han: The nephrotoxic action of Russell's viper (*Vipera russelli*) venom. Toxicon 1990; 28:461–467.
35. Thamaree S, Sitprija V, Tongvongchai S, Chaiyabutr N: Changes in renal hemodynamics induced by Russell's viper venom: effects of indomethacin. Nephron 1994; 67:209–213.
36. Tungthanathanich P, Chaiyabutr N, Sitprija V: Effect of Russell's viper (*Vipera russelli siamensis*) venom on renal hemodynamics in dogs. Toxicon 1986; 24:365–371.
37. Acott CJ: Acute renal failure after envenomation by the common brown snake. Med J Aust 1988; 149:709–710.

38. Vijeth SR, Dutta TK, Shahapurkar J: Correlation of renal status with hematologic profile in viperine bite. Am J Trop Med Hyg 1997; 56:168–170.

39. Win A, Khin PPK, Baby H, et al: Renal involvement in Russell's viper bite patients without disseminated intravascular coagulation. Trans R Soc Trop Med Hyg 1998; 92:322–324.

40. Sutherland SK, Coulter AR, Harris RD: Rationalisation of first aid measures for the elapid snakebite. Lancet 1979; 1:183–186.

41. Futrell, JM: Loxoscelism. Am J Med Sci 1992; 304:261–267.

42. Sezerino UM, Zannin M, Coelho LK, et al: A clinical and epidemiological study of *Loxosceles* spider envenoming in Santa Catarino, Brazil. Trans R Soc Trop Med Hyg 1998; 92: 546–548.

43. Maretic Z: Latrodectism: variations in clinical manifestations provoked by *Latrodectus* species of spiders. Toxicon 1983; 21:457–466.

44. Vetter RS, Visscher PK, Camazine S: Mass envenomation by honey bees and wasps. West J Med 1999; 170:223–227.

45. Barss P: Renal failure and death after multiple stings in Papua, New Guinea: ecology, prevention and management of attacks by vespid wasps. Med J Aust 1989; 151:659–663.

46. Haberman E: Bee and wasp venoms. Science 1972; 177:314–322.

47. Kolecki P: Delayed toxic reaction following massive bee envenomation. Ann Emerg Med 1999; 33:114–116.

48. Nance L, Bauer P, Lelarge P, et al: Multiple European wasp stings and acute renal failure. Nephron 1992; 61:477.

49. Chen WY, Yen TS, Cheg JT, et al: Acute renal failure due to ingestion of raw bile of grass carp (*Ctenopharyngodon idellus*). J Formos Med Assoc 1976; 75:149–157.

50. Centers for Disease Control and Prevention: Acute hepatitis and renal failure following ingestion of raw carp gallbladders—Maryland and Pennsylvania, 1991 and 1994. JAMA 1995; 274:604.

51. Department of Internal Medicine, Department of Pathology, Department of Biochemistry, Second Hospital of Beijing Medical University. Poisoning caused by gallbladder of black carp. [Chinese] J New Med Drugs 1974; 12:31–34.

52. Lin CT, Huang PC, Yen TS, et al: Partial purification and some characteristic nature of a toxic fraction of the grass carp bile. Chin Biochem Soc 1977; 6:1.

53. Ng HL, Kum KP: Common ichthyogallotoxic fishes in China. Donwuxue Zazhi 1977; 3:28–29.

54. Lim PS, Lin JL, Hu SA, Huang CC: Acute renal failure due to the ingestion of the gallbladder of the grass carp: report of 3 cases with review of the literature. Ren Fail 1993; 15:639–644.

55. Chan TYK, Chan JCN, Tomlinson B, Critchley JAJH: Chinese herbal medicines revisited: a Hong Kong perspective. Lancet 1993; 34a:1532–1534.

56. Chan TYK, Chan AYW, Critchley JAJH: Hospital admissions due to adverse reactions to Chinese herbal medication. J Trop Med Hyg 1992; 95:296–298.

57. Lu LX: Lei-Gong-Teng: In: Yan ZH, ed: *Textbook of Chinese Medical Herbs*. Beijing: People's Medical Publishing House; 1991:304.

58. *Pharmacopoeia of People's Republic of China*. Vol. 1. 5th ed. Beijing: People's Med Publishing House; 1995:124.

59. Zhou FJ, Lu HW, Nie CF: Acute renal failure caused by *Aristolochia manshuriensis Kom* poisoning: case reports and animal experiment [Chinese]. Chin J Nephrol 1988; 4:223.

60. Liu JY, Zeng HJ: A case report of death caused by acute renal failure due to ingestion of *Aristolochia manshuriensis Kom* decoction. [Chinese]. Chin J Clin Materia Medica 1994; 19:692.

61. Depierreux M, Damme BV, Houte KV, et al: Pathologic aspects of a newly described nephropathy related to the prolonged use of Chinese herbs. Am J Kidney Dis 1994; 24:172–180.

62. Nortier JL, Martinez MC, Schmeiser HH, et al: Urothelial carcinoma associated with the use of a Chinese herb (*Aristolochia fangchi*). N Engl J Med 2000; 342:1686–1692.

63. Cosyns JP, Goebbels KM, Liberton V, et al: Chinese herbs nephropathy-associated slimming regimen induces tumors in the stomach but no interstitial nephropathy in rats. Arch Toxicol 1998; 72:738–743.

64. Colson CR, De Greef KE, Duymelinck C, et al: Role of serotonin in the development of Chinese herbs nephropathy. J Am Soc Nephrol 1998; 9:593A.

65. Huang N: Clinical analysis of 31 cases of *Tripterygium wilfordii Hook f* poisoning. [Chinese]. Chin J Intern Med 1982; 21:363–364.

66. Jiang YS, Zhao SP: Analysis of 15 cases of acute renal failure caused by *Tripterygium wilfordii Hook f* poisoning. [Chinese]. Bull Hunan Med College 1987; 12:290–291.

67. Pillans PI: Toxicity of herbal products. N Z Med J 1995; 108:469–471.

CHAPTER 31

Osmotic Nephropathy

Priya Visweswaran Balakrishnan ▪ Thomas D. DuBose, Jr.

DEFINITION

Osmotic nephropathy is a distinct pathologic entity that may result in acute renal failure (ARF) following the intravenous administration of high doses of hyperosmolar substances such as mannitol, sucrose, intravenous immunoglobulin G (IVIG), dextran, starch, and inulin. This disorder has also been reported after the administration of radiocontrast material when mannitol was used for prophylaxis against contrast nephropathy. Indeed, because recent studies have demonstrated that mannitol does not prevent contrast nephropathy,[1] and with the knowledge that mannitol may itself cause ARF, the use of mannitol before, during, or after procedures involving radiocontrast agents should be avoided.

SCOPE OF THE PROBLEM

The incidence of osmotic nephropathy as the cause of ARF has not been defined. Since this disorder is appreciated rarely, the true incidence is probably underestimated.

HISTORICAL PERSPECTIVE (Table 31–1)

Osmotic nephrosis was initially described by Helmholz,[2] who noted swelling of cytoplasmic vacuoles in proximal tubular cells after injecting rabbits with hypertonic sucrose. Subsequently, renal biopsy findings in patients who received sucrose as an osmotic diuretic agent[3, 4] confirmed the relevance of these observations. An in-depth description of this pathologic entity was based on studies in rats following administration of high doses of intravenous hyperosmolar solutions of glucose, mannitol, or dextran.[5] Later, light and electron microscopic studies of proximal convoluted tubule cells were conducted after intravenous administration of mannitol, hypertonic glucose, and dextran. The term *osmotic nephrosis* was introduced to indicate that proximal tubular epithelial cells were substantially vacuolized. It was not determined, however, if these vacuoles contained the injected substance. Numerous vacuoles packed the cytoplasm of the proximal tubular epithelial cells and were almost always uniform in size. Periodic acid–Schiff (PAS) and hematoxylin-eosin stains revealed expanded proximal convoluted tubules, some of which exhibited obliteration of the tubule lumen. The cytoplasm was pale and the brush border was flattened. Vacuolization was noted to be more prominent when mannitol was injected than when a comparable amount of glucose was injected.

DIFFERENTIAL DIAGNOSIS

Although a somewhat similar pattern of cytoplasmic vacuolization may also be seen with cyclosporine nephrotoxicity,[6] the degree of vacuolization is generally much more extensive and uniform after mannitol intoxication. Moreover, the arteriolar hyalinization typical of chronic cyclosporine nephrotoxicity is not observed in osmotic nephropathy. Studies in rats have revealed potentiation of the degree of vacuolization when mannitol and cyclosporine were administered concomitantly.[7] Nevertheless, such potentiation has not been confirmed in human studies.[8]

REVIEW OF CLINICAL AND PATHOLOGIC MANIFESTATIONS OF INDIVIDUAL AGENTS
Mannitol

Mannitol is an osmotic diuretic and obligate extracellular solute. This agent is widely used to (1) reduce

TABLE 31–1. Review of Osmotic Nephrosis Literature: Mannitol and IVIG

AUTHOR (REFERENCE NUMBER)	DESCRIPTION OF STUDY	YEAR
Maunsbach et al[5]	Intramuscular and subcutaneous injections of hypertonic solutions such as mannitol caused vacuolization of proximal tubular epithelial cells. First English language article describing this effect. (Referenced are five German and French papers describing same.)	1962
Brunner et al[7]	In rats, combined infusion of cyclosporine and mannitol had a much more nephrotoxic effect than either agent alone. Tubular vacuolization was slight with either agent but pronounced when both are infused	1986
Dorman et al[10]	Photomicrographs of urinary sediment showing vacuolated tubular epithelial cells after massive mannitol administration and vacuolization seen in tubules on kidney biopsy	1990
Visweswaran et al[17]	Case report of mannitol-induced acute renal failure with review of the literature	1997
Khalil et al[37]	Case report of IVIG-induced acute renal failure that demonstrated unique urine cytology	2000
Ahsan[45]	Review of all cases of IVIG-induced acute renal failure reported in the literature	1998

IVIG, intravenous immunoglobulin G.

intracranial edema resulting from trauma, surgery, or hemorrhage; (2) reduce intraocular pressure in acute angle-closure glaucoma; or (3) prevent and treat dialysis-disequilibrium syndrome.[9, 10] Mannitol has also been recommended, along with volume expansion and sodium bicarbonate, for the prevention of myoglobin-induced acute renal injury.[11] Intravenous mannitol infusion before vascular clamp release and before the initiation of cyclosporine has been suggested for the prevention of post-transplant ARF.[12, 13] Such applications may require high doses of mannitol that may, paradoxically, induce ARF.[10] In earlier uncontrolled studies mannitol was reported to reduce the nephrotoxicity of radiocontrast agents in patients with chronic renal insufficiency.[9] On the basis of this report and other evidence that suggested a possible beneficial effect of mannitol in preventing cell swelling,[14] mannitol was recommended in the setting of early or impending ARF. More recent controlled studies, however, have failed to substantiate a beneficial prophylactic effect for patients at risk for contrast nephropathy.[1] Indeed, intravenous saline administration was observed to impart a beneficial effect in preventing contrast nephropathy, whereas furosemide and mannitol had a deleterious effect.[1] It has been assumed that altered vascular reactivity in response to mannitol can explain the absence of renal protection in diabetic patients who were given mannitol to prevent radiocontrast nephropathy.[15] The incidence of ARF was much higher in patients who received mannitol, dopamine, or atrial natriuretic peptide compared with those who received only intravenous normal saline in this setting.[15]

CLINICAL MANIFESTATIONS

Typically mannitol-induced ARF occurs in the setting of administration of large cumulative doses of this agent. The mean reported dose of mannitol that precipitated ARF in patients with previously compromised kidney function was 295 g.[10] In contrast, in individuals with previously normal baseline kidney function, the mean total dose of mannitol that precipitated ARF was 626 g over 2 to 5 days.[10] In patients who are concomitantly on cyclosporine, the amount of mannitol necessary to precipitate ARF appears to be much less. Laboratory findings include rapidly rising creatinine and blood urea nitrogen levels, which typically decline slowly once mannitol is discontinued.[10] An elevated serum potassium level is common when intoxication results from higher doses because of the solvent-drag phenomenon associated with mannitol. Early in the course of infusion, however, hypokalemia may be observed. Hyponatremia, hypobicarbonatemia, hypocalcemia, hypophosphatemia, and acidosis are other features of mannitol excess.[16] Hypocalcemia and hypophosphatemia may result from increased urinary excretion.

The urinalysis may reveal tubular epithelial cells with vacuolization (see section on intravenous immunoglobulin).[10] Urine chemistries, including electrolytes, the fractional excretion of sodium, and the renal failure index are unreliable because mannitol is an osmotic diuretic.[16] Clinical features of intracellular dehydration include lethargy, stupor, and deterioration of mental function.[10] In severe cases, signs of acute congestive heart failure and pulmonary edema with hypotension, pulmonary rales, dyspnea, and decreased urine output are seen.[10]

In the presence of nephrotoxicity the serum level of mannitol may be extremely high (>1000 mg/dL). Overdose may be recognized more readily by the accompanying increase in serum osmolality, which is best appreciated by calculating the osmolal gap.[16] Every effort should be made to keep the osmolal gap below 55 mOsm/kg H_2O, because values in this range are associated with a lower incidence of ARF.[16] The serum concentration of mannitol [mannitol] may be estimated using the expression:

$$[\text{Mannitol}] = \text{Osmolal gap} \times \frac{182}{10}$$

where 182 represents the molecular weight of mannitol. In general, mannitol, especially in large doses, should not be administered to patients with chronic renal insufficiency.

KIDNEY BIOPSY

To document osmotic nephropathy unequivocally, a percutaneous kidney biopsy with light and electron microscopy is necessary. The typical features seen on light microscopy in a case reported recently by the authors[17] are displayed in Figure 31–1. The markedly expanded proximal convoluted tubules, some with obliterated lumina, and the uniform distributing of vacuoles in the cytoplasm are pathognomonic for osmotic nephrosis. These findings on biopsy recapitulate the features reported previously in toxicity studies in animals.[2, 5]

PATHOPHYSIOLOGY

Mannitol, a 6-carbon alcohol prepared by the reduction of dextrose,[8] is metabolically inert and is excreted unchanged in the urine.[18] In 1940, Smith and associates showed that mannitol clearance correlated directly with the glomerular filtration rate (GFR) in humans.[18] Mannitol has myriad effects on tubular transport and hemodynamics, including (1) osmotic inhibition of water reabsorption in the proximal tubule; (2) reduction in the concentration gradient for passive absorption of NaCl in the thin ascending limb of Henle's loop; and (3) increase in renal blood flow.[16] The GFR may be augmented (by extracellular volume expansion and increased renal plasma flow) or reduced (by increased intratubular pressure and efferent arteriolar dilation).[16] Recent evaluation of mannitol pharmacokinetics reveals that the elimination half-life of mannitol varies with GFR and the volume of distribution. Variation in GFR probably explains the wide variation in the $t_{1/2}$ (39 to 103 minutes) after administration of standard doses (0.6 g/kg).[10]

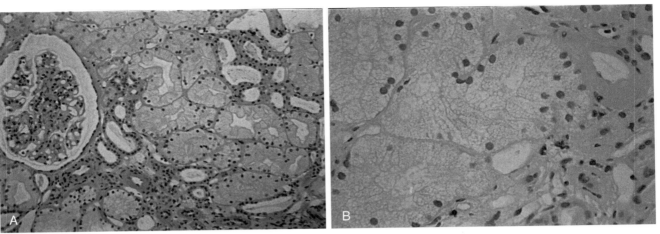

FIGURE 31–1 ▪ Percutaneous biopsy of the kidney, light microscopy. *A*, Periodic acid–Schiff-stained section with markedly expanded proximal convoluted tubules, which in some examples have obliterated lumina. Note the pale cytoplasm and flattened brush border (×200). *B*, Hematoxylin-eosin–stained section of proximal tubules, which display uniform distribution of vacuoles in cytoplasm (×400).

Congestive heart failure was the first described manifestation of mannitol toxicity. Early studies revealed that if mannitol was used in high doses as a diagnostic aid in ARF, it could exacerbate the condition.[19] Subsequently, it was observed that mannitol caused dose-dependent renal vasoconstriction.[20] Studies of animals given high doses of hyperosmolar agents have shown that numerous isometric vacuoles are present in the cytoplasm of the proximal tubules.[5] These tubular vacuoles are presumed to contain the osmotic agent, which may have entered the tubular epithelial cell by pinocytosis.[5] Such a mechanism of cell injury has also been proposed for sucrose (see later), which causes a similar syndrome. Studies in dogs reveal that although the proximal tubular cells contained vacuoles, the tubule lumen was not compromised and the proximal intratubular pressure was not elevated, even during the nadir of renal function.[21] Taken together, these findings suggested that there was more than an anatomic component to this event.[7, 21] In addition, the fact that the ARF was so often reversible after the initiation of hemodialysis also suggests that the pathology is more likely to be pathophysiologic in origin.[10] In this regard it has been proposed that mannitol causes ARF because of activation of tubuloglomerular feedback in response to the increase in tubule fluid osmolality delivered to the macula densa.[22] In a rat micropuncture study, however, mannitol alone, when used to increase the osmolality of tubule fluid to 400 mOsm/L, did not decrease the single-nephron GFR until NaCl was added to the solution.[23] Thus, an increase in the tubular osmolality in conjunction with the increase in NaCl delivery to the macula densa could activate the tubuloglomerular feedback system and decrease single-nephron GFR.

It has also been proposed that the osmotic diuresis indicated by mannitol causes prerenal failure by depleting intravascular volume.[21] Concomitant administration of diuretics (furosemide or acetazolamide) or other potentially nephrotoxic agents such as cyclosporine, increases the likelihood of mannitol-induced renal failure.[6, 7, 24–27] As described earlier, cyclosporine and mannitol together may elicit more intense afferent arteriolar vasoconstriction, resulting eventually in tubular injury.[28]

Thus, mannitol-induced ARF is a complex pathophysiologic process that may occur as a result of several possible mechanisms. Confounding factors include concomitant administration of other nephrotoxic agents, volume depletion, and preexisting renal disease (especially diabetes), all of which have the capacity to potentiate the nephrotoxicity of mannitol.

Intravenous Immunoglobulin G

CLINICAL MANIFESTATIONS

Over the past two decades IVIG administration has been used in the management of primary immunodeficiency syndrome, pediatric acquired immunodeficiency syndrome, infections in low-birth-weight infants, bone marrow transplant recipients, chronic lymphocytic leukemia, idiopathic thrombocytopenic purpura, Kawasaki disease, and demyelinating polyneuropathy. The uses for IVIG may also include any condition that may require plasmapheresis (such as thrombotic thrombocytopenic purpura or hemolytic-uremic syndrome). Several cases have been reported recently of ARF following administration of IVIG.[29–33] The clinical features are indistinguishable from those described earlier for mannitol.

PATHOPHYSIOLOGY

The proposed mechanisms of IVIG-induced renal injury include osmotic injury to the tubular epithelium in response to the hyperosmolality of the sucrose vehicle,[29, 30, 32, 33] renal artery vasoconstriction, and ischemic renal damage.[34]

It has been postulated that renal injury occurs because of incorporation of sucrose into the phagolysosomes of tubular epithelial cells by pinocytosis.[29, 34, 35] Because there is little extragastrointestinal metabolism of sucrose in mammals,[34] retained sucrose in phagolysosomes could lead to cell enlargement through osmosis. This results in rupture and coalescence of the phagolysosomes, creating visible vacuoles. Although this theory has been challenged because of the lack of demonstrable PAS staining within the vacuoles, the presence of radiolabeled sucrose (sucrose-^{14}C) in association with lysosomal acid phosphatase within vacuoles has been reported.[34] The presence of histologic changes in the proximal tubules of the kidney indicative of osmotic injury, in the absence of immunoglobulin deposition in the glomeruli or the interstitium, has attracted attention to the sucrose content of IVIG preparations.[31] Recent studies have suggested that IVIG compounds containing high sucrose concentrations are more likely to cause osmotic nephrosis and attendant renal dysfunction than preparations with lower sucrose concentrations.[30] When glycine-containing immunoglobulin G, rather than sucrose-containing IgG, is used, the likelihood of osmotic nephrosis is much less.[36]

KIDNEY BIOPSY

Kidney biopsies from affected patients show swelling and vacuolization of the epithelial cells lining the proximal convoluted tubules. These findings are similar to the features displayed in Figure 31–1 for mannitol.[29–33] Occasional apoptotic cells have also been described within the tubules.[31]

URINE CYTOLOGY

The urine from a patient with ARF following administration of high-dose sucrose-containing IVIG was recently reported to contain, by cytology, multivacuo-

lated, foamy tubular cells (Fig. 31–2).[37] The differential diagnosis of such cells in the urine includes mycobacterial and fungal infections, xanthogranulomatous pyelonephritis, malakoplakia, urothelial cells with degenerative changes, and low-grade renal cell carcinoma. Special stains were useful to exclude infections. When the urine specimen was stained using Papanicolaou and Diff-Quik methods, vacuolated epithelioid cells were observed. However, the vacuoles did not stain with either PAS or oil red-O stains. Also, no other inflammatory cells were seen. Additionally, the presence of a positive immunoperoxidase stain for cytokeratin verified the tubular origin of these cells.[37] Electron microscopy revealed that the cells were filled with electrolucent vacuoles, scant protoplasmic processes, and sparse cytoplasmic organelles composed primarily of mitochondria (Fig. 31–3). These abnormal cells slowly disappeared from the urine 1 week after IVIG was stopped.[37]

Other Substances That Have Caused Osmotic Nephrosis

Osmotic nephrosis has also been reported with administration of dextran 40[38] (to expand extracellular fluid in burned patients), and hydroxyethyl starch,[39] which has been used as a preservative for renal allografts and as a plasma volume expander in potential cadaveric kidney donors. Other substances such as saccharose, gelatin,[39] glycerol[40] and inulin,[41] and iodinated contrast material[42] also have the potential to cause osmotic nephrosis, but their use in sufficiently high doses is rare.

DIAGNOSIS AND TREATMENT

Patients at high risk to develop osmotic nephrosis include the elderly, patients with diabetes mellitus,

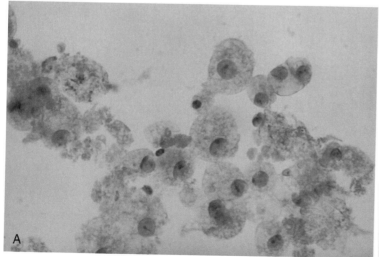
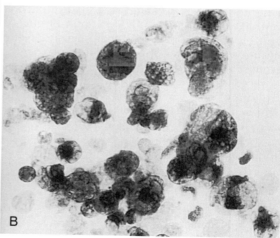

FIGURE 31–2 ■ *A,* The voided urine specimen (obtained on day 2 of hospitalization) showing clusters of bland, epithelioid cells with small nuclei, multivacuolated cytoplasm, and inconspicuous nucleoli mimicking macrophages. Neither inflammatory infiltrates nor necrosis are present in the background (Papanicolaou stain, original magnification ×40). *B,* Positive immunostaining for cytokeratin confirms the epithelial nature of the multivacuolated cells (Immunostain, original magnification ×40).

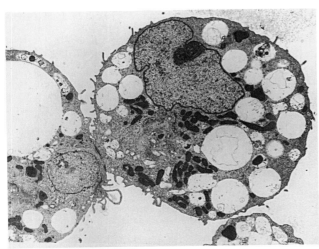

FIGURE 31–3 ▪ Electron microscopy of urinary sediment reveals that the cytoplasm of the epithelial cells was filled with many clear vacuoles of various sizes. Notice that the adjacent cell membranes of two of the cells are joined (original magnification ×6200).

preexisting renal dysfunction due to other causes (especially volume depletion[26]) or the concomitant use of other nephrotoxicants. Higher doses of osmotic agents are more likely to predispose an individual to nephrotoxicity, although the highest tolerable dose is highly variable.

The most valuable tool in making the diagnosis of osmotic nephrosis-induced ARF is maintaining a high index of clinical suspicion for, and being alert to, the possibility that osmotic nephrosis may occur in these specific clinical situations when high doses of osmotic agents, especially mannitol, or sucrose, are administered.

During the period that a patient is on an osmotic agent, there should be regular monitoring of serum concentrations of sodium, potassium, calcium, phosphate, serum osmolality, the osmolal gap, and the hourly urine output.[17] A rise in the osmolal gap above 55 mOsm/L suggests an overwhelming accumulation of the osmotic agent. This should prompt immediate cessation of the agent.

The measurement of urinary tubular enzyme markers such as N-acetyl-beta-glucosaminidase, alanine aminopeptidase, alpha₁-microglobulin, or Tamm-Horsfall protein to detect renal tubular injury has not been a reliable means of predicting onset of ARF and offers no value in making the diagnosis.[43, 44] Osmotic nephrosis is confirmed by kidney biopsy or urine cytology, if the characteristic isometric vacuoles are present in tubular cells.[37]

When present, osmotic nephrotoxicity can be treated successfully by discontinuing the agent and by restoring extracellular fluid volume. Recovery may occur spontaneously but may take as long as 14 days.[17, 37] At the onset of recovery an osmotic diuresis may be observed concomitant with a decline in the osmolal gap.[17] Hemodialysis may be required in the interim. IVIG-sucrose–induced osmotic nephrosis may be prevented or reversed by hemodialysis if applied early.[45] Although there have been case reports of death occurring, partly as a result of osmotic nephrosis–induced ARF,[21] there is no evidence to suggest progression to end-stage renal disease if the patient survives. Peritoneal dialysis may effectively remove sucrose, but there are no reports available suggesting its efficacy. Likewise, the effectiveness of continuous dialysis has not been reported.

There have been no controlled experiments or trials to demonstrate whether additional therapy allows for more rapid resolution of ARF induced by an osmotic agent. However, plasmapheresis for dextran 40–induced osmotic nephrosis with ARF has been reported.[38] In this case, plasmapheresis was associated with initiation of a spontaneous diuresis accompanied by resolution of the ARF. It is likely that in this case the timing of the plasma exchange coincided fortuitously with peak plasma concentrations of sucrose, allowing for its effective removal.

In summary, monitoring of the osmolar gap should prevent the development of osmotic nephrosis. Alternatively, either mannitol or sucrose should be discontinued immediately if ARF develops. Renal replacement therapy, preferably as acute intermittent hemodialysis, may be necessary in the interim if extracellular fluid volume expansion does not correct the azotemia. Recovery of renal function within 3 to 14 days is anticipated. End-stage renal disease following documented osmotic nephrosis has not been reported.

REFERENCES

1. Solomon R, Werner C, Mann D, et al: Effects of saline, mannitol, and furosemide on acute decreases in renal function induced by radiocontrast agents. N Engl J Med 1994; 331:1416–1420.
2. Helmholz HF: Renal changes in rabbits resulting from intravenous injection of hypertonic solution of sucrose. J Pediatr 1933; 3:144–157.
3. Anderson WAD: Sucrose nephrosis and other types of renal tubular injuries. South Med J 1941; 34:257–262.
4. Rigdon RH, Cardwell ES: Renal lesions following the intravenous injection of a hypertonic solution of sucrose: a clinical and experimental study. Arch Intern Med 1942; 69:670–690.
5. Maunsbach AB, Madden SC, Latta H: Light and electron microscopic changes in proximal tubules of rats after administration of glucose, mannitol, sucrose, or dextran. Lab Invest 1962; 6:421–432.
6. Mihatsch MJ, Thiel G, Basler V, et al: Morphological patterns in cyclosporine-treated renal transplant recipients. Transplant Proc 1985; 17(4 Suppl 1):101–116.
7. Brunner FP, Hermle M, Mihatsch MJ, et al: Mannitol potentiates cyclosporine nephrotoxicity. Clin Nephrol 1986; 25:S130–S136.
8. Biesenbach G, Zagormik J, Kaiser W, et al: Severe tubulopathy and kidney graft rupture after coadministration of mannitol and cyclosporin. Nephron 1992; 62:93–96.
9. Nissenson AR, Weston RE, Kleeman CR: Mannitol. West J Med 1979; 131:277–284.
10. Dorman HR, Sondheimer JH, Cadnapaphornchai P: Mannitol-induced acute renal failure. Medicine 1990; 69:153–159.
11. Thadhani R, Pascual M, Bonventre JV: Acute renal failure. N Engl J Med 1996; 334:1448–1460.
12. Lauzurica R, Teixido J, Serra A, et al: Hydration and mannitol reduce the need for dialysis in cadaveric kidney transplant recipients treated with cyclosporin A. Transplant Proc 1992; 24:46–47.
13. van Valenburg PLJ, Hoitsma AJ, Tiggeler RG, et al: Mannitol as indispensable constituent of an intraoperative hydration protocol for the prevention of acute renal failure after renal cadaveric transplantation. Transplantation 1987; 44:784–788.

14. Flores J, DiBona DR, Beck CH, et al: The role of cell swelling in ischemic renal damage and the protective effect of hypertonic solute. J Clin Invest 1972; 51:118–126.

15. Weisberg LS, Kurnik PB, Kurnik BRC: Risk of radiocontrast nephropathy in patients with and without diabetes mellitus. Kidney Int 1994; 45:259–265.

16. Rabetoy GM, Fredricks MR, Hostettler CF: Where the kidney is concerned, how much mannitol is too much? Ann Pharmacother 1993; 27:25–28.

17. Visweswaran P, Massin EK, DuBose TD Jr: Mannitol-induced acute renal failure. J Am Soc Nephrol 1997; 8:1028–1033.

18. Smith WW, Finkelstein N, Smith HW: Renal excretion of hexitols and their derivatives and of endogenous creatinine-like chromogen in dog and man. J Biol Chem 1940; 135:231–250.

19. Aviram A, Pfau A, Czackes JW, et al: Hyperosmolality with hyponatremia, caused by inappropriate administration of mannitol. Am J Med 1967; 42:648–650.

20. Temes SP, Lilien OM, Chamberlain W: A direct vasoconstrictor effect of mannitol on the renal artery. Surg Gynecol Obstet 1975; 141:223–226.

21. Stuart FP, Torres E, Fletcher R, et al: Effects of single, repeated, and massive mannitol infusion in the dog: structural and functional changes in the kidney and brain. Ann Surg 1970; 172:190–204.

22. Goldwasser P, Fotino S: Acute renal failure following massive mannitol infusion: appropriate response of tubuloglomerular feedback? Arch Intern Med 1984; 144:2214–2216.

23. Briggs JP, Schnermann J, Wright FS: Failure of tubule fluid osmolarity to affect feedback regulation of glomerular filtration. Am J Physiol 1980; 239:F427–F432.

24. Whelan TV, Bacon ME, Madden M, et al: Acute renal failure associated with mannitol intoxication. Arch Intern Med 1984; 144:2053–2055.

25. Horgan KJ, Ottaviano YL, Watson AJ: Acute renal failure due to mannitol intoxication. Am J Nephrol 1989; 9:106–109.

26. Weaver A, Sica DA: Mannitol-induced acute renal failure. Nephron 1987; 45:233–235.

27. Plouvier B, Baclet J, deConinck P: Une association nephrotoxique: mannitol et furosemide. Nouv Presse Med 1981; 10:1744–1745.

28. Hogstrom B, Hietala SO, Rooth P: In vivo fluorescence microscopy of microcirculation in the renal cortex of mice: III. Effects of mannitol and iohexol infusions after pretreatment with cyclosporin A. Acta Radiol 1993; 34:500–504.

29. Ahsan N, Palmer BF, Wheeler D, et al: Intravenous immunoglobulin–induced osmotic nephrosis. Arch Intern Med 1994; 154:1985–1987.

30. Ahsan N, Wiegand LA, Abendroth CS, et al: Acute renal failure following immunoglobulin therapy. Am J Nephrol 1996; 16:532–536.

31. Cantu TG, Hoehn-Saric EW, Burgess KM, et al: Acute renal failure associated with immunoglobulin therapy. Am J Kidney Dis 1995; 25:228–234.

32. Rault R, Piraino B, Johnston JR, et al: Pulmonary and renal toxicity of intravenous immunoglobulin. Clin Nephrol 1991; 36:83–86.

33. Tan E, Hajinazarian M, Bay W, et al: Acute renal failure resulting from intravenous immunoglobulin therapy. Arch Neurol 1993; 50:137–139.

34. Schwartz SL, Johnson CB: Pinocytosis as the cause of sucrose nephrosis. Nephron 1971; 8:246–254.

35. Janigan DT, Santamaria A: A histochemical study of swelling and vacuolization of proximal tubular cells in sucrose nephrosis in the rat. Am J Pathol 1960; 39:175–193.

36. Hansen-Schmidt S, Silomon J, Keller F: Osmotic nephrosis due to high-dose immunoglobulin therapy containing sucrose (but not with glycine) in a patient with immunoglobulin A nephritis. Am J Kidney Dis 1996; 28:451–453.

37. Khalil M, Shin HYS, Tan A, et al: Macrophage-like vacuolated renal tubular cells in the urine of a patient with intravenous immunoglobulin therapy: a case report. Acta Cytol 2000; 44:86–90.

38. Ferraboli R, Malheiro PS, Abdulkader RC, et al: Anuric acute renal failure caused by dextran 40 administration. Ren Fail 1997; 19:303–306.

39. Cittanova ML, Leblanc I, Legendre C, et al: Effect of hydroxyethyl starch in brain-dead kidney donors on renal function in kidney transplant patients. Lancet 1996; 348:1620–1622.

40. Ackermann RH: Effects of parenteral infusion of glycerol on glycerol kinase and adenosine triphosphate in rat kidneys. Res Exp Med (Berl) 1975; 166:251–263.

41. Kief H, Hajdu P, Engelbart K: Reabsorptive vacuolization (so-called osmotic nephrosis) after inulin. Frankf Z Pathol 1967; 77:12–19.

42. Moreau JF, Droz D, Sabto J, et al: Osmotic nephrosis induced by water-soluble triiodinated contrast media in man: a retrospective study of 47 cases. Radiology 1975; 115:329–336.

43. Lanza V, Guglielmo L, Sapio M, et al: Evaluation of the liberation of urinary necrosis enzymes (NAG-AP) after administration of plasma expanders: study of dextran-40, hydroxyethyl starch, and polymerized gelatin. Boll Soc Ital Biol Sper 1989; 65:1155–1161.

44. Dehne MG, Muhling J, Sablotzki A, et al: Effect of hydroxyethyl starch solution on kidney function in surgical intensive care patients. Anasthesiol Intensivmed Notfallmed Schmerzther 1997; 32:348–354.

45. Ahsan N: Intravenous immunoglobulin–induced nephropathy: a complication of IVIG therapy. J Nephrol 1998; 1:157–161.

CHAPTER 32

Acute Renal Failure Associated With Recreational Drug Use

John H. Turney

Thou hast the keys of Paradise, oh just, subtle, and mighty opium.

"Confessions of an English Opium Eater"
Thomas de Quincy (1785–1859)

INTRODUCTION

Use and abuse of recreational drugs are probably as old as mankind itself (ethanol, khat, mushrooms, opium, cocaine), and the need for chemically aided relaxation, alteration of perception, and mood modification seems almost universal. Of interest to the nephrologist, internist, and intensivist is the propensity for substance abuse to cause acute renal failure (ARF), either directly or indirectly (Tables 32–1 and 32–2).

The illicit nature of recreational drug use makes it difficult to determine the extent of the problem, but it is undoubtedly widespread and common. Epidemiologic studies are further confounded by the shifting nature of drug usage, with patterns changing according to availability, cost, and fashion, so that there may be sudden localized upsurges, or habits may drift across age groups or social classes. Thus, there have been peaks and troughs of abuse of barbiturates, amphetamines, cocaine, and heroin, with a recent upsurge of the use of the latter, mainly by inhalation. Surveys in the United States indicate that there were 13 million illicit drug users in 1996, of whom 2 million

TABLE 32–1. Acute Renal Failure Syndromes Associated With Recreational Drugs

SYNDROME	CAUSE
Rhabdomyolysis	Pressure (crush)
	Coma, restraint
	Seizures and so on
	Muscle activity
	Vasoconstriction
	Microembolization
	Hyperthermia
Vasculitis	Serotonin syndrome
	Neuroleptic malignant syndrome
Interstitial nephritis	
Renal infarction	
Tubular toxicity	
Indirect effects	Hepatic failure
	Disseminated intravascular coagulation
	Infections
	Bacterial endocarditis
	HIV/AIDS
	Tetanus
	Septicemia

TABLE 32–2. Acute Renal Failure Syndromes Associated With Specific Drugs

DRUG	SYNDROME	ETIOLOGIC MECHANISMS
Amphetamines	Rhabdomyolysis	Coma (crush syndrome)
		Hyperthermia
		Serotonin syndrome
	Vasculitis	
Cocaine	Rhabdomyolysis	Muscle activity
		Direct myotoxicity
		Hyperthermia
		Neuroleptic malignant syndrome
Heroin	Rhabdomyolysis	Coma (crush syndrome)
Ethanol	Rhabdomyolysis	Coma (crush syndrome)
		Myotoxicity
		Hypophosphatemia
		Acid/base and electrolyte disorders
		Interaction with other drugs (NSAID, acetaminophen)
Barbiturates	Rhabdomyolysis	
Phencyclidine	Rhabdomyolysis	Coma (crush syndrome)
		Coma (crush syndrome)
		Seizures and so on
		Restraint
		Hyperuricemia

regularly used cocaine (down from a peak of 5.7 million in 1985).[1] In some age groups, recreational drug use is very high and an integral part of some countercultures. For example, upward of 40% of university undergraduates admitted to at least some use of "ecstasy" as part of the culture of clubs, dances, and "raves." If the extent of recreational drug use is imprecise, it is difficult to know what proportion of users experience significant medical problems. In 1995, there were 531,800 drug-related emergency department visits in the United States, more than half of which were overdoses and 143,000 related to cocaine.

This chapter surveys and collates the recent literature on recreational drugs and ARF, which is based largely on case reports.

AMPHETAMINES AND RELATED COMPOUNDS

Amphetamine-like compounds are substituted phenylisopropylamines, some of which are naturally occurring. Originally developed as bronchodilators, amphetamines rapidly achieved widespread use as stimulants and anorectics but increasingly became drugs of abuse for their stimulant and euphoric effects. Amphetamines are easily manufactured, and this has led to the synthesis of derivatives with additional hallucinogenic properties, particularly by methoxyl group substitution on the basic phenyl ring at the 3,4 position. These newer agents include 3,4-methylenedioxymethamphetamine (MDMA, "ecstasy"), 3,4-methylenedioxyamphetamine (MDA), 3,4-methylenedioxyethamphetamine (MDEA, "eve"), and 2,5-dimethoxy-4-methylamphetamine (DOM). These "designer" drugs are increasingly widely used, but the pattern of use varies, with MDMA being consumed at dances (or "raves") in Britain and Europe but at parties or alone in the United States, a factor that may be relevant to the different patterns of toxicity seen in different countries.[2] The precise mode of action of amphetamine and its derivatives and the pharmacologic mechanisms of toxicity are far from clear, largely because of their complicated and diverse effects. They work primarily as sympathomimetics by increasing postsynaptic catecholamines, which occurs by blocking presynaptic uptake and storage, and reducing catecholamine destruction, which occurs by inhibiting mitochondrial monoamine oxidase. The sympathomimetic action explains the cardiovascular effects, but many of the central nervous system and toxic effects may be the result of serotonin release or reuptake blockade. As with all recreational drugs, amphetamines are not supplied in pure form or in standard dosage and are often taken in combination with other substances, many of which also have potent vasoactive or psychoactive properties. The role of adulterants in toxicity associated with amphetamines is impossible to assess but may be relevant to the comparative rarity of reports of ARF with these agents, which are extremely commonly used. It is doubtful whether there is a pharmacologic basis to individual susceptibility to toxicity. MDMA has nonlinear pharmacokinetics, with a small increase in dose resulting in a large increase in blood levels. None of three individuals with MDMA-associated fulminant hepatic failure had deficiency of the cytochrome P-450 2D6 (CYP2D6) enzyme,[3] making it unlikely that slow metabolism is the cause of individual susceptibility to toxicity. More MDMA-related deaths have occurred in the United Kingdom than in the United States, probably because of its use in the former at "rave" dances, characterized by prolonged, violent dancing in hot, overcrowded clubs with little opportunity for rehydration.[3]

Although there are reports of ARF apparently directly due to nephrotoxicity of MDMA[4] and acute interstitial nephritis with amphetamine,[5] most ARF results from rhabdomyolysis, with a few reports of renal vasculitis. Hallucinogen-associated rhabdomyolysis has many causes and may result from coma[6–10] or seizures or other violent muscular activity,[9, 11–17] but in several instances the extent of the rhabdomyolysis appears to be greater than the extent of the reported direct muscle injury, leading to the suggestion that amphetamine-induced vasoconstriction may cause generalized patchy muscle ischemia and necrosis.[10, 17] Indeed, there is nuclear imaging evidence[18] of generalized rhabdomyo-

lysis in a case of ARF following amphetamine overdose. However, hyperpyrexia is a consistent feature in most, if not all, cases of rhabdomyolysis associated with amphetamines[9, 19–21]; MDMA, MDA, MDEA[13–15, 19, 22–33]; and related hallucinogens.[7, 19] Fatal ARF is usually associated with disseminated intravascular coagulation,[7, 13, 14, 22, 24, 25, 28, 30–33] shock, multiorgan failure,[9, 14, 28, 32] and hepatic necrosis.[3, 30, 31] Fulminant hepatic failure appears to be a feature of the use of MDMA and its analogues and may occur with or without hyperpyrexia. The importance of hyperthermic, rather than exertional, muscle damage is illustrated by the illuminating case of ecstasy-induced rhabdomyolysis and ARF with astronomically high creatine kinase levels in a paraplegic subject.[32] The mechanism of hyperpyrexia is not entirely clear. Although some liken it to exertional heatstroke,[28, 30] this appears not to be the case. An explanation more in keeping with the known pharmacologic effects[29] is that amphetamines (especially the methoxy-substituted phenethylamines such as MDMA or MDA) precipitate the serotonin syndrome, which itself causes the adverse effects, including rhabdomyolysis and secondary ARF, mainly via hyperpyrexia.[34, 35] That the serotonin syndrome is the primary mechanism of toxicity is indirectly supported by reports indicating the ineffectiveness of dantrolene in the treatment of hyperpyrexia and its consequence.[28, 29, 32, 33] The most rational treatment of the amphetamine-intoxicated patient that prevents serious adverse consequences should be cooling, rehydration, cardiovascular and respiratory support, and sedation with benzodiazepines or chlormethiazole.[29]

A possible relationship between amphetamines and vasculitis has long been suggested[36] but remains controversial. There are several reports of amphetamine-associated polyarteritis nodosa, both with[37] and without[38] positive hepatitis B serology, and in the latter case the arteritis dramatically worsened with resumption of amphetamine abuse. Malignant hypertension was a prominent feature in both these cases and in a further MDMA-related renal vasculitis.[39] Renal necrotizing angiitis and ARF have been temporally related to MDMA exposure,[39, 40] and in one of these cases the patient went on to develop a scleroderma-like illness,[41] similar to a case reported in association with cocaine.[42] The reports of renal vasculitis are greatly outnumbered by cases of amphetamine-associated cerebral vasculitis,[43, 44] demonstrated both radiologically and histologically, which provide convincing evidence that amphetamine and its analogues may rarely cause vasculitis, irrespective of the route of administration. The vasculitis may represent a hypersensitivity reaction and may respond to immunosuppressive therapy.

The α-adrenergic effects of amphetamines may sometimes cause acute bladder outflow obstruction.[45] Finally, three cases of ARF have been reported in association with phenylpropanolamine,[46, 47] a sympathomimetic agent with close structural affinity to amphetamine, which has been widely used in diet pills. The reports again suggest a multifactorial etiology, including rhabdomyolysis, for ARF.

COCAINE

It is estimated that 11.3% of the US population has used cocaine, with 1.3% using it at least monthly. As cocaine may cause a variety of medical problems, the health care burden is considerable.[48] Cocaine (benzoylmethylecgonine) is an ester of benzoic acid and the complex alcohol 2-carbomethoxy,3-hydroxytropane, and is the extract of the leaves of the shrub *Erythroxylon coca*. The pharmacology and toxicology of cocaine are complex.[49–51] Cocaine hydrochloride is water-soluble and taken orally or by injection. "Freebase" and "crack" are cocaine alkaloids, manufactured in different ways, that are not water soluble but form a stable vapor when heated. All "street" cocaine contains adulterants, many of which are pharmacologically active or toxic.[52] Cocaine is frequently taken with other substances, the most frequent combination being with ethanol, which results in an important metabolic interaction, with some cocaine being esterified to cocaethylene, which is equipotent to the parent drug in blocking dopamine reuptake. The increasing use of alkaloid cocaine has resulted in a great increase in the number of acute hospital visits, predominantly for cardiopulmonary, neurologic, or psychiatric toxicity, alone or in combination. About 10% of patients require hospital admission, but the overall acute mortality is less than 1%. Cocaine is possibly now the major cause of stroke and myocardial disease in young adults.[53]

Rhabdomyolysis is by far the most common cause of cocaine-associated ARF[51, 54–74] and may occur with either of the forms of cocaine and with any route of administration. The causes of rhabdomyolysis are complex and may differ among individuals, but they include hyperpyrexia, ischemia due to vasoconstriction, seizures, coma, direct myotoxicity, and the effects of adulterants, such as strychnine,[75] arsenic, amphetamines, and phencyclidine. Rhabdomyolysis appears to be a specific effect of cocaine, the severity being determined by dose and individual susceptibility. Myoglobinuric ARF may occur on repeated exposure to cocaine.[60, 67] Elevated creatinine kinase levels are found in as many as 53% of hospital attendees,[76] the levels being proportional to the degree of intoxication, as reflected by the degree of physical activity.[77] Most patients with elevated creatine kinase levels do not display muscle symptoms, so the presence of rhabdomyolysis and hence the risk of ARF at first presentation can be determined only by laboratory investigation. The risk of developing ARF is related to the level of the admission creatine kinase.[77] Rhabdomyolysis is usually generalized,[70] without localizing symptoms, and this most likely occurs in the cases that are caused by hyperpyrexia.[19, 54, 56–59, 63–66, 72, 78, 79] Cocaine-induced hyperpyrexia has the features of the neuroleptic malignant syndrome[35, 48, 72, 80–82] and may result in rhabdomyolysis, disseminated intravascular coagulation, ARF, and hepatic necrosis,[58, 59, 64, 66, 78, 79] with multiorgan system failure developing as the result of hyperthermia and carrying a high mortality, reportedly[58, 60, 66, 72] between 25% and 85%.

There are a few reports of nonmyoglobinuric ARF, one of which could find no risk factors for the severe, reversible renal dysfunction, and postulated intense renal vasoconstriction as the cause.[83] Other cases had the features of Henoch-Schönlein purpura,[84] hemolytic-uremic syndrome,[85] and scleroderma crisis.[42] These cases have in common a significant vasculitic element.

HEROIN AND OTHER OPIATES

Heroin (diacetylmorphine) is the most widely abused opium derivative, and its consumption continues to increase as the result of greater availability and falling prices.[1] Increasing purity means that it is no longer necessary to inject heroin, which can be smoked or snorted. While this may result in a decline in the medical complications of parenteral drug abuse (eg, infections), inhalation of heroin does not decrease the toxicity of the drug. Heroin is a short-acting, lipid-soluble narcotic that rapidly crosses the blood-brain barrier, where it is deacylated to the active metabolites 6-monoacetyl morphine and morphine. All opiates may be abused and may also be admixed with other drugs (eg, heroin-cocaine "speedballs").

Rhabdomyolysis, almost invariably due to crush injury from prolonged coma, is by far the most common cause of heroin-associated ARF, and nontraumatic rhabdomyolysis resulting from heroin- or alcohol-induced coma accounts for 3% to 7% of all cases of ARF,[6, 86, 87] and 30% to 80% of cases of rhabdomyolysis[71, 87, 88] in some series. Rhabdomyolysis occurs in about 10% of all hospital admissions for acute drug intoxication.[89, 90] Acute renal failure due to coma-induced rhabdomyolysis has been widely reported with heroin.[6, 86, 91, 92] Overdosage of methadone, a long-acting diphenylheptane narcotic often used to aid the patient in withdrawal from heroin addiction, may also result in coma, rhabdomyolysis, and ARF,[93] as indeed may occur with overdoses of other opiates.[94] Narcotic-induced rhabdomyolysis may result in acute, life-threatening hyperkalemia,[95] and narcotic overdose may cause severe hypoxic tissue damage with myonecrosis and ARF.[96, 97] There are many reports of heroin-related rhabdomyolysis[92, 98, 99] with ARF in patients without prolonged coma. In these cases, the rhabdomyolysis is frequently generalized, rather than localized to pressure areas, and may result from direct myotoxicity of heroin or its adulterants. It is probable that heroin-induced myoglobinuric ARF is so common that it is under-reported, but nevertheless it constitutes a major nephrologic problem. There appear to be no reports of renal vasculopathy, other than a case of hemolytic-uremic syndrome and vasculitis coinciding with an injection of heroin.[100]

PHENCYCLIDINE

Phencyclidine (PCP) was originally developed as an anesthetic agent and is widely smoked or ingested as a hallucinogen (as is its structural analogue ketamine) either alone or in deliberate or accidental combination with a wide variety of other drugs, including marijuana and cocaine.[49, 50] Increasing dosage results in agitated or violent behavior, muscle rigidity, seizures, coma, hyperthermia, and hypotension. The isometric muscle contractions, seizures, violent behavior, and hyperthermia may all cause rhabdomyolysis, which is the cause of almost all the cases of PCP-related ARF.[101–103] The majority of patients are young males exhibiting organic brain syndromes, of whom almost half are comatose. Exaggerated muscle activity and acute dystonic motor reactions are usual in those with myoglobinuria, and indeed a rise in creatine kinase is seen in 70% of patients hospitalized for PCP intoxication,[104] with significant rhabdomyolysis in about 2.5%, of whom 40% develop ARF,[101] with about half being oliguric. Mortality in PCP-associated ARF has been reported at about 10%. From at least some of the reports, it is clear that the majority of cases developing myoglobinuric ARF have required physical restraint,[101–103] which might very well exacerbate the muscle damage from the violent muscular activity, and, indeed, physical restraint has been implicated in other cases of psychedelic drug–associated rhabdomyolysis.[11] The risk of myoglobinuric renal failure would also have been increased by the previously advocated treatment regimen of urinary acidification in the (probably mistaken) attempt to increase PCP excretion, but which would encourage tubular precipitation of myoglobin and urate.[105] In fact, treatment with rehydration alone, with or without urinary alkalinization, may prevent many cases of ARF.[101] The role of uric acid in the development of ARF in association with rhabdomyolysis remains unclear. In patients in which it is recorded, the level of urate in PCP-related rhabdomyolysis is extremely high,[101, 103, 106] and there is a report of acute uric acid nephropathy with PCP-induced thrashing of the limbs but without seizures and with only a modest rise in creatine kinase.[106] Clearly, the role of uric acid in causing myoglobinuric ARF is of interest, but in practical terms it does not influence the conventional treatment with rehydration, mannitol, and bicarbonate. Hyperthermia associated with PCP probably results from intense physical activity and may cause hepatic necrosis and ARF.[19, 107]

BARBITURATES

Barbiturates are sedative-hypnotic drugs, the pharmacologic characteristics of which are determined by the substituted radicals on the parent barbituric acid molecule.[49, 50] All barbiturates have been abused at some time, often in combination with other substances. Barbiturate overdose and abuse was in vogue in the 1950s and 1960s and became less popular, but there appears to have been a recent upsurge in usage. Barbiturate overdose results in deep coma and respiratory depression and is frequently complicated by pressure-induced rhabdomyolysis,[6, 71, 86, 108, 109] which may be associated with characteristic bullous skin lesions over pressure points.[110]

ETHANOL AND OTHER ALCOHOLS

The drinking of alcohol is almost ubiquitous, and alcohol excess is the most common substance-related cause of hospital visits. Acute and chronic excessive alcohol consumption may result in metabolic, nutritional, and neuromuscular effects that may indirectly lead to acute renal dysfunction. Nevertheless, ARF is surprisingly infrequent in view of the widespread use and abuse of alcohol but may occur secondary to alcoholic liver disease, pancreatitis, or rhabdomyolysis.

Alcoholic ketoacidosis is frequently observed in chronic alcohol abuse, results from the accumulation of β-hydroxybutyrate and lactate, and is multifactorial in origin, being associated with malnutrition and vitamin deficiency. It is usually associated with electrolyte disturbances, particularly hypokalemia and hypophosphatemia, the latter often being dramatically exacerbated by rehydration treatment of the acidosis[111] because of reentry of phosphate into the cells. The profound hypophosphatemia is a potent cause of rhabdomyolysis,[112, 113] which may secondarily lead to ARF. The hypophosphatemia in chronic alcoholics may also result from tubular dysfunction,[114] possibly resulting from localized toxicity of acetaldehyde generated by the oxidation of ethanol by renal alcohol dehydrogenase.[115] The reduction in electrolytes is exacerbated by alcohol-induced diuresis caused by inhibition of antidiuretic hormone.[115] The situation may be worsened by the consumption of large volumes of beer, which has a sodium content of 2 mmol/L or less and may cause hyponatremia and hypo-osmolality. The electrolyte and acid-base disorders contribute to the development of chronic alcoholic myopathy, which predisposes to the development of rhabdomyolysis with myoglobinuric renal failure if the patient's system is stressed by binge drinking, vigorous exercise,[116] seizures or delirium,[117] or coincident medical or surgical events.[118] In these cases, there is a marked rise in the creatine kinase level but usually no localized muscle swelling or pain, unlike cases of ARF due to pressure-induced rhabdomyolysis (crush syndrome) during alcoholic coma,[6, 71, 86, 88, 91, 117, 119, 120] which is often complicated by the compartment syndrome.[38] When urate levels have been reported in alcohol-related rhabdomyolysis, they have been exceedingly high, and it is possible that both urate and myoglobin contribute to the development of ARF.[119] Alcohols other than ethanol are considerably more toxic and are available illicitly. They are also available as constituents of household products, so they may be consumed deliberately when ethanol is unavailable, inadvertently, or with suicidal intent. Consequently, there are occasional reports of myoglobinuric ARF resulting from consumption of methanol[121] and isopropyl (rubbing) alcohol.[122]

Ethanol may potentiate the toxicity of other drugs, particularly acetaminophen. Both are metabolized by the microsomal P-450–dependent enzyme system, specifically the CYP3E1 enzyme, which is induced in chronic drinkers and so may possibly increase the production of the toxic metabolites of acetaminophen. Acute renal failure has been described in alcoholics with hepatic necrosis induced by therapeutic doses of acetaminophen,[123, 124] with rhabdomyolysis,[125] and with possible direct acetaminophen nephrotoxicity.[126]

Perhaps the most intriguing ethanol-drug interaction is the syndrome of flank pain and ARF resulting from binge drinking and subsequent consumption of nonsteroidal anti-inflammatory drugs (NSAIDs).[127–132] Although there have been a number of well-documented cases, this must be a rare cause of ARF, as NSAIDs are widely available and are a commonly sold treatment for hangover symptoms. Ibuprofen has been most frequently implicated, but this may simply reflect its availability, as the syndrome is not unique to this particular NSAID. The unusual associated symptom of flank pain, presumably of renal origin, has not been explained. It is probable that the ARF results from vasomotor nephropathy due to NSAID-induced vasoconstriction in the presence of dehydration caused by alcohol-induced diuresis, vomiting, and decreased fluid intake. Dehydration is a recognized risk factor for acute NSAID nephrotoxicity,[133] but although this mechanism would explain the acute renal dysfunction (in the documented absence of rhabdomyolysis or other risk factors), it appears not to explain the associated flank pain. There remain a few cases of alcohol-related severe, acute renal dysfunction in which causes other than direct ethanol nephrotoxicity appear to have been excluded.[134]

SOLVENTS

Inhalation of volatile hydrocarbons, particularly toluene-based solvents, glues, and paints, for their euphoric and intoxicating effects is a common form of substance abuse, especially among the young. Hospitalization usually results from muscle weakness, gastrointestinal symptoms, or neuropsychiatric problems.[135] Metabolic abnormalities are usual in hospitalized individuals, including hypokalemia, hypophosphatemia, and metabolic acidosis.[135, 136] The metabolic acidosis may be associated with hyperchloremia and normal anion gap, features of renal tubular acidosis, or a high anion gap. The acidosis and, perhaps, the excess urinary electrolyte loss result from the production of hippuric acid, which is derived from glycine conjugation of benzoic acid, the oxidation product of toluene. Rhabdomyolysis with or without renal dysfunction[135] presumably results from the profound hypokalemia and hypophosphatemia[112, 113] but may reflect myocyte membrane damage by the highly lipid-soluble solvents. Acute renal failure has been reported in isolation[137] or associated with hepatocellular dysfunction.[138] These cases share a number of features, including pyuria or hematuria, and rapid recovery of renal function within 1 to 5 days. Solvent abuse may also cause acute tubulointerstitial nephritis,[139] which may lead to nonrecovery of independent renal function because of interstitial fibrosis.[140]

PERFORMANCE-ENHANCING DRUGS

Rhabdomyolysis may occur in body builders as the result of exertion[141] or thermal trauma[142] but has also been reported as a consequence of the use of anabolic steroids for performance enhancement,[143] and stanozolol has also been implicated in acute tubular necrosis secondary to severe cholestasis in another athlete.[144] In theory, the creatine supplements for enhancing physical performance might be expected to confer some protection to muscles at least against anoxic damage. In normal volunteers, creatine has no renal effects.[145] Nevertheless, there are reports of transient modest declines in renal function associated with the recreational use of creatine for fitness enhancement: in one case as the result of acute tubulointerstitial nephritis[146] and, in another, with pre-existing focal segmental glomerulosclerosis but normal renal function.[147]

ACUTE RENAL EFFECTS OF ADULTERANTS, MODE OF ADMINISTRATION, AND DRUG-RELATED INFECTIONS

Illicit drugs are rarely obtainable in pure form, usually having been adulterated or "cut" with other substances of similar physical appearance. Adulterants may be psychoactive drugs such as phenylpropanolamine,[52] inert talc, sugars, or starch, or potentially toxic chemicals such as quinine, arsenic, or strychnine. Because of its sweet taste and effects similar to ethanol, ethylene glycol has been used to adulterate, among others, white wine, and this may potentially cause severe acidosis and ARF. It is rarely possible to identify adulterants, and their role in the toxicity of recreational drugs is far from clear. Only in cases related to strychnine contamination of cocaine[75] has ARF been proved to be due to adulterants. However, renal dysfunction is well documented after the parenteral administration of oral or inhaled substances. In these cases, the toxicity largely may be due to the nondrug components. Thus, starch or talc from tablets dissolved or suspended in water and then injected are unlikely to cause significant renal dysfunction, but the self-injection of water containing suspended drugs may cause rhabdomyolysis. It is probable that the nondrug components of injected dextropropoxyphene capsules resulted in disseminated intravascular coagulation and ARF.[148] Intravenous injection of a solution prepared by heating marijuana in water may cause hypotension and ARF.[149]

Temazepam is a benzodiazepine hypnotic abused by injection of the dissolved oral preparations. This practice continued after the gelatin capsules were replaced by temazepam tablets, resulting in a number of cases of rhabdomyolysis, compartment syndrome, and ARF requiring dialysis following intra-arterial injection of a suspension of the tablets in heated water.[150, 151] The rhabdomyolysis resulted from microembolization in the distribution of the injected artery, and not infrequently limb or digit amputation was required. It must be assumed that the microemboli consisted of both the temazepam crystals, which are virtually insoluble in water, and the inert substances contained within the tablets.

Inadvertent ingestion of toxic Cortinarius mushrooms in place of hallucinogenic "magic" mushrooms (*Psilocybe* species) may lead to ARF,[152] which in one case progressed to end-stage renal failure resulting from interstitial fibrosis.[153] The misidentification of the mushroom species resulted in the ingestion of toxic orellanine rather than the psychedelic LSD-like psilocybin.

Intravenous drug abusers are at great risk for infections, such as tetanus, hepatitis, HIV/AIDS, bacterial endocarditis, or other bacterial sepsis, which may themselves cause ARF by rhabdomyolysis, septicemia, or acute glomerulonephritis.[154, 155]

DRUG-RELATED RENOVASCULAR DISEASE

Not surprisingly for such potent vasoactive substances, the use of cocaine and, to a lesser extent, amphetamines and marijuana has been associated with myocardial and cerebral vasoconstriction, thrombosis, and infarction. Chronic cocaine use has been suggested as a significant cause of accelerated hypertension and end-stage renal disease[156] due to severe renal arteriosclerosis,[157–159] probably related to the suggested effect of cocaine in inducing accelerated atherosclerosis.[160] Despite this, reports of acute renovascular effects are sparse. Renal infarction temporally related to intravenous cocaine[161–163] or heavy marijuana use[164] has been reported but has been associated with at worst only mild and transient acute renal dysfunction.

ACUTE TUBULOINTERSTITIAL NEPHRITIS

Acute renal failure due to acute interstitial nephritis associated with recreational drug use has been rarely reported, but whether this is due to actual rarity or under-recognition is unclear. Interstitial nephritis has been reported in association with crack cocaine,[165] amphetamine,[5] heroin,[166] diazepam,[167] solvents,[139, 140] and the nutrition- or performance-enhancing product creatine[146] and possibly related to granulomas caused by parenteral injection of oral narcotic preparations.

REFERENCES

1. NIDA, NIDA Infofax: Nationwide Trends. Washington, DC: National Institute on Drug Abuse; 1998.
2. Henry JA: Ecstasy and the dance of death. BMJ 1992; 305:5–6.
3. Schwab M, Seyringer E, Brauer RB, et al: Fatal MDMA intoxication. Lancet 1999; 353:593–594.
4. Fahal IH, Sallormi DF, Yaqoob M, et al: Acute renal failure after ecstasy. BMJ 1992; 305:29.
5. Foley RJ, Kapatkin K, Verani R, et al: Amphetamine-induced acute renal failure. South Med J 1984; 77:258–259.
6. Grossman RA, Hamilton RW, Morse BM, et al: Non traumatic rhabdomyolysis and acute renal failure. N Engl J Med 1974; 291:807–811.
7. Klock JC, Boerner U, Becker CE: Coma, hyperthermia, and bleeding associated with massive LSD overdose: a report of eight cases. Clin Toxicol 1975; 8:191–203.
8. Terada Y, Shinohara S, Matui N, et al: Amphetamine-induced myoglobinuric acute renal failure. Jpn J Med 1988; 27:305–308.
9. Lan KC, Lin YF, Yu FC, et al: Clinical manifestations and prognostic features of acute methamphetamine intoxication. J Formos Med Assoc 1998; 97:528–533.
10. Woodard ML, Brent LD: Acute renal failure, anterior myocardial infarction, and atrial fibrillation complicating ephedrine abuse. Pharmacotherapy 1998; 18:656–658.
11. Mercieca J, Brown EA: Acute renal failure due to rhabdomyolysis associated with use of a straightjacket in lysergide intoxication. BMJ 1984; 288:1949–1950.
12. Briscoe JG, Curry SC, Gerkin RD, et al: Pemoline-induced choreoathetosis and rhabdomyolysis. Med Toxicol Adverse Drug Exp 1988; 3:72–76.
13. Campkin NTA, Davies UM: Another death from ecstasy. J R Soc Med 1992; 85:61.
14. Henry JA, Jeffreys KJ, Dawling S: Toxicity and deaths from 3,4-methylene-dioxymethamphetamine ("ecstasy"). Lancet 1992; 340:384–387.
15. Barrett PJ, Taylor GT: "Ecstasy" ingestion: a case report of severe complications. J R Soc Med 1993; 86:233–234.
16. Sperling LS, Horowitz JL: Methamphetamine-induced choreoathetosis and rhabdomyolysis. Ann Intern Med 1994; 121:986.
17. Cartledge JJ, Chow WM, Stewart PA: Acute renal failure after amphetamine presenting with loin pain. Br J Urol 1998; 81:160–161.
18. Kao C-H, Liao S-Q, Wang S-J, et al: Tc-99m PYP imaging in amphetamine intoxication associated with nontraumatic rhabdomyolysis. Clin Nucl Med 1992; 17:101–102.
19. Rosenberg J, Pentel P, Pond S, et al: Hyperthermia associated with drug intoxication. Crit Care Med 1986; 14:964–969.
20. Chan P, Chen JH, Lee MH, et al: Fatal and nonfatal methamphetamine intoxication in the intensive care unit. Clin Toxicol 1994; 32:147–155.
21. Chan T, Evans S, Clark R: Drug-induced hyperthermia. Crit Care Clin 1997; 13:785–808.
22. Simpson DL, Rumack BH: Methylenedioxymethamphetamine: clinical description of overdose, death, and review of pharmacology. Arch Intern Med 1981; 141:1507–1509.
23. Brown C, Osterloh J: Multiple severe complications from recreational ingestion of MDMA ("ecstasy"). JAMA 1987; 258:780–781.
24. Chadwick IS, Curry PD, Linsley A, et al: Ecstasy, 3,4-methylenedioxymethamphetamine (MDMA), a fatality associated with coagulopathy and hyperthermia. J R Soc Med 1991; 84:371.
25. Screaton GR, Singer M, Cairns HS, et al: Hyperpyrexia and rhabdomyolysis after MDMA ("ecstasy") use. Lancet 1992; 339:677–678.
26. Singarajah C, Lavies NG: An overdose of ecstasy: a role for dantrolene. Anaesthesia 1992; 47:686–687.
27. Woods JD, Henry JA: Hyperpyrexia induced by 3,4-methylenedioxyamphetamine ("Eve"). Lancet 1992; 340:305.
28. Watson JD, Ferguson C, Hinds CJ, et al: Exertional heat stroke induced by amphetamine analogues: does dantrolene have a place? Anaesthesia 1993; 48:1057–1060.
29. Green AR, Cross AJ, Goodwin GM: Review of the pharmacology and clinical pharmacology of 3,4-methylenedioxymethamphetamine (MDMA or "ecstasy"). Psychopharmacology (Berl) 1995; 119:247–260.
30. Milroy CM, Clark JC, Forrest ARW: Pathology of deaths associated with "ecstasy" and "eve" misuse. J Clin Pathol 1996; 49:149–153.
31. Ellis AJ, Wendon JA, Portmann B, et al: Acute liver damage and ecstasy ingestion. Gut 1996; 38:454–458.
32. Hall AP, Lyburn ID, Spears FD, et al: An unusual case of ecstasy poisoning. Intensive Care Med 1996; 22:670–671.
33. Dar KJ, McBrien ME: MDMA-induced hyperthermia: report of a fatality and review of current therapy. Intensive Care Med 1996; 22:995–996.
34. Demirkiran M, Jankovic J, Dean JM: Ecstasy intoxication: an overlap between serotonin syndrome and neuroleptic malignant syndrome. Clin Neuropharmacol 1996; 19:157–164.
35. Bertorini TE: Myoglobinuria; malignant hyperthermia, neuroleptic malignant syndrome and serotonin syndrome. Neurol Clin 1997; 15:649–671.
36. Citron BP, Halpern M, McCarron M, et al: Necrotizing angiitis associated with drug abuse. N Engl J Med 1970; 283:1003–1011.

37. Heazlewood VJ, Bochner F, Craswell PW: Hallucinogenic drug induced vasculitis. Med J Aust 1981; 1:359–360.
38. Rifkin SI: Amphetamine-induced angiitis leading to renal failure. Southern Med J 1977; 70:108–109.
39. Woodrow G, Harnden P, Turney JH: Acute renal failure due to accelerated hypertension following ingestion of 3,4-methylenedioxymethamphetamine ("ecstasy"). Nephrol Dial Transplant 1995; 10:399–400.
40. Bingham C, Beaman M, Nicholls AJ, et al: Necrotizing renal vasculopathy resulting in chronic renal failure after ingestion of methamphetamine and 3,4-methylenedioxymethamphetamine ("ecstasy"). Nephrol Dial Transplant 1998; 13:2654–2655.
41. Woodrow G, Turney JH: Ecstasy-induced renal vasculitis. Nephrol Dial Transplant 1999; 14:798.
42. Lam M, Ballou SP: Reversible scleroderma crisis after cocaine use. N Engl J Med 1992; 326:1435.
43. Brust JCM: Vasculitis owing to substance abuse. Neurol Clin 1997; 15:945–957.
44. Lie JT: Classification and histopathologic spectrum of central nervous system vasculitis. Neurol Clin 1997; 15:805–819.
45. Bryden AA, Rothwell PJW, O'Reilly PH: Urinary retention with misuse of "ecstasy." BMJ 1995; 310:504.
46. Duffy WB, Senekjian HO, Knight TE, et al: Acute renal failure due to phenylpropanolamine. South Med J 1981; 74:1548–1549.
47. Swenson RD, Golper TA, Bennett WM: Acute renal failure and rhabdomyolysis after ingestion of phenylpropanolamine-containing diet pills. JAMA 1982; 248:1216.
48. Warner EA: Cocaine abuse. Ann Intern Med 1993; 119:226–235.
49. Haddad LM, Shannon MW, Winchester JF: *Clinical Management of Poisoning and Drug Overdose.* 3rd ed. Philadelphia: WB Saunders; 1998.
50. Hardman JG, Goodman LS, Gilman A, Limbird LE, eds: *The Pharmacological Basis of Therapeutics.* 9th ed. New York: McGraw-Hill; 1996.
51. Boghdadi MS, Henning RJ: Cocaine: pathophysiology and clinical toxicology. Heart Lung 1997; 26:466–483.
52. Shannon M: Clinical toxicity of cocaine adulterants. Ann Emerg Med 1988; 17:1243–1247.
53. Mouhaffel AH, Madu EC, Satmary WA, et al: Cardiovascular complications of cocaine. Chest 1995; 107:1426–1434.
54. Merigian KS, Roberts JR: Cocaine intoxication: hyperpyrexia, rhabdomyolysis and acute renal failure. Clin Toxicol 1987; 25:135–148.
55. Herzlich BC, Arsura EL, Pagala M, et al: Rhabdomyolysis related to cocaine abuse. Ann Intern Med 1988; 109:335–336.
56. Menashe PI, Gottlieb JE: Hyperthermia, rhabdomyolysis, and myoglobinuric renal failure after recreational use of cocaine. South Med J 1988; 81:379–380.
57. Lombard J, Wong B, Young JH: Acute renal failure due to rhabdomyolysis associated with cocaine toxicity. West J Med 1988; 148:466–468.
58. Roth D, Alarcon FJ, Fernandez JA, et al: Acute rhabdomyolysis associated with cocaine intoxication. N Engl J Med 1988; 319:673–677.
59. Guerin JM, Lustman C, Barbotin-Larrieu F: Cocaine-associated acute myoglobinuric renal failure. Am J Med 1989; 87:248.
60. Parks JM, Reed G, Knochel JP: Cocaine-associated rhabdomyolysis. Am J Med Sci 1989; 297:334–336.
61. Pogue VA, Nurse HM: Cocaine-associated acute myoglobinuric renal failure. Am J Med 1989; 86:183–186.
62. Singhal P, Horowitz B, Qinones MC, et al: Acute renal failure following cocaine abuse. Nephron 1989; 52:76–78.
63. Anand V, Siami G, Stone WJ: Cocaine-associated rhabdomyolysis and acute renal failure. South Med J 1989; 82:67–69.
64. Bauwens JE, Boggs JM, Hartwell PS: Fatal hyperthermia associated with cocaine use. West J Med 1989; 150:210–212.
65. Singlial PC, Rubin RB, Peters A, et al: Rhabdomyolysis and acute renal failure associated with cocaine abuse. Clin Toxicol 1990; 28:321–330.
66. Silva MO, Roth D, Reddy KR, et al: Hepatic dysfunction accompanying acute cocaine intoxication. J Hepatol 1991; 12:312–315.
67. Horst E, Bennett RL, Barrett O: Recurrent rhabdomyolysis in association with cocaine use. South Med J 1991; 84:269–270.

68. Castano JG, Ramallo VG, Miguez AM, et al: Rabdomiolisis y consuma de cocaina: presentacion de 13 casos. An Med Intern (Madrid) 1992; 9:340–342.
69. Lucatello A, Sturani A, Cocchi R, et al: Dopamine plus furosemide in cocaine-associated acute myoglobinuric renal failure. Nephron 1992; 60:242–243.
70. McCrea MS, Rust RJ, Cook DL, Stephens BA: Cocaine-induced rhabdomyolysis: findings on bone scintigraphy. Clin Nucl Med 1992; 17:292–293.
71. Veenstra J, Smit WM, Krediet RT, et al: Relationship between elevated creatine phosphokinase and the clinical spectrum of rhabdomyolysis. Nephrol Dial Transplant 1994; 9:637–641.
72. Daras M, Kakkouras L, Tuchman AJ, et al: Rhabdomyolysis and hyperthermia after cocaine abuse: a variant of the neuroleptic malignant syndrome? Acta Neurol Scand 1995; 92:161–165.
73. Lampley EC, Williams S, Myers SA: Cocaine-associated rhabdomyolysis causing renal failure in pregnancy. Obstet Gynecol 1996; 87:804–806.
74. Horowitz BZ, Panacek EA, Jouriles NJ: Severe rhabdomyolysis with renal failure after intranasal cocaine use. J Emerg Med 1997; 15:833–837.
75. Boyd RE, Brennan PT, Deng J-F, et al: Strychnine poisoning: recovery from profound lactic acidosis, hyperthermia, and rhabdomyolysis. Am J Med 1983; 74:507–512.
76. Counselman FL, McLaughlin EW, Kardon EM, et al: Creatine phosphokinase elevation in patients presenting to the emergency department with cocaine-related complaints. Am J Emerg Med 1997; 15:221–223.
77. Brody SV, Wrenn KD, Wilber MM, et al: Predicting the severity of cocaine-associated rhabdomyolysis. Ann Emerg Med 1990; 19:1137–1143.
78. Kanel GC, Cassidy W, Shuster L, et al: Cocaine-induced liver cell injury: comparison of morphological features in man and in experimental models. Hepatology 1990; 11:646–651.
79. Nolte KB: Rhabdomyolysis associated with cocaine abuse. Hum Pathol 1991; 22:1141–1145.
80. Becker BN, Ismal N: The neuroleptic malignant syndrome and acute renal failure. J Am Soc Nephrol 1994; 4:1406–1416.
81. Callaway CW, Clark RF: Hyperthermia in psychostimulant overdose. Ann Emerg Med 1994; 24:68–75.
82. Welt CV, Mash DC, Karachi S: Cocaine-associated agitated delirium and the neuroleptic malignant syndrome. Am J Emerg Med 1996; 14:425–428.
83. Leblanc M, Hebert M-J, Mongeau J-G: Cocaine-induced acute renal failure without rhabdomyolysis. Ann Intern Med 1994; 121:721–722.
84. Chevalier X, Rostoker G, Larget-Piet B, et al: Henoch-Schönlein purpura with necrotizing vasculitis after cocaine snorting. Clin Nephrol 1995; 43:348–349.
85. Tumlin JA, Sands JM, Someren A: Hemolytic-uremic syndrome following "crack" cocaine inhalation. Am J Med Sci 1990; 299:366–371.
86. Koffler A, Friedler RN, Massry SG: Acute renal failure due to nontraumatic rhabdomyolysis. Ann Intern Med 1976; 85:23–28.
87. Woodrow G, Brownjohn AM, Turney JH: The clinical and biochemical features of acute renal failure due to rhabdomyolysis. Ren Fail 1995; 17:467–474.
88. Gabow PA, Kaehny WD, Kelleher SP: The spectrum of rhabdomyolysis. Medicine 1982; 61:141–152.
89. Larpin R, Vincent A, Perret C: Morbidite et mortalite hospitalieres de l'intoxication aigue par les opiaces. Presse Med 1990; 19:1403–1406.
90. Villalba Garcia MV, Lopez Glez-Cobos C, Garcia Castano J, et al: Rabdomiolisis en intoxicaciones agudas. An Med Intern 1994; 11:119–122.
91. Cadnapaphornchai P, Taher S, McDonald FD: Acute drug-associated rhabdomyolysis: an examination of its diverse renal manifestations and complications. Am J Med Sci 1980; 280:66–72.
92. Nicholls K, Niall JF, Moran JE: Rhabdomyolysis and renal failure: complications of narcotic abuse. Med J Aust 1982; 2:387–389.
93. Hojs R, Sinkovic A: Rhabdomyolysis and acute renal failure following methadone abuse. Nephron 1992; 62:362.
94. Blain PG, Lane RJM, Bateman DN, et al: Opiate-induced rhabdomyolysis. Hum Toxicol 1985; 4:71–74.

95. Kiely PD, Weavind GP: Opiate abuse manifesting as hyperkalemic cardiac arrest. J R Soc Med 1993;86:114–115.
96. Otero A, Esteban J, Martinez J, et al: Rhabdomyolysis and acute renal failure as a consequence of heroin inhalation. Nephron 1992; 62:245.
97. Melandri R, Re G, Lanzarini C, et al: Myocardial damage and rhabdomyolysis associated with prolonged hypoxic coma following opiate overdose. Clin Toxicol 1996; 34:199–203.
98. Gibb WRG, Shaw IC: Myoglobinuria due to heroin abuse. J R Soc Med 1985; 78:862–863.
99. Annane D, Teboul JL, Richard C, et al: Severe rhabdomyolysis related to heroin sniffing. Intensive Care Med 1990; 16:410.
100. Peces R, Diaz-Corte C, Baltar J, et al: Haemolytic-uremic syndrome in a heroin addict. Nephrol Dial Transplant 1998; 13:3197–3199.
101. Akmal M, Valdin JR, McCarron MM, et al: Rhabdomyolysis with and without acute renal failure in patients with phencyclidine intoxication. Am J Nephrol 1981; 1:91–96.
102. Lahmeyer HH, Stock PG: Phencyclidine intoxication, physical restraint, and acute renal failure. J Clin Psychiatry 1983; 44:184–185.
103. Patel R, Connor G: A review of thirty cases of rhabdomyolysis-associated acute renal failure among phencyclidine users. J Toxicol Clin Toxicol 1986; 23:547–556.
104. McCarron MM, Schultze BW, Thompson GA, et al: Acute phencyclidine intoxication: incidence of clinical findings in 1,000 cases. Ann Emerg Med 1981; 10:237–242.
105. Artzer D, Patak RV, Weigmann TB: PCP intoxication: management of associated renal failure. J Kansas Med Soc 1983; 84:384–385.
106. Patel R: Acute uric acid nephropathy: a complication of phencyclidine intoxication. Postgrad Med J 1982; 58:783–785.
107. Armen R, Kanel G, Reynolds T: Phencyclidine-induced malignant hyperthermia causing submassive liver necrosis. Am J Med 1984; 77:167–172.
108. Bogaerts Y, Lameire N, Ringoir S: The compartment syndrome: a serious complication of acute rhabdomyolysis. Clin Nephrol 1982; 17:206–211.
109. Vukanovic S, Hauser H, Curati WL: Myonecrosis induced by drug overdose: pathogenesis, clinical aspects, and radiological manifestations. Eur J Radiol 1983; 3:314–318.
110. Mandy S, Ackerman AB: Characteristic traumatic skin lesions in drug-induced coma. JAMA 1970; 213:253–256.
111. Wrenn KD, Slovis CM, Minion GE, et al: The syndrome of alcoholic ketoacidosis. Am J Med 1991; 91:119–128.
112. Knochel JP: Neuromuscular manifestations of electrolyte disorders. Am J Med 1982; 72:521–535.
113. Singhal PC, Kumar A, Desroches L, et al: Prevalence and predictors of rhabdomyolysis in patients with hypophosphatemia. Am J Med 1992; 92:458–463.
114. de Marchi S, Cecchin E, Basile A, et al: Renal tubular dysfunction in chronic alcohol abuse—effects of abstinence. N Engl J Med 1993; 329:1927–1934.
115. Vamvakas S, Teschner M, Bahner U, et al: Alcohol abuse: potential role in electrolyte disturbances and kidney diseases. Clin Nephrol 1998; 49:205–213.
116. Zajaczkowski T, Potjan G, Wojewski-Zajaczkowski E, et al: Rhabdomyolysis and myoglobinuria associated with violent exercise and alcohol abuse: report of two cases. Int Urol Nephrol 1991; 23:517–525.
117. Haapanen E, Partanen J, Pellinen TJ: Acute renal failure following nontraumatic rhabdomyolysis. Scand J Urol Nephrol 1988; 22:305–308.
118. Saltissi D, Parfrey PS, Curtis JR, et al: Rhabdomyolysis and acute renal failure in chronic alcoholics with myopathy unrelated to acute alcohol ingestion. Clin Nephrol 1984; 21:294–300.
119. Robertson C, Paton JYL: Acute renal failure after a beer-drinking binge. BMJ 1980; 1:938–939.
120. Haapanen E, Pellinen TJ, Partanen J: Acute renal failure caused by alcohol-induced rhabdomyolysis. Nephron 1984; 36:191–193.
121. Grufferman S, Morris D, Alvarez J: Methanol poisoning complicated by myoglobinuric renal failure. Am J Emerg Med 1985; 3:24–26.
122. Juncos L, Taguchi JT: Isopropyl alcohol intoxication. JAMA 1968; 204:732–733.
123. Kaysen GA, Pond SM, Roper MH, et al: Combined hepatic and renal injury in alcoholics during therapeutic use of acetaminophen. Arch Intern Med 1985; 145:2019–2023.
124. Keaton MR: Acute renal failure in an alcoholic during therapeutic acetaminophen ingestion. South Med J 1988; 81:1163–1166.
125. Riggs JE, Schochet SS, Parmar JP: Rhabdomyolysis with acute renal failure and disseminated intravascular coagulation: association with acetaminophen and ethanol. Milit Med 1996; 161:708–709.
126. Drenth JPH, Frenken LAM, Wuis EW, et al: Acute renal failure associated with paracetamol ingestion in an alcoholic patient. Nephron 1994; 67:483–485.
127. Elasser GN, Lopez L, Evans E, et al: Reversible acute renal failure associated with ibuprofen ingestion and binge drinking. J Fam Pract 1988; 27:221–222.
128. Blau EB: Ibuprofen and ethanol overdose-induced acute tubular necrosis. Wisconsin Med J 1987; 86:23–24.
129. Wen S-F, Parthasarathy R, Iliopoulos O, et al: Acute renal failure following binge drinking and nonsteroidal antiinflammatory drugs. Am J Kidney Dis 1992; 3:281–285.
130. Johnson GR, Wen S-F: Syndrome of flank pain and acute renal failure after binge drinking and nonsteroidal anti-inflammatory drug ingestion. J Am Soc Nephrol 1995; 5:1647–1652.
131. Gaizin M, Brunet P, Burtey S, et al: Necrose tubulaire apres prise d'antiinflammatoire non steroidien et intoxication ethylique aigue. Nephrologie 1997; 18:113–115.
132. Tsuboi N, Yoshida H, Shibamura K, et al: Acute renal failure after binge drinking of alcohol and nonsteroidal antiinflammatory drug ingestion. Intern Med 1997; 36:102–106.
133. Blackshear JL, Davidman M, Stillman MT: Identification of risk for renal insufficiency from nonsteroidal anti-inflammatory drugs. Arch Intern Med 1983; 143:1130–1134.
134. Hirsch DJ, Jindal KK, Trillo A, et al: Acute renal failure after binge drinking. Nephrol Dial Transplant 1994; 9:330–331.
135. Streicher HZ, Gabow PA, Moss AH, et al: Syndromes of toluene sniffing in adults. Ann Intern Med 1981; 94:758–762.
136. Carlisle E, Donnelly SM, Vasuvattakul S, et al: Glue-sniffing and distal renal tubular acidosis: sticking to the facts. J Am Soc Nephrol 1991; 1:1019–1027.
137. Will AM, McLaren EH: Reversible renal damage due to glue sniffing. BMJ 1981; 283:525–526.
138. Gupta RK, van der Meulen J, Johny KV: Oliguric acute renal failure due to glue sniffing. Scand J Urol Nephrol 1991; 25:247–250.
139. Taverner D, Harrison DJ, Bell GM: Acute renal failure due to interstitial nephritis induced by "glue-sniffing" with subsequent recovery. Scott Med J 1988; 33:246–247.
140. Russ G, Clarkson AR, Woodroffe AJ, et al: Renal failure from "glue sniffing." Med J Aust 1981; 2:121–122.
141. Doriguzzi C, Palmucci L, Mongini T, et al: Body building and myoglobinuria: report of three cases. BMJ 1988; 296:826–827.
142. Cook JA, Hill JM, Turney JH: Rhabdomyolysis and a "greenhouse effect." Lancet 1990; 336:1136–1137.
143. Hageloch W, Appell HJ, Weicker H: Rhabdomyolyse bei bodybuilder unter anabolika-einnahme. Sportverletzung-Sportschaden 1988; 2:122–125.
144. Yoshida EM, Kaum MA, Shaikh JF, et al: At what price glory? Severe cholestasis and acute renal failure in an athlete abusing stanozolol. Can Med Assoc J 1994; 151:791–793.
145. Poortmans JR, Francaux M: Renal dysfunction accompanying oral creatine supplements. Lancet 1998; 352:234.
146. Koshy KM, Griswold E, Schneeberger EE: Interstitial nephritis in a patient taking creatine. N Engl J Med 1999; 340:814–815.
147. Pritchard N, Kalra P: Renal dysfunction accompanying oral creatine supplements. Lancet 1998; 351:1252–1253.
148. Fisch HP, Wands J, Yeung J, et al: Pulmonary edema and disseminated intravascular coagulation after intravenous abuse of D-propoxyphene (Darvon). South Med J 1972; 65:493–495.
149. Farber SJ, Huertas VE: Intravenously injected marijuana syndrome. Arch Intern Med 1976; 136:337–339.
150. Scott RW, Going J, Woodburn KR, et al: Intra-arterial temazepam. BMJ 1992; 304:1630.
151. Jenkinson DF, Pusey CD: Rhabdomyolysis and renal failure after intra-arterial temazepam injection. Nephrol Dial Transplant 1994; 9:1334–1335.

152. Franz M, Regele H, Kirchmair M, et al: Magic mushrooms: hope for a "cheap high" resulting in end-stage renal failure. Nephrol Dial Transplant 1996; 11:2324–2327.

153. Raff E, Halloran PF, Kjellstrand CM: Renal failure after eating "magic" mushrooms. Can Med Assoc J 1992; 147:1339–1341.

154. Montseny J-J, Meyrier A, Kleinknecht D, et al: The current spectrum of infectious glomerulonephritis. Medicine 1995; 74:63–73.

155. Peraldi MN, Maslo C, Akposso K, et al: Acute renal failure in the course of HIV infection: a single-institution retrospective study of ninety-two patients and sixty renal biopsies. Nephrol Dial Transplant 1999; 14:1578–1585.

156. Dunea G, Arruda JAL, Bakir AA, et al: Role of cocaine in end-stage renal disease in some hypertensive African Americans. Am J Nephrol 1995; 15:5–9.

157. Fogo A, Superdock KR, Atkinson JB: Severe arteriosclerosis in the kidney of a cocaine addict. Am J Kidney Dis 1992; 5:513–515.

158. di Paolo N, Fineschi V, di Paolo M, et al: Kidney vascular damage and cocaine. Clin Nephrol 1997; 47:298–303.

159. van der Woude FJ, Waldherr R: Severe renal arterio-arteriolo-sclerosis after cocaine use. Nephrol Dial Transplant 1999; 14:434–435.

160. Langrier RO, Bement CL, Peny LE: Arteriosclerotic toxicity of cocaine. Natl Inst Drug Abuse Res Monogr 1988; 88:325–336.

161. Sharff JA: Renal infarction associated with intravenous cocaine use. Ann Emerg Med 1984; 13:1145–1147.

162. Wohlman RA: Renal artery thrombosis and embolization associated with intravenous cocaine injection. South Med J 1987; 80:928–930.

163. Kramer RK, Turner RC: Renal infarction associated with cocaine use and latent protein C deficiency. South Med J 1993; 86:1436–1438.

164. Lambrecht GL, Malbrain ML, Coremans P, et al: Acute renal infarction and heavy marijuana smoking. Nephron 1995; 70:494–496.

165. Alvarez D, Nzerue C-M, Daniel JF, et al: Acute interstitial nephritis induced by crack cocaine binge. Nephrol Dial Transplant 1999; 14:1260–1262.

166. McAllister CJ, Horn R, Havron A, et al: Granulomatous interstitial nephritis: a complication of heroin abuse. South Med J 1979; 72:162–165.

167. Sadjadi SA, McLaughlin K, Shah RM: Allergic interstitial nephritis due to diazepam. Arch Intern Med 1987; 141:579–580.

CHAPTER 33

Acute Renal Failure and Nonsteroidal Anti-Inflammatory Drugs

Garabed Eknoyan

INTRODUCTION

Nonsteroidal anti-inflammatory drugs (NSAIDs) are among the most useful therapeutic agents introduced in the past century. Their principal use derives from their effectiveness as anti-inflammatory agents coupled with variable analgesic properties. While their principal utility has been in the treatment of rheumatologic diseases and musculoskeletal disorders, their analgesic properties have allowed for the development of potent derivatives that have proved useful as substitutes for opiates in the relief of postoperative pain. As a result of their effectiveness, NSAIDs became one of the most commonly prescribed drugs shortly after their introduction. Their overall safety profile led to their availability on a nonprescription basis as over-the-counter (OTC) drugs in 1984 and has resulted in an additional and considerable increase in the number of individuals who consume NSAIDs. It is estimated that approximately 20% of the general population in the United States uses NSAIDs at some time for acute musculoskeletal complaints, and that 10% to 15% of older individuals consume NSAIDs regularly.[1]

The therapeutic effect of NSAIDs is due to their ability, but variable capacity, to limit the formation of prostaglandins (PGs) by interfering with the cyclooxygenase activity of prostaglandin endoperoxide synthetase (cyclooxygenase, COX), the first enzyme in the biosynthesis of PGs from arachidonic acid, and consequently to decrease the production of PGs at sites of inflammation.[2] It is this mode of action that also accounts for their potential adverse effects at various body sites where PGs serve important protective functions, primarily in the gastrointestinal tract and the kidneys. While the prevalence of their nephrotoxicity is unknown and appears to be relatively low, their extensive use places a significant number of individuals at risk, particularly in some 20% of NSAID users whose underlying clinical conditions, superimposed complications, or concomitant use of other drugs predispose them to the detrimental effects of prostaglandin inhibition.[3-7] To the extent that the untoward effects of NSAIDs on the kidney are reversible following their discontinuation, it is essential to be familiar with the renal effects of NSAIDs and to identify the subgroups of the population who are susceptible to the detrimental effects of NSAIDs on renal function.

RENAL EFFECTS OF NSAIDs

The renal effects of NSAIDs derive from their variable inhibitory action on COX activity at specific regions within the renal parenchyma, where it accounts for the local production of PGs with autacoid action at distinct anatomic sites in the kidney (Table 33–1). The regional action of the various PGs, especially PGI_2 and PGE_2, exert a variety of physiologic effects that are crucial for the maintenance of renal function in situations in which the systemic hemodynamic balance is compromised either by actual volume depletion (hemorrhage, fluid sequestration, sodium depletion) or by reduced effective intravascular volume (congestive heart failure, liver cirrhosis, nephrotic syndrome, arteriovenous shunts).[8, 9]

In the cortex, PGI_2 is the more common form of prostaglandin produced in the vasculature and glomerular capillaries and is important in the regulation of renal blood flow (RBF), vascular tone, glomerular filtration rate (GFR), and juxtaglomerular renin release. In the glomeruli, the mesangial and epithelial cell production of PGs affects glomerular flow, ultrafiltration, and response to inflammatory cytokines. In the medulla, PGE_2 is the more common form of prostaglandin produced in the tubules and interstitial cells and is important in the modulation of medullary blood flow and the tubular handling of salt and water. The tubular production of PGs is most copious in the collecting duct, where, in addition to sodium modulation, they counteract the action of antidiuretic hormone (ADH). In the macula densa, PGE_2 production regulates the release of renin. The tubular production of PGs is relatively lower in the thick ascending limb of the loop of Henle and minimal in the proximal tubule, where it regulates sodium absorption. The medullary interstitial cell production of PGE_2 and PGF_2 is important in the modulation of medullary blood flow.[5, 8, 10]

The production of PGs is regulated by two separate isoforms of COX with a differential regulation of expression: a constitutive COX-1 isoform considered to produce PGs involved in rapid physiologic responses to circulating hormones such as angiotensin II, catecholamines, ADH, and atrial natriuretic factor; and an inducible COX-2 isoform involved secondarily in prolonged physiologic reactions to cytokines, endotoxins, growth factors, or mitogens.[2, 11] Both enzymes are integral membrane proteins that are encoded by separate genes located on separate chromosomes but are 60% identical within species. Their kinetic properties are very similar albeit coupled to different signaling pathways. It is the inducible COX-2 isoform whose expression is increased during inflammation that accounts for the main therapeutic anti-inflammatory ef-

TABLE 33–1. Localization and Effect of Prostaglandins on Kidney Function and Consequences of Their Inhibition by NSAIDs

SITE	COX ISOFORM	PROSTAGLANDIN	RESPONSE	EFFECT OF NSAIDs	
				Functional	Clinical
Vasculature					
Arteries	1	$PGI_2 > PGE_2$	Vasodilate	↓↓ RBF, ↓ GFR	ARF
Afferent arteriole	1	$PGI_2 > PGE_2$	Vasodilate	↓↓ RBF, ↓ GFR	ARF
Efferent arteriole	1	$PGI_2 > PGE_2$	Vasodilate	↓ Gcp, ↓ GFR	ARF
Glomerulus					
Capillary tuft (mesangium)	1	$PGI_2 > PGE_2$	Vasodilate / Maintain K_f	↓↓ GFR, ↓ RBF	ARF
Podocytes	2	$PGE_2 > PGI_2$	Maintain K_f	↓↓ GFR	ARF / Proteinuria
Tubules					
Proximal	2	Minimal	?	?	?
Thick ascending limb	2	$PGE_2 > PGI_2$	↓ Na^+ reabsorption / Vasodilate	↑ Na^+ reabsorption / ↓ Blood flow	Edema / Ischemia
Macula densa	2	PGE_2	↑ Renin		↑ $[P_K]$ / ↓ $[P_{Na}]$
Collecting duct	1	$PGE_2 > PGI_2$	↓ ADH activity / ↓ Na reabsorption	↑ ADH activity / ↑ Na^+ reabsorption	Edema
JG Apparatus	1,2	$PGE_2 > PGI_2$	↑ Renin / Autoregulation	↓ RAS / ↓ GFR	↑ $[P_K]$ / ARF
Interstitial Cells					
Outer medulla	1	$PGI_2 > PGE_2$	Vasodilate / ↓ ADH activity	↓↓ Blood flow / ↑ ADH activity	ARF, RPN / ↓ $[P_{Na}]$
Papilla	2	$PGE_2 > PGI_2$	Vasodilate / ↓ ADH activity	↓↓ Blood flow / ↑ ADH activity	RPN / ↓ $[P_{Na}]$

ADH, antidiuretic hormone; *ARF*, acute renal failure; *COX*, cyclooxygenase; *Gcp*, glomerular capillary pressure; *GFR*, glomerular filtration rate; *JG*, juxtaglomerular apparatus; *NSAID*, nonsteroidal anti-inflammatory drug; *PG*, prostaglandin; *P_K*, plasma potassium concentration; *RAS*, renin angiotensin system; *RBF*, renal blood flow; *RPN*, renal papillary necrosis.

fects of NSAIDs and that is the target of the new preferential COX-2 inhibitory NSAIDs.[11–14]

Although there seem to be some differences among the species examined, immunoreactive COX-1 has been localized in the renal vasculature, arterioles, glomeruli, collecting ducts, and medullary interstitial cells but not in the proximal or distal tubules, the loop of Henle, or the macula densa.[11–15] In the renal vasculature, COX-1 is expressed constitutively in the endothelial and smooth muscle cells. Of the various organs examined for COX-2, the kidneys constitutively express the relatively highest, albeit low, concentrations of the COX-2 messenger ribonucleic acid, which has been localized to the macula densa of the juxtaglomerular apparatus, to a subset of the epithelial cells of the cortical thick ascending limb, and to the papillary interstitial cells.[15–18] Up-regulation of COX-2 expression in the macula densa has been shown following chronic sodium restriction and in an experimental model of renovascular hypertension.[15, 18] No COX-2 has been detected in the arterioles, glomeruli, or collecting ducts.[15] It would seem, therefore, that COX-2 accounts for PGs that are important in the tubular regulation of sodium and potassium and the release of renin, while COX-1 accounts for PGs with vasodilatory and anti-ADH activity.[15–19]

The long-term renal effect of the new selective COX-1–sparing NSAIDs remains to be determined. In studies of their effect on the gastrointestinal tract, they appear to result in fewer ulcers but are not entirely free from adverse effects, relative to nonselective agents.[20] In a volume-depleted rat model, a COX-2 selective NSAID, unlike indomethacin, did not reduce the RBF or alter the renovascular response to angiotensin II.[21] However, a transient reversible effect on urinary biomarkers of a renal effect of COX-2 inhibitors has been shown,[22] and they do not seem to spare the kidney as they do the gastrointestinal tract.[23]

While the relative role of COX-1 or COX-2 inhibition in NSAID-induced nephrotoxicity is not clear and independent of these important biochemical considerations, it must be emphasized that the adverse renal effects of NSAIDs is different from those of other nephrotoxic drugs that exert a direct toxic action on the kidney. By contrast, the adverse renal effects of NSAIDs are indirect ones caused by the therapeutic action of blocking cyclooxygenase activity and, thereby, temporarily reducing the counter-regulatory protective action of PGs in the kidney. In essence, it is a potentially reversible and implicitly preventable nephrotoxic effect.

ACUTE RENAL FAILURE

Under normal conditions, PGs contribute little to the maintenance of renal function. Consequently, while an acute hemodynamic effect of NSAIDs on normal kidney function can be demonstrated experimentally, it is transient in nature and invariably reversible with no demonstrable residual nephrotoxic action.[5] It is under conditions of hemodynamic stress, when the renin-angiotensin system is activated and the sympathetic system stimulated, that the kidney becomes increasingly dependent on the counter-regulatory protective effects of PGs to maintain renal function. While the actions of increased release of PGs on the kidney are varied (see Table 33–1), their principal effect is on the control of vascular tone. Consequently, during vasoconstriction induced by angiotensin II, catecholamines, or endothelin, NSAID-mediated inhibition of the counter-regulatory vasodilatory action of PGs results in a fall in RBF and GFR. This accounts for the false sense of security inferred from acute and long-term studies of the effects of NSAIDs on renal function in otherwise stable individuals. The limitation of such studies derives from the exclusion of subjects who are in a prostaglandin-dependent state for the protection of renal function. Perhaps a good example of this is illustrated from studies that failed to show an effect of indomethacin on renal function in healthy subjects during stress induced by exercise at 80% maximal oxygen consumption for 30 minutes, a condition associated with increases in sympathetic outflow and renin-angiotensin activation.[24] However, when healthy subjects were studied after 3 days of a low-sodium (10 mEq/day) diet and dehydration (1.6% loss of dry weight) induced by light exercise in a hot environment (40°C), a condition that caused measurable decreases in baseline RBF and GFR, the administration of ibuprofen did result in an added significant decrease in renal function.[25] The same considerations apply to the renal effects of NSAIDs with selective COX-2 action. In normal older subjects on a sodium diet of 200 mEq/day, a selective COX-2 inhibitor, rofecoxib, resulted in acute limited sodium retention and reduced potassium excretion similar to indomethacin, without the transient drop in GFR associated with indomethacin.[26] However, in salt-restricted (50 mEq/day) subjects, another selective COX-2 inhibitor, celecoxib, caused the same transient decrease in RBF and GFR as the nonselective inhibitor naproxen.[27] It would seem, therefore, that increased selectivity for COX-2, or sparing of COX-1, does not protect the kidney in volume-depleted prostaglandin-dependent states.

Ischemic Injury

The clinical equivalent of these experimental observations is that of subjects with compromised effective intravascular fluid volume (diuretic-induced, sepsis, congestive heart failure, nephrotic syndrome, liver cirrhosis) or impaired renal function (diabetic nephropathy, lupus nephritis, hypertensive nephrosclerosis) who persistently show a decrease in RBF and GFR following the administration of NSAIDs.[5, 28–30] As observed clinically and demonstrated experimentally, these detrimental effects of NSAIDs on renal function are reversible when the drugs are discontinued.[5] Several studies have confirmed these observations and identified the predisposing risk factors and subjects at risk for the untoward effects of NSAIDs (Table 33–2). As shown in Figure 33–1, if the changes in renal function are appreciated early and NSAIDs discontinued, the RBF and GFR will return to baseline.[31] However, if they go

TABLE 33–2. Risk Factors That Predispose to NSAID-Induced ARF

Underlying clinical condition
  Congestive heart failure
  Cirrhosis of the liver
  Nephrotic syndrome
  Chronic renal insufficiency
  Obstructive nephropathy
  Sickle cell disease
  Acute glomerulonephritis
  Active lupus nephritis
Patient-related
  Age >65
  Reduced drug metabolism
  Hypoalbuminemia
Superimposed complications
  Sepsis
  Hemorrhage
  ↓ Extracellular fluid volume (diarrhea, vomiting, fluid
    sequestration, heavy sweating)
Coadministered drug interactions
  Diuretics
  Angiotensin-converting enzyme inhibitors
  Cyclosporine
NSAID-related
  COX-inhibitory potency
  COX isoform sparing effect
  Dose
  Duration of NSAID use
  Longer duration of action
  Chemical structure

COX, cyclooxygenase; *NSAID*, nonsteroidal anti-inflammatory drug.

undetected and the stressful systemic hemodynamic condition persists and increases in severity, prolonged and unremitting renal vasoconstriction results in progressive ischemic injury. This occurs in its most dramatic form when more than one of the stressful underlying predisposing conditions coexists in the same patient, such as an older patient in heart failure on diuretics who presents with an acute inflammatory arthritis and is given NSAIDs. In this setting, the change in renal function can be dramatic but remains reversible. The acute renal failure (ARF) is nonoliguric, and the fractional excretion of sodium is low (<1%). However, if the initial reversible adverse effect is not appreciated, progressive ARF occurs, oliguria supervenes, and dialysis for renal replacement therapy becomes necessary.[29, 32] While there are no reliable figures for this serious eventuality, its incidence from reported cases is low, and this seems to be the case in 10% to 12% of cases of NSAID-induced ARF.[5, 7, 33] Even then, the condition is reversible following discontinuation of the NSAIDs, although occasional rare cases of permanent renal damage have been reported.[5, 7, 9, 34]

As might be expected, these critical situations tend to occur in hospitalized sick patients and account for the relatively higher occurrence of NSAID-induced ARF in the hospital setting. It is not unexpected then that among drug-induced ARF cases encountered in hospitals, NSAID-induced ARF ranks alongside aminoglycoside-induced ARF in incidence and severity.[35] In the ambulatory setting, case control studies show that predisposed individuals who use NSAIDs have higher

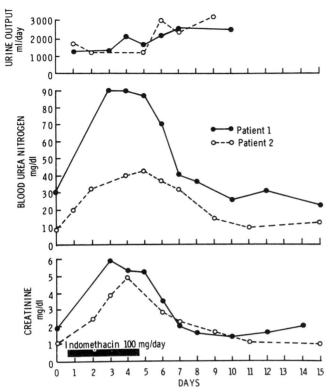

FIGURE 33–1 ■ The clinical course of indomethacin-induced nonoliguric acute renal failure. Note the rapid increments in blood urea nitrogen and creatinine levels and their improvement following indomethacin discontinuation, as well as the continued urine output of over 1 L/day during the deterioration of renal function. The higher urine output following cessation of indomethacin is probably due to urea diuresis and increased intravenous fluid administration. (From O'Meara ME, Eknoyan G: Acute renal failure associated with indomethacin administration. South Med J 1980; 73:587; with permission.)

levels of common laboratory markers of renal dysfunction, and that it is chronic users, particularly those on concomitant diuretic drugs, who account for the increased risk of elevated levels of serum creatinine.[36] It is the unforeseen superimposition of volume depletion (diarrhea, vomiting, aggravation of cardiomyopathy, increased use of diuretics) in these individuals that accounts for the relatively less common occurrence of ARF in community settings.

Nephrotic Syndrome and Tubulointerstitial Nephritis

Another cause of ARF encountered with chronic NSAID use in the community setting is that of a distinct syndrome of renal insufficiency and massive proteinuria.[37] Although the sudden onset of nephrotic syndrome is the presenting feature of these patients, and nephrotic-range proteinuria and renal failure coexist in the majority of such cases, some 15% to 20% of them have nephrotic syndrome or ARF alone. The structural hallmarks noted on renal biopsy of such cases are those of acute tubulointerstitial nephritis

(TIN) and minimal-change nephropathy,[37, 38] but cases of membranous glomerulonephropathy have been reported also.[39] Unlike hemodynamically induced ARF, this is an idiosyncratic hypersensitivity reaction with no identifiable risk factors. While hypersensitivity is the basis of this syndrome, the onset of acute TIN is variable and delayed, usually occurring several months after institution of NSAID therapy. Common markers of hypersensitivity (fever, rash, eosinophilia) are rare and may be noted in fewer than 20% of cases. The exact incidence of this form of ARF is unknown but has been estimated at 1 in 5300 patient-years of NSAID use.[28] It is more common with the use of propionic acid derivatives (fenoprofen > ibuprofen > naproxen), indicating a contributory role of NSAID chemical structure to its cause. The lesions usually occur in the elderly, the mean age of individuals who develop this unique syndrome being about 65, with more than half the cases encountered in those who are older than 64 years of age.[32, 39] This may reflect the greater use of NSAIDs in the elderly rather than an age-related predilection. As a rule, there is prompt resolution of the nephrotic-range proteinuria following cessation of NSAIDs, with a slower resolution of the renal insufficiency and residual modest proteinuria. In some, it may take up to a year for these abnormalities to resolve. Instances of the failure to recover renal function have been reported.[40] Treatment with steroids has not been effective.[41]

Renal Papillary Necrosis

Much less common as a cause of NSAID-induced ARF is the rare occurrence of acute renal papillary necrosis (RPN).[42] In the majority of cases, RPN is due to ischemic necrosis of the relatively underperfused renal papillae.[43] Most of the normal medullary blood flow serves the countercurrent multiplier. Medullary nutrient flow is provided by a gradually diminishing number of capillaries that arise from the vasa rectae. Maintenance of medullary blood flow is dependent on PGs produced by medullary and papillary interstitial cells under stress conditions that induce renal vasoconstriction.[20, 26] NSAID-induced inhibition of prostaglandin biosynthesis, which decreases total renal perfusion, results in a preferential redistribution of blood flow to the cortex, with the consequent renal vasoconstriction being most marked in the papillary tips.[3, 8] The papillary interstitial cells are the first site of injury in analgesic nephropathy, and inhibition of PG biosynthesis by these cells is probably relevant to the RPN induced by NSAIDs.[6, 43] As a result, under severe stress conditions (dehydration, volume depletion), the use of NSAIDs can result in acute papillary necrosis, which occasionally causes ARF due to bilateral obstruction of the ureters, a condition that renders the kidneys all the more prostaglandin-independent.[44] The presenting symptoms are those of obstruction due to sloughing of the necrotic papillae, with associated symptoms of renal colic. Prompt diagnosis and removal or passage of the obstructing necrotic papillae results in reversal of the ARF. Residual renal dysfunction is unusual, because the lesion affects only a few of the several (7–10) papillae in each kidney, and only a few of the nephrons (15%) have loops of Henle that extend to the papillae. As such, only a few of the papillae slough, and the residual unaffected cortical nephrons compensate for the lost nephrons.[45] Whether the incidence of RPN will be changed by the increased use of selective COX-2 inhibitors because of their effect on the papillary interstitial cells (see Table 33–1) remains to be determined.

FLUID AND ELECTROLYTE DISTURBANCES

NSAID-induced prostaglandin inhibition also affects the renal handling of sodium, potassium, and water. Although these effects usually occur in the course of chronic NSAID use, they deserve attention, because they are probably indicative of potential susceptibility to the detrimental hemodynamic effect of NSAIDs on renal function in more stressful prostaglandin-dependent states.[46]

Some degree of sodium retention occurs in about one fourth of all individuals treated with NSAIDs. The sodium retention stems from direct inhibition of the tubular modulation of sodium by PGs and from the reduced RBF coupled with a redistribution of RBF from the medulla to the cortex. This tends to occur shortly after initiation of NSAID use and is usually of moderate severity, resulting in a weight gain of 1 to 2 kg, with clinically detectable edema present in fewer than 5% of cases.[7, 26–29]

An increment in serum potassium occurs in 15% of chronic NSAID users. Inhibition of prostaglandin-mediated renin release with consequent decreased aldosterone production (hyporeninemic hypoaldosteronism) accounts for the diminished potassium excretion in such individuals.[7, 23, 29] Its occurrence in those with avid sodium retention reflects an additional role for the diminished distal delivery of sodium, as well as that of increased macula densa COX-2 expression induced by salt restriction.[47, 48] It is more likely to occur in individuals with reduced baseline renal function who have underlying hyporeninemic hypoaldosteronism (diabetic nephropathy, lupus nephritis), those on angiotensin-converting enzyme inhibitor therapy, and individuals receiving potassium supplements.[49]

Much less common is the rare occurrence of hyponatremia, caused by inhibition of PGs that counteract the distal tubular action of ADH.[46] In individuals using NSAIDs, an increased effect of ADH on urine concentration can be demonstrated experimentally. In the occasional cases in which hyponatremia has been encountered clinically, the patient was elderly, receiving another drug that inhibits free water clearance (thiazide diuretics), and ingesting large amounts of water.[50]

INTERACTIVE AND SPECIAL CONSIDERATIONS

The term NSAIDs has been used in its generic sense heretofore. This is justifiable because, in the final anal-

ysis, their effect on renal function seems to be quite uniform. However, subtle differences do exist, because the available compounds differ in their chemical structure and capacity to inhibit cyclooxygenase. The importance of chemical structure is evident from the variability with which NSAIDs cause ARF resulting from acute TIN, as mentioned earlier. Another, and perhaps more important, determinant of their hemodynamic effects may be their variable capacity to inhibit cyclooxygenase activity in vitro (meclofenamate > diclofenac > ibuprofen > naproxen > indomethacin > piroxicam > ketorolac >> aspirin), which may account for the greater occurrence of ARF in association with the use of the more potent COX-inhibitory agents and those with a longer duration of action (oxicams > pyrazolones > heterocyclic acetic acids > propionic acids > arylacetic acids).[2, 5, 51] In this regard, the relative safety of sulindac is likely due to the fact that it is a prodrug that is converted to its active form less well in the kidneys but, much like other NSAIDs, can affect renal function in the prostaglandin-dependent kidney.[5, 7, 29] However, in vitro differences among the NSAIDs are difficult to demonstrate clinically, because their effects then depend on the dose of the NSAID used, the age of the patient, interaction with coadministered drugs, and the heterogeneity of underlying clinical conditions (see Table 33–2), each of which has been an important contributory variable in reported cases of ARF attributed to NSAIDs.

In terms of the dose of NSAIDs, there is convincing evidence from controlled studies on otherwise healthy subjects that the larger the dose of NSAIDs, the greater is the demonstrable effect on renal function.[5, 7] The age of the patient is an equally important factor. Apart from the fact that the elderly are more likely to use NSAIDs, older individuals are more predisposed to the adverse hemodynamic effects of NSAIDs, because of age-associated decrements in baseline renal function; the prevalence of comorbid conditions that affect renal hemodynamics, such as congestive cardiomyopathy, diabetes, and hypertension; and the greater likelihood of these patients being on concomitant drugs that affect renal function, such as diuretics, angiotensin-converting enzyme inhibitors (ACEIs), and other antihypertensive agents. Other important contributors may be the difficulty of detecting early renal dysfunction in the elderly and the likelihood of continued NSAID use despite significant losses of renal function. This is because the age-related decrements in GFR are paralleled by reductions in muscle mass and, therefore, reduced production of creatinine. Because creatinine production falls with aging at about the same rate as that of GFR, the serum creatinine level remains within the normal range.[32] A trend toward clinically detectable increments in serum creatinine begins to occur after age 75.[52] As a result, despite reductions in GFR of about 50% between the third and seventh decade of life, there is no accompanying increase in the creatinine level.[32, 53] As such, an increase in creatinine from 0.8 to 1.2 mg/dL, indicating a 50% loss of renal function in an older individual, would go unnoticed because the creatinine level is considered within the normal range. In such a person, the impending onset of NSAID-induced ARF would go undetected, and the drug continued until more severe ARF becomes established. This may be the reason that NSAIDs, in the elderly, account for more than 10% of all cases of ARF and for more than 40% of all cases of drug-induced ARF.[33] Thus, and especially in the elderly, it is the directional changes in serum creatinine that should be monitored, rather than changes in the absolute level reported by the laboratory.

Coadministered Drugs

Several groups of coadministered drugs that predispose to NSAID-induced ARF deserve special mention. The first group consists of diuretics that induce a reduction in intravascular volume and thereby produce a prostaglandin-dependent state caused by the stimulated release of angiotensin and catecholamines. The second group consists of the ACEIs that deprive the individual of the protection provided by angiotensin II–mediated efferent vasoconstriction that increases intracapillary glomerular pressure and thereby maintains GFR when total RBF is reduced. In addition, by suppressing aldosterone production, ACEIs increase the likelihood of NSAID-induced hyperkalemia.[49] Two other coadministered drugs that aggravate hyperkalemia are heparin, which suppresses aldosterone production, and beta-blockers, which suppress the epinephrine-induced cellular uptake of potassium. The third agent deserving comment is cyclosporine, which, because of its vasoconstrictive action, renders the kidney prostaglandin-dependent. The concomitant use of cyclosporine with indomethacin has been reported to be successful in the treatment of recurrent nephrotic syndrome caused by focal segmental glomerulosclerosis following renal transplantation, and the use of cyclosporine with NSAIDs has proven beneficial in severe cases of rheumatoid arthritis. However, the reduction in GFR has been shown to be more severe when the two agents are used concomitantly than that observed with either agent alone.[54–56]

The underlying clinical state of prostaglandin dependence is especially important in NSAID-induced decrements in GFR. That these comorbid conditions include congestive cardiomyopathy, nephrotic syndrome, and cirrhosis of the liver has been well established.[5, 7, 57, 58] Among patients with these condition, it is those with the greatest capacity for sodium retention (ie, greater activation of the renin-angiotensin system and ADH) who are more prone to NSAID-induced ARF. Thus, patients with liver cirrhosis and ascites are more susceptible, as are those with significant hypoalbuminemia due to cirrhosis or nephrotic syndrome.[52, 53] The concomitant use of diuretics in these patients increases their likelihood of developing ARF.[7]

Equally susceptible are patients with reduced renal function. Kidney disease is associated with greater dependence on PGs to maintain RBF and GFR.[5, 7, 60] An added decrement in renal function following the institution of NSAID therapy has been reported to

occur in as many as one third of patients with underlying kidney disease.[5, 7, 9] Among patients with kidney disease, those with systemic lupus erythematosus seem to be particularly prone to such an eventuality, perhaps because of the greater use of NSAIDs to treat the arthralgias in these patients and the greater activation of renal PGs in active lupus erythematosus.[5, 7, 61] Another clinical condition is sickle cell disease, in which the ability to maintain GFR depends on prostaglandin-induced afferent vasodilatation. A significant drop in GFR occurs following the administration of NSAIDs to patients with sickle cell disease.[62] It is relevant to mention in this regard that in streptozocin-induced diabetic rats, whose baseline afferent arteriolar constriction in response to increases in perfusion pressure was low, administration of ibuprofen restored the response to normal,[63] indicating the possible role of PGs in the afferent dilatation of the diabetic kidney. Finally, postoperative patients who have increased levels of circulating angiotensin, catecholamines, and ADH are in a prostaglandin-dependent vasoconstrictive state that makes them especially susceptible to NSAIDs. The use of ketorolac for the relief of postoperative pain renders these individuals especially susceptible to NSAID-induced ARF.[32, 64]

PREVENTION

Although the adverse effects of NSAIDs on the kidney are well demonstrated and must be a matter of concern, their overall anti-inflammatory and analgesic benefits outweigh the associated risk of ARF, which is relatively low.[65] The occurrence of NSAID-induced ARF can best be considered an overlap phenomenon, rather than merely a simple direct cause and effect (Fig. 33–2). It is when a series of aggravating conditions, each of which individually predisposes to a reduction in GFR (see Table 33–2), coexist in the same individual, and when the additional early reduction in GFR induced by NSAIDs goes undetected, that ARF supervenes. Thus, it is usually the elderly patient, with an underlying predisposing condition (congestive heart failure, nephrotic syndrome, liver cirrhosis) and with volume depletion due to drugs (diuretics) or superimposed stress (diarrhea, vomiting, sepsis), who is susceptible to NSAID-induced ARF. Increased awareness of this combination of conducive events and avoidance or discontinuation of NSAIDs, should any increment in creatinine occur, allows preservation of renal function. Even when mild ARF develops, it remains reversible following discontinuation of NSAIDs (see Fig. 33–1). It is only when the problem goes undetected and the administration of NSAID is continued that ARF becomes severe enough to necessitate renal replacement therapy. Even in cases of ARF due to NSAID-induced acute TIN, the renal lesions seem to abate when the causative agent is discontinued. Thus, with proper use, careful monitoring, and preventive measures, the occasional occurrence of NSAID-induced ARF can be further reduced. To this end, it is prudent to do the following:

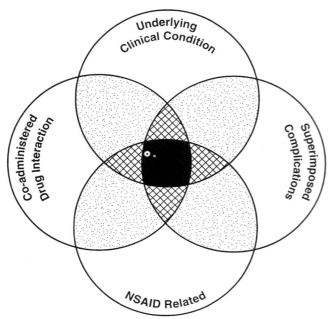

FIGURE 33–2 ■ Schematic representation of the overlap phenomenon conducive to NSAID-induced acute renal failure (ARF). The propensity for ARF increases when more than one of the risk factors listed in Table 33–2, each of which can predispose to a loss of renal function, coexist in the same individual. Not shown in this diagram, but of special importance, is the age of the patient. The central black region indicates those at greatest risk, because of the overlap of all four risk factors. The risk is relatively lower in the cross-striped regions with overlap of three risk factors, less in the dotted regions with overlap of two risk factors, and lowest when only one risk factor exists, in which case the severity of the condition becomes the determinant for increased risk.

- Monitor renal function on an ongoing basis. Early monitoring following initiation of NSAID therapy is essential in susceptible individuals (see Table 33–2) but does not imply that the problem will not occur with long-term use.
- Be concerned about any increment above baseline serum creatinine, even if the reported value is within the normal laboratory range, and more closely monitor renal function in such conditions. When in doubt, the NSAID agent can be discontinued and reversibility of renal function verified.
- Monitor renal function following the institution of any new drug, especially diuretics and ACEIs.
- Be aware that patients who show the fluid and electrolyte effects of NSAIDs (salt retention, hyperkalemia) are likely to be more susceptible to the hemodynamic effect of NSAIDs and therefore require closer monitoring of renal function.
- Instruct patients of the adverse effects of NSAIDs on renal function and to discontinue their use if supervening conditions of volume depletion, such as diarrhea, vomiting, or exercise-induced dehydration, occur.
- Limit the duration of NSAID use and restrict it to specific conditions for which safer analgesics have been ineffective.

REFERENCES

1. Hall WD: NSAIDs and renal function in older people. J Am Geriatr Soc 1999; 47:626.
2. Smith WL, DeWitt DL: Biochemistry of prostaglandin endoperoxide H synthetase-1 and synthetase-2 and their differential susceptibility to nonsteroidal anti-inflammatory drugs. Semin Nephrol 1995; 15:179.
3. Dunn MJ: Nonsteroidal anti-inflammatory drugs and renal function. Annu Rev Med 1984; 35:411.
4. Clive DM, Staff JS: Renal syndromes associated with nonsteroidal anti-inflammatory drugs. N Engl J Med 1984; 310:563.
5. Murray MD, Brater DC: Renal toxicity of the nonsteroidal anti-inflammatory drugs. Annu Rev Pharmacol Toxicol 1993; 32:435.
6. Eknoyan G: Current status of chronic analgesic and nonsteroidal anti-inflammatory drug nephropathy. Curr Opin Nephrol Hypertension 1994; 3:182.
7. Whelton A: Nephrotoxicity of nonsteroidal anti-inflammatory drugs: physiologic foundations and clinical implications. Am J Med 1999; 106:13S.
8. Schlondorff D: Renal prostaglandin synthesis: sites of production and specific actions of prostaglandins. Am J Med 1986; 81(suppl 2B):1.
9. Schlondorff I: Renal complications of nonsteroidal anti-inflammatory drugs. Kidney Int 1993; 44:643.
10. Bonvalet IP, Pradelles P, Forman N: Segmental synthesis and actions of prostaglandins along the nephron. Am J Physiol 1987; 253:F377.
11. Vane JR, Bakhle YS, Botting RM: Cyclooxygenases 1 and 2. Annu Rev Pharmacol Toxicol 1998; 38:97.
12. Laneuville O, Breuer DK, DeWitt DL, et al: Differential inhibition of human endoperoxide H synthetases-1 and -2 by nonsteroidal anti-inflammatory drugs. J Pharmacol Exp Ther 1994; 271:927.
13. Khan KN, Venturini CM, Bunch RT, et al: Interspecies differences in renal localization of cyclooxygenase isoforms: implications in nonsteroidal anti-inflammatory drug–related nephrotoxicity. Toxicol Pathol 1998; 26:612.
14. Lipsky PE: The clinical potential of cyclooxygenase-2 specific inhibitors. Am J Med 1999; 106(5B):51S.
15. Harris RC, McKanna JA, Akai Y, et al: Cyclooxygenase-2 associated with the macula densa of rat kidney and increases in salt retention. J Clin Invest 1994; 94:2504.
16. O'Neill GP, Ford-Hutchinson AW: Expression of mRNA for cyclooxygenase-1 and cyclooxygenase-2 in human tissues. FEBS Lett 1993; 330:156.
17. Guan Y, Chang M, Chow W, et al: Cloning, expression and regulation of rabbit cyclooxygenase-2 in renal medullary interstitial cells. Am J Physiol 1997; 273:F18.
18. Hartner A, Goppelt-Struebe M, Hilgers KF: Coordinate expression of cyclooxygenase-2 and renin in the rat kidney in renovascular hypertension. Hypertension 1998; 31:201.
19. Komhoff M, Gröne HJ, Klein T, et al: Localization of cyclooxygenase-1 and -2 in adult and fetal human kidney: implication for renal function. Am J Physiol 1997; 272:F460.
20. Peterson WL, Cryer B: COX-1–sparing NSAIDs: is the enthusiasm justified? JAMA 1999; 282:1961.
21. Gans K, Galbraith W, Roman RJ, et al: Anti-inflammatory and safety profile of DuP 697, a novel orally effective prostaglandin synthesis inhibitor. J Pharmacol Exp Ther 1990; 254:180.
22. Porter GA, Norton TL, Legg V: Using urinary biomarkers to evaluate renal effects of a COX-2 NSAID in volunteers. Ren Fail 1999; 21:311.
23. Breyer MD: COX-2–selective NSAIDs and renal function: gain without pain? Kidney Int 1999; 55:738.
24. Walker RJ, Fawcett JP, Flannery EM, et al: Indomethacin potentiates exercise-induced reduction in renal hemodynamics in athletes. Med Sci Sports Exerc 1994; 26:1302.
25. Farquhar WB, Morgan AL, Zambraski EJ, et al: Effects of acetaminophen and ibuprofen on renal function in the stressed kidney. J Appl Physiol 1999; 86:598.
26. Catella-Lawson F, McAdam B, Morrison BW, et al: Effects of specific inhibition of cyclooxygenase-2 on sodium balance, hemodynamics, and vasoactive eicosanoids. J Pharmacol Exp Ther 1999; 289:735.

27. Rossat J, Maillard M, Nussberger J, et al: Renal effects of selective cyclooxygenase-2 inhibition in normotensive salt-depleted subjects. Clin Pharmacol Ther 1999; 66:76.

28. Palmer BF: Renal complications associated with nonsteroidal anti-inflammatory agents. J Invest Med 1995; 43:516.

29. Palmer BF, Henrich WL: Clinical acute renal failure with nonsteroidal anti-inflammatory drugs. Semin Nephrol 1995; 15:214.

30. Pugliese F, Cinoti GA: Nonsteroidal anti-inflammatory drugs (NSAIDs) and the kidney. Nephrol Dial Transplant 1997; 12:386.

31. O'Meara ME, Eknoyan G: Acute renal failure associated with indomethacin administration. South Med J 1980; 73:587.

32. Ailabouni W, Eknoyan G: Nonsteroidal anti-inflammatory drugs and acute renal failure in the elderly: a risk benefit assessment. Drugs Aging 1996; 9:341.

33. Lamiere N, Matthys E, Vanholder R, et al: Causes and prognosis of acute renal failure in elderly patients. Nephrol Dial Transplant 1987; 2:316.

34. Garella S, Maurese RA: Renal effects of prostaglandins and clinical adverse effects of nonsteroidal anti-inflammatory agents. Medicine 1984; 68:165.

35. Davidman M, Olson P, Kohen J, et al: Iatrogenic renal disease. Arch Intern Med 1991; 151:1809.

36. Field TS, Gurwitz JH, Glynn RJ, et al: The renal effects of nonsteroidal anti-inflammatory drugs in older people: findings from the established populations for epidemiologic studies of the elderly. J Am Geriatr Soc 1999; 47:507.

37. Kleinknecht D: Interstitial nephritis, the nephrotic syndrome, and chronic renal failure secondary to nonsteroidal anti-inflammatory drugs. Semin Nephrol 1995; 15:228.

38. Shankel SW, Johnson DC, Clark PS, et al: Acute renal failure and glomerulopathy caused by nonsteroidal anti-inflammatory drugs. Arch Intern Med 1992; 152:986.

39. Radford MG, Holley KE, Grande JP: Reversible membranous nephropathy associated with the use of nonsteroidal anti-inflammatory drugs. JAMA 1996; 276:466.

40. Lam G, Kjellstrand C: Sudden catastrophic renal failure from nonsteroidal anti-inflammatory drugs (NSAIDs). J Am Soc Nephrol 1994; 3:399.

41. Porile J, Bakris G, Garella S: Acute interstitial nephritis with glomerulopathy due to NSAID agents: a review of its clinical spectrum and effects of steroid therapy. J Clin Pharmacol 1990; 30:468.

42. Atta MG, Whelton A: Acute renal papillary necrosis induced by ibuprofen. Am J Ther 1997; 4:55.

43. Eknoyan G: Renal papillary necrosis. In Greenberg A, ed: *Primer on Kidney Diseases*. 2nd ed. San Diego: Academic Press; 1998:345.

44. Seibert K, Masferrer JL, Needleman F, et al: Pharmacological manipulation of cyclo-oxygenase-2 in the inflamed hydronephrotic kidney. Br J Pharmacol 1996; 117:1016.

45. Eknoyan G, Quinbi WY, Grissom RT, et al: Renal papillary necrosis: an update. Medicine 1982; 61:55.

46. Murray MD, Nazaridis EN, Brizendine E, et al: The effects of nonsteroidal antiinflammatory drugs on electrolyte homeostasis and blood pressure in young and elderly persons with and without renal insufficiency. Am J Med Sci 1997; 314:80.

47. Yang T, Singh I, Pham H, et al: Regulation of cyclooxygenase expression in the kidney by dietary salt intake. Am J Physiol 1997; 274:F481.

48. Harding P, Sigmon DH, Alfie ME, et al: Cyclooxygenase-2 mediates increased renal renin content induced by low sodium diet. Hypertension 1997; 29:297.

49. Seelig C, Maloley P, Campbell J: Nephrotoxicity associated with concomitant ACE inhibitor and NSAID therapy. South Med J 1990; 83:1144.

50. Clark BA, Shannon RP, Rosa RM, et al: Increased susceptibility to thiazide-induced hyponatremia in the elderly. J Am Soc Nephrol 1994; 5:1106.

51. Mitchell JA, Akarasereenont P, Thiemermann C, et al: Selectivity of nonsteroidal anti-inflammatory drugs as inhibitors of constitutive and inducible cyclooxygenase. Proc Soc Natl Acad Sci 1993; 90:11693.

52. Robbins J, Wahl P, Savage P, et al: Hematological and biochemical laboratory values in older Cardiovascular Health Study participants. J Am Geriatr Soc 1995; 43:855.

53. Anderson S, Brenner BM: The aging kidney structure, function, mechanisms and therapeutic implications. J Am Geriatr Soc 1987; 35:590.

54. Altman RD, Perez GO, Sfakianakis GN: Interaction of cyclosporine A and nonsteroidal anti-inflammatory drugs on renal function in patients with rheumatoid arthritis. Am J Med 1992; 93:396.

55. Kooijmans-Coutinbo MF, Tegzess AM, Bruijn JA, et al: Indomethacin treatment of recurrent nephrotic syndrome and focal segmental glomerulosclerosis after renal transplantation. Nephrol Dial Transplant 1993; 8:469.

56. Ludwin D, Alexopoulou I: Cyclosporine A nephropathy in patients with rheumatoid arthritis. Br J Rheumatol 1993; 32(suppl 1):60.

57. Toto RD, Anderson SA, Brown-Cartwright D, et al: Effects of acute and chronic NSAIDs in patients with renal insufficiency. Kidney Int 1986; 80:760.

58. Gentilini P: Cirrhosis, renal function and NSAIDs. J Hepatol 1993; 19:200.

59. Blackshear JL, Davidman M, Stillman MT: Identification of risk for renal insufficiency from nonsteroidal anti-inflammatory drugs. Arch Intern Med 1983; 43:1130.

60. Patrono C, Pierucci A: Renal effects of nonsteroidal anti-inflammatory drugs in chronic glomerular disease. Am J Med 1986; 81:71.

61. Tomasoni S, Noris M, Zapella S, et al: Upregulation of renal and systemic cyclooxygenase-2 in patients with active lupus nephritis. J Am Soc Nephrol 1998; 9:1202.

62. Allon M, Lawson L, Echman JR, et al: Effects of nonsteroidal anti-inflammatory drugs on renal function in sickle cell anemia. Kidney Int 1988; 34:500.

63. Hayashi K, Epstein M, Loutzenhiser R: Impaired myogenic responsiveness of the afferent arteriole in streptozotocin-induced diabetic rats: role of eicosanoid derangements. J Am Soc Nephrol 1992; 2:1578.

64. Feldman HI, Kimnan JL, Berlin JA, et al: Parenteral ketorolac: the risk for acute renal failure. Ann Intern Med 1997; 126:193.

65. Murray MD, Brater DC, Tierney WM, et al: Ibuprofen-associated renal impairment in a large general internal medicine practice. Am J Med Sci 1990; 299:222.

CHAPTER 34

Acute Renal Failure Associated With Occupational and Environmental Settings

Peter H. Bach

INTRODUCTION

Humans are exposed to a range of chemicals that adversely affect the kidney. Many of these are medicines, but there are also a considerable number of occupational and environmental substances that can cause acute renal failure (ARF) (Table 34–1). As is common with such relationships, some are well defined, but many are poorly investigated, and some substances are associated with a limited number of case reports. It is against this background that a selection of environmental and occupational nephrotoxins are considered. This chapter has been formulated to help provide an understanding of how some of these molecules exert their effects, if known, and also to catalogue several less well investigated agents. Mechanistic investigations should provide the basis for better rational clinical management.

There is a compelling relationship between ARF and a series of chemical insults.[1–13] Indeed, environmental substances and occupational exposure have long been recognized[14] as factors that cause or contribute to ARF.[15–19] In the case of medicines, substance, dose, and consequences are well defined and properly documented. Proving the relationship between environmental and occupational chemical exposure and

ARF is not always easy. Many uncertainties are associated with exposure to these substances, in which exposure levels vary considerably (and generally cannot be reliably measured), and many products contain mixtures that, at best, may be poorly defined. In the case of plant substances, toxic constituents also vary seasonally and within the same season between plants grown in different locales. It is therefore most difficult to identify which agent or agents have caused or contributed to ARF. Often, individuals are exposed to several potential nephrotoxins over a period of time, which is known to reduce renal functional reserve and make them more sensitive to certain types of nephrotoxic insult.

HEAVY METALS

The heavy metals were among the earliest known molecules that cause ARF, and they have also been investigated intensively as models that provide the mechanistic basis of the lesion. Despite the well-known toxicity of these substances and the strict legislation that limits exposure of individuals to them, they continue to cause ARF, especially in developing countries. Also, researchers are continually uncovering new aspects of these molecules associated with their nephrotoxicity. These data provide depth to our understanding of the cellular and molecular processes that underlie ARF.

Mercury-Induced Acute Renal Failure

Mercury exists in the form of mercury vapor (Hg^0), ionized inorganic mercury (Hg^{1+}, Hg^{2+}), and organic mercury compounds. Excessive exposure to inorganic mercury compounds, either through inhalation of elemental mercury vapor, ingestion of divalent mercury salts, or the use of skin-lightening cosmetics containing mercury, may lead to significant kidney injury, including ARF. Inhaled mercury vapor leads to the deposition of mercury in the kidney. The kidney is also the major site of deposition of mercury from mercurous and mercuric mercury compounds and organomercurials, such as methyl mercury. In the past, mercury has been regarded as a highly selective proximal tubular toxin that mediated its effects by binding to cellular sulfhydryl groups[20] and affecting glomerular function.[21] More recently, it has become appreciated that mercury forms a complex with sulfhydryl-containing

TABLE 34–1. Environmental Nephrotoxic Agents

TYPE	AGENT
Organic solvents	Ethylene glycol
	Diethylene glycol
	Propylene glycol
	Carbon tetrachloride
	Chloroform
	Trichloroethylene
Heavy metals	Antimony
	Arsenic
	Bismuth
	Cadmium
	Copper
	Gold
	Lead
	Inorganic mercury
	Organic mercury salts
	Uranium
Insecticides and herbicides	Chlorinated hydrocarbons
	Organophosphorus compounds
	Bipyridium compounds
	Pentachlorophenol
Biologicals	Mycotoxins
	Snake and spider venoms
	Mushrooms

ligands, which are filtered in the glomeruli and degraded into Hg^{2+}-cysteine in the proximal tubules by the combined action of γ-glutamyl transpeptidase and dipeptidase present in the epithelial cells. These organometallic molecules probably gain easiest access to the proximal tubular cells and mediate directly toxic effects. Changes in the glomerular filtration rate are associated with direct effects on this region of the kidney and perturbation of vasoconstrictors, angiotensin II, and endothelin-1 and with the decreased action of the vasodilator nitric oxide.[22] The nephroprotection associated with aminoguanidine (a nitric oxide synthase inhibitor) confirms that induction of inducible nitric oxide synthase exacerbates proximal tubule epithelial cell damage,[23] but the mechanism is not clear. The involvement of endothelin-1 and nitric oxide in the pathogenesis of mercury-induced ARF does offer the potential to better modulate these mediators of renal blood flow associated with mercury poisoning.

Poisoning with inorganic mercury, once a common cause of ARF and tubular necrosis,[24] is still seen today. There have been reported cases of metallic mercury vapor–induced[25] ARF, which is likely to be very significant in those countries where gold amalgams are processed as part of the "underground economy." Treatment consists of intravenous chelation therapy and the promotion of diuresis. The available chelating agents include British anti-Lewisite (dimercaprols; BAL, 2,3-dimercapto-1-propanol or dimercaprol), penicillamine, 2,3-dimercaptopropane-1 sulfonate (DMPS), and dimercaptosuccinic acid (DMSA).[26]

Arsenic-Induced Acute Renal Failure

Arsenic is used in insecticides, ant poisons, weed killers, wallpaper, antifouling paint, ceramics, wood preservatives, and glass. The inorganic arsenicals, such as arsenic trioxide, are more toxic than the organic compounds. Absorption follows inhalation or ingestion. The soluble compounds are readily absorbed via skin and mucous membranes and are excreted primarily in the urine. Repeated doses are cumulative. Toxicity results when arsenic combines with sulfhydryl enzymes and interferes with cellular oxidative processes. When arsenic is ingested in large amounts, the initial symptoms include a dry, burning sensation in the mouth and throat. Crampy abdominal pain, severe vomiting, and diarrhea follow the initial symptoms. Vertigo, delirium, and coma are quite obvious manifestations of central nervous system involvement. Death may be caused by circulatory collapse and liver and renal failure. Hemodialysis has been found to be effective treatment for the renal failure. British anti-Lewisite (BAL) is valuable in the treatment of acute arsenic poisoning.

Arsine-Induced Acute Renal Failure

Arsine (AsH_3) is a colorless gas. It has a garlic-like or fishy smell but does not burn the eyes, nose, or throat. Inhalation is the major route of exposure. Arsine gas is formed when arsenic-containing materials react with water or acids. Accidental exposures have occurred during refining of ores (eg, lead, copper, zinc, iron, and antimony ores) that are contaminated with arsenic. Arsine is used as a dopant in the semiconductor industry and in the manufacture of crystals for fiberoptics and computer chips. It has minor uses in galvanizing, soldering, etching, and lead plating.[27] This compound has been reported to cause ARF in humans under a number of different circumstances,[28–31] all associated with a profound hemolysis (Table 34–2).

The signs and symptoms of acute arsine poisoning are usually delayed for 2 to 24 hours, depending on the intensity of exposure. After absorption by the lungs, arsine enters red blood cells and inhibits red cell catalase, which leads to accumulation of hydrogen peroxide. Hydrogen peroxide, in turn, destroys red cell membranes and causes the massive intravascular hemolysis that develops within hours and continues for up to 96 hours following exposure. Haptoglobin levels decline rapidly. Plasma free hemoglobin rises, with concentrations greater than 2 g/dL reported. Anemia develops; peripheral blood smears show anisocytosis, poikilocytosis, red-cell fragments, basophilic stippling, and ghost cells.

Renal failure caused by acute tubular necrosis is a significant sequela of arsine exposure. Hemoglobinuria is thought to be the major insult, but a direct toxic effect of arsine or deposition of the arsine-hemoglobin-haptoglobin complex may also play a role. Urinalysis shows large amounts of methemoglobin, protein, and hemoglobin without intact erythrocytes. The urine may be colored (ie, brown, red, orange). Oliguria or anuria may develop within 24 to 48 hours.

If hemolysis develops, 50 to 100 mEq of sodium bicarbonate may be added to 1 L of 5% dextrose in 0.25 normal saline and administered intravenously at a rate that maintains urine output at 2 to 3 mL/kg per hour in an attempt to promote urinary alkalization. Maintenance of an alkaline urine (ie, pH > 7.5) is recommended until the urine is hemoglobin free. Although BAL (dimercaprol) and other chelating agents are useful in arsenic poisoning, they are not effective antidotes for arsine poisoning. Blood transfusions may be necessary if hemolysis causes severe anemia.

TABLE 34–2. Causes of Pigment Nephropathy

Hemoglobinuria
  Aniline
  Arsine
  Creosol
  Naphthalene
  Nitrobenzene
  Phenol
  Sodium chlorate
  Toluene
Myoglobinuria
  Carbon monoxide
  Mercuric chlorate

Other Heavy Metals

Other heavy metals shown to produce clinical ARF include antimony, bismuth, copper, and gold. Bismuth compounds were once prepared as therapeutic agents. Copper may be ingested in fungicide-contaminated feed grains or in water from copper-containing heaters. Gold has been implicated as a rare cause of ARF.

SOLVENTS

In an industrial environment, workers are often exposed to a number of different solvents, and it may be difficult to identify which component or components are toxic. Short-term exposure to solvents, such as halogenated hydrocarbons, petroleum distillates, ethylene glycol, ethylene glycol ethers, and diethylene glycol, may cause renal tubular necrosis and ARF,[14, 17, 18] and similar effects are reported in addicts who have inhaled solvent vapors (eg, toluene).[32–33]

Ethylene Glycol–Induced Acute Renal Failure

Ethylene glycol is an oxygenated hydrocarbon. It is the main component in antifreeze and may be present in agents such as lacquers and deicers. It is colorless and odorless and has a sweet taste, and may be ingested as a substitute for alcohol. More commonly, however, ingestion is unintentional. It is converted to glycolaldehyde, with further metabolism to glycolic acid and glycoxylate and eventual irreversible oxidation to oxalate[34] (Fig. 34–1). The initial reaction is dependent on alcohol dehydrogenase. Aldehyde dehydrogenase rapidly converts glycolaldehyde to glycolate. The rate-limiting step is the conversion of glycolic acid to glyoxylic acid. This reaction is slow and accounts for the accumulation of glycolate in the blood and contributes to the metabolic acidosis. Pyridoxine deficiency may limit the metabolism of glyoxylate to glycine and thereby may promote its accumulation. A small proportion of glyoxylate is rapidly metabolized to oxalate. This alters the ratio of NAD to NADH and promotes the production of lactic acid. The liver is the primary site of metabolism, although approximately 20% of the ethylene glycol is excreted unchanged in the urine. About 1% of the ethylene glycol appears in the urine as oxalic acid.

The initial manifestations of ethylene glycol poisoning involve the central nervous system and generally occur within 0.5 to 12 hours of ingestion, which coincides with the greatest amount of aldehyde production. Alterations in mental status, seizures, and coma may occur. Approximately 12 to 24 hours after ingestion, cardiopulmonary symptoms in the form of arrhythmias and pulmonary edema predominate. The renal manifestations follow at 24 to 72 hours after ingestion. Calcium oxalate crystals are deposited in the epithelium of the proximal tubule and may produce hydronephrosis. Toxic metabolites of ethylene glycol probably contribute to the renal toxicity, which is

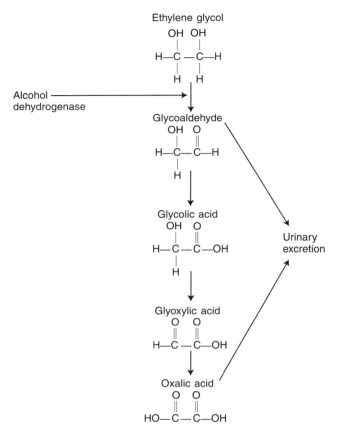

FIGURE 34–1 ■ The major pathway for the metabolism of ethylene glycol. The first step in this pathway is catalyzed by alcohol dehydrogenase. Thus, inhibitors of alcohol dehydrogenase prevent the metabolism of ethylene glycol to toxic metabolites. (From Barceloux DG, Krenzelok EP, Olson K, Watson W: American Academy of Clinical Toxicology Practice Guidelines on the treatment of ethylene glycol poisoning. Clin Toxicol 1999; 37:537–560; with permission.)

characterized by oliguria, ARF, kidney and flank pain,[35] and an overwhelming acidosis aggravated by the production of lactate.

The direct measurement of serum ethylene glycol concentrations is the definitive method for diagnosing ethylene glycol poisoning. However, the diagnosis should be considered when examination of the urine reveals alcohol-like intoxication without the odor of alcohol, coma with a severe metabolic acidosis and a large anion gap, or massive calcium oxalate crystalluria. The presence of an elevated osmolar gap suggests that significant concentrations of ethylene glycol may be present. Also, since the metabolism of ethylene glycol produces organic acids, the ensuing metabolic acidosis is characterized by the presence of a large anion gap, with glycolic acid as its major constituent. Crytalluria occurs and is associated with the presence of needle-shaped crystals of calcium oxalate monohydrate or octahedral "envelopes" of calcium oxalate dihydrate. The latter is more specific for ethylene glycol toxicity. Severe hypocalcemia may be suspected when a prolonged QT interval is present on the electrocardiogram. Hypocalcemia is caused by the chelation of calcium ions by oxalate.

In the absence of treatment, the lethal dose of ethylene glycol is 2 mL/kg or approximately 150 mL for an adult. This represents 0.1 g/kg of oxalic acid. In a child, as little as 15 mL of a concentrated ethylene glycol solution can be fatal. The simultaneous ingestion of ethyl alcohol and ethylene glycol decreases the oxidation of the latter and modifies its toxicity. Treatment is designed to correct the acidosis, prevent the manifestations of hypocalcemia, supply adequate thiamine and pyridoxine, and inhibit the metabolism of ethylene glycol and remove it and its products by means of a forced diuresis and hemodialysis. At one time, intravenous treatment with ethyl alcohol was given in a loading dose of 0.6 to 1.0 g/kg over 1 hour, followed by a sustained infusion of 10 to 12 g/h to maintain the blood level at 100 mg/dL. This therapy was effective by virtue of ethylene glycol's competition with alcohol dehydrogenase. Fomepizole, or 4-methylpyrazole, has an affinity for alcohol dehydrogenase that is 8000 times greater than ethanol and has been used effectively to prevent the metabolism of ethylene glycol.[36–38] A loading dose of 15 mg/kg is administered, followed by doses of 10 mg/kg every 12 hours for four doses, then 15 mg/kg every 12 hours until serum ethylene glycol concentrations have fallen below 20 mg/dL. These recommendations are based on the American Academy of Clinical Toxicology's practice guidelines on the treatment of ethylene glycol poisoning[39] and are summarized in Tables 34–3 and 34–4.

Other Glycols

Other potentially toxic glycols include ethylene glycol dinitrate, propylene glycol, ethylene dichloride, and diethylene glycol. *Diethylene glycol* has been used in the past as a medicinal vehicle in an elixir of sulfanilamide. It is a potent tubular toxin and was responsible for a number of cases of anuric ARF in children in Haiti in 1996 when diethylene glycol (DEG)–contaminated glycerin was used in the manufacture of acetaminophen syrup.[40] *Propylene glycol* is a solvent that is used in many oral, injectable, and topical medications. Although uncommon, ARF may be caused by propylene glycol and is attributable to proximal renal tubular cell injury.[41]

Mixed Solvents

Acute renal failure following overexposure to aliphatic hydrocarbons in diesel fuel and solvents is probably underrecognized,[17] as are the effects of heavy exposure to upholsterer's glue and other solvent-containing material.[42] There is relatively little known about the underlying processes, which are often explained in terms of multiorgan failure. There is, however, a case report involving only the kidney in a patient after immersion in seawater polluted by diesel oil.[43] This suggests that ARF associated with toxic doses of hydrocarbon may affect only the kidney.

HALOGENATED ORGANIC MOLECULES

Halogenated organic molecules include solvents and agrochemical products. Acute exposure to halogenated pesticides and herbicides has generally decreased in recent years, because of the heightened awareness of their potential dangers. Many halogenated chemicals cause nephrotoxicity in experimental animals and in humans because of their common pathways of metabolism via either cytochrome P-450 or glutathione conjugation. Chloroform and carbon tetrachloride are examples of cytochrome P-450–mediated activation, and dihaloethanes and hexachloro-1,3-butadiene undergo glutathione conjugation followed by activation.[44–46]

Carbon Tetrachloride

Carbon tetrachloride is a halogenated hydrocarbon. It has been used as an industrial solvent and as a household cleaning agent. It is soluble in alcohol, and both hepatic and renal toxicities increase if alcohol is consumed during the period of exposure. Acute renal failure may occur as the consequence of ingestion, although it is usually the result of inhalation of the toxic vapor of carbon tetrachloride. The interval between exposure and medical care often exceeds 24 hours, and a reduction in urine volume may not be apparent for 7 to 10 days. During this time, individuals may be free from symptoms, but they are more likely to complain of vomiting, abdominal pain, constipation, diarrhea, or fever. The oliguria lasts 1 to 2 weeks. Analysis of the urine reveals that more red blood cells and protein are present in this condition than in other forms of nephrotoxic ARF. Treatment with *N*-acetylcysteine has been advocated (300 mg/kg).[47] Recovery is expected.

Carbon tetrachloride–induced ARF is still being reported in terms of liver toxicity and effects on other organs,[48] especially in countries where the levels of occupational and industrial hygiene have not been well developed or controlled. Such effects are especially marked in individuals who have also been exposed to isopropyl alcohol, as this is metabolized to acetone, a major potentiator of carbon tetrachloride toxicity.[49–51]

TABLE 34–3. Indications for Treatment of Ethylene Glycol Poisoning With an Antidote

1. Documented plasma ethylene glycol concentration > 20 mg/dL
   OR
2. Documented recent (hours) history of ingesting toxic amounts of ethylene glycol and osmol gap > 10 mOsm/L
   OR
3. History or strong clinical suspicion of ethylene glycol poisoning and at least two of the following criteria:
   A. Arterial pH < 7.3
   B. Serum bicarbonate < 20 mEq/L
   C. Osmol gap > 10 mOsm/L
   D. Urinary oxylate crystals present

From Barceloux DG, Krenzelok EP, Olson K, Watson W: American Academy of Clinical Toxicology Practice Guidelines on the treatment of ethylene glycol poisoning. Clin Toxicol 1999; 37:537–560; with permission.

TABLE 34–4. Practice Guidelines for the Treatment of Potentially Serious Ethylene Glycol Ingestions

TREATMENT	INDICATIONS
Gut decontamination	1. Consider gastric aspiration and lavage if < 1 h after ingestion. 2. Activated charcoal if mixed ingestion.
Initial laboratory tests	*Blood:* Complete blood count, electrolytes, magnesium, calcium, osmolality, ethanol, and ethylene glycol. If alcoholic ketoacidosis is suspected, obtain serum lactate, β-hydroxybutyrate. *Urine:* Urinalysis with microscopy for crystals.
General use of an antidote	1. For indications, see Table 34–3. 2. Administration of the antidote should continue until the ethylene glycol is undetectable or ethylene glycol < 20 mg/dL and the patient is asymptomatic with normal pH.
Indications for the administration of fomepizole, rather than ethanol	1. Ingestion of multiple substances with depressed level of consciousness. 2. Altered consciousness. 3. Lack of adequate intensive care staffing or laboratory support to monitor ethanol administration. 4. Relative contraindication to ethanol.* 5. Critically ill patient with an anion gap acidosis of unknown etiology and potential exposure to ethylene glycol. 6. Patients with active hepatic disease.
Indications for the administration of ethanol, rather than fomepizole	1. Fomepizole unavailable. 2. Hypersensitivity to fomepizole.
Indications for hemodialysis	1. Severe metabolic acidosis (<7.25–7.3) unresponsive to therapy. 2. Renal failure. 3. Ethylene glycol > 50 mg/dL unless fomepizole is being administered and patient is asymptomatic with normal arterial pH.
Supportive care	1. Correct fluid balance. 2. Correct pH <7.3 with intravenous bicarbonate. 3. Replacement of magnesium and administration of thiamine and pyridoxine in depleted patients. 4. Monitor acid-base status; urine output and serum creatinine. 5. Calcium replenishment only for symptomatic hypocalcemia or intractable seizures. 6. Monitor patients receiving an ethanol infusion in an ICU or similar setting capable of providing close monitoring of metabolic acidosis, vital signs, serum abnormalities (glucose, electrolytes), and serum ethanol.

*Ethanol should be administered cautiously to young children because of the risk of hypoglycemia.

From Barceloux DG, Krenzelok EP, Olson K, Watson W: American Academy of Clinical Toxicology Practice Guidelines on the treatment of ethylene glycol poisoning. Clin Toxicol 1999; 37:537–560; with permission.

Carbon tetrachloride toxicity is the result of CYP-450–mediated activation, which takes place in the liver and can also occur in the kidney.[52] In addition to the potential for a direct toxic mechanism, there is also evidence that severe rhabdomyolysis resulting from liver failure following carbon tetrachloride intoxication could also play a role in ARF.[53]

Chloroform

Chloroform is used chiefly as a refrigerant and as an aerosol propellant and in the synthesis of fluorinated resins. It is also produced during the chlorination of water. Although its primary effect is on the central nervous system and liver, it is also nephrotoxic. Chloroform may be transformed into a toxic product by microsomal metabolism. On this basis, the ingestion of diets high in polybrominated biphenyls, known to be inducers of microsomal enzyme activity, enhances chloroform nephrotoxicity.

Trichloroethylene

Trichloroethylene is an aromatic hydrocarbon chemically related to both carbon tetrachloride and chloroform and shares with them the propensity for liver and kidney damage. It has a number of industrial applications and has been used as an anesthetic agent for obstetric patients. Acute renal failure has followed inhalation by "solvent sniffers" and has been seen in those using cleaning solutions containing this agent.

Toluene

Toluene is an aromatic hydrocarbon that has widespread use as an organic solvent. Those who have sniffed toluene-containing substances, such as model glues, have demonstrated the potential for renal toxicity. The maximal allowable concentration of toluene is far exceeded when these compounds are inhaled from paper bags. Although the renal damage is generally mild, severe defects in the individual's ability to excrete an acid load have been noted.

PESTICIDES, INSECTICIDES, HERBICIDES, AND FUNGICIDES

Nephrotoxicity has been associated with the use of two major categories of insecticides: the organophosphorus compounds such as *parathion* and the chlorinated hydrocarbons such as *chlordane*. Bipyridium compounds have been used as herbicides. Acute renal failure has been reported with the glyphosphate surfactant herbicide Roundup (Monsanto, St. Louis).[54] The herbicide 2,4-dichlorophenoxyacetic acid has been associated with hypocalcemia and hyperphosphatemia.[55]

Renal uptake occurs in the proximal tubule via the organic acid transport system.[56] The ingestion or parenteral injection of *paraquat* (1,1'dimethyl-4-4'-bipyridium) has a mortality rate of up to 70%. After it is absorbed into the systemic circulation, approximately 85% of the paraquat is excreted unchanged by the kidney. Toxic doses of paraquat cause ARF, with damage to proximal renal epithelial cells. When ARF occurs, plasma levels of paraquat rise, leading to its accumulation in vital organs, such as the lungs.

Chloroanilines

Chloroanilines are widely used chemical intermediates in dye, agricultural chemical, and industrial compound manufacture. They have been shown to be highly nephrotoxic, for example, in rodents, but there are no reported cases of ARF in humans, possibly owing to the fact that they are less toxic when administered orally.[57]

1,2-Dibromoethane

1,2-Dibromoethane was once a widely used insecticide, fumigant, nematocide, fungicide, and an additive in leaded gasoline. Despite its well-established and almost guaranteed fatal hazard,[58] managed recovery has been reported.[59] 1,2-Dibromoethane is metabolized to a direct-acting toxin, as shown by kidney autoradiography in the *cynomolgus monkey*, in which products of 1,2-dibromoethane–derived metabolism bound preferentially to liver and kidney tubules, and this binding was localized to the sites where tissue lesions had been observed in humans.[60] 1,2-Dibromoethane is conjugated by glutathione S-transferases and oxidized by cytochrome P-450 to form one or more reactive metabolites.[61] Depending on the dose, these metabolites deplete glutathione in liver and kidney and then bind to essential biological macromolecules[62] and also bind DNA.[61]

NATURAL TOXINS

Nature provides some of the most toxic molecules known to humans, many of which affect the kidney, but most often these have been involved in chronic toxicity following multiple exposures. Also, a number of natural toxins cause ARF.

Animal Toxins

INSECTS

There are a number of reports of envenomations by African "killer" bees that resulted in rhabdomyolysis, hemolysis, and ARF,[63, 64] and, in addition, some evidence that there may be a direct effect of venom on the renal tubules.[65]

REPTILES

A bite from Russell's viper (*Vipera russellii*) is the commonest cause of ARF in several south Asian countries.[66] The venom contains peptides and proteins, including a number of phospholipases, which cause hemolysis, rhabdomyolysis, pre-synaptic neurotoxicity, vasodilatation, and release of endogenous autacoids. Shock and renal failure develop rapidly, and although specific antivenom controls bleeding and clotting disorders, it does not reverse nephrotoxicity and shock.[66]

MARINE SPECIES

Jellyfish (*Physalia physalis*) venom contains polypeptides and enzymes with toxic and antigenic properties that have the potential to cause ARF.[67] Bile from a number of aquatic species is potently nephrotoxic. For example, grass carp (*Ctenopharyngodon idella*) bile and gallbladder cause ARF in humans and death in laboratory rodents.[68, 69] Bile extract causes a prompt fall in systemic arterial blood pressure and cardiac output, and an increase in urinary excretion of water and salts, which, together with the potential to cause hemolysis, are thought to be responsible for renal functional damage.[69] Ingestion of the gallbladder of *Labeo rohita*, a freshwater fish commonly found in India, has also caused a significant number of deaths in the past. Currently, there are no experimental data on the nephrotoxic components likely to be responsible for such effects, nor any data on their effects on the cardiovascular-renal axis.[70]

Botanical and Plant-Derived Materials

Plant and plant-derived materials have long been associated with ARF, and examples of "one-of-a-kind" case reports are extensive. For example, there are limited clinical data indicating that both the latex of *pokok ipoh* (*Antiaris toxocaria*) and the root bark of *akar ipoh* (*Strychnos* species) used for blowpipe dart poisoning cause rhabdomyolysis ARF.[71] Consumption of the tubers of *Gloriosa superba* (which contains colchicine) has also been reported to cause ARF and hematologic abnormalities.[72]

The role of botanicals in renal injury is probably under-estimated, as shown by the fatalities associated with the use of traditional herbal remedies in east,[73] central[74] and southern[75] Africa. In these regions, fatalities are especially high in children and following the use of plant decoctions as abortifacients.[75, 76] However, in busy hospitals, where there is a high incidence of malnutrition and tropical disease, death is often attributed to other causes, and, even if ethnomedicines are suspected, there is little probability that an attempt will be made to ascertain whether herbal medications have been used.

HEMLOCK

The ingestion of wildfowl that have eaten hemlock buds causes rhabdomyolysis, myoglobinuria, acute tubular necrosis, and ARF,[77, 78] in addition to the neurotoxic effects associated with such poisonings. The earliest reference to this phenomenon is in the Bible, in Numbers 11:31–34:

> There sprang up a wind from the Lord, which drove quails in from the west, and they were flying all around the camp for the distance of a day's journey, three feet above the ground. The people were busy gathering quails all that day and night, and all next day, and even those who got least gathered ten homers of them. They spread them out to dry all about the camp. But the meat was scarcely between their teeth, and they had not so much as bitten it, when the Lord's anger flared up against the people and he struck them with a severe plague. The place came to be called Kibroth-hattaavah, because there they buried the people who had been greedy for meat.[79]

There are data to suggest that rhabdomyolysis following hemlock ingestion is associated with conline (an alkaloid of *Conium maculatim*), rather than cicutoxin (active principle of water hemlock)[77]; however, such poisoning appears to be rare. Usually, intoxication occurs by the ingestion of stems, leaves, roots, or fruits, mistakenly chosen as edible vegetables.

ATRACTYLOSIDE-CONTAINING PLANTS

A number of plants (eg, *Callilepsis laureola* and *Atractylis gummifera-L*) in Europe along the Aegean[80] and in developing countries[76, 81–84] are used as traditional ethnomedicines, where they often cause fatalities, especially in children. *Callilepsis laureola* (impila), a member of the family Compositae, is a perennial herb grown in the grasslands of southern Africa. It has been used by the local people in infusions for a wide variety of illnesses. Chewing and ingesting parts of the plant result in impila poisoning, with ARF occurring in the majority of severe cases. Death is associated with hepatic and renal necrosis,[80–82, 84–88] with the latter affecting both the convoluted tubule and the loop of Henle.[89] This condition accounts for 1500 deaths per annum in Kwa-Zulu Natal, South Africa,[82] and 1200 per annum in Tunis.[90]

Atractyloside, a diterpenoid glycoside, is the common toxin found in these plants, which is well known to competitively inhibit the adenine nucleoside carrier in mitochondria, blocking oxidative phosphorylation, which eventually leads to cellular necrosis. The perturbation of intermediary metabolism is thought to explain changes in intermediary metabolism (eg, hyperglycemia, which is followed by a hypoglycemic phase and then acidosis), which precedes toxic effects in liver and kidney.

There is uncertainty regarding the sensitivity of humans to atractyloside.[91, 92] Organ injury seemingly occurs in humans exposed to oral doses of atractyloside in the μg/kg range. This level of exposure is enough to cause severe kidney damage.[81, 84, 88] By contrast, clinical symptoms and target organ toxicity of laboratory and domestic species typically follow exposure to single intraperitoneal doses of 10 to 200 mg/kg.[81, 85, 92] Direct comparison between humans and experimental animals is complicated by the lack of reliable data on the quantities of atractyloside ingested by humans, and its plasma and organ concentrations. At present, there is no information to suggest whether the presence of malnutrition or tropical disease somehow increases the human sensitivity to the toxic effects of atractyloside. Until these data are available, humans must be considered to be much more sensitive to this plant toxin than are either laboratory or domestic animals.[92]

Atractyloside appears to target the proximal tubule as the result of selective transport into these cells, where the high mitochondrial component is essential for renal function.[92] The molecular basis of atractyloside-induced proximal tubular necrosis and centrilobular necrosis is not fully understood. There are data[91] to suggest that the targeting of liver and kidney involves more than one mechanism. The most likely mechanism of atractyloside toxicity involves alteration in mitochondrial function with a subsequent loss of cellular energy.[93]

Treatment of atractyloside poisoning is purely systemic, and there are no antidotes for acute poisoning. However, preliminary in vitro studies by Obatomi and Bach suggest that appropriate therapeutic interventional strategies could limit toxicity by blocking the selective transport of atractyloside into proximal renal cells through the administration of probenecid. There is also the possibility that the use of dithiothreitol and verapamil could reduce the severity of atractyloside toxicity in vivo, based on the protection of proximal renal cells by the use of an in vitro[93] system.

DJENKOL BEANS

The djenkol bean (*Pithecellobium jiringa*, family Mimosaceae) is widely consumed as food in Southeast Asia. Djenkol beans have long been associated with ARF.[94, 95] The clinical presentation includes abdominal pain, nausea, vomiting, dysuria, proteinuria, hematuria, and oliguria that may progress to anuria and ARF with focal tubular necrosis[96] in severe cases.

The toxicity has been attributed to djenkolic acid, which experimentally decreases urinary output and causes celluria and mild to severe ATN with some glomerular cell necrosis, in rats and mice, but does not cause renal failure per se.[97] Djenkolic acid is an analogue of thiazolidine-4-carboxylic acid, a cyclic cysteine-formaldehyde condensation product, which has been used clinically for treatment of liver disease and related gastrointestinal disturbances.[98] The nephrotoxicity of djenkol beans may be more complex, because acute overdose of thiazolidine-4-carboxylic acid in humans causes neurotoxicity and limited metabolic acidosis. Severe hypoglycemia is possible, but hyperglycemia is rare.[99] Most importantly, no indication of nephrotoxicity has been reported.[99] This suggests that the role of djenkolic acid in ARF is questionable or, at least, it is more complex than has been suggested by designating this molecule the proximate toxin. One possible factor could be the pH-dependent solubility of L-djenkolic acid, which could explain both its nephrotoxicity and its propensity to form crystal and calculi.[100]

MUSHROOM NEPHROTOXINS

Fungi are ubiquitous and poisonous, and therefore they have been linked to fatalities throughout the world. Acute mushroom poisonings are well known. The effect of fungal ingestion on the renal system is less well established, although it is known that various species of mushrooms contain nephrotoxic compounds that may result in irreversible renal failure.[101] At times, a specific nephrotoxin can be detected in renal biopsy material by thin-layer chromatography.[102] Gastrointestinal symptoms herald the onset of toxicity within hours of ingestion and may continue for several days, followed by the appearance of ARF. With hemodialysis and supportive care, renal function can be expected to return.[103]

Cortinarius Genus

In the last few years, there have been a number of case records of patients poisoned by Cortinarius orellanus.[104] The origins were diverse and included attempted suicide,[105] food poisoning,[106] and inexperienced collectors thinking they were using hallucinogenic "magic mushrooms."[107] All individuals showed the classic "Orellanus syndrome" in which ARF develops after a symptom-free period ranging from 2 to 21 days. Renal biopsy showed both nonspecific histopathologic findings[107] and an interstitial nephritis. Renal effects are caused by a direct-acting nephrotoxin, orellanine, which is generally lethal if appropriate treatment, such as hemodialysis, is not given. Often, renal injury is followed by the need for peritoneal dialysis and renal transplantation.[105, 108] The limited usefulness of plasma exchange in Cortinarius speciosissimus poisoning is probably related to the long latency between ingestion and the occurrence of the first renal symptoms,[109] and even 10 days after ingestion of the mushrooms plasma has contained small but measurable concentrations of orellanine.[105]

Orellanine is a semiquinone ([2,2'-bipyridine]-3,3',4,4'-tetrol-1,1'-dioxide) that has also been reported to be found in C. henrici and C. orellanus and five Cortinarius species from the subgenus Leprocybe, section Orellani. In addition to orellanine, the close analogues orellinine and orelline have also been reported. Orellanine is absent, however, from D. cinnamomea and C. splendens, which have previously been claimed to be toxic and assumed to contain orellanine.[110] Semiquinones (which are formed from compounds such as phenacetin and acetaminophen) undergo redox cycling, as a result of which they generate free radicals and cause significant local cellular injury where they accumulate.[111]

Cortinarius speciocissimus also causes interstitial nephritis[112] but contains no orellanine.[113, 114] This heightens the concept that a range of related toxins may work individually or together to cause renal injury. This also underscores the need for the clinician to consider interstitial nephritis of unknown etiology as possibly resulting from intoxication with a mushroom when he or she undertakes the differential diagnosis of ARF.

Amanita Genus

Mushroom poisoning leading to ARF is rare in North America, but both Cortinarius species and Amanita smithiana have been identified as causing ARF in the Pacific northwest.[115] Amanita proxima is a rarely consumed mushroom but has recently been reported to cause nonfatal ARF,[116, 117] the effects of which appear to have been dose related. Acute renal failure has also been associated with the acute hepatitis caused by Amanita phalloides,[118] which is most often linked only to other major organ failure.

These mushrooms contain amatoxins, a group of octopeptides that have been identified as the principal toxins. The amatoxins can irreversibly inhibit RNA polymerase, which results in cellular necrosis.[119] Amanita poisoning is characterized by a latent period of about 12 hours between ingestion and the initial phase of the intoxication, which begins with nausea, vomiting, abdominal pain, and watery diarrhea. These signs subside after a few hours, and the patient enters a symptom-free period that may last up to 3 days. Hepatic and renal lesions develop afterward. Renal involvement is manifested as oliguric ARF. However, hepatic damage is more prominent and is often the cause of death.[120, 121] Renal pathology shows tubular necrosis involving mainly the proximal convoluted tubules.[122]

Acute renal failure has also been associated with immune hemolysis after repeated ingestion of cooked Paxillus involutus caused by antibodies against the fungus circulating in sensitized patients.[123, 124]

MYCOTOXINS

Despite the marked and highly selective nephrotoxicity of a number of mycotoxins, there is a paucity of reports on their acute clinical toxicity. Ochratoxin A is a mycotoxin produced by at least 10 species of Penicillium and eight of Aspergillus. These mycotoxins contaminate cereals (eg, those made of corn, wheat, and beans) during the storage process. Ochratoxin A is nephrotoxic and is responsible for porcine nephropathy. It has been implicated as a potential factor in Balkan nephropathy, and has been shown to induce interstitial nephritis and tubular necrosis.[125] It produces proximal tubular injury with glycosuria, no or low proteinuria, proximal tubular cell karyomegalic lesions, and nonspecific interstitial lesions. Interestingly, several mysterious deaths of archeologists that occurred after they opened Egyptian tombs have been suspected to be secondary to inhalation of mycotoxin. In these cases, nonoliguric ARF due to the inhalation of ochratoxin of Aspergillus ochraceus resulted in biopsy-proven tubular necrosis.[125, 126]

CONCLUSIONS

Chemicals will always provide unique models for constructing an understanding of the cellular and molecular processes that underlie renal injury. Indeed, there are many occupational and environmental chemicals that cause ARF. In some cases (eg, mercury), these substances have been investigated for decades, but novel aspects of renal cellular changes have been and will continue to be uncovered that demonstrate a multiplicity of factors underlying the cascade of events that lead to renal failure. Gaining knowledge and understanding of renal injury is likely to be an ongoing process, even when well-known compounds, such as the heavy metals, are investigated. There is little doubt that these lesions will serve as models from which we can learn more about cell signaling as well as up-regulation and down-regulation of genes in the different cell types that are affected by such injury. All additional understanding derived from these investigations will be relevant to ARF caused by disease processes, medicines, and chemicals.

The need for more experimental investigations is far greater for compounds, such as atractyloside, that are responsible for the death of children in developing countries. Here, an understanding of the mechanism of injury could provide a rational basis for blocking toxicity and facilitating better therapeutic management and intervention, rather than relying purely on systemic treatment. There is an important need to more fully assess the effects of mushroom toxins, venoms, and fish bile, which are extremely toxic and for which systemic management does not always have a successful clinical outcome.

There will always be examples in which limited case reports, inability to reproduce animal models, and the influence of other factors provide those interesting "one of" examples of occupational and environmental nephrotoxins. These examples may remain rare and poorly understood events. Or, they may provide the basis for carefully designed and executed investigations that will open new vistas in our understanding of the kidney in health and disease, illuminate the processes underlying ARF, and help establish ways in which therapeutic intervention can be developed.

ACKNOWLEDGMENTS

I am grateful to Kerry Henderson for providing library support and Alan Johnston for useful comments.

REFERENCES

1. Solez K: *Acute Renal Failure.* New York: Marcel Dekker; 1991.
2. Goligorsky MS, Stein JH, eds: *Acute Renal Failure: New Concepts and Therapeutic Strategies. Contemporary Issues in Nephrology.* Vol. 30. Edinburgh: Churchill Livingstone; 1995.
3. Abuelo JG, ed: *Renal Failure: Diagnosis and Treatment. (Developments in Nephrology.* Vol. 37.) Dordrecht: Kluwer Academic Publishers; 1995.
4. Lazarus JM, Brenner BM, eds: *Acute Renal Failure.* 3rd ed. Edinburgh: Churchill Livingstone; 1993.
5. Guglielminotti J, Guidet B: Acute renal failure in rhabdomyolysis. Minerva Anesthesiol 1999; 65:250–255.
6. Visweswaran P, Guntupalli J: Rhabdomyolysis. Crit Care Clin 1999; 15:415–428.
7. Nissenson AR: Acute renal failure: definition and pathogenesis. Kidney Int 1998; 66(suppl):S7–S10.
8. Baliga R, Ueda N, Walker PD, Shah SV: Oxidant mechanisms in toxic acute renal failure. Am J Kidney Dis 1997; 29:465–477.
9. Heyman SN, Fuchs S, Brezis M: The role of medullary ischemia in acute renal failure. New Horiz 1995; 3:597–607.
10. Wardle EN: Acute renal failure and multiorgan failure. Nephron 1994; 66:380–385.
11. Andreoli SP: Reactive oxygen molecules, oxidant injury and renal disease. Pediatr Nephrol 1991; 5:733–742.
12. Farrugia E, Larson TS: Drug-induced renal toxicity: help in recognizing offending agents. Postgrad Med 1991; 90:241–244, 247–248.
13. Reubi FC: Pathogenesis and renal function in acute toxic nephropathies. Contrib Nephrol 1978; 10:1–14.
14. Editorial: Consensus statement on the health significance of nephrotoxicity. Toxicol Lett; 1989; 46:1–11.
15. Lote CJ, Harper L, Savage COS: Mechanisms of acute renal failure. Br J Anaesth 1996; 77:82–89.
16. Finn WF: Environmental toxins and renal disease. J Clin Pharmacol 1983; 23:461–472.
17. Landry JF, Langlois S: Acute exposure to aliphatic hydrocarbons: an unusual cause of acute tubular necrosis. Arch Intern Med 1998; 158:1821–1823.
18. Roy AT, Brautbar N, Lee DB: Hydrocarbons and renal failure. Nephron 1991; 58:385–392.
19. Abuelo GJ: Renal failure caused by chemicals, foods, plants, animal venoms, and misuse of drugs: an overview. Arch Intern Med 1990; 150:505–510.
20. Houser MT, Milner LS, Kolbeck PC, et al: Glutathione monoethyl ester moderates mercuric chloride–induced acute renal failure. Nephron 1992; 61:449–455.
21. Wolfert AI, Laveri LA, Reilly KM, et al: Glomerular hemodynamics in mercury-induced acute renal failure. Kidney Int 1987; 32:246–255.
22. Yanagisawa H: Mecuric chloride–induced acute renal failure and its pathophysiology. [Article in Japanese.] Nippon Eiseigaku Zasshi 1998; 52:618–623.
23. Yanagisawa H, Nodera M, Wada O: Inducible nitric oxide synthase expression in mercury chloride–induced acute tubular necrosis. Ind Health 1998; 36:324–330.
24. Troen P, Seymour A, Kaufman SA, Katz KH: Mercuric bichloride poisoning. N Engl J Med 1951; 244:459–463.
25. Aguado S, de Quiros IF, Marin R, et al: Acute mercury vapour intoxication: report of six cases. Nephrol Dial Transplant 1989; 4:133–136.
26. Bluhm RE, Bobbit RG, Welch LW, Wood AJ: Elemental mercury vapour toxicity, treatment, and prognosis after acute, intensive exposure in chloralkali plant workers. Part I: History, neuropsychological findings and chelator effects. Hum Exp Toxicol 1992; 11:201–210.
27. Fowler BA, Weissberg JB: Arsine poisoning. N Engl J Med 1974; 291:1171–1174.
28. Rogge H, Fassbinder W, Martin H: Arsine (AsH₃) poisoning: hemolysis and kidney failure]. [Article in German.] Dtsch Med Wochenschr 1983; 108:1720–1725.
29. Phoon WH, Chan MO, Goh CH, et al: Five cases of arsine poisoning. Ann Acad Med Singapore 1985; 13(suppl 2):394–398.
30. Wilkinson SP, McHugh P, Horsley S, et al: Arsine toxicity aboard the Asia freighter. BMJ 1975; 3:559–563.
31. Parish GG, Glass R, Kimbrough R: Acute arsine poisoning in two workers cleaning a clogged drain. Arch Environ Health 1979; 34:224–227.
32. Lauwerys R, Bernard A, Viau C, Buchet JP: Kidney disorders and hematotoxicity from organic solvent exposure. Scand J Work Environ Health 1985; 1(suppl 11):83–90.
33. Ehrenreich T: Renal disease from exposure to solvents. Ann Clin Lab Sci 1977; 7:6–16.
34. Gabow PA, Clay K, Sullivan JR, et al: Organic acids in ethylene glycol intoxication. Ann Intern Med 1986; 105:16–20.
35. Kruse J: Ethylene glycol intoxication. J Intensive Care Med 1992; 7:234–243.

36. Baud F, Galliot M, Astier A, et al: Treatment of ethylene glycol poisoning with intravenous 4-methylpyrazole. N Engl J Med 1988; 319:97–100.
37. Jacobsen D, McMartin K: 4-Methylpyrazole: present status. Clin Toxicol 1996; 34:379–381.
38. Shannon M: Toxicology reviews: Fomepizole: a new antidote. Pediatr Emerg Care 1998; 14:170–172.
39. Barceloux DG, Krenzelok EP, Olson K, Watson W: American Academy of Clinical Toxicology Practice Guidelines on the treatment of ethylene glycol poisoning. Clin Toxicol 1999; 37:537–560.
40. Anonymous: Fatalities associated with ingestion of diethylene glycol-contaminated glycerin used to manufacture acetaminophen syrup: Haiti, November 1995–June 1996. MMWR Mor Mortal Wkly Rep 1996; 45:649–650.
41. Yorgin PD, Theodorou AA, Al-Uzri A, et al: Propylene glycol–induced proximal renal tubular cell injury. Am J Kidney Dis 1997; 30:134–139.
42. Knight AT, Pawsey CG, Aroney RS, et al: Upholsterers' glue associated with myocarditis, hepatitis, acute renal failure and lymphoma. Med J Aust 1991; 154:360–362.
43. Li FK, Yip PS, Chan KW, et al: Acute renal failure after immersion in seawater polluted by diesel oil. Am J Kidney Dis 1999; 34:E26.
44. David NJ, Wolman R, Milne FJ, van Niekerk I: Acute renal failure due to trichloroethylene poisoning. Br J Ind Med 1989; 46:347–349.
45. Shafer N, Shafer R: Tetrachloroethylene: a cause of permanent kidney damage. Med Trial Tech Q 1982; 28:387–395.
46. Lock EA: Mechanism of nephrotoxic action due to organohalogenated compounds. Toxicol Lett 1989; 46:93–106.
47. Ochoa Gomez FJ, Lisa Caton V, Saralegui Reta I, Monzon Marin JL: Carbon tetrachloride poisoning. Anales de Medicina Interna 1996; 13:393–394.
48. Casas E, Martinez Ara J, Valencia ME, et al: Carbon tetrachloride poisoning: a report of 3 cases. [Article in Spanish.] An Med Interna 1989; 9:486–488.
49. Folland DS, Schaffner W, Ginn HE, et al: Carbon tetrachloride toxicity potentiated by isopropyl alcohol. JAMA 1976; 236:1853–1856.
50. Ochoa Gomez FJ, Lisa Caton V, Saralegui Reta I, Monzon Marin JL: Carbon tetrachloride poisoning. [Article in Spanish.] An Med Interna 1996; 8:393–394.
51. Deng JF, Wang JD, Shih TS, Lan FL: Outbreak of carbon tetrachloride poisoning in a color printing factory related to the use of isopropyl alcohol and an air conditioning system in Taiwan. Am J Ind Med 1987; 12:11–19.
52. IARC: Carbon tetrachloride. IARC Monogr Eval Carcinog Risks Hum 1999; 71(Pt 2):401–432.
53. Nehoda H, Wieser C, Koller J, et al: Recurrent liver failure with severe rhabdomyolysis after liver transplantation for carbon tetrachloride intoxication. Hepatogastroenterology 1998; 45:191–195.
54. Talbot AR, Shiaw MH, Huang JS, et al: Acute poisoning with a glyphosate-surfactant herbicide (Round-up): a review of 93 cases. Hum Exp Toxicol 1991; 10:1–8.
55. Kancir CB, Anderson C, Olesen AS: Marked hypocalcemia in a fatal poisoning with chlorinated phenoxy acid derivatives. Clin Toxicol 1988; 26:257–264.
56. Berndt WO, Koschier F: In vivo uptake of 2,4-dichlorophenoxyacetic acid (2,4-D) and 2,4,5-trichlorophenoxyacetic acid (2,4,5-T) by renal cortical tissue of rabbits and rats. Toxicol Appl Pharmacol 1973; 26:559–570.
57. Lo HH, Valentovic MA, Brown PI, Rankin GO: Effect of chemical form, route of administration and vehicle on 3,5-dichloroaniline–induced nephrotoxicity in the Fischer 344 rat. J Appl Toxicol 1994; 14:417–422.
58. Letz GA, Pond SM, Osterloh JD, et al: Two fatalities after acute occupational exposure to ethylene dibromide. JAMA 1984; 252:2428–2431.
59. Prakash MS, Sud K, Kohli HS, et al: Ethylene dibromide poisoning with acute renal failure: first reported case with nonfatal outcome. Ren Fail 1999; 21:219–222.
60. Brandt I, Brittebo EB, Kowalski B, Lund BO: Tissue binding of 1,2-dibromoethane in the cynomolgus monkey (Macaca fascicularis). Carcinogenesis 1987; 8:1359–1361.
61. Ploemen JP, Wormhoudt LW, Haenen GR, et al: The use of human in vitro metabolic parameters to explore the risk assessment of hazardous compounds: the case of ethylene dibromide. Toxicol Appl Pharmacol 1997; 143:56–69.
62. Mann AM, Darby FJ: Effects of 1,2-Dibromoethane on glutathione metabolism in rat liver and kidney. Biochem Pharmacol 1985; 34:2827–2830.
63. Hommel D, Bollandard F, Hulin A: Multiple African honeybee stings and acute renal failure. Nephron 1998; 78:235–236.
64. Beccari M, Castiglione A, Cavaliere G, et al: Unusual case of anuria due to African bee stings. Int J Artif Organs 1992; 15:281–283.
65. Spielman FJ, Bowe EA, Watson CB, Klein EF Jr: Acute renal failure as a result of Physalia physalis sting. South Med J 1982; 75:1425–1426.
66. Warrell DA: Snake venoms in science and clinical medicine. 1. Russell's viper: biology, venom and treatment of bites. Trans R Soc Trop Med Hyg 1989; 83:732–740.
67. Burnett JW, Calton GJ, Burnett HW: Jellyfish envenomation syndromes. J Am Acad Dermatol 1986; 14:100–106.
68. Lim PS, Lin JL, Hu SA, Huang CC: Acute renal failure due to ingestion of the gallbladder of grass carp: report of 3 cases with review of literature. Ren Fail 1993; 15:639–644.
69. Chen CF, Yen TS, Chen WY, et al: The renal, cardiovascular and hemolytic actions in the rat of a toxic extract from the bile of the grass carp (Ctenopharyngodon idellus). Toxicon 1984; 22:433–439.
70. Sahoo RN, Mohapatra MK, Sahoo B, Das GC: Acute renal failure associated with freshwater fish toxin. Trop Geogr Med 1995; 47:94–95.
71. Ho LM, Cheong I, Jalil HA: Rhabdomyolysis and acute renal failure following blowpipe dart poisoning. Nephron 1996; 72:676–678.
72. Mendis S: Colchicine cardiotoxicity following ingestion of Gloriosa superba tubers. Postgrad Med J 1989; 65:752–755.
73. Otieno LS, McLigeyo SO, Luta M: Acute renal failure following the use of herbal remedies. East Afr Med J 1991; 68:993–998.
74. Lowenthal MN, Jones IG, Mohelsky V: Acute renal failure in Zambian women using traditional herbal remedies. J Trop Med Hyg 1974; 77:190–192.
75. Seedat YK: Acute renal failure among Blacks and Indians in South Africa. S Afr Med J 1978; 54:427–431.
76. Seedat YK, North-Coombes D, Sewdarsen M: Acute renal failure in Indian and Black patients. S Afr Med J 1975; 49:1907–1910.
77. Rizzi D, Basile C, Di Maggio A, et al: Clinical spectrum of accidental hemlock poisoning: neurotoxic manifestations, rhabdomyolysis, and acute tubular necrosis. Nephrol Dial Transplant 1991; 6:939–943.
78. Scatizzi A, Di Maggio A, Rizzi D, et al: Acute renal failure due to tubular necrosis caused by wildfowl-mediated hemlock poisoning. Ren Fail 1993; 15:93–96.
79. Blythe WB: Hemlock poisoning, acute renal failure, and the Bible. Ren Fail 1993; 15:653.
80. Georgiou M, Sianidou L, Hatzis T, et al: Hepatotoxicity due to Atractylis gummifera-L. Toxicol Clin Toxicol 1988; 26:487–493.
81. Bhoola KDN: A clinico-pathological and biochemical study of the toxicity of Callilepsis laureola (impila). Doctor of Medicine Thesis. University of Natal, Durban, 1983.
82. Hutchings A, Terblanche SE: Observations on the use of some known and suspected toxic Liliiflorae in Zulu and Xhosa medicine. S Afr Med J 1989; 75:62–69.
83. Schteingart CD, Pomilio AB: Atractyloside, toxic compound from Wedelia glauca. J Nat Prod 1984; 47:1046–1047.
84. Seedat YK, Hitchcock PJ: Acute renal failure from Callilepsis laureola. S Afr Med J 1971; 45:832–833.
85. Carpenedo F, Luciani S, Scaravilli F, et al: Nephrotoxic effect of atractyloside in rats. Arch Toxicol 1974; 32:169–180.
86. Caravaca-Magarinos F, Cubero-Gomez JJ, Arrobasvaca M: Renal and hepatic injuries in human intoxication with Atractylis gummifera. Nefrologia 1985; 5:205–210.
87. Hedili A, Warnet JM, Thevenin M, et al: Biochemical investigation of Atractylis gummifera L. hepatotoxicity in the rat. Arch Toxicol Suppl 1989; 13:312–315.
88. Wainwright J, Schonland MM, Candy HA: Toxicity of Callilepsis laureola. S Afr Med J 1977; 52:313–315.

89. Seedat YK, Hitchcock PJ: Acute renal failure from *Callilepsis laureola*. S Afr Med J 1978; 54:832–838.
90. Kechrid C, el Ouakdi M, Ben Abdallah T, et al: The first thirty months of kidney transplantation in Tunisia. [Article in French.] Nephrologie 1990; 11:157–160.
91. Obatomi DK, Brant S, Anthonypillai V, Bach PH: Toxicity of atractyloside in precision-cut rat and porcine renal and hepatic tissue slices. Toxicol Appl Pharmacol 1998; 148:35–45.
92. Obatomi DK, Bach PH: Biochemistry and toxicology of the diterpenoid glycoside atractyloside. Food Chem Toxicol 1998; 36:335–346.
93. Obatomi DK, Bach PH: Atractyloside nephrotoxicity: in vitro studies with suspension of rat renal fragments and precision-cut cortical slices. In Vitro Molec Toxicol 2000;13:25–36.
94. Yong M, Cheong I: Jering-induced acute renal failure with blue urine. Trop Doct 1995; 25:31.
95. H'ng PK, Nayar SK, Lau WM, Segasothy M: Acute renal failure following jering ingestion. Singapore Med J 1991; 32:148–149.
96. Segasothy M, Swaminathan M, Kong NCT, et al: Djenkol bean poisoning (Djenkolism): an unusual cause of acute renal failure. Am J Kidney Dis 1995; 25:63–66.
97. Areekul S, Kirdudom P, Chaovanapricha K: Studies on djenkol bean poisoning (djenkolism) in experimental animals. Southeast Asian J Trop Med Public Health 1976; 7:551–558.
98. Weber HU, Fleming JF, Miquel J: Thiazolidine-4-carboxylic acid, a physiologic sulfhydryl antioxidant with potential value in geriatric medicine. Arch Gerontol Geriatr 1982; 1:299–310.
99. Efthymiou ML, Jouglard J: Thiazolidine carboxylic acid toxicity: a review of 78 cases. [Article in French.] Nouv Presse Med 1982; 11:509–512.
100. Areekul S, Muangman V, Bohkerd C, Saenghirun C: Southeast Asian djenkol bean as a cause of urolithiasis. J Trop Med Public Health 1978; 9:427–432.
101. Holzl B, Regele H, Kirchmair M, Sandhofer F: Acute renal failure after ingestion of *Cortinarius speciocissimus*. Clin Nephrol 1997; 48:260–262.
102. Rohrmoser M, Kirchmair M, Feifel E, et al: Orellanine poisoning: rapid detection of the fungal toxin in renal biopsy material. J Toxicol Clin Toxicol 1997; 35:63–66.
103. Leathem AM, Purssell RA, Chan VR, Kroeger PD: Renal failure caused by mushroom poisoning. J Toxicol Clin Toxicol 1997; 35:67–75.
104. Bednarova V, Bodlakova B, Pelclova D, Sulkova S: Mushroom poisoning by *Cortinarius orellanus*. [Article in Czech.] Cas Lek Cesk 1999; 138:119–121.
105. Delpech N, Rapior S, Cozette AP, et al: Outcome of acute renal failure caused by voluntary ingestion of *Cortinarius orellanus*. [Article in French.] Presse Med 1990; 19:122–124.
106. Bouget J, Bousser J, Pats B, et al: Acute renal failure following collective intoxication by *Cortinarius orellanus*. Intensive Care Med 1990; 16:506–510.
107. Calvino J, Romero R, Pintos E, et al: Voluntary ingestion of *Cortinarius* mushrooms leading to chronic interstitial nephritis. Am J Nephrol 1998; 18:565–569.
108. Holmdahl J, Mulec H, Ahlmen: Acute renal failure after intoxication with *Cortinarius* mushrooms. J Hum Toxicol 1984; 3:309–313.
109. Busnach G, Dal Col A, Perrino ML, et al: Plasma exchange in acute renal failure by *Cortinarius speciosissimus*. Int J Artif Organs 1983; 1(suppl 6):73–74.
110. Oubrahim H, Richard JM, Cantin-Esnault D, et al: Novel methods for identification and quantification of the mushroom nephrotoxin orellanine: thin-layer chromatography and electrophoresis screening of mushrooms with electron spin resonance determination of the toxin. J Chromatogr A 1997; 758:145–157.
111. Yamada K, Fukushima T: Mechanism of cytotoxicity of paraquat. II. Organ specificity of paraquat-stimulated lipid peroxidation in the inner membrane of mitochondria. Exp Toxicol Pathol 1993; 45:375–380.
112. Nolte S, Hufschmidt C, Steinhauer H, et al: Terminal renal failure caused by interstitial nephritis following mushroom poisoning by *Cortinarius speciosissimus*. [Article in German.] Monatsschr Kinderheilkd 1987; 135:280–281.
113. Holzl B, Regele H, Kirchmair M, Sandhofer F: Acute renal failure after ingestion of *Cortinarius speciocissimus*. Clin Nephrol 1997; 48:260–262.
114. Tidman M, Sjostrom P: Acute renal failure caused by mushroom poisoning with *Cortinarius speciosissimus*. [Article in Swedish.] Lakartidningen 1992; 89:2763–2764.
115. Warden CR, Benjamin DR: Acute renal failure associated with suspected *Amanita smithiana* mushroom ingestions: a case series. Acad Emerg Med 1998; 5:808–812.
116. de Haro L, Jouglard J, Arditti J, David JM: Acute renal insufficiency caused by *Amanita proxima* poisoning: experience of the Poison Center of Marseille. [Article in French.] Nephrologie 1998; 19:21–24.
117. Leray H, Canaud B, Andary C, et al: *Amanita proxima* poisoning: a new cause of acute renal insufficiency. [Article in French.] Nephrologie 1994; 15:197–199.
118. Bourgeois J, Bourgeois N, Gelin M, et al: Acute hepatitis and poisoning by *Amanita phalloides*. [Article in French.] Acta Gastroenterol Belg 1992; 55:358–363.
119. Vetter J: Toxins of *Amanita phalloides*. Toxicon 1998; 36:13–24.
120. Lampe KF: Toxic fungi. Annu Rev Pharmacol Toxicol 1997; 19:85–104.
121. Chen ZY, Liao LS: Renal damages caused by the common mushrooms [Chinese.] Chin J Nephrol 1993; 9:107–108.
122. Fiume L, Marinozzi V, Nardi F: The effects of amanitine poisoning on the mouse kidney. Br J Exp Pathol 1969; 50:196–204.
123. Winkelmann M, Borchard F, Stangel W, Grabensee B: Fatal immunohaemolytic anaemia after eating the mushroom *Paxillus involutus*. [Article in German.] Dtsch Med Wochenschr 1982; 107:1190–1194.
124. Winkelmann M, Stangel W, Schedel I, Grabensee B: Severe hemolysis caused by antibodies against the mushroom *Paxillus involutus* and its therapy by plasma exchange. Klin Wochenschr 1986; 64:935–938.
125. Di Paolo N, Guarnieri A, Garosi G, et al: Inhaled mycotoxins lead to acute renal failure. Nephrol Dial Transplant 1994; 4(suppl 9):116–120.
126. Di Paolo N, Guarnieri A, Loi F, et al: Acute renal failure from inhalation of mycotoxins. Nephron 1993; 64:621–625.

MANAGEMENT OF ACUTE RENAL FAILURE

CHAPTER 35

Recovery From Acute Renal Failure

William F. Finn

INTRODUCTION

Acute renal failure (ARF) is an important illness in both industrialized and less developed countries. Indeed, it has been estimated that ARF may affect as many as 5% of hospitalized patients and 30% of patients in intensive care units.[1] To prevent this condition from developing into one of chronic renal failure, attention needs to be directed toward the factors that influence recovery. It is generally accepted that the rate and extent of recovery from both postischemic and nephrotoxic ARF are inversely related to the severity of the initial injury. With that in mind, the management of patients with ARF should start with efforts aimed at minimizing the impact of the initial injury and avoiding the situations known to accentuate the decline in renal function. With the ultimate goal set at full structural and functional recovery and the prevention of chronic, irreversible changes, it is helpful to review the classic phases of ARF, because treatment plans are different at each stage of disease.

PHASES OF ACUTE RENAL FAILURE

The clinical course of ARF was originally separated into several distinct phases: the onset phase, the oliguric phase, and the recovery phase, with the latter category subdivided into a diuretic phase and a phase of functional recovery[2] (Table 35–1). As a result of changes in the patient population and the complex nature of modern medical care, these phases are now frequently indistinct. This is most obvious in two groups: those whose urine output is not decreased and who present with nonoliguric ARF, and those in whom the pattern of recovery is altered by pharmacologic agents or dialytic treatment. Thus, it is more reasonable to discuss the clinical course of ARF in terms of the initial phase, the maintenance phase, and the recovery phase.[3] This is based on the understanding that nonoliguric and oliguric ARF can be considered to be variations of a similar condition, with the difference in urine flow rates indicative of differences in the degree of tubular epithelial injury and the residual level of the glomerular filtration rate (GFR)[4] (Fig. 35–1).

Initial Phase

The initial phase of ARF begins with the period of ischemia or exposure to the nephrotoxic agent and continues until there is a clinically definable change in renal function. An alteration in urine output, an increase in the blood urea nitrogen (BUN) level, or an increase in the serum creatinine concentration (S_{Cr}) most often indicates this. During the initial phase, a transition zone of variable length may be present during which the progression to established ARF might be modified or even interrupted.[5, 6] The length of the initial phase is variable and depends largely on the nature and severity of the renal insult, ie, the renal response to ischemia or nephrotoxic agents may be immediate or delayed. In the case of an ischemic insult, the initial phase may be brief. In contrast, obvious changes in renal function resulting from the administration of a nephrotoxic agent, eg, an aminoglycoside, may not be apparent for a week or more.

Maintenance Phase

The maintenance phase of ARF is also variable in degree and duration. During this time, the patient may be oliguric, defined as a urine output of less than 400 to 500 mL per day. A reduction in urine volume to less than 100 mL per day is generally considered to be equivalent to anuria and suggests alternative diagnoses such as urinary tract obstruction or bilateral cortical

TABLE 35–1. Pathophysiologic Abnormalities in Stages of Acute Renal Failure

CLINICAL PHASE	PATHOPHYSIOLOGIC CORRELATES
Initial phase	Tubular epithelial cell injury
	Vasoconstriction
Maintenance phase	Tubular obstruction
	Passive backflow of filtrate
	Secondary vasoconstriction
	Medullary congestion
	Changes in glomerular capillary ultrafiltration coefficient
Early recovery phase	Restoration of tubular epithelial cell integrity
Phase of functional recovery	Vasodilation
	Nephron recruitment

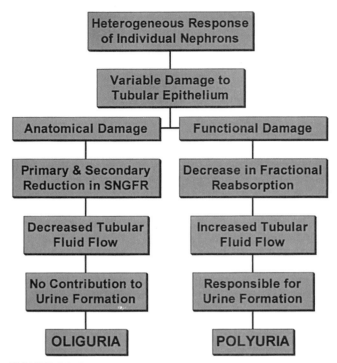

FIGURE 35–1 ■ Schema of interrelated events responsible for the functional abnormalities following an hour of complete unilateral renal artery occlusion in the rat. Individual nephron response to ischemia or nephrotoxic agents may determine whether acute renal failure is oliguric or polyuric.

necrosis. With increased frequency, the urine output is not reduced (nonoliguric ARF) and may even be increased (polyuric ARF). Whatever the pattern of urine output, there are a number of changes in the composition of the urine that confirm the decline in renal clearance of urea (C_{Urea}) and creatinine (C_{Cr}) and are indicative of abnormalities in renal tubular epithelial cell function. Suffice it to say that in this phase the urine elaborated more closely resembles that of an ultrafiltrate of plasma and gives the appearance that there has been little modification by tubular reabsorptive or secretory processes. The maintenance phase lasts for approximately 1 to 3 weeks. There is, however, wide variation in this time period. The decline in renal function may be of short duration, as may occur following exposure to radiocontrast agents, or it may persist for 2 months or more with considerable hope of recovery.

Early Recovery Phase

EARLY RECOVERY PHASE IN OLIGURIC ACUTE RENAL FAILURE

In patients who are oliguric, the onset of the early recovery phase is marked by an increase in urine flow, which may be gradual or sudden. In either case, subsequent increases in flow rates can be anticipated over a period of hours or days. Once established, the daily increase in urine flow proceeds at a relatively constant rate. The initial increase in urine volume may[7, 8] or may not[2] be preceded by an increase in the urine urea (U_{Urea}) and creatinine concentrations (U_{Cr}) or by a fall in the urine sodium concentration (U_{Na}). If the latter does not occur, sodium losses during the early recovery phase may be considerable. If not monitored at frequent intervals and replaced promptly, the clinical condition will be complicated by the hemodynamic consequences of volume depletion, and renal recovery may be delayed or interrupted.[9]

The magnitude of the natriuresis and diuresis probably represents an inability of regenerating tubules to reabsorb sodium and water normally. Studies of the molecular basis of the natriuresis observed during this time have shown abnormalities to exist in proximal tubule and ascending limb of Henle sodium transporters.[10] During the early recovery phase, the urine osmolality remains low and is not modified by the administration of vasopressin. This defect in urinary concentrating ability may also be related to a reduction in the sodium transporters. In this case, the limitation in active sodium transport reduces the osmotic gradient between the medullary interstitium and tubular fluid, thus limiting water reabsorption. In addition, since osmotic water permeability across the tubular epithelium is chiefly dependent on aquaporin (AQP) water channels,[11] it is not surprising that following ischemic injury, a reduction of AQP-2 protein is involved in the loss of urinary concentrating ability.[12]

The excretion of urea and other nitrogenous compounds lags behind that of salt and water as reflected by the continual rise in the plasma concentrations of these substances for several days after the onset of the diuresis. Consequently, uremic symptoms requiring dialysis may develop despite the dramatic increase in urine flow. Functional recovery can be anticipated as long as the urine volume continues to rise toward appropriate values. If, however, there is an initial increase in urine volume, followed by a plateau during which the urine volume remains constant, complete recovery is less likely. At times, the rate of recovery may be predicted by the length of the oliguric phase. A pattern of slow recovery with small incremental increases in the GFR may follow longer periods of oliguria. With shorter periods of oliguria, recovery may be more rapid, with larger daily increases in the GFR.

EARLY RECOVERY PHASE IN NONOLIGURIC ACUTE RENAL FAILURE

In nonoliguric ARF, changes in urine volume may not be a useful index of recovery. Instead, the onset of recovery is heralded by an improvement in markers of renal clearance and tubular function. The latter may include a return of the ability to concentrate the urine and a decrease in the fractional excretion of sodium (FE_{Na}). An increase in urinary concentration, as judged by an increase in urine specific gravity or osmolarity, is most often a result of an increase in the urinary excretion of urea (U_{Urea}) and creatinine (U_{Cr}). Even without a change in urine volume, the increases in U_{Urea} and U_{Cr} are indicative of an increase in the renal clearance of these substances. At the same time, the FE_{Na}, which is generally elevated in nonoliguric patients as well as those with oliguria, may decline. Any improvement of these indices is a useful indicator of early recovery.

Phase of Functional Recovery

After several days, the early recovery phase merges into a phase of functional recovery in which the GFR increases and tubular function is restored. When the GFR increases to a value of approximately 7 mL/min, the S_{Cr} level may reach a plateau. However, because the C_{Urea} is from 40% to 60% of the C_{Cr}, it can be expected that the BUN will continue to increase until the C_{Cr} approaches 10 to 12 mL/min or more. Thereafter, gradual reductions in the BUN and S_{Cr} occur. The rapidity with which they fall can be related to the severity of the initial injury, the time and magnitude of the preceding diuresis, improvement in urinary compositional changes, and the metabolic state of the individual. The kidneys of the patients who are markedly catabolic and whose endogenous nitrogen loads are high, take a longer period of time to clear these substances from the blood.

Occasionally, the failure of the GFR to improve at the expected interval is related to the superimposition of a state of intravascular volume depletion owing to the failure to replace urinary sodium losses or the loss of volume with dialysis. For this reason, it is helpful to measure the U_{Na} level periodically and to calculate the FE_{Na} level along with the C_{Urea} and C_{Cr}. The return of the ability to conserve sodium in the absence of an improvement in the GFR suggests that the slope of the recovery phase has been flattened by superimposed intravascular volume contraction, perhaps because of aggressive ultrafiltration during dialysis treatments. As recovery occurs, the return of tubular function can be demonstrated by the ability to vary urine flow in response to hydration, although the response is delayed. Similarly, in response to sodium chloride loading, as recovery occurs, U_{Na} levels may rise along with an increase in urine flow. Likewise, the U_{Na} level may fall with sodium restriction.

RESIDUAL DEFECTS

The extent to which renal function recovers is influenced by the presence or absence of preexisting renal disease, the age of the patient at the time of the acute episode, and, as mentioned, the severity of the ARF itself. Because nonoliguric ARF is generally considered to be reflective of less serious injury than oliguric ARF, recovery is anticipated to be more complete. In nonoliguric ARF, there is evidence of less severe tubular injury as judged by a higher urine-to-plasma urea ratio, a less severe defect in tubular sodium reabsorption, and retention of the secretory capacity of the proximal and terminal tubular segments.[13] A less severe reduction in both the C_{Urea} and

the C_{Cr} leads to lower values for the maximal level to which the BUN and S_{Cr} rise, a decrease in the duration of the azotemia, and a decrease in the requirement for dialysis.[14]

In either case, as recovery occurs, there is a considerable amount of discordance in the return of function of individual nephron units, ie, not all nephrons recover at the same time or to the same extent. The level to which the GFR returns depends on the number of nephrons that recover and the absolute level of function in each. While it is hoped that a full complement of nephrons are present, this is often not the case.

In the patients with ARF who do not succumb to their underlying illness or to one of the many complications, recovery of life-sustaining renal function can be expected. However, the degree of recovery is often incomplete, and renal function does not return in many cases. In a few patients, regressive changes occur after an initial phase of improvement, with the development of chronic, irreversible renal failure. Indeed, end-stage renal disease resulting from ARF is not uncommon. For example, in one large study of 1095 patients with severe ARF, the overall survival was only 59.5%. Of these, 16.2% remained dependent on long-term dialysis. Of interest, several patients recovered sufficient renal function to become independent of dialysis 6 to 21 months after the onset of ARF.[15] With regard to the number of deaths in patients with ARF, it has been appreciated for some time that the mortality rate in nonoliguric patients is substantially lower than in those who are oliguric.[16] The difference is related to the fact that the nonoliguric patients have a significantly lower incidence of complications than that of oliguric patients,[17] as a result of a decrease in the severity of the ARF.

Functional Defects

Recovery of renal function appears to be complete in only one third of the patients who survive, and the remainder may regain only 60% of normal function.[18–22] A few continue to exhibit a more severe depression of renal function with C_{Cr} as low as 20 mL/min. Occasionally, renal function slowly deteriorates after the initial improvement. This occurs most often when the original return of renal function has been poor. The S_{Cr} level at recovery tends to be higher in patients requiring longer periods of dialysis support, although there does not appear to be a relationship between the cause of the renal failure and the degree of residual function obtained.[21, 22] In a representative study of 125 patients who survived an episode of ARF, at 1 year, 62.4% had complete recovery, 31.2% had partial recovery, and 6.4% had no recovery. At 5 years, the GFR was greater than 80 mL/min in 56.8%, greater than 15 mL/min in 32%, and less than 15 mL/min in 11.2%[23] (Fig. 35–2). Recovery is delayed in older patients and in those whose oliguric period is prolonged.[24]

Several tubular defects have been reported to persist for months to years following recovery. The most

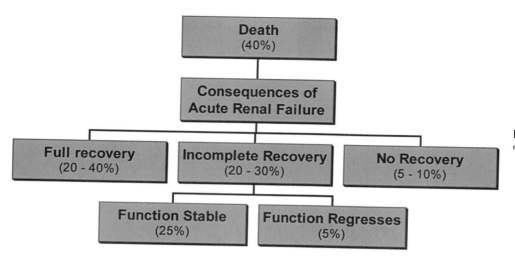

FIGURE 35–2 ■ Consequences of acute renal failure.

prominent defect is in the ability to maximally concentrate the urine.[20] This has occasionally been associated with the presence of nocturia. The inability to achieve a urinary pH of less than 5.4 has been observed in as many as one third of the patients.[18] Hypertension and proteinuria are inconsistent findings. In addition, the kidney size may be less than normal in 10% to 13% of patients following recovery.

The rate of return of renal function tends to be slower in patients who ultimately have permanent defects. In patients who completely recover, renal function returns to normal within 2 to 6 months, while, with few exceptions, patients with a diminished clearance at the end of 1 year can be expected to continue to have impaired function.[20] Routine urinalysis has not been found to be helpful in identifying patients destined to have impaired clearances. A positive correlation between the intensity of the renal image obtained using iodohippurate sodium 131 and the extent of recovery has been demonstrated. In certain patients, the image acquired after the administration of ^{99m}Tc-mercaptoacetyltriglycine (MAG3) may be an accurate prognosticator of recovery.[25]

The age of the patient appears to be an important determinant of the extent of recovery, that is, patients whose recovery is incomplete tend to be on average nearly two decades older than those who recover completely. Patients more than 40 years of age may regain at most 75% of the expected levels of renal function for their age group. It has been noted that the patients who fail to achieve an S_{Cr} level of less than 2 mg/dL tend to be 60 years of age or older. Indeed, the clinical outcome is significantly worse in elderly patients with regard to mortality, the need for chronic dialytic treatment, and the likelihood of complete recovery.[26]

Even in children, residual defects can be demonstrated.[27] Glomerular function is abnormal in a significant number of children who have apparently recovered completely from ARF. This is thought to be a consequence of the destruction of a proportion of the total nephron population, predominantly those located in the superficial layers of the cortex. With the exception of the occasional finding of microscopic

hematuria, the urine sediment appears normal. Tubular function, including proximal and distal sodium reabsorption and tubular reabsorption of phosphate, glucose, and amino acids return to normal, as does urinary concentrating and diluting ability.[28]

Anatomic Defects

In the late phase of functional recovery, the microscopic examination of renal tissue may be characterized by the presence of interstitial edema or fibrosis; tubular dilation with flattened epithelium, epithelial regeneration, and tubular debris (Fig. 35–3). Interstitial infiltrates may also be present, although glomerular and vascular changes are minimal.[20] The tubular epithelial cells give the appearance of being incompletely differentiated. As recovery progresses, the interstitial edema subsides, and a diffuse interstitial nephritis may develop that later becomes focal.[29] At this juncture, there may be divergence in the pattern of recovery. Death of nephrons may occur with subsequent tubular atrophy and hyalinization of glomeruli. Conversely, almost complete structural and functional recovery occurs if tubular changes were absent or mild. Residual abnormalities in glomeruli are often present.[20] These include thickening and splitting of the basement membranes, capsular adhesions, periglomerular fibrosis, and hyalinized glomeruli.

In the kidneys that show persistent functional defects, the degree of structural abnormalities may be directly related to the length of time it takes for recovery to become evident. In these kidneys, the most common feature is either diffuse or focal interstitial fibrosis, along with varying degrees of tubular atrophy.[30] Indeed, it appears that complete tubular atrophy occurs in some groups of nephrons, whereas in others, complete recovery with secondary compensatory hypertrophy takes place (Figs. 35–4, 35–5, 35–6). Unfortunately, in the presence of severe diffuse interstitial fibrosis, progression to chronic renal failure can be seen. It should be noted that the phenotypic characteristics of glomerular mesangial cells resemble both fi-

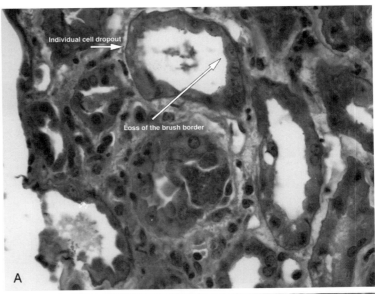

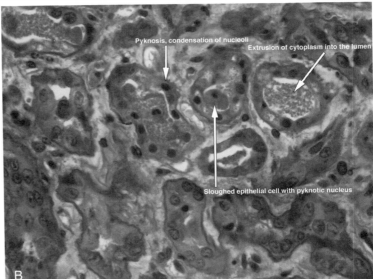

FIGURE 35–3 ■ Light micrographs of a percutaneous renal biopsy specimen obtained during the early recovery phase from ischemic injury following renal transplantation. *A,* Individual cell dropout can be seen along with the absence of the brush border membrane. *B,* Tubular lumina contain sloughed epithelial cells with pyknotic nucleus and extruded cytoplasm. *C,* Mitotic activity is apparent. Also seen is a reactive epithelial cell with large nucleoli. (Courtesy of Dr. David Thomas.)

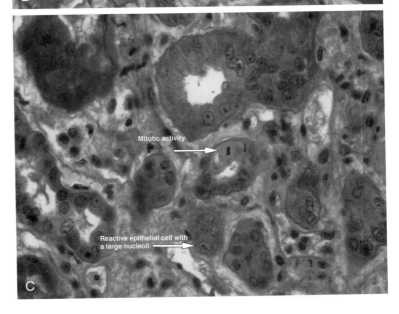

broblasts and muscle cells, and as a result, they have been referred to as myofibroblasts. In some experimental models, an increase in the number of macrophages can be seen in areas of markedly advanced interstitial fibrosis. It has been suggested that the macrophages contribute to the development of myofibroblasts, leading to the augmented fibrosis observed during the recovery phase.[31]

MODIFICATION OF CLINICAL COURSE

The annual incidence of ARF in unselected populations approaches 200 patients per million inhabitants. Notably, the incidence is five times higher in the elderly than in younger people,[24] although, even in the latter group, differences occur. For example, while the yearly incidence of ARF in children has been reported to be 8 per million per total population, the incidence in the neonate and infant population is much higher and is comparable to that in the adult.[32] Accepting the proposition that prevention is the primary objective, once this goal is no longer attainable, attention must be directed at achieving prompt and complete recovery. In this regard, anything that can be done to mini-

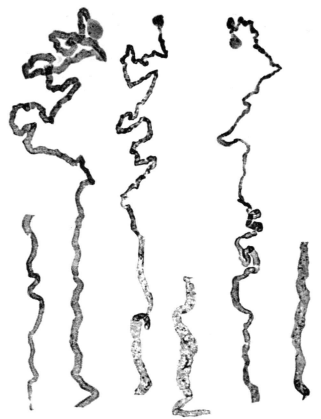

FIGURE 35–5 ■ Mosaic photomicrographs of proximal tubules from control and postischemic kidneys of rats studied 24 hours following 60 minutes of unilateral complete renal artery occlusion. Nephrons from *left* to *right* are from the contralateral normal kidney, and the outer, and middle cortex from the postischemic kidney. There is now acute diffuse tubular necrosis involving virtually every proximal tubule with the appearance of "swan-neck" deformities in some proximal tubular segments. Disruptive lesions appear in greater number. A squamate appearance in microdissected preparations was the result of a plate-like separation of necrotic tubular epithelial cells.

mize the initial injury or prevent secondary complications is desirable.

Minimization of Initial Injury

The immediate concern in the management of patients with ARF is to eliminate the possibility that the acute decline in renal function is a result of correctable conditions such as volume depletion or urinary tract obstruction. With this accomplished, attention can be directed toward lessening the initial impact of ischemic or nephrotoxic injury. The intent has been to reestablish urine flow with the use of diuretics, to restore renal perfusion by treatment with vasodilators, and to preserve tubular epithelial cell integrity by the administration of cytoprotective agents (Table 35–2). Unfortunately, in most cases the anticipated benefit has not been realized.

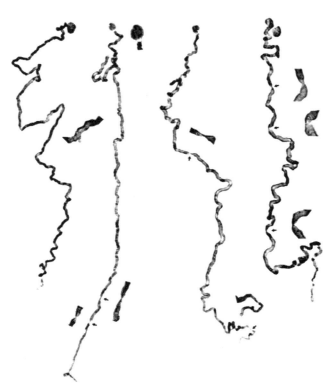

FIGURE 35–4 ■ Mosaic photomicrographs of proximal tubules from control and postischemic kidneys of rats studied 2 to 3 hours following 60 minutes of unilateral complete renal artery occlusion. Nephrons from *left* to *right* are from the contralateral normal kidney and the outer, middle, and inner cortex from the postischemic kidney. All show typical disruptive or tubulorrhexic lesions, especially in the proximal tubules *(arrows)*. There is randomness of distribution of the disruptive lesions. Some of the proximal tubules appear normal.

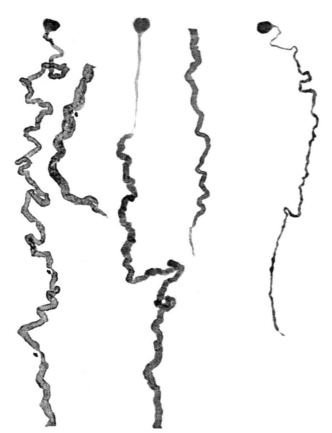

FIGURE 35–6 ■ Mosaic photomicrographs of proximal tubules in postischemic kidneys of rats studied 1, 2, and 4 weeks following 60 minutes of unilateral complete renal artery occlusion. At one week *(left)*, a common finding is dilation of pars recta of proximal tubules. Pars convoluta appears normal or atrophic. At two weeks *(middle)*, atrophy is present in many nephrons. At four weeks *(right)*, there are some atrophic proximal tubules. At this time, there is differential or selective hyperplasia of the pars recta in most nephrons.

RESTORATION OF URINE FLOW: DIURETIC AGENTS

Osmotic Diuretics

Mannitol. Mannitol is a simple sugar. When given intravenously it is not metabolized but is freely filtered by the glomeruli into the tubular fluid, where it acts as an osmotic diuretic. The six theoretical reasons why mannitol might ameliorate ARF[33] include (1) intratubular casts may be flushed out by an increase in tubule flow; (2) renal blood flow (RBF) may increase as the result of a decline in renal vascular resistance (RVR); (3) vascular congestion may be reduced by preventing hypoxic cell swelling; (4) erythrocyte aggregation may be prevented; (5) mitochondria function may be protected; and (6) free radical damage may be minimized.

While there is much anecdotal evidence in favor of a beneficial role for mannitol, there are no prospective, randomly allocated studies in which its effects are compared with those of volume expansion alone. Moreover, when mannitol is used in an attempt to prevent ARF, an excessively high plasma mannitol concentration (>1050 mg/dL) may induce ARF. To prevent this, the plasma concentration of mannitol can be estimated using the osmolal gap, ie, the difference between the calculated osmolality and the measured osmolality. Patients with marked mannitol accumulation (an osmolal gap of >60 to 75 mOsm/kg) appear to be at highest risk for toxicity.[34]

Loop Diuretics

Furosemide. There are four theoretical reasons why loop diuretics such as furosemide might be beneficial in the treatment of ARF[33]: (1) loop diuretics produce a resting state in cells of the thick ascending limb of Henle by inhibiting the $Na^+/2Cl^-/K^+$ transporter; (2) loop diuretics increase tubule flow rate; (3) loop diuretics inhibit tubuloglomerular feedback by blocking chloride flux at the macula densa; and (4) loop diuretics reduce RVR and increase RBF. Despite the fact that the administration of furosemide as a bolus or by continuous infusion may be followed by an increase in urine flow or even polyuria,[35] additional data are needed to support the position that loop diuretics shorten the period of renal dysfunction or reduce the need for dialysis.[36] There is no firm evidence that the mortality rate is lowered.[37] Indeed, studies on the role of loop diuretics in patients with ARF are largely retrospective, anecdotal, and poorly controlled.

It is important to point out that the observation that patients with nonoliguric ARF generally have a better prognosis than that of those with oliguric ARF is true only for those in whom nonoliguric ARF occurs spontaneously. There is little evidence that the chance of recovery in established ARF is improved by administration of diuretics and the pharmacologic conversion from oliguria to nonoliguria. As an example, in a prospective, randomized, placebo-controlled, double-blind study of patients with ARF, despite the fact that patients given a loop diuretic had a significant rise in urine flow, there were no differences in renal recovery, the need for dialysis, or death. Although as a group, nonoliguric patients (≥50 mL/h) had a significantly lower mortality than that of oliguric patients (<50 mL/h), this was due to the fact that the nonoliguric patients were less ill and had less severe renal failure at the time of entry into the study.[38]

TABLE 35–2. Summary of Therapy and Goals in the Initial Phase of Acute Renal Failure

THERAPY	GOAL
Volume expansion/hydration	Increase in renal blood flow
	Prevention of tubular epithelial cell injury
Diuretics	Restoration of urine flow
Osmotic diuretics	
Loop diuretics	
Vasoactive agents	Restoration of renal perfusion
Dopamine	
Atrial natriuretic peptide	
Cytoprotective agents	Preservation of cell integrity
Free radical scavengers	
Xanthine oxidase inhibitors	
Calcium channel blocking agents	
Prostaglandins	

RESTORATION OF RENAL PERFUSION: VASOACTIVE AGENTS

Dopamine

There are two different dopaminergic agent receptors (DA-1 and DA-2) of interest. Dopamine, a nonselective dopaminergic agent, is chemically related to epinephrine and norepinephrine. It acts primarily on alpha$_1$- and beta$_1$-adrenergic receptors. At dosages higher than 5 mg/kg body weight per minute, dopamine increases systemic vascular resistance and induces renal vasoconstriction, a response that is mediated by activation of alpha-adrenergic receptors. When infused in lower doses (0.5 to 3.0 mg/kg body weight per minute), dopamine stimulates dopaminergic receptors with dilation of renal and splanchnic vasculature. In the kidney, dopamine dilates both the interlobular arteries and the afferent and efferent arterioles. Dopamine is also a natriuretic hormone that decreases sodium reabsorption, primarily in the proximal tubule. This rate of administration is often called "renal-dose" or "low-dose" dopamine, and is thought to minimize the spillover stimulation of other adrenergic receptors.

Dopamine is commonly used in critically ill patients at risk for developing ARF and in those whose renal function is already decreased. While it often increases urine output and sodium excretion, the evidence is inconclusive that low doses of dopamine avert the onset or ameliorate the course of ARF in critically ill patients.[39] When critically examined, the changes in renal function that were thought to be in response to low-dose dopamine infusion may be no different from those that occurred spontaneously with placebo infusion.[40] Nonetheless, many believe that the use of low-dose dopamine has reduced the incidence of postoperative ARF[41] and, in particular, ARF following cardiac surgery, vascular surgery, and liver transplantation.[42] A therapeutic renal effect has been observed in selected cases of oliguric ARF and shock.

There are arguments for[43] and against[39] the use of renal dose dopamine to prevent or treat ARF.[44] In general, the results of studies in humans are inconsistent and disappointing for both prevention and treatment.[39, 45] Indeed, there is no proof of a consistent, substantial, and reproducible benefit of the use of low-dose dopamine in either preventing or treating ARF in humans.

Recently, the results of a multicenter, randomized, double-blind, placebo-controlled trial of low-dose dopamine infusion have been reported.[46] This study was undertaken in intensive care unit patients at risk of ARF (Fig. 35–7) and was designed to assess whether dopamine attenuated the rise in S_{Cr}. The administration of low-dose dopamine by continuous intravenous infusion to these critically ill patients did not confer clinically significant protection from renal dysfunction (Fig. 35–8).

Consequently, until controlled trials are conducted, there seems to be little justification for the routine administration of dopamine in patients at risk for renal failure in the absence of specific indications.[47]

There is, however, hope that the use of selective DA-1 receptor agonists such as fenoldopam will be helpful in patients with ARF. DA-1 receptor agonists decrease renovascular resistance, leading to an increase in RBF and GFR. In addition, they lead to a decrease in renal sodium reabsorption and an increase in urine output.[48–50] An advantage over nonselective dopaminergic agents is that the selective DA-1 receptor agonists do not stimulate DA-2 or alpha$_1$- and beta$_1$-adrenergic receptors.[48] There are, however, no reported studies of the use of DA-1–selective agents for the prevention or treatment of ARF in humans.[51]

Atrial Natriuretic Peptide

The natriuretic peptide family[52] includes atrial natriuretic peptide (cardiodilan/atrial natriuretic peptide [CCD/ANP]), known as A-type natriuretic peptide; brain natriuretic peptide (BNP), known as B-type natriuretic peptide; and C-type natriuretic peptide (CNP). A 126–amino acid precursor of CCD/ANP (CDD/ANP-1-126) is synthesized in the heart and cleaved into its circulating form, a 28–amino acid carboxy fragment (CDD/ANP-99-126). The biological effects of ANP are

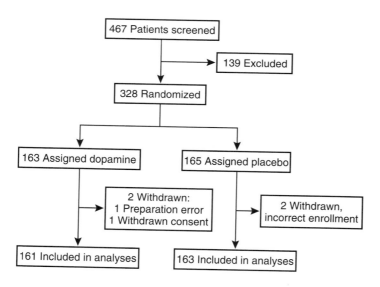

FIGURE 35–7 ■ Trial profile. Two groups of patients with renal dysfunction were well matched for illness severity and other clinical characteristics. Dopamine was infused continuously at 2 μg/kg/min. The control group received the equivalent volume of placebo. (From Australian and New Zealand Intensive Care Society [ANZICS] Clinical Trial Group: Low-dose dopamine in patients with early renal dysfunction: a placebo-controlled randomized trial. Lancet 2000; 356:2139–2143; with permission.)

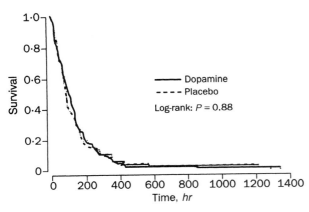

FIGURE 35–8 ■ Kaplan-Meier curve of the time to recovery of normal renal function. When patients who stopped dopamine or placebo because of resolution of renal dysfunction were separately analyzed, no differences in time to recovery were found. (From Australian and New Zealand Intensive Care Society [ANZICS] Clinical Trial Group: Low-dose dopamine in patients with early renal dysfunction: a placebo-controlled randomized trial. Lancet 2000; 356:2139–2143; with permission.)

mediated by the generation of intracellular 3', 5'-cyclic guanosine monophosphate (cGMP). In addition to renal tubular effects that result in an increase in salt and water excretion, ANP stimulates afferent arteriolar dilation and efferent arteriolar constriction, causing an increase in GFR. In experimental studies, ANP substantially reduced the severity of ARF associated with ischemic insults but was less effective for nephrotoxic injury. In clinical trials, however, ANP has not been shown to be as effective. Even in renal transplant patients whose allograft has sustained ischemic injury, there has been a failure of ANP to lower RVR or increase GFR despite a progressive elevation of endogenous plasma ANP levels and evidence of enhanced cGMP generation.[53] Renal tubular effects have been equally difficult to establish in this setting as a relationship between plasma ANP levels and total or fractional sodium excretion or free water clearance has not been evident.[54] In contrast to the studies using cardiodilan/atrial natriuretic peptide, when alpha-human (1-28) ANP was infused into the renal artery at the time of renal transplantation, a decreased incidence of ARF and a reduced need for hemodialysis were noted.[55]

Urodilan (URO; CDD/ANP-95-126) is a 32–amino acid peptide that differs from CDD/ANP-99-126 by only four amino acids.[56] Urodilan is synthesized in the kidney, exerts its renal effects in a paracrine fashion, and can be found in urine. After its secretion from cells in the distal tubule, it interacts with receptors located at the luminal surface of collecting duct epithelial cells, resulting in increased diuresis and natriuresis. When urodilan is given intravenously, its diuretic and natriuretic effects are more evident than those achieved by cardiodilan/atrial natriuretic peptide. A beneficial effect of urodilan in patients suffering from

ARF following organ transplantation has been reported.[56, 57]

Anaritide (hANP, ANP-4-28; auriculin) is a synthetic atrial natriuretic peptide. Early human trials in patients with ARF suggested a beneficial effect on C_{Cr} and a reduction in the need for dialysis.[58] A subsequent multicenter trial in patients with ARF did not show an improvement in the overall rate of dialysis-free survival, although it was thought that anaritide may have improved dialysis-free survival in patients with oliguria.[59] Unfortunately, these findings could not be confirmed,[60] and it can be concluded that the trials failed to show a clinically relevant benefit.[61, 62]

PRESERVATION OF CELL INTEGRITY: CYTOPROTECTIVE AGENTS

Calcium Channel Blocking Agents

Changes in the concentration and compartmentalization of intracellular calcium are closely related to ischemia-reperfusion injury and to the transition from reversible cell injury to cell death.[63] Under normal conditions, free calcium in the cytosol of the cell is maintained at low levels compared with that in the calcium-rich extracellular fluid. In contrast, irreversibly injured cells contain high levels of calcium. The extent to which these levels rise can be correlated with the severity of the histologic damage.

The intracellular concentration and distribution of calcium can be altered during and following ischemia via several mechanisms. First, with the depletion of oxygen and the fall in ATP levels, the ability of cells to export calcium by ATP-dependent pumps is reduced. In addition, calcium sequestration by mitochondria and the endoplasmic reticulum is also energy-dependent, and the cell's capacity to compensate for an influx of calcium might be limited. Second, a significant quantity of calcium is complexed to soluble substances such as ATP, citrate, and glutamate. The decrease in pH that occurs when organs are rendered ischemic decreases the affinity of calcium for these substances and therefore can result in the release of calcium as free ions. Third, lipid peroxidation induced by free radicals renders cell membranes permeable to calcium.

When calcium accumulates, several interrelated reactions proceed. First, calcium activates phospholipases that remove fatty acids from membranes and potentiate the damaging effects of free radicals. Calcium-activated phospholipases also control the release of arachidonic acid from the membrane and influence the production of various prostaglandins. Second, the activation of phospholipases by calcium contributes to mitochondrial damage and limits the cell's capacity for ATP synthesis. Third, a calcium-activated protease may favor the formation of xanthine oxidase and promote free radical formation. Calcium channel blocking agents have been used to prevent ARF associated with ischemic injury,[64] radiocontrast exposure,[65] drug-induced toxic nephropathies,[66] and cadaveric renal transplantation.[67, 68]

Oxygen Free Radical Scavengers and Xanthine Oxidase Inhibitors

A significant portion of the damage sustained by the ischemic kidney occurs, not during the period of ischemia, but rather during and following reperfusion.[69] Exposure of the previously ischemic kidney to molecular oxygen (O_2) during reperfusion elicits the production of reactive oxygen radicals. These free radicals have one or more unpaired electrons in their outer shells, and as they attempt to restore normal electron pairing in their orbitals, they interact with other molecules and produce secondary tissue damage.

Superoxide radical (O_2^-) formation results from electron transfer processes, such as those in mitochondria and the endoplasmic reticulum, from NADPH-requiring enzymes of macrophages, and from the action of xanthine oxidase. Under the influence of superoxide dismutase, two molecules of O_2^- form hydrogen peroxide (H_2O_2) and O_2. Various peroxidases, such as catalase and glutathione peroxidase, inactivate H_2O_2. In the presence of transition metals, such as iron, however, the highly reactive hydroxyl radical ($OH^\cdot$) is produced from O_2^- and H_2O_2. Superoxide-radical–induced cytotoxicity appears to be dependent largely on the subsequent production of $OH^\cdot$. Histidine, tryptophan, ascorbate, and alpha-tocopherol are natural $OH^\cdot$ scavengers. Uric acid can act as an $OH^\cdot$ scavenger as well, but it also has the capacity to bind iron and to influence the formation of $OH^\cdot$.

With reperfusion of the previously ischemic kidney, a sudden increase in free radical activity can overwhelm protective mechanisms and promote the peroxidation of polyunsaturated fatty acids in the membranes of cells, mitochondria, and lysosomes. In this way, permeability is increased, transport processes are altered, and a series of self-perpetuating adverse events is set into motion. These adverse events sometimes involve changes in intracellular calcium concentration and distribution and abnormalities in prostaglandin synthesis. In addition, there has been accumulating evidence of a role for reactive oxygen metabolites in the pathogenesis of nephrotoxic ARF.[70]

Much of the free radical production during the reperfusion period results from the activity of the enzyme xanthine oxidase following its proteolytic conversion from xanthine dehydrogenase. Hypoxanthine produced from ATP breakdown during ischemia is oxidized to xanthine and, subsequently, uric acid by xanthine oxidase during and after reperfusion. During these reactions, superoxide radicals and hydrogen peroxide are produced from molecular oxygen. The decrease in cellular ATP levels associated with ischemia is accompanied by an increase in the dephosphorylated degradation products of adenine nucleotides and in the intracellular accumulation of hypoxanthine.

The xanthine oxidase inhibitor allopurinol is effective in reducing ischemic injury in laboratory animals.[71] Several mechanisms for explaining this effect have been proposed. First, the conversion of hypoxanthine to xanthine and uric acid is irreversible, so this reaction has the potential of removing purine metabolites from the pool available for the resynthesis of AMP, ADP, and ATP.[72] Second, it has been suggested that the rate of decline in ATP levels could be reduced by xanthine oxidase inhibition to the extent that the conversion of hypoxanthine to xanthine to uric acid was the rate-limiting reaction. Third, xanthine oxidase activity is an important component of free-radical generation and it has been proposed that the major benefit of xanthine oxidase inhibition is to decrease the formation of oxygen free radicals.[73]

Prostaglandins

The normal balance between the production of prostacyclin (PGI_2), PGE_2, and thromboxane (TXA_2) may be markedly altered during renal ischemia. An increase in cellular calcium is thought to activate phospholipases, which in turn promote the release of arachidonic acid from cell membranes. As a result of the lipid peroxidation from the action of oxygen free radicals, PGI_2 synthesis is inhibited and TXA_2 synthesis is stimulated. It has been proposed that the combination of an increase in PGI_2 and a decrease in TXA_2 is important in minimizing renal ischemic injury.[74] PGI_2 possesses cytoprotective properties and can decrease the severity of postischemic ARF.[75] Along this line, it would be expected that cyclooxygenase inhibitors that block conversion of endoperoxide to both TXA_2 and PGI_2 would not be effective, whereas thromboxane synthetase inhibitors, which not only inhibit TXA_2 synthesis but also stimulate PGI_2 production, are beneficial. Indeed, a series of dibenzoxepin derivatives exerting both thromboxane synthase inhibitory and thromboxane receptor antagonist activities has demonstrated a significant protective effect in an experimental model of ARF.[76]

Prevention of Secondary Injury

A major concern during the maintenance phase is to prevent secondary renal injury. This is of concern because of the findings that residual renal function may decline at the initiation of hemodialysis.[77] Also, fresh areas of tubular necrosis have been found in biopsies from patients with ARF receiving hemodialysis treatments despite the fact that the tissue samples were obtained much later after the original injury.[78] Also in support of the notion that secondary injury may occur is the observation that there may be an increase in the urinary concentration of the proximal tubule lysosomal enzyme N-acetyl-β-D-glucosaminidase in association with hemodialysis treatments.[79] The list of the factors that may contribute to secondary renal injury is contained in Table 35–3.

AUTOREGULATION OF RENAL BLOOD FLOW

Acute renal failure is associated with loss of the capacity to autoregulate RBF.[80, 81] Consequently, any reduction in arterial blood pressure results in a proportionate decrease in RBF. The mechanism underlying the loss of autoregulatory capacity is not known. It

TABLE 35–3. Potential Factors Contributing to Secondary Renal Injury in the Maintenance Phase of Acute Renal Failure

THERAPY	FACTOR
Hemodialysis	Biocompatible vs. bioincompatible membranes
Hypotension	Loss of autoregulatory capability
Nephrotoxins	Increase sensitivity vs. acquired resistance
Diuretics and sodium restriction	Volume depletion and prerenal azotemia

has been ascribed to abnormalities in tubuloglomerular feedback, to vascular defects in smooth muscle contraction, and to intrinsic properties of the autonomic nervous system. The impairment in autoregulation is of some consequence to the patient with ARF whose baseline RBF is already depressed. At this time, recurrent renal ischemia might induce fresh episodes of tubular necrosis or prevent healing of established, preexisting lesions. Paradoxically, hemodialysis treatments may account for much of the episodic hypotension that is observed during the treatment of patients with ARF, and it has been suggested that further damage could occur as a result.[78]

ROLE OF HEMODIALYSIS MEMBRANES

A controversy has arisen concerning the possibility that inflammatory reactions to the hemodialysis membranes themselves may be responsible for some of the secondary changes noted previously. Dialyzer membranes are composed of unmodified cellulose, modified cellulose, or synthetic materials. Unmodified cellulose membranes are derived from processed cotton or wood products. They can be made of regenerated cellulose that has been treated with ammonia and cupric oxide, called cuprammonium cellulose or cuprophane, cuprammonium rayon, or saponified cellulose ester. Free hydroxyl groups along their surface are thought to cause various side effects, including the release of histamine, thromboxane, interleukin-1, and tumor necrosis factor, along with changes in leukocyte activity. These membranes have thrombogenicity greater than that of the synthetic membranes and promote activation of the alternative pathway of complement. Complement-dependent granulocyte activation during hemodialysis causes neutrophil degranulation and protease release, the production of reactive oxygen species, and the modulation of granulocyte cell adhesion molecules.[82] These membranes are included under the term "bioincompatible."

Modified or substituted cellulose is a cellulose polymer that comes in two types: cellulose acetate membranes, which have acetate bonded to the free hydroxyl groups, and modified cellulose (hemophan) membranes that have tertiary amino compounds bound to the hydroxyl groups. As a result, the modified cellulose membranes have substantially lower complement- and leukocyte-activating potential than cuprophane membranes. Synthetic membranes are not cellulose based and include thermoplastics such as polyacrylonitrile (PAN), polysulfone, and polymethylmethacrylate (PMMA). They have been found to be more "biocompatible" than the cellulose types, and their middle molecule clearance is much greater.

It is by virtue of their enhancement of cytokine release, complement activation, or neutrophil stimulation that the membranes included under the term bioincompatible may perpetuate continued renal injury or prolong recovery.[83] Although the results of animal studies have supported the position that activation of neutrophils[84] or complement[85] negatively influences the severity or resolution of ischemic renal injury, they have not fully established a link between exposure to complement-activating cellulosic dialysis membranes and delayed recovery from ischemic injury.[86, 87]

Nonetheless, several prospective clinical studies comparing bioincompatible cellulosic membranes with biocompatible artificial membranes have reported improved survival rate and better recovery of renal function with the use of the latter. In an early study of 52 patients with postoperative ARF, it was observed that those randomized to receive dialysis using cuprophane membranes had a lower survival rate, required more dialysis sessions, and had a delay in recovering from ARF when compared with patients treated with a biocompatible membrane.[88] Likewise, in a series of 72 patients with various medical categories of ARF, it was found that the recovery of renal function was significantly greater and the number of dialysis treatments prior to recovery of renal function was significantly smaller in the group treated with a biocompatible PMMA compared with those treated with a bioincompatible cuprophane membrane.[89] When various subgroups were analyzed it was noted that the survival rate was significantly higher only among the patients dialyzed with the biocompatible membrane who were nonoliguric at the onset of the ARF. Similar conclusions were reached by others[90] in a prospective, multicenter study. Again, differences in outcome related to the type of membrane used were noted. Once again these differences were particularly prominent among the patients with ARF who were nonoliguric at the initiation of the study. Of interest is the fact that in this study a larger fraction of patients became oliguric after starting dialysis with a bioincompatible membrane compared with those who started dialysis with a biocompatible membrane. In agreement with prior observations, oliguria at the onset of dialysis had an adverse effect on both the survival and the recovery of renal function even in patients dialyzed with biocompatible membranes.[91]

A significant decline in mortality related to the choice of dialysis membranes was found in a study[92] comparing the influence of sepsis on the outcome of ARF. Of 58 patients receiving dialysis with a bioincompatible cuprophane membrane, 79% died, while of 111 patients treated with bioincompatible synthetic membranes, 55% died. In a different study,[93] a difference in mortality rate was not observed among 87 patients treated with bioincompatible cuprophane membranes compared with 18 patients treated with biocompatible synthetic membranes (42% vs. 38%). However, the median time for resolution of the ARF was reduced from 15.4 days to 10.9 days by the use of the synthetic membranes. Finally, it has been argued that on the basis of data from a retrospective multicenter study, the choice of the dialysis membrane should be at least as important and possibly more so than was the choice between daily and alternate-day dialysis.[94]

These studies have come under intense criticism for a number of reasons[95–98] and stand in contrast to others that have not shown differences related to the choice of dialysis membranes. For example, in 57 intensive care unit (ICU) patients with ARF who were alternatively assigned either a cuprophane or a synthetic membrane, there were no differences in mortality (72% vs. 64%) or the number of dialysis treatments required prior to recovery (6.4 vs. 6.0).[99] Similarly, the results of a 4-year prospective study of 363 ICU patients likewise found no difference in mortality (71% vs. 80%).[100] In a study involving 13 tertiary-care hospitals, 84 patients were treated with cellulosic membranes and 50 patients treated with synthetic membranes. The mortality rate was 59.5% in the former and 60% in the latter.[101] Also, in a prospective, randomized, multicenter trial of 180 patients with dialysis-dependent ARF, the largest study to date, 86 patients were treated with cuprophane membranes and 84 with PMMA membranes. There were no differences between the two groups in recovery of renal function and survival.[102]

These studies have also been criticized[103] for various reasons. One study[99] called into question the unequal distribution of causes of ARF, and another study[100] questioned the retrospective analysis of risk factors and the inability to determine the distribution of risk factors known to affect outcome from ARF. Also, the use of APACHE II scores, as an index of illness at the time of inclusion in the study,[101] has been thought inappropriate. These criticisms, however, cannot be applied to two studies in patients who developed ARF following cadaveric renal transplantation. In a prospective trial comparing cuprophane with PMMA membranes, 36 uncomplicated cases of ARF caused by ischemic injury were randomized into two groups of 18 each.[104] There were no differences in patient characteristics, mean time to recovery, or the average number of hemodialysis treatments required. Similar findings were found in a separate prospective study.[105] Patients were again randomized into two treatment groups to receive hemodialysis with either a bioincompatible cuprophane membrane or a biocompatible polysulfone membrane. The two groups did not differ according to patient characteristics, the number of hemodialysis sessions required prior to the recovery of renal function, the number of oliguric days, or the number of hospital days.

In addition to the previously mentioned results, there are several studies that have compared substituted cellulose membranes with synthetic membranes. In one such study, no significant differences in mortality rates in patients treated with cellulose acetate versus PMMA were described.[106] In a separate prospective, randomized study, the outcome of ARF patients dialyzed either with substituted cellulose membrane or with a biocompatible synthetic membrane was compared. Patients were randomized to one of three dialysis membranes: low-flux polysulfone, high-flux polysulfone, and meltspun cellulose diacetate. There were no significant differences among the three groups for patient survival, the time necessary for recovery of renal function, or the number of dialysis sessions required before recovery of renal function. Multivariate analysis showed that survival was significantly influenced only by the severity of the disease state, and not by the nature of the dialysis membrane or the presence of oliguria.[107]

ACQUIRED RESISTANCE TO INJURY

It is hard to reconcile the previous discussion with the curious biological phenomenon wherein tissues exposed to one insult acquire resistance to a second. Indeed, an increased tolerance of the kidney to superimposed insults has been demonstrated in several experimental settings that include ischemic injury, oxidant stress, hypoxia, and various forms of nephrotoxic injury. At this point, it is necessary to emphasize that a distinction should be made between the effects of mild and severe injury. When cell injury is mild (ie, sublethal), additional ischemic or nephrotoxic stress acts synergistically to result in overt ARF. It is only in the situation in which cell injury is severe that cytoprotective adaptive changes take place. For example, in rats with glycerol-induced ARF, subsequent injury from mercuric chloride is attenuated in direct proportion to the severity of the initial glycerol-induced damage, that is, the more severe the initial renal insufficiency, the milder the renal insufficiency following subsequent mercuric chloride administration. Based on the data presented, it is likely that factors related to the regenerative process are involved in the protection from repeated renal insults.[108] It is tempting to speculate that these considerations contribute to the difficulty in determining whether or not the use of biocompatible hemodialysis membranes are preferred in some patients with ARF, particularly those with less severe injury, as judged by the lack of oliguria.

The acquired resistance of the kidney to secondary injury is a well-known phenomenon. In 1912, Suzuki[109] called attention to the fact that the sensitivity of regenerated epithelium in the presence of repeated uranium poisoning is remarkably decreased. In 1916, MacNider[110] found that a specific type of regenerated convoluted tubular epithelium was resistant to injury from uranium, whereas normal convoluted tubular epithelium failed to show this resistance. Later, he put forward the thesis that repair could be accomplished by two processes: first, by regeneration of convoluted tubular cells from similar cells in the same location and, second, by regeneration from different cells derived from other areas of the nephron. MacNider favored the latter explanation.[111]

It was later found that rats recovering from glycerol-induced myohemoglobinuric ARF did not develop a second attack of renal failure when reinjected with glycerol[112] or given other nephrotoxins.[113] Even more striking observations have been made in rats with severe ARF due to the aminoglycoside gentamicin. Despite its continued administration, renal function was found to improve. This recovery occurred even though the regenerating tubular epithelial cells regained the capacity to transport gentamicin, as evidenced by the restoration of renal cortical concentrations to levels that were previously associated with nephrotoxicity.[114]

A second form of resistance to primary ischemic and nephrotoxic injury is found in young animals. For example, weanling rats, as opposed to adult rats, are relatively resistant to the nephrotoxic effects of aminoglycoside antibiotics.[115] This is notable because certain characteristics of the tubular epithelial cells of the young kidney are shared with the regenerating cells of the adult kidney. In each case, the cells remain relatively immature for long periods of time. Not only is there a decreased susceptibility to injury of the young kidney but also an increase in the rate of recovery. Thus, weanling rats have a greater capacity for tubular epithelial cell repair than do their adult counterparts.[114] Along these lines, it has been suggested that in addition to the brisk hyperplastic response of the kidney from young animals, a decrease in the amount of apoptosis might contribute to the phenomenon of acquired resistance.[115]

A third form of resistance is that conferred by the prior administration of endotoxin, a procedure that confers resistance to tissue damage in a number of models of organ injury. Since enhanced tissue oxidative stress is a feature of endotoxin-associated injury, the beneficial effect conferred by endotoxin may be dependent on the up-regulation of antioxidant defenses[116] in renal tubular epithelial cells.[117]

A common occurrence in acquired resistance is a decrease in membrane lipid peroxidation that occurs with repeated insults. Thus, proximal tubule segments isolated from rats previously injected with glycerol show a 50% decrease in membrane lipid peroxidation.[118] This may be the result of a number of changes in phospholipid composition, secondary increases in the supply of antioxidants,[119] or a decrease in mitochondrial free-radical generation with a down-regulation of proximal tubule H_2O_2 and hydroxyl radical ($OH^·$) expression.[120] The up-regulation of antioxidant defenses may effectively serve to decrease oxidant-mediated tissue injury.[121, 122] Lipid peroxidation is a component of gentamicin-induced ARF, and it has been suggested that a secondary increase in antioxidant activity may partially explain the acquired resistance to secondary injury during gentamicin administration.[123] Alternatively or in addition, there may be a decrease in the generation of reactive oxygen metabolites by mitochondria with down-regulation of proximal tubule H_2O_2 and $OH^·$.[124] It has also been suggested that the acquired resistance to secondary injury might be mediated by heat-shock proteins[125, 126] which, at the same time, may serve to protect against apoptosis.[127]

RECOVERY OF RENAL FUNCTION

Factors Initiating Recovery

The specific events necessary for initiation of recovery are not completely understood. Cellular injury provokes a reparative process involving gene transcription and cell cycle modulation, all of which are under the influence of various growth factors and other cytokines and which may be modified by pharmacologic agents or dietary manipulation (Table 35–4). As cell injury subsides and recovery begins, a number of physiologic changes follow. These include a decrease in RVR, an increase in RBF, the restoration of tubular function, and, ultimately, an improvement in GFR. Each of these factors has been judged to be of primary importance in initiating functional recovery.

Changes in Renal Blood Flow During Recovery

There are two lines of evidence that support the notion that changes in RVR and RBF are of fundamental importance in initiating recovery. The first line of evidence relates to the observed changes in the production or concentration of intrarenal vasoactive substances that seem to precede recovery. For example, changes in the activity of the renin-angiotensin system,[128] alterations in the renal synthesis of prostaglandins, and variation in the urinary concentrations of kallikrein[129] all occur prior to changes in urine flow rates.

The second line of evidence follows from the observation that in the oliguric patient an increase in urine volume may occur prior to evidence of the return of tubular function.[130, 131] Thus, serial monitoring of U/P_{Urea}, U/P_{Cr} and U/P_{Na} ratios during the transition to the early diuretic phase may show little improvement. Furthermore, during the early diuretic phase, the GFR may increase in parallel with the increase in RBF, supporting the notion that the return of glomerular filtration precedes the return of tubular function. Increases in the U/P_{Urea} and U/P_{Cr} ratios and normalization of the U/P_{Na} ratio follow the improvement in RBF and GFR.

Changes in Tubular Function During Recovery

The pattern just described may not be universally observed. In some patients, tubular function improves

TABLE 35–4. Summary of Therapy and Goals in the Recovery Phase of Acute Renal Failure

THERAPY	GOAL
Pharmacologic agents	Accelerate regeneration
Dietary manipulations	Stimulate hypertrophy
	Retard atrophy
Growth factors	Promote hyperplasia
	Prevent apoptosis

before an increase in urine output.[7] A progressive fall in U_{Na} and an increase in U_K have been observed with an increase in U_{Urea}. These are not static effects, for appropriate changes in urine composition may occur in response to hemodynamic stress, such as that related to hemodialysis sessions.

In postischemic ARF in the rat[132] there is widespread tubular epithelial cell injury and intense preglomerular vasoconstriction. As recovery occurs, there is very early evidence of tubular epithelial cell regeneration as judged by an increase in ³H-thymidine uptake and accelerated DNA synthesis. The restoration of tubular transport mechanisms is marked by a return of the ability to secrete organic acids such as para-aminohippurate (PAH) and to reabsorb sodium. This leads to an increase of the extraction ratio of PAH (E_{PAH}) and a decrease in the FE_{Na}. This is followed by an initial increase in the C_{Cr} in association with a substantial rise in urine volume, in the absence of any significant elevation in RBF. The later more sustained rise in the C_{Cr} occurs in parallel with a progressive increase in RBF. Thus, recovery occurs in a biphasic pattern with the early phase marked by the restoration of the anatomic and functional integrity of the tubular epithelium and the later phase marked by progressive vasodilatation.

In patients with postischemic ARF following renal transplantation, E_{PAH} is significantly reduced at a time when renal plasma flow (RPF) is only slightly depressed and GFR is markedly reduced. Failure to increase E_{PAH} is associated with a sustained reduction in GFR. Even in those with recovering ARF, E_{PAH} remained below normal control values.[133] It should be noted that the use of the PAH clearance (C_{PAH}) to estimate RPF according to the formula: RPF = C_{PAH} ÷ E_{PAH} is dependent upon an accurate measure of E_{PAH}. RBF is then calculated from the formula: RBF = RPF ÷ (1-Hct).

Nephron Recruitment

This inability to achieve normal values for E_{PAH} may be a result of a decrease in the relative capacity of all nephrons to transport PAH or a consequence of a reduction in the total nephron mass. Indeed, as recovery occurs, there appears to be a considerable amount of discordance in the return of function of individual nephrons. That is, not all nephrons recover at the same time or to the same extent.[134, 135] In has been observed in micropuncture studies of individual nephron function during recovery from experimental ARF in the rat that recovery occurs with the recruitment of increasing numbers of functioning nephrons. In these studies, normal values of single nephron glomerular filtration rate (SNGFR) were measured despite a persistent reduction in the whole-kidney GFR. Since the number of functioning nephrons can be derived from the relationship GFR/SNGFR, this indicated that some nephrons recover before others and that the extent of recovery depends on the number of nephrons that eventually recover[136] (Fig. 35–9). This agrees with studies showing that following recovery from ARF the number of functioning glomeruli is reduced by as much as 30% in the superficial cortex and by 80% in the juxtamedullary cortex.[137]

HYPERTROPHY, HYPERPLASIA, AND APOPTOSIS

A reduction in renal function stimulates both hypertrophy (an increase in the size of existing cells) and hyperplasia (an increase in the number of cells). When the reduction in renal function occurs in a normal host, such as with a unilateral nephrectomy, the remaining kidney undergoes hypertrophy. With ischemic or nephrotoxic injury to tubular epithelial cells, hyperplasia predominates and, indeed, is the desired goal. In addition, apoptotic changes occur, either in response to exuberant cell proliferation as a part of organ remodeling or as a consequence of external factors relating to the regulation of the cell cycle (Fig. 35–10). There are several factors that influence the extent of renal hypertrophy and hyperplasia, some of which may be manipulated so as to influence the rate or extent of recovery.

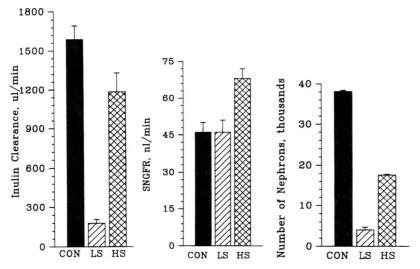

FIGURE 35–9 ■ Eight weeks following 60 minutes of unilateral complete renal artery occlusion in the rat. The number of nephrons is calculated from the inulin clearance and the single nephron glomerular filtration rate. The results obtained in control rats (CON) are compared to those obtained in rats maintained on low-salt (LS) and high-salt (HS) diets. Substantial differences in the pattern of recovery are noted.

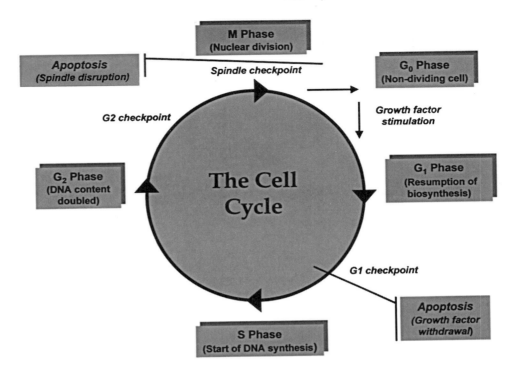

FIGURE 35–10 ▪ A schematic representation of the cell cycle. Apoptotic changes may take place at more than one point.

Compensatory Hypertrophy

As recovery occurs, the overall GFR may return to or toward normal despite histologic evidence of tubular atrophy. This suggests that the filtration rate of some or all of the nephrons that have recovered is greater than normal and that hypertrophy of these nephrons has occurred. Indeed, the kidney recovering from acute injury may undergo hypertrophy with an increase in kidney size apparent during the maintenance phase. This hypertrophy is reversible once renal function returns.

The hallmark of compensatory growth is a substantial increase in the cellular content of RNA and protein. Alterations in DNA synthesis occur but are much less pronounced, so that both the RNA:DNA and the protein:DNA ratios increase. Since ribosomal RNA constitutes more than 85% of total RNA in the kidney, the characteristic growth-induced increase in the renal RNA:DNA ratio results from an increase in ribosome number. The principal loci are the renal tubular cells of the cortex. As has been noted, in the kidney recovering from injury, the nephron population is heterogeneous. Some nephrons do not recover, others recovery incompletely, and still others exhibit hypertrophic changes.

Hyperplasia

In the adult kidney, cell division is normally quite low but may increase up to tenfold after acute injury.[138] Indeed, in the mammalian kidney, regeneration after injury is associated with the activation of certain genes and the release of growth factors that are necessary for cell growth. This has raised the hope that tubular regeneration and functional recovery in established ARF may be accelerated by the administration of various growth factors or other pharmacologic agents. It is important to point out that in addition to stimulating proliferation of surviving tubular epithelial cells, any intervention must promote cell differentiation in such a manner that the result is a fully functional lining epithelium. At the same time, the degree of apoptosis must be regulated to prevent the permanent loss of cells and associated structures.[139]

GROWTH FACTORS

During acute renal injury, there are alterations in the expression of several growth factors and their receptors in the kidney. These polypeptide cytokines are present in renal tissue and regulate kidney development, growth, and function. They are fundamental participants in the repair processes after renal injury where they act in an autocrine or paracrine fashion.[140–142] Receptors for various growth factors have been found in renal tubular epithelial cells, medullary interstitial cells, and glomeruli.[140, 143, 144] In addition, there are other locally produced growth factors that may serve as mediators of renal regeneration after acute injury just as they regulate nephrogenesis and differentiation during renal development.

Growth factors act through several mechanisms that include altered cell-cycle regulation. For example, in cultured cells, administration of one or a mixture of growth factors to quiescent cells initiates progression through the cell cycle and cell division. Growth factors also promote cellular repair in cells that have undergone sublethal injury and may limit injury by decreasing the factors that induce damage.[138] They influence the differentiation of recovered cells, initiate or promote protein and lipid biosynthesis, improve renal hemodynamics, and serve other functions. Lastly, they may inhibit programmed cell death or apoptosis.[139] In a number of experimental models of acute renal injury, administration of exogenous growth factors has effectively decreased the degree of renal insufficiency as measured by the peak S_{Cr} level and has hastened renal recovery as measured by the duration of time required to return to the baseline S_{Cr}[143] level with acceleration of both structural and functional recovery.

EPIDERMAL GROWTH FACTOR

Epidermal growth factor (EGF) is capable of stimulating the proliferation of tubular epithelial cells and is one of the many signals involved in the hyperplastic response induced by renal injury[145] (Table 35–5). Epidermal growth factor is produced in the kidney along with its precursor, preproEGF. Once released from its precursor, it acts in an autocrine or paracrine fashion to promote cell growth.[146] In normal kidneys, EGF is localized to the ascending limb of Henle and the distal convoluted tubule, and antibodies to EGF receptor react with distal tubules and collecting ducts.[147] However, binding sites for EGF have been found in the pars recta, the proximal convoluted tubule, the cortical collecting duct, and the outer medullary collecting duct, as well as in the glomeruli. With renal ischemia, there is an increase in EGF receptor density and binding and a modification of preproEGF mRNA synthesis. In animals following ischemic injury, renal immunoreactive EGF levels increase and a peak in EGF levels precedes the peak in tubular regeneration,[145] suggesting a causal relationship. In postischemic kidneys, EGF can be identified in proximal tubular epithelial cells with EGF receptors localized in the basolateral membrane.

In patients with ARF, a significant positive correlation between urinary EGF levels and C_{Cr} has been described. This has led to the proposal that the measurement of urinary EGF may be useful in the diagnosis of ARF, in monitoring recovery,[148] and as a marker of the severity of the renal injury.[149]

TABLE 35–5. Characteristics of Epidermal Growth Factor

Potent mitogen produced in the kidney
Stimulates tubular cell proliferation
Binding sites in various portions of the renal tubules
Autocrine pathway regulates distal tubular cell repair
Paracrine pathway regulates proximal tubular cell repair
Stimulates the production of IGF-I
With renal ischemic injury:
   Prolonged reduction of EGF excretion
   Reduction in prepro-EGF mRNA
   Increase in EGF receptor density
   Increase in the binding of EGF in the postischemic kidneys
Exogenous EGF in rats after renal ischemic injury
   Enhances renal tubular cell regeneration
   Accelerates the recovery of renal function

EGF, epidermal growth factor; *IGF-I,* insulin growth factor-I.

TABLE 35–6. Characteristics of Insulin-Like Growth Factors

Synthesized in the kidneys
Regulate various metabolic and growth processes
Found in the medullary collecting duct and thin loop of Henle
IGF-I receptors present on proximal tubule cells
Implicated in the compensatory hypertrophy following:
   Unilateral nephrectomy
      IGF-I gene expression is stimulated
      Renal concentration of IGF-I elevated
   High protein diets
      Serum IGF-I levels increase
Implicated in the regeneration of tubular cells after ischemic
   injury in rats:
IGF-I immunoreactivity is transiently expressed
regenerative cells express IGF-I peptide and IGF-I mRNA
better correlated to cell differentiation than cell division

IGF-I, insulin-like growth factor-I.

INSULIN-LIKE GROWTH FACTORS

The insulin-like growth factors (IGF-I and IGF-II) bind to a family of IGF-binding proteins[150] and are capable of promoting cellular growth and differentiation through paracrine or autocrine actions (Table 35–6). Moreover, the circulating hormone also displays activity. High-affinity cell surface receptors are present in various tubular segments. For example, IGF-I receptors are present in proximal tubular epithelial cells, and IGF-I can be found in the medullary collecting duct and in the parts of the thin loop of Henle located in the medulla.

IGF-I dilates the resistance-regulating microvasculature, increases GFR, and promotes tubular phosphate and possibly sodium absorption. IGF-I also plays a role in the compensatory hypertrophy of the kidney that follows unilateral nephrectomy and the hypertrophy that accompanies a high-protein diet.[151]

With ischemic injury, low IGF-binding protein levels and high IGF-I receptor numbers effectively increase IGF-I bioavailability and enhance the reparative actions of both local and circulating IGF-I.[152] In response, there is an increase in the expression of ischemia-induced genes with enhanced DNA synthesis and an accelerated rate of tubular epithelial cell regeneration.[153–155] In rats with ARF, IGF-I increases recovery of renal function, enhances formation of new renal tubular cells, lowers protein degradation, increases protein synthesis in skeletal muscle, and reduces net catabolism.[156, 157] In radiocontrast-induced ARF in the rat, there is selective necrosis of the medullary thick ascending limbs, leading to a significant change in the amount of and in the distribution of IGF-1, its binding protein, and its mRNA.[158]

In addition to its mitogenic effects, IGF-I may enhance recovery through its hemodynamic effects or because of direct metabolic and antiapoptotic action on injured renal tubular epithelial cells.[159] IGF-I peptide and mRNA have been found in the cytoplasm of the epithelial cells of proximal tubules in patients with ARF with improving renal function. In these patients, the greater the intensity of the staining of IGF-I peptide and mRNA, the more favorable the prognosis.[160] Various alterations in serum and urinary IGF binding proteins in patients with ARF have also been described.[161]

Recombinant human insulin-like growth factor-I (rhIGF-I)[155] has been shown to significantly enhance functional and histologic recovery in rats with nephrotoxic[162] or postischemic ARF.[159] This may be the result of the known hemodynamic effects and a result of direct metabolic, mitogenic, and antiapoptotic actions on injured tubules. While rhIGF-I has been safely used in persons at risk for ARF, clinical trials in patients with ARF have been indeterminate or negative.[163] In one multicenter, clinical trial, there were no differences in the changes from baseline values of the GFR, C_{Cr}, daily urine volume, serum urea nitrogen, creatinine, albumin, or transferrin in patients treated with rhIGF-I compared with those receiving a placebo.[164]

HEPATOCYTE GROWTH FACTOR

Hepatocyte growth factor (HGF) is a potent mitogen for mature hepatocytes and is an important hepatotropic factor involved in liver regeneration (Table 35–7). It is known to have mitogenic and morphogenic activities for various other epithelial cells, including those of the kidney.[165] Indeed, it is thought to play an essential role in renal tubular repair and regeneration following injury.[166] Both HGF mRNA and HGF protein are expressed in renal interstitial cells, presumably endothelial cells and macrophages, but not in tubular epithelial cells. Each has been shown to increase markedly in models of nephrotoxic and ischemic ARF,[167] and as tubular regeneration ceases, their activity returns to normal levels. The intravenous injection of human recombinant HGF in experimental nephrotoxic ARF stimulates DNA synthesis of renal tubular cells in vivo, attenuates the increases in BUN and S_{Cr},[168] and accelerates recovery.

Of interest is the fact that in rats, partial hepatectomy, a maneuver designed to increase the endogenous synthesis of growth factors, accelerates recovery of renal function and decreases the number of necrotic tubules following glycerol-induced ARF.[169] HGF also protects renal epithelial cells from undergoing apoptotic cell death. Thus, HGF may not only activate tubular repair processes but also serve to ameliorate the initial injury by protecting renal epithelial cells from undergoing apoptosis.[166] Notably, serum HGF concentrations have been found to be strikingly elevated in ARF patients compared with normal subjects and others with chronic renal failure.[170] Also, a marked increase in urine HGF has been observed in patients with ARF. Hepatocyte growth factor excretion tended to correlate with disease severity, and levels have been found to return to control values in recovering patients.[171]

ANGIOTENSIN II

It has long been known that the rate of growth in rats increases progressively as the NaCl content of the diet increases.[172] A more curious relationship exists between NaCl intake and the growth and development of the kidney.[173] NaCl feeding increases both normal and compensatory renal growth in the rat.[174] Moreover, an excess intake of NaCl has been linked to renal hyperplasia[174–176] and an increase in renal mass in normal rats.[177] Replacement of drinking water with 1% NaCl solution,[165] injection of NaCl solution,[166] or feeding an NaCl-enriched diet results in hyperplasia[178] and an increased mitotic index in renal tubular epithelial cells. Increases in the kidney weight–to–body weight ratio, the total protein content, the total DNA content, and the number of nuclei have been found in rats fed a high-NaCl diet when compared with rats on a low-NaCl diet.[179] In weanling rats, the kidney weight–to–body weight ratio can be increased by the ingestion of a high-NaCl diet and decreased with a low-NaCl diet.[180] In mature rats, growth can be stimulated by a unilateral nephrectomy. When this is combined with an increased NaCl intake, the rate of cell proliferation accelerates.[181]

Recovery from ischemic injury is also associated with a rapid growth phase, and it has been observed that the sodium content of the diet affects the extent of recovery.[182] In rats fed a low-salt diet after the period of ischemia, following a limited period of recovery, function regresses, with the gradual loss of individual nephron function. By contrast, in rats fed a high-salt diet, recovery is facilitated, and the number of nephrons regaining function increases with time. Histologic sections from these kidneys show marked mitotic activity and active tubular epithelial-cell regeneration. Furthermore, ^{3}H-thymidine uptake in the postischemic kidneys from rats fed a high-salt diet is greater than that in the kidneys of rats fed a low-salt diet (Fig. 36–11).

The differences in outcome that are results of dietary changes are clear indications that the outcome is not predetermined at the time of the initial injury. The fact that the dietary changes involve variation in NaCl intake is consistent with the notion that stimula-

TABLE 35–7. Characteristics of Hepatocyte Growth Factor

Potent hepatotropic factor for liver regeneration
Mitogenic activity for various epithelial cells, including renal tubular epithelial cells
May play essential role in renal tubular repair and regeneration following injury
Activity increases with nephrotoxic and ischemic injury
Activity subsides as tubular regeneration ceases
Exogenous administration suppresses cisplatin and HgCl$_2$–induced increases in BUN and S$_{Cr}$ levels
Exogenous administration stimulates DNA synthesis of renal tubular cells after HgCl$_2$ administration and unilateral nephrectomy and induces reconstruction of the normal renal tissue structure in vivo
Partial hepatectomy accelerates recovery of renal function after glycerol-induced ARF
Protects renal epithelial cells from undergoing apoptotic cell death

ARF, acute renal failure; *BUN,* blood urea nitrogen; *HgCl$_2$,* mercuric chloride; *S$_{Cr}$,* serum creatinine.

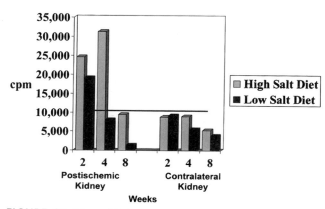

FIGURE 35–11 ■ ³H-thymidine incorporation in kidneys, 2, 4, and 8 weeks following 60 minutes of unilateral complete renal artery occlusion in the rat. Animals were maintained on low-salt (LS) or high-salt diets. Substantial differences in the hyperplastic response to renal injury are noted.

tion or suppression of the renin-angiotensin system or alteration in the type or degree of receptor expression is an important determinant of recovery. In this regard, it has come to be appreciated that angiotensin II (ATII) is important in the regulation of cell growth and differentiation (Table 35–8). This is particularly true in the fetal kidney, where the renin-angiotensin system is highly expressed during early kidney development and is essential in the modulation of growth and differentiation.[183]

Angiotensin II exerts its effect through two major classes of receptors, designated AT1 and AT2. The ratio and location of these receptor subtypes change throughout the period of renal development and may be altered in the kidney recovering from ARF. AT1 receptor activation is associated with the stimulation of growth factors, cytokines, and arachidonic acid products, along with the regulation of cell migration and adhesion.[184] In response to these stimuli, epithelial cells exhibit distinct patterns of growth behavior with hypertrophy of proximal tubule segments and proliferation of more distal segments. The growth-promoting effect of the AT1 receptor is counteracted by the antiproliferative actions of the AT2 receptor. Angiotensin 1 and AT2 receptors seem to exert counteracting effects on cellular growth and differentiation. Stimulation of AT2 receptors leads to an inhibition of cell

proliferation, induces cell differentiation, and influences the processes of both apoptosis and cell regeneration.[185] Thus, ATII exerts different growth-modulating actions, depending on the presence or absence of AT1 or AT2 receptor subtypes on a given cell.[186] For example, the AT2 subtype is highly expressed in fetal tissues but appears to be silent in adult tissue.[187] Nevertheless, disease states in adult tissues often result in expression of phenotypic changes resembling the embryonic pattern,[188] raising the possibility that AT2 receptors could be expressed in the renal tubular epithelia cells recovering from ischemic or nephrotoxic injury.

The kidney is highly susceptible to rapid fibrosis,[189] and in many ways ATII can be considered a profibrotic molecule.[190] In large part, this may be due to the fact that proximal tubular epithelial cells produce angiotensin at a concentration that exceeds systemic concentrations by approximately 100-fold.[191] Local tissue AT1 receptor stimulation is accompanied by increased production of the cytokine transforming growth factor-beta (TGFβ).[192–195] It plays a major role in stimulating synthesis of many extracellular matrix components and in inhibiting matrix degradation, finally leading to renal scarring. The contribution of ATII to the tubule loss, interstitial fibrosis, and glomerular sclerosis has been assessed in uninephrectomized rats recovering from acute renal ischemia. Treatment with an ATII receptor blocker did not prevent tubule loss or interstitial fibrosis during the early phase of recovery from acute ischemia, but treatment with an angiotensin-converting enzyme inhibitor did largely prevent the late development of glomerular injury.[196] It has been shown that ATII induces oxidative stress in vivo, which contributes to renal injury. In this regard, ATII induces renal heme oxygenase activity caused by up-regulation of heme oxygenase-1 (HO-1) in renal proximal tubules. Angiotensin II directly induces HO-1 in renal proximal epithelial cells in vitro.[197]

There is evidence that the direct cellular effects of ATII can promote renal injury that culminates in fibrotic renal disease.[198–200] The accumulation of intracellular matrix accompanying progressive tubulointerstitial fibrosis may be related to ATII stimulation of various profibrotic molecules[201] or the inhibition of extracellular matrix degradation, as may occur with induction of plasminogen activator inhibitor-1 (PAI-1) via the AT1 receptor.[202] Angiotensin II may be involved in the process of apoptosis (Fig. 35–12).

Thyroxine

The administration of thyroid hormone to animals with ARF has been reported to be protective and to promote recovery.[203–207] These actions derive from the physiologic and metabolic effects of thyroid hormone on the kidney. The physiologic effects include increased RPF and GFR and increased tubular reabsorptive and secretory ability. The metabolic effects include increased protein synthesis, glucose uptake, and amino acid uptake by renal tubular epithelial cells.[208] Thyroid hormones also enhance renal compensatory growth

TABLE 35–8. Angiotensin II: Features of Growth Factors

Enhances tubular epithelial cell proliferation in the presence of EGF or PDGF
Capable of promoting cellular hypertrophy
Induces the expression of various cellular oncogenes
Binds to specific cell surface receptors on tubular epithelial cells
Activates many of the intracellular signaling pathways
Associated with cell growth
Stimulates Na⁺, H⁺ pump activity in proximal tubular epithelial cells

EGF, epidermal growth factor; *PDGF,* platelet-derived growth factor.

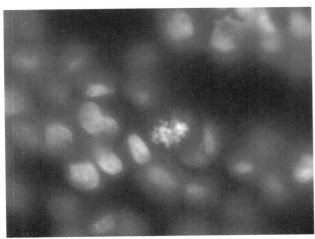

FIGURE 35–12 ■ LLC-PK₁ cells in culture incubated with angiotensin II demonstrating apoptotic changes.

through a direct action or indirectly by interacting with growth factors or glucocorticoids. The major action of thyroid hormone appears to be on the inner mitochondrial membrane to promote the entry of ADP to allow its conversion to ATP. The action of thyroid hormone on the kidney may depend on local conversion of thyroxine to triiodothyronine. In ARF, the damaged kidney may not be able to accomplish this deiodination step, making exogenous thyroid hormone more important. Notably, in the early phase of ARF, patients may have reduced plasma concentrations of both free and total T3 and reduced concentrations of free and total T4.[209]

In a prospective, randomized, placebo-controlled, double-blind trial of thyroxine in patients with ARF, a defined course of thyroxine was administered to determine if the course or mortality of clinical ARF could be improved. Baseline thyroid function, including T3, T4, rT3, and thyroid stimulating hormone (TSH) levels, were typical of patients with euthyroid sick syndrome. Thyroxine resulted in a progressive and sustained suppression of TSH levels in the treated group but had no effect on the percentage requiring dialysis, the percentage recovering renal function, or time to recovery. In fact, mortality was higher in the thyroxine group than the control group and correlated with suppression of TSH.[210]

Apoptosis

Unfortunately, recovery from ARF may be accompanied or followed by atrophy of some or all of the previously damaged tissue.[211] For example, in laboratory animals, tubular atrophy[212, 213] with interstitial fibrosis and segmental glomerular tuft abnormalities may be found as a delayed consequence of ischemic injury. A similar pattern has been observed in clinical forms of ARF. These changes certainly limit the extent of functional recovery[212] and are likely to be responsible for the secondary loss of renal mass when recovery

is incomplete.[213] This is an extremely important observation, because it may give some insight into the progressive decline in renal function that occurs in patients with other forms of renal injury.

The mechanisms that promote atrophy and serve to diminish renal mass in these circumstances involve apoptotic cell death. This is an active process under molecular control that is characterized by several morphologic changes that differ from those equated with cell death due to necrosis. They include plasma and nuclear membrane blebbing and widespread condensation of chromatin with the formation of crescent-like caps at the periphery of the nucleus[214] (Fig. 35–13). Chromatin is cleaved at nucleosomal intervals by an endogenous endonuclease resulting in DNA fragments[214, 215] of 180 base pairs or multiples thereof.[216] Eventually, the cells degenerate and break up into plasma membrane–bound vesicles called "apoptotic bodies." These undergo phagocytosis by macrophages and neighboring cells without inducing an inflammatory response.[217] Necrosis, in contrast, results in an early loss of plasma membrane integrity, the release of various injurious substances from the cytosol, and an inflammatory reaction in the surrounding tissue that is readily detected morphologically. It is notable that apoptotic cell death is not necessarily a pathologic event, for it occurs normally during embryogenesis[218] when the metanephric mesenchyme recedes as the ureteric bud develops.

Classically, renal cell loss after ischemic injury has been attributed to cellular necrosis.[219] It is now apparent that both necrosis and apoptosis are present with postischemic and nephrotoxic ARF. The relative contribution of one versus the other depends on several factors, including the severity of the initial insult, the sensitivity of the affected cells, the nature of the response to one or more renal growth factors, and the loss of cell-matrix or cell-cell adhesive interactions. Also, within the kidney there are some cells that are particularly vulnerable to ischemic and nephrotoxic injury. The outer zone of the outer medulla is most susceptible to ischemic damage. Within this zone, the epithelial cells of the proximal straight tubule and, to some extent, the epithelial cells of the thick ascending limb of the loop of Henle[220] are more apt to show necrotic changes while at the same time other tubular epithelial cells follow the pathway toward apoptosis.

It is generally considered that after injury there are two periods of increased apoptotic activity.[221] The first period occurs early after the initial insult and may actually contribute to the extent of cell loss. The second period occurs days later and follows a period of hyperplasia. Now, apoptosis is more closely associated with the deletion of unneeded cells as the result of excessive hyperplasia. In this way, apoptosis may be considered as a normal component of the restorative process of both glomeruli and tubules after renal injury.[222] Apoptotic cells have been found following the administration of a variety of nephrotoxins, ranging from antibacterial agents[223] and heavy metals[224, 225] to alkylating agents[226] and mycotoxins.[227] In addition, apoptotic cells may be found in the kidney following

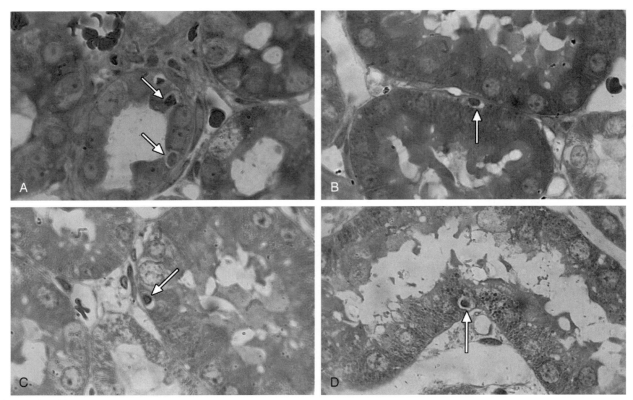

FIGURE 35–13 ■ Histologic evidence of the apoptosis of postischemic kidney from rats on a low-salt diet. *A* and *B*, One week after unilateral renal ischemia. *C* and *D*, Two weeks after unilateral renal ischemia. *Arrows* indicate apoptotic bodies (H&E).

hypoxic[228] and ischemic[229, 230] injury and in association with renal artery stenosis[231] and ureteral obstruction[232, 233] and with various other causes of tubular epithelial cell damage.[217, 231, 232, 234]

While this remodeling has been thought to facilitate the return to a normal structural and functional state, this is not always the case. Evidence exists that apoptosis is an important determinant of the atrophy found in a number of circumstances in other organs[232] when there is uniform tissue shrinkage without total architectural disorganization.[235–238] There is also substantial morphologic, biochemical, and molecular evidence that apoptosis is an important determinant of the extent of renal atrophy following postischemic and nephrotoxic injury.[237] In both clinical[239] and experimental nephrotoxic ARF,[240, 241] apoptotic changes are prominent.

It appears that there is a third period of apoptotic cell death that may determine whether or not there will be progressive tissue loss and eventual renal atrophy (Fig. 35–14). Thus, a reduction in apoptotic cell death and enhanced cell regeneration may have an important role in the attenuation of postischemic ARF in both experimental and clinical settings. For this reason, it has been suggested that any minimization of the chronic changes that result from acute injury depends on a reduction in apoptotic cell death in concert with enhanced cell regeneration.[242]

For example, following a period of unilateral renal ischemia, apoptotic cells, along with the "ladder" pattern of DNA fragments, appear soon after reperfusion

and increase in number thereafter.[240] Strikingly, removal of the contralateral kidney at 48 hours reduces the number of apoptotic cells and the extent of DNA fragmentation and allows recovery to continue.

Apoptosis is a process that is under both extracellular and intracellular regulatory control. Various exogenous cytokines function as either survival factors or lethal factors, with the latter activating specific cell death receptors or damaging cells independent of receptor activation. Endogenous proteins encoded by the protooncogene B-cell lymphoma/leukemia gene product-2 (Bcl-2) family are important intracellular factors.[243] The Bcl-2 family consists of proapoptotic and antiapoptotic genes, and the balance in expression between these gene lineages influences the death or survival of a cell. Also crucial to this process are various caspases, some of which are directly involved in apoptosis in such a manner that their inhibition can prevent cell death.[244]

Bcl-2 is crucial for normal development in the kidney, with a deficiency in Bcl-2–producing malformations resulting in renal failure and death. Ischemia-induced ARF is associated with up-regulation of antiapoptotic proteins in the damaged distal tubule and occasionally up-regulation in the proximal tubule.

Distal tubular epithelial cells, protected by the anti–cell death action of the Bcl-2 genes, may be able to produce growth factors that have a further reparative or protective role via an autocrine mechanism in the distal segment and a paracrine mechanism in the proximal cells. Both EGF and IGF-1 are also up-regulated

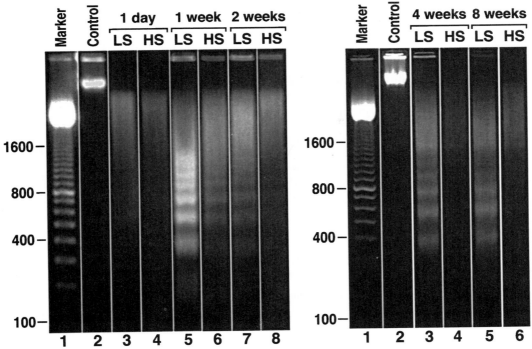

FIGURE 35–14 ▪ Agarose gel electrophoresis of DNA fragments isolated from control and postischemic kidneys. DNA extracted from control kidneys showed no signs of apoptotic ladder pattern. DNA extracted from postischemic kidneys from rats on a low-salt diet for 1 day, 1, 2, 4, or 8 weeks after ischemia, and postischemic kidneys from rats on a high-salt diet for 1 day, 1, 2, 4, or 8 weeks after ischemia, showed the typical laddering pattern.

in the surviving distal tubules and are detected in the surviving proximal tubules, where these growth factors are not usually synthesized.[245]

There are a number of other factors to consider, including the role of osteogenic protein-1 (OP-1) (bone morphogenetic protein-7), which is responsible for the induction of nephrogenic mesenchyme during embryonic kidney development. In its absence, mice die of renal failure within the first day of postnatal life. When used for the treatment of ARF in rats, recombinant human OP-1 reduces programmed cell death during the period of recovery.[246] In some situations, receptor-mediated events induced by tumor necrosis factor-alpha (TNFα) may play a role in ARF-associated apoptosis.[247] Also, various protooncogenes may regulate and modify apoptotic cell death. For example, the process of DNA fragmentation, characteristic of apoptosis, is associated with the abnormal expression of immediate early genes, such as Fas and Fas-ligand in the plasma membrane, cytoplasmic proteases,[248] such as interleukin-1 beta–converting enzyme, and various stress-activated protein kinases.[249]

RENAL COUNTERBALANCE

The theory of renal counterbalance was first described more than 80 years ago.[250–253] It was based on the well-known observation that injury to a kidney was followed by compensatory changes in the opposite kidney, which tended to minimize the loss in overall renal function. It was believed that this response was not necessarily advantageous, because once the adjustment occurred, it persisted even though the injured kidney retained the potential for recovery. In other words, the hypertrophy of the normal kidney suppressed recovery of the injured kidney. Furthermore, it was suggested that the redistribution of function contributed to the development of atrophic changes in the injured kidney. Thus, the theory of renal counterbalance involved elements of both compensatory hypertrophy and what was termed *disuse atrophy*. The concept of disuse atrophy proved difficult to establish and was later challenged[254] in such a fashion that other implications of the counterbalance theory were questioned, namely, that the presence of a normal kidney inhibits the recovery of an injured kidney and that the redistribution of function ultimately results in atrophy of the damaged kidney.

Unilateral renal injury, whether caused by ureteral obstruction or ischemia, is often followed by a significant reduction in renal function and some degree of tubular atrophy. Each of these abnormalities can be modified by a reduction in the function of the contralateral kidney. The mechanism by which this occurs is unknown. However, it seems apparent that a stimulus for growth of the previously damaged kidney is necessary for full recovery to occur and that in its absence there is progressive atrophy.

It was originally thought that counterbalance described a relationship between a hypertrophic kidney and an injured kidney and required the presence of both. However, it is quite possible that a similar relationship exists in instances of bilateral disease when the injury does not involve all nephrons to the same extent. If so, a vicious cycle may be established in which the least-damaged nephrons, which are first to recover, later hypertrophy. This internal redistribution of function may not only suppress the recovery of the most severely injured nephrons but also promote their eventual atrophy. Ultimately, the continued hypertrophy and hyperperfusion of the functioning nephrons may lead to sclerotic changes within their glomeruli. The net effect is an eventual and progressive decline in whole kidney function. Prevention of the initial atrophy appears to be possible and, if accomplished, would be expected to interrupt the cycle and preserve renal function.

REFERENCES

1. Edelstein CL, Ling H, Schrier R: The nature of renal cell injury. Kidney Int 1997: 51:1341–1351.
2. Swann RC, Merrill JP: Clinical course of acute renal failure. Medicine 1953; 32:215–292.
3. Finn WF: Postischemic acute renal failure: initiation, maintenance, and recovery. Invest Urol 1980; 17:427–431.
4. Rahman SN, Conger JD: Glomerular and tubular factors in urine flow rates of acute renal failure patients. Am J Kidney Dis 1994; 23:788–793.
5. Eliahou HE, Bata A: The diagnosis of acute renal failure. Nephron 1965; 2:287–295.
6. Luke RG, Briggs JD, Allison ME, Kennedy AC: Factors determining response to mannitol in acute renal failure. Am J Med Sci 1970; 259:168–174.
7. Meroney WH, Rubini ME: Kidney function during acute tubular necrosis: clinical studies and theory. Metabolism 1959; 9:1.
8. Iseri LT, Batchelor, Boyle AJ, Myers GB: Studies of fluid, electrolyte, and nitrogen balance in acute renal failure. Arch Intern Med 1952; 89:188.
9. Lam M, Kaufman CE: Fractional excretion of sodium as a guide to volume depletion during recovery from acute renal failure. Am J Kidney Dis 1995; 6:18–21.
10. Wang Z, Rabb H, Haq M, et al: A possible molecular basis of natriuresis during ischemic-reperfusion injury in the kidney. J Am Soc Nephrol 1998; 9:605–613.
11. Nielsen S, Kwon TH, Christensen BM, et al: Physiology and pathophysiology of renal aquaporins. J Am Soc Nephrol 1999; 10:647–663.
12. Jung JS, Lee RH, Koh SH, Kim YK: Changes in expression of sodium cotransporters and acquaporin-2 during ischemia-reperfusion injury in rabbit kidney. Ren Fail 2000; 22:407–421.
13. Myers BD, Hilberman M, Spencer RJ, Jamison RL: Glomerular and tubular function in nonoliguric acute renal failure. Am J Med 1982; 72:642–649.
14. Danovitch G, Carvounis C, Weinstein E, Levenson S: Nonoliguric acute renal failure. Isr J Med Sci 1979; 15:5–8.
15. Bhandari S, Turney JH: Survivors of acute renal failure who do not recover renal function. QJM 1996; 89:415–421.
16. Stene JK: Renal failure in the trauma patient. Crit Care Clin 1990; 6:111–119.
17. Anderson RJ, Linas SL, Berns AS, et al: Nonoliguric acute renal failure. N Engl J Med 1977; 296:1134–1138.
18. Briggs JD, Kennedy AC, Young LH, et al: Renal function after acute tubular necrosis. BMJ 1986; 3:513–516.
19. Lewers DT, Matthew TH, Maher JF, Schreiner GE: Long-term follow up of renal function and histology after acute tubular necrosis. Ann Intern Med 1970; 73:523–529.
20. Price JDE, Palmer RA: A functional and morphological follow-up study of acute renal function. Arch Intern Med 1960; 105:114–122.
21. Finkenstaedt JT, Merrill JP: Renal function after recovery from acute renal failure. N Engl J Med 1956; 254:1023–1026.
22. Lowe LG: The late prognosis in acute tubular necrosis: an interim follow-up report on 14 patients. Lancet 1952; 1:1086–1088.
23. Bonomini V, Stefoni S, Vangelista A: Long-term patient and renal prognosis in acute renal failure. Nephron 1984; 36:169.
24. Kleinknecht D, Pallot JL: Epidemiology and prognosis of acute renal insufficiency in 1997: recent data. Nephrologie 1998; 19:49–55.
25. Tulchinsky M, Dietrich TJ, Eggli DF, Yang HC: Technetium-99m-MAG3 scintigraphy in acute renal failure after transplantation: a marker of viability and prognosis. J Nucl Med 1997; 38:475–478.
26. Baraldi A, Ballestri M, Rapana R, et al: Acute renal failure of medical type in an elderly population. Nephrol Dial Transplant 1998; 13(suppl 70):25–29.
27. Shaw NJ, Brocklebank JT, Dickinson DF, et al: Long-term outcome for children with acute renal failure following cardiac surgery. Int J Cardiol 1991; 31:161.
28. Georgaki-Angelaki HN, Steed DB, Chantler C, Haycock GB: Renal function following acute renal failure in childhood: a long-term follow-up study. Kidney Int 1989; 35:84–89.
29. Muehrcke RC: Acute Renal Failure: Diagnosis and Management. St. Louis: CV Mosby: 1969; 58–81.
30. Muehrcke RC, Rosen S, Pirani CL, Kark RM: Renal lesions in patients recovering from acute renal failure [abstract]. J Lab Clin Med 1964; 64:888.
31. Yamate J, Ishida A, Tsujino K, et al: Immunohistochemical study of rat renal interstitial fibrosis induced by repeated injection of cisplatin, with special reference to the kinetics of macrophages and myofibroblasts. Toxicol Pathol 1996; 24:199–206.
32. Moghal NE, Brocklebank JT, Meadow SR: A review of acute renal failure in children: incidence, etiology and outcome. Clin Nephrol 1998; 49:91–95.
33. Shilliday I, Allison MEM: Diuretics in acute renal failure. Ren Fail 1994; 16:3–17.
34. Oken DE: Renal and extrarenal considerations in high-dose mannitol therapy. Ren Fail 1984; 16:147–159.
35. Brown CB, Ogg CS, Cameron JS: High-dose furosemide in acute renal failure: a controlled trial. Clin Nephrol 1981; 15:90–96.
36. Kleinknecht D, Ganeval D, Gonzalez-Duque LA, Fermanian J: Furosemide in acute oliguric renal failure: a controlled trial. Nephron 1976; 17:51–58.
37. Cantarovich F, Locatelli A, Fernandez JC, et al: Furosemide in high doses in the treatment of acute renal failure. Postgrad Med J 1971; 47(suppl):13–17.
38. Shilliday IR, Quinn KJ, Allison ME: Loop diuretics in the management of acute renal failure: a prospective, double-blind, placebo-controlled, randomized study. Nephrol Dial Transplant 1997; 12:2592–2596.
39. Cottee DBF, Saul WP: Is renal dose dopamine protective or therapeutic? No. Crit Care Med 1996; 12:687–695.
40. Baldwin L, Henderson A, Hickman P: Effect of postoperative low-dose dopamine on renal function after elective major vascular surgery. Ann Intern Med 1994; 120:744–747.
41. Salem MG, Crooke JW, McLoughlin GA, et al: The effect of dopamine on renal function during aortic cross clamping. Ann R Coll Surg Engl 1988; 71:9–12.
42. Polsen RJ, Park GR, Lindop MJ, et al: The prevention of renal impairment in patients undergoing orthotopic liver grafting by infusion of low-dose dopamine. Anaesthesia 1987; 42:15–19.
43. Carcoana OV, Hines RL: Is renal dose dopamine protective or therapeutics? Yes. Crit Care Med 1996; 12:677–685.
44. Szerlip HM: Renal-dose dopamine: fact and fiction. Ann Intern Med 1991; 115:153–154.
45. Denton MD, Chertow GM, Brady HR: "Renal-dose" dopamine for the treatment of acute renal failure: scientific rationale, experimental studies and clinical trial. Kidney Int 1996; 50:4–14.
46. Australian and New Zealand Intensive Care Society (ANZICS) Clinical Trials Group: Low-dose dopamine in patients with early renal dysfunction: a placebo-controlled randomized trial. Lancet 2000; 356:2139–2143.
47. Chertow GM, Sayegh MH, Allgren RL, Lazarus JM: Is the administration of dopamine associated with adverse or favorable outcomes in acute renal failure? Auriculin Anaritide Acute Renal Failure Study Group. Am J Med 1996; 101:49–53.

48. Lokhandwala MF: Effects of dopamine receptor agonists on cardiovascular and renal function. In Vincent JL, ed: *Update in Intensive Care and Emergency Medicine.* New York: Springer-Verlag; 1991:74–90.
49. Murphy MB, McCoy CE, Weber RR, et al: Augmentation of renal blood flow and sodium excretion in hypertensive patients during blood pressure reduction by intravenous administration of the dopamine agonist fenoldopam. Circulation 1987; 76:1312–1318.
50. Allison NL, Dubb JW, Ziemniak JA, et al: The effect of fenoldopam, a dopaminergic agonist, on renal hemodynamics. Clin Pharmacol Ther 1987; 41:282–288.
51. Singer I, Epstein M: Potential of dopamine A-1 agonists in the management of acute renal failure. Am J Kidney Dis 1998; 31:743–755.
52. Levin ER, Gardner DG, Samson WK: Natriuretic peptides. N Engl J Med 1998; 339:321–328.
53. Vinot O, Bialek J, Canaan-Kuhl S, et al: Endogenous ANP in postischemic acute renal allograft failure. Am J Physiol 1995; 269:F125–F133.
54. Plum J, Scholtz W, Grabensee B: Atrial natriuretic peptide in renal transplantation. Horm Res 1996; 46:74–82.
55. Gianello P, Carlier M, Jamart J, et al: Effect of 1–28 alpha-h atrial natriuretic peptide on acute renal failure in cadaveric renal transplantation. Clin Transplant 1995; 9:481–489.
56. Meyer M, Stief CG, Becker AJ, et al: The renal paracrine peptide system: possible urologic implications of urodilan. World J Urol 1996; 14:375–379.
57. Kuse ER, Meyer M, Constantin R, et al: Urodilatin (INN: ularitide): a new peptide in the treatment of acute renal failure following liver transplantation. Anaesthesist 1996; 45:351–358.
58. Rahman SN, Kim GE, Mathew AS, et al: Effects of atrial natriuretic peptide in clinical acute renal failure. Kidney Int 1994; 45:1731–1738.
59. Allgren RL, Marbury TC, Rahman SN, et al: Anaritide in acute tubular necrosis. N Engl J Med 1997; 336:828–834.
60. Allgren RL: Update on clinical trials with atrial natriuretic peptide in acute tubular necrosis. Ren Fail 1998; 20:691–695.
61. Brenner RM, Chertow GM: The rise and fall of atrial natriuretic peptide for acute renal failure. Curr Opin Nephrol Hypertens 1997; 6:474–476.
62. Kurnik BR, Allgren RL, Genter FC, et al: Prospective study of atrial natriuretic peptide for the prevention of radiocontrast-induced nephropathy. Am J Kidney Dis 1998; 31:674–680.
63. Schrier RW, Burke TJ: Calcium-channel blockers in experimental and human acute renal failure. Adv Nephrol 1980; 17:287–300.
64. Lumlertgul D, Hutdagoon P, Sirivanichai C, Keoplung M: Beneficial effects of intrarenal verapamil in human acute renal failure. Ren Fail 1989–1990; 11:201–208.
65. Bakris GL, Burnett JC: A role for calcium in radiocontrast-induced reductions in renal hemodynamics. Kidney Int 1985; 27:465–468.
66. Barros EJG, Boim MA, Ajzen H, et al: Glomerular hemodynamics and hormonal participation in cyclosporin nephrotoxicity. Kidney Int 1987; 32:19–25.
67. Duggan KA, Macdonald GJ, Charlesworth JA, Pussel BA: Verapamil prevents post-transplant oliguric renal failure. Clin Nephrol 1985; 24:289–291.
68. Wagner K, Albrecht S, Neumayer HH: Prevention of posttransplant acute tubular necrosis by the calcium antagonist diltiazem: a prospective randomized study. Am J Nephrol 1987; 7:287–291.
69. McCord JM: Oxygen-derived free radicals in post-ischemic tissue injury. N Engl J Med 1985; 312:159–163.
70. Baliga R, Ueda N, Walker PD, Shah SV: Oxidant mechanisms in toxic acute renal failure. Am J Kidney Dis 1997; 29:465–477.
71. Cunningham SK, Keaveny TV, Fitzgerald P: Effect of allopurinol on tissue ATP, ADP, and AMP concentrations in renal ischemia. Br J Surg 1974; 61:562–565.
72. Macoviak JA, McDougall IR, Bayer MF, et al: Significance of thyroid dysfunction in human cardiac allograft procurement. Transplantation 1987; 43:824–826.
73. Hansson R, Gustafsson B, Jonsson O, et al: Effects of xanthine oxidase inhibition on renal circulation after ischemia. Transplant Proc 1982; 14:51–58.
74. Lelcuk S, Alexander F, Kobzik L, et al: Prostacyclin and thromboxane A2 moderate postischemic renal failure. Surgery 1985; 98:207–212.
75. Finn WF, Hak LJ, Grossman SH: Protective effect on prostacycline on postischemic acute renal failure. Kidney Int 1987; 132:479–487.
76. Ohshima E, Sato H, Obase H, et al: Dibenzoxepin derivatives: thromboxane A2 synthase inhibition and thromboxane A2 receptor antagonism combined in one molecule. J Med Chem 1993; 36:1613–1618.
77. Solez K, Morel-Moroger L, Sraer JD: The morphology of "cute tubular necrosis" in man: analysis of 57 renal biopsies and a comparison with the glycerol model. Medicine 1979; 58:362–376.
78. Conger JD: Does hemodialysis delay recovery from acute renal failure? Semin Dial 1990; 3:146–148.
79. Fink JC, Cooper MA, Zager RA: Hemodialysis exacerbates enzymuria in patients with acute renal failure: brief report. Ren Fail 1996; 18:947–950.
80. Williams RH, Thomas CE, Navar LG, Evan AP: Hemodynamic and single nephron function during the maintenance phase of ischemic acute renal failure in the dog. Kidney Int 1981; 19:503–515.
81. Conger JD, Robinette JB, Kelleher SP: Nephron heterogeneity in ischemic acute renal failure. Kidney Int 1984; 26:422–429.
82. Himmelfarb J, Hakim RM: The use of biocompatible dialysis membranes in acute renal failure. Adv Ren Replace Ther 1997; 4(suppl 1):72–80.
83. Schulman G, Hakim R: Hemodialysis membrane biocompatibility in acute renal failure. Adv Ren Replace Ther 1994; 1:75–82.
84. Linas SL, Whittenberg D, Parsons PE, Repine JE: Mild renal ischemia activates primed neutrophils to cause acute renal failure. Kidney Int 1992; 42:610–616.
85. Schulman G, Fogo A, Gung A, et al: Complement activation retards resolution of acute ischemic renal failure in the rat. Kidney Int 1991; 40:1069–1074.
86. Kranzlin B, Reuss A, Gretz N, et al: Recovery from ischemic acute renal failure: independence from dialysis membrane type. Nephron 1996; 73:644–651.
87. Kranzlin B, Gretz N, Kirschfink M, Mujais SK: Dialysis in rats with acute renal failure: evaluation of three different dialyzer membranes. Artif Organs 1996; 20:1162–1168.
88. Schiffl H, Lang SM, König A, et al: Biocompatible membranes in acute renal failure: prospective case controlled study. Lancet 1994; 344:570–572.
89. Hakim RM, Wingard RL, Parker RA: Effect of the dialysis membrane in the treatment of patients with acute renal failure. N Engl J Med 1994; 331:1338–1342.
90. Himmelfarb J, Tolkoff-Rubin N, Chandran P, et al: A multicenter comparison of dialysis membranes in the treatment of acute renal failure requiring dialysis. J Am Soc Nephrol 1998; 9:257–266.
91. Parker RA, Himmelfarb J, Tolkoff-Rubin N, et al: Prognosis of patients with acute renal failure requiring dialysis: results of a multicenter study. Am J Kidney Dis 1998; 32:432–433.
92. Neveu H, Kleinknecht D, Brivet F, Loivat PH, Landis P, and the French Study Group on Acute Renal Failure: Prognostic factors in acute renal failure due to sepsis: results of a prospective multicenter study. Nephrol Dial Transplant 1996; 11:293–299.
93. Splendiani G, Mazzarella V: Is the choice of membrane important for patients with acute renal failure requiring hemodialysis? Artif Organs 1996; 20:281.
94. Schiffl H, Lang S, Haider M: Biocompatibility of dialyzer membranes may have a negative impact on outcome of acute renal failure, independent of the dose of dialysis delivered: a retrospective multicenter analysis. ASAIO J 1998; 44:M418–M422.
95. Jacobs C: Membrane biocompatibility in the treatment of acute renal failure: what is the evidence in 1996? Nephrol Dial Transplant 1997; 12:38–42.
96. Shaldon S: Biocompatible membranes in acute renal failure. Lancet 1996; 347:205–206.
97. Shaldon S: Biocompatible membranes in acute renal failure: prospective case controlled study. Nephrol Dial Transplant 1997; 12:235–236.

98. Papadimitriou M, Papagianni A, Diamantopoulou D, et al: Acute renal failure: which treatment modality is the best? Ren Fail 1998; 20:651–661.

99. Kurtal H, von Herrath D, Schafer K: Is the choice of membrane important for patients with acute renal failure requiring hemodialysis? Artif Organs 1995; 19:391–394.

100. Cosentino F, Chaff C, Piedmonte M: Risk factors influencing survival in ICU acute renal failure. Nephrol Dial Transplant 1994; 9(suppl 4):179–182.

101. Liano F, Pascual J, and the Madrid Acute Renal Failure Study Group: Epidemiology of acute renal failure: a prospective multicenter, community based study. Kidney Int 1996; 50:811–818.

102. Jorres A, Gahl GM, Dobis C, et al: Hemodialysis membrane biocompatibility and mortality of patients with dialysis-dependent acute renal failure: a prospective randomized multicentre trial. International Study Group. Lancet 1999; 354:1137–1141.

103. Vanholder R, Lameire N: Does biocompatibility of dialysis membranes affect recovery of renal function and survival? Lancet 1999; 354:1316–1318.

104. Valeri A, Radhakrishnan J, Ryan R, Powell D: Biocompatible dialysis membranes and acute renal failure: a study in postoperative acute tubular necrosis in cadaveric renal transplant recipients. Clin Nephrol 1996; 46:402–409.

105. Romao JE Jr, Abensur H, de Castro MC, et al: Effect of dialyser biocompatibility on recovery from acute renal failure after cadaver renal transplantation. Nephrol Dial Transplant 1999; 14:709–712.

106. Assouad M, Tseng S, Dunn K, et al: Biocompatibility of dialyzed membrane is important in the outcome of acute renal failure [abstract]. J Am Soc Nephrol 1996; 7:1437.

107. Gastaldello K, Melot C, Kahn RJ, et al: Comparison of cellulose diacetate and polysulfone membranes in the outcome of acute renal failure: a prospective randomized study. Nephrol Dial Transplant 2000; 15:224–230.

108. Backenroth R, Schuger L, Wald H, Popovtzer MM: Glycerol-induced acute renal failure attenuates subsequent HgCl₂-associated nephrotoxicity: correlation of renal function and morphology. Ren Fail 1998; 20:15–26.

109. Suzuki T: Zur Morphologie der Nierensekretion unter physiologischen und pathologischen Bedingungen. Jena: Fischer; 1912.

110. MacNider W deB: A pathological study of the naturally acquired chronic nephropathy of the dog. Part I. J Med Res 1916; 34:177–230.

111. MacNider W deB: The functional and pathological response of the kidney in dogs subjected to a second subcutaneous injection of uranium nitrate. J Exp Med 1929; 49:411–434.

112. Hayes JM, Boonshaft B, Maher JF, et al: Resistance to glycerol-induced hemoglobinuric acute renal failure. Nephron 1970; 7:155–164.

113. Oken DE, Mende CW, Taraba T, Flamenbaum W: Resistance to acute renal failure afforded by prior renal failure: examination of the role of renal renin content. Nephron 1975; 15:131–142.

114. Gilbert DN, Houghton DC, Bennett WM, et al: Reversibility of gentamicin nephrotoxicity in rats: recovery during continuous drug administration. Proc Soc Exp Biol Med 1979; 160:99–103.

115. Fernandez-Repollet E, Finn WF, Yang JJ, Diaz L: Role of age in gentamicin nephrotoxicity [abstract]. J Am Soc Nephrol 1992; 3:723.

116. Sano K, Fujigaki Y, Ikegaya N, et al: The roles of apoptosis in uranyl acetate–induced acute renal failure. Ren Fail 1998; 20:697–701.

117. Vogt BA, Shanley TP, Croatt A, et al: Glomerular inflammation induces resistance to tubular injury in the rat: a novel form of acquired, heme oxygenase–dependent resistance to renal injury. J Clin Invest 1996; 98:2139–2145.

118. Zager RA: Heme protein–induced tubular cytoresistance: expression at the plasma membrane level. Kidney Int 1995; 47:1336–1345.

119. Kim G, Gazarian M, Verjee Z, John D: Acute renal insufficiency in ibuprofen overdose. Pediatr Emerg Care 1995; 11:107–108.

120. Zager RA, Burkhart K: Decreased expression of mitochondrial-derived H₂O₂ and hydroxyl radical in cytoresistant proximal tubules. Kidney Int 1997; 52:942–952.

121. Vogt BA, Alam J, Croatt AJ, et al: Acquired resistance to acute oxidative stress: possible role of heme oxygenase and ferritin. Lab Invest 1995; 72:474–483.

122. Vogt BA, Shanley TP, Croatt A, et al: Glomerular inflammation induces resistance to tubular injury in the rat. A novel form of acquired, heme oxygenase-dependent resistance to renal injury. J Clin Invest 1996; 98:2139–2145.

123. Ishizuka S: An experimental study on the pathogenetic role of acquired resistance to acute renal failure: enzymochemical investigation. Jpn J Nephrol 1996; 38:65–73.

124. Zager RA, Burkhart K: Decreased expression of mitochondrial-derived H₂O₂ and hydroxyl radical in cytoresistant proximal tubules. Kidney Int 1997; 52:942–952.

125. Mizuno S, Fujita K, Furuya R, et al: Association of HSP73 with the acquired resistance to uranyl acetate–induced acute renal failure. Toxicology 1997; 117:183–191.

126. Furuya R, Kumagai H, Hishida A: Acquired resistance to rechallenge injury with uranyl acetate in LLC-PK1 cells. J Lab Clin Med 1997; 129:347–355.

127. Samali A, Cotter TG: Heat shock proteins increase resistance to apoptosis. Exp Cell Res 1996; 223:163–170.

128. Haley WE, Johnson JW: Measurement of urinary renin activity by radioimmunoassay: sequential studies in acute renal failure in man. Nephron 1978; 20:273–285.

129. Funaki N, Kuroda M, Sudo J, Takeda R: Urinary prostaglandins and kallikrein in the course of acute renal failure. Prostaglandins Leukot Med 1982; 9:387–399.

130. Bull GM, Joekes AM, Lowe KG: Renal function studies in acute tubular necrosis. Clin Sci 1950; 9:379–404.

131. Marshall D, Hoffman WS: The nature of the altered renal function in lower nephron nephrosis. J Lab Clin Med 1949; 34:31–39.

132. Finn WF, Chevalier RL: Recovery from postischemic acute renal failure in the rat. Kidney Int 1979; 16:113–123.

133. Corrigan G, Ramaswamy D, Kwon O, et al: PAH extraction and estimation of plasma flow in human postischemic acute renal failure. Am J Physiol 1999; 277:F312–F318.

134. Oken DE, DiBona GF, McDonald FD: Micropuncture studies on the recovery phase of myohemoglobinuric acute renal failure in the rat. J Clin Invest 1970; 49:730–737.

135. Karlberg L, Kallskog O, Norlen BJ, Wolgast M: Postischemic renal failure: intrarenal blood flow and functional characteristics in the recovery phase. Acta Physiol Scand 1982; 115:1–10.

136. Finn WF: Enhanced recovery from postischemic acute renal failure: micropuncture studies in the rat. Circ Res 1980; 46:440–448.

137. Kallskog O, Hellstrom I, Rissler K, Wolgast M: Long-term recovery of superficial and deep glomeruli after acute renal failure evoked by warm ischemia. Ren Physiol 1985; 8:328–337.

138. Harris RC: Growth factors and cytokines in acute renal failure. Adv Ren Replace Ther 1997; 4(2 suppl 1):43–53.

139. Abbate M, Remuzzi G: Acceleration of recovery in acute renal failure: from cellular mechanisms of tubular repair to innovative targeted therapies. Ren Fail 1996; 18:377–388.

140. Schena FP: Role of growth factors in acute renal failure. Kidney Int Suppl 1998; 66:S11–S15.

141. Humes HD: Potential molecular therapy for acute renal failure. Cleve Clin J Med 1993; 60:166–168.

142. Wagener OE, Lieske JC, Toback FG: Molecular and cell biology of acute renal failure: new therapeutic strategies. New Horiz 1995; 3:634–649.

143. Humes HD, Lake EW, Liu S: Renal tubule cell repair following acute renal injury. Min Electrolyte Metab 1995; 21:353–365.

144. Hirschberg R, Ding H: Growth factors and acute renal failure. Semin Nephrol 1998; 18:191–207.

145. Schaudies RP, Nonclercq D, Nelson L, et al: Endogenous EGF as a potential renotropic factor in ischemia-induced acute renal failure. Am J Physiol 1993; 265:F425–F434.

146. Schaudies RP, Johnson JP: Increased soluble EGF after ischemia is accompanied by a decrease in membrane-associated precursors. Am J Physiol 1993; 264:F523–F531.

147. Taira T, Yoshimura A, Iizuka K, et al: Expression of epidermal growth factor and its receptor in rabbits with ischemic acute renal failure. Virchows Arch 1996; 427:583–588.

148. Taira T, Yoshimura A, Iizuka K, et al: Urinary epidermal growth

factor levels in patients with acute renal failure. Am J Kidney Dis 1993; 22:656–661.

149. Chen L, Liu W: Effect of asphyxia on urinary epidermal growth factor levels in newborns. J Tongji Med Univ 1997; 17:144–146.

150. Lee DY, Park SK, Yorgin PD, et al: Alteration in insulin-like growth factor–binding proteins (IGFBPs) and IGFBP-3 protease activity in serum and urine from acute and chronic renal failure. J Clin Endocrinol Metab 1994; 79:1376–1382.

151. Hirschberg R, Adler S: Insulin-like growth factor system and the kidney: physiology, pathophysiology, and therapeutic implications. Am J Kidney Dis 1998; 31:901–919.

152. Tsao T, Wang J, Fervenza FC, et al: Renal growth hormone–insulin-like growth factor-1 system in acute renal failure. Kidney Int 1995; 47:1658–1668.

153. Hammerman MR, Miller SB: Effects of growth hormone and insulin-like growth factor I on renal growth and function. J Pediatr 1997; 131:S17–S19.

154. van Bommel E, Bouvy ND, So KL, et al: Acute dialytic support for the critically ill: intermittent hemodialysis versus continuous arteriovenous hemodiafiltration. Am J Nephrol 1995; 15:192–200.

155. Ding H, Kopple JD, Cohen A, Hirschberg R: Recombinant human insulin-like growth factor-I accelerates recovery and reduces catabolism in rats with ischemic acute renal failure. J Clin Invest 1993; 91:2281–2287.

156. Kopple JD: The nutrition management of the patient with acute renal failure. JPEN J Parenter Enteral Nutr 1996; 20:3–12.

157. Ding H, Kopple JD, Cohen A, Hirschberg R: Recombinant human insulin-like growth factor-I accelerates recovery and reduces catabolism in rats with ischemic acute renal failure. J Clin Invest 1993; 91:2281–2287.

158. Symon Z, Fuchs S, Agmon Y, et al: The endogenous insulin-like growth factor system in radiocontrast nephropathy. Am J Physiol 1998; 274:F490–F497.

159. Hirschberg R, Ding H: Mechanism of insulin-like growth factor-1–induced accelerated recovery in experimental ischemic acute renal failure. Min Electrolyte Metab 1998; 24:211–219.

160. Nishiki M, Murakami Y, Kawaguchi M, et al: Renal expression of insulin-like growth factor-l in acute renal failure: a preliminary report. Clin Nephrol 1999; 52:148–151.

161. Lee DY, Park SK, Yorgin PD, et al: Alteration in insulin-like growth factor–binding proteins (IGFBPs) and IGFBP-3 protease activity in serum and urine from acute and chronic renal failure. J Clin Endocrinol Metabol 1994; 79:1376–1382.

162. Friedlaender M, Popovtzer MM, Weiss O, et al: Insulin-like growth factor-1 (IGF-1) enhances recovery from HgCl₂-induced acute renal failure: the effects on renal IGF-1, IGF-1 receptor, and IGF-binding protein-1 mRNA. J Am Soc Nephrol 1995; 5:1782–1791.

163. Wang S, Hirschberg R: Role of growth factors in acute renal failure. Nephrol Dial Transplant 1997; 12:1560–1563.

164. Hirschberg R, Kopple J, Lipsett P, et al: Multicenter clinical trial of recombinant human insulin-like growth factor I in patients with acute renal failure. Kidney Int 1999; 55:2423–2432.

165. Vargas GA, Hoeflich A, Jehle PM: Hepatocyte growth factor in renal failure: promise and reality. Kidney Int 2000; 57:1426–1436.

166. Liu Y, Sun AM, Dworkin LD: Hepatocyte growth factor protects renal epithelial cells from apoptotic cell death. Biochem Biophys Res Comm 1998; 246:821–826.

167. Kawaida K, Matsumoto K, Shimazu H, Nakamura T: Hepatocyte growth factor prevents ARF and accelerates renal regeneration in mice. Proc Natl Acad Sci USA 1994; 91:4357–4361.

168. Igawa T, Matsumoto K, Kanda S, et al: Hepatocyte growth factor may function as a renotropic factor for regeneration in rats with acute renal injury. Am J Physiol 1993; 265:F61–F69.

169. Homsi E, Pires de Oliveira Dias E, Figueiredo JF, Gontijo JA: Accelerated recovery of glycerol-induced acute renal failure in rats with previous partial hepatectomy. Exper Nephrol 1998; 6:551–556.

170. Libetta C, Rampino T, Esposito C, et al: Stimulation of hepatocyte growth factor in human acute renal failure. Nephron 1998; 80:41–45.

171. Taman M, Liu Y, Tolbert E, Dworkin LD: Increased urinary

172. Grunert RR, Meyer JH, Phillips PH: The sodium and potassium requirements of the rat for growth. J Nutr 1950; 42:609–618.

173. Gross RJ, Ditmer JE: Compensatory Renal Hypertrophy: Problems and Prospects. In: Nowinski WW, Goss RJ, eds: Compensatory Renal Hypertrophy. New York: Academic Press; 1969:299.

174. Reville P, de Laharpe F, Koll-Back MH: Enhancement of renal compensatory hypertrophy by hyperadrenocorticism and its modulation by nutritional factors. Horm Metab Res 1982; 13:487–493.

175. Hall CE, Hall O: Comparative effectiveness of glucose and sucrose in enhancement of hypersalimentation and salt hypertension. Proc Soc Exp Biol Med 1966; 123:370–374.

176. Moraski R: Renal hyperplasia in the intact rat. Proc Soc Exp Biol Med 1966; 1221:838–840.

177. Binet L, Dejours P, Lacaisse A: Action du chlorure de sodium alimentaire sur le development ponderal du rein chez le rat. CR de la Soc de Biol 1950; 144:84.

178. Lalich JJ, Paik WC, Pradham B: Epithelial hyperplasia in the renal papilla of rats: induction in animals fed excess sodium chloride. Arch Pathol 1974; 97:29–32.

179. McCormick CP, Rauch AL, Buckalew VM Jr: Differential effect of dietary salt on renal growth in Dahl salt-sensitive and salt-resistant rats. Hypertension 1989; 13:122–127.

180. Solomen S, Romero C, Moore L: The effect of age and salt intake on growth and renal development of rats. Arch Int Physiol Boitel 1972; 80:871–882.

181. Tingle LE, Cameron IL: Cell proliferation response in several tissues following combined unilateral nephrectomy and high-salt diet in mice. Tex Rep Biol Med 1973; 31:537.

182. Finn WF: Recovery From Acute Renal Failure. In: Lacers JM, Brenner BM, eds: Acute Renal Failure. 3rd ed. New York: Churchill Livingstone; 1993.

183. Harris JM, Gomez RA: Renin-angiotensin system genes in kidney development. Microsc Res Tech 1997; 39:211–221.

184. Hsueh WA, Do YS, Anderson PW, Law RE: Angiotensin II in cell growth and matrix production. Adv Exp Med Biol 1995; 377:217–223.

185. Chung O, Kuhl H, Stoll M, Unger T: Physiological and pharmacological implications of AT1 versus AT2 receptors. Kidney Int Suppl 1998; 67:S95–S99.

186. Stoll M, Meffert S, Stroth U, Unger T: Growth or antigrowth: angiotensin and the endothelium. J Hypertens 1995; 13:1529–1534.

187. Capponi AM: Distribution and signal transduction of angiotensin II AT1 and AT2 receptors. Blood Press Suppl 1996; 2:41–46.

188. Gomez RA, Norwood VF: Developmental consequences of the renin-angiotensin system. Am J Kidney Dis 1995; 26:409–431.

189. Border WA, Noble NA: Interactions of transforming growth factor-beta and angiotensin II in renal fibrosis. Hypertension 1998; 31:181–188.

190. Peters H, Noble NA: Angiotensin II and L-arginine in tissue fibrosis: more than blood pressure. Kidney Int 1997; 51:1481–1486.

191. Wolf G: Angiotensin as a renal growth promoting factor. Adv Exp Med Biol 1995; 377:225–236.

192. Wolf G, Ziyadeh FN: Renal tubular hypertrophy induced by angiotensin II. Semin Nephrol 1997; 17:448–454.

193. Wolf G: Link between angiotensin II and TGF-beta in the kidney. Miner Electrolyte Metab 1998; 24:174–180.

194. Harris RC, Martinez-Maldonado M: Angiotensin II–mediated renal injury. Miner Electrolyte Metab 1995; 21:328–335.

195. Noble NA, Border WA: Angiotensin II in renal fibrosis: should TGF-beta rather than blood pressure be the therapeutic target? Semin Nephrol 1997; 17:455–466.

196. Pagtalunan ME, Olson JL, Meyer TW: Contribution of angiotensin II to late renal injury after acute ischemia. J Am Soc Nephrol 2000; 11:1278–1286.

197. Haugen EN, Croatt AJ, Nath KA: Angiotensin II–induced renal oxidant stress in vivo and heme oxygenase-1 in vivo and in vitro. Kidney Int 2000; 58:144–152.

198. Levy BI: The potential role of angiotensin II in the vasculature. J Hum Hypertens 1998; 12:283–287.

199. Diamond JR, Ricardo SD, Klahr S: Mechanisms of interstitial

fibrosis in obstructive nephropathy. Semin Nephrol 1998; 18:594–602.

200. Wolf G: Angiotensin II is involved in the progression of renal disease: importance of nonhemodynamic mechanisms. Nephrologie 1998; 19:451–456.

201. Basile DP: Is angiotensin II's role in fibrosis as easy as PAI-1? Kidney Int 2000; 58:460–461.

202. Nakamura S, Nakamura I, Ma L, Vaughan DE: Plasminogen activator inhibitor-1 expression is regulated by the angiotensin type 1 receptor in vivo. Kidney Int 2000; 58:251–259.

203. Siegel NJ, Gaudio KM, Katz LA, et al: Beneficial effects of thyroxin on recovery from toxic acute renal failure. Kidney Int 1984; 25:906–911.

204. Cronin RE, Newman JA: Protective effects of thyroxin but not parathyroidectomy on gentamicin nephrotoxicity. Am J Physiol 1985; 248:F332–F339.

205. Cronin RE, Brown DM, Simonsen R: Protection by thyroxin in nephrotoxic acute renal failure. Am J Physiol 1986; 251:F408–F416.

206. Sutter PM, Thulin G, Siegel NJ: Beneficial effect of thyroxin in the treatment of ischemic acute renal failure. Pediatr Nephrol 1988; 2:1–7.

207. Negri AL, Alvarez C, Fernandez MC, et al: Accelerated recovery from toxic acute renal failure with thyroxin: stimulation of renal phospholipid biosynthesis. Ren Fail 1994; 16:19–26.

208. Capasso G, De Santo NG, Kinne R: Thyroid hormones and renal transport: cellular and biochemical aspects. Kidney Int 1987; 32:443–451.

209. Hronek I, Hronkova B, Davenport A, Mackenzie JC: Thyroid hormone levels in acute renal failure. Ren Fail 1993; 15:47–49.

210. Acker CG, Singh AR, Flick RP, et al: A trial of thyroxine in acute renal failure. Kidney Int 2000; 57:293–298.

211. Koletsky S: Effects of temporary interruption of renal circulation in rats. Arch Pathol 1954; 58:592–603.

212. Fox M: Progressive renal fibrosis following tubular necrosis: an experimental study. J Urol 1967; 97:196–202.

213. Finn WF: Enhanced recovery from postischemic acute renal failure: micropuncture studies in the rat. Circ Res 1980; 46:440–448.

214. Wyllie AH, Kerr JFR, Currie AR: Cell death: the significance of apoptosis. Int Rev Cytol 1980; 68:251–305.

215. Ucker DS: Cytotoxic T lymphocytes and glucocorticoids activate an endogenous suicide process in target cells. Nature (London) 1987; 327:62–64.

216. Arends MJ, Morris RG, Wyllie AH: Apoptosis: the role of the endonuclease. Am J Pathol 1990; 136:593–608.

217. Kerr JFR, Wyllie AH, Currie AR: Apoptosis: a basic biological phenomenon with wide-ranging implications in tissue kinetics. Br J Cancer 1972; 26:239–257.

218. Buttyan R, Olsson CA, Pintar J, et al: Induction of the TRPM-2 gene in cells undergoing programmed death. Mol Cell Biol 1989; 9:3473–3481.

219. Schumer M, Colombel MC, Sawczuk IS, et al: Morphologic, biochemical, and molecular evidence of apoptosis during the reperfusion phase after brief periods of renal ischemia. Am J Pathol 1992; 140:831–838.

220. Gobe G, Willgoss D, Hogg N, et al: Cell survival or death in renal tubular epithelium after ischemia-reperfusion injury. Kidney Int 1999; 56:1299–1304.

221. Shirnizu A, Yamanaka N: Apoptosis and cell desquamation in repair process of ischemic tubular necrosis. Virchows Arch B Cell Pathol 1993; 64:171–180.

222. Savill J: Apoptosis and renal injury. Curr Opin Nephrol Hypertens 1995; 4:263–269.

223. Dharnidharka VR, Nadeau K, Cannon CL, et al: Ciprofloxacin overdose: acute renal failure with prominent apoptotic changes. Am J Kidney Dis 1998; 31:710–712.

224. Takeda M, Fukuoka K, Endou H: Cisplatin-induced apoptosis in mouse proximal tubular cell line. Contrib Nephrol 1996; 118:24–28.

225. Sano K, Fujigaki Y, Ikegaya N, et al: The roles of apoptosis in uranyl acetate–induced acute renal failure. Ren Fail 1998; 20:697–701.

226. Takeda T: A patholomorphological study on damage and repair

227. Seegers JC, Bohmer LH, Kruger MC, et al: A comparative study of ochratoxin A–induced apoptosis in hamster kidney and HeLa cells. Toxicol Appl Pharmacol 1994; 129:1–11.

228. Jaffe R, Ariel I, Beeri R, et al: Frequent apoptosis in human kidneys after acute renal hypoperfusion. Exp Nephrol 1997; 5:399–403.

229. Olsen TS, Olsen HS, Hansen HE: Tubular ultrastructure in acute renal failure in man: epithelial necrosis and regeneration. Virchows Arch A Pathol Anat Histopathol 1985; 406:75–89.

230. Olsen S, Burdick JF, Keown PA, et al: Primary acute renal failure ("acute tubular necrosis") in the transplanted kidney: morphology and pathogenesis. Medicine 1989; 68:173–187.

231. Gobe GC, Axelsen RA, Searle JW: Cellular events in experimental unilateral ischemic renal atrophy and in regeneration after contralateral nephrectomy. Lab Invest 1990; 63:770–779.

232. Gobe GC, Axelsen RA: Genesis of renal tubular atrophy in experimental hydronephrosis in the rat: role of apoptosis. Lab Invest 1987; 56:273–281.

233. Kennedy WA, Stenberg A, Lackgren G, et al: Renal tubular apoptosis after partial ureteral obstruction. J Urol 1994; 152:658–664.

234. Racusen LC: Biology of disease: alterations in tubular epithelial cell adhesion and mechanisms of acute renal failure. Lab Invest 1989; 67:173–187.

235. Kerr JF: Shrinkage necrosis: a distinct mode of cellular death. J Pathol 1971; 105:13–20.

236. Wyllie AH, Kerr JFR, Currie AR: Adrenocortical cell deletion: the role of ACTH. J Pathol 1973; 111:85–94.

237. Wyllie AH, Kerr JFR, Currie AR: Cell death: the significance of apoptosis. Int Rev Cytol 1980; 68:251–305.

238. Pound AW, Walker NI: Involution of the pancreas after ligation of the pancreatic duct. I. A histological study. Br J Exp Pathol 1981; 62:547–558.

239. Dharnidharka VR, Nadeau K, Cannon CL, et al: Ciprofloxacin overdose: acute renal failure with prominent apoptotic changes. Am J Kidney Dis 1998; 31:710–712.

240. Takeda T: A patholomorphological study on damage and repair process of tubuli after renal ischemia. Jpn J Nephrol 1996; 38:493–501.

241. Megyesi J, Safirstein RL, Price PM: J Clin Invest 1998; 101:777–782.

242. Nakajima T, Miyaji T, Kato A, et al: Uninephrectomy reduces apoptotic cell death and enhances renal tubular cell regeneration in ischemic ARF in rats. Am J Physiol 1996; 271:F846–F853.

243. Hammerman MR: Growth factors and apoptosis in acute renal injury. Curr Opin Nephrol Hypertens 1998; 7:419–424.

244. Ortiz A: Apoptotic regulatory proteins in renal injury. Kidney Int 2000; 58:467–485.

245. Gobe G, Zhang XJ, Cuttle L, et al: Bcl-2 genes and growth factors in the pathology of ischemic acute renal failure. Immunol Cell Biol 1999; 77:279–286.

246. Vukicevic S, Basic V, Rogic D, et al: Osteogenic protein-1 (bone morphogenetic protein-7) reduces severity of injury after ischemic acute renal failure in rat. J Clin Invest 1998; 102:202–214.

247. Lieberthal W, Koh JS, Levine JS: Necrosis and apoptosis in acute renal failure. Semin Nephrol 1998; 18:505–518.

248. Ueda N, Kaushal GP, Shah SV: Recent advances in understanding mechanisms of renal tubular injury. Adv Ren Replace Ther 1997; 4(suppl 1):17–24.

249. Safirstein R: Renal stress response and acute renal failure. Adv Ren Replace Therapy 1997; 4(suppl 2):38–42.

250. Hinman F: Experimental hydronephrosis: repair following ureterocystoneostomy in white rats with complete ureteral obstruction. J Urol 1919; 3:147–174.

251. Hinman F: Renal counterbalance: an experimental and clinical study with reference to the significance of disuse atrophy. Trans Am Assoc Genitourinary Surg 1922; 15:241–392.

252. Hinman F: The condition of renal counterbalance and the theory of renal atrophy of disease. J Urol 1943; 49:392–400.

253. Hinman F: Renal counterbalance. AMA Arch Surg 1926; 12:1105–1223.

254. Joelson JJ, Beck CS, Moritz AR: Renal counterbalance. Arch Surg 1929; 19:673–711.

CHAPTER 36

Inflammatory Cells in Renal Damage and Regeneration

Dirk K. Ysebaert ▪ Kathleen E. De Greef ▪ Marc E. De Broe

INTRODUCTION

Acute renal failure (ARF) is a common renal disease affecting about 5% of all hospitalized patients. ARF still carries a very high mortality of more than 50%, and there has been almost no significant change in mortality over the last four decades.[1-3] The kidney is highly vulnerable to the deleterious effects of renal hypoperfusion (ischemia) and to many toxic substances or a combination of both. Renal ischemia-reperfusion (I-R) injury is the major cause of ARF in the native[4] as well as in the transplanted kidney.[5] Although numerous substances have been tested, there is no specific treatment for this devastating clinical syndrome, reflecting, in part, the relatively poor understanding of the pathophysiology of this disease.[4]

Although the decline in renal function may be very pronounced and protracted, it is remarkable that the acutely injured kidney has a striking capacity to restore function. As opposed to chronic renal failure, in the majority of cases of ARF the kidney regains complete functionality in the absence of interstitial inflammation and fibrosis. The regeneration process responsible for this functional and morphologic recovery is one of the major research topics in nephrology.[6] A manifest and intriguing effect during acute tubular necrosis (ATN) and repair is the prompt appearance, immediately following injury, and disappearance of inflammatory cells when the regeneration is complete. Both detrimental and regenerative ("clean-up" function-potential) are terms that have been ascribed to these cells.[7] Although the literature on the possible role of these interstitial leukocytes is abundant, their exact initiating and resolving mechanisms, and their effect on early and final outcome of ARF, are still unclear. This chapter discusses the infiltrating network of leukocytes as a major participant in the successful or unsuccessful regeneration process after ARF, including the different approaches that can be followed to investigate the role of these cells in ARF.

A better understanding of the repair mechanisms is critical to the creation and implementation of effective therapies.[8] This chapter discusses the types of leukocytes involved, their appearance at different points in time during the course of ARF, and their possible roles in both injury and repair.

LEUKOCYTES AFTER ACUTE RENAL FAILURE

Leukocyte infiltration in response to ischemic or toxic injury is a well-known phenomenon, which is not only present in models of chronic renal failure but also is particularly very pronounced in ARF. Despite much attention to the role attributed to leukocytes in renal injury, the composition and the kinetics of this infiltrate in relation to the evolution of the pathology are still not clearly defined. Ischemia-reperfusion injury, perhaps best studied in the heart, is clearly associated with an increase in infiltrating neutrophils, as depletion of these phagocytes diminishes myocardial injury. In the kidney, polymorphonuclear leukocytes (PMNs) recruited during reperfusion have long been considered critical mediators of the early parenchymal injury in ischemic ARF.[8] However, there is still a lack of clear evidence demonstrating that the number of PMNs have a critical role on their own in the initiation or outcome of ARF.[9] On the other hand, the presence of monocytes-macrophages and T cells in experimental models as well as in clinical renal pathology seems to be consistent (Table 36–1).[10-23] Depending on the renal insult, the kinetics of this mononuclear infiltrate (monocytes-macrophages and T-cells) may vary as well as the participation of other leukocytes (eg, B cells, PMNs). Only in situations of pyelonephritis and ureteric obstruction is there a distinct PMN infiltration. It is remarkable that macrophages and both subsets of T lymphocytes remain localized predominantly in the zone of most severe injury. Provided that the insult is not sustained, this infiltrate remains as long as, but no longer than, the duration of the process restoring renal tubular morphology.[24]

Renal injury after ischemia appears to be a consequence not only of tissue hypoxia from interrupted blood supply but also of the process of reperfusion leading to an active inflammatory response, consisting of the recruitment of leukocytes from the peripheral circulation and of the proliferation of resident interstitial cells. This process is triggered by sublethal or even lethal injured endothelial and proximal tubular cells through the release of cytokines and chemokines that promote cellular infiltration.

The recruitment of leukocytes to the side of injury consists of a series of coordinated steps (Fig. 36–1). The following adhesion cascade can be divided into four sequential steps of tethering, triggering, strong adhesion, and transendothelial migration. This complex process is mediated by different major leukocyte adhesion molecules and their ligands (Table 36–2). After the initial insult, an array of chemoattractants, cytokines, and complement is released, generated by the local inflammatory area, activating the endothelium and the leukocytes. Leukocyte–endothelial cell

TABLE 36–1. Interstitial Leukocytes in Clinical and Experimental Acute Renal Failure

EXPERIMENTAL MODELS FOR ARF	INJURED NEPHRON SEGMENT	MONONUCLEAR CELLS					PMN	PLATELETS
		Macrophages	T cells		B cells	NK cells		
			Th	Ts/c				
Ischemia-reperfusion[10, 11]	PST (S3), TAL (PCT)	+ +	+ +	+	−	?	+ +/?	?
Gentamicin[12]	PCT	+ +	+	+	?	?	?	?
Mercuric chloride[13]	PST (S3)	+ +	+ +	+	−	−	−	−
Cisplatinum[14]	PST (S3)	?	?	?	?	?	+ +/?	?
Lithium chloride[15]	DCT, CD	+	±	?	?	?	?	?
Cyclosporin A[16]	PCT, PST	+ +	+		+	?	−	?
Adriamycin nephrosis[17]	Proximal	+ +	?	+	?	?	?	?
5-ASA[18]	—	+	+	+	+	?	−	?
PAN-nephrosis[19]	Glomerular + proximal	+ +	±	+	?	?	?	?
Protein-overloaded proteinuria[20]	Proximal	+ +	±	+	?	?	−	?
Urethral obstruction[21]	Distal	+ +	+	+	−	?	+ + +	?
Pyelonephritis[22]	Variable	?	−		?	?	+ + +	?
5/6 Nephrectomy[23]	—	+ +	+		−	−	−	?

+ +, + = present; ± = probably present; − = not present; ? = unclear.

5-ASA, oral megalamine; *NK,* natural killer; *PMN,* polymorphonuclear cells; *PAN,* puromycin of aminonucleoside; *PST,* proximal straight tubule; *PCT,* proximal convoluted tubule; *DCT,* distal convoluted tubule; *CD,* collecting duct; *TAL,* thick ascending limb.

adherence depends on adhesion molecules both on the leukocyte and on the endothelial cell. Up-regulation of local and systemic cytokines, such as tumor necrosis factor-alpha (TNF-α), interleukin-1 (IL-1), IL-2, and IL-8,[25, 26] provides a possible mechanism of up-regulation of intercellular adhesion molecule-1 (ICAM-1),[27, 28] and others such as E-selectin and P-selectin,[10] in postischemic-toxic renal tissue. Ischemia-reperfusion is associated with complement activation and increased levels of lipid mediators, such as leukotrienes and platelet-activating factor (PAF), which are chemotactic for neutrophils.[29, 30] When the endothelium becomes activated by cytokines (triggering), there is rapid translocation of integrins from cytoplasmic granules to the plasma membrane of the endothelial cell. Tethering interactions between the leukocyte and endothelial cell slow down the leukocyte, mediated by selectins and their ligands. Firm adhesion between the endothelium and the leukocyte takes place, mediated by integrins and intercellular adhesion molecules. Adherent and activated leukocytes, among them PMNs in particular, release reactive oxygen species, myeloperoxidase (MPO), proteases, elastases, leukotrienes, and other enzymes that damage the ischemic tissue directly, en-

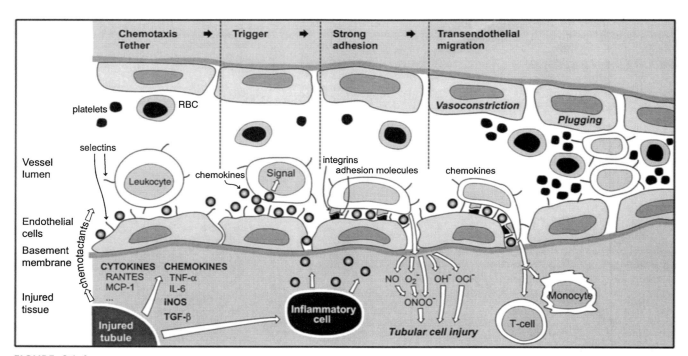

FIGURE 36–1 ■ Sequential steps in the activation, adhesion, and infiltration of leukocytes to endothelium and interstitium. *IL-6,* interleukin-6; *iNOS,* inducible nitric oxide synthase; *MCP-1,* monocyte chemotactic protein-1; *RANTES,* regulated on T-cell activation, normal T-cell expressed and secreted; *TGF-β,* transforming growth factor-β; *TNF-α,* tumor necrosis factor-α.

TABLE 36–2. Classification, Cellular Distribution, Ligands, and Target Cells for Major Leukocyte Adhesion Molecules

MAJOR FAMILIES	INDIVIDUAL MEMBERS	ALTERNATE NOMENCLATURE	CELLULAR DISTRIBUTION	LIGANDS ON TARGET CELLS	TARGET CELLS
Lectins	L-selectin	LAM-1, LECCAM-1, MEL-14, Leu-8, TQ-1, DREG.56	Leukocytes	Glycoproteins, glycolipids	Endothelial cells, other?
	P-selectin	CD62, GMP140, PADGEM, LECCAM-3	Platelets, endothelial	Glycoproteins, glycolipids	Granulocytes, monocytes, T-cell subsets, some cancer cells
	E-selectin	ELAM-1, LECCAM-2	Endothelial	Glycoproteins, glycolipids	Neutrophils, monocytes, lymphocyte subsets, some cancer cells
Carbohydrate ligands for selectins	Sulfated polysaccharides (GlyCAM-1)	Sgp50, mucin-like	Endothelium	L-selectin	Lymphocytes, other?
	Oligosaccharides (sialyl lewis[s])	SLe[x]	Granulocytes, monocytes, lymphocytes	E-selectin P-selectin	Endothelium, platelets
Integrins	VLA-4 (b-1)	LPAM-2	Monocytes, lymphocytes, eosinophils	VCAM-1 fibronectin	Endothelium, epithelial, mesangial, vascular, smooth muscle
	CD11a/CD18 (b-2)	LFA-1, TA-1	Leukocytes	ICAM-1, ICAM-2	Endothelial, epithelial, mesangial, vascular, smooth muscle
	CD11b/CD18 (b-2)	Mac-a, Mo1, OKM1, gp160	Granulocytes, monocytes	ICAM-1, C3bi, fibrinogen, other	Endothelial, epithelial, mesangial, vascular, smooth muscle
	CD11c/CD18 (b-2)	P150,95; LeuM5	Granulocytes, monocytes	Not characterized	Endothelial, mesangial
Ig-like	ICAM-1	CD54	Endothelial, epithelial, mesangial, smooth muscle, some cancer cells	CD11a/CD18 CD11b/CD18	Most leukocytes
	ICAM-2		Endothelial	CD11a/CD18	Most leukocytes
	VCAM-1	INCAM 110	Endothelial, epithelial, mesangial, smooth muscle	VLA-4	Monocytes, lymphocytes, eosinophils
	PECAM-1	EndoCAM, CD31	Endothelial, platelets, some leukocytes	PECAM-1	Some leukocytes, endothelial, platelets

From Brady HR: Leukocyte adhesion molecules and kidney diseases. Kidney Int 1994; 45:1285–1300; with permission.

hance additional inflammatory cell infiltration, and increase vasoconstriction.[31] These substances, together with leukotriene B$_4$ and PAF, generated by the infiltrating cells, increase vascular permeability and up-regulate adhesion molecule expression, thereby promoting further inflammation. In addition, interaction of neutrophils and other leukocytes with the endothelium may cause capillary plugging, which can interfere with the restitution of blood flow to areas of the kidney on reperfusion, even though total renal blood flow is restored ("no-reflow phenomenon").[32] Adhesion and subsequent transendothelial migration take place preferentially at peculiar sites in blood vessels, namely, the postcapillary venules.[33, 34] After strong adhesion, flattening of the leukocyte occurs, followed by a migration step. Migration through the basement membrane takes place by the release of proteases, produced by the emigrating leukocyte.

Proliferation of leukocytes in the interstitium is the secondary mechanism by which leukocytes accumulate in the renal interstitium. Such in-situ proliferation of interstitial macrophages was clearly demonstrated by double immunohistochemical staining (proliferating cell nuclear antigen [PCNA] and ED-1 cell staining) in the renal interstitium in an experimental model of toxic injury.[35, 36]

TYPES OF INFLAMMATORY CELLS

Inflammatory Cells in Injury (0–24 h)

After severe warm ischemia-reperfusion injury of the rat kidney, pronounced ATN can be noticed after 24 hours in the absence of a marked cellular infiltrate. In this very early, critical period postischemia, important MPO activity can be noticed, which most authors interpret as a reflection of significant PMN infiltration.[27, 28, 37] Polymorphonuclear cells recruited during reperfusion have long been implicated as critical mediators of the early renal parenchymal injury in ischemic ARF.[8] These assumptions were supported not only by MPO assay but also by other enzymatic criteria, such as chloroacetate esterase[25, 38–40] or labeling techniques (eg, [111]indium labeling[41]), all considered specific for PMN infiltration. Neutrophilic presence, however, investigated by others using hematoxylin and eosin (H&E) staining, revealed only a few neutrophils in glomeruli, medullary rays, and the outer strip of the outer medulla (OSOM).[11, 42] These so-called PMN-specific staining techniques (eg, MPO, chloroacetate esterase), however, do not distinguish the difference between macrophages and PMNs.[9] Indeed, the presence of macrophages after renal injury can not be ignored: significant monocyte-macrophage adhesion-infiltration (ED-1 staining) occurred at the OSOM already at 12 to 24 hours postischemia (Fig. 36–2). Also, the observation that monocytes and macrophages infiltrated the ischemic kidney within the first 24 hours, their number being 12 to 25 times higher than the present number of PMNs, contributes to solving the controversy about the number of PMNs in postische-

mic injury. The highly significant correlation between the interstitial macrophages and the renal functional impairment has refocused attention on the importance of macrophages in renal injury.[43] Macrophages, like PMNs, are capable of secreting a wide array of reactive oxygen species, nitric oxide, MPO, proinflammatory cytokines, and growth factors. Indeed, monocytes and macrophages also contribute to the initial ischemic damage not only by production of reactive oxygen species but also by production of MPO when activated.[44, 45] Hence, the MPO content of postischemic tissue reflects the presence of PMNs as well as activated residential interstitial macrophages and freshly emigrated monocytes-macrophages in inflamed tissue.[46, 47] The relationship between these accumulated cells and the onset of ARF is still a matter for debate. In any case, this observation has serious implications when one uses enzymatic tests such as MPO content in renal postischemic tissue as the sole indicator of PMN infiltration. The same holds true for other so-called cell-specific stains for PMNs, such as chloroacetate esterase,[25, 38–40] specific Mabs for PMNs (eg, as HIS-48),[48] and labeling techniques (eg, [111]indium labeling[41]); none of these methods has proved to be specific for this particular cell type and can cross-react with monocytes-macrophages. Hematoxylin and eosin staining (morphology of cell nucleus) remains the gold standard for identification of PMNs, while MPO assays or chloroacetate esterase (Leder) staining should be regarded as tools for quantitating both PMNs and monocytes-macrophages. These observations explain the conflicting results in the literature concerning the presence of PMNs in I-R syndrome: using routine (H&E) histologic stains, infiltration of the renal parenchyma by PMNs seemed not to be a prominent feature of human postischemic ARF or experimental ARF, whereas studies using the previously mentioned, so-called specialized stains for PMNs, based on enzymatic or on physiologic criteria, suggest robust PMN recruitment to ischemic kidney.[4, 9]

The suggestion that both PMNs and macrophages contribute to the MPO activity of postischemic kidney still does not explain the early MPO activity observed in the first 12 hours after the start of reperfusion,[27, 28] measured in the absence of a significant increased presence of inflammatory cells. Indeed, macrophages begin to infiltrate the postischemic kidney only 8 to 12 hours after reperfusion, a time when the MPO activity has already reached its maximal level. It could be argued that in the first phase PMNs and monocytes-macrophages do not infiltrate early after reperfusion but adhere to the activated endothelium only long enough to release their enzymes (eg, MPO). In this respect, MPO activity is more reflective, in fact, of the activation of the adhering inflammatory cells and of residential interstitial macrophages, resulting from postischemic chemotactic and other cytokine activation, than of infiltration itself. It could be argued that in this first critical phase, these activated inflammatory cells adhere to the vascular endothelium and simply block or slow down the vascular flow in the capillary network,[8] and thereafter reenter the systemic circula-

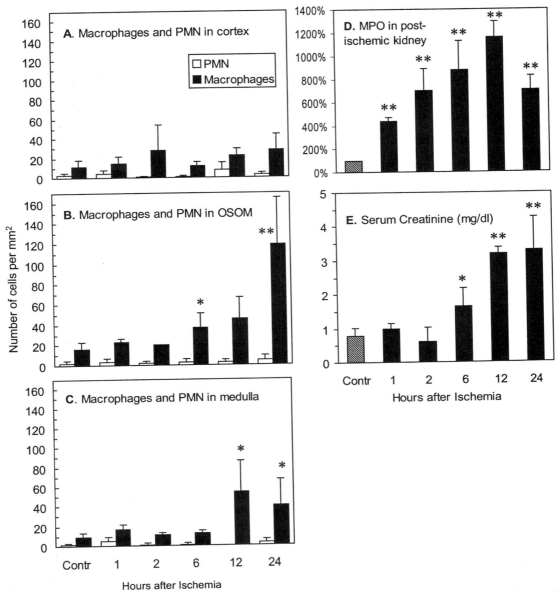

FIGURE 36–2 ■ Early PMN-macrophage accumulation post I-R versus renal function and renal MPO-assay during the first 24 hours post I-R. *A–C,* Relationship of monocyte-macrophage and neutrophil adhesion-infiltration in cortex, OSOM, and medulla. *Dark bars* indicate the number of monocytes-macrophages/mm². *Light bars* indicate the number of PMNs/mm². *D,* MPO activity in postischemic kidney (*dark bars*), normalized to the protein content of the supernatant, expressed as the percentage of levels in kidneys subjected to sham surgery (*striped bar*). *E,* Renal function as measured by the serum creatinine level (mg/dL) in postischemic animals (*dark bars*) versus controls without ischemia (*striped bar*). * indicates $P < 0.05$; ** indicates $P < 0.01$. (Adapted from Ysebaert DK, De Greef KE, Ghielli M, et al: Identification and kinetics of leukocytes after severe ischemia/reperfusion renal injury. Nephrol Dial Transplant 2000; 15:1562–1574; with permission.)

tion ("hit-and-run" phenomenon). In a later phase, firm adhesion and diapedesis take place, generating the classic infiltration and proliferation observed in many conditions (eg, ischemia, corrosive mercuric chloride [HgCl₂], obstruction). Hence, the beneficial functional effect of antiadhesion therapy with, for example, antibodies to ICAM-1 and leukocyte function–associated antigen 1 (LFA-1) seems to have its explanation early at the level of the microcirculation or at the level of inflammatory cell activation, but not necessarily at the level of the interstitial infiltrate, becoming apparent only at the time the functional recovery is already operational. In conclusion, new evidence indicates that the activation and adherence of the inflammatory cells very early after I-R seem to be more important in exacerbating postischemic damage than the phenomenon of infiltration itself. This appealing paradigm needs further investigation.

Inflammatory Cells During Regeneration (1–14 Days)

As outlined previously, a manifest effect during ATN and repair is the increased presence of inflammatory cells and the occurrence of interstitial edema. The presence of monocytes-macrophages and T cells in experimental models as well as in clinical renal pathology seems to be consistent (see Table 36–1). Depending on the renal pathology, the kinetics of this mononuclear infiltrate (monocytes-macrophages and T cells) may vary, as well as the participation of other leukocytes (eg, B cells, PMNs). Their exact initiating and resolving mechanisms and their effect on the early and final outcomes of ARF need further study.

Although many data are available concerning the overall cellular infiltrate after injury, only scarce information can be found on the presence, number, and time course of the different subsets of these infiltrating (and proliferating) leukocytes. A mixed mononuclear-cell (macrophage and CD4⁺ cell) infiltration of the kidney within a few days after I-R was described after warm ischemia of 45°C[10, 49] and after experimental cold ischemia,[10] but there is limited information about the different topographic localizations. In the latter and in many other studies, no important neutrophilic infiltration was mentioned, while even very recently, other researchers, using enzymatic tests and membrane markers, have described mainly neutrophilic infiltration.[25, 40, 50] The identification and quantification of the interstitial leukocytes in the rat kidney after ischemia-reperfusion injury demonstrated a sequential accumulation of monocytes-macrophages and helper T cells, a few suppressor-cytotoxic T cells, and no B cells (Fig. 36–3). The total number of neutrophils remained low in this model of renal I-R injury.[11] This mononuclear leukocyte infiltrate is most prominent at the time of full regeneration but after functional recovery. Interestingly, these observations are very similar to those noted after gentamicin or mercuric chloride toxicant-induced ARF (Fig. 36–4).[12, 13]

The fact that a mononuclear leukocyte infiltrate is most prominent at the site of the most injured tissue, and at the time of full regeneration suggests that it has a role in the repair process after ARF.[11] The macrophages in this mononuclear cell infiltrate can be regarded as phagocytes, acting as important scavengers of apoptotic cells or necrotic debris.[4] These infiltrating inflammatory cells may also be a source of growth-stimulating substances,[12, 51] suggesting a role in the repair process after ARF. Indeed, in the repair process, much research has been focused on the endogenously produced growth factors as major mediators of tubular epithelial cell proliferation. However, in different experimental models of ARF, an early decrease of renal epidermal growth factor (EGF) and insulin-like growth factor-1 (IGF-1), at both the mRNA and the protein level, frequently has been shown, while increases in other growth factors could not be demonstrated.[12] Exogenous administration of IGF-1 was moderately active in the prevention of postoperative renal dysfunction in high-risk patients,[52] as was EGF in post–I-R ARF in rats.[53] The inaccessibility of the up-regulated receptors for endogenously produced growth factors has encouraged research to seek alternative origins of the signals that induce renal regeneration. Here is a possible particular role for the infiltrating leukocyte, attracted by the injured proximal tubular cell, which is the source of chemokines released after sublethal or lethal injury. The role of the macrophage in wound healing is well known, because wound healing has been shown to be retarded in macrophage depletion[54] and enhanced in rodents with local macrophage injections.[55]

The existence of a regenerative potential provided by the network of infiltrating mononuclear leukocytes is supported by studies on tissue repair in different fields. Activated mononuclear cells can produce various kinds of growth factors able to promote epithelialization, angiogenesis, and extracellular matrix turnover, all of which are necessary for the realization of the different steps of wound repair.[56, 57] Evidence exists that macrophages and T lymphocytes produce different growth factors, for example, transforming growth factor-alpha (TGF-α; stimulation of epithelialization), fibroblast growth factor (stimulation of epithelialization), PAF (angiogenesis), and TGF-β (extracellular matrix turnover).[58] The delivery of these factors locally at the site of injury may create a microenvironment in which high growth factor concentration can exert its effect on renal tubular cells, so that regeneration would not depend solely on the ability of residential cells to produce and release sufficient amounts of growth-promoting substances.

Long-Term Effects of Persistent Inflammatory Cells (14 Days–3 Months)

The kidney exhibits a remarkable ability to recover from acute (ischemic) injury. When injury is severe and protracted, however, kidney function may not completely return to normal.[59] While wound repairs usually are self-limited and tightly controlled by homeostatic mechanisms that regulate fibrosis, this regu-

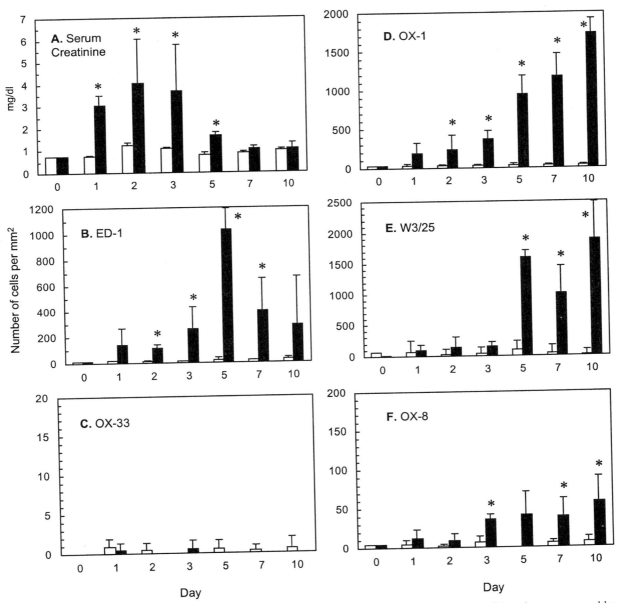

FIGURE 36–3 ▪ Renal function versus renal interstitial infiltrate during the first 10 days post I-R. *A,* Renal function as measured by serum creatinine level (mg/dL) in postischemic animals (*dark bars*) versus controls (uni-nephrectomy without ischemia) (*light bars*). * indicates $P <$ 0.05. *B–F,* Leukocyte infiltrate expressed as number/mm². *Dark bars* indicate post–I-R animals, after warm ischemia of 60°C on the remaining left kidney. *Light bars* indicate control animals without ischemia. * indicates $P < 0.05$. *ED-1,* macrophages; *OX-33,* B cells; *OX-1,* panleukocytes; *W3/25,* CD4⁺ helper T cells (and macrophages); *OX-8,* CD8⁺ suppressor-cytotoxic T cells. (Adapted from Ysebaert DK, De Greef KE, Ghielli M, et al: Identification and kinetics of leukocytes after severe ischemia/reperfusion renal injury. Nephrol Dial Transplant 2000; 15:1562–1574; with permission.)

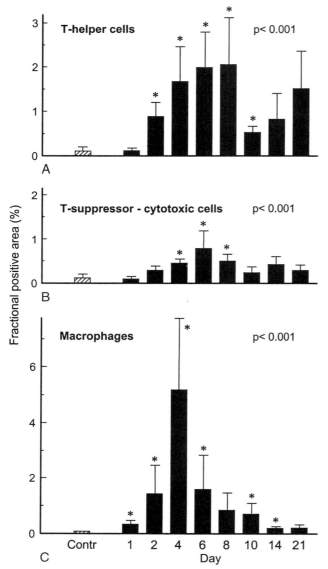

FIGURE 36–4 ■ Interstitial infiltrate in mercuric chloride–treated rats (single injection 2.5 mg/kg SC; control rats received saline) during the first 21 days. Analysis of cellular infiltration in six randomly chosen fields from outer stripe of outer medulla (OSOM). *A,* Fractional positive area taken by CD4$^+$ cells (helper T cells and macrophages). *B,* Fractional positive area taken by CD8$^+$ cells (suppressor-cytotoxic T cells). *C,* Fractional positive area taken by ED-1 cells (macrophages). (Adapted from Verstrepen WA, Nouwen EJ, Zhu MG, et al: Time course of growth factor expression in mercuric chloride acute renal failure. Nephrol Dial Transplant 1995; 10:1361–1371; with permission.)

of tubular damage and of interstitial infiltration. As a consequence, tubular cells can become activated and begin to express several cytokines–growth factors, adhesion molecules, and extracellular matrix components, creating a profibrogenic milieu.[60] Overproduction of these matrix components results in fibrosis, which ultimately leads to permanent loss of normal integrity and function of the kidney. In a more recently acquired perception, this fibrotic process is the result of a disturbed balance between quite normal extracellular matrix (ECM) production and the up-regulated expression of inhibitors of ECM degradation, plasminogen activator inhibitor type 1 (PAI-1), and tissue inhibitor of matrix metalloproteinase type 1 (TIMP-1).[62]

There is a considerable amount of evidence that infiltrating cells participate in this process. Studies in postischemic unique rat kidneys have shown that incomplete recovery from acute and protracted injury may be followed by progressive renal injury, with widespread segmental glomerulosclerosis and tubulointerstitial disease, together with proteinuria.[49] A prominent feature of this tubulointerstitial disease is a persistent, mixed mononuclear infiltrate, consisting of ED1$^+$ macrophages and CD4$^+$ lymphocytes (but not CD8$^+$ cells). This infiltrating network of mononuclear leukocytes is a major participant in the successful or unsuccessful regeneration process after ARF. Despite an intervening period during which apparently complete resolution of the initial insult has occurred, mechanisms contributing to chronic injury had been initiated: the temporal relationship of macrophage infiltration, together with their derived products (monocyte chemotactic protein-1 [MCP-1], IL-1, IL-6, TGF-β), suggests that these cells contribute to the development of subsequent injury to the kidney. Certainly, the increased deposition of extracellular matrix by tubular cells, fibroblasts, and also by macrophages, through TGF-β up-regulation, results in the formation of fibrogenous tissue, partially replacing the original functional tissue[53] (Fig. 36–5).

In humans, this process is also illustrated by the observation that impairment of graft function immediately after transplantation ("delayed graft function"), due to mixed ischemic and toxic etiology, is associated with an increased risk of chronic graft failure.[5, 63] This tubulointerstitial disease is characterized by tubular atrophy, patchy interstitial fibrosis, and modest infiltration of mononuclear cells, features of injury that are regularly associated with chronic renal disease.

ROLE OF INFLAMMATORY CELLS IN POST–ARF INJURY AND REGENERATION

The accumulation of mononuclear leukocytes in the renal interstitium is a striking observation in ARF. Whereas interstitial disease, recognized by the persistent interstitial accumulation of leukocytes, is a better predictor of chronic renal failure and developing fibrosis, ARF resulting from other causes distinguishes itself by the prompt appearance of mononuclear leukocytes, followed by the disappearance of this infiltrate

lation process deteriorates, for reasons that are yet unclear, during episodes of persistent inflammation. Also, in the kidney, fibrosis is particularly devastating when it appears and persists as a sequela to persistent inflammation post–ARF injury.[60]

It is thought that this progressive loss of kidney function results from a pathogenic process that is independent of the original etiology, functioning as a final common pathway.[61] Initially, this common final pathway is characterized by the triggering of the induction

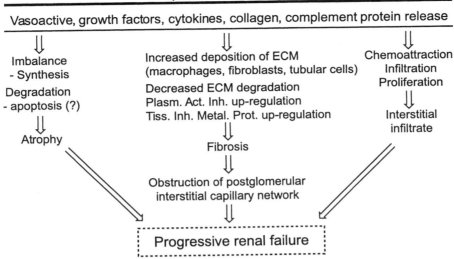

Acute severe/protracted post I/R or toxic ARF

Vasoactive, growth factors, cytokines, collagen, complement protein release

Imbalance
- Synthesis
Degradation
- apoptosis (?)

⇓

Atrophy

Increased deposition of ECM
(macrophages, fibroblasts, tubular cells)
Decreased ECM degradation
Plasm. Act. Inh. up-regulation
Tiss. Inh. Metal. Prot. up-regulation

⇓

Fibrosis

Chemoattraction
Infiltration
Proliferation

⇓

Interstitial
infiltrate

Obstruction of postglomerular
interstitial capillary network

⇓

Progressive renal failure

FIGURE 36–5 ■ Mechanisms of tubulointerstitial injury in progressive renal diseases after acute severe or protracted ARF. *ECM,* extracellular matrix. *ECM,* extracellular membrane; *Plasm Act Inh,* Plasminogen activator inhibitor; *tiss inh metal prot,* tissue inhibitor metalloproteinese. (Adapted from Fine LG, Ong AC, Norman JT: Mechanisms of tubulo-interstitial injury in progressive renal diseases. Eur J Clin Invest 1993; 23:259-265; with permission.)

when regeneration is complete. The role of these leukocytes is still a controversial issue. Until recently, this leukocyte infiltrate, particularly the PMNs among them, was mostly regarded as a damaging event, exacerbating I-R damage. Indeed, activated leukocytes directly injure endothelial and renal tubular cells by releasing a number of potent oxidants, like peroxynitrite and hypochlorous acid[64] (see Fig. 36–1). In addition to causing oxidant injury, leukocytes may also contribute indirectly to tubular injury by exacerbating the medullary hypoperfusion that follows an ischemic or toxic insult to the kidney.[65] Activated leukocytes can also exacerbate intrarenal vasoconstriction by releasing a number of vasoactive factors, including thromboxane A_2, leukotriene B_4, and PAF.[66] On the other hand, the existence of a regenerative potential provided by the network of inflammatory mononuclear leukocytes is supported by studies on tissue repair in different fields: infiltrating leukocytes as important scavengers of apoptotic cells or necrotic cellular debris and as a possible source of growth-stimulating substances,[12, 51] suggesting a role in the repair process after ARF.

Hence, with respect to the treatment of ARF, it is worthwhile to investigate whether it is beneficial to impede or to enhance the infiltration of these inflammatory cells as a whole or only certain subsets of these leukocytes. Recent breakthroughs in leukocyte adhesion molecule research have prompted reevaluation of the role of leukocytes in the pathophysiology of ischemic ARF.[4]

To investigate whether the inflammatory cells in the kidney play a biological role in the process of damage or regeneration or both, several methods are employed to prevent their interstitial accumulation (Table 36–3). One method used frequently was the removal of leukocytes from the circulation and from tissues (depletion). In order to evaluate the pathophysiologic role of infiltrating neutrophils, studies using antineu-

trophil serum have demonstrated a pathogenic role of neutrophils.[37, 67] Ex vivo studies of ischemic kidneys have also demonstrated a deleterious role for neutrophils.[41] However, other studies with antineutrophil serum have failed to demonstrate a pathogenic role for neutrophils.[38, 42] The studies that showed a protective effect of neutrophil depletion were characterized by induction of extremely low neutrophil counts, while studies that did not show renal protection reduced neutrophils to even a lesser extent. Thus, even small numbers of neutrophils can apparently exert significant deleterious action. The controversy regarding the role of neutrophils is certainly ongoing. Although many conclusions on the role of PMNs in ischemic damage are based on the use of such polyclonal antineutrophil serum, there are concerns about the specificity of this polyclonal antineutrophil serum. The effects of a heterologous antiserum do not seem to be limited to the single cell type used as an immunogen.

TABLE 36–3. Methods for Investigating the Role of Infiltrating Inflammatory Cells in Renal Injury-Regeneration

Experimental approaches
  depletion of
    leukocytes (pan-leukocytes)
    subsets of leukocytes
  athymic rats
  antiadhesion approach:
    antibodies to adhesion molecules (eg, ICAM-1, LFA-1)
    antisense oligonucleotides for ICAM-1
    ICAM-1 knockout mice
  B7-CD28 costimulatory pathway
  anti-inflammatory therapy:
    α-melanocyte–stimulating hormone
    osteogenic protein-1

ICAM-1, intercellular adhesion molecule-1; *LFA*-1, leukocyte function–associated antigen-1.

Administration of antineutrophil serum results in a 50% to 70% decrease of monocytes within 12 hours.[68] Most studies in which an antineutrophil serum was used lack data concerning the effect on other cell types.[9] In addition, even monoclonal antibodies, which are considered to be specific for PMNs (eg, HIS-48, RP1, and RP3), react with epitopes on macrophages.[11] So, when using polyclonal or monoclonal antibodies, their cell specificity should be examined carefully before drawing definite conclusions.

Other selective approaches were undertaken to obtain selective leukocyte subset depletion, using monoclonal antibodies against target molecules present on one subtype of the leukocyte population. Although efficient depletion of CD8$^+$ cells (cytotoxic and suppressor T lymphocytes) prevented infiltration of these cells into the renal interstitium, neither the development nor the resolution of the ARF was influenced in a corrosive mercuric chloride (HgCl$_2$) toxic model.[69] Attempts to deplete CD4$^+$ cells (helper T lymphocytes) in the same HgCl$_2$ toxic model achieved only partial depletion, insufficient to prevent renal interstitial infiltration and to influence ARF.

An alternative to experimentally T lymphocyte–depleted euthymic rats is the use of athymic animals, autosomal recessive mutants by which the gene defect results in a defective growth of hair and the absence of the thymus. T lymphocytes inhibit the vascular response to injury, as larger, induced vascular lesions were observed in athymic rats.[70] Protection against gentamicin and HgCl$_2$ nephrotoxicity was reported in athymic rats, but not in euthymic controls.[71] This effect could be explained by possible growth-repressing and matrix-reducing effects of activated lymphocytes on renal fibroblasts.[72] Nevertheless, results obtained from athymic animals should be handled cautiously, because the extrathymic maturation of T cells partially compensates for the deficiency in aging athymic animals, and the T-cell deficiency does not permit discrimination between the different T-lymphocyte subsets.

Evidence of a critical role for mononuclear cells (T cells and macrophages) in ARF comes from blocking one of the costimulatory pathways necessary for T-cell activation. The costimulatory signal provided by binding of T-cell surface receptor CD28 and its natural ligands B7 and CTLA-4, expressed also on antigen-presenting cells (eg, macrophages), can be blocked by CTLA-4 Ig, a recombinant fusion protein (cytotoxic T-lymphocyte antigen immunoglobulin) containing the extracellular domain of human CTLA-4, a homologue of CD28. Blocking this B7-CD28 costimulation pathway, which results in T-cell anergy, in a model of renal cold ischemia[73, 74] ameliorated renal dysfunction and decreased mononuclear cell infiltration. The protective effect of blocking T-cell costimulatory activity, in the absence of the immune stimulus provided by alloantigens, suggests that the T-cell monocyte-macrophage activation cascade may be critical in the very early phase of ischemic renal injury, possibly at the leukocyte-endothelial activation level. Indeed, endothelial cells can initiate both primary and secondary responses and, because of the ability of these cells to provide costimulatory signals to circulating T cells and other cells, they may serve as the initial antigen-presenting cell in the immune responses in peripheral tissues.[75]

Developments in cell adhesion biology have demonstrated the diverse and important roles of cell adhesion in health and disease. Different approaches have been used to prevent leukocyte-endothelial adherence and subsequently transendothelial migration: monoclonal antibodies against adhesion molecules (eg, anti–LFA-1, anti–ICAM-1, anti-CD18, anti–MAC-1), ICAM-1 knockout animals, antisense oligonucleotides against ICAM-1, and so on. Dramatic tissue protection has been observed in ischemic models of heart,[76] muscle,[77] and brain[78] by blockade of diverse leukocyte adhesion molecules. The presumed mechanism of protection by interruption of the ICAM-1 pathway has been the blockade of emigration of inflammatory cells to postischemic tissue. However, ICAM-1 has also been shown to mediate other functions, such as signal transduction and antigen presentation.[79, 80] From the growing series of studies examining the role of leukocyte adhesion molecules in renal ischemic and now toxic injury, it is clear that leukocyte adhesion molecules CD11a/CD18,[27, 81] CD11b/CD18,[81] and especially ICAM-1 in a more prominent role,[27, 28, 41, 82, 83] have been shown to mediate renal I-R injury in both rat and mouse models. The administration of antisense oligonucleotides to ICAM-1 mRNA had similar effects.[50] Unlike the case in other organs, L-selectin does not appear to mediate leukocyte recruitment to postischemic kidney or tubular damage.[80]

The results of these experiments, using the antiadhesion approach, have to be considered cautiously, because of the wide distribution of adhesion molecules and their ligands on different leukocyte subsets, endothelial cells, and brush borders of the proximal tubular cells. Although blockade of leukocyte adhesion-infiltration can be obtained efficiently with an antiadhesion approach, several reasons might explain its beneficial functional effects. It is possible that, as in the important early endothelial adhesion and activation of adherent leukocytes, the adhesive events critical for the subsequent tubular obstruction in ATN also occur early post I-R, explaining the beneficial effect of anti–adhesion-infiltration therapy in ATN. This is illustrated by the protective effect of RGD peptides in preventing tubular obstruction in the ischemic rat kidney. The RGD binding sites, however, are found not only at the apical site of tubular epithelia but also on the intimal surface of blood vessels in these ischemic kidneys.[84] Hence, the decrease in "infiltrated" leukocytes might simply be an epiphenomenon. Adhesion molecules may provoke intravascular obstruction by adhesion and "sticking" of leukocytes to the endothelial wall. In addition, not only cell-endothelium adhesion but also cell-cell aggregates, mediated by adhesion molecules, may contribute to a mechanical no-reflow phenomenon and inadequate restoration of the blood flow post I-R. Adhesion molecules may enhance cell-cell adhesion of sloughed epithelial cells in the tubular lumen, promoting intratubular obstruction and impaired glomerular filtration.[32] Antiadhesion molecules may inhibit cell-cell contacts and may prevent the necessary costimulation of leukocytes, resulting in the absence of chemoattractants or nonresponsiveness of leukocytes. Moreover, leukocyte adhesion promotes cellular biosynthesis of lipoxygenase products during leukocyte–glomerular cell interactions, probably by enhancing the exchange of arachidonic acid metabolites between leukocytes and glomerular cells. Therefore, agents that block adhesion may inhibit the generation of lipid mediators at sites of inflammation and consequently inhibit recruitment of leukocytes.[83] Hence, the beneficial effect of administration of antiadhesion molecules may be the consequence of a decrease of potent vasoconstrictive agents and thereby overcome the reduced renal blood flow and the glomerular filtration rate. In any case, the functional protective effects of the anti–adhesion-infiltration approach remains a solid observation that, however, cannot be completely explained yet, certainly not by the anti-infiltration effect alone. Better insights into these mechanisms are necessary to unravel the pathophysiology of ARF.

Additional insights can come from the comparison of ischemic versus toxicant-mediated ARF: renal dysfunction following exposure to HgCl₂[13] or the antineoplastic agent cisplatin[14] is characterized by ATN at the S3 segment–OSOM of the nephron and an interstitial infiltrate, similar to the situation following I-R.[10, 11] Single injection of anti–ICAM-1 Mab could prevent renal functional decline in post–I-R ARF[27] and cisplatin-mediated toxic ARF,[14] concomitant with less pronounced renal injury and infiltration. In contrast, treatment with anti–ICAM-1 and anti–LFA-1 Mabs in a HgCl₂ toxic model clearly resulted in the prevention of leukocyte infiltration-proliferation but did not influence ARF functionally or morphologically.[85] This observation provides arguments that the functional protective effects of the anti–adhesion-infiltration approach cannot be explained entirely by the anti-infiltration effect alone. Hemodynamic disturbances at the peritubular microcirculation are evident in post–I-R ARF and also in cisplatin-mediated renal injury,[86, 87] while frank alterations in renal hemodynamics are absent in the HgCl₂ toxic model[88] (Fig. 36–6). Again, this observation provides evidence that the critical role of leukocytes in postischemic or toxicant-mediated ARF occurs at the level of intravascular activation and endothelial adhesion, resulting in a vasoactive response and altered vascular permeability, rather than at the level of interstitial infiltration.

After it was shown that anti–ICAM-1 antibodies reduced delayed graft function (DGF),[3, 27] it seemed logical to use this approach in the prophylaxis and treatment of acute rejection in human renal transplantation by influencing the leukocyte infiltration and the T-cell activation that requires ICAM-1 as a costimu-

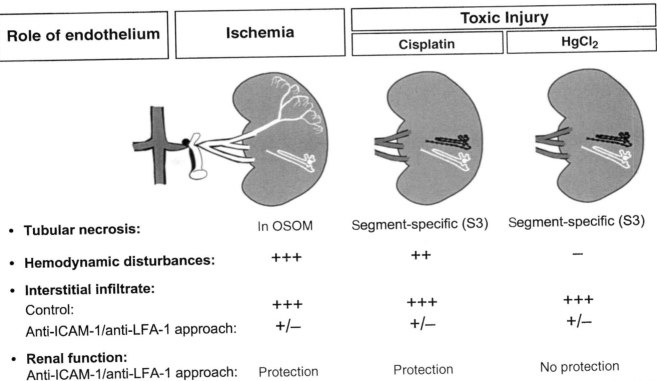

FIGURE 36–6 ■ Comparison of ischemic- versus toxicant-mediated ARF. Renal dysfunction following exposure to mercuric chloride (HgCl₂) or the antineoplastic agent cisplatin is characterized by ATN at the S3 segment–OSOM of the nephron and an interstitial infiltrate, a situation similar to the one that occurs after I-R. A single injection of anti–ICAM-1 mAb could prevent renal functional decline in post–I-R ARF and cisplatin-mediated toxic ARF concomitant with a less pronounced renal injury and infiltration, in contrast with the situation in the HgCl₂ toxic model, in which it prevented leukocyte infiltration-proliferation but did not influence ARF. *ICAM-1,* intercellular adhesion molecule-1; *LFA-1,* leukocye function–associated antigen-1; *OSOM,* outer surface of outer medulla.

latory molecule. In preclinical studies with primates, enlimomab, an anti–ICAM-1 monoclonal antibody, was indeed effective as prophylaxis and treatment of allograft rejection and vascular damage; however, leukocyte infiltration was not reduced.[89] A phase I trial with short-term induction of murine anti–ICAM-1 Mab seemed to reduce the risk of delayed graft function,[90] but the first human multicenter trial with the same short-term induction of murine anti–ICAM-1 Mab, however, did not reduce the rate of acute rejection or DGF.[91] On the other hand, a phase I multicenter trial using anti–LFA-1 (the ICAM-1 ligand) as induction therapy in renal transplants demonstrated reduced acute rejection and a tendency for the prevention of DGF.[92] It is clear that the concept of anti–ICAM-1 therapy in renal transplantation needs further investigation: the use of combined anti-adhesion antibody preparations and ICAM-1 antisense oligonucleotides may improve the therapeutic result.

The importance of the inflammatory response in ARF is also illustrated by the dramatic protective effect of anti-inflammatory peptides, such as α-melanocyte stimulating hormone (α-MSH)[25] and osteogenic protein-1.[40] These peptides have broad anti-inflammatory effects acting on the production of many chemoattractant cytokines and the expression of different leukocyte adhesion molecules. Using such a general approach, it is difficult to unravel the role of certain leukocyte subsets.

In summary, because of the lack of appropriate methodology for the specific depletion of a particular leukocyte subset, the exact role of the different accumulated leukocytes at the site of injury is far from completely understood. Currently, more general approaches such as anti-adhesion and anti-costimulation approaches will lead to better understanding of the pathophysiology of ARF.

CONCLUSION

Acute renal injury is accompanied by an important inflammatory reaction. There is no evidence that neutrophils do infiltrate the ischemic-toxic–injured kidney. The most prominent infiltrate is a mixed mononuclear infiltrate, consisting of initial monocytes-macrophages, later followed by T cells, mainly CD4[+] cells. This infiltrate is most prominent at the time of maximal regeneration activity following functional recovery. Hence, reasonable doubt exists as to whether this cellular infiltrate is important in exacerbating postischemic damage. Regardless of cell type, the very early endothelial adhesion, perhaps more important than the infiltration itself, seems of utmost importance for functional outcome. Intravascular activation and adhesion of neutrophils-macrophages play an important role in acute ischemic (but not in every toxic) injury, because its prevention by antiadhesion approaches results in functional protection.

When ARF is not too severe, the kidney has the remarkable capacity for full functional recovery and morphologic regeneration, whereby the infiltrate completely disappears. In case of protracted injury and when this infiltrate persists, it contributes substantially toward the development of fibrosis and chronic renal dysfunction.

REFERENCES

1. Thadhani R, Pascual M, Bonventre JV: Acute renal failure. N Engl J Med 1996; 334:1448–1460.
2. Nolan CR, Anderson RJ: Hospital acquired acute renal failure. J Am Soc Nephrol 1998; 9:710–718.
3. Brady H, Singer G: Acute renal failure. Lancet 1995; 346:1533–1540.
4. Rabb H, O'Meara YM, Maderna P, et al: Leukocytes, cell adhesion molecules and ischemic acute renal failure. Kidney Int 1997; 51:1463–1468.
5. Shoskes DA, Halloran PF: Delayed graft function in renal transplantation: etiology, management, and long-term significance. J Urol 1996; 155:1831–1840.
6. Toback FG: Regeneration after acute tubular necrosis. Kidney Int 1992; 41:226–246.
7. Ghielli M, Verstrepen WA, Nouwen EJ, De Broe ME: Inflammatory cells in renal regeneration. Ren Fail 1996; 18:355–375.
8. Bonventre JV: Mechanisms of ischemic acute renal failure. Kidney Int 1993; 43:1160–1178.
9. De Greef K, Ysebaert D, Ghielli M, et al: Neutrophils and ischemia/reperfusion injury: a review. J Nephrol 1998; 11:2–13.
10. Takada M, Nadeau KC, Shaw GD, et al: The cytokine-adhesion molecule cascade in ischemia/reperfusion injury of the rat kidney: inhibition by a soluble P-selectin ligand. J Clin Invest 1997; 99:2682–2690.
11. Ysebaert DK, De Greef KE, Ghielli M, et al: Identification and kinetics of leukocytes after severe ischemia/reperfusion renal injury. Nephrol Dial Transplant 2000; 15:1562–1574.
12. Verstrepen WA, Nouwen EJ, Xiao SY, De Broe ME: Altered growth factor expression during toxic proximal tubular necrosis and regeneration. Kidney Int 1993; 43:1267–1279.
13. Verstrepen WA, Nouwen EJ, Zhu MQ, et al: Time course of growth factor expression in mercuric chloride acute renal failure. Nephrol Dial Transplant 1995; 10:1361–1371.
14. Kelly KJ, Meehan S, Colvin RB, et al: Protection from toxicant-mediated injury in the rat with anti-CD54 antibody. Kidney Int 1999; 56:922–931.
15. Zhu MQ, De Broe ME, Nouwen EJ: Vimentin expression and distal tubular damage in the rat kidney. Exp Nephrol 1996; 4:172–183.
16. Duymelinck C, Dauwe SEH, Nouwen EJ, et al: Cholesterol feeding accentuates the cyclosporine-induced elevation of renal plasminogen activator inhibitor type 1. Kidney Int 1997; 51:1818–1830.
17. Bertani T, Cutillo F, Zoja C, et al: Tubulointerstitial lesions mediate renal damage in adriamycin glomerulopathy. Kidney Int 1986; 30:488–496.
18. De Broe ME, Stolear JC, Nouwen EJ, Elseviers MM: 5-Aminosalicylic acid (5-ASA) and chronic tubular nephritis in patients with chronic inflammatory bowel disease: is there a link? Nephrol Dial Transplant 1997; 12:1839–1841.
19. Eddy A, Mitchell V: Acute tubulointerstitial nephritis with aminonucleoside nephrosis. Kidney Int 1988; 33:14–23.
20. Eddy A, McCulloch L, Adams J, Liu E: Interstitial nephritis induced by protein overload proteinuria. Am J Pathol 1989; 135:719–733.
21. Schreiner GF, Harris KPG, Purkerson ML, Klahr S: Immunological aspects of acute ureteral obstruction: immune cell infiltrate in the kidney. Kidney Int 1988; 34:487–493.
22. Glauser MP, Meylan P, Bille J: The inflammatory response and tissue damage: the example of renal scars following acute renal infection. Pediatr Nephrol 1987; 1:615–622.
23. Kliem V, Johnson RJ, Alpers CE, et al: Mechanisms involved in the pathogenesis of tubulointerstitial fibrosis in 5/6 nephrectomized rats. Kidney Int 1996; 49:666–678.
24. Ghielli M, Verstrepen WA, De Greef K, et al: Inflammatory cells in renal pathology. Néphrologie 1998; 19:59–67.

25. Chiao H, Kohda Y, McLeroy P, et al: α-Melanocyte–stimulating hormone protects against renal injury after ischemia in mice and rats. J Clin Invest 1997; 99:1165–1172.

26. Goes N, Urmson J, Ramassar V, Halloran PF: Ischemic acute tubular necrosis induces an extensive local cytokine response: evidence for induction of interferon-γ, transforming growth factor-β1, granulocyte-macrophage colony-stimulating factor, interleukin-2 and interleukin-10. Transplantation 1995; 59:565–572.

27. Kelly KJ, Williams WW, Colvin RB, Bonventre JV: Antibody to intercellular adhesion molecule 1 protects the kidney against ischemic injury. Proc Natl Acad Sci USA 1994; 91:812–816.

28. Kelly KJ, Williams WW, Colvin RB, et al: Intercellular adhesion molecule-1–deficient mice are protected against ischemic renal injury. J Clin Invest 1996; 97:1056–1063.

29. Takano T, Brady HR: The endothelium and glomerular inflammation. Curr Opin Nephrol Hypertens 1995; 4:277–286.

30. Heinzelmann M, Mercer-Jones MA, Passmore JC: Neutrophils and renal failure. Am J Kidney Dis 1999; 34:384–399.

31. Lieberthal W: Biology of ischemic and toxic renal tubular cell injury: role of nitric oxide and the inflammatory response. Curr Opin Nephrol Hypertens 1998; 7:289–295.

32. Bonventre JV, Colvin RB: Adhesion molecules and renal disease. Curr Opin Nephrol Hypertens 1996; 5:254–261.

33. Adams DH, Shaw S: Leukocyte-endothelial interactions and regulation of leukocyte migration. Lancet 1994; 343:831–836.

34. Brady HR: Leukocyte adhesion molecules and kidney diseases. Kidney Int 1994; 45:1285–1300.

35. Lan HY, Nickolic-Patterson DJ, Mu W, Atkins RC: Local macrophage proliferation in the progression of glomerular and tubulointerstitial injury in rat anti-GBM glomerulonephritis. Kidney Int 1995; 48:753–763.

36. Verstrepen WA, Ghielli M, Dauwe S, et al: Local macrophage proliferation in rat mercuric chloride acute renal failure. Abstract Book of the European Dialysis and Transplantation Association 36, 1996.

37. Klausner JM, Paterson IA, Goldman G, et al: Postischemic renal injury is mediated by neutrophils and leukotrienes. Am J Physiol 1989; 256:F794–F802.

38. Paller MS: Effect of PMN depletion on ischemic renal injury. J Lab Clin Invest 1989; 133:379–386.

39. Willinger CC, Schramek H, Pfaller K, Pfaller W: Tissue distribution of neutrophils in postischemic acute renal failure. Virchows Archiv B Cell Pathol 1992; 62:237–243.

40. Vukicevic S, Basic V, Rogic D, et al: Osteogenic protein-1 reduces severity of injury after ischemic acute renal failure in rat. J Clin Invest 1998; 102:202–214.

41. Linas SL, Wittenburg D, Parsons PE, Repine JE: Ischemia increases neutrophil retention and worsens acute renal failure: role of oxygen metabolites and ICAM-1. Kidney Int 1995; 48:1584–1591.

42. Thornton MA, Winn R, Alpers CE, Zhager RA: An evaluation of the neutrophil as the mediator of in vivo renal ischemia-reperfusion injury. Am J Pathol 1988; 135:509–515.

43. Nickolic-Patterson DJ, Lan HY, Hill PA, Atkins RC: Macrophages in renal injury. Kidney Int 1994; S45:S79–S82.

44. Bos A, Wever R, Roos D: Characterization and quantification of the peroxidase in human monocytes. Biochem Biophys Acta 1978; 525:37–44.

45. Heinecke JW, Li W, Daehnke HL, Goldstein JA: Dityrosine, a specific marker of oxidation, is synthesized by the myeloperoxidase-hydrogen peroxidase system of human neutrophils and macrophages. J Biol Chem 1993; 268:4069–4077.

46. Bradley PP, Priebat DA, Christensen RD, Rothstein G: Measurement of cutaneous inflammation: estimation of neutrophil content with enzyme marker. J Invest Dermatol 1982; 78:206–209.

47. Barone FC, Hillegass LM, Tzimas MN, et al: Time-related changes in myeloperoxidase activity and leukotriene B4 receptor binding reflect leukocyte influx in cerebral focal stroke. Mol Chem Neuropathol 1995; 24:13–30.

48. Van Goor H, Fidler V, Weening J, Grond J: Determinants of focal and segmental glomerulosclerosis in the rat after renal ablation. Lab Invest 1991; 64:754–765.

49. Azuma H, Nadeau K, Takada M, et al: Cellular and molecular predictors of chronic renal dysfunction after initial ischemia/ reperfusion injury of a single kidney. Transplantation 1997; 64:190–197.

50. Haller H, Dragun D, Miethke A, et al: Antisense oligonucleotides for ICAM-1 attenuate reperfusion injury and renal failure in the rat. Kidney Int 1996; 50:473–480.

51. Humes H: Potential molecular therapy for acute renal failure. Cleve Clin J Med 1993; 60:166–168.

52. Franklin SC, Moulton M, Sicard GA, et al: Insulin-like growth factor 1 preserves renal function postoperatively. Am J Physiol 1997; 272:F257–F259.

53. Fine LG, Ong AC, Norman JT: Mechanisms of tubulo-interstitial injury in progressive renal diseases. Eur J Clin Invest 1993; 23:259–265.

54. Leibovich SJ, Ross R: The role of the macrophage in wound repair: a study with hydrocortisone and antimacrophage serum. Am J Pathol 1975; 78:71–100.

55. Danon D, Kowatch MA, Roth GS: Promotion of wound repair in old mice by local injection of macrophages. Proc Natl Acad Sci USA 1989; 86:2018–2020.

56. Kunt TK: Basic principles of wound healing. J Trauma 1990; 30:S122–S128.

57. Strutz F, Neilson EG: The role of lymphocytes in the progression of interstitial disease. Kidney Int 1994; 45:S106–S110.

58. Cromack DT, Porras-Reyees B, Mutoe TA: Current concepts in wound healing: growth factors and macrophage interaction. J Trauma 1990; S12:S129–S133.

59. Finn WF: Recovery From Acute Renal Failure. In: Lazarus JM, Brenner BM, eds: Acute Renal Failure. 3rd ed. New York: Churchill Livingstone; 1993:553–596.

60. Okada H, Strutz F, Danoff T, Neilson EG: Possible pathogenesis of renal fibrosis. Kidney Int 1996; 54:S37–S38.

61. Remuzzi G, Ruggeneti P, Benigni A: Understanding the nature of renal disease progression. Kidney Int 1997; 51:2–15.

62. Duymelinck C, Dauwe S, Nouwen EJ, et al: Cholesterol feeding accentuates the cyclosporine-induced elevation of renal plasminogen activator inhibitor type I (PAI-1) in rats. Kidney Int 1997; 51:1818–1830.

63. Tilney NL, Guttman RD: Effects of initial renal ischemia/reperfusion injury on the transplanted kidney. Transplantation 1997; 64:945–947.

64. Eiserich JP, Hrsitova M, Cross CE, et al: Formation of nitric oxide–derived inflammatory oxidants by myeloperoxidase in neutrophils. Nature 1998; 391:393–396.

65. Brezis M, Rosen S: Hypoxia of the renal medulla: its implications for disease. N Engl J Med 1995; 332:647–655.

66. Kelly KJ, Tolkoff-Rubin N, Rubin R, et al: An oral platelet activating factor antagonist, Ro-24-4736, protects the rat kidney from ischemic injury. Am J Physiol 1996; 271:F1061–F1067.

67. Hellberg PO, Kalskog OK: Neutrophil mediated post-ischemic tubular leakage in the rat kidney. Kidney Int 1989; 36:555–561.

68. Simpson DM, Ross R: Effects of heterologous antineutrophil serum in guinea pigs. Am J Pathol 1971; 65:79–102.

69. Ghielli M, Verstrepen WA, Dauwe SE, et al: Selective depletion of CD8 positive leukocytes does not alter mercuric chloride induced acute renal failure. Exp Nephrol 1997; 5:69–81.

70. Hansson GK, Holm J, Holm S, et al: T lymphocytes inhibit the vascular response to injury. Proc Natl Acad Sci USA 1991; 88:10530–10534.

71. Vaamonde CA, Pardo V, Fajardo C, et al: The nude rat is protected against gentamycin nephrotoxicity (abstract). J Am Soc Nephrol 1992; 3:713.

72. Kitamura A, Kitamura M, Nagasawa R, et al: Renal fibroblasts are sensitive to growth-repressing and matrix-reducing factors from activated lymphocytes. Clin Exp Immunol 1993; 91:516–520.

73. Takada M, Chandraker A, Nadeau KC, et al: The role of the B7 costimulatory pathway in experimental cold ischemia/reperfusion injury. J Clin Invest 1997; 100:1199–1203.

74. Chandraker A, Takada M, Nadeau KC, et al: CD28-B7 blockade in organ dysfunction secondary to cold ischemia/reperfusion injury. Kidney Int 1997; 52:1678–1684.

75. Hancock WW, Sayegh MH, Zheng XG, et al: Costimulatory function of CD40L, CD80, and CD86 in vascularized cardiac allograft rejection. Proc Natl Acad Sci USA 1996; 93:13967–13972.

76. Ma XL, Lefer DJ, Lefer AM, Rothlein R: Coronary endothelial and cardiac protective effects of a monoclonal antibody to intercellular adhesion molecule-1 in myocardial ischemia and reperfusion. Circulation 1992; 86:937–946.
77. Seekamp A, Till GO, Mulligan MS, et al: Role of selectins in local remote tissue injury following injury and reperfusion. Am J Pathol 1994; 144:592–598.
78. Connolly ES, Winfree CJ, Springer TA, et al: Cerebral protection in homozygous null ICAM-1 mice after middle cerebral artery occlusion: role of neutrophil adhesion in the pathogenesis of stroke. J Clin Invest 1996; 97:209–216.
79. Jevnikar AM, Wuthrich RP, Takei F: Differing regulation and function of ICAM-1 and class II antigens on renal tubular cells. Kidney Int 1990; 38:417–425.
80. Rabb H, Postler G: Leukocyte adhesion molecules in ischemic renal injury: kidney specific paradigms? Clin Exp Pharmacol Physiol 1998; 25:286–291.
81. Rabb H, Mendiola CC, Dietz J, et al: Role of CD11a and CD11b in ischemic acute renal failure in rats. Am J Physiol 1994; 267:F1052-F1058.
82. Rabb H, Mendiola CC, Saba SR, et al: Antibodies to ICAM-1 protect the kidney in severe ischemic reperfusion injury. Biochem Biophys Res Commun 1995; 211:67–73.
83. Brady HR, Papayianni A, Serhan CN: Leukocyte adhesion promotes biosynthesis of lipoxygenase products by transcellular routes. Kidney Int 1994; 45S:S90–S97.
84. Romanov V, Noiri E, Czerwinski G, et al: Two novel probes reveal tubular and vascular Arg-Gly-Asp (RGD) binding sites in the ischemic rat kidney. Kidney Int 1997; 52:93–102.
85. Ghielli M, Dauwe S, De Greef K, et al: Prevention of macrophage infiltration by anti-LFA-1/anti-ICAM-1 monoclonal antibodies does not alter mercuric chloride–induced acute renal failure. Nephrol Dial Transplant 1998; 13:A51.
86. Winston JA, Safirstein R: Reduced renal blood flow in early cisplatin-induced acute renal failure in the rat. Am J Physiol 1985; 249:F490–F496.
87. Luke DR, Vadiei K, Lopez-Berenstein G: Role of vascular congestion in cisplatin-induced acute renal failure in the rat. Nephrol Dial Transplant 1992; 71:1–7.
88. Conger JD, Falk SA: Glomerular and tubular dynamics in mercuric chloride acute renal failure. J Lab Clin Med 1986; 107:281–289.
89. Cosimi AB, Conti D, Delmonico FL, et al: In vivo effects of monoclonal antibody to ICAM-1 (CD54) in nonhuman primates with renal allografts. J Immunol 1990; 144:4604.
90. Haug CE, Colvin RB, Delmonico FL, et al: A phase I trial of immunosuppression with anti-ICAM-1 (CD54) Mab in renal allograft recipients. Transplantation 1993; 55:766.
91. Salmela K, Wramner L, Ekberg H, et al: A randomized multicenter trial of the ICAM-1 monoclonal antibody (enlimomab) for the prevention of acute rejection and delayed onset of graft function in cadaveric renal transplantation. Transplantation 1999; 67:729–736.
92. Hourmant M, Bedrossion J, Durand D, et al: A randomized multicenter trial comparing leukocyte-function associated antigen-1 monoclonal antibody with rabbit antithymocyte globulin as induction treatment in first kidney transplantations. Transplantation 1996; 62:1565.

CHAPTER 37

Nutritional Support in Patients With Acute Renal Failure

Wilfred Druml

INTRODUCTION

All patients require adequate nutrition to maintain protein stores, to correct preexisting and disease-related deficits in lean body mass, and to prevent "hospital-acquired" malnutrition. The objectives of nutritional support for patients with acute renal failure (ARF) are not greatly different from those for patients with other acute catabolic conditions. However, the principles of nutritional support for patients with ARF differ from those for patients with chronic renal failure (CRF), because diets or infusions for satisfying the minimal requirements for patients with ARF are not necessarily sufficient for patients with ARF.

The primary goals of nutrition in patients with ARF and, accordingly, the composition of nutritional regimens have changed considerably during the last several decades. In the predialysis era and the early years of hemodialysis, severe or total restriction of nutrients was recommended. Subsequently, in analogy with the treatment of CRF, "minimal requirements" were used, and later there was a period of more liberal hyperalimentation with little regard given to impaired renal function. With increasing knowledge of the pathophysiology and the metabolic alterations that specifically occur in ARF and a better understanding of nutrient requirements in patients with various degrees of stress and hypercatabolism, nutritional therapy now is adapted to the specific needs of the individual patient with ARF.

With the implementation of modern nutritional support, the requirements are met for all nutrients necessary for the preservation of lean body mass and the stimulation of immunocompetence, reparative functions, and wound healing in patients who, in most instances, have acquired ARF, among other complications. However, at the same time that the specific metabolic alterations and demands of ARF are dealt with, the consequences of impaired excretory renal function and the alterations in nutrient balance induced by renal replacement therapy also have to be taken into consideration.

For many years, parenteral nutrition was the preferred method of nutritional support in patients with ARF, and most investigations have been performed with a parenteral nutrient supply. There can be no doubt that enteral nutrition has become a primary type of nutritional support for patients with ARF, but, unfortunately, little systematic research has been conducted in this field. Nevertheless, enteral and parenteral nutrition should not be viewed as alternatives to each other but, rather, as complementary methods of nutritional support, because in many patients it is not possible to meet requirements by the enteral route alone, and supplementary or even total parenteral nutrition (TPN) may become necessary.

Despite the difficulty in demonstrating the clear-cut effects of nutritional interventions, especially of parenteral nutrition, on prognosis in critically ill patients, there can be no doubt that nutritional therapy is one of the cornerstones of modern critical care medicine. Preexisting or hospital-acquired malnutrition has been identified as an important factor in the persistently high mortality in acutely ill patients with ARF. Moreover, it is increasingly recognized that individual nutritional substrates can exert specific metabolic effects on various physiologic functions, such as immunocompetence. Clinical nutrition is gradually transforming from mere provision of energy and nitrogen to a more specific and qualitative type of metabolic intervention.

In this chapter, the metabolic alterations induced by ARF and by renal replacement therapy are summarized, requirements of individual nutrients in patients with ARF are analyzed, compositions of parenteral and enteral diets are discussed, and clinical experience regarding the use of various nutritional regimens are reviewed. This knowledge and information is mandatory for defining an optimal program of nutritional therapy in the extremely heterogeneous group of patients with ARF.

METABOLIC ENVIRONMENT IN PATIENTS WITH ACUTE RENAL FAILURE

Acute renal failure is associated with a broad pattern of disturbances of physiologic functions that exert a pronounced impact on morbidity and mortality.[1] The metabolic consequences of ARF play a crucial role among these disturbances. Certainly, in many instances, ARF is not an isolated event, but a complication of sepsis, trauma, or multiple-organ failure, so it is difficult to ascribe specific metabolic alterations to ARF per se. Thus, metabolic changes in most patients are determined by the acute uremic state plus the underlying disease process or by complications such as severe infections and organ dysfunction, and the type and intensity of renal replacement therapy. Nevertheless, it must be recognized that the acute loss of excretory renal function not only affects water, electrolyte, and acid-base metabolism but also has a profound effect on the *milieu intérieur*, with specific and distinct alterations in protein and amino acid, carbohydrate, and lipid metabolism.[2, 3]

Energy Metabolism

In experimental animals, ARF decreases oxygen consumption, even when hypothermia and acidosis are corrected.[4] An impairment of oxidative phosphorylation was implicated as the cause of this "uremic hypometabolism." In humans, only a slightly decreased—if at all—energy expenditure was observed, and only in patients with advanced chronic uremia.[5]

Similarly, in patients with uncomplicated ARF, oxygen consumption is within the range of healthy subjects.[5, 6] However, in patients with sepsis or multiple organ dysfunction syndrome (MODS) and associated ARF, oxygen consumption is increased by approximately 20% to 30% compared with subjects who have uncomplicated ARF.[5, 6] Thus, energy expenditure in patients with ARF is determined by the underlying disease, rather than by the acutely uremic state. Remarkably, in multiple organ failure syndrome (MOFS), oxygen consumption was significantly higher in patients who did not have impairment of renal function than in those with ARF.[7]

Taken together, these data indicate that when uremia is well controlled by hemodialysis or hemofiltration, there is little if any change in energy metabolism in ARF. Oxygen consumption is determined mainly by the underlying disease and, in contrast with several other acute disease processes, ARF has a tendency to decrease, rather than to increase, energy expenditure.

The pattern of oxidation of individual substrates, especially lipids and glucose, in ARF is similar to that in other acute diseases.[5] The oxidation of fatty acids was increased and the carbohydrate oxidation reduced (at least after overnight fast). This preferential oxidation of fat may reflect insulin resistance or decreased hepatic glycogen stores in ARF.

Protein and Amino Acid Metabolism

One of the main characteristics of metabolic alterations in ARF is activation of protein catabolism, with excessive release of amino acids from skeletal muscle and a sustained negative nitrogen balance.[8, 9] Muscle protein degradation and amino acid catabolism are activated.[10] There is not only an acceleration of protein breakdown but also defective muscular utilization of amino acids for protein synthesis.[11] Amino acid transport into skeletal muscle is impaired in ARF.[12, 13] This abnormality can be linked to both insulin resistance and a generalized defect in ion transport in uremia; both the activity and the receptor density of the sodium pump are abnormal in adipose cells and muscle tissue.[14]

Amino acids are redistributed from muscle tissue to the liver. Hepatic extraction of amino acids from the circulation, hepatic gluconeogenesis, and ureagenesis

all are increased.[15] In the liver, protein synthesis and secretion of acute phase proteins are also stimulated.[16]

AMINO ACID POOLS AND AMINO ACID UTILIZATION IN ACUTE RENAL FAILURE

As a consequence of these metabolic alterations, imbalances in amino acid pools in plasma and in the intracellular compartment occur in ARF, and a typical plasma amino acid pattern is induced.[17] Plasma concentrations of cysteine, taurine, methionine, and phenylalanine are elevated, but levels of valine and leucine are decreased in patients with ARF.

Moreover, the elimination of amino acids from the intravascular space is altered. As expected from the stimulation of hepatic extraction of amino acids observed in animal experiments, overall amino acid clearance and clearance of most glucoplastic amino acids are enhanced (Fig. 37–1). In contrast, the clearance of phenylalanine, proline, and, remarkably, valine is decreased in ARF.[17, 18]

CAUSES OF PROTEIN CATABOLISM IN ACUTE RENAL FAILURE

The causes of hypercatabolism in ARF are complex and manifold, consisting of a combination of nonspecific mechanisms induced by the acute disease process, acidosis, the underlying illness and associated complications, specific effects induced by the acute loss of

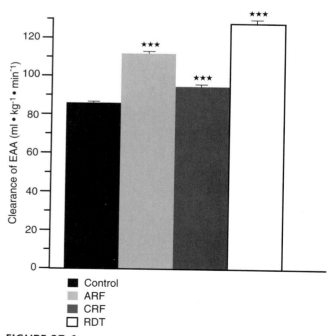

FIGURE 37–1 ■ Clearance of essential amino acids (except tryptophan) plus histidine and arginine after intravenous infusion in healthy control subjects (n = 5), patients with acute renal failure (n = 6), patients with compensated chronic renal failure (n = 6), and patients undergoing regular hemodialysis therapy (n = 6). $P < 0.001$ of patient groups vs. controls. (Adapted from Druml W, Fischer M, Liebisch BB, et al: Elimination of amino acids in renal failure. Am J Clin Nutr 1994; 60:418–423; with permission.)

renal function, and the type and intensity of renal replacement therapy (Table 37–1).

A dominant mechanism of accelerated protein breakdown is the stimulation of hepatic gluconeogenesis from amino acids. In healthy subjects, but also in patients with CRF, hepatic gluconeogenesis from amino acids is readily and completely suppressed by exogenous glucose infusion.[19, 20] In contrast, in ARF, hepatic glucose formation is only decreased but not halted by exogenous substrate supply: even during glucose infusion, gluconeogenesis from amino acids persists.[21]

These findings have important implications for nutritional support in patients with ARF, because it is impossible to achieve a positive nitrogen balance in a patient with ARF during the acute phase of disease. Protein catabolism cannot be suppressed merely by provision of conventional nutritional substrates alone, and in order to effectively suppress protein catabolism, alternative means for preserving lean body mass must be identified.

The stimulation of muscular protein catabolism and enhanced hepatic gluconeogenesis is mediated by a glucocorticoid-dependent pathway. In the experimental situation, increased protein catabolism from ARF animals is normalized by either adrenalectomy or pretreatment with glucocorticoid receptor–blocking agents.[22–24]

An important stimulus of muscle protein catabolism in ARF is insulin resistance. In muscle, the maximal rate of insulin-stimulated protein synthesis is depressed by ARF, and protein degradation is increased even in the presence of insulin.[11] Results from experimental animals suggest a common defect in protein and glucose metabolism: tyrosine release from muscle (as a measure of protein catabolism) is highly correlated with the ratio of lactate release to glucose uptake.[11] Thus, an inefficient intracellular energy metabolism stimulates protein breakdown and interrupts the normal control of protein turnover.

Acidosis was identified as a major factor in muscle protein breakdown. Metabolic acidosis activates catabolism of protein and oxidation of amino acids independently of azotemia.[25, 26] In a manner similar to that in CRF and despite the fact that these findings have not been uniformly confirmed,[27] there is evidence that increased muscle protein degradation and amino acid catabolism can be mitigated by correcting metabolic acidosis in ARF as well.[10, 28]

Several additional catabolic factors are operative in ARF. The secretion of catabolic hormones (catecholamines, glucagon, glucocorticoids),[29, 30] the presence of hyperparathyroidism (which is also frequently present in ARF),[31] the suppression or decreased sensitivity of growth factors,[32] and the release of proteases from activated leukocytes[33, 34] can stimulate protein breakdown. In addition, the release of inflammatory mediators such as tumor necrosis factor-α (TNF-α) and interleukins has been shown to mediate hypercatabolism in acute disease states.[35]

Moreover, the type and frequency of renal replacement therapy affects protein metabolism in patients with ARF. Aggravation of protein catabolism is mediated, certainly in part, by the loss of nutritional substrates, but there are findings suggesting that in addition both an activation of protein breakdown and an inhibition of muscular protein synthesis are induced by hemodialysis[36](see later).

Finally, another factor of major relevance to the clinical situation is that inadequate nutrition contributes to the loss of lean body mass in ARF. In experimental animals, starvation potentiates the catabolic response of ARF.[37] In the clinical situation, malnutrition was identified as a major determinant in the evolution of complications and of the prognosis in patients with ARF.[38–40]

EFFECTS OF METABOLIC FUNCTIONS OF THE KIDNEY ON PROTEIN AND AMINO ACID METABOLISM IN ACUTE RENAL FAILURE

Protein and amino acid metabolism in ARF is also affected by impairment of multiple metabolic functions of the kidney itself. Various amino acids are synthesized or converted by the kidneys and released into the circulation: arginine, cysteine, methionine (from homocysteine), tyrosine, and serine.[41] Thus, loss of renal functions can contribute to the altered amino acid pools in ARF, and several amino acids, which conventionally are termed nonessential, such as arginine or tyrosine, might become conditionally indispensable in ARF.[42, 43]

In addition, the kidney is an important organ of protein degradation. Multiple peptides are filtered and catabolized at the tubular brush border, with the constituent amino acids being reabsorbed and recycled into the metabolic pool. In renal failure, catabolism of peptides, such as peptide hormones, is retarded.[44] This is also the case for insulin, and insulin requirements decrease in diabetic patients after the development of ARF.[45]

With the increased use of dipeptides as a source of amino acids such as glutamine and tyrosine, which are not stable or soluble in aqueous solutions in artificial nutrition, this metabolic function of the kidney may also gain in importance with regard to the utilization of nutritional substrates. However, most dipeptides currently evaluated as nutritional substrates for example,

TABLE 37–1. Factors Contributing to Protein Catabolism in Acute Renal Failure

Impairment of metabolic functions by uremic toxins
Endocrine factors
  Insulin resistance
  Increased secretion of catabolic hormones (catecholamines, glucagon, glucocorticoids)
  Hyperparathyroidism
  Suppression of release/resistance to growth factors
Acidosis
Acute phase reaction: systemic inflammatory response syndrome (activation of cytokine network)
Release of proteases
Inadequate supply of nutritional substrates
Loss of nutritional substrates (renal replacement therapy)

as sources of glutamine or tyrosine, contain alanine or glycine in the N-terminal position and are also rapidly hydrolyzed in the presence of renal dysfunction.[44, 46]

POTENTIAL METABOLIC INTERVENTIONS FOR CONTROLLING CATABOLISM

Excessive mortality in ARF is strongly correlated with the extent of hypercatabolism. Unfortunately, there has been no identification of effective methods of reducing or stopping catabolism in the clinical situation. Potentially, hypercatabolism can be modified at three levels of metabolic intervention:

Substrate Level. As discussed earlier, it is impossible in patients with ARF to halt hypercatabolism and persisting hepatic gluconeogenesis simply by providing conventional nutritional substrates.[20, 21, 35] It remains to be demonstrated that novel nutritional substrates such as glutamine and structured triglycerides exert a more pronounced anticatabolic effect in patients with ARF.

Endocrine Level. Endocrine interventions include therapy with hormones (insulin, insulin-like growth factor [IGF-I], recombinant human growth hormone [rHGH]) and hormone antagonists (eg, antiglucocorticoids).[23, 35] In rats with ischemic ARF, IGF-I not only accelerated recovery from renal failure but also improved nitrogen balance.[47] However, available clinical results are rather disappointing. A multicenter study using IGF-I in patients with ARF was terminated prematurely, because of a lack of effect.[48] Growth hormone was withdrawn for the treatment of critical illness because an increase in mortality became apparent during rHGH therapy in critically ill patients, many of whom also had ARF.[49]

Mediator Level. Cytokines, such as the interleukins and TNF-α mediate excessive release of amino acids from skeletal muscle and activation of hepatic amino acid extraction in acute disease states. Therapies for limiting an overwhelming release or action of inflammatory mediators (eg, antagonists of thromboxane, of platelet-activating factor, and of interleukins, antibodies to TNF-α, and soluble TNF-α receptors) are under experimental evaluation.[35] It should be recognized also that nutritional factors such as amino acids (glutamine, glycine, arginine) and polyunsaturated fatty acids can modify the inflammatory response and affect the release of mediators.[50]

Some of these novel therapeutic strategies offer promising perspectives, but none of them has entered clinical routine. Certainly, the mystery of accelerated breakdown in ARF has not been elucidated, and it is highly improbable that a single factor is responsible for hypercatabolism in ARF or that a single agent can reverse accelerated protein degradation.

Carbohydrate Metabolism

Usually, ARF is associated with hyperglycemia. An important cause of elevated blood glucose concentrations is insulin resistance.[51-53] Plasma insulin concentration is elevated, maximal insulin-stimulated glucose uptake by skeletal muscle is decreased by 50%, and muscular glycogen synthesis is impaired. However, insulin concentrations that cause half-maximal stimulation of glucose uptake is normal, which points to a postreceptor defect, rather than impaired insulin sensitivity, as the cause of defective glucose metabolism in ARF.[53]

A second feature of glucose metabolism in ARF is accelerated hepatic gluconeogenesis, mainly from conversion of amino acids released during protein catabolism. Hepatic extraction of amino acids, their conversion to glucose, and urea production all are increased in ARF.[15, 21, 54] As discussed earlier, in contrast with the nonuremic state and CRF, hepatic gluconeogenesis cannot be suppressed by exogenous glucose infusions in ARF.[19, 21]

Alterations in glucose and protein metabolism in ARF are interrelated, and many factors that activate protein catabolism contribute to impairment of glucose metabolism (see Table 37–1).[11] Again, the stimulation of muscle protein catabolism and enhanced hepatic gluconeogenesis are mediated by a glucocorticoid-dependent pathway. In the experimental situation, increased glucose formation by hepatocytes in ARF animals is normalized by incubation with glucocorticoid receptor–blocking agents.[23] Metabolic acidosis also affects glucose metabolism in ARF by further deteriorating glucose tolerance.[51]

Finally, metabolism of insulin is grossly abnormal in ARF. Endogenous insulin secretion is reduced in the basal state and during glucose infusion.[55] The kidney is a main organ of insulin disposal, and so insulin degradation is decreased in ARF. But not only is there a reduction of renal insulin degradation in ARF but also, surprisingly, insulin catabolism by the liver is consistently reduced.[55] The resulting elevation in plasma insulin concentration may explain the normal blood glucose levels in several patients with ARF.

Lipid Metabolism

Acute renal failure is also associated with profound alterations in lipid metabolism. The triglyceride content of plasma lipoproteins, especially very low density lipoprotein (VLDL) and low density lipoprotein (LDL), is increased, while total cholesterol and, in particular, high density lipoprotein (HDL)-cholesterol is decreased.[56-58] Additionally, concentrations of apoproteins AI, AII, and B become abnormal.

The major cause of lipid abnormalities in ARF is an impairment of lipolysis. The activities of both lipolytic systems, peripheral lipoprotein lipase and hepatic triglyceride lipase, are decreased to less than 50% of normal (Fig. 37–2).[59] Compared with healthy subjects, the kinetics of lipolytic activity after heparin stimulation are altered, and inactivation is accelerated in ARF patients. Metabolic acidosis contributes also to the impairment of lipolysis in ARF by further inhibiting lipoprotein lipase.[60]

Whether an increased hepatic triglyceride secretion contributes to the hypertriglyceridemia of ARF re-

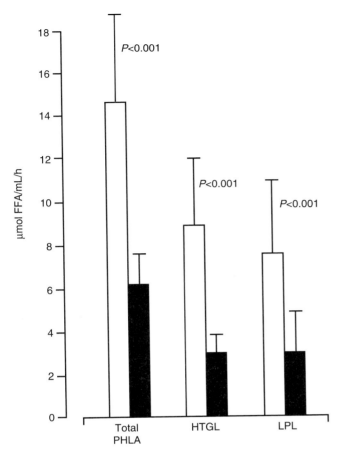

FIGURE 37–2 ▪ Maximal postheparin lipolytic activity (PHLA), hepatic triglyceride lipase (HTGL), and peripheral lipoprotein lipase (LPL) in healthy subjects (n = 10, *open bars*) and subjects with acute renal failure (n = 8, *closed bars*). P < 0.001. (Adapted from Druml W, Zechner R, Magometschnigg D, et al: Post-heparin lipolytic activity in acute renal failure. Clin Nephrol 1985; 23:289–293; with permission.)

mains a subject of controversy. Animal experiments have yielded conflicting results, VLDL secretion being increased, normal, or decreased in ARF rats.[61–63] In ARF, plasma triglyceride levels do not correlate with triglyceride clearance or postheparin lipolytic activity, suggesting that, in contrast with that found in CRF, hepatic triglyceride synthesis might be increased, at least in some patients.[64]

Changes in lipid metabolism develop rapidly; an impairment of fat elimination (as a function of lipolysis) becomes apparent within 48 to 96 hours after renal shutdown. A creatinine clearance of 30 to 50 mL/min appears to represent the critical threshold for the development of these metabolic alterations.[64]

Despite this impairment of lipolysis, oxidation of fatty acids is not affected by ARF. During infusion of labeled long-chain fatty acids, CO_2 production from lipids in healthy subjects was comparable with that in patients with ARF.[65]

Particles of artificial fat emulsions for parenteral nutrition are degraded in a manner similar to that with endogenous VLDL. Thus, the nutritional consequence of the impaired lipolysis in ARF is a delayed

elimination of intravenously infused lipid emulsions (see later).[56, 57] Elimination half-life is doubled, and the clearance of conventional fat emulsions is reduced by more than 50% in ARF.

Carnitine does not participate in the development of lipid abnormalities in ARF. In contrast with CRF, plasma carnitine levels are increased in ARF.[64] This might be mediated by both increased release from muscle tissues during catabolism and activated hepatic carnitine synthesis.[66]

Electrolytes

POTASSIUM

Hyperkalemia is frequently observed in patients with ARF, but it should be recognized that elevation of the plasma potassium level is caused not only by impaired renal excretion but also by increased release during accelerated protein catabolism and the altered distribution between intracellular and extracellular spaces[67] (Table 37–2). Several factors contribute to a decrease in the cellular uptake of potassium (the uremic state per se, acidosis, drugs such as digitalis, glycosides, or beta-blocking agents), and thus potassium tolerance of the organism is impaired, and the rise in plasma potassium level is augmented during exogenous intake.[14, 67] However, with modern infusion therapy and nutritional support, excessive hyperkalemia is rarely observed, and in fewer than 5% of the cases hyperkalemia is the leading indication for initiation of extracorporeal therapy.[68]

It must be noted that some patients with ARF may, in fact, present with decreased serum potassium concentration.[68] Furthermore, during the course of disease, nutritional support with low electrolyte content may cause hypokalemia in a considerable number of patients. Potassium depletion may aggravate tissue injury and the severity of metabolic disturbances and can precipitate ARF.[69, 70]

PHOSPHATE

Serum phosphate may increase in uremic patients not only because of a impaired renal excretion but

TABLE 37–2. Causes of Hyperkalemia and Hyperphosphatemia in ARF

Hyperkalemia
  Decreased renal elimination
  Increased release during catabolism
    2.38 mmol/g N
    0.36 mmol/g glycogen
  Decreased cellular uptake/increased release
  Metabolic acidosis
    0.6 mmol/L rise—0.1 decrease in pH
Hyperphosphatemia
  Decreased renal elimination
  Increased release from bone
  Increased release during catabolism
    2 mmol/g N
  Decreased cellular uptake/utilization or increased release from
    cells

also because of increased release from cells during catabolism, enhanced gastrointestinal adsorption, decreased metabolic utilization, and augmented mobilization from bone (see Table 37–2). Thus, the type of underlying disease and the degree of hypercatabolism also determine the occurrence and extent of electrolyte abnormalities.

However, in ARF, decreased plasma phosphate levels are much more common than hyperphosphatemia and, in fact, many patients with ARF may present with hypophosphatemia at the time of admission.[68] During the diuretic phase of ARF (and especially, after renal transplantation), phosphate-free continuous renal replacement therapy, and artificial nutrition with low phosphate content, hypophosphatemia may develop in a considerable number of patients.[71] Even if hyperphosphatemia is present at the time of admission of the patient, hypophosphatemia can develop during phosphate-free alimentation within several days.[72, 73] Both phosphate depletion and hyperphosphatemia may predispose to the development of ARF and can retard the recovery of renal function.[74–76]

CALCIUM

The majority of patients with ARF are hypocalcemic, usually with a diminution of both protein-bound and ionized fractions. The precise causes of hypocalcemia are only partially understood. Hypoalbuminemia, hyperphosphatemia, citrate anticoagulation, reduced formation of 1, 25(OH)$_2$ vitamin D$_3$ with reduced calcium adsorption from the gastrointestinal tract, and, potentially, skeletal resistance to the calcemic effect of parathyroid hormone all may contribute to the condition.[31]

Hypercalcemia may develop with high dialysate calcium concentrations, immobilization, acidosis, or hyperparathyroidism, because parathyroid hormone is also elevated in ARF.[31, 77, 78] In ARF caused by rhabdomyolysis, persistent elevations of serum calcitriol may result in a rebound hypercalcemia during the diuretic phase.[79] Acute hypercalcemia per se can cause ARF by inducing acute nephrocalcinosis, arterial calcifications, and interstitial nephritis.

MAGNESIUM

Elevations of serum magnesium are rarely encountered in patients with ARF. Symptomatic hypermagnesemia may develop only during increased magnesium intake or infusion. Hypomagnesemia, on the other hand, may be seen more frequently, such as during the use of magnesium-free substitution fluids for hemofiltration, during citrate anticoagulation, in the presence of associated gastrointestinal disorders, and during the diuretic phase of ARF and after renal transplantation.[80] Moreover, several nephrotoxic drugs, such as cisplatin, aminoglycosides, and amphotericin B, may cause renal magnesium wasting. In transplant recipients treated with cyclosporine, hypomagnesemia is seen in as many as 100% of patients.[81]

Micronutrients

VITAMINS

Serum levels of water-soluble vitamins usually are low in ARF patients mainly because of losses induced by renal replacement therapy.[82, 83] Nutritional status before hospital admission and the type and duration of underlying disease determine vitamin body stores. A deficiency of pyridoxine (vitamin B$_6$) was linked to abnormal amino acid and lipid metabolism in uremia and depletion of thiamine (vitamin B$_1$) during continuous hemofiltration, and inadequate exogenous supplementation may result in perturbations in energy metabolism and in lactic acidosis.[84] Thiamine deficiency per se can promote tubular injury.[85] On the other hand, the potential of inducing toxic effects by overdose is low for water soluble vitamins. An exception is vitamin C, an excess supply of which should be avoided. Ascorbic acid is metabolized via oxalic acid, and any exaggerated intake potentially may induce a secondary oxalosis, which can precipitate the development or retard the resolution of ARF.[86]

Of the fat soluble vitamins, it is the activation of vitamin D$_3$ that is decreased in patients with ARF, and plasma levels of 25(OH) vitamin D and 1,25(OH)$_2$ vitamin D are severely depressed despite the fact that the metabolic clearance rate of calcitriol is also reduced.[31, 87]

Vitamin K pools mostly are normal or even elevated in ARF patients.[31] This may be linked to an increase in the concentration of plasma lipoproteins with which phyllochinone is transported in the blood stream. With additional exogenous vitamin K supplementation, toxic effects may occur; high-dose vitamin K administration was implicated as the cause of a prolonged nonoliguric ARF in a renal transplant recipient.[88] Vitamin K deficiency is much less frequent and is reported mainly in patients receiving certain antibiotics that may reduce intestinal vitamin K production.[89] The prolonged plasma half-life of the drug or of its metabolites in the presence of ARF can contribute to vitamin K depletion.

Metabolism of vitamin A was investigated in detail in experimental ARF.[90] Hepatic release of retinol and of retinol-binding protein into the circulation is increased. The kidney plays a major role in the breakdown of the transport protein and, thus, renal catabolism is decreased, resulting in elevated vitamin A plasma levels in ARF. In contrast, in the clinical situation, a severe depression of plasma concentration of retinol, despite normal levels of retinol-binding protein, is present in ARF.[31]

Similarly, plasma and intraerythrocyte concentrations of antioxidative vitamin E (α-tocopherol) are reduced by more than 50% in patients with ARF.[31] Again, type and severity of underlying disease can modulate vitamin status, and in patients with associated multiple organ dysfunctions, plasma levels of vitamin E have been found to be profoundly decreased.[91]

TRACE ELEMENTS

The available information on trace element metabolism in ARF is limited and, in part, conflicting, and it has not been possible to draw a consistent picture of the metabolic characteristics of trace elements in ARF. The cause and stage of underlying disease must be considered in the interpretation of specific observations.[92] Many of the reported findings, such as decreases in the plasma concentrations of iron and zinc or increases in copper levels indicate unspecific alterations within the spectrum of "acute phase reaction" and do not necessarily reflect deficiency or toxicity states.[93] Geographic and therapeutic factors, such as the content of tap water, the type of therapy, and, especially, the highly variable contamination of infusion-dialysis-hemofiltration fluids with trace elements may profoundly affect trace element balance.[94]

Selenium concentrations in plasma and erythrocytes have been found to be decreased in ARF and CRF patients, and selenium deficiency has been implicated in accelerated lipid peroxidation, impaired immune function, and cardiomyopathy.[91, 95, 96] In critically ill patients, selenium replacement improved clinical outcome and reduced the incidence of ARF requiring extracorporeal renal replacement therapy.[97] Similarly, it was suggested that zinc requirements may be increased in critically ill patients.

The high protein binding of most trace elements does not allow them to be eliminated by renal replacement therapies.[82, 96] Moreover, with supplementation of trace elements in patients with ARF, one must keep in mind the possibility of inducing toxic effects, because during parenteral administration in renal failure the two main regulatory functions in trace element homeostasis, intestinal absorption and renal excretion, are circumvented.[98, 99]

NUTRITIONAL ANTIOXIDANTS

Several micronutrients, such as retinol, vitamin C, vitamin E, and selenium are part of the organism's defense mechanisms against oxygen free radical–induced injury. In experimental ARF, deficiency of antioxidants (decreased vitamin E or selenium status) exacerbates ischemic renal injury, worsens the course, and increases mortality, whereas repletion of antioxidant status exerts the opposite effect.[100–102] A severely compromised antioxidant status has been found in patients with ARF.[91] This is not the reflection of an acute disease process only: in patients with multiple organ dysfunction syndrome (MODS), plasma concentrations of nutritional antioxidants are profoundly decreased. However, when patients with ARF were compared with patients who did not have ARF, the decrease in plasma selenium and in glutathione peroxidase (GSH-Px) activity and the increase in plasma concentrations of lipid perioxidation products were even more pronounced in subjects with accompanying renal dysfunction.[91]

METABOLIC IMPACT OF EXTRACORPOREAL THERAPY

The effects of hemodialysis therapy on metabolism are manifold. Protein catabolism during dialysis is caused not only by substrate losses but also by activation of protein breakdown, mediated by the release of leukocyte-derived proteases or inflammatory mediators (TNF-α and interleukins) induced by blood membrane interactions or endotoxin.[103] Potentially, dialysis also induces an inhibition of muscular protein synthesis.[104] Several water-soluble substances, such as amino acids and vitamins, are lost during hemodialysis, and it has been suggested that generation of reactive oxygen species is augmented during treatment.[105]

Newer renal replacement modalities and in particular, continuous renal replacement therapies (CRRT), such as continuous (arteriovenous or venovenous) hemofiltration and continuous hemodialysis, have gained wide application in the management of patients with ARF and especially in critically ill patients. These CRRTs are associated with a broad pattern of metabolic consequences in addition to renal replacement (Table 37–3).[106, 107]

One major effect is the elimination of small and medium-sized molecules. In the case of amino acids, the sieving coefficient is within the range of 0.8 to 1.0, so amino acid losses can be estimated from the volume of the filtrate and the average plasma concentrations. Usually, this accounts for a loss of approximately 0.2 g/L filtrate and, depending on the filtered volume, results in a total loss of 5 to 15 g amino acids per day, representing about 10% to 15% of amino acid intake.[108–111] Amino acid losses during continuous hemofiltration and continuous hemodialysis are of comparable magnitude.[112]

Similarly, water-soluble vitamins, such as folic acid, vitamin B_6, and vitamin C are eliminated during CRRT.[82, 83] A daily intake higher than that usually recommended is required for the maintenance of plasma concentrations of these vitamins in patients with ARF.

With the high molecular size cut-off of membranes used in hemofiltration, small proteins, such as peptide hormones (insulin, catecholamines, and, potentially, cytokines and mediators) are filtered. In view of their short plasma half-life, hormone losses are minimal and probably not of pathophysiologic importance.[113] Depending on the type of therapy and the membrane

TABLE 37–3. Metabolic Effects of Continuous Renal Replacement Therapy

Amelioration of uremic intoxication ("renal replacement")
plus
Heat loss
Excessive load of substrates (eg, lactate, glucose)
Loss of nutrients (eg, amino acids, vitamins)
Loss of electrolytes (eg, phosphate, magnesium)
Elimination of short-chain proteins (eg, hormones, mediators?)
Metabolic consequences of bioincompatibility (induction/activation of mediator cascades, stimulation of protein catabolism?)

material used, protein losses can vary between 1.2 and 7.5 g/day.[114]

By cooling of the extracorporeal circuit and infusion of substitution fluids that are not prewarmed, CRRT can be associated with a considerable heat loss, accounting for 350 to 700 kcal/day. On the other hand, hemofiltration fluids contain lactate as anions, oxidation of which can compensate in part for the heat loss.[115]

Glucose balance during CRRT obviously is dependent on the glucose concentration of the substitution fluid. Solutions designed for peritoneal dialysis should no longer be used, because of the associated excessive glucose uptake.[116] Glucose concentrations should range between 1 and 2 g/dL to maintain a zero glucose balance.

Uptake of lactate, the organic anion present in most substitution fluids, during CRRT can be considerable and within the magnitude of endogenous lactate turnover. During disease states associated with increased lactate formation (eg, cardiogenic shock) or decreased lactate clearance (liver insufficiency), bicarbonate-based substitution fluids should be used to prevent excessive increases in plasma lactate concentrations.

In patients with ARF treated with CRRT, nutrition solutions must be given during extracorporeal therapy. Nutrition should also be provided during intermittent therapeutic modalities. The endogenous clearance of amino acids is in the range of 80 to 1800 mL/min and thus exceeds dialytic clearance 10 to 100 times (Fig. 37–3), so infusion results in minimal increases in plasma amino acid concentrations; consequently, only

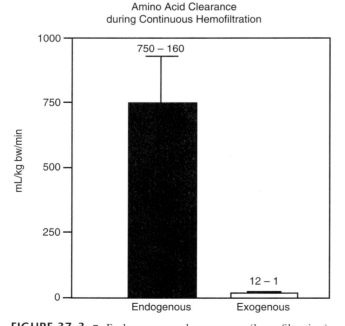

Amino Acid Clearance during Continuous Hemofiltration

FIGURE 37–3 ■ Endogenous and exogenous (hemofiltration) clearance of amino acids (mean + SEM of 18 amino acids) during continuous hemofiltration therapy and infusion of amino acids. (Adapted from Druml W: Nutritional considerations in the treatment of acute renal failure in septic patients. Nephrol Dial Transplant 1994; 9(suppl 4):219–223; with permission.)

a small fraction of the infused amino acids are removed, in addition to the basal amino acid elimination.[17, 18, 111] Thus, nutrition infused during hemodialysis CRRT does not augment amino acid losses substantially, and only about 10% to 15% of the amino acids given are lost in the dialysate-hemofiltrate.[111, 117]

IMPACT OF METABOLIC AND NUTRITIONAL INTERVENTIONS ON RENAL FUNCTION AND COURSE OF ACUTE RENAL FAILURE

Starvation accelerates protein breakdown and impairs protein synthesis in the kidney, whereas refeeding exerts the opposite effects.[118] In the experimental animal, provision of amino acids or TPN accelerates tissue repair and recovery of renal function.[119] In patients, however, this has been much more difficult to prove, and only one study has reported on a positive effect of TPN on the resolution of ARF.[120]

Infusion of amino acids raised renal cortical protein synthesis as evaluated by ^{14}C-leucine incorporation and depressed protein breakdown in rats with mercuric chloride–induced ARF.[121] Intravenous amino acids enhanced renal cortical phospholipid synthesis, suggesting an accelerated membrane formation in regenerating cells.[122] On the other hand, in a similar model of ARF, infusions of varying quantities of essential amino acids (EAA) and nonessential amino acids (NEAA) did not provide any protection of renal function and, in fact, increased mortality.[123] Nevertheless, on balance, available evidence suggests that provision of substrates can stimulate wound healing and tissue regeneration and possibly also renal tubular repair.

The infusion of amino acids before or during ischemia or nephrotoxicity may enhance tubular damage and accelerate loss of renal function in rat models of ARF.[124] In part, this "therapeutic paradox"[125] from amino acid alimentation in ARF is related to the increase in metabolic work for transport processes when oxygen supply is limited, with resulting aggravation of ischemic injury.[126] Similar observations have been made with excess glucose infusion during renal ischemia.[127] Continuous infusion of amino acids does not enhance renal oxygen consumption in humans.[128] Nevertheless, during the insult phase of ARF, the "ebb phase" immediately after trauma, shock, major operations, and so on, any excess nutritional intake should be avoided (see later).

Basic amino acids, such as lysine and arginine, may interfere with proximal tubular functions, resulting in proteinuria, but amino acids do not exert intrinsic nephrotoxic effects.[129] Infusion of an amino acid solution adapted to the metabolic alterations of ARF raises plasma levels of amino acids marginally, eliminates concentration peaks, and limits the probability of inducing untoward side effects.

Some amino acids exert a protective effect. Glycine, in particular, and, to a lesser degree, alanine can limit tubular injury in ischemic and nephrotoxic models of ARF.[130] The mechanisms of these effects remain to be elucidated. Arginine (possibly by producing nitric oxide) reportedly acts to preserve renal perfusion and tubular function during both nephrotoxic and ischemic injury, whereas inhibitors of nitric oxide synthase exert an opposite effect.[131, 132]

The adverse effects of a high-protein diet on morbidity and mortality in CRF, with mention of possible consequences for ARF, were also addressed in multiple studies. A high protein intake prior to an ischemic insult accelerated renal damage and increased mortality in ARF rats.[133, 134] A high-protein diet given to rats before and during gentamicin injections did not affect muscular protein synthesis but accelerated protein degradation.[135] In a further study, protein restriction during the 10 days before ischemic renal failure exerted a protective effect during the first days after induction of ARF but delayed further recovery from renal failure.[136] In sharp contrast, in a nephrotoxic ARF model, a high-protein diet preserved renal function and improved survival.[137]

Both parenterally infused amino acids and enterally given amino acids or protein increase both renal perfusion and excretory renal function (renal functional reserve).[138] Whether this effect can be utilized to improve renal function in patients with ARF remains unknown. Intravenous amino acids improved renal plasma flow ($+ 25\%$) and glomerular filtration rate in cirrhotic patients with functional renal failure.[139] Preliminary data suggest that amino acid infusions can help to conserve diuresis, increase glomerular filtration, and reduce requirements for diuretics in patients with ARF.[140] Moreover, it has been shown in animal experiments that enteral nutrition improves renal perfusion and function and increases survival.[141, 142]

Various other endocrine-metabolic interventions (eg, thyroxine, rHGH, epidermal growth factor [EGF], insulin-like growth factor-1 [IGF-1], hepatocyte growth factor [HGF]) have been shown to accelerate regeneration after experimental ARF.[47, 143–145] In the rat, IGF-1 accelerated recovery from ischemic ARF and improved nitrogen balance, and in a preliminary clinical study in perioperative patients, it prevented the development of renal dysfunction.[47, 146] However, the efficacy of these interventions was not confirmed in clinical studies. Administration of triiodothyronine, which potentially acts through up-regulation of EGF receptor expression, not only was ineffective in human ARF but also increased mortality.[147] Similarly, therapy with rHGH augmented mortality in critically ill patients,[49] and a multicenter study using IGF-I was terminated because of a lack of effect.[48] To date, HGF has not been evaluated in humans.[145]

IMPACT OF ACUTE RENAL FAILURE ON THE GASTROINTESTINAL TRACT

During the last decade, enteral nutrition has become the standard modality for nutritional support in critically ill patients and, thus, also of patients with ARF.[148] Among the multiple well-documented advantages of enteral nutrition, the most important is the fact that provision of luminal nutrients is mandatory to maintain gastrointestinal functions, such as immunologic functions (mucous and secretory IgA production, proliferation of gut-associated lymphoid tissue), motility, bile flow, and, especially, support of the barrier function of the intestinal mucosa. Enteral nutrition helps to preserve the structural integrity of the mucosal layer, to prevent the development of mucosal ulcerations and the translocation of bacteria, and the evolution of systemic infections. Moreover, in experimental ARF, it was shown that enteral nutrition augments not only mesenteric perfusion but also renal plasma flow and can improve renal function.[141, 142]

Knowledge of the impact of acute disease processes and also of ARF on various intestinal functions thus has gained importance for the practice of enteral alimentation. In patients with CRF and subjects undergoing regular hemodialysis therapy, a broad pattern of alterations in intestinal function (eg, gastric emptying and intestinal motility, and digestive and absorptive functions), in biliary and pancreatic secretions, and in bacterial flora have been described.[148, 149] Upper gastrointestinal bleeding has been an important cause of morbidity in ARF patients before the introduction of ulcer prophylaxis.[149] The impact of ARF on various gastrointestinal functions, however, remains poorly characterized.

In patients with MODS, various gastrointestinal functions are affected. As an example, there is a decrease in exocrine pancreatic secretions, depending on the severity of the disease process.[150] How this affects utilization of enterally administered nutrients remains to be clarified. Moreover, gastrointestinal motility is impaired in many critically ill patients. Various factors, such as the underlying disease (eg, pancreatitis or abdominal surgery), circulatory support with catecholamines, and continuous analgesic therapy using opiates all can contribute. Serum creatinine was a strong predictor of an impairment of gastric emptying in intensive care patients and thus ARF might, in fact, exert specific effects on various functions of the gastrointestinal tract.[151]

NUTRIENT REQUIREMENTS IN ACUTE RENAL FAILURE AND PATIENT CLASSIFICATION

The optimal intake of nutrients in patients with ARF is influenced more by the nature of the illness causing ARF, the extent of catabolism, and the type and frequency of dialysis than by the renal dysfunction per se. In most clinical situations, daily requirements exceed the minimal intake recommended for stable CRF patients or the recommended daily allowances (RDA) for normal subjects. Patients with ARF are an extremely heterogeneous group of subjects with widely differing nutrient requirements. It should be noted also that, in an individual patient, requirements can vary considerably during the course of disease.

Energy Requirements

As previously described, ARF per se has little impact on an organism's oxygen consumption, and energy requirements are determined more by the underlying illness than by the ARF. Energy requirements have been grossly overestimated in the past. Energy intakes of more than 50 kcal/kg BW per day (ie, about 100% above basic energy expenditure [BEE]) have been advocated in patients with ARF to achieve a positive nitrogen balance.[152] However, the adverse effects and dangers of exaggerated nutrient intakes are increasingly recognized, and energy substrate supply should cover but certainly not exceed the actual energy consumption.[153] Complications, if any, from slightly underfeeding may, in fact, be less deleterious than those from overfeeding.[154]

A direct measurement of the energy requirements of the individual patient is usually not available. Few institutions perform indirect calorimetry or pulmonary thermodilution catheterism. Nevertheless, the calculation of energy requirements according to a standard formula can provide an acceptable estimate of oxygen consumption. This includes the calculation of BEE and multiplication with a "stress factor," but not the additional multiplication by 1.3 (as recommended in the past) (Table 37–4).

Thus, patients with ARF should receive 25 to 30 kcal/kg BW per day. Even in hypermetabolic conditions such as sepsis or MODS, energy expenditure rarely is higher than 130% of calculated BEE, and energy intake should not exceed 35 kcal/kg BW per day.[5–7] This is in accordance with general guidelines for energy intake in critically ill patients.[155, 156] In the critically ill patient, nitrogen loss cannot be attenuated merely by increasing energy intake.[157]

Amino Acid and Protein Requirements in Patients With Acute Renal Failure

Unfortunately, only a few studies have attempted to define the optimal intake for protein or amino acids

TABLE 37–4. Estimation of Energy Requirements

Calculation of basic energy expenditure (BEE) (Harris Benedict equation):
  Males: 66.47 + (13.75 × BW) + (5 × height) − (6.76 × age)
  Females: 655.1 + (9.56 × BW) + (1.85 × height) − (4.67 × age)
The average BEE is approximately 25 kcal/kg BW/day
Stress factors for correcting calculated energy requirement for hypermetabolism:
  Postoperative (no complications): 1.0
  Long bone fracture: 1.15–1.30
  Cancer: 1.10–1.30
  Peritonitis/sepsis: 1.20–1.30
  Severe infection/multiple trauma: 1.20–1.40
  Burns: 1.20–2.00
  (approximately BEE + % burned body surface area)

Corrected energy requirements (kcal/day) = BEE × stress factor.
BW, body weight.

in ARF. In nonhypercatabolic patients during the polyuric phase of ARF, a protein intake of 0.97 g/kg BW per day was required for a positive nitrogen balance.[158] A similar number (1.03 g/kg BW/day) was concluded from a study in which, unfortunately, energy intake was not kept constant.[152] In the polyuric recovery phase in patients with sepsis-induced ARF, a nitrogen intake of 15 g/day (averaging an amino acid intake of 1.3 g/kg BW/day) as compared with 4.4 g/day (about 0.3 g/kg amino acids) was superior in amelioration of nitrogen balance.[159]

In a randomized double-blind trial in 23 catabolic ARF patients, Feinstein and coworkers[160] compared the infusion of 21 g of EAAs (averaging 0.25 g/kg BW/day) with infusion of the same amount of EAA plus 21 g of NEAAs (a further group received glucose alone). There were no differences in recovery of renal function or survival among the groups investigated. Urea appearance tended to be higher with increased amino acid intake. Nevertheless, the authors suggest that greater quantities of energy and both essential and nonessential amino acids should be given in hypercatabolic patients with ARF.

In a similar study of a limited number of patients, the same authors compared patients receiving 21 g of EAA with a group receiving EAAs and NEAAs in an amount equaling or even slightly exceeding urea nitrogen appearance of the previous day (on average 76 g amino acids/day).[161] In patients with the higher amino acid intake, urea appearance was higher but nitrogen was less negative (−3.0 vs. −5.2 g N/day; not significant).

More recent studies have tried to evaluate protein and amino acids requirements in critically ill patients with ARF on CRRT. Kierdorf and coworkers[162] found that in these hypercatabolic patients provision of 1.5 g amino acids/kg BW per day was more effective in reducing nitrogen loss than infusion of 0.7 g (−3.4 vs. −8.1 g N/day). However, an increase in amino acid intake to 1.74 g/kg BW per day did not further ameliorate nitrogen balance (−3.2 g N/day). Chima and coworkers[163] evaluated the protein catabolic rate, urea nitrogen appearance, and total nitrogen appearance in 19 critically ill patients. A mean protein catabolic rate of 1.7 g/kg BW per day was observed, and it was concluded that protein needs in these patients range between 1.4 g and 1.7 g/kg BW per day. Similarly, Macias and coworkers[164] have measured a protein catabolic rate of 1.4 g/kg BW per day. There was an inverse relationship between protein and energy provision and protein catabolic rate, and nitrogen deficit was less in the patients receiving nutritional support. Again, a protein intake of 1.5 to 1.8 g/kg BW per day was recommended. Finally, Bellomo and coworkers[165] compared a protein intake of 1.2 g/kg BW per day with an intake of 2.5 g/kg BW per day in critically ill patients with ARF on CRRT. When patients were given this excessive amount of protein, there was some improvement in nitrogen balance (−5.5 g/day vs. −1.92 g/day, not significant), but at the cost of augmented urea generation rate and the need for more aggressive renal replacement therapy.

Thus, unless renal insufficiency is brief and there is no associated catabolic illness, the intake of protein or amino acids should not be lower than 0.8 g/kg BW per day. Nevertheless, again it should be emphasized, that hypercatabolism cannot be overcome by increasing protein or amino acid intake.[20, 166] Patients with ARF should receive 1.2 g to 1.5 g protein–amino acids (maximum)/kg BW per day; again, this is in accordance with more general recommendations for critically ill patients.[157, 167] Any exaggerated protein intake, as recommended in some studies,[165] has no proven benefit and simply stimulates the formation of urea and other nitrogenous waste products, increases the required intensity of renal replacement therapy, and, potentially, may aggravate uremic complications.

For patients treated with hemodialysis-continuous hemofiltration and those undergoing peritoneal dialysis, an extra protein-amino acid intake of 0.2 to 0.3 g/kg BW per day (again to a maximum of 1.3 to 1.5 g/kg BW/day) should be provided to compensate for losses occurring during therapy.[107–109, 111]

ASSESSMENT OF PROTEIN CATABOLISM

Virtually all nitrogen arising from amino acids liberated during protein degradation is converted to urea. Thus, the degree of protein catabolism can be judged clinically by calculating the urea nitrogen appearance rate (UNA) (Table 37–5). When UNA is multiplied by 6.25 it can be converted to protein equivalents. Muscle contains about 20% protein; thus, multiplying the estimated protein loss by 5 yields an approximation of the loss of muscle mass. Obviously, UNA is not a "true" rate of protein catabolism, because it does not take into account the high endogenous rate of protein turnover (3 to 4 g of protein/kg BW/day in adults).

In patients with renal insufficiency, the urea produced is not excreted completely but accumulates in body fluids. Urea is distributed equally in total body water (about 60% of BW); thus, changes in the urea pool can be easily calculated. Besides urea in urine, nitrogen losses in other body fluids (eg, gastrointestinal or choledochal losses) must be added to the net change in urea pool. In addition, non–urea nitrogen must be taken into account. These losses do not vary substantially with the diet and can be estimated to be 0.031 g of nitrogen/kg BW per day.[168] If this value is

TABLE 37–5. Estimating the Extent of Protein Catabolism

Urea Nitrogen Appearance (UNA) (g/day)
 = urinary urea nitrogen excretion
 + change in urea nitrogen pool
 = (UUN × V) + (BUN$_2$ − BUN$_1$) 0.006 × BW + (BW$_2$ − BW$_1$) × BUN$_2$/100
If there are substantial GI losses, add urea nitrogen in secretions:
 = volume of secretions × BUN$_2$
Net protein breakdown (g/day) = UNA × 6.25
Muscle loss (g/day)   = UNA × 6.25 × 5

UUN, urinary urea nitrogen concentration; *V,* urinary volume; *BUN$_1$* and *BUN$_2$,* BUN in mg/dL on days 1 and 2; *BW$_1$* and *BW$_2$,* body weight in kg on days 1 and 2.

added to UNA, total waste nitrogen production can be estimated. When nitrogen intake from the diet or parenteral nutrition is known, nitrogen balance can be calculated.

Electrolytes

As discussed earlier, derangements in the electrolyte balance in patients with ARF are affected by a broad spectrum of factors beyond renal failure, including the type of underlying disease and degree of hypercatabolism, the type and frequency of renal replacement therapy, and also the type and composition of nutritional support.

Electrolyte requirements vary considerably among patients and also can change fundamentally during the course of the disease in a particular patient. In nonoliguric patients, in subjects on CRRT, and during the polyuric phase of ARF, electrolyte requirements can increase considerably. Nutritional support, especially parenteral nutrition with low electrolyte contents, can cause hypophosphatemia and hypokalemia, respectively, in a large number of patients.[71, 73] Thus, in patients with ARF, the evaluation of electrolyte requirements on a day-to-day basis and the frequent adjustment of intake is even more crucial than for other substrates that are administered.

Micronutrients

Balance studies on micronutrients (vitamins, trace elements) in ARF are not available, and no scientifically based recommendations can be given for this patient group (see previous discussion). Requirements for water-soluble vitamins are expected to be increased in patients with ARF, because of losses associated with renal replacement therapy.[82, 83] As an example, depletion of thiamine (vitamin B$_1$) during continuous hemofiltration and inadequate supply may result in lactic acidosis and heart failure.[84] Malnutrition with depletion of vitamin body stores and underlying disease in ARF can further increase the requirements for vitamins. An exception is ascorbic acid (vitamin C); as a precursor of oxalic acid, the intake should be kept below 200 mg/day, because any excess supply can precipitate secondary oxalosis or even induce ARF or retard resolution of ARF.[86]

Despite the fact that fat-soluble vitamins are not lost during hemodialysis-CRRT, their requirements are increased in ARF.[31] An exception is vitamin K, plasma concentrations of which are within the normal range in ARF. Most commercial multivitamin preparations for parenteral infusion contain the recommended daily allowances of vitamins and can be safely used in ARF patients.

For supplementation of trace elements, one should keep in mind that parenteral infusion in patients with renal failure bypasses the two main regulators of trace-element homeostasis: gastrointestinal absorption and renal excretion. This increases the risk of toxicity.[98]

Parenteral zinc supplementation can increase the febrile response during the acute-phase reaction.[99] The requirement for selenium, the cofactor of glutathione peroxidase, might be increased. Supplementation of selenium can augment the oxygen radical scavenger system of the organism and, at least potentially, prevent the development of renal dysfunction and improve survival in critically ill patients (see previous discussion).[97]

Patient Classification

Ideally, a nutritional program should be designed for each individual patient with ARF. In clinical practice, it has proved useful to distinguish three groups of ARF patients based on the extent of protein catabolism associated with the underlying disease and the resulting levels of nutrient requirements (Table 37–6).

GROUP I

The patients in this group include those without excess catabolism and a UNA of less than 6 g of nitrogen above nitrogen intake per day. ARF is usually caused by nephrotoxins, such as aminoglycosides or contrast medium. These patients rarely exhibit major nutritional problems and, in most cases, can be fed orally, with the prognosis for recovery of renal function and survival excellent.

GROUP II

Group II patients have a moderate hypercatabolism and a UNA exceeding nitrogen intake 6 to 12 g of nitrogen/day. Affected patients frequently suffer from complicating infections or moderate injury in association with ARF. Tube feeding or intravenous nutritional support are generally required, and dialysis-hemofiltration often becomes necessary to limit waste product accumulation.

GROUP III

The patients in group II are those in whom ARF occurs in association with severe trauma, burns, or overwhelming infections and, in many instances, in whom ARF is a component of MODS. The UNA is markedly elevated, that is, more than 12 g of nitrogen above nitrogen intake. Treatment strategies are usually complex and include enteral-parenteral nutrition, hemodialysis–continuous hemofiltration, plus blood pressure and ventilatory support. To reduce catabolism and avoid protein depletion, high nutrient requirements must be met, and dialysis is used to maintain fluid balance and blood urea nitrogen (BUN) level below 80 to 100 mg/dL. Mortality in this group of patients exceeds 60% to 80%. It is not the loss of renal function that accounts for the poor prognosis, but mainly the superimposed hypercatabolism and the severity of underlying illness.

SUBSTRATES AND DIETS FOR PARENTERAL AND ENTERAL NUTRITION

Substrates for Parenteral Nutrition

CARBOHYDRATES

Glucose should be used as the main energy substrate for parenteral nutrition because it can be utilized by all organs even under hypoxic conditions. In contrast to earlier recommendations, glucose intake must be restricted to less than 5 g/kg BW per day. Higher intakes are not used for energy but do promote

TABLE 37–6. Patient Classification and Nutrient Requirements in Patients With ARF

	EXTENT OF CATABOLISM		
	Mild	Moderate	Severe
Excess urea appearance (above N intake)	>5 g	5–10 g	>10 g
Clinical setting (examples)	Drug toxicity	Elective surgery ± infection	Severe injury or sepsis
Mortality	20%	60%	>80%
Dialysis/hemofiltration frequency	Rare	As needed	Frequent
Route of nutrient administration	Oral	Enteral and/or parenteral	Enteral and/or parenteral
Energy recommendations (kcal/kg BW/day)	25	25–30	25–35
Energy substrates	Glucose	Glucose + fat	Glucose + fat
Glucose (g/kg BW/day)	3.0–5.0	3.0–5.0	3.0–5.0 (max. 7.0)
Fat (g/kg/BW/day)		0.5–1.0	0.8–1.2
Amino acids/protein (g/kg/day)	0.6–1.0	0.8–1.2	1.0–1.5
	EAA (+NEAA)	EAA + NEAA	EAA + NEAA
Nutrients used oral/enteral	Food	Enteral formulas Glucose 50%–70% + fat emulsions 10% or 20%	Enteral formulas Glucose 50%–70%
parenteral		EAA + specific NEAA solutions (general or "nephro") Multivitamin and multi–trace element preparations	

BW, body weight; EAA, essential amino acids; NEAA, nonessential amino acids.

lipogenesis with fatty infiltration of the liver, excessive carbon dioxide production, and hypercapnia.[169, 170] Since ARF impairs glucose tolerance, insulin is frequently necessary to maintain normoglycemia. Insulin, however, does not increase oxidative glucose disposal, and insulin dosage should be limited to a maximum of 4 U/h, or glucose infusions should be reduced.[171] Because of the many well-characterized side effects of even short-term hyperglycemia, blood glucose levels must be maintained within the physiologic range.[172-174]

Energy requirements cannot be met by glucose infusion alone, so a portion of the energy should be supplied by lipid emulsions. The most suitable means of providing the energy requirements in critically ill patients is not glucose or lipids, but glucose and lipids.[175-177, 178]

Other carbohydrates, including fructose, sorbitol, and xylitol, which are available in some countries (but not the United States), should be avoided because of potential adverse metabolic effects.

FAT EMULSIONS

Advantages of intravenous lipids include a high specific energy content, a low osmolality, provision of essential fatty acids to prevent deficiency syndromes, a lower frequency of hepatic side effects, and reduced carbon dioxide production, which is especially relevant in patients with respiratory failure. It should be kept in mind that lipids not only provide an energy substrate but also act as important structural components of cell membranes and as precursors of regulatory molecules, such as hormones, prostanoids, and leukotrienes. Addition of a lipid emulsion to intravenous nutrition promoted weight gain and body composition and improved the uremic state in rats.[179]

Changes in lipid metabolism associated with ARF should not prevent the use of lipid emulsions. Instead, the amount infused should be adjusted to meet the patient's capacity to utilize lipids. Usually, 1 g fat/kg BW per day does not increase plasma triglycerides substantially, so about 20% to 25% of energy requirements can be met.[64] Lipids should not be administered to patients with hyperlipidemia (plasma triglycerides >350 mg/dL), activated intravascular coagulation, acidosis (pH <7.20), impaired circulation, or hypoxemia.

Parenteral lipid emulsions usually contain long-chain triglycerides, mostly derived from soybean oil. Recently, fat emulsions containing a mixture of long- and medium-chain triglycerides have been introduced for intravenous use. Proposed advantages include a faster elimination from the plasma, due to a higher affinity for the lipoprotein lipase enzyme, the complete, rapid, and carnitine-independent metabolism, and a triglyceride-lowering effect. However, in patients with ARF, the use of medium-chain triglycerides does not augment lipolysis, and the elimination of parenterally infused triglycerides is equally retarded (Fig. 37–4).[58]

AMINO ACID SOLUTIONS FOR PARENTERAL NUTRITION IN ACUTE RENAL FAILURE

The most controversial question regarding parenteral nutrition in patients with ARF is the type of amino acid solution to be used: either solutions of exclusively EAAs, solutions of EAAs plus NEAAs in standard proportions as used in nonuremic patients,

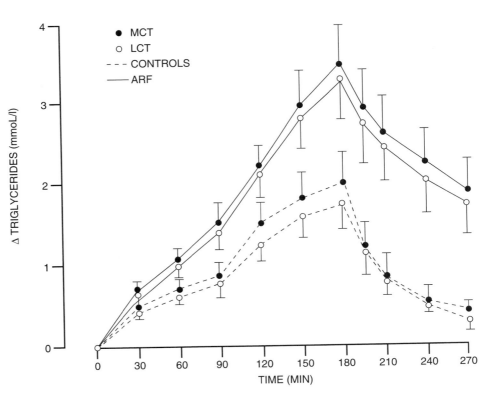

FIGURE 37–4 ■ Increase in plasma triglycerides above basal concentrations in healthy subjects (n = 6, *solid lines*) and patients with acute renal failure (n = 7, *dashed lines*) during infusion of a lipid emulsion containing exclusively long-chain triglycerides (LCT; *open circles*) or a mixture of LCT and medium-chain triglycerides (50:50) (MCT; *closed circles*). P < 0.01 for rise of triglyceride levels during both types of lipid emulsions; patients vs. controls. (Adapted from Druml W, Fischer M, Sertl S, et al: Fat elimination in acute renal failure: long chain vs. medium-chain triglycerides. Am J Clin Nutr 1992; 55:468–472; with permission.)

or specifically designed "nephro" solutions of different proportions of EAAs and specific NEAAs that might become "conditionally essential" in ARF (Table 37–7).

The use of solutions of EAAs alone is based on principles established for treating CRF patients with a low-protein diet and an EAA supplement. This may be inappropriate, because the metabolic adaptations to low-protein diets present in response to CRF may not occur in patients with ARF, and there are fundamental differences in the goals of nutritional therapy between the two groups of patients. Consequently, infusion solutions of EAA may be suboptimal for the following reasons:

- Amino acid requirements, as evaluated by modern isotope turnover techniques, are likely to be considerably higher than suggested from tests carried out in the 1940s.
- Certain amino acids designated as NEAAs for healthy subjects may become conditionally indispensable in sick patients (eg, histidine, arginine, tyrosine, serine, cysteine);[3, 43, 180] Arginine-free amino acid solutions can cause life-threatening complications, such as hyperammonemia, coma, and acidosis in patients with ARF.[181, 182]
- Changes in amino acid metabolism caused by ARF (or hypercatabolism) can result in serious imbalances of plasma amino acid concentrations during infusions of EAA.[18]

- Infusion of more than 0.6 g EAAs/kg per day simply leads to conversion of infused amino acids to waste products.
- Use of EAAs to synthesize NEAAs has no obvious advantage and wastes energy.
- A complete amino acid mixture may improve net nitrogen retention more than an EAA solution.[183]

Taken together, solutions including both EAAs and NEAAs in standard proportions or in special proportions designed to counteract the metabolic changes of renal failure ("nephro" solutions) should be used in nutritional support in patients with ARF. Provision of 0.6 g EAAs/kg per day may be sufficient for noncatabolic patients, but those requiring a higher level should receive a mixture of EAAs and NEAAs and, especially including the amino acids that might become conditionally essential in ARF.

Because of the low water solubility of tyrosine, dipeptides containing tyrosine (such as glycyltyrosine) are contained in some of the modern "nephro" solutions as a tyrosine source[43, 44, 184] (see Table 37–7). One should be aware of the fact that the amino acid analogue N-acetyl tyrosine, which in the past was often used as a tyrosine source, cannot be converted into tyrosine in humans and might even stimulate protein catabolism.[43]

Despite considerable investigation, there is no persuasive evidence that amino acid solutions enriched in branched-chain amino acids (BCAA) exert a clinically

TABLE 37–7. Amino Acid Solutions for the Treatment of ARF

	DOSE REQUIREMENT	RENAMIN (CLINTEC)	AMINESS (CLINTEC)	AMINOSYN RF (ABBOTT)	NEPHR-AMINE (MCGAW)	NEPHOTECT (FRESENIUS)
Amino acids (g/L)		65	52	52	54	100
(= g/%)		6.5%	5.2%	5.2%	5.4%	10%
Volume (mL)		500	400	1000	1000	500
mOsm/L		600	416	475	435	908
Nitrogen (g/L)		10	8.3	8.3	6.5	16.3
Essential amino acids (g/L)						
Isoleucine	1.40	5.00	5.25	4.62	5.60	5.80
Leucine	2.20	6.00	8.25	7.26	8.80	12.80
Lysine-acetate/HCl	1.60	4.50	6.00	5.35	6.40	12.00
Methionine	2.20	5.00	8.25	7.26	8.80	2.00
Phenylalanine	2.20	4.90	8.25	7.26	8.80	3.50
Threonine	1.00	3.80	3.75	3.30	4.00	8.20
Tryptophan	0.50	1.60	1.88	1.60	2.00	3.00
Valine	1.60	8.20	6.00	5.20	6.40	8.70
Nonessential amino acids (g/L)						
Alanine		5.60				
Arginine		6.30		6.00		6.20
Glycine		3.00				8.20
Histidine		4.20	4.12	4.29	2.50	6.30*
Proline		3.50				9.80
Serine		3.00				3.00
Tyrosine		0.40				7.60
Cysteine		—			0.20	3.00†
Electrolytes (mEq/L)						0.40
Acetate		60	50	105	44	71
Sodium					5	
Potassium				5.4		
Chloride		31			3	

*Tyrosine is included as dipeptide (glycl-L-tyrosine).
†Glycine in part is component of the dipeptide.

significant anticatabolic effect. In patients with ARF, there is very limited experience with BCAA. A parenteral supplement of BCAA in patients with ARF failed to exert any effect on nitrogen balance or plasma concentrations of plasma proteins.[185] Similarly, in a study comparing a BCAA-enriched amino acid solution and a standard amino acid solution in critically ill patients with ARF treated with CRRT, no amelioration of nitrogen balance and plasma protein concentrations was observed.[186]

It was suggested that glutamine, an amino acid that traditionally was termed nonessential, exerts important metabolic functions in regulating nitrogen metabolism, supporting immunologic functions and preserving the gastrointestinal barrier and, thus, may become conditionally indispensable in catabolic illness.[50, 187] For glutamine supplementation in patients with ARF, only limited information is available. Glutamine supplementation in animals with postischemic ARF decreased survival rate.[188] This, however, may not appropriately reflect the clinical situation, in which, obviously, any excess nitrogen is removed during renal replacement therapy. In a study comparing standard parenteral nutrition with a nutritional solution enriched with glutamine in critically ill patients, long-term survival was improved in patients receiving glutamine.[189] In a post hoc analysis, the improvement in prognosis was most pronounced in patients with ARF (4/24 survivors without glutamine, 14/23 with glutamine, $P < 0.02$, personal communication).

Since free glutamine is not stable in aqueous solutions, glutamine-containing dipeptides are used as a glutamine source in parenteral nutrition.[190] It must be recognized that the utilization of dipeptides in part is dependent on intact renal function, and renal failure may impair hydrolysis and, during high-dose therapy with glycylglutamine, the dipeptide may accumulate in the plasma compartment.[44, 46]

ELECTROLYTES

Electrolyte concentrates should be added to the nutrition solution as required. It must be remembered that the infusion of glucose or amino acids causes a shift of potassium and phosphate into the cells, potentially causing hypokalemia or hypophosphatemia, respectively, in a considerable number of patients. If phosphate is added to "all-in-one" solutions, organic phosphates (glycerophosphate, glucose-1-phosphate) must be used to avoid incompatibilities with other ions in the solution. Divalent ions (calcium, magnesium) can impair the stability of fat emulsions and should be used with caution in lipid-containing nutrition solutions. Again, organic salts of divalent ions, such as calcium gluconate, should be used to avoid precipitation of insoluble salts.

MICRONUTRIENTS

It is not feasible to supply vitamins individually; thus standard multivitamin preparations for intravenous application should be used for parenteral nutrition, and these can be safely added to the nutrition solution. Extra vitamin C (>200 mg/day) should be avoided. As detailed earlier, trace-element supplementation should be restricted in ARF to avoid inducing toxic effects. Again, combinations of multiple trace elements for intravenous use can be used as admixtures to nutritional solutions.

Diets for Enteral Nutrition

The basic difficulty in designing an enteral diet for patients with ARF is to address not only the broad spectrum of clinical problems but also the extreme diversity of individual needs that often prevents the use of commercially available enteral diets. It must be stressed that none of these diets have been specifically developed for subjects with ARF. Essentially, three types of enteral formulas can be used in ARF patients, as described in the following paragraphs.[148]

(SEMI-) ELEMENTAL POWDER DIETS CONTAINING MAINLY ESSENTIAL AMINO ACIDS

The concept of a low-protein diet supplemented with EAAs designed in the 1960s for oral nutrition in patients with CRF was extended in analogy to enteral nutrition in patients with ARF. These diets (Table 37–8) contain the eight classic EAAs plus histidine and, thus, are not complete and must be supplemented with energy substrates, vitamins, and trace elements. The major disadvantages of these kinds of enteral diets are not only the limited spectrum of nutrients, but also the high osmolality of the nutrient solution and problems associated with powder diets. These formulations can be used as a dietary supplement, but if total enteral nutrition becomes necessary, these diets should be replaced by more complete formulas.

STANDARD (HIGH-MOLECULAR) ENTERAL FORMULAS DESIGNED FOR NONUREMIC PATIENTS

In many intensive care patients with ARF, standard enteral formulas are given if enteral nutrition is instituted.[148] The disadvantages of these conventional diets are the fixed composition of the nutrients, which prevents the possibility of adaptation to individual needs; the amount and type of protein; and the high content of electrolytes, especially potassium and phosphate. Nevertheless, these diets are frequently used in patients with ARF, at least in supplementary enteral nutrition. Whether diets enriched with specific substrates, such as glutamine, arginine, nucleotides, and ω-3 fatty acids ("immunonutrition"), can exert beneficial effects also in patients with ARF remains to be shown.[191]

SPECIFIC ENTERAL FORMULAS ADAPTED TO THE METABOLIC ALTERATIONS OF UREMIA

Two basic technical concepts have been followed in designing a specialized enteral diet for patients with

TABLE 37–8. Enteral Diets for Patients With Renal Failure

	TRAVASORB RENAL* (CLINTEC)	SALVIPEPTIDE† NEPHRO (CLINTEC)	SURVIMED RENAL‡ (FRESENIUS)	REPLENA§ (SUPLENA) (ROSS)	RENALCAL‖ (NESTLE)	NEPRO¶ (ROSS)	NOVA SOURCE RENAL# (NOVARTIS)	MAGNACAL RENAL** (MEAD JOHNSON)
Volume (mL)	1000	1000	1000	1000	1000	1000	1000	1000
Calories (kcal)	1333.3	2000	1320	2000	2000	2000	2000	2000
(cal/mL)	1.35	2	1.32	2	2	2	2	2
Protein:fat:carbohydrate	7:12:81	8:22:70	6:10:84	6:43:51	6.9:35:58.1	14:43:43	15:45:40	15.3:45:40
Nitrogen (g)	3.42	6.4	3.32	4.8	5.9	11.2	12.2	11.8
Kcal/g N	389:1	313:1	398:1	417:1	360:1	179:1	164:1	169:1
Nonprotein	363:1	288:1	374:1	393:1	340:1	154:1	140:1	144:1
Osmol (mOsm/kg)	590	507	600	600	600	635	700	570
Protein (g)	22.9	40	20.8	30	34.4	69.9	74	75
EAA (%)	60	23			67			
NEAA (%)	30	20			33			
Hydrolysate (%)		23	100					
Total protein (%)		34		100		100		100
Carbohydrate (g)	270.5	350	276	256	290.4	215.78	200	200
Monosaccharide and disaccharide (%)	100	3		10		12		
Oligosaccharide (%)		8						
Polysaccharide (%)		69	100	90		88		
Fat (g)	17.7	48	15.2	95.7	82.4	95.6	100	101
LCT (%)	30	50	70	100	30	100	86	80
Ess. FA (%)	18	31	52	22		20		
MCT (%)	70	50	30		70		14	20
Sodium (mmol/L)	N/A	7.2	15.2	34	N/A	36.1	43.5	35
Potassium (mmol/L)	N/A	1.5	8	29	N/A	27	20.8	32
Phosphorus (mg/L)	N/A			728	N/A	695	650	800
Vitamins	a	a	a	a	a	a	a	a
Trace elements	b	a	a	a	a	a	a	a

*Powder diet: 3 bags + 810 mL water = 1050 mL.
†Powder diet (1 × component I + 1 × component II + 350 mL water) × 2 = 1000 mL.
‡Powder diet 4 bags + 800 mL water = 1000 mL.
§Ready-to-use liquid diet, taurine + carnitine − supplement, 8 fl oz cans.
‖Ready-to-use liquid diet, 250 mL cans.
¶Ready-to-use liquid diet, taurine + carnitine − supplement, 8 fl oz cans.
#Ready-to-use liquid diet, 8 fl oz Tetra Brik Paks; 1000 mL; RTH = Ready to Hang.
**Ready-to-use liquid diet, 8 fl oz cans.
  a, 2000 kcal/d for RDI of vitamins and trace elements; *b,* have to be supplied; *EAA,* essential amino acids; *NEAA,* nonessential amino acids; *FA,* fatty acids; *LCT,* long-chain triglycerides; *MCT,* medium-chain triglycerides; *N/A,* information not available; *RDI,* recommended daily intake for vitamins and minerals.

renal failure: modular (elemental) powder diets and ready-to-use (high-molecular) preparations. Unfortunately, again, these diets have been designed for nutritional therapy in either CRF patients or subjects undergoing chronic hemodialysis therapy. These diets include the following:

• Modular (elemental) diets composed of "energy" and "protein" components. With these diets, the problems of variations in individual requirements can, at least in part, be circumvented, and the diet can be somewhat adapted to the needs of a specific patient by altering the number and types of components. From a theoretical standpoint, this presents a promising concept of enteral diets for renal failure patients. The main disadvantages of these powder diets are the time-consuming preparation and the risk of contamination.
• Ready-to-use (high-molecular) liquid diets. Available preparations have been designed as a supplement for patients with compensated CRF and are characterized by a reduced protein content and low electrolyte concentrations (see Table 37–8). A second type of preparation has been adapted to the nutrient

requirements of patients undergoing regular hemodialysis therapy with a higher protein component, but again with a reduced electrolyte content (see Table 37–8). Several of these diets contain other additions, such as taurine or carnitine, and have a high specific energy content ranging from 1.5 to 2.0 kcal/mL. The formulas with a moderate protein content present the most reasonable approach to enteral nutrition in hypercatabolic intensive care patients with ARF.

EXPERIENCE WITH NUTRITIONAL SUPPORT IN ACUTE RENAL FAILURE

Clinical Experience With Parenteral Nutrition

Only a limited number of systematic clinical studies have been conducted on nutritional support in ARF, and few were prospective and fulfilled minimal requirements in study design with respect to patient numbers, definition of end points, and stratification of groups. Early investigations attempted to define the effect of nutritional support, including amino acids, compared with glucose infusions alone.[120, 160, 192, 193] Subsequent studies addressed the question of whether EAAs only or EAAs and NEAAs should be provided and sought to determine what level of nitrogen intake would be preferential in ARF[161, 194–196, 197] (see previous discussion). The majority of investigations have generated conflicting or inconclusive results with respect to outcome.

In a highly quoted study using a double-blind protocol, Abel and coworkers[120] compared a "renal-failure solution," including 16 g of EAAs, with the infusion of glucose alone. A significantly higher percentage of ARF patients receiving the "renal failure fluid" survived, and this was more apparent in high-risk patients, in those requiring dialysis, and in those who developed pneumonia, generalized sepsis, or a major gastrointestinal hemorrhage. There was also a tendency for a shorter overall duration of renal dysfunction. The finding that especially high-risk patients with ARF benefit from nutritional intervention was confirmed in noncontrolled studies.[40, 198]

Baek and coworkers[192] compared the treatment with a fibrin hydrolysate (containing EAAs and NEAAs) and glucose with glucose alone in patients who had ARF. In the treatment group, morbidity and mortality were lower. Leonard and coworkers[193] treated patients with ARF with either EAAs and glucose or glucose alone and found that the rise in BUN level was significantly reduced in the nutrition group, but survival and duration of renal failure were unaffected.

Studies that aimed at defining optimal nitrogen intake in ARF have been detailed previously. Various investigations have compared infusions of EAAs only versus EAAs and NEAAs in patients with ARF, but rarely were infusion solutions isocaloric or isonitrogenic. In a randomized, controlled study in a limited number of patients, Feinstein and coworkers[161] compared, in a double-blind protocol, three types of nutrition in ARF: (1) glucose alone, (2) glucose and the "safe intake" of EAAs (14 g), or (3) glucose and EAAs + NEAAs (33 g). Although there were no differences in the rapidity or incidence of recovery of renal function or in the rate of survival among the three treatment groups, nitrogen balance and outcome tended to be improved in patients receiving EAA.

Comparing provision of 2 g of nitrogen as EAAs with 4 g of nitrogen as EAAs and NEAAs, Freund and coworkers[196] showed a dramatic advantage for EAAs only, but the control group consisted of data from an earlier investigation.[120] In a crossover study, parenteral nutrition regimen with 15 to 20 g of EAAs or 20 to 40 g of EAAs and NEAAs were evaluated.[194] The UNA was higher during EAA and NEAA administration, but there was also a tendency toward an improvement in nitrogen balance with the higher nitrogen intake. Finally, Mirtallo and coworkers[195] compared an infusion containing 28 g of EAAs with that containing 33 g of EAAs and NEAAs. There were no differences in UNA and no changes in renal function or survival. Patients,

however, were not catabolic (they were in positive nitrogen balance) and did not require dialysis.

Taken together, the results of these studies suggest that the sicker a patient is, the more he or she benefits from a nutritional intervention; that nutrition, including amino acid in patients with ARF, is superior to glucose alone, especially in high-risk patients; and that hypercatabolic patients should receive both EAAs and NEAAs. Moreover, in critically ill patients with ARF undergoing continuous renal replacement therapies, a higher amino acid or protein intake may be necessary to maintain nitrogen balance.

A well-known difficulty in providing nutritional support is the demonstration of beneficial effects with respect to survival.[199, 200] This problem certainly is not confined to patients with ARF but extends to all critically ill subjects.[201] Patients with ARF are extremely heterogeneous, with a highly variable clinical course and a broad pattern of associated complications; outcome depends on the severity of underlying illness and the degree of associated catabolism but does not directly depend on the impairment of renal function. Nutrition is just a single component in a complex pattern of therapeutic interventions. However, there can be no question that every patient needs nutrition; it is only the optimal composition of the nutritional regimen that remains to be specified.

Clinical Experience With Enteral Nutrition in Acute Renal Failure

In sharp contrast to daily practice in most intensive care units where enteral nutrition has become a standard type of nutritional support, systematic studies on enteral nutrition in patients with ARF are virtually nonexistent.[202] The results of animal experiments that suggest an improvement in renal perfusion and renal function in ARF after enteral nutrition have currently not been confirmed in clinical studies.[141, 142] Most available investigations have focused instead on the feasibility and tolerance of enteral diets in patients with CRF and undergoing chronic hemodialysis therapy, and information regarding nutritional efficiency is rarely provided.[148]

Fiaccadori and coworkers[202] evaluated the adequacy of nutrient intake of, the nutritional effects of, and the tolerance for a ready-to-use renal enteral formula with a moderate protein content in 14 noncatabolic patients with ARF undergoing bi-daily hemodialysis therapy during a total of 209 treatment days. Nutrient intake of more than 90% of calculated needs was achieved within 64 hours, biochemical and immunologic nutritional indexes improved, nitrogen balance became positive in several patients, and tolerance for the diet was good.

A protein-restricted formula (see Table 37–8) was tested in 18 patients with CRF during 4 weeks. The patients ate normally and added the supplement at a rate of 10 kcal/kg BW per day.[203] With this combination, energy and protein intakes were raised to the recommended level in patients undergoing regular dialysis treatment. Blood chemistry remained stable in all patients, and gastrointestinal tolerance was good. A diet with a higher protein content was designed for patients undergoing hemodialysis and was tested in 79 subjects undergoing regular hemodialysis treatment during 21 days, as the primary source of nutrition delivered at two rates, 28 and 35 kcal/kg BW per day, respectively.[204] Tolerance was good, and nitrogen balance became positive. The sodium content of the diet was not sufficient, and sodium chloride supplementation was required. Several subjects became hypercalcemic, an observation that was also repeatedly seen during enteral nutrition with standard diets.

NUTRITIONAL STRATEGIES IN ACUTE RENAL FAILURE

General Considerations

- *What patient needs nutritional support?* The decision to initiate nutritional support is influenced by the following:

The patient's ability to cover nutritional requirements by eating.

The nutritional status of the patient as well as the type of underlying illness and the degree of accompanying catabolism. In any patient with evidence of malnourishment, nutritional therapy should be initiated regardless of whether the patient is likely to eat. If a well-nourished patient is to resume a normal diet within 5 days, no specific nutritional support is necessary.

The degree of accompanying catabolism. In patients with underlying diseases associated with excess protein catabolism, nutritional support should be initiated early.

Specific risk constellations (eg, immunosuppression, chemotherapy, or agranulocytosis).

- *When should nutrition be started?* The timing of nutritional support is determined again by the nutritional status and the degree of catabolism. The higher the level of malnutrition is and the more pronounced the degree of catabolism is, the earlier nutrition should be initiated. The decision should be made early in the course of disease to avoid the development of deficiencies and of hospital-acquired malnutrition. During the acute phase of ARF (within the first 24 to 48 hours after trauma or surgery), nutritional support should be withheld. Infusions of large quantities of amino acids or glucose during this "ebb phase" can increase tissue oxygen requirements and may aggravate tubular damage and the degree of renal functional loss.
- *At what degree of renal dysfunction should the nutritional regimen be adapted to renal failure?* Animal experiments have demonstrated that protein synthesis is decreased after a fall in renal function below 30% of normal.[205] Similarly, in studies in patients with CRF, impairment of glucose tolerance and lipid abnormalities occurred when creatinine clearance fell below 40 mL/min.[206] Thus, at a serum creatinine level

above 3 mg/dL or creatinine clearance below 40 mL/min, nutritional regimens should be designed to counteract the specific metabolic abnormalities of ARF.

- *Is enteral or parenteral nutrition the most appropriate means of providing nutritional support in patients with ARF?* Enteral feeding is the preferred type of nutritional support for all patients, including those with ARF. Nevertheless, in a high portion of patients with ARF, parenteral nutrition as total or supplementary nutrition becomes necessary to meet nutritional requirements.
- *In a patient with multiple organ dysfunction syndrome, which organ determines the type of nutritional support?* With the exception of severe hepatic failure, ARF is the major determinant of an adaptation of the composition of a nutritional regimen.
- *How should nutritional support be started?* Because of the broad spectrum of derangements in substrate utilization and intolerance to various nutrients, both parenteral and enteral nutrition should be started at a low rate and then gradually increased over several days until requirements are met.

Nutrient Administration

ORAL FEEDING

In all patients who can tolerate them, oral feedings should be used, but usually this is restricted to nonhypercatabolic patients with single-organ dysfunction. Calories are provided by simple carbohydrates (sugar, jellies, sweets) at regular intervals. Initially, 40 g of high-quality protein per day is given (0.6 g/kg BW/day) and subsequently is gradually increased to 0.8 g/kg BW per day as long as BUN remains below 100 mg/dL. For patients treated with hemodialysis, protein intake should be increased to 1.0 to 1.2 g/kg per day to make up for amino acids lost during dialysis plus the potential catabolic effects of dialysis. For peritoneal dialysis patients, protein intake should be raised to 1.2 to 1.4 g/kg per day to counteract losses of both amino acids and protein. A supplement of water-soluble vitamins is recommended, but vitamin C intake should be limited to 200 mg/day.

ENTERAL NUTRITION

Without any doubt, enteral nutrition must be utilized as the first-line route of nutrient application in artificial nutrition in patients with ARF. Enteral nutrition is the first and most important means of supporting intestinal function in intensive care patients.[207] Nevertheless, in the critically ill patient with ARF, it is frequently impossible to cover nutrient requirements exclusively by the enteral route, and supplementary or, even, total parenteral nutrition may become necessary. Enteral nutrition and parenteral nutrition should be viewed as complementary types of nutritional support. It should be recognized that even when intestinal motility is severely compromised and nutritional requirements cannot be met by the enteral route, provision of even small amounts of enteral diets given regularly (ie, 6 × 50 to 100 mL/day) can help to maintain intestinal function.[208]

Feeding Tubes

Soft, fine-bore feeding tubes should be used exclusively to prevent the development of pressure ulcerations in the esophagus. Usually, it is sufficient that the tip of the tube is positioned in the stomach. In patients with impaired gastric emptying and vomiting due to gastroparesis, persistent duodenogastric or gastroesophageal reflux, or impairment of intestinal motility by drugs, such as sedation or catecholamines, the tip of the tube should be advanced into the small intestine, preferably into the jejunum.[209] In these patients, a second lumen tube should be positioned in the stomach for gastric decompensation.

Percutaneous endoscopic gastrostomy (PEG) should be considered for any prolonged enteral nutritional support, such as that in the nursing home setting, for confused patients and subjects with neurologic disabilities, and for mechanical obstruction in the upper gastrointestinal tract, as well as for patients admitted for a prolonged stay in critical care units.

Enteral Nutrient Administration

The techniques of enteral nutrition in patients with renal failure are identical to those employed in other patient groups. Feeding solutions can be administered intermittently or continuously into the stomach or continuously into the jejunum, preferably by pump. If solutions are given continuously, the stomach should be aspirated every 4 to 6 hours until adequate gastric emptying and intestinal peristalsis are established. This practice prevents vomiting and reduces the risk of bronchopulmonary aspiration and development of pneumonia.

To avoid the development both of gastrointestinal side effects, such as osmotic diarrhea (especially diets with free amino acids and a high osmolality), and of metabolic complications, the infusion should be started at a low rate and the amount and concentration of the solution gradually should be increased over several days until nutritional requirements are met. The gradual increase in nutrient infusion helps to ensure adequate utilization of nutrients and at the same time avoids metabolic derangements in patients with reduced tolerance to many nutrients. Undesired but potentially treatable side effects include nausea, vomiting, abdominal distention, and cramping and diarrhea.

Again, it should be stressed that even in patients with impaired gastrointestinal motility, as is frequently encountered in patients with ARF, with impairment of gastric emptying, or duodenogastric reflux, small amounts of enteral nutrients should be provided to help to maintain intestinal functions.[208]

PARENTERAL NUTRITION

Parenteral nutrition should not be viewed as an alternative, but rather as a complementary method of nutritional support, because in many patients with ARF, it is often not possible to meet nutritional requirements by the enteral route alone.[210] Moreover, ARF frequently occurs in patients with severe gastrointestinal dysfunction, such as those with pancreatitis and in hypercatabolic patients with multiple organ dysfunction, so a total or a supplementary parenteral nutrient supply may become necessary.

Fluids are usually restricted in ARF; thus nutritional solutions are hyperosmolar and must be infused through central venous catheters to avoid damage to peripheral veins. Special venous catheters used as an infusion port, for temporary dialysis access, and for measurements of central venous pressure are frequently employed but require attentive care in order to limit the significant risk of infections. Ideally, a separate venous line should be used for parenteral nutrition.

Parenteral Solutions

Solutions with amino acids, glucose, and lipids plus additions of vitamins, trace elements, and electrolytes contained in a single bag have become the standard means of providing parenteral nutrition ("all-in-one" solutions, total nutritional admixtures)[211] (Table 37–9). The stability of fat emulsions in such mixtures should be tested. If hyperglycemia is present, insulin can be added to the solution or administered separately.

To ensure maximal nutrient utilization and to avoid metabolic derangements such as a mineral imbalance, hyperglycemia, or an excessive increase in BUN level, the infusion should be started at a low rate (providing about 50% of requirements) and gradually increased over several days. The nutritional solution should be infused continuously over 24 hours to ensure optimal substrate utilization and to avoid marked changes in substrate concentrations.

COMPLICATIONS OF NUTRITIONAL SUPPORT

The gastrointestinal side effects of enteral nutrition are similar in ARF patients and nonuremic subjects but can occur at a higher frequency in ARF patients, mainly because of the impairment of gastrointestinal motility in the presence of ARF. Similarly, technical problems and infectious complications originating from the central venous catheter, and chemical incompatibilities of parenteral nutrition, do not differ from those observed in other patient groups.

However, metabolic complications of artificial nutrition are frequently encountered in patients with ARF, because tolerance for volume load is limited, electrolyte derangements can develop rapidly, and the utilization of several nutrients is altered. Any exaggerated protein or amino acid intake results in excessive BUN (and waste product) accumulation. Glucose intolerance and decreased fat clearance can cause hyperglycemia and hypertriglyceridemia.

Most complications are related to an excess intake of substrates (hyperglycemia, fatty infiltration of the

TABLE 37–9. Renal Failure Fluid–All-in-One Solution*

COMPONENT		QUANITY	REMARKS
Glucose	40%–70%	500 mL	In the presence of severe insulin resistance, switch to $D_{30}W$
Fat emulsion	10%–20%	500 mL	Start with 10%, switch to 20% if triglycerides are <350 mg/dL
Amino acids	6.5%–10%	500 mL	General or special "nephro" amino acid solutions, including EAA and NEAA
Water-soluble vitamins†		Daily	Limit vitamin C intake to <200 mg/day
Fat-soluble vitamins†		Daily	
Trace elements†		Twice weekly	Caveat: toxic effects
Electrolytes		As required	Caveat: hypophosphatemia or hypokalemia after initiation of total parenteral nutrition
Insulin		As required	Added directly to the solution or given separately

*All-in-one solution with all components contained in a single bag. Infusion rate initially 50% of requirements, to be increased over a period of 3 days to satisfy requirements.
†Combination products containing the recommended daily allowances.
$D_{30}W$, 30% dextrose in water; *EAA*, essential amino acid; *NEAA*, nonessential amino acid.

liver, increased carbon dioxide production, hypertriglyceridemia, hyperkalemia, accelerated BUN increase) or the development of deficiencies (eg, of minerals, vitamins, or essential fatty acids). Many side effects can be minimized by gradually increasing the infusion rate, by limiting the infusion to supply requirements, and by combining glucose with lipids.

MONITORING OF NUTRITIONAL THERAPY

Because of the reduced tolerance for nutrients in ARF and the associated high frequency of metabolic complications, nutritional therapy in patients with ARF requires a tighter schedule of monitoring than it does in other patient groups. Table 37–10 summarizes laboratory tests for monitoring nutritional support and avoiding the development of metabolic complications. The frequency of testing depends on the metabolic stability of the patient. In particular, plasma glucose, potassium, and phosphate should be monitored repeatedly after the start of nutritional therapy.

CONCLUSIONS

All patients require adequate nutrition to maintain protein stores and to correct preexisting or disease-

TABLE 37–10. A Minimal Suggested Schedule for Monitoring of Nutritional Support

	PATIENT METABOLICALLY	
VARIABLES	Unstable	Stable
Blood glucose, potassium	1–6 times daily	Daily
Osmolality	Daily	1 time weekly
Electrolytes (sodium, chloride)	Daily	3 times weekly
Calcium, phosphate, magnesium	Daily	3 times weekly
BUN/BUN rise/day	Daily	Daily
UNA	Daily	2 times weekly
Triglycerides	Daily	2 times weekly
Blood gas analysis/pH	Daily	1 time weekly
Ammonia	2 times weekly	1 time weekly
Transaminases + bilirubin	2 times weekly	1 time weekly

BUN, blood urea nitrogen; *UNA*, urinary nitrogen appearance.

related deficits in lean body mass. In ARF patients, it is not the impairment of renal function per se that determines the decision to initiate nutritional support, but rather the nutritional status, the type and severity of underlying disease, and the degree of associated hypercatabolism. However, in a patient who has acquired ARF and who needs nutritional support, the nutritional regimen has to be adapted to the complex metabolic sequelae of impaired renal function and of renal replacement therapies and to the associated impairment of tolerance for various nutrients.

Increasing understanding of the pathophysiology of these metabolic changes, better definitions of nutritional requirements, and advances in the techniques of parenteral and enteral nutrition have greatly improved the success of nutritional therapy. Dietary restrictions and concepts based on the principles of treating CRF patients have been largely abandoned in favor of an approach directed at meeting nutrient requirements, but one that also respects the specific metabolic alterations in ARF and the loss of excretory renal function.

Enteral nutrition has become the preferred route of nutritional support also in patients with ARF. Even small amounts of luminally provided nutrients can help to support intestinal function, and especially the barrier function against translocation of intestinal bacteria. Enteral and parenteral nutrition techniques must be viewed as complementary means of nutritional support, because in many patients nutritional requirements can be met only by a combination of both techniques.

Unfortunately, the optimal nutritional regimen has not been defined, and nutritional support has not convincingly reduced morbidity and mortality in ARF patients. The poor prognosis in ARF patients is related to the severity of the underlying illness and the associated complications and hypercatabolism, respectively. Nutritional therapy, like renal replacement therapy, should be viewed as a means of supporting the patient until the underlying illness is controlled, and hypermetabolism is reversed. For future advances, nutritional therapy must leave behind the merely quantitatively oriented approach of just covering nitrogen and energy requirements and move toward a more qualitative type of metabolic intervention, taking advantage of the specific effects of various nutrients on various physiologic functions (eg, effects on protein metabolism or on immunologic function) to improve the efficiency of nutritional support in patients with ARF.

REFERENCES

1. Levy EM, Viscoli CM, Horwitz RI: The effect of acute renal failure on mortality. JAMA 1996; 275:1489–1494.
2. Druml W: Nutritional Support in Acute Renal Failure. In: Mitch WE, Klahr S: *Nutrition and the Kidney*. Boston: Little Brown; 1998:314–345.
3. Druml W, Mitch WE: Metabolic abnormalities in acute renal failure. Semin Dial 1996; 9:484–490.
4. Om P, Hohenegger M: Energy metabolism in acutely uremic rats. Nephron 1980; 25:249–253.
5. Schneeweiss B, Graninger W, Stockenhuber F, et al: Energy metabolism in acute and chronic renal failure. Am J Clin Nutr 1990; 52:596–601.
6. Bouffard Y, Viale JP, Annat G, et al: Energy expenditure in the acute renal failure patient mechanically ventilated. Intensive Care Med 1987; 13:401–406.
7. Soop M, Forsberg E, Thörne A, Alvestrand A: Energy expenditure in postoperative multiple organ failure with acute renal failure. Clin Nephrol 1989; 31:139–143.
8. Druml W: Protein metabolism in acute renal failure. Miner Electrolyte Metab 1998; 24:47–54.
9. Mitch WE: Amino acid release from the hindquarter and urea appearance in acute uremia. Am J Physiol 1981; 241:E415–E419.
10. Price SR, Reaich D, Marinovic AC, et al: Mechanisms contributing to muscle wasting in acute uremia: activation of amino acid catabolism. J Am Soc Nephrol 1998; 9:439–443.
11. Clark AS, Mitch WE: Muscle protein turnover and glucose uptake in acutely uremic rats. J Clin Invest 1983; 72:836–845.
12. Arnold WE, Holliday MA: Tissue resistance to insulin stimulation of amino acid uptake in acutely uremic rats. Kidney Int 1979; 16:124–129.
13. Maroni BJ, Haesemeyer RW, Kutner MH, Mitch WE: Kinetics of system A amino acid uptake by muscle: effects of insulin and acute uremia. Am J Physiol 1990; 258:F1304–F1310.
14. Druml W, Kelly RA, Mitch WE, May RC: Abnormal cation transport in uremia. J Clin Invest 1988; 81:1197–1203.
15. Fröhlich J, Schölmerich J, Hoppe-Seyler G, et al: The effect of acute uremia on gluconeogenesis in isolated perfused rat livers. Eur J Clin Invest 1974; 4:453–458.
16. Lacy WW: Uptake of individual amino acids by the perfused rat liver: effects of acute uremia. Am J Physiol 1970; 219: 649–653.
17. Druml W, Bürger U, Kleinberger G, et al: Elimination of amino acids in acute renal failure. Nephron 1986; 42:62–67.
18. Druml W, Fischer M, Liebisch B, et al: Elimination of amino acids in renal failure. Am J Clin Nutr 1994; 60:418–423.
19. DeFronzo RA, Smith D, Alvestrand A: Insulin action in uremia. Kidney Int 1983; 24(suppl 16):S102–S114.
20. Shaw JFH, Wildbore M, Wolfe RR: Whole body protein kinetics in severely septic patients: the response to glucose infusion and total parenteral nutrition. Ann Surg 1987; 205:288–292.
21. Cianciaruso B, Bellizzi V, Napoli R, et al: Hepatic uptake and release of glucose, lactate and amino acids in acutely uremic dogs. Metabolism 1991; 40:261–290.
22. Schaefer RM, Weipert J, Moser M, et al: Reduction of urea generation and muscle protein degradation by adrenalectomy in acutely uremic rats. Nephron 1988; 48:149–153.
23. Schaefer RM, Teschner M, Riegel W, Heidland A: Reduced protein catabolism by the antiglucocorticoid RU 38486 in acutely uremic rats. Kidney Int 1989; 36(suppl 27):S208–S211.
24. Schaefer RM, Riegel W, Stephan E, et al: Normalization of enhanced hepatic gluconeogenesis by the antiglucocorticoid RU 38486 in acutely uremic rats. Eur J Clin Invest 1990; 20: 35–40.
25. Mitch WE, May RC, Maroni BJ, Druml W: Protein and amino acid metabolism in uremia: influence of metabolic acidosis. Kidney Int 1989; 36(suppl 27):S205–S207.
26. May RC, Kelly RA, Mitch WE: Mechanisms for defects in muscle protein metabolism in rats with chronic uremia: the influence of metabolic acidosis. J Clin Invest 1987; 79:1099–1103.
27. Kuhlmann MK, Shahmir E, Maasarani E, et al: New experimental model of acute renal failure and sepsis in rats. JPEN 1994; 18:477–485.
28. Olbricht CJ, Huxman-Nägeli D, Koch KM: Urea generation during continuous arteriovenous hemofiltration (CAVH) with lactate- versus bicarbonate based substitution fluids. Nieren- und Hochdruckkrankh. 1992; 21:410A.
29. Kokot F, Kuska J: The endocrine system in patients with acute renal insufficiency. Kidney Int 1976; 10(suppl 6):S26–S31.
30. Levitan D, Massry SG, Romoff MS, Campese VM: Autonomic nervous system dysfunction in patients with acute renal failure. Am J Nephrol 1982; 2:213–217.
31. Druml W, Schwarzenhofer M, Apsner R, Hörl WH: Fat soluble vitamins in acute renal failure. Miner Electrolyte Metab 1998; 24:220–226.
32. Tsao T, Wang J, Fervenza FC, et al: Renal growth hormone–insulin like growth factor-I system in acute renal failure. Kidney Int 1995; 47:1658–1668.
33. Hörl WH, Heidland A: Enhanced proteolytic activity: cause of protein catabolism in acute renal failure. Am J Clin Nutr 1980; 33:1423–1427.
34. Hörl WH, Gantert C, Auer LA, Heidland A: In vitro inhibition of protein catabolism by alpha 2-macroglobulin in plasma from a patient with posttraumatic acute renal failure. Am J Nephrol 1982; 2:32–34.
35. Wilmore DW: Catabolic illness: strategies for enhancing recovery. N Engl J Med 1991; 325:695–702.
36. Bergström J: Factors causing catabolism in maintenance hemodialysis patients. Min Electrolyte Metab 1992; 18:280–283.
37. Baliga R, George VT, Ray PE, Holiday MA: Effects of reduced renal function and dietary protein on muscle protein synthesis. Kidney Int 1991; 39:831–836.
38. McMurray SD, Luft FC, Maxwell DR: Prevailing patterns and predictor variables in patients with acute tubular necrosis Arch Intern Med 1978; 138:950–955.
39. Mault JR, Bartlett RH, Dechert RE, et al: Starvation: a major contributor to mortality in acute renal failure. Trans Am Soc Artif Intern Organs 1983; 29:390–394.
40. Fiaccadori E, Lombardi M, Leonardi S, et al: Prevalence and clinical outcome of malnutrition in acute renal failure. J Am Soc Nephrol 1999; 10:581–593.
41. Mitch WE, Chesney RW: Amino acid metabolism by the kidney. Miner Electrolyte Metab 1983; 9:190–202.
42. Laidlaw SA, Kopple JD: Newer concepts of indispensable amino acids. Am J Clin Nutr 1987; 46:593–605.
43. Druml W, Roth E, Lenz K, et al: Phenylalanine and tyrosine metabolism in renal failure. Kidney Int 1989; 36(suppl 27):S282–S286.
44. Druml W, Lochs H, Roth E, et al: Utilization of tyrosine dipeptides and acetyl-tyrosine in normal and uremic humans. Am J Physiol 1991; 260:E280–E285.
45. Naschitz JE, Barak C, Yeshurun D: Reversible diminished insulin requirement in acute renal failure. Postgrad Med J 1983; 59:269–271.
46. Hübl W, Druml W, Roth E, Lochs H: Importance of liver and kidney for the utilization of glutamine-containing dipeptides in man. Metabolism 1994; 43:1104–1107.
47. Ding H, Kopple JD, Cohen A, Hirschberg R: Recombinant human insulin-like growth factor-1 accelerates recovery and reduces catabolism in rats with ischemic acute renal failure. J Clin Invest 1993; 91:2281–2287.
48. Hirschberg R, Kopple J, Lipsett P, et al: Multicenter clinical trial of recombinant human insulin-like growth factor-I in patients with acute renal failure. Kidney Int 1999; 55:2423–2432.
49. Takala J, Ruokonen E, Webster NR, et al: Increased mortality associated with growth hormone treatment in critically ill adults. N Engl J Med 1999; 341:785–792.
50. Spittler A, Winkler S, Götzinger P, et al: Influence of glutamine on the phenotype and function of human monocytes. Blood 1995; 86:1564–1569.

51. Weisinger J, Swenson RS, Greene W, et al: Comparison of the effects of metabolic acidosis and acute uremia on carbohydrate tolerance. Diabetes 1972; 21:1109–1115.

52. Mondon CE, Dolkas CB, Reaven GM: The site of insulin resistance in acute uremia. Diabetes 1978; 27:572–576.

53. May RC, Clark AS, Goheer MA, Mitch WE: Specific defects in insulin-mediated muscle metabolism in acute uremia. Kidney Int 1985; 28:490–497.

54. Fröhlich J, Hoppe-Seyler G, Schollmeyer P, et al: Possible sites of interaction of acute renal failure with amino acid utilization for gluconeogenesis in isolated perfused rat liver. Eur J Clin Invest 1977; 7:261–268.

55. Cianciaruso B, Sacca L, Terracciano V, et al: Insulin metabolism in acute renal failure. Kidney Int 1987; 23(suppl 27):109–112.

56. Druml W, Laggner A, Widhalm K, et al: Lipid metabolism in acute renal failure. Kidney Int 1983; 24(suppl 16):139–142.

57. Druml W, Laggner AN, Lenz K, et al: Lipid metabolism and lipid utilization in renal failure. Infusionsther Klin Ernahr 1983; 10:206–212.

58. Druml W, Fischer M, Sertl S, et al: Fat elimination in acute renal failure: long-chain versus medium-chain triglycerides. Am J Clin Nutr 1992; 55:468–472.

59. Druml W, Zechner R, Magometschnigg D, et al: Post-heparin lipolytic activity in acute renal failure. Clin Nephrol 1985; 23:289–293.

60. Zimmermann E, Hohenegger M: Lipid metabolism in uremic and nonuremic acidosis. Nephron 1979; 24:217–222.

61. Nitzan M: Hepatic lipogenesis in acute uremic syndrome. Nutr Metab 1971; 13:292–297.

62. Gregg R, Mondon CE, Reaven EP, Reaven RM: Effect of acute uremia on triglyceride kinetics in the rat. Metabolism 1976; 25:1557–1565.

63. Hohenegger M, Schuh H: Triacylglycerol secretion and fatty acid synthesis by the liver in acute uremic rats. Exp Pathol 1984; 25:89–95.

64. Druml W: Lipid metabolism and amino acid metabolism in acute renal failure. Klin Ernähr 1987; 28:1–99. (In Serman)

65. Adolph M, Eckart J, Metges C, et al: Oxidative utilization of lipid emulsions in septic patients with and without acute renal failure. Clin Nutr 1995; 14(suppl 2):35A.

66. Wanner C, Riegel W, Schaefer RM, Hörl WH: Carnitine and carnitine esters in acute renal failure. Nephrol Dial Transplant 1989; 4:951–956.

67. Allon M: Hyperkalemia in endstage renal disease: mechanisms and management. J Am Soc Nephrol 1995, 6:1134–1142.

68. Druml W, Lax F, Grimm G, et al: Acute renal failure in the elderly 1975–1990. Clin Nephrol 1994; 41:342–349.

69. Hörl WH, Schaefer RM, Haag M, Heidland A: Acute uremia following dietary potassium depletion. Miner Electrolyte Metab 1986; 12:218–225.

70. Cronin RE, Thompson JR: Role of potassium in the pathogenesis of acute renal failure. Miner Electrolyte Metab 1991; 17:100–105.

71. Kurtin P, Kouba J: Profound hypophosphatemia in the course of acute renal failure. Am J Kidney Dis 1987; 10:346–349.

72. Kleinberger G, Gabl F, Gassner A, et al: Hypophosphatemia during parenteral nutrition in patients with renal failure. Wien Klin Wochenschr 1978; 90:169–172.

73. Marik PE, Bedigian MK: Refeeding hypophosphatemia in critically ill patients in an intensive care unit. Arch Surg 1996; 131:1043–1047.

74. Lumlertgul D, Harris DCH, Burke TJ, Schrier RW: Detrimental effects of hypophosphatemia on the severity and progression of ischemic acute renal failure. Miner Electrolyte Metab 1986; 12:204–209.

75. Dobyan DC, Bulger RE, Eknoyan G: The role of phosphate in the potentiation and amelioration of acute renal failure. Miner Electrolyte Metab 1991; 17:112–115.

76. Haas M, Öhler L, Watzke H, et al: The spectrum of acute renal failure in tumor lysis syndrome. Nephrol Dial Transpl 1999; 14:776–779.

77. Pietrek J, Kokot F, Kuska J: Serum 25-hydroxyvitamin D and parathyroid hormone in patients with acute renal failure. Kidney Int 1978; 13:178–185.

78. Saha H, Mustonen J, Pietila K, Pasternack A: Metabolism of calcium and vitamin D_3 in patients with acute tubulointerstitial nephritis. Nephron 1993; 63:159–163.

79. Akmal M, Bishop JE, Telfer N, et al: Hypocalcemia and hypercalcemia in patients with rhabdomyolysis with and without acute renal failure. J Clin Endocrinol Metab 1986; 63:137–142.

80. Al-Ghamdi SMG, Cameron ECC, Sutton RAL: Magnesium deficiency: pathophysiologic and clinical overview. Am J Kidney Dis 1994; 24:737–752.

81. Shaah GM, Kirschenbaum MA: Renal magnesium wasting associated with therapeutic agents. Miner Electrolyte Metab 1991; 17:58–64.

82. Story DA, Ronco C, Bellomo R: Trace element and vitamin concentrations and losses in critically ill patients treated with continuous venovenous hemofiltration. Crit Care Med 1999; 27:220–223.

83. Fortin MC, Amyot SL, Geadah D, Leblanc M: Serum concentrations and clearances of folic acid and pyridoxal-5-phosphate during venovenous continuous renal replacement therapy. Intensive Care Med 1999; 25:594–598.

84. Madl CH, Kranz A, Liebisch B, et al: Lactic acidosis in thiamine deficiency. Clin Nutr 1993; 12:108–111.

85. Bakker SJL, Yin M, Koostra G: Tissue thiamine and carnitine deficiency as a possible cause of acute tubular necrosis after renal transplantation. Transplant Proc 1996; 28:314–315.

86. Alkhunaizi AM, Chan L: Secondary oxalosis: a cause of delayed recovery of renal function in the setting of acute renal failure. J Am Soc Nephrol 1996; 7:2320–2326.

87. Hsu CH, Patel S, Young EW, Simpson RU: Production and metabolic clearance of calcitriol in acute renal failure. Kidney Int 1988; 33:530–535.

88. Chung YC, Huang MT, Chang CN, et al: Prolonged nonoliguric acute renal failure associated with high-dose vitamin K administration in a renal transplant recipient. Transplant Proc 1994; 26:2129–2131.

89. Lipsky JJ: Vitamin K deficiency. J Intensive Care Med 1992; 7:328–336.

90. Gerlach TH, Zile MH: Effect of retinoic acid and apo-RBP on serum retinol concentration in acute renal failure. FASEB J 1991; 5:86–92.

91. Metnitz PGH, Fischer M, Bartnes S, et al: Impact of acute renal failure on antioxidant status in patients with multiple organ failure. Acta Anaesthesiol Scand 2000; 44:236–240.

92. Okada A, Takagi Y, Nezu R, et al: Trace element metabolism in parenteral and enteral nutrition. Nutrition 1995; 11:106–113.

93. Shenkin A: Trace elements and inflammatory response: implications for nutritional support. Nutrition 1995; 11:100–105.

94. Jetton MM, Sullivan JF, Burch RE: Trace element contamination of intravenous solutions. Arch Intern Med 1976; 136:782–784.

95. Chauhan DP, Gupta PH, Nampoothiri MRN, et al: Determination of erythrocyte superoxide dismutase, catalase, glucose-6-phosphate dehydrogenase, reduced glutathione, and malonyldialdehyde in uremia. Clin Chim Acta 1982; 123:153–159.

96. König JS, Fischer M, Bulant E, et al: Antioxidant status in patients on chronic hemodialysis therapy: impact of parenteral selenium supplementation. Wien Klin Wochenschr 1997; 109:13–19.

97. Angstwurm MW, Schottdorf J, Schopohl J, Gaertner R: Selenium replacement in patients with severe systemic inflammatory response syndrome improves clinical outcome. Crit Care Med 1999; 27:1807–1813.

98. Besunder JB, Smith PG: Toxic effects of electrolyte and trace mineral administration in the intensive care unit. Crit Care Clin 1991; 7:659–693.

99. Braunschweig C, Sowers M, Koracevich D, et al: Parenteral zinc supplementation in adult humans during the acute phase response increases the febrile response. J Nutr 1997; 127:70–79.

100. Nath KA, Paller MS: Dietary deficiency of antioxidants exacerbates ischemic injury in the rat kidney. Kidney Int 1990; 38:1109–1117.

101. Kim SY, Kim CH, Yoo HJ, Kim YK: Effects of radical scavengers and antioxidants on ischemic acute renal failure in rabbits. Ren Fail 1999; 21:1–11.

102. Zurovsky Y, Gispaan I: Antioxidants attenuate endotoxin-induced acute renal failure in rats. Am J Kidney Dis 1995; 25:51–57.

103. Bergström J: Factors causing catabolism in maintenance hemodialysis patients. Min Electrolyte Metab 1992; 18:280–283.
104. Gutierrez A, Alvestrand A, Bergström J: Membrane selection and muscle protein catabolism. Kidney Int 1992; 42(suppl 38):S86–S90.
105. Jackson P, Loughrey CM, Lightbody JH, et al: Effects of hemodialysis on total antioxidant capacity and serum antioxidants in patients with chronic renal failure. Endocrinol Metab 1995; 41:1135–1138.
106. Frankenfeld DC, Reynolds HN: Nutritional effects of continuous hemodiafiltration. Nutrition 1995; 11:388–393.
107. Druml W: Metabolic aspects of continuous renal replacement therapies. Kidney Int 1999; 56(suppl 72):S56–S61.
108. Davies SP, Reaveley DA, Brown EA, Kox WJ: Amino acid clearances and daily losses in patients with acute renal failure treated by continuous arteriovenous hemodialysis. Crit Care Med 1991; 19:1510–1515.
109. Davenport A, Roberts NB: Amino acid losses during continuous high-flux hemofiltration in the critically ill patient. Crit Care Med 1989; 17:1010–1015.
110. Frankenfeld DC, Badellino MM, Reynolds N, et al: Amino acid loss and plasma concentration during continuous hemofiltration. JPEN 1993; 17:551–561.
111. Druml W: Nutritional considerations in the treatment of acute renal failure in septic patients. Nephrol Dial Transplant 1994; 9(suppl 4):219–223.
112. Maxvold NJ, Smoyer WE, Custer JR, Bunchman TE: Amino acid loss and nitrogen balance in critically ill children with acute renal failure: a prospective comparison between classical hemofiltration and hemofiltration with dialysis. Crit Care Med 2000; 28:1161–1165.
113. Bellomo R, McGrath B, Boyce N: In vivo catecholamine extraction during continuous hemodiafiltration in inotrope-dependent patients. Trans Am Soc Intern Organs 1991; 37:324–325.
114. Mokrzycki MH, Kaplan AA: Protein losses in continuous renal replacement therapies. JASN 1996; 7:2259–2263.
115. Teoh KH, Mickle DAG, Weisel RD, et al: Improving myocardial metabolic and functional recovery after cardiac arrest. J Thorac Cardiovasc Surg 1988; 95:788–798.
116. Monaghan R, Watters JM, Clancey SM, et al: Uptake of glucose during continuous arteriovenous hemofiltration. Crit Care Med 1993; 21:1159–1163.
117. Wolfson M, Jones MR, Kopple JD: Amino acid losses during hemodialysis with infusion of amino acids and glucose. Kidney Int 1982; 21:500–506.
118. Rabkin R, Tsao T, Shi JD, Mortimore G: Amino acids regulate kidney cell protein breakdown. J Lab Clin Med 1991; 117:505–510.
119. Toback FG: Regeneration after acute tubular necrosis. Kidney Int 1992; 41:226–246.
120. Abel RM, Beck CH, Abbott WM, et al: Improved survival from acute renal failure after treatment with intravenous essential amino acids and glucose: results of a prospective double-blind study. N Engl J Med 1973; 288:695–699.
121. Toback FG, Dodd RC, Maier ER, Havener LJ: Amino acid administration enhances renal protein metabolism after acute tubular necrosis. Nephron 1983; 33:238–243.
122. Toback FG, Teegarden DE, Havener LJ: Amino acid–mediated stimulation of renal phospholipid biosynthesis after acute tubular necrosis. Kidney Int 1979; 15:542–547.
123. Oken DE, Sprinkel M, Kirschbaum BB, Landwehr DM: Amino acid therapy in the treatment of experimental acute renal failure in the rat. Kidney Int 1980; 17:14–23.
124. Zager RA, Venkatachalam MA: Potentiation of ischemic renal injury by amino acid infusion. Kidney Int 1983; 24:620–625.
125. Zager RA: Amino acid hyperalimentation in acute renal failure: a potential therapeutic paradox. Kidney Int 1987; 32(suppl 22):S72–S75.
126. Brezis M, Rosen S, Spokes K, et al: Transport-dependent anoxic cell injury in the isolated perfused rat kidney. Am J Pathol 1984; 116:327–341.
127. Moursi M, Rising CL, Zelenock GB, D'Alecy LG: Dextrose administration exacerbates acute renal ischemic damage in anesthetized dogs. Arch Surg 1987; 122:790–794.
128. Brundin T, Wahren J: Renal oxygen consumption, thermogenesis, and amino acid utilization during IV infusion of amino acids in man. Am J Physiol 1994; 267:E648–E655.
129. Racusen LC, Finn WF, Whelton A, Solez K: Mechanisms of lysine-induced acute renal failure in rats. Kidney Int 1985; 32:517–522.
130. Heyman SN, Rosen S, Silva P, et al: Protective action of glycine in cisplatin nephrotoxicity. Kidney Int 1991; 40: 273–279.
131. Schramm L, Heidbreder E, Lopau K, et al: Influence of nitric oxide on renal function in toxic renal failure in the rat. Miner Electrolyte Metab 1996; 22:168–173.
132. Wakabayashi Y, Kikawada R: Effect of l-arginine on myoglobin-induced acute renal failure in the rabbit. Am J Physiol 1996; 270:F784–F789.
133. Andrews PM, Bates SB: Dietary protein prior to renal ischemia dramatically affects postischemic kidney function. Kidney Int 1986; 29:995–1003.
134. Ichikawa I, Purkenson ML, Yates J, Klahr S: Dietary protein intake conditions the degree of renal vasoconstriction in acute renal failure caused by ureteral obstruction. Am J Physiol 1985; 249:F54–F61.
135. Baliga R, Shah SV: Effects of dietary protein intake on muscle protein synthesis and degradation in rats with gentamicin-induced acute renal failure. J Am Soc Nephrol 1991; 1:1230–1235.
136. Seguro AC, Shimizu MHM, Campos SB, Rocha AS: The effect of protein restriction on the severity and recovery from ischemic renal failure. Ren Fail 1990; 12:249–255.
137. Andrews PM, Chung EM: High dietary protein regimens provide significant protection from mercury nephrotoxicity in rats. Toxicol Appl Pharmacol 1990; 105:288–304.
138. Elsayed AA, Haylor J, Elnahas AM: Differential effects of amino acids on the isolated perfused rat kidney. Clin Sci 1990; 79:381–386.
139. Badalamenti S, Gines P, Arroyo V, et al: Effects of intravenous amino acid infusion and dietary protein on kidney function in cirrhosis. Hepatology 1990; 11:379–386.
140. Singer P, Bursztein S, Segal A, et al: Reduced morbidity in acute renal failure with high rates of amino acid infusion. Clin Nutr 1990; 9(suppl):23A.
141. Roberts PR, Black KW, Zaloga GP: Enteral feeding improves outcome and protects against glycerol-induced acute renal failure in the rat. Am J Respir Crit Care Med 1997; 156:1265–1269.
142. Mouser JF, Hak EB, Kuhl DA, et al: Recovery from ischemic acute renal failure is improved with enteral compared with parenteral nutrition. Crit Care Med 1997; 25:1748–1754.
143. Michael UF, Logan JL, Meeks LA: The beneficial effects of thyroxine on nephrotoxic acute renal failure in the rat. JASN 1991; 1:1236–1240.
144. Coimbra TM, Cieslinski DA, Humes HD: Epidermal growth factor accelerates renal repair in mercuric chloride nephrotoxicity. Am J Physiol 1990; 259:F438–F443.
145. Vargas GA, Hoeflich A, Jehle PM: Hepatocyte growth factor in renal failure: promise and reality. Kidney Int 2000; 57:1426–1436.
146. Franklin SC, Moulton M, Sicard GA, et al: Insulin-like growth factor I preserves renal function postoperatively. Am J Physiol 1997; 272:F257–F259.
147. Acker CG, Singh AR, Flick RP, et al: A trial of thyroxine in acute renal failure. Kidney Int 2000; 57:293–298.
148. Druml W, Mitch WE: Enteral Nutrition in Renal Disease. In: Rombeau JL, Rolandelli RH, eds: Enteral and Tube Feeding. Philadelphia: WB Saunders; 1997:439–461.
149. Kang JY: The gastrointestinal tract in uremia. Dig Dis Sci 1993; 28:257–268.
150. Tribl B, Madl C, Mazal P, et al: Exocrine pancreatic function in critically ill patients: septic shock versus nonseptic patients. Crit Care Med 2000; 28:1393–1398.
151. Barnert J, Dumitrascu D, Neeser G, et al: Gastric emptying of a liquid meal in intensive care unit patients. Gastroenterology 1998; 114:A865.
152. Spreiter SC, Myers BD, Swenson RS: Protein-energy requirements in subjects with acute renal failure receiving intermittent hemodialysis. Am J Clin Nutr 1980; 33:1433–1437.
153. Alexander JW, Gonce SJ, Miskell PW: A new model for studying nutrition in peritonitis: the adverse effect of overfeeding. Ann Surg 1989; 209:334–340.

154. Taveroff A, McArdle AH, Rybka WB: Reducing parenteral energy and protein intake improves metabolic homeostasis after bone marrow transplantation. Am J Clin Nutr 1991; 54:1087–1092.

155. Cerra FB, Benitez MR, Blackburn GL, et al: Applied nutrition in ICU patients: a consensus statement of the American College of Chest Physicans. Chest 1997; 111:769–778.

156. Hunter DC, Jaksic T, Lewis D, et al: Resting energy expenditure in the critically ill: estimations versus measurement. Br J Surg 1988; 75:875–878.

157. Frankenfeld DC, Smith JS, Cooney RN: Accelerated nitrogen loss after traumatic injury is not attenuated by achievement of energy balance. JPEN 1997; 21:324–329.

158. Hasik J, Hryniewiecki L, Baczyk K, Grala T: An attempt to evaluate minimum requirements for protein in patients with acute renal failure. Pol Arch Med Wewn 1979; 61:29–36.

159. Lopez-Martinez J, Caparros T, Perez-Picouto F: Nutrition parenteral en enfermos septicos con fracaso renal agudo en fase poliurica. Rev Clin Esp 1980; 157:171–178.

160. Feinstein EI, Blumenkrantz MJ, Healy M, et al: Clinical and metabolic response to parenteral nutrition in acute renal failure: a controlled double-blind study. Medicine 1981; 60:124–137.

161. Feinstein EI, Kopple JD, Silberman H, Massry SG: Total parenteral nutrition with high or low nitrogen intakes in patients with acute renal failure. Kidney Int 1983; 26(suppl 16):S319–S323.

162. Kierdorf H, Kindler J, Sieberth HG: Nitrogen balance in patients with acute renal failure treated by continuous arteriovenous hemofiltration. Nephrol Dial Transplant 1986; 1:72.

163. Chima CS, Meyer L, Hummell AC, et al: Protein catabolic rate in patients with acute renal failure on continuous arteriovenous hemofiltration and total parenteral nutrition. JASN 1993; 3:1516–1521.

164. Macias WL, Alaka KJ, Murphy MH, et al: Impact of nutritional regimen on protein catabolism and nitrogen balance in patients with acute renal failure. JPEN 1996; 20:56–62.

165. Bellomo R, Seacombe J, Daskalakis M, et al: A prospective comparative study of moderate versus high protein intake for critically ill patients with acute renal failure. Ren Fail 1997; 19:111–120.

166. Greig PD, Elwyn DH, Askanazi J, et al: Parenteral nutrition in septic patients: effect of increasing nitrogen intake. Am J Clin Nutr 1987; 46:1040–1047.

167. Larsson J, Lenmarken C, Martensen J, et al: Nitrogen requirements in severely injured patients. Br J Surg 1990; 77:413–416.

168. Maroni BJ, Steinman T, Mitch WE: A method for estimating nitrogen intake of patients with chronic renal failure. Kidney Int 1986; 27:58–63.

169. Burke JF, Wolfe RR, Mullany CJ, et al: Glucose requirements following burn injury. Ann Surg 1979; 190:274–285.

170. Askanazi J, Elwyn DH, Silberberg PA, et al: Respiratory distress secondary to a high carbohydrate load. Surgery 1980; 87:596–598.

171. Wolfe RR, Allsop JR, Burke JF: Glucose metabolism in man: response to intravenous glucose infusion. Metabolism 1979; 28:210–220.

172. Flakoll PJ, Hill JO, Abumrad NN: Acute hyperglycemia enhances proteolysis in normal man. Am J Physiol 1993; 265:E715–E721.

173. Hennessey PJ, Black CT, Andrassy RJ: Nonenzymatic glycosylation of immunoglobulin G impairs complement fixation. JPEN 1991; 15:60–64.

174. Björnsson ES, Urbanavicius V, Eliasoson B, et al: Effects of hyperglycemia on interdigestive gastrointestinal motility in humans. Scand J Gastroenterol 1994; 29:1096–1104.

175. Bresson JL, Bader B, Rocchiccioli F, et al: Protein-metabolism kinetics and energy-substrate utilization in infants fed parenteral solutions with different glucose-fat ratios. Am J Clin Nutr 1991; 54:346–350.

176. Schneeweiss B, Graninger W, Ferenci P, et al: Short-term energy balance in patients with infections: carbohydrate-based versus fat-based diets. Metabolism 1992; 41:125–130.

177. Tappy L, Schwarz JM, Schneiter P, et al: Effects of isoenergetic glucose-based or lipid-based parenteral nutrition on glucose metabolism, de novo liponeogenesis, and respiratory gas exchange in critically ill patients. Crit Care Med 1998; 26:860–867.

178. Druml W, Fischer M, Ratheiser K: Utilization of intravenous lipids in critically ill patients with sepsis without and with hepatic failure. JPEN 1998; 22:217–223.

179. Wennberg A, Norbeck HE, Sterner G, Lundholm K: Effects of intravenous nutrition on lipoprotein metabolism, body composition, weight gain and uremic state in experimental uremia in rats. J Nutr 1991; 121:1439–1446.

180. Laidlaw SA, Kopple JD: Newer concepts of indispensable amino acids. Am J Clin Nutr 1987; 46:593–605.

181. Grazer RE, Sutton JM, Friedstrom S, McBarron FD: Hyperammonemic encephalopathy due to essential amino acid hyperalimentation. Arch Intern Med 1984; 144:2278–2279.

182. Nakasaki H, Katayama T, Yokoyama S, et al: Complication of parenteral nutrition composed of essential amino acids and histidine in adults with renal failure. JPEN 1993; 17:86–90.

183. Teraoka S, Kawai T, Hayashi T, et al: Nutritional Management in Acute Renal Failure: Problems of Conventional Amino Acid Preparation and Investigation on Optimal Composition of Amino Acids for Uremic Subjects. In: Aochi O, Amaha K, Takeshita H, eds: Intensive and Critical Medicine. Amsterdam: Elsevier Publishers; 1990:539–556.

184. Smolle KH, Kaufmann P, Fleck S, et al: Influence of a novel amino acid solution (enriched with the dipeptide glycyl-tyrosine) on plasma amino acid concentration of patients with acute renal failure. Clin Nutr 1997; 16:239–246.

185. Pelosi G, Proietti R, Aecangeli A, et al: Total parenteral nutrition infusate: an approach to its optimal composition in post-trauma acute renal failure. Resuscitation 1981; 9:45–51.

186. Kierdorf HP: The nutritional management of acute renal failure in the intensive care unit. New Horizons 1995; 3:699–707.

187. Neu J, Shenoy V, Chakrabarti R: Glutamine nutrition and metabolism: where do we go from here? FASEB J 1996; 10:829–837.

188. Imai E, Yamanoto S, Isaka Y, et al: Delay of recovery from renal ischemic injury by administration of glutamine. JASN 1991; 2:648A.

189. Griffiths RD, Jones CJ, Palmer TEA: Six-month outcome of critically ill patients given glutamine-supplemented parenteral nutrition. Nutrition 1997; 13:295–302.

190. Fürst P, Stehle P: The potential use of dipeptides in clinical nutrition. Nutr Clin Pract 1993; 8:106–114.

191. Bower RH, Cerra FB, Bershadsky B, et al: Early enteral administration of a formula (Impact) supplemented with arginine, nucleotides, and fish oil in intensive care unit patients: results of a multicenter, prospective, randomized, clinical trial. Crit Care Med 1995; 23:436–449.

192. Baek S-M, Makabali GG, Bryan-Brown CW, Kusek J: The influence of parenteral nutrition on the course of acute renal failure. Surg Gynecol Obstet 1975; 141:405–408.

193. Leonard CD, Luke RC, Siegel RR: Parenteral essential amino acids in acute renal failure. Urology 1975; 6:154–157.

194. Blackburn GL, Etter G, Mackenzie T: Criteria for choosing amino acid therapy in acute renal failure. Am J Clin Nutr 1978; 31:1841–1853.

195. Mirtallo JM, Schneider PJ, Mavko K, et al: A comparison of essential and general amino acid infusions in the nutritional support of patients with compromised renal function. JPEN 1982; 6:109–113.

196. Freund H, Atamian S, Fischer JE: Comparative study of parenteral nutrition in renal failure using essential and nonessential amino acid containing solution. Surg Gynecol Obstet 1980; 151:652–656.

197. Proietti R, Pelosi G, Santori R, et al: Nutrition in acute renal failure. Resuscitation 1983; 10:159–166.

198. Milligan SL, Luft FC, McMurray SD, Kleit SA: Intra-abdominal infection and acute renal failure. Arch Surg 1978; 113:467–472.

199. Naylor DC, Detsky AS, O'Rourke K, Fonberg E: Does treatment with essential amino acids and hypertonic glucose improve survival in acute renal failure? A meta-analysis. Ren Fail 1988; 10:141–152.

200. Sponsel H, Conger JD: Is parenteral nutrition therapy of value in acute renal failure? Am J Kidney Dis 1995; 25:96–102.

201. Heyland DK, MacDonald S, Keefe L, Drover JW: Total parenteral nutrition in the critically ill: a meta-analysis. JAMA 1998; 280:2013–2019.

202. Fiaccadori E, Leonardi S, Lombardi M, et al: Enteral nutrition in patients with acute renal failure: nutritional effects and adequacy of nutrient intakes. JASN 1996; 7:1372A.

203. Cockram DB, Moore LW, Acchiardo SR: Response to an oral nutritional supplement for chronic renal failure patients. J Renal Nutr 1994; 4:78–85.

204. Cockram DB, Hensley MK, Rodriguez M, et al: Safety and tolerance of medical nutritional products as a sole source of nutrition in people on hemodialysis. J Ren Nutr 1998; 8:25–33.

205. Baliga R, George VT, Ray PE, Holiday MA: Effects of reduced renal function and dietary protein on muscle protein synthesis. Kidney Int 1991; 39:831–836.

206. Grützmacher P, Radke HW, Schifferdecker E, et al: Early changes of plasma lipid status and glucose tolerance during the course of chronic renal failure. Contrib Nephrol 1984; 41:332–336.

207. Deitch EA: The role of intestinal barrier failure and bacterial translocation in the development of systemic infection and multiple organ failure. Arch Surg 1990; 125: 403–404.

208. Sax HG, Illig KA, Ryan CK, Hardy DJ: Low-dose enteral feeding is beneficial during total parenteral nutrition. Am J Surg 1996; 171:587–590.

209. Abernathy GB, Heizer WD, Holcombe BJ, et al: Efficacy of tube feeding in supplying energy requirements of hospitalized patients. JPEN 1989; 13:336–339.

210. Montecalvo MA, Steger KA, Farber HW, et al: Nutritional outcome and pneumonia in critical care patients randomized to gastric versus jejunal tube feedings. Crit Care Med 1992; 20:1377–1387.

211. Campos ACL, Paluzzi M, Meguid MM: Clinical use of total nutritional admixtures. Nutrition 1990; 6:346–356.

CHAPTER 38

Multiple Organ System Failure

Dieter Kleinknecht

INTRODUCTION

Multiple organ failure is now the main cause of death in intensive care units (ICUs).[1-3] Despite the use of sophisticated techniques of resuscitation and a better care of critically ill patients, an increasing number of these patients develop progressive deterioration of several organs, often unresponsive to therapeutic efforts.

Sepsis is the major cause of organ failure in ICUs, but a variety of noninfectious conditions may also be responsible; for example, acute pancreatitis, severe trauma, major surgery, hypovolemic shock, and burns.[4] Moreover, organ failure can be reproduced experimentally by a number of endogenous mediators of inflammation that exert a complex of interrelated effects among individual organs, the injury of one organ precipitating the failure of another.[4]

DEFINITIONS

The terms *organ system failure* (OSF)[5] and *multiple organ system failure* (MOSF)[6] were introduced in the early 1980s to describe not a specific entity, but a syndrome characterized by the development of abnormalities affecting one or more organs in critically ill patients. This syndrome can emerge during infectious or noninfectious conditions.

The criteria used to define abnormalities of organ function are widely dissimilar from one study to another and are based on the concept of failure, a dichotomous event that is either present or absent. Some authors note that there is a continuum of physiologic derangements, ranging from a mild organ *dysfunction*, such as a moderate increase in the serum creatinine level, to an obvious organ *failure*, such as oliguric acute renal failure (ARF) that requires dialysis.[4] The term *multiple organ dysfunction syndrome* (MODS) was therefore proposed, defined as the "presence of altered organ function in an acutely ill patient such that homeostasis cannot be maintained without intervention."[4]

Thus, the acronym MODS describes a pattern of multiple and progressive symptoms and signs that are thought to be pathogenetically related and potentially reversible. This process is dynamic rather than static, its expression varying over time. MODS can be primary, as a direct result of the insult, or secondary, as the consequence of a host *systemic inflammatory response* (SIRS), whether infectious or not.[4, 7]

Until recently, there was no clear consensus on the best description of organ dysfunction or failure. In ICU patients, Knaus and coworkers[5] first considered five failing organ systems, including cardiovascular, respiratory, renal, hematologic, and neurologic failure (Table 38–1). Definitions of OSF were based on objective quantifiable variables. With one exception, criteria were independent of therapy. For instance, renal failure (acute) was present if the patient had one or more of the following during a 24-hour period, regardless of other values: urine output <480 mL/24 h or <160 mL/8 h; serum BUN ≥100 mg/dL; and serum creatinine ≥3.5 mg/dL. Patients receiving chronic hemodialysis prior to hospital admission were excluded. Each patient was followed until recovery from all OSF, death, or for 7 days.

Fagon and coworkers[8] added hepatic dysfunction and the presence of infection to the five organs mentioned previously that could fail. Hepatic and gastrointestinal dysfunction were also added by other investigators[9-11] (see Table 38–1).

Tran and coworkers[12] proposed a scale of dysfunction, or MOSF score, representing the sum of the most abnormal daily recording of seven individual OSFs (graded from 0 to 2). The parameters recorded included not only clinical and biochemical markers but also some disease categories, such as acalculous cholecystitis and stress ulcer and the need for mechanical support (ventilation, dialysis) and pharmacologic support (inotropes). The Sepsis-related Organ Failure Assessment (SOFA) score of Vincent and coworkers[13] also expresses grading of severity of disease and includes in its scale the need for therapy.

All these scores are based on a personal 5- to 7-point ordinal scale, which may or may not[14] include respiratory failure. More details can be found in the original published reports or in general reviews.[15, 16] Recent scoring systems are more sophisticated than the earlier systems, but their use may help to better quantify the disease progression or the influence of therapy.

EPIDEMIOLOGY AND PROGNOSIS

Multiple organ system failure develops in 40% to 50% of patients admitted to ICUs,[5, 17] most of the cases being due to an infectious process. Mortality of patients with MOSF ranges between 30% and 100%, and is significantly related to the number of failing organs.[2, 5, 6, 9, 17]

In his pioneering work, Knaus and coworkers[5] showed that in ICU patients, striking increases in mortality were associated with an increase in the number and duration of OSFs. Mortality in patients with OSF

TABLE 38–1. Current Scores Used to Evaluate MOSF and MODS in ICU Patients

AUTHORS	CARDIOVASCULAR	RESPIRATORY	RENAL	HEMATOLOGIC	NEUROLOGIC	HEPATIC	GASTROINTESTINAL	INFECTION
Knaus et al[5]	+	+	+	+	+			
Tran et al[10]	+	+	+	+	+	+	+	
Fagon et al[8]	+	+	+	+	+	+		+
Hebert et al[9]	+	+	+	+	+	+	+	
Marshall et al[11]	+	+	+	+	+	+	+	
Chertow et al[14]*	+		+	+	+	+	+	
Vincent et al[13]†	+	+	+	+	+	+		

*ARF patients requiring dialysis.
†Sepsis-related Organ Failure Assessment (SOFA) score.

of three or more organs persisting for more than 3 days was 98% and reached 100% after 4 days. This high proportion of deaths was not found in further studies published by this same group[18] (Table 38–2). Significant risk factors for developing OSF included older age, a pre-existing severe chronic disease, and a nonoperative diagnosis, particularly sepsis, as was hospital admission for septic shock or cardiac arrest.[5]

Similar results were presented by Rauss and coworkers.[19] Patients with three or more OSFs after the first ICU day had a mortality rate ranging between 93% and 100%. Isolated neurologic failure (coma) had the highest mortality (40%), compared with an average of 20% mortality for any other single OSF. Various combinations of other OSFs had little independent correlation with outcome.

Using a scale of 0 to 4 for each organ dysfunction, Marshall and coworkers[11] found that their score allowed excellent discrimination, as reflected in areas under the receiving operating characteristic (ROC) curve. Intensive care unit mortality was strongly influenced by the degree of organ dysfunction present at the time of ICU admission and, most importantly, after ICU admission.

Many reports dealing with ARF patients confirm these findings[3, 20–24] (see Table 38–2). The criteria of Knaus and coworkers[5] were used in a 6-month prospective study on 360 patients with ARF hospitalized in 20 ICUs.[3, 25, 26] Univariate analysis showed a significant relationship between the number of failed organs and sex; a septic origin of ARF; oliguria; prothrombin time; mechanical ventilation; the mean values of two severity scoring indexes, SAPS and APACHE II; and the hospital mortality. The mean number of OSFs was higher in nonsurvivors than in survivors, whether the values were recorded at admission or at inclusion. With the use of multivariate analysis, OSF at inclusion was a significant predictor of hospital mortality, as were ARF occurring during ICU stay, oliguria, hospitalization prior to ICU admission, ARF of septic origin, previous altered health status, and an older age.[3] Hospital mortality was higher in patients with septic shock (79%) than in those with nonseptic ARF (45%). Interestingly, mortality was also higher in septic ARF if, in addition to ARF, two organs were failing, but the difference was no longer significant if three or more organs failed. These results suggest that a high number of failing organs have more prognostic value than the origin of ARF, whether septic or not.[26]

In a retrospective study, Groeneveld and coworkers[27] were unable to show a relationship between mortality and organ failure (including hepatic and gastrointestinal failure) developing after the onset of ARF. Only cardiovascular failure complicating ARF predicted death. However, in the 10% of patients without OSF, both before and after the onset of ARF, all survived, whereas in patients with OSF, either before or after ARF, mortality was 70%. Prior pulmonary and cardiovascular failure increased the risk of death by 2.3 and 2.5, respectively.

TABLE 38–2. In-Hospital Mortality (%) in ICU Patients According to the Number of Failing Organs

AUTHORS	PATIENTS, n	TYPE OF PATIENTS	TIME OF ASSESSMENT	NUMBER OF FAILING ORGANS					
				1	2	>2	3	4	5
Knaus et al[5]	5677	Medical/surgical	Day 1*	22	52	80			
			Day 5*	40	56	100			
Lohr et al[20]	126	ARF/dialysis	Day 1 of dialysis	56	70	—	81	100	94
Maher et al[21]	90	ARF/dialysis	?	—	33	—	54	88	—
Rauss et al[19]	5248	Medical/surgical	Day 1*	37†	64†	82			
			Day 5*	48†	72†	97			
Fagon et al[8]	1070	Medical/surgical	Admission	10	17	—	32	65	76
Marshall et al[4]	692	Surgical	Day 1*	7	26	—	48	69	83
Kleinknecht et al[3]	360	ARF	Inclusion	46	62	90			
Zimmerman et al[18]	7703	Medical/surgical	Day 1*	23	52	85			
			Day 5*	37	68	86			

*When organ dysfunction was present.
†Patients older than 65.

The incidence of renal dysfunction in MODS seems to be increasing. Kierdorf and Seeliger[23] found that the frequency of ARF in MODS was significantly higher during the period 1981 to 1988 (78.4%) compared with the period 1966 to 1980 (54.1%), without change in mortality.

CLINICAL MANIFESTATIONS

In MOSF, organ failure may be due to the primary event, infectious or not, or to the inflammatory and noninflammatory host response. If this response is inadequate, exaggerated, or impaired, as occurs in immunocompromised subjects, SIRS may develop (see previous discussion), even without documented infection.[1] Therefore, the clinical picture may vary extensively, with the failing organ or organs often not involved in the initial event. In addition, in most cases, there is a lag period between this event and the development of SIRS or MOSF.[1, 23] In general, the respiratory system is the first organ to fail, followed by cardiovascular, hepatic, intestinal, and renal dysfunction or failure.[2, 6, 27, 28] However, in patients with severe diseases, such as those with septic shock, most organ failures occur early and almost simultaneously.

Cardiovascular Dysfunction

In septic conditions, circulatory failure (septic shock) occurs in half of the cases and is an important contributor to MOSF. Nevertheless, there is a continuum between mild hypotension and progressive severe hypovolemia.[2] At the initial acute phase, hypovolemia is due both to arterial and venous dilatation and to leakage of plasma into the extravascular space. As a compensatory mechanism for maintaining normal blood pressure, systemic vascular resistances increase. Pulmonary-artery oxygenation is decreased, resulting in an impairment of oxygen delivery to hypoperfused tissues.[29] Correction of hypovolemia by massive fluid infusion is followed by tachycardia, an increase in cardiac output, a decrease in peripheral resistances, and an elevation in pulmonary-artery oxygen, a syndrome sometimes called hyperdynamic shock, or hypermetabolic organ failure.[2] Persistent low-grade fever, leukocytosis, hyperglycemia, hyperlactatemia, and increased urea production are associated features.

Despite normal cardiac output, there is usually an early and acute myocardial dysfunction, with reduced left and right ventricular ejection fraction, and increased end-diastolic and end-systolic volumes of both ventricles.[29] These abnormalities may reverse in surviving patients if sepsis can be cured. There is experimental evidence that myocardial depressant factors are liberated during sepsis, including various cytokines such as tissue necrosis factor (TNF), interleukin-1 (IL-1), and IL-6.

Pulmonary Dysfunction

Acute lung injury complicates sepsis in about 40% of cases. In the most severe forms, an acute respiratory distress syndrome (ARDS) may occur with progressive dyspnea, hyperventilation, use of auxiliary respiratory muscles, and cyanosis. Hypoxemia and hypercapnia are then common. Radiographic films show diffuse alveolar infiltrates. Mechanical ventilation is promptly required,[2, 29] and its need is currently used as a marker of respiratory failure.[5, 8, 9, 19, 22, 25] Other investigators have selected the Po_2/Fio_2 ratio as the best descriptor of respiratory dysfunction.[11, 13]

This acute lung injury is due to an increased pulmonary microvascular leakage of protein-rich fluid, related to epithelial alveolar and endothelial damage. It is worth recalling that pulmonary failure may be facilitated or prolonged by excessive salt and water overload.

Renal Dysfunction

An increase in serum creatinine and a drop in the glomerular filtration rate (GFR) are frequent in sepsis and septic shock, because of hypotension and intrarenal microvascular disturbances (see Chapter 21). Renal dysfunction is usually preceded by cardiovascular and pulmonary failure. Oliguria is common but nonoliguric forms of ARF are increasingly recognized.[3, 26] A normal urine output does not preclude the need for dialysis.

There has been an emphasis on the role of nonhemodynamic factors in the pathogenesis of ARF during sepsis, including the release of cytokines and of various vasoactive substances, the activation of circulating leukocytes secreting proteases and free oxygen radicals, and the lesions related to reperfusion after temporary hypoperfusion.[2, 30]

The influence of previous chronic renal diseases is controversial. Tran and colleagues[12] found that preexisting chronic renal failure did not predispose patients with sepsis to ARF. On the other hand, Thijs and coworkers[2] stated that in such patients the kidneys tend to be the first organ to fail. In any case, many investigators did not find any difference in mortality between ICU patients who had pre-existing renal failure and those who did not.[11, 25, 26]

In a number of patients, kidney failure is a late event. In a series of 100 ARF patients studied prospectively, Kierdorf and Seeliger[23] showed that ARF requiring dialysis occurred, as a mean, 7 days after the underlying insult. In all cases, ARF was part of MODS. In addition, patients who developed late ARF were more often oliguric and had a higher mortality rate than those with early ARF. Kleinknecht and coworkers[3] found similar results in ARF patients, whether they required dialysis or not.

Neurologic Dysfunction

Encephalopathy may occur early in severe sepsis, sometimes as the sole manifestation of infection, particularly in elderly people. The symptoms and signs range from mild disorientation to confusion, focal signs, and seizures. Many studies use the Glasgow Coma Score as a quantitative measure of neurologic deficit.[5, 8, 9, 11–13, 19, 22, 25] The mortality rate increases as the Glasgow Coma Score decreases.[11]

The pathogenesis of septic encephalopathy includes cerebral hypoperfusion, hypoxemia, cerebral edema, focal thrombosis or bleeding, and a possible effect of mediators on the blood-brain barrier.[31]

Hematologic Dysfunction

An increase of leukocytes, or transient leukopenia, or both, is usually included in the definition of hematologic dysfunction,[5, 8, 9, 11, 19, 25] as well as thrombocytopenia, mainly related in MOSF to disseminated intravascular coagulation (DIC). Disseminated intravascular coagulation results from an increase in thrombin and fibrin production and an activation of both extrinsic and intrinsic pathways of coagulation, probably facilitated by endothelial injury. Prothrombin time or partial thromboplastin time are prolonged, fibrinogen level is decreased, and fibrin degradation products are present in serum. Petechiae and mucosal hemorrhage are then common features.

Liver Dysfunction

Liver dysfunction occurs early and frequently in MOSF. It may be limited to a moderate rise in liver enzymes or extended to frank jaundice in severe forms.[2] In most reports, hyperbilirubinemia is included in the definition of liver dysfunction or failure,[8, 9, 11–13] sometimes associated with an increase in serum alkaline phosphatase.[8, 9] Typically, the increase in serum bilirubin occurs in the conjugated fraction, a prominent rise in its unconjugated fraction being the rule if hemolysis is an associated feature.

The pathogenesis of liver dysfunction in MOSF is multifactorial and includes, to various degrees, liver ischemia, injury to hepatocytes and endothelial cells due to endotoxin and mediators liberated during sepsis, parenteral nutrition, massive transfusions, and the consequences of renal failure.[2] Hepatic abscesses are exceptionally well documented. Some reports emphasize that pre-existing liver disease may predispose patients to the development of MOSF or impair its resolution.[22]

Gastrointestinal Dysfunction

Sepsis may lead to a decrease in splanchnic perfusion and to lesions of the digestive tract, thereby aggravating hypovolemia. Splanchnic ischemia may damage its barrier function, favoring plasma leakage and bacterial translocation. Stress ulcers may be observed, but are now less common in ICU patients.[32]

Most investigators withdraw gastrointestinal dysfunction from their score, because of the great number of primary digestive diseases requiring an admission in ICU and the difficulty to find reliable descriptors of this organ failure.[5, 8, 11, 13, 25]

PATHOPHYSIOLOGY

There is much experimental and clinical evidence that MOSF, especially in septic conditions, results from microcirculatory ischemia of vital organs and from the systemic, excessive inflammatory host response called SIRS. In this situation, a wide variety of mediators and products are released, inducing cellular alterations and eventually tissue damage and MOSF.[1, 2, 28, 29, 33] The principal mediators and cellular mechanisms thought to be involved in this cascade are listed in Table 38–3. A very complex interplay seems to occur between all these factors, whose precise action remains in part unknown. Some have opposite effects, for example, prostaglandins and thromboxanes, nitric oxide and endothelin, and pro-inflammatory cytokines (IL-1, IL-6, and IL-8) and anti-inflammatory cytokines (IL-4 and IL-10).

Recently, emphasis has been placed on the role of endothelial lesions and of adhesion molecules, mainly intracellular adhesion molecules (ICAM) and endothelial leukocyte adhesion molecules (ELAM). These molecules attach to endothelial cells and attract granulocytes, macrophages, and platelets, resulting in a release of a number of cytotoxic substances, such as TNF, responsible for cell detachment and tissue damage.[2] Once initiated, this process is often self-perpetuating, whether the original event has been controlled or not (Fig. 38–1). This has led to therapeutic trials in order to inhibit the formation or action of the involved mediators.

TREATMENT

Considering the poor prognosis of MOSF, the most important goal is to prevent its occurrence.[1] The prin-

TABLE 38–3. Principal Mediators Thought to Be Involved in MOSF and MODS

Cytokines	Interleukins, IL-1, IL-6, IL-8, TNF
Complement system	C3a, C4a, C5a
Arachidonic acid derivatives	Prostaglandins, leukotrienes, thromboxanes
Coagulation factors	Contact system, extrinsic coagulation pathway, fibrinolytic system, platelets
Cellular	Neutrophil and macrophage activation, endothelial injury
Adhesion molecules	ICAM, ELAM, VCAM
Hormones	Catecholamines, steroids, insulin, glucagon, thyroxin, growth hormone, endorphins
Other factors	Nitric oxide, endothelin, oxygen free radicals, myocardial depressant factor, histamine, serotonin, fibronectin, PAF, proteinases, neuropeptides, and so on

ELAM, endothelial leukocyte adhesion molecules; *ICAM,* intracellular adhesion molecules; *PAF,* platelet activating factor; *VCAM,* vascular cell adhesion molecules.

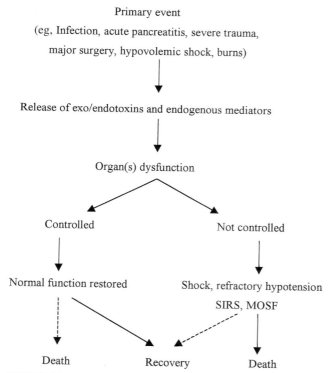

FIGURE 38–1 ■ Schematic of sequence of events leading to multiple organ system failure.

ciples of management can be found in excellent reviews.[1, 16, 29, 33] An outline of these principles is given in Table 38–4.

Prevention

The first objective in prevention is to maintain adequate tissue perfusion in high-risk patients, particularly in the perioperative period.[16] This is difficult to achieve, since it requires both optimal ventilation and

TABLE 38–4. Management of Patients With MOSF and MODS

Prevention
  Treat promptly:
    Infection
    Hemorrhage
    Hypotension
    Trauma
    Low oxygen delivery
  Provide adequate nutritional support
  Use selective decontamination of the digestive tract?
  Avoid or minimize nosocomial infection
Management
  Use conservative measures:
    Maintain adequate intravascular volume and glomerular
      filtration rate
    Supply sufficient oxygen delivery and renal support
    Use enteral feeding as soon as possible
    Avoid nephrotoxic agents
  Use antibodies to endotoxin, mediators, adhesion molecules,
    proteases??

the maintenance of normal cardiac output and its distribution within each vital organ. Intravascular volume repletion with artificial colloids is of paramount importance. There is some evidence that maintaining a supranormal oxygen delivery in ICU patients does not change mortality.[34]

Infection control is mandatory. The source of infection should be eradicated by appropriate antibiotic therapy or surgical drainage, or both.[29] Prevention of infection includes handwashing in current care of ICU patients, isolation of immunocompromised patients, withdrawal of useless catheters and cannulae,[35, 36] and specific treatments such as early fixation of bone and pelvic fractures, and débridement of necrotic tissue in burns and, according to some authors, in acute pancreatitis.[16, 33] Such measures can minimize nosocomial infections, which significantly affect prognosis.[25, 26]

The purpose of selective decontamination of the digestive tract is to decrease the incidence of bacterial translocation and of gram-negative sepsis,[37] but up until now the results have seemed inconclusive.[33]

Patients with pre-existing malnutrition are more prone to developing sepsis, cardiogenic shock, and acute respiratory failure.[12, 38, 39] The provision of adequate nutritional support, preferably by the enteral route, may reduce the incidence of these complications.

Medical Management

Once MOSF has developed, supportive measures are urgently needed. The aim is to ensure adequate intravascular volume, to maintain sufficient tissue perfusion pressure, including renal perfusion, and to supply nearly normal oxygen delivery. The simultaneous control of infection and the treatment of the portal of entry should not be underestimated. This strategy can best be conducted in ICUs.[29]

Volume expansion can be obtained by administering whole blood, artificial colloid, and crystalloid solutions, according to the specific situation. Currently, there is no definitive argument for the preferential use of a given fluid in the treatment of septic conditions. However, some studies have reported a significant reduction in mortality in patients with septic shock who were treated with aggressive hemodynamic support.[29]

After restoration of normovolemia, persistent hypotension may require vasopressor therapy. Under careful monitoring, dopamine and norepinephrine are often prescribed to increase vasomotor tone, and dobutamine is preferred for the improvement of cardiac performance.[33]

Supplying sufficient oxygen delivery is the most difficult goal, requiring both optimal mechanical ventilation and optimal cardiac output. Regular monitoring of blood gases and serum lactate, and perhaps tonometric measurement of gastric mucosal pH,[16] are considered to be helpful measures. Unfortunately, there is no consensus as to what extent cardiac output and its regional distribution should be optimized. The management of ARDS requires specific measures detailed elsewhere.[16, 33]

Renal protection is best ensured by the maintenance of blood pressure and of an adequate intravascular volume, and by avoiding nephrotoxic agents whenever possible. In this setting, it is of no help to rely solely on vasoactive agents, since mortality in ARF patients has not been improved by the use of any of them.[40] Some of these agents may even be harmful. Thus, in a multicenter controlled trial conducted in critically ill patients with acute tubular necrosis, atrial natriuretic peptide (anaritide) improved dialysis-free survival in patients with oliguria, but appeared to worsen it in patients without oliguria.[41]

If dialysis is required, continuous hemofiltration or hemodialysis, or a combination of both, is now preferred to intermittent dialysis.[42, 43] Few prospective studies, if any, have shown a decrease in mortality with the use of continuous dialysis techniques. In some prospective trials, the use of biocompatible membranes seemed to improve prognosis in ARF patients, but this issue has been questioned,[44] and it is not known whether these results may be applicable to the subset of patients with MOSF. Further trials are awaited.

As already stated, early enteral feeding should be encouraged, even if no clear-cut benefit has yet been demonstrated in a general ICU population.[33]

In humans, attempts to inhibit the formation or action of mediators in septic conditions have been rather disappointing, including the use of antibodies to lipid A, endotoxin, TNF, IL-1, adhesion molecules, and proteases.[29] This is not surprising, considering the great number of mediators involved. Studies attempting to modulate the immune response or to interrupt the pathogenetic sequence at multiple points are underway.

REFERENCES

1. Murray MJ, Coursin DB: Multiple organ dysfunction syndrome. Yale J Biol Med 1993; 66:501.
2. Thijs LG, Groeneveld ABJ, Hack CE: Multiple Organ Failure in Septic Shock. In: Rietschel ET, Wagner H, eds: Pathophysiology of Septic Shock: Current Topics in Microbiology and Immunology. Berlin: Springer-Verlag; 1996:209.
3. Kleinknecht D, Landais P, Brivet F, Loirat P, The French Study Group on Acute Renal Failure: Prognosis and mortality in patients with multiple organ failure (MOSF). Renal Fail 1996; 18:347.
4. Bone RC, Balk RA, Cerra FB, et al: Definitions for sepsis and organ failure and guidelines for the use of innovative therapies in sepsis. Chest 1992; 101:1644.
5. Knaus WA, Draper EA, Wagner DP, Zimmerman JE: Prognosis of acute organ-system failure. Ann Surg 1985; 202:685.
6. Fry DE, Pearlstein L, Fulton RL, Hiram CP: Multiple system organ failure: the role of uncontrolled infection. Arch Surg 1980; 115:136.
7. Rangel-Frausto MS, Pittet D, Costigan M, et al: The natural history of the systemic inflammatory response syndrome (SIRS): a prospective study. JAMA 1995; 273:117.
8. Fagon JY, Chastre J, Novara A, et al: Characterization of intensive care unit patients using a model based on the presence or absence of organ dysfunctions and/or infection: the ODIN model. Intensive Care Med 1993; 19:137.
9. Hebert PC, Drummond AJ, Singer J, et al: A simple multiple system organ failure scoring system predicts mortality of patients who have sepsis syndrome. Chest 1993; 104:230.
10. Tran DD, Cuesta MA, Van Leeuwen PAM, et al: Risk factors for multiple organ system failure and mortality in critically injured patients. Surgery 1993; 114:21.
11. Marshall JC, Cook DJ, Christou NV, et al: Multiple organ dysfunction score: a reliable descriptor of a complex clinical outcome. Crit Care Med 1995; 23:1638.
12. Tran DD, Van Onselem EBH, Wensink AJF, Cuesta MA: Factors related to multiple organ system failure and mortality in a surgical intensive care unit. Nephrol Dial Transplant 1994; 9(suppl 4):172.
13. Vincent JL, Moreno R, Takala J, et al: The SOFA (sepsis-related organ failure assessment) score to describe organ dysfunction/failure. Intensive Care Med 1996; 22:707.
14. Chertow GM, Christiansen CL, Cleary PD, et al: Prognostic stratification in critically ill patients with acute renal failure requiring dialysis. Arch Intern Med 1995; 155:1505.
15. Brivet F: Multiorgan Failure and Acute Renal Failure. In: Cantarovich F, Rangoonwala B, Verho M, eds: Progress in Acute Renal Failure. Bridgewater, NJ: Hoechst-Marion Roussel, 1998:129.
16. Singer M: Management of multiple organ failure: guidelines but no hard-and-fast rules. J Antimicrob Chemother 1998; 41 (suppl A):103.
17. Tran DD, Groeneveld ABJ, Van der Meulen J, et al: Age, chronic disease, sepsis, organ system failure, and mortality in a medical intensive care unit. Crit Care Med 1990; 18:474.
18. Zimmerman JE, Knaus WA, Wagner DP, et al: A comparison of risks and outcomes for patients with organ system failure: 1982–1990. Crit Care Med 1996; 24:1633.
19. Rauss A, Knaus WA, Patois E, Le Gall JR, The French Multicentric Group of ICU Research: Prognosis for recovery from multiple organ system failure: the accuracy of objective estimates of chances for survival. Med Decis Making 1990; 10:155.
20. Lohr JW, McFarlane MJ, Grantham JJ: A clinical index to predict survival in acute renal failure patients requiring dialysis. Am J Kidney Dis 1988; 11:254.
21. Maher ER, Robinson KN, Scoble JE et al: Prognosis of critically ill patients with acute renal failure: APACHE II score and other predictive factors. Quart J Med 1989; 72:857.
22. Cosentino F, Chaff C, Piedmonte M: Risk factors influencing survival in ICU acute renal failure. Nephrol Dial Transplant 1994; 9(suppl 4):179.
23. Kierdorf HP, Seeliger S: Acute renal failure in multiple-organ dysfunction syndrome. Kidney Blood Press Res 1997; 20:164.
24. Liano F, Junco E, Madero R, Pascual J, Verde E, Madrid Acute Renal Failure Study Group: The spectrum of acute renal failure in the intensive care unit compared with that seen in other settings. Kidney Int 1998; 53(suppl 66):S16.
25. Brivet FG, Kleinknecht DJ, Loirat P, Landais P, The French Study Group on Acute Renal Failure: Acute renal failure in intensive care units: causes, outcome, and prognostic factors of hospital mortality: a prospective multicenter study. Crit Care Med 1996; 24:192.
26. Neveu H, Kleinknecht D, Brivet F, Loirat P, Landais P, The French Study Group on Acute Renal Failure: Prognostic factors in acute renal failure due to sepsis: results of a prospective multicenter study. Nephrol Dial Transplant 1996; 11:293.
27. Groeneveld ABJ, Tran DD, Van der Meulen J, et al: Acute renal failure in the medical intensive care unit: predisposing, complicating factors and outcome. Nephron 1991; 59:602.
28. Deitch EA: Multiple organ failure: pathophysiology and potential future therapy. Ann Surg 1992; 216:117.
29. Parrillo JE: Pathogenetic mechanisms of septic shock. N Engl J Med 1993; 328:1471.
30. Groeneveld ABJ: Pathogenesis of acute renal failure during sepsis. Nephrol Dial Transplant 1994; 9(suppl 4):47.
31. Bolton CF, Young GB, Zochodne DW: The neurologic complications of sepsis. Ann Neurol 1993; 33:94.
32. Cook DJ, Fuller HD, Guyatt GH, et al: Risk factors for gastrointestinal bleeding in critically ill patients. N Engl J Med 1994; 330:377.
33. Rosser DM, Singer M: Multiple organ dysfunction in the intensive therapy unit. Nephrol Dial Transplant 1995; 10:S105.

34. Hayes MA, Timmins AC, Yau EH, et al: Elevation of systemic oxygen delivery in the treatment of critically ill patients. N Engl J Med 1994; 330:1717.

35. Vincent JL, Bihari DJ, Suter PM, et al: The prevalence of nosocomial infection in intensive care units in Europe: results of the European Prevalence of Infection in Intensive Care (EPIC) study. JAMA 1995; 274:639.

36. Pearson ML: Hospital infection control practices advisory committee. Guidelines for prevention of intravascular device-related infections. Infect Control Hosp Epidemiol 1996; 17:438.

37. Cockerill FR, Muller SR, Anhalt JP, et al: Prevention of infection in critically ill patients by selective decontamination of the digestive tract. Ann Intern Med 1992; 117:545.

38. Bagley JS, Wan JMF, Georgieff M, et al: Cellular nutrition in support of early multiple organ failure. Chest 1991; 100:182S.

39. Fiaccadori E, Lombardi M, Leonardi S, et al: Prevalence and clinical outcome associated with preexisting malnutrition in acute renal failure: a prospective cohort study. J Am Soc Nephrol 1999; 10:581.

40. Conger J: Prophylaxis and treatment of acute renal failure by vasoactive agents: the fact and the myths. Kidney Int 1998; 53(suppl 64):S23.

41. Allgren RL, Marbury TC, Rahman SN, et al: Anaritide in acute tubular necrosis. N Engl J Med 1997; 336:828.

42. Van Bommel E, Bouvy ND, So KL, et al: Acute dialytic support for the critically ill: intermittent versus continuous arteriovenous hemodiafiltration. Am J Nephrol 1995; 15:192.

43. Grootendorst AF, Bouman CSC, Hoeben KHN, et al: The role of continuous renal replacement therapy in sepsis and multiorgan failure. Am J Kidney Dis 1996; 28(suppl 3):S50.

44. Jacobs C: Membrane biocompatibility in the treatment of acute renal failure: what is the evidence in 1996? Nephrol Dial Transplant 1997; 12:38.

CHAPTER 39

Dialysis: Continuous Versus Intermittent Renal Replacement Therapy in the Treatment of Acute Renal Failure

Claudio Ronco ▪ Rinaldo Bellomo

INTRODUCTION

Acute renal failure (ARF) can occur in hospitalized patients as the result of several pathologic events. While the classic form of ARF caused by exogenous toxins is less frequent, new causes of renal impairment are frequently seen in intensive care and surgical settings.

Renal hypoperfusion is one of the main causes of ARF in patients undergoing abdominal or cardiac surgery. Furthermore, ARF is frequently seen as part of a more complex syndrome, such as multiple organ failure and sepsis. In the latter case, the patient's severity scores are at the highest levels, and they are frequently under different life support treatments (eg, mechanical ventilation, cardiac mechanical support, and hemodialysis).

Acute renal failure as a single pathologic entity is generally treated with intermittent or daily hemodialysis and has a favorable outcome in a high percentage of cases.[1, 2] The isolated renal disorder is mostly followed in renal wards, and renal replacement therapy permits the patient to overcome the transient period of oliguria until renal recovery has taken place. In contrast, patients with multiple organ dysfunction, infectious complications, or sepsis have a poor prognosis, and mortality is very high. In these patients, hemodialysis or peritoneal dialysis may sometimes be contraindicated, or they may even present potential hazards.[2-4] To overcome these problems, continuous renal replacement therapies (CRRTs) have been in use since 1977.[5, 6] The slow and gentle nature of the therapy, together with its remarkable clinical effectiveness, has made continuous renal replacement modalities a successful therapy for critically ill patients with ARF.

The aim of an adequate renal replacement therapy in intensive care is the effective substitution of renal function with minimal incidence of complications. The adequacy of dialysis in the critically ill patient is determined by a number of variables, including blood chemistry control, restoration and maintenance of homeostasis, appropriate nutrition, and fluid balance control. Tolerance is defined by a good hemodynamic response to fluid withdrawal, by minimal interaction between the artificial circulation and the patient and, finally, by minimal or absent unwanted effects.

The heterogeneity of the patient population[7-12] makes it nearly impossible to evaluate the impact of different dialytic strategies in the absence of very large multicenter studies. The variability in illness severity, the "bounded physiologic chaos" inherent in intensive care unit (ICU) therapeutic interventions, and the small numbers of cases obtained in single institutions further aggravate the problem of defining adequacy in this setting.

Although the problem of improving patient outcome is still one of the major unsolved issues in this field, progress has been made in several directions. We now have several safe, effective, and flexible forms of renal replacement therapy that allow for personalization of therapy and for a problem-oriented approach.[13-20] At the same time, illness severity scores have been developed and validated,[21-24] although they seem to be inadequate to describe the condition of the patient with complicated ARF. Nevertheless, such scores now make it possible to make more accurate comparisons of populations of critically ill patients among different ICUs or within the same institution. Ventilator techniques, hemodynamic manipulations, and approaches to the management of sepsis are increasingly performed according to consensus principles.[25-28] The ability to organize multicenter studies is increasing because of recent advances in telecommunications. These changes open the door to the possibility of testing the concept of adequacy of dialysis for ARF in the near future. At present, however, any discussion of the concept of adequacy of dialysis in the critically ill patient with ARF has to rely on indirect data and physiologic principles. Such principles are helpful in defining "a priori" the necessary properties of an adequate renal replacement therapy.

REQUIREMENTS FOR ADEQUATE RENAL REPLACEMENT IN THE INTENSIVE CARE UNIT

The first, indirectly established principle in the management of critically ill patients is that the degree of physiologic derangement in the first 24 hours after admission to the ICU (but also thereafter) "drives" prognosis. This principle has been widely tested and demonstrated by multiple studies in thousands of ICU patients.[21-28] A corollary of this principle is that early correction or prevention of any physiologic derangement is a very important therapeutic goal in critical care medicine. Acute renal failure should be no exception. Adequate therapy, therefore, means renal replacement therapy that is applied early to prevent hyperkalemia, hyponatremia, uremia, acidosis, and pulmonary and peripheral edema. It also means a therapy that does not generate derangement of its own.

The second principle is that the adequacy of any artificial organ support in the ICU is measured by how closely such support mimics the flexibility, versatility, and efficacy of the organ system it seeks to substitute. This is true for mechanical ventilation, cardiac assistive devices, and artificial oxygenators. It should also be true of any artificial kidney.

The third principle is that the use of any artificial organ support should not delay the recovery from injury of the native organ.

The fourth principle is that any organ replacement therapy should have absent or minimal proinflammatory effects, particularly in the setting of multiorgan system failure.

The conclusion of this discussion leads to the point that any renal replacement method should aim at a complete restoration of the homeostatic equilibrium that is normally guaranteed by the function of native kidneys.

CHARACTERIZATION OF THE PATIENT

To adequately treat ARF in the complicated setting of ICU, we must analyze the nature and the complexity of the critically ill patient. The typical features of the multiple organ dysfunction syndrome (MODS) can be summarized as follows: the syndrome is one of the major causes of death in intensive care; patients are on different life support systems and maintenance of homeostatic parameters become extremely complex; vasoactive drugs are utilized to counterbalance hemodynamic instability or shock; mechanical ventilation or extracorporeal CO_2 removal is often required to sustain tissue oxygenation; cardiac support is frequently achieved not only with inotropic drugs but also with mechanical devices. Acute renal failure is a common finding in this complex clinical picture. Finally, humoral and cellular mediators of inflammation are generally present in tissues and systemic circulation at very high levels of concentration.

Under such circumstances, an effective renal replacement therapy must provide adequate blood purification from uremic toxins; correction of fluid, electrolyte, and acid-base derangement; protection of the kidneys from further injury; and, if possible, accelerate recovery of renal function. The possibility of protecting the kidney from inflammatory insults is under discussion, but it is certainly an appealing concept to explore.

RENAL REPLACEMENT STRATEGIES

The clinical pattern and the history of patients affected by MODS have changed over the years. For a long time, these patients were unable to survive for more than a few hours, and renal replacement was not even instituted, or it was instituted only at the last minute. Subsequently, with the advent of different life support systems, critically ill patients could be maintained at a level of stability sufficient to permit the institution of renal replacement therapy. The final outcome did not change significantly, and in some cases it appeared worse. This observation may be justified by the fact that sicker patients are treated with resuscitation procedures that were not applicable in the past. Therefore, a population of patients with higher severity scores is now treated with renal replacement therapies. In these cases, both hemodialysis and peritoneal dialysis display some limitations and appear inadequate. Nevertheless, these therapies have been the sole possible approach for many years and, in many cases, are still considered the standard for renal replacement in ARF. In 1977, Peter Kramer described a new treat-

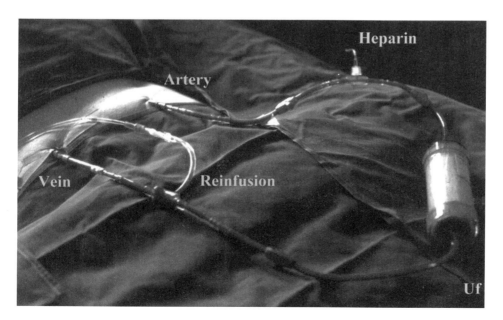

FIGURE 39–1 ■ The extracorporeal circuit in continuous arteriovenous hemofiltration. No pumps are used.

ment that he named continuous arteriovenous hemo-filtration (CAVH).[5] This treatment was based on a highly permeable hemofilter connected to an artery and a vein by modified hemodialysis bloodlines. The arteriovenous pressure gradient moved the blood through the extracorporeal circuit, and no pumps were utilized (Fig. 39–1). Slow continuous production of ultrafiltrate was achieved, and substitution fluid was administered in postdilution mode to maintain the patient's fluid balance. The advantage of this technique was the simplicity and the possibility that it could be performed in almost every hospital, even in the absence of an organized hemodialysis service.

The technique very soon displayed some limitations, and for this reason it was subsequently modified, and newer options were made available. The use of a blood pump with a venovenous blood access became popular and the arteriovenous approach was almost completely abandoned. At the same time, the hemofilters were equipped with a second port in the ultrafiltrate compartment, thus permitting the countercurrent circulation of dialysate. With these modifications, the treatment was named continuous hemodialysis or continuous hemodiafiltration. All these modifications are today available as routine treatments, and special machines have also been designed to facilitate the clinical application of these techniques (Fig. 39–2).

The authors have utilized some of this new equipment both in hemofiltration and in hemodiafiltration, using single-pass or even recirculation techniques. Sterile fluid bags are used both as a replacement solution and as a dialysate to be circulated countercurrent to blood flow in high-flux, hollow-fiber dialyzers. The machines are equipped with a weighing system and pumps for the dialysate inlet and outlet flow.[29–32] Urea and creatinine clearances as high as 60 L/24 h can be

achieved with these systems. Larger molecules are also cleared at high speed because of the high convective transport. As an example, inulin clearances up to 36 to 48 L/24 h have been obtained. Several companies have now undertaken the effort to build newly conceived machines, based on the principle that specifically designed equipment should be used in intensive care patients as an alternative to classic, more sophisticated dialysis machines. The approach is a user-friendly interface, beyond which the sophisticated complexity of the machine is maintained with advanced functions. Self-priming procedures and self-loading of the circuit are some of the new features that contribute to the simplicity of use of the machine even by personnel who have not been completely trained for standard hemodialysis.

EFFICIENCY IN CONTINUOUS AND INTERMITTENT THERAPIES

When continuous hemofiltration is utilized, solute clearance is equal to the amount of ultrafiltrate obtained. In CAVH, if one assumes a maximal clearance of 16 L/24 h, in a given patient with a blood urea nitrogen concentration (BUN) of 100 mg/dL, 16 g of urea nitrogen can be removed daily. When severely catabolic patients are involved, higher amounts of ultrafiltrate are needed to control azotemia, and continuous venovenous hemofiltration (CVVH) is frequently used. Under such conditions, clearances of up to 36 to 48 L/24 h are required, and the use of a blood pump in the circuit permits the achievement of the desired level of efficiency. Urea is even more effectively removed when a countercurrent flow of dialysate is utilized in the circuit, and diffusion is added to convec-

Last Generation of Machines for CRRT

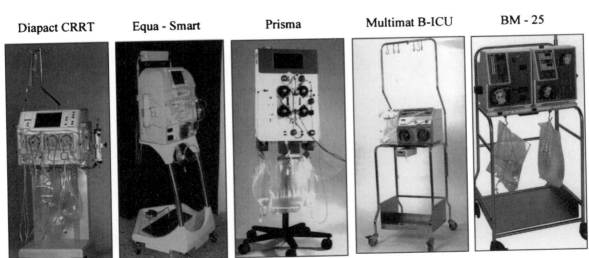

Diapact CRRT   Equa - Smart   Prisma   Multimat B-ICU   BM - 25

FIGURE 39–2 ■ Different machines for continuous renal replacement therapies available on the market. From *left* to *right*: Diapact, B. Braun, Melsungen, Germany; Equa-Smart, Medica, Mirandola, Italy; Prisma, Hospal-Cobe, Lyon, France; Multimat B-ICU, Bellco, Mirandola, Italy; BM-25, Baxter CVG, Irvine, California, USA.

tion, thus obtaining a treatment-defined CAVHD (continuous hemodialysis) or CAVHDF (continuous hemodiafiltration). A system derived from the chronic hemodialysis in which filtration and back-filtration take place in a highly permeable dialyzer during several hours of recirculation of sterile bicarbonate dialysate has also been used (continuous high-flux dialysis [CHFD]). Maximal utilization of the used fluid is achieved since the 20 L batch is discarded only when urea nitrogen has been equilibrated with the patient's blood levels. Clearances of up to 60 to 70 L/d can be obtained for urea, while larger molecules can be cleared at a rate of 36 to 40 L/d. The weighing system of the machine allows for accurate and precise fluid control in the patient.

Improved clearances can also be achieved with higher filtration rates in continuous hemofiltration. This is frequently achieved with predilution techniques. In this case, however, a careful measurement of solute clearance corrected for predilution must be done in order to obtain the exact calculation of the efficiency of the system.

Despite lower clearance, continuous therapies are more efficient in removing urea nitrogen compared with intermittent daily hemodialysis (Fig. 39–3). The explanation depends on the stable concentration profile of urea in blood during continuous therapies. On the contrary, during intermittent hemodialysis, the treatment is very efficient in the first hour, but the amount of solute removal decreases significantly later on. In fact, despite maintenance of high clearance, the solute concentration in blood is lowered and the relevant amount of solute removal decreases. Additionally, a remarkable rebound in concentration after dialysis can be observed in intermittent treatments, showing that a certain degree of solute sequestration in peripheral tissues is present (Table 39–1).

TABLE 39–1. Quantitative Blood Purification: Example of 24-Hour Kinetics

VARIABLE	HEMODIALYSIS	CVVH
K, mL/min	200	20
Urea [C]o, mg/dL	120	70
Urea [C]t, mg/dL	30	65
Tx time, min	240	1440
Kt/V	1.5	1.5
Total clearance, L	48	48
Urea removed, g	18	33.6
Rebound, %	22	0

CLINICAL ASPECTS

The complexity of the patient with ARF with associated multiple organ failure suggests that continuous therapies should probably be utilized as a first choice treatment in intensive care unit settings. In the meantime, clinical conditions other than ARF, such as congestive heart failure, respiratory distress syndrome, cerebral edema, may also benefit from these forms of treatment when oliguria is present or early signs of renal insufficiency are associated.

The patient with severe hemodynamic instability cannot be controlled with intermittent treatments such as hemodialysis or hemodiafiltration carried out for 3 to 4 hours per day. On the other hand, peritoneal dialysis can be inadequate in obtaining the ultrafiltration volumes and solute clearances necessary to control overhydration and severe catabolism. The slow continuous fluid removal achieved with continuous therapies such as CAVH-CVVH or CAVHD-CVVHD (continuous, venovenous hemodialysis) is generally well tolerated, and an optimal status of hydration can generally be reached over an extended period of time

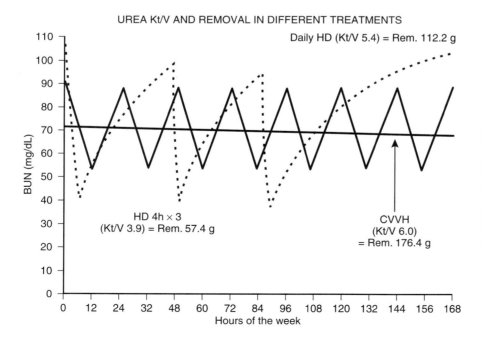

UREA Kt/V AND REMOVAL IN DIFFERENT TREATMENTS

Daily HD (Kt/V 5.4) = Rem. 112.2 g

HD 4h × 3
(Kt/V 3.9) = Rem. 57.4 g

CVVH
(Kt/V 6.0)
= Rem. 176.4 g

BUN (mg/dL)

Hours of the week

FIGURE 39–3 ■ Urea kinetics in continuous hemofiltration and daily hemodialysis. Despite a higher clearance and higher daily Kt/V value, intermittent hemodialysis removes less urea nitrogen per week. The explanation lies in the stable concentration profile of urea nitrogen during continuous therapy, compared with intermittent treatments. Furthermore, patients on intermittent hemodialysis spend a remarkable number of hours per day with a higher degree of uremic intoxication because of higher levels of uremic toxins.

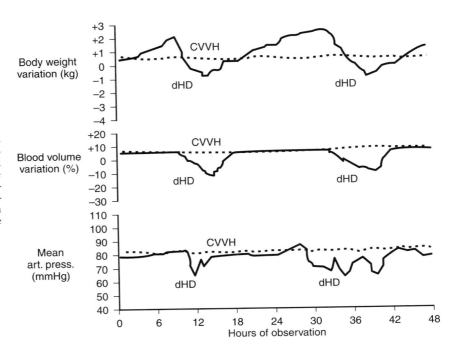

FIGURE 39–4 ▪ Hemodynamic instability is frequently observed during intermittent hemodialysis. The process of ultrafiltration obtained within a few hours leads to a reduction of the circulating blood volume and hypotensive episodes. This is not the case in continuous therapies, in which a slow progressive ultrafiltration is accompanied by a continuous refilling of the intravascular fluid volume.

with excellent cardiovascular tolerance and steady-state hemodynamic parameters.

On-line measurement of relative blood volume changes during treatment has demonstrated that even at relatively low ultrafiltration rates (25 mL/min), a significant drop in circulating blood volume can be observed in intermittent treatments. This phenomenon is not observed in continuous treatments (Fig. 39–4). Variations in blood volume during intermittent treatments are accompanied by episodes of hypotension and tachycardia and are related to a discrepancy between the rate of filtration and the rate of intravascular refilling (Fig. 39–5). These effects are less evident or even absent when continuous ultrafiltration is performed gently and slowly over an extended period of time. Assuming a certain fluid intake and a consequent fluid accumulation in the oligoanuric patient, the rate of fluid removal in continuous therapies is scaled down by one order of magnitude compared with that required for intermittent hemodialysis (Fig. 39–6). This results in an improved cardiovascular stability during continuous therapies at similar levels of daily fluid balance. This aspect may be of remarkable importance in the phase of recovery from ARF. The recovering

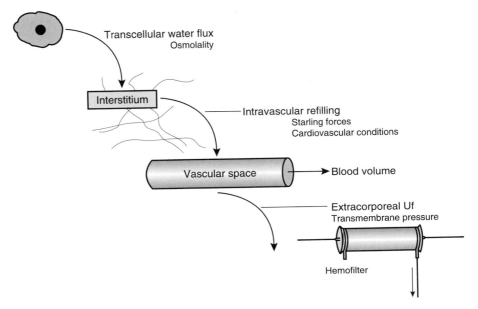

FIGURE 39–5 ▪ The process of ultrafiltration must cope with the rate of intravascular refilling from interstitium and intracellular space. The final objective is to maintain circulating blood volume.

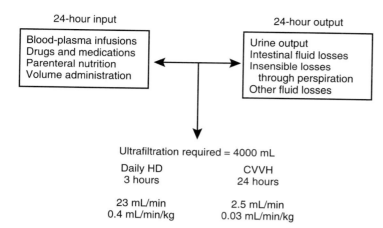

70-kg PATIENT WITH ARF: FLUID BALANCE REQUIREMENT

FIGURE 39-6 ■ Typical fluid balance over a 24-hour period in an oligoanuric patient and ultrafiltration rates required in intermittent hemodialysis and continuous venovenous hemofiltration.

kidney is extremely sensitive to variations in perfusion pressure and blood flow. Based on the previously mentioned observations, intermittent treatments not only may be inadequate for maintenance of steady hemodynamics and sufficient renal perfusion but also may contribute to further damage to the renal parenchyma, perpetuating the ischemic insult and the consequent anuria. On the other hand, CRRT may be well tolerated and may contribute to a constant and progressive recovery of the kidney by preventing major hemodynamic alterations.

The slow continuous nature of CRRT seems to present particular benefits for patients with severe cardiac contractility failure. Several mechanisms have been considered important in the amelioration of the hemodynamic conditions of patients with congestive heart failure treated with continuous hemofiltration. These include the improvement of the ventricular filling pressures, the reduction of preload, the maintenance of the blood volume, modulation of the renin angiotensin axis, the reduction of afterload, and the possible clearance of myocardial depressant substances. Another factor considered to be important is the possibility of a dissociation between sodium and water transport during hemofiltration techniques. By modifying the volume and composition of the replacement solution, it is in fact possible to remove water and sodium selectively, thus obtaining the desired independent balances. This, together with the isotonic composition of the ultrafiltrate, may lead to continuous vascular refilling and an improved hemodynamic condition with full control of the patient's hydration.

Continuous therapies can also effectively correct various forms of acidosis. In fact, whereas intermittent hemodialysis produces dramatic alkalinization during treatment but with rebound of acidosis frequently observed (the same effect is seen for urea removal), continuous therapies are slowly but continuously acting and result in a steady-state concentration of both uremic solutes and organic acids in blood (Fig. 39–7). Bicarbonate and organic anions (considered alkaline equivalents) are lost in the ultrafiltrate. If no replacement is provided and the patient will just lose weight,

blood pH does not change because of the parallel volume contraction. If, on the other hand, replacement fluid is administered, the concentration of buffers (lactate or bicarbonate) in the substitution fluid must be carefully prescribed to obtain the desired acid-base correction. Once a given level of bicarbonate is reached, any increment in bicarbonate level in blood results in a parallel increase of bicarbonate losses in the ultrafiltrate. Thus, in continuous therapies, a steady state is reached, and the desired bicarbonate level depends on the daily acid production, the amount of fluid exchanged in hemofiltration, and the concentration of buffer in the substitution fluid. Oral supplementation may also be considered an important factor.

In patients with cerebral edema, intermittent treatments may worsen the clinical condition, because of a postdialytic influx of fluid in both the gray matter and the white matter. The authors analyzed the behavior of the brain density in patients undergoing different forms of renal replacement therapy. In patients with chronic renal failure, brain density decreases after intermittent hemodialysis with an influx of water in the tissue. This effect leads to a normalization of the brain tissue that shows a severe dehydration in the predialytic phase.[33, 34] Other studies have confirmed that patients with ARF frequently show baseline values for brain density to be nearly normal or slightly decreased. Intermittent hemodialysis further decreases brain density values, leading to a condition of transient postdialytic edema. The alterations induced by intermittent treatments are not observed with continuous therapies, and the latter can therefore be utilized to maximal advantage in these patients (Fig. 39–8).[35]

Several mechanisms have been proposed to explain the improvement in acute respiratory distress syndrome (ARDS) patients treated with continuous hemofiltration. The continuous fluid withdrawal from the interstitium resulting from progressive vascular refilling represents a major advantage. However, the modulation of the vascular inflammation, thanks to the clearance or adsorption of specific proinflammatory substance onto the membrane, has been recently hy-

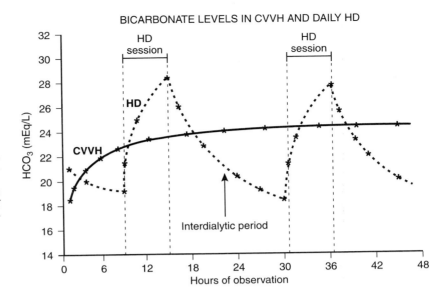

FIGURE 39-7 ▪ Bicarbonate kinetics in continuous venovenous hemofiltration (CVVH) and daily hemodialysis (HD). Intermittent treatments provide a sudden correction of acidosis with a transient period of alkalemia. After dialysis has ceased, the patient experiences a rapid rebound of bicarbonate, returning to a condition of definite acidosis. This has been shown to affect protein metabolism, albumin levels, and enzyme function. A stable correction of acidosis is reached in continuous hemofiltration because of a constant infusion of buffer via the replacement solution.

pothesized. This mechanism has also been invoked as an interesting possibility for patients with SIRS (systemic immunoresponse syndrome) or septic shock. A typical case is shown in Figure 39-9. The patient was suffering from a nontraumatic rhabdomyolysis and a sepsis-induced multiple organ dysfunction. The degree of overhydration was modest, and oliguria was present for a few days. Despite this, a severe impairment of oxygen exchanges could be detected, and the patient was placed on hemofiltration. After a few hours of zero balance hemofiltration, the clinical picture started to improve. The norepinephrine requirement was dramatically decreased and the pulmonary condition significantly improved, as depicted in Figure 39-9. It seems that hemofiltration is doing something more than just removing water or urea, which may have to

do with a possible modulation of the immune function or a potential limitation of the status of systemic acute inflammation.

THE CONCEPT OF RENAL SUPPORT

The current era of critical care practice has witnessed the evolution of challenging new trends. Today, serious manifestations may arise in transplanted patients owing to surgical or medical complications, immunosuppressive therapy, and renal failure.

Clinically important infection or acute sepsis may occur in these patients alone or as a major complication of ARF. Roughly 50% of such infections are caused by gram-negative bacteria, and, of these cases, 10% to

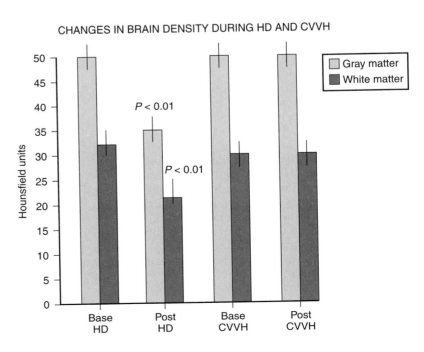

FIGURE 39-8 ▪ Changes in brain density observed in patients undergoing continuous and intermittent therapies. Although a stable condition of hydration is maintained by continuous hemofiltration, a remarkable influx of water in the brain tissue is observed after a short intermittent dialysis session.

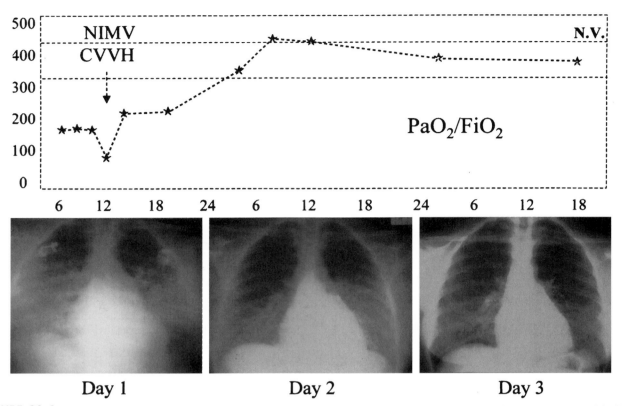

FIGURE 39–9 ■ The clinical pattern of a septic patient with multiple organ dysfunction. The patient begins treatment with CVVH (continuous venovenous hemofiltration) and NIMV (noninvasive mechanical ventilation), and the ratio PaO_2/FiO_2 improves dramatically. The improvement is also noted in subsequent chest radiographs.

20% may result in a documented period of bacteremia, hemodynamic instability, and organ dysfunction. High mortality is reported for such severe pathologic conditions.

The magnitude of this problem has made sepsis and its treatment a prominent public and scientific issue. Sepsis is a frequently associated gram-negative infection. Bacterial lipopolysaccharides (LPS), released from the gram-negative cell wall, possess a wide range of biologic activities and appear to be the main causative factors in sepsis-induced ARF. The mechanisms of LPS-induced tissue injury are complex. Hemodynamic changes—namely, the protracted hypotension—play a primary role but not an exclusive one in the causation of the fall in glomerular filtration rate (GFR) of the transplanted kidney.

Recently, several studies have provided evidence of inflammatory mediators being of relevance in determining the structural and functional changes capable of establishing ARF. Eicosanoids, cytokines (tumor necrosis factor [TNF], and interleukins [IL] such as IL-1, IL-6, IL-8), endothelin (ET), and platelet-activating factors (PAF) all may contribute to the fall of renal blood flow (RBF) and GFR during sepsis. The biologic properties of these mediators alone or in combination may account for the metabolic and hemodynamic changes in sepsis.

Evidence that excesses of TNF-α, or IL-1β, or both, may be involved in the development or sepsis-induced multiple organ dysfunction raises the possibility that removal of these cytokines from the circulation of clinically ill patients may be of benefit. In studies by Bellomo and coworkers,[36] CVVH was shown to remove significant amounts of proinflammatory mediators. We have found clearances of 30.7 L/d and 36.1 L/d for TNF-α, and for IL-1β a total excretion rate of 14.1 ng/d and 1.06 ng/d. Excretion was mainly by ultrafiltrate, although in other studies we have also demonstrated significant absorption capacity of cytokines and autocoids by hydrophobic membranes.[37]

However, several aspects need to be clarified before the extracorporeal removal of cytokines can be unanimously accepted as clinically relevant. Possible advancements in extracorporeal therapies utilized for critically ill patients should take into account the need for (1) the higher convective rates, (2) the type of reinfusate, and (3) the removal of protein-bound cytokines.

Advances have been made showing the positive effects on hemodynamics of high-volume hemofiltration techniques[38] (Fig. 39–10) or even plasmafiltration techniques coupled with adsorption.[39] Cytokines are insufficiently removed with standard techniques; thus the newer techniques, based on a higher convective rate or on a more permeable membrane, seem to succeed in controlling the peaks of the septic inflammation. There are, however, other possible considerations that may limit the enthusiasm for cytokine-removing techniques. Monocytes taken from septic patients are, in fact, exhausted; these cells do not respond adequately

IMPACT OF VOLUME EXCHANGE ON HEMODYNAMICS DURING HEMOFILTRATION IN SEPTIC SHOCK

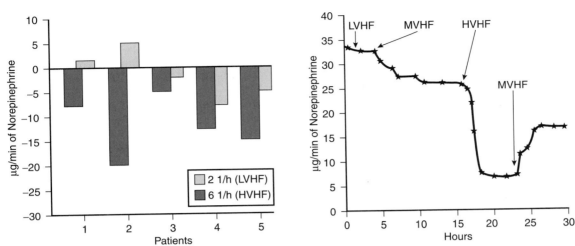

FIGURE 39–10 ■ *Right panel,* The hemodynamic response to variations in ultrafiltration rate during low-volume hemofiltration (LVHF = 1 L/h), middle-volume hemofiltration (MVHF = 3 L/h), and high-volume hemofiltration (HVHF = 6 L/h). At the same time, the norepinephrine requirement for the maintenance of blood pressure is shown in the *left panel.*

by secreting TNF-α if incubated with endotoxin in vitro. Interestingly, when the patient has been treated for hours with plasmafiltration coupled with adsorption, the monocytes recover the capacity to produce TNF-α in response to an in vitro stimulus with endotoxin. Furthermore, if normal monocytes are incubated with endotoxin and the plasma of the patient before the treatment, the production of TNF is inhibited; this is not the case if the plasma used for incubation is that taken after the treatment with the adsorption procedure.[39]

In conclusion, it seems that instead of looking for a "magic bullet" against the septic syndrome and one of the thousands of factors involved in the systemic inflammation, hemofiltration and derived techniques, because of their continuity and their mechanisms, may provide a "magic shield" against the excess of proinflammatory or anti-inflammatory mediators spilled over into the circulation. Because this is a poussées phenomenon, it may be useful to provide continuous coverage by hemofiltration, so that the peaks of immune system derangement are prevented. In this case, the action of the extracorporeal therapy becomes more of a modulation of the inflammatory cascade than a simple system to remove a particular cytokine.

All these considerations suggest the use of CRRT in the very early phase of ARF. There is still no scientific evidence that this approach is justified. However, the absence of evidence is not evidence of absence, and the clinician working every day in the ICU battlefield, the clinical opportunity to begin early with CRRT becomes more and more useful and beneficial. If the patient's organs can be protected at least in part by this system, a new era may begin for the septic syndrome, and clinicians can try to prevent patients from developing multiple organ failure.[40]

CONCLUSIONS

While isolated ARF can be advantageously treated with standard intermittent treatments, CRRTs appear to be the appropriate treatment in patients with ARF complicated by different clinical problems. In patients with ARF and other organ system failure, they appear to be the only possibility of obtaining positive results from extracorporeal therapy. Finally, if adequate modulation of chemical mediators of the septic syndrome could be achieved with these treatments, the whole concept of "renal protection" or "renal support" would be exploited, and a real possibility of preventing or shortening ARF would probably be in the hands of clinicians. There is no question, however, that continuous therapies seem to meet the criteria for adequacy that we have proposed in the introduction. Such treatments should be provided to all patients in which standard therapies represent less benefit or even a potential hazard.

REFERENCES

1. Knochel J: Biochemical, Electrolyte, and Acid-Base Disturbances in Acute Renal Failure. In: Brenner BM, Lazarus JM, eds: *Acute Renal Failure.* Philadelphia: WB Saunders; 1983:568–585.
2. Lien J, Chan V: Risk factors influencing survival in acute renal failure treated by hemodialysis. Arch Intern Med 1985; 145:2067.
3. Henderson LW, Besarab A, Michaels A, Bluemle LW Jr: Blood purification by ultrafiltration and fluid replacement (diafiltration). Trans ASAIO 1967; 17:216–221.
4. Silverstein ME, Ford CA, Lysaght MT, Henderson LW: Treatment of severe fluid overload by ultrafiltration. N Engl J Med 1974; 291:747.
5. Kramer P, Wigger W, Rieger J: Arteriovenous hemofiltration: a new and simple method for treatment of overhydrated patients resistant to diuretics. Klin Wochenschr 1977; 55:1121.
6. Lauer A, Saccggi A, Ronco C, et al: Continuous arteriovenous

hemofiltration in the critically ill patient. Ann Intern Med 1983; 99:455.

7. Lien J, Chan V: Risk factors influencing survival in acute renal failure treated by hemodialysis. Arch Intern Med 1985; 145:2067–2069.

8. Groeneveld ABJ, Tran DD, van der Meulen J, et al: Acute renal failure in the medical intensive care unit: predisposing complicating factors and outcome. Nephron 1991; 59:602–610.

9. Wheeler DC, Feehally J, Walls J: High-risk acute renal failure. QJM 1986; 61:977–984.

10. Lange HW, Aeppli DM, Brown DC: Survival of patients with acute renal failure requiring dialysis after open heart surgery: early prognostic indicators. Am Heart J 1987; 113: 1138–1143.

11. Spiegel DM, Ullian ME, Zerbe GO, Berl T: Determinants of survival and recovery in acute renal failure patients dialyzed in intensive care unit. Am J Nephrol 1991; 11:44–47.

12. Chew SL, Lins RL, Daelemans R, De Boer ME: Outcome in acute renal failure. Nephrol Dial Transplant 1993; 8:101–107.

13. Ronco C, Brendolan A, Bragantini L, et al: Continuous arteriovenous hemofiltration. Contrib Nephrol 1985; 48:70–78.

14. Geronemus R, Schneider N: Continuous arteriovenous hemodialysis: a new modality for treatment of acute renal failure. Trans Am Soc Artif Intern Organs 1984; 30:610–613.

15. Bellomo R, Parkin G, Love J, Boyce N: Management of acute renal failure in the critically ill with continuous hemovenous hemodiafiltration. Ren Fail 1992; 14:183–186.

16. Wendon J, Smithies M, Sheppard A, et al: Continuous high-volume venovenous hemofiltration in acute renal failure. Intensive Care Med 1989; 15:358–363.

17. McDonald BR, Mehta RL: Decreased mortality in patients with acute renal failure undergoing continuous arteriovenous hemodialysis. Contrib Nephrol 1991; 93:51–56.

18. Hakim RM: Clinical implications of hemodialysis membrane biocompatibility. Kidney Int 1993; 44:484–494.

19. Schiffe H, Lang SM, Koenig A, et al: Biocompatible membranes in acute renal failure: prospective case-controlled study. Lancet 1994; 344:570–572.

20. Knaus WA, Draper EA, Wagner DP, Zimmerman JE: APACHE II: a severity of disease classification system. Crit Care Med 1985; 13:818–829.

21. Knaus WA, Wagner DA, Draper EA, et al: The APACHE II prognostic system: risk predictions of hospital mortality for critically ill hospitalized adults. Chest 1991; 100:1619–1636.

22. Le Gall J-R, Lameshow S, Saulnier F: A new simplified acute physiology score (SAPS II) based on a European/North American multicenter Study. JAMA 1993; 270: 2957–2963.

23. Lameshaw S, Teres D, Klar J, et al: Mortality probability models (MPM II) based on an international cohort of intensive care unit patients. JAMA 1993; 270:2478–2486.

24. The ACCP/SCCM Consensus Conference Committee: Definitions for sepsis and organ failure and guidelines for the use of innovative therapies in sepsis. Chest 1992; 101:1644–1655.

25. European Society of Intensive Care Medicine Expert Panel: The use of the pulmonary artery catheter. Intensive Care Med 1991; 17:I–VIII.

26. Bidani A, Tzounakis AE, Cardenas VJ, Zwischenberger JB: Permissive hypercapnia in acute respiratory failure. JAMA 1994; 272:957–962.

27. Slutsky AS: Consensus conference on mechanical ventilation. Part I. Intensive Care Med 1994; 20:64–79.

28. Slutsky AS: Consensus conference on mechanical ventilation. Part II. Intensive Care Med 1994; 20:150–162.

29. Ronco C: Continuous renal replacement therapies for the treatment of acute renal failure in intensive care patients. Clin Nephrol 1993; 40:187–198.

30. Ronco C: Continuous renal replacement therapies in the treatment of acute renal failure in intensive care patients. Part 1. Theoretical aspects and techniques. Nephrol Dial Transplant 1994; 9(suppl 4):191–200.

31. Ronco C: Continuous renal replacement therapies in the treatment of acute renal failure in intensive care patients. Part 2. Clinical indications and prescription. Nephrol Dial Transplant 1994; 9(suppl 4):201–209.

32. Grootendorst AF, van Bommel EFH, van der Hoven B, et al:. High volume hemofiltration improves right ventricular function in endotoxin-induced shock in the pig. Intensive Care Med 1992; 18:235–240.

33. La Greca G, Dettori P, Biasioli S, et al: Brain density studies during dialysis. Lancet 1980; 2:582.

34. La Greca G, Biasioli S, Chiaramonte S, et al: Studies on brain density in hemodialysis and peritoneal dialysis. Nephron 1982; 31:146–150.

35. Ronco C, Bellomo R, Brendolan A, et al: Study on brain density changes during continuous renal replacement in critically ill patients with acute renal failure: continuous hemofiltration versus intermittent hemodialysis. J Nephrol 1999; 12:173–178.

36. Bellomo R, Tipping P, Boyce N: Continuous venovenous hemofiltration with dialysis removes cytokines from the circulation of septic patients. Crit Care Med 1993; 21:522–526.

37. Ronco C, Tetta C, Lupi A, et al: Removal of platelet-activating factor in experimental continuous arteriovenous hemofiltration. Crit Care Med 1995; 1:99–107.

38. Bellomo R, Baldwin I, Cole L, Ronco C: Preliminary experience with high-volume hemofiltration. Kidney Int 1998; 53(suppl 66):182–185.

39. Tetta C, Cavaillon JM, Camussi G, et al: Continuous plasma filtration coupled with adsorption. Kidney Int 1998; 53(suppl 66):186–189.

40. Ronco C, Ghezzi PM, Bellomo R, Brendolan A: New perspectives in the treatment of acute renal failure. Blood Purif 1999; 17:166–172.

CHAPTER 40

Predictive Factors and Scoring

Fernando Liaño ▪ Julio Pascual

INTRODUCTION

Acute renal failure (ARF) is a syndrome with multiple etiologies and is associated with a high mortality rate, about 50% in general series[1–15] and about 70% to 80% in patients treated in intensive care units (ICU).[16–29] The incidence of ARF is high, nearly 200 cases per million adult population in developed countries.[15] In addition to the human toll, the financial resources necessary for the treatment of patients with ARF are considerable.[30–32] Because of concern for both the individual patient and society in general, a thorough analysis of the factors associated with the ability to predict outcome is necessary. However, caution must be used when one considers the available data from the literature, mainly because of differences in the following:

- Definitions of ARF (eg, different serum creatinine concentrations [S_{Cr}]) have been used; some studies include only dialysis-treated patients; many authors use ARF synonymously with acute tubular necrosis (ATN)
- Type of ARF considered (eg, homogeneous or case-mixed patient population)
- Setting in which the ARF develops (eg, community vs. hospital cases)
- Place in which ARF is treated (eg, ICU vs. other hospital areas)
- Treatment modalities used
- Other considerations[33]

For these reasons, all the factors presented in Table 40–1 must be considered when one reviews the outcome of patients with ARF.

The prognosis in patients with ARF is not uniform. It varies according to the pathophysiologic origin of each type of ARF and the underlying processes (Table 40–2). At the present time, ARF due to ATN is the most frequent and severe form of ARF in developed countries, both in general series[15] and in the ICU setting.[28] For this reason, the following section focuses on predictive aspects related to this entity, excluding ATN following kidney transplantation.[64, 65]

BACKGROUND

Concepts

Prognosis is an estimation of the future based on present data. In general, as in the setting of ARF, the present data are the factors or variables influencing outcome. Whereas outcome is the real evolution of the

patient, prognosis is the expected outcome.[66] Although other factors influence prognosis, probably one of the most important is the severity of the ARF. In this sense, all these concepts—prognosis, outcome, and severity—depend on each other (Fig. 40–1, *top*), and this explains why the terms *prognostic indexes, severity indexes,* and *scoring systems* are usually used synonymously. The concept of prognosis in ARF has usually been linked with the vital outcome of the patient. Although some studies deal with the risk of developing ARF[67–73] and the functional outcome of these patients,[28, 39, 74–76] in the near future these two topics along with the quality of life[77] of the surviving patients will be more frequently taken into consideration (see Fig. 40–1, *bottom*).

Historical Perspective

Three historical periods and thus three prognostic approaches may be distinguished in the effort of the medical community to determine the prognosis of patients with ARF. The first approach is the *classic, or heuristic,* which derives from the hypocratic era. While the approach is extremely easy to follow and is potentially useful for individual prognosis, it has two main disadvantages: first, it is limited by the physician's own

TABLE 40–1. Factors to Consider in the Analysis of Outcome in ARF Patients

FACTORS	COMMENTS
ARF definition	Great variability among authors
Demographic aspects	Mainly age
Etiology of ARF	Syndrome classification
Patient's original disease	Related to the specific outcome of the patient's underlying disease
Complications developed in the course of the ARF	For example, adult respiratory distress syndrome and sepsis
Associated clinical conditions	For example, oliguria, hypotension, and coma
Place of ARF development	Community- or hospital-acquired ARF
Setting of ARF treatment	Intensive care unit or other hospital areas
Severity of ARF	Measured with prognostic estimators
World geographic area	Related to economic power and medical development of each country. Also there could be specific types of ARF
Treatments	Could modify the expected outcome

TABLE 40–2. Mortality Rates in Several ARF Situations

	MORTALITY, %	REFERENCES
According to the ARF Type		
Prerenal	20–52	28, 29, 34–36
ATN		
General series	45–50	1–15
ICU series	54–80	16–29
AIN	0–37	10, 12, 15, 34
AGN (primary and secondary)	19–27	15, 37, 38
Vasculitis	6–50	12, 15, 34, 39
Total acute renal artery occlusion	53	33
Obstructive ARF	3–27	14, 15, 28, 34, 35
With malignant neoplasia	49	15
Without malignant neoplasia	0	15
Related to the Underlying Disease		
Myeloma	72	40
Hematologic malignancies	72–86	41, 42
After bone marrow transplantation	46	43
AIDS	60	44
Aortic aneurysm surgery	48	45
Atheroembolic disease	25–60	46–48
HUS (adults)	25–30 (at 3 months)	49–51
Cortical necrosis (India)	87	52
Pregnancy	2–28	53–55
Burns (dialysis-requiring)	82	56
Nontraumatic rhabdomyolysis	21	57
Pancreatitis	70–81	58–59
Community-acquired bacteremia	53	60
Rocky Mountain spotted fever	52	61
Idiopathic nephrotic syndrome		62
Adult	19	
Child	0	
Ethylene glycol intoxication	17	63

and also that many scores have some degree of complexity when applied in daily clinical practice. A fourth period will spring up in the near future. Ideally, at that time we will be able, by the use of simple score systems, to estimate an exact individual prognosis, as well as to predict both the quality of life of our patients and their functional outcomes. Although separated by didactic reasons, the first three approaches to prognosis just discussed are and will continue to be simultaneously applied in practice.

Mortality in Acute Renal Failure

After an initial reduction of the mortality rate in ARF from 90% to 50% caused by the introduction of dialysis years ago, the mortality rate has remained disappointingly high.[78] Moreover, it seems that the mortality rate has increased during a 40-year period starting in 1951. This conclusion was reached by Kierdorf and Sieberth[79] on the basis of an analysis of the outcome in a total of 32,996 patients with ARF reported in 258 published papers. The increase in mortality has occurred despite the theoretic availability—at least in developed countries—of a better therapeutic armamentarium (mainly antibiotics, vasoactive drugs, and nutritional support), a deeper knowledge of dialysis techniques, and wider access to intensive care and nephrologic facilities.[33, 66] This improvement in supportive measures allows the physician to keep alive, for longer periods of time, patients who otherwise would

experience, and second, it is not measurable and consequently unsuitable for use in a group of patients. The *traditional period* started with the 20th century and witnessed the beginning of the measurement of medical experience by the use of simple mathematical tools applied to isolated variables. Although this approach to prognosis is easy to do and suitable for risk stratification, it has one major disadvantage: only one variable can be correlated with outcome, when in fact many factors, both favorable and unfavorable, interact with each other and play a significant role in determining outcome. The *present period* began coincidentally with the expansion of computer facilities, which allowed the use of sophisticated statistical packages and consequently the application of multivariate regression analysis. With these powerful tools, we are able to study the influence not only of a single variable on outcome but also of several variables and, even, the interrelationship among the measured variables. This approach is the best for ARF and ICU patients who have many variables influencing prognosis. It is also suitable both for risk stratification and, with certain precautions that are discussed later, for individual prognosis; however, it is not useful for trigger decisions. The major inconveniences of these approaches to prognosis are that the development of prognostic scores is cumbersome

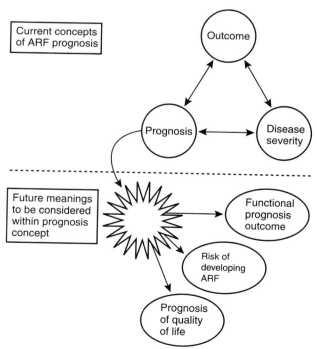

FIGURE 40–1 ■ The *top* of the figure shows the usual concept of prognosis and its relationship with outcome and severity of the ARF. On the *bottom* of the figure are other concepts of prognosis that should be considered in the future.

have died. A complementary explanation of the increase in mortality rate may be that the patients now treated are usually older,[33] sicker,[80, 81] and more likely to be treated quite aggressively. Nevertheless, despite this disappointing impression, Druml and coworkers reached a more positive conclusion.[24] They reported that in elderly people with ARF, there was a significant decrease in mortality from 70% in the period from 1973 through 1982 to 54% in the period from 1983 to 1990, and that this took place despite a greater need for mechanical ventilation and a higher incidence of sepsis in the second period. Notably, the APACHE II score was similar in both of the two time periods. Similar findings have been reported by McCarthy.[82] He observed that the hospital mortality rate among ARF patients treated in an ICU setting in two different periods (1977–1979 vs. 1991–1992) decreased from 68% to 48%. Whereas, in the past, functional recovery of the ARF caused by ATN seemed to be the rule if the patient survived,[39] at present, the number of patients needing chronic dialysis support after an ARF episode has increased, at least among those treated in an ICU setting.[25, 82]

FACTORS INFLUENCING OUTCOME IN ARF PATIENTS

General Factors

The main general factors influencing outcome in ARF are illustrated in Figure 40–2. The previous health condition in humans is dependent on two aspects: age and comorbid processes. Age has two essential implications in ARF. The first is that older age predisposes to the development of ARF in adult populations.[14, 15, 83–85] The second is that advanced age has a detrimental effect on outcome in ARF patients. This fact was observed either in studies using univariate[7, 12, 13, 17, 86–91] or multivariate analysis.[11, 13, 20, 26, 70, 87–92] In fact, in the studies that used a multivariate approach, age was the third most frequent factor influencing prognosis. It was preceded only by mechanical ventilation and hypotension.[66] There are, however, some studies that did not find age to be an adverse variable on outcome.[8–10, 27, 72, 93–99] The authors analyzed both mortality and severity using the Individual Severity Index (ISI) in three groups of patients with ARF. Group 1 included 103 patients, 80 years of age and older; group 2 included 256 patients, aged 65 to 79 years old; and group 3 included people younger than age 65. We observed that neither mortality nor severity was statistically different among the groups.[98] It is of note, however, that two important variables included in the ISI (ie, the number of patients with jaundice and the number of patients needing mechanical ventilation) were significantly lower in the oldest group. These observations suggest that age is a very important factor contributing to both the severity and the outcome of ARF in very old patients. Among the other demographic aspects, male sex has been only rarely associated with a worse

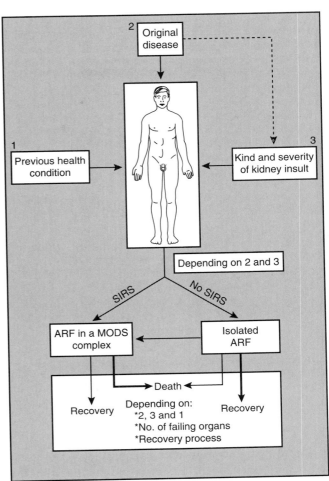

FIGURE 40–2 ▪ Outcome of acute renal failure. Two groups of factors play a role in ARF outcome. The first includes factors that affect the patient: (1) previous health condition (age and comorbid processes); (2) initial disease, usually the direct or indirect (eg, treatments) cause of kidney failure; and (3) the kind and severity of kidney injury. While No. 1 is a conditioning effect element, Nos. 2 and 3 trigger the second group of factors: the response of the patient to the insult. If this response includes a systemic inflammatory response syndrome (SIRS) similar to that usually seen in the intensive care patients (eg, sepsis, pancreatitis, burns), a multiple organ dysfunction syndrome (MODS) frequently appears, and consequently the outcome is associated with a higher fatality rate (*thick line, left*). On the contrary, if SIRS does not develop and isolated ARF predominates, death (*thin line, right*) is less frequent than survival (*thick line, right*). (From Liaño F, Pascual J: Acute Renal Failure: Causes and Prognosis. In: Berl T, Bonventre JV, Schrier RW, eds: Atlas of Diseases of the Kidney. Vol. 1. Philadelphia: Current Medicine; 1999; with permission.)

outcome than that in females.[87, 99] There is no research reporting outcome differences based on race.

The prognostic systems used in intensive care medicine have for a long time included the comorbid processes as factors influencing prognosis in ICU patients,[100–105] whereas it is only recently that these factors have been considered among the nephrologic scores.[28] However, the available data suggest that a reasonably good prognostic estimation in ARF patients could be made using both systems, including the comorbid factors (APACHE III) or not (ISI).[106]

The original disease of the patient seems to be one of the major factors contributing to outcome in ARF. It is obvious that a patient with diarrhea who develops ARF has a better prognosis than the patient with leukemia who develops ARF. The fact that the primary disease of the patient is the main cause of death is also reported in the literature.[10, 13, 15, 107, 108]

The type and severity of the kidney insult play a crucial role in outcome. As an example, ATN caused by an ischemic insult usually carries a worse prognosis (mortality 50%–70%) than that observed in ATN secondary to nephrotoxins (survival rates approaching 80%).[7, 12, 13, 15, 109]

In the last several decades, there has been a shift in the clinical spectrum of ARF with a move from an isolated kidney dysfunction to ARF appearing in the setting of a multiple organ dysfunction syndrome (MODS).[29, 110] Among other reasons, it seems that the development of medicine itself has contributed to this fact. Nowadays kidney insults, mainly those related to aggressive surgery, are of greater intensity than those in the past. Additionally, intensive care medicine allows patients to be kept alive for longer periods than the time expected previously. Both events, by promoting a systemic inflammatory response syndrome, may predispose to the development of MODS, in which the kidney is one of the organs that fails. If the patient's response is of lower intensity, isolated ARF with a lower mortality rate occurs (see Fig. 40–2).[29, 66]

Clinical and Biochemical Factors

The presence of the following clinical situations has been related to a worse outcome in ARF patients: (1) mechanical ventilation,[2, 8, 11–13, 15, 17, 21, 25–27, 70, 89–93, 95, 96, 99, 111–115] (2) low perfusion status (identified as persistent arterial hypotension, need of inotropic drugs, or cardiovascular failure),[2, 4, 11, 13, 19, 69, 70, 87, 90–93, 95, 96, 113–117] (3) sepsis,[7, 12, 13, 19, 25, 26, 28, 88, 91–93, 95, 111, 13–118] (4) jaundice or hepatic failure,[11, 13, 25, 27, 91, 92, 99, 116] (5) coma or disturbance of consciousness,[2, 8, 13, 15, 87, 93, 95, 99] (6) oliguria,[4, 6–8, 10, 13–17, 19, 26, 28, 69, 92, 94, 99] (7) need of dialysis,[13, 15, 26, 28, 88, 119] (8) hemorrhage,[4, 25, 118] and (9) disseminated intravascular coagulation.[11, 25] The presence of one of the first five items mentioned in ARF patients is associated with a mortality of about 70% to 80% in most of the published series. Mortality for oliguria is close to 60%. A surgical origin[7, 8, 10–13, 19, 86, 95] of the ARF implies a worse outcome than that observed in medical cases. ARF secondary to a toxic insult has an even better outcome (see previous discussion).

Among the analytical factors studied, a negative effect on outcome of ARF patients has been reported for high levels of serum creatinine (S_{Cr})[17, 27, 87, 92, 93] or BUN,[11, 27, 93, 97] metabolic acidosis,[92, 99] low leukocyte and platelet counts,[27] hypoalbuminemia,[91, 99] and low prothrombin time.[91] Hypokalemia,[10, 24] metabolic alkalosis,[10] or hypophosphatemia[24] have a negative effect in elderly patients. Some authors are in disagreement in the case of S_{Cr}[15, 25, 69, 97, 99] and BUN levels,[69] and of leukocyte and platelet counts.[92] Although hyperka-

lemia is still an emergency in some ARF patients, it is not a factor influencing the outcome of a group of patients. Other analytical parameters have been reviewed by Chew and coworkers.[120] In summary, the influence of clinical variables on outcome is more important than that of analytical ones.[33]

Other Aspects Conditioning Outcome

In the past, it was well established that the number of complications appearing in the course of ARF contribute to a worsening of the outcome.[7, 10, 88, 89, 93, 107] Sepsis and respiratory, cardiovascular, and hepatic failure were the more usual complications among the most frequently reported ones in older research. At present, there has been a conceptual change. Investigators now usually deal with the number of organs in failure, rather than with ARF complications. A wide agreement has been established in this respect; that is, the higher the number of organs in failure, the higher the mortality.[23, 26, 28, 29, 70, 90, 96, 111, 113, 121, 122]

Another important point to be considered is that the development of ARF worsens the prognosis of other diseases or processes.[68] Chertow and coworkers[112] have provided evidence of this point. They prospectively analyzed 43,642 patients who underwent coronary bypass or valvular heart surgery between 1987 and 1994. Acute renal failure that needed dialysis developed in 460 patients. Outcome was clearly different: mortality among those patients who developed ARF was 63.7%, in contrast to the 4.3% observed in patients without this complication.

Acute renal failure developing in the hospital has a worse outcome than that starting in the community setting.[15] Iatrogenic cases associated with diagnostic or therapeutic maneuvers produce severe forms of ATN. On the other hand, a great number of the ARF cases developing in the community are secondary to obstructive processes that have a better outcome.[14, 15] Similarly, among the ARF patients treated in an ICU setting, those who already had ARF when admitted to the ICU had a better prognosis than patients who developed ARF after their ICU admission.[28] A worse outcome has also been observed when either a nephrologic consultation has not been made or there has been a delay in carrying out the consultation.[14, 123] Although the type of treatment could potentially play a role in the outcome of ARF patients, unfortunately the data in support of this is sparse. Among the new therapeutic measures available at present, such as the administration of dopamine,[124] atrial natriuretic peptide,[125] or growth factors,[126] only the use of biocompatible membranes seems to be associated with a better outcome,[127] and even this position is not fully accepted.[128] Finally, it should be remembered that ARF itself plays a role in the outcome of patients having this condition.[15, 129, 130] In a cohort analysis, Levy and coworkers[129] demonstrated that after adjusting for differences in comorbidity, ARF was associated with an odds ratio of dying of 5.5. Also in the Madrid Study, a mortality rate of about 20% was observed both in the

ICU and the non-ICU settings in patients in whom the kidney was the only organ in failure.[29] Similar results have been reported by Vincent and coworkers.[130]

MEASURING THE SEVERITY OF ACUTE RENAL FAILURE

Prediction of outcome is unquestionably important in ARF patients. It also helps the physician in his or her decisions about the medical management of this critical situation. Additionally, an exact tool for measuring ARF severity allows the following: (1) estimation of the severity of disease in a particular group of patients and consequently comparison of the management of ARF in different settings and at other hospitals; (2) adequate classification of patients according to the severity of illness (an essential maneuver in assessing the effectiveness of a specific treatment); (3) a method for the individual physician to measure whether there is any agreement between the real outcome and the estimated evolution of the disease process; and (4) a means of checking whether the resources devoted to the treatment of these patients are being used correctly.[131]

At the present time, estimations of the severity of ARF can be accomplished using either the general ICU scores or the specific ARF scores. Ideally, both approaches should have several characteristics. They should be (1) *efficient,* with a high sensitivity and specificity; (2) *carried out early,* so that a prognosis can be made as soon as possible in the clinical course, preferably at the time of the patient's referral; (3) *simple* and easy to do; (4) *inexpensive* (cost-free); (5) *reproducible,* so that the score can be reproduced in settings outside of the place where it was designed; (6) *universal,* that is, the index should work well both in severely ill patients and in those who are less severely ill; (7) *dynamic,* in that the method should work well at different moments along the course of the patient's disease; and (8) able to identify the patients who have any possibility of survival.[131] In the paragraphs that follow, these concepts are considered for each of the prognostic systems analyzed. However, it should be taken into account from this moment that at our present level of knowledge, no treatment can be denied to or discontinued in any ARF patient based solely on prognostic estimations. Nevertheless, these estimations can be of help in counseling patients and their families.[132]

THE ICU PROGNOSTIC SCORES

The APACHE (acute physiology and chronic health evaluation) system is the scoring system that has undergone the most changes since its appearance in 1981.[133] Initially, it had 34 acute physiologic variables derived from the major physiologic systems that a panel of experts considered possible to influence patient outcome. Each variable has a score according to the patient's clinical situation. The sum of all the variables provides the final acute physiologic score (APS)

thought to represent the severity of the illness. Severe disease significantly reduces the probability of survival during acute illness; thus, a chronic health category was incorporated into to the score. An age score was also added. Unfortunately, its use in the clinical practice was cumbersome because of the number of variables under consideration. To solve this problem, APACHE II was developed in a population of 5030 ICU patients treated in the United States and published in 1985.[100] No patients undergoing cardiac surgery were included in this population. The APS was reduced to 12 simple variables considered within the first 24 hours of admission to the ICU, and the chronic health score was transformed into a quantitative score. The authors also described a quantitative equation that considered the APACHE II score value, the performance or not of postemergency surgery, and a diagnostic category weight that allows physicians to predict individual risk of death, but unfortunately only in selected groups of patients. Unlike its score, the APACHE II equation has not been well accepted.

APACHE III, the latest version of this prognostic system,[101] was developed with the use of data from 17,440 unselected adult patients from 40 medical and surgical ICUs in the United States. The APACHE III consists of two options. The first is an APACHE III score, which can provide initial risk stratification for severely ill hospitalized patients within independently defined patient groups. The second is an APACHE III predictive equation. APACHE III is calculated with the use of a new APS with 17 variables, a new age score, and a new chronic health evaluation score, in which seven comorbid processes are considered. The use of the APACHE III score is inexpensive, but this is not so for its equation.

The Simplified Acute Physiological Score (SAPS)[102] was developed in France to obtain a prognostic system that would be easier to use than the initial APACHE. This system included only 13 physiologic variables obtained during the first 24 hours after the ICU admission. A second version of this score, SAPS II, was developed later in 13,152 patients treated in European and American ICUs.[103] Seventeen variables selected by a logistic regression model are considered in this version: 12 physiologic variables, age, type of admission (scheduled surgical, unscheduled surgical, or medical), and three underlying disease variables (acquired immunodeficiency syndrome, metastatic cancer, and hematologic malignancy). Some of the advantages of this score are that it is not time-consuming and that it requires neither special venous nor arterial samples.

The Mortality Prediction Model (MPM) was designed with the same purpose as the SAPS[104] through a multiple logistic regression analysis that identified seven prognostic variables collected on ICU admission and at 24 and 48 hours thereafter.

A new version of this model, MPM II,[105] is composed of two models, the MPM II admission model (MPM II$_0$) and the MPM II 24-hour model (MPM II$_{24}$), both of which estimate the probability of death at hospital discharge. The MPM II$_0$ allows us to do this at the time of the patient's admission to the ICU, by using 15 categorical variables, including age and ARF. The MPM II_0, unlike most other indexes or scoring systems, permits us to estimate the probability of death before ICU treatments can have an influence on outcome. The MPM II_{24} was designed as a calculation for the more severely ill patients who remain in the ICU for 24 hours or longer. It contains five variables from MPM II_0 and eight variables collected at 24 hours. Two of these variables are associated with renal function impairment; a serum creatinine concentration higher than 2 mg/dL and a urine output lower than 150 mL per 8 hours. The MPM II allows a better prediction than MPM. These observations demonstrate that predictive models need to be adapted to changes occurring in the ICU environment. Because MPM_0 measures the severity of a patient's condition before the ICU treatment can introduce any bias, the authors of this system consider it to be the best baseline measure to apply when comparing different ICUs or monitoring quality of care in a single ICU.

In general, the new versions of the previously mentioned scores are better calibrated and have a better goodness of fit than the old ones,[134] as was the case of APACHE III for ARF patients.[106] However, in some processes, such as gastrointestinal diseases and surgical patients, older versions could be preferable.[135] It seems also that contemporary versions of different prognostic models have a similar predictive power.[28, 135, 136] In any case, bias caused by translation, conversion of different units, definition ambiguities, or other problems should be avoided when using these systems.[137]

Another family of prognostic systems in the ICU setting is that of the Organ System Failure Scores. It is formed by four members, the first being the Organ System Failure Score (OSF-score) developed by Knaus and coworkers.[138] The clinician calculates it by considering the presence or absence of a failure in five organ systems: cardiovascular, respiratory, renal, hematologic, and neurologic. Thus, the score range is between 0 and 5. With its use, the authors were able to demonstrate how the mortality rate increased in relation to the number of OSFs. For example, a mortality rate of 22%, 52%, and 80% was found in patients having 1, 2, and 3 or more OSFs, respectively. They also demonstrated that for any OSF-score higher than 1 and lasting more than 1 day, the mortality rate increased. The major advantage of the OSF-score is its simplicity, while its major inconvenience is that it is a dichotomous system unable to grade the failure of an organic system. It is a good score for measuring the severity of disease in a group of patients. For this purpose, it has been used in ARF-related studies.[28]

The Multiple Organ Dysfunction Score (MOD-score[139] was developed from 612 patients treated in a Canadian ICU. Similarly to OSF, the MOD-score works as a severity index at ICU admission. Later during the ICU stay, it correlates well with outcome, measuring to some extent the evolution of the patient's situation (improvements and complications). Unlike the OSF-score,[138] which, as previously stated, is a dichotomous system, the MOD-score has the advantage of allowing a graded scale for each organ dysfunction considered

in the model. In this prognostic index, six organic systems are considered. They are (1) the respiratory system (PaO_2/FiO_2), (2) the renal system (serum creatinine concentration), (3) the hepatic system (serum bilirubin concentration), (4) the hematologic system (platelet count), (5) the central nervous system (Glasgow Coma Scale [GCS]), and (6) the cardiovascular system. The latter is evaluated through a new variable developed by the authors, the pressure-adjusted heart rate (pressure-adjusted heart rate = heart rate × central venous pressure/mean arterial pressure). Each one of these systems has a range of 0 to 4 points. Consequently, the MOD-score could vary from 0 to 24. After a logistic analysis, the authors of the MOD-score pointed out that incremental increases in scores over the course of the ICU stay have a higher outcome prediction than that of the other admission severity indexes usually used. This new score system, which in its developmental population included 61 patients with severe ARF, needs to be tested in other settings.

The Logistic Organ Dysfunction System (LODS) was developed by Le Gall and coworkers[140] with the same population as that used for developing SAPS II. The data of 10,547 patients were used for developing the system, whereas 2605 constituted the validation sample. Using 12 physiologic variables, LODS defines dysfunction in six organ systems: neurologic system (GCS), cardiovascular system (heart rate and systolic blood pressure), renal system (urea and creatinine levels and urine output), pulmonary system (ventilation/continuous positive airway pressure status and PaO_2/FiO_2 ratio), hematologic system (white blood cell and platelets counts), and hepatic system (bilirubin levels and prothrombin time). The variables, which are recorded as the worst value in the first 24-hour period in the ICU, takes a value of 0 points when organ dysfunction is absent, or 1, 3, or 5 for different organ derangements in the case of neurologic, cardiovascular, or renal systems, according to the degree of organ dysfunction. In the case of the pulmonary and hematologic systems, there are only two levels for measuring organic dysfunction, recorded as 1 or 3. Hepatic dysfunction has only a degree of dysfunction scored as 1 point. Consequently the resulting LOD-score ranges from 0 to 22 points. LOD-score is useful for patients' stratification. Also, applying a logistic regression equation using the LOD-score as the single variable, this prognostic system allows prediction of the probability of death of a patient. However, it should be borne in mind that this system, which is well calibrated, does not differentiate between patients with ARF and those having chronic renal failure. To our knowledge it has not been tested in ARF patients

The Sepsis-related Organ Failure Assessment (SOFA) score was developed by the European Society of Intensive Care Medicine in 1643 patients with sepsis,[141] but could be applied in other ICU patients.[130] In this score, six organic systems are evaluated through the following variables: respiration (PaO_2/FiO_2), coagulation (platelets count), liver (bilirubin levels), cardiovascular (hypotension or use of vasoactive drugs), central nervous system (GCS), and renal (creatinine concentration or urine volume). Each variable ranges from a 0 score (normal function) to 4 for the most abnormal dysfunction in each organ. So, the SOFA-score could range from 0 to 24. The SOFA-score was created with the intention of evaluating morbidity, not the risk of mortality. However, as would be expected, it has been observed that the higher the SOFA-score, the higher the mortality, both for each organ system as well as for the whole of the organs involved in the score.[130] This score has two main advantages: it is extremely simple to do, and it can provide a measurement of the patient's morbidity along their clinical course. It seems to work well in ARF patients.[142]

SPECIFIC PROGNOSTIC SCORES IN ACUTE RENAL FAILURE

In 1982, multiple regression analysis started to be used in the ARF field and this methodology has been used in at least 30 articles. Some of them are focused in the probability of developing ARF.[49, 50, 61, 67, 68, 71, 112] The others deal with outcome prognosis.[8, 9, 11, 13, 20, 25, 28, 41, 70, 85, 88–93, 95, 96, 99, 115, 121, 143, 144] Unfortunately, there is no uniformity among these studies: Only a few of them analyzed general series of ARF patients,[8, 9, 11, 13, 88, 89, 95] some are centered on ARF patients treated in an ICU setting,[25, 28, 70, 91, 92, 96, 99, 143] and others only study ARF patients treated by dialysis.[11, 25, 41, 85, 89, 90, 92–96, 121, 143] Additionally, only some of them are prospective,[8, 13, 28, 90–92, 96, 99] and others did not give a prognostic estimation early in the clinical course of the patients.[8, 9, 11, 20, 70, 85, 88, 89, 96, 115] Also, few authors have checked the result of their developmental score in a control population.[8, 13, 85, 143]

It is of note that, in spite of the high number of specific ARF prognostic scores and unlike the general ICU prognostic systems (see the section on ICU prognostic scores), only three of the specific ARF indexes, the individual severity index (ISI),[13, 145] the Stuivenger Hospital ARF score (SHARF score),[91] and the Cleveland Clinic Foundation (CCF) have had more than one version.[143, 99]

In general, every prognostic system is developed with the hope that it will be of use in places other than that in which it was developed. However, when looking at this aspect in the ARF scores, we found the following: (1) Some of the prognostic systems published before 1996 have never been analyzed, to our knowledge, in other places;[9, 11, 20, 25, 41, 70, 89, 115] and (2) Others systems[8, 85, 88, 95, 96] have not worked well when tested in other settings.[106, 146] (3) Only a few, notably ISI[13, 147] and CCF score[99, 143] have worked well in other places.[15, 91, 147] The Barton's score[92] ran well at the same place at a later time period.[148] (4) For those ARF prognostic systems published since 1996,[28, 90, 91, 99, 121, 144] there has not been time to study them yet.

Recently two articles have been published in which the expression "simple prognostic index" appeared in the title.[90, 121] Both of them, using multivariate analysis, studied 94 and 102 ARF patients, respectively, who needed dialysis in an ICU setting. In both cases, the authors did not obtain a prognostic equation. How-

ever, they arrived at similar conclusions: the outcome was related to the number of adverse variables: The higher the number, the worse the prognosis. It seems as if the circle is closing. However, these data have been known for a long time.[1, 7, 10, 23, 25, 26, 29, 88, 89, 92, 93, 96, 107, 111, 113] In our opinion, a factor that could contribute either to not getting good prognostic equations or simply to not getting an equation at all is the number of patients included in the sample. In fact a small number of patients, lower than 100,[20, 70, 85, 89, 90] and sometimes lower than 50,[41, 68, 93, 115] were used by many researchers to obtain ARF prognostic scores.

ICU SCORES OR SPECIFIC ARF SYSTEMS?

Among the general ICU scores, APACHE II is the one that is used world-wide in the ARF setting.[149] These scores have been used for the randomization of ARF patients at the same level of risk in different clinical trials,[80, 127, 150–152] as well as for comparing the severity of ARF at different periods of time.[80] No cost predictions in ARF patients have been done, and none of these systems have been applied for treatment decisions.

However, APACHE II has some drawbacks. In fact, we should keep in mind that it was developed with only 192 patients having renal or urologic diseases,[100] much fewer than those considered for developing some of the specific ARF scores.[13, 28, 88, 91, 92, 99, 143] Also, it is noteworthy that APACHE II has been used for stratifying groups of ARF patients before dialysis.[127, 150–152] The results of these studies should be considered with caution, because several authors indicate that APACHE II is not a good predictor of mortality when calculated at the time of starting with the dialysis treatment.[96, 153] Also, some prospective studies have demonstrated that APACHE II, measured at the ICU admission time, is not a good predictor for ARF patients.[28, 96, 154] In this respect, Brivet and coworkers[28] have shown that the most adequate moment to use a prognostic score is when ARF begins, as was done in the logistic estimation of prognosis developed by them,[28] in the ISI,[13] and in the SHARF score.[91] Recently, Douma and coworkers[106] demonstrated that APACHE III is a better prognostic estimator for ARF than APACHE II, SAPS, MPM systems, and the Rasmussen, Lohr, and Schaefer scores.

Although the information referring to the use of the new OSF-score family in ARF is scarce, preliminary data using SOFA seem hopeful.[142] Future research using those systems will be welcome.

On the other hand, even in the world of intensive care medicine, there is a call to use specific prognostic systems more than general ones.[155] Until now, the ISI has been the only one among the specific ARF indexes studied that has proved to work well outside the place at which it was developed, both for individual prognosis and risk stratification.[15, 91, 106, 142, 147] It works as well as APACHE III in ARF patients, and it is very much easier to manage[106] (Fig. 40–3). For these reasons, in

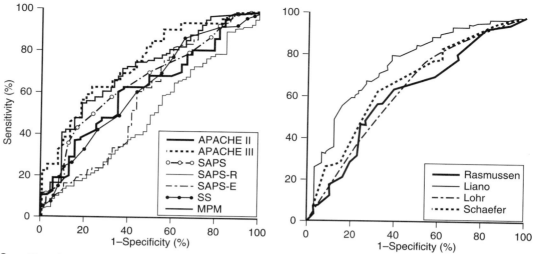

FIGURE 40–3 ■ The observed (—) and predicted (- - -) mortality in each quintile of risk for two general prognostic models (APACHE III, Mortality Prediction Model) and two ARF-specific models (Liaño, Schaefer). (From Douma CE, Redekop WK, Van Der Meulen JHP, et al: Predicting mortality in intensive care patients with acute renal failure treated with dialysis. J Am Soc Nephrol 1997; 8:111–117; with permission.)

the next section the authors present the general scope of this index.

Finally, Braitman and Davidoff[156] have published findings that can help clinicians in deciding which specific prognostic index is suitable for use in a particular patient.

THE INDIVIDUAL SEVERITY INDEX

The ISI prospective index compared, for the first time in the nephrologic literature, both multiple logistic and linear regression analysis.[145] Although both of the equations obtained worked well, the linear equation was finally chosen, mainly due to its simplicity. A new version of this prognostic system was later developed and validated in 328 ATN patients.[13] The ISI provides us with an easy linear equation that allows estimation of the probability of death of an individual patient, and works well both in severe and moderate ARF patients. The system also allows clinicians to stratify the risk of a group of patients by the calculation of the severity index (SI), which is nothing other than the arithmetical mean of the individual prognosis of each patient (ISI). The ROC (receiver operating characteristic) curve of this system is similar to that of APACHE III[106] (Fig. 40–4). Calculation of the equation is very simple:

$$ATN\text{-}ISI = 0.032 \ (age \ decades) - 0.086 \ (sex) - 0.109 \ (nephrotoxic) + 0.109 \ (oliguria) + 0.116 \ (hypotension) + 0.122 \ (jaundice) + 0.150 \ (coma) - 0.154 \ (consciousness) + 0.182 \ (assisted \ respiration) + 0.21.$$

Where sex means male; *hypotension* is defined as systolic blood pressure lower than 100 mm Hg for more than 10 h regardless of the use or not of vasoactive drugs; *jaundice* is understood as a concentration of bilirubin higher than 2 mg/dL; deep *coma*, if pres-

ent, is defined as a Glasgow Coma Scale <5; *consciousness* represents normal consciousness; and *assisted respiration* indicates need of mechanical support. The numbers preceding these keys denote the contribution of each one to the prognosis and are the factor for multiplying the clinical variables; 0.21 is the equation constant. Each variable takes a value of 1 (presence) or 0 (absence), with the exception of age, which takes the value of the patient's decade. As can be seen, it is not necessary to resort to complex techniques for calculation, because a simple card with the equation values and a piece of paper are all that are necessary.

Another important aspect of this system lies in the fact that it allows the establishment of a discriminative cut-off point of 0.9 above which no patient has survived, with the exception of a cirrhotic patient who later received a liver transplant. Until now, no patient has been taken off treatment, and treatment has not been denied to a patient based on the results of the equation. However, as said before, the results are useful for patients or family counseling.

SUMMARY

Researchers have come a long way in the study of the factors contributing to outcome in ARF patients. At present, the measure of the ARF severity could be done using both ICU and specific ARF scores. Among the first of these measures APACHE III seems to be the one of choice, but the OSF scores promise to be very useful. Among the second group, ISI has proved to be the best, although several scores recently published are waiting for additional study. In the future, new indexes—to measure outcome, the risk for developing ARF, the functional outcome, and quality of life of surviving patients—will be developed.

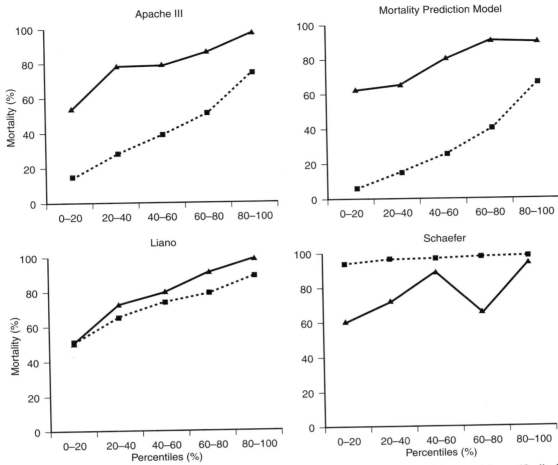

FIGURE 40–4 ▪ ROC curve analysis for seven general mortality prediction models (*left panels*) and four models specifically developed for patients with acute renal failure (*right panels*). (From Douma CE, Redekop WK, Van Der Meulen JHP, et al: Predicting mortality in intensive care patients with acute renal failure treated with dialysis. J Am Soc Nephrol 1997; 8:111–117; with permission.)

REFERENCES

1. Kiley JE, Powers SR, Beebe RT: Acute renal failure: eighty cases of acute tubular necrosis. N Engl J Med 1960; 262:481–485.
2. Lunding M, Steiness I, Thaysen JH: Acute renal failure due to tubular necrosis: immediate prognosis and complications. Acta Med Scand 1964; 176:103–119.
3. Hall JW, Johnson WJ, Maher FT, et al: Immediate and long-term prognosis in acute renal failure. Ann Intern Med 1970; 73:515–521.
4. Kleinknecht D, Jungers P, Chanard J, et al: Factors influencing immediate prognosis in acute renal failure with special reference to prophylactic hemodialysis. Adv Nephrol 1971; 1:207–230.
5. Kennedy AC, Burton JA, Luke RG, et al: Factors affecting the prognosis in acute renal failure: a survey of 251 cases. QJM 1973; 42:73–86.
6. Anderson RJ, Linas SL, Berns AS, et al: Nonoliguric acute renal failure. N Engl J Med 1977; 296:1134–1138.
7. McMurray SD, Luft FC, Maxwell DR, et al: Prevailing patterns and predictor variables in patients with acute tubular necrosis. Arch Intern Med 1978; 138:950–955.
8. Rasmussen HH, Pitt EA, Ibels LS, et al: Prediction of outcome in acute renal failure by discriminant analysis of clinical variables. Arch Intern Med 1985; 145:2015–2018.
9. Corwin HL, Teplick RS, Schreiber MJ, et al: Prediction of outcome in acute renal failure. Am J Nephrol 1987; 7:8–12.
10. Lameire N, Matthys E, Vanholder R, et al: Causes and prognosis of acute renal failure in elderly patients. Nephrol Dial Transplant 1987; 2:316–322.
11. Montoliu J, Campistol JM, Cases A, et al: Mortalidad y factores pronósticos de supervivencia en la insuficiencia renal aguda grave que requiera diálisis. Nefrología 1989; 9:152–158.
12. Turney JH, Marshall DH, Brownjhon AM, et al: The evolution of acute renal failure, 1956–1988. QJM 1990; 273:83–104.
13. Liaño F, Gallego A, Pascual J, et al: Prognosis of acute tubular necrosis: an extended prospectively contrasted study. Nephron 1993; 63:21–31.
14. Feest TG, Round A, Hamad S: Incidence of severe acute renal failure in adults: results of a community-based study. BMJ 1993; 306:481–483.
15. Liaño F, Pascual J, and the Madrid Acute Renal Failure Study Group: Epidemiology of acute renal failure: a prospective, multicenter, community-based study. Kidney Int 1996; 50:811–818.
16. Wilkins RG, Faragher EB: Acute renal failure in an intensive care unit: incidence, prediction and outcome. Anaesthesia 1983; 38:628–634.
17. Wheeler DC, Feehally J, Walls J: High-risk acute renal failure. QJM 1986; 61:977–984.
18. Barlett RH, Mault JR, Dechert RE, et al: Continuous arteriovenous hemofiltration: improved survival in surgical acute renal failure. Surgery 1986; 100:400–408.
19. Maher ER, Robinson KN, Scoble JE, et al: Prognosis of critically ill patients with acute renal failure: APACHE II score and other predictive factors. QJM 1989; 72:857–866.
20. Berisa F, Beaman M, Adu D, et al: Prognostic factors in acute renal failure following aortic aneurysm surgery. QJM 1990; 76:689–698.
21. Spiegel DM, Ulian ME, Zerbe GO, et al: Determinants of

survival and recovery in acute renal failure patients dialyzed in intensive-care units. Am J Nephrol 1991; 11:44–47.

22. Storck M, Hartl WH, Zimmerer E, et al: Comparison of pump-driven and spontaneous continuous hemofiltration in postoperative acute renal failure. Lancet 1991; 337:452–455.

23. Baldyca AP, Paganini EP, Chaff C, et al: Acute dialytic support of the octogenarian: is it worth it? ASAIO J 1993; 39:M795–M808.

24. Druml W, Lax F, Grimm G, et al: Acute renal failure in the elderly 1975–1990. Clin Nephrol 1994; 41:342–349.

25. Chertow GM, Christiansen CL, Cleary PD, et al: Prognostic stratification in critically ill patients with acute renal failure requiring dialysis. Arch Intern Med 1995; 155:1505–1511.

26. Neveu H, Kleinknecht D, Brivet F, et al: Prognostic factors in acute renal failure due to sepsis: results of a prospective multicentre study. Nephrol Dial Transplant 1996; 11:293–299.

27. Paganini EP, Halstenberg WK, Goormastic M: Risk modeling in acute renal failure requiring dialysis: the introduction of a new model. Clin Nephrol 1996; 46:206–211.

28. Brivet FG, Kleinknecht D, Loirat PH, et al: Acute renal failure in intensive care units: causes, outcome, and prognostic factors of hospital mortality: a prospective, multicenter study. Crit Care Med 1996; 24:192–198.

29. Liaño F, Junco E, Pascual J, et al: The spectrum of acute renal failure in the intensive care unit: a comparison with the acute renal failure seen in other settings. Kidney Int 1998; (suppl 66):516–524.

30. Gilbertson AA, Smith JM, Mostafa SM: The cost of an intensive care unit: a prospective study. Intensive Care Med 1991; 17:204–209.

31. Hamel MB, Phillips RS, Davis RB, et al: Outcomes and cost-effectiveness of initiating dialysis and continuous aggressive care in seriously ill hospitalized adults. Ann Intern Med 1997; 127:195–202.

32. Daly K, Bihari D: Assessment of Outcome From Acute Renal Failure. In: Ronco C, Bellomo R, eds: Critical Care Nephrology. Dordrecht: Kluwer Academic Publishers; 1998;153–161.

33. Liaño F, Pascual J: Outcomes in acute renal failure. Semin Nephrol 1998; 18:541–550.

34. Kleinknecht D: Epidemiology of Acute Renal Failure in France Today. In: Bihari D, Neild G, eds: Acute Renal Failure in the Intensive Therapy Unit. London: Springer-Verlag; 1990:13–22.

35. Liaño F: Fracaso renal agudo: revisión de 202 casos. Aspectos pronósticos. Nefrología 1984; 4:181–190.

36. Sánchez-Rodríguez L, Martin-Escobar E, Garía-Martín F, et al: Aspectos epidemiológicos del fracaso renal agudo en el área sanitaria de Cuenca. Nefrología 1992; 12(suppl 4):87–91.

37. Frost L, Pedersen RS, Ostgaard SE, et al: Short- and long-term outcome in a consecutive series of 419 patients with acute dialysis–requiring renal failure. Scand J Urol Nephrol 1993; 27:453–462.

38. Montseny JJ, Meyrier A, Kleinknecht D, et al: The current spectrum of infectious glomerulonephritis: experience with 76 patients and review of the literature. Medicine 1995; 74:63–73.

39. Kjellstrand CM, Ebben J, Davin T: Time of death, recovery of renal function, development of chronic renal failure and need for chronic hemodialysis in patients with acute renal failure. Trans Am Soc Artif Intern Organs 1981; 28:45–50.

40. Pasquali S, Casanova S, Zucchelli A, et al: Long-term survival in patients with acute and severe renal failure due to multiple myeloma. Clin Nephrol 1990: 34:247–254.

41. Lanore JJ, Brunet F, Pochard F, et al: Hemodialysis for acute renal failure in patients with hematologic malignancies. Crit Care Med 1991; 19:346–351.

42. Harris KPG, Hattersley JM, Feehally J, et al: Acute renal failure associated with haematological malignancies: a review of 10 years experience. Eur J Haematol 1991; 47:119–122.

43. Gruss E, Bernis C, Tomas JF, et al: Acute renal failure in patients following bone marrow transplantation: prevalence, risk factors, and outcome. Am J Nephrol 1995; 15:473–479.

44. Rao TKS: Acute renal failure syndrome in human immunodeficiency infection. Semin Nephrol 1998; 18:378–395.

45. Olsen TS: Renal failure after operation for abdominal aortic aneurysm in elderly patients. Geriatr Nephrol Urol 1993; 3:87–91.

46. Thadhani RI, Camargo CA, Xavier RJ, et al: Atheroembolic renal failure after invasive procedures. Medicine 1995; 74:350–358.

47. Scolari F, Bracchi M, Valzorio B, et al: Cholesterol atheromatous embolism: an increasing recognized cause of acute renal failure. Nephrol Dial Transplant 1996; 11:1607–1612.

48. Mayo RR, Swartz RD, Michigan AA: Redefining the incidence of clinically detectable atheroembolism. Am J Med 1996; 100:524–529.

49. Matsumae T, Takebayashi S, Naito S: The clinico-pathological characteristics and outcome in hemolytic-uremic syndrome of adults. Clin Nephrol 1996; 45:153–162.

50. Colon PJ, Howell DN, Macik G, et al: The renal manifestations and outcome of thrombotic thrombocytopenic purpura/hemolytic uremic syndrome in adults. Nephrol Dial Transplant 1995; 10:1189–1193.

51. Melnyk AM, Solez K, Kjellstrand CM: Adult hemolytic-uremic syndrome. Arch Intern Med 1995; 155:2077–2084.

52. Prakash J, Tripathi K, Pandey LK, et al: Spectrum of renal cortical necrosis in acute renal failure in eastern India. Postgrad Med J 1995; 71:208–210.

53. Ventura JE, Villa M, Mizraji R, et al: Acute renal failure in pregnancy. Ren Fail 1997; 19:217–220.

54. Alexopoulos E, Tambokoudis P, Bili H, et al: Acute renal failure in pregnancy. Ren Fail 1993; 15:609–613.

55. Naqvi R, Akhtar F, Ahmed E, et al: Acute renal failure of obstetrical origin during 1994 at one center. Ren Fail 1996; 18:681–683.

56. Leblanc M, Thibèault Y, Querin S: Continuous hemofiltration and hemodiafiltration for acute renal failure in severely burned patients. Burns 1997; 23:160–165.

57. Woodrow G, Brownjhon AM, Turney JH: The clinical and biochemical features of acute renal failure due to rhabdomyolysis. Ren Fail 1995; 17:467–474.

58. Frost L, Pedersen RS, Ostgaard SE, et al: Prognosis in acute pancreatitis complicated by acute renal failure requiring dialysis. Scand J Urol Nephrol 1990; 24:257–260.

59. Tran DD, Oe PL, de Fijter CWH, et al: Acute renal failure in patients with acute pancreatitis: prevalence, risk factors and outcome. Nephrol Dial Transplant 1993; 8:1079–1084.

60. Rayner BL, Willcox PA, Pascoe MD: Acute renal failure in community-acquired bacteremia. Nephron 1990; 54:32–35.

61. Conlon PJ, Procop GW, Fowler V, et al: Predictors of prognosis and risk of acute renal failure in patients with Rocky Mountain spotted fever. Am J Med 1996; 101:621–626.

62. Loghman-Adham M, Siegler RL, Pysher TJ: Acute renal failure in idiopathic nephrotic syndrome. Clin Nephrol 1997; 47:76–80.

63. Hylander B, Kjellstrand CM: Prognostic factors and treatment of severe ethylene glycol intoxication. Intensive Care Med 1996; 22:546–552.

64. Pérez-Fontán M, Rodríguez-Carmona A, Bouza P, et al: The prognostic significance of acute renal failure after renal transplantation in patients treated with cyclosporin. QJM 1998; 91:27–40.

65. Marcén R, Orofino L, Pascual J, et al: Delayed graft function does not reduce the survival of renal transplant allografts. Transplantation 1998; 66:461–466.

66. Liaño F, Pascual J: Acute Renal Failure: Causes and Prognosis. In: Berl T, Bonventre JV and Schrier RW, ed: Atlas of Diseases of the Kidney. Vol. 1. Philadelphia: Current Medicine; 1999; 8.1–8.16.

67. Rasmussen HH, Ibels LS: Acute renal failure: multivariate analysis of causes and risk factors. Am J Med 1982; 73:211–218.

68. Shusterman N, Strom BL, Murray TG, et al: Risk factors and outcome of hospital-acquired acute renal failure: a clinical epidemiologic study. Am J Med 1987; 83:65–71.

69. Menashe PI, Ross SA, Gottlier JE: Acquired renal insufficiency in critically ill patients. Crit Care Med 1988; 16:1106–1109.

70. Groeneveld ABJ, Tran DD, Van der Meulen J, et al: Acute renal failure in the medical intensive care unit: predisposing, complicating factors and outcome. Nephron 1991; 59:602–610.

71. Jochimsen F, Schäfer JH, Maurer A, et al: Impairment of renal function in medical intensive care: predictability of acute renal failure. Crit Care Med 1990; 18:480–485.

72. Kaufman J, Dahkal M, Patel B, et al: Community-acquired acute renal failure. Am J Kidney Dis 1991; 17:191–198.

73. Novis BK, Roizen MF, Aronson S, et al: Association of preoperative risk factors with postoperative acute renal failure. Anesth Analg 1994; 78:143–149.

74. Bonomini V, Stefani S, Vangelista A: Long-term and renal prognosis in acute renal failure. Nephron 1984; 36:169–172.

75. Spurney RF, Fulkerson WJ, Schwab SJ: Acute renal failure in critically ill patients: prognosis for recovery of kidney function after prolonged dialysis support. Crit Care Med 1991; 19:8–11.

76. Abdulkader R, Malheiro P, Daher E, et al: Late evaluation of glomerular filtration rate, proteinuria, and urinary acidification after acute tubular necrosis. Ren Fail 1992; 14:57–61.

77. Gopal I, Bhonagiri S, Ronco C, et al: Out of hospital outcome and quality of life in survivors of combined acute multiple organ and renal failure treated with continuous venovenous hemofiltration/hemodiafiltration. Intensive Care Med 1997; 23:766–772.

78. Kolff WJ: First clinical experience with artificial kidney. Ann Intern Med 1965; 62:608–619.

79. Kierdorf H, Sieberth HG: Continuous treatment modalities in acute renal failure. Nephrol Dial Transplant 1995; 10:2001–2008.

80. Turney JH: Why is mortality persistently high in acute renal failure? Lancet 1990; 335:971.

81. Routh GS, Briggs JD, Mone JG, et al: Survival from acute renal failure with and without multiple organ dysfunction. Postgrad Med J 1980; 56:244–247.

82. McCarthy JT: Prognosis of patients with acute renal failure in the intensive-care unit: a tale of two eras. Mayo Clin Proc 1996; 71:117–126.

83. Pascual J, Liaño F, Ortuño J: The elderly patient with acute renal failure. J Am Soc Nephrol 1995; 6:144–153.

84. Epstein M: Aging and the kidney. J Am Soc Nephrol 1996; 7:1106–1122.

85. Macias-Nuñez JF, López-Novoa JM, Martínez-Maldonado JM: Acute renal failure in the aged. Semin Nephrol 1996; 16:330–338.

86. Balslov JT, Jorgensen HE: A survey of 499 patients with acute anuric renal insufficiency. Am J Med 1963; 34:753–764.

87. Cioffi WG, Ashikaga T, Gamelli RL: Probability of surviving postoperative acute renal failure: development of a prognostic index. Ann Surg 1984; 200:205–211.

88. Bullock ML, Umen AJ, Finkelstein M, et al: The assessment of risk factors in 462 patients with acute renal failure. Am J Kidney Dis 1985; 5:97–102.

89. Lien J, Chan V: Risk factors influencing survival in acute renal failure treated by hemodialysis. Arch Intern Med 1985; 145:2067–2069.

90. Cantarovich F, Verho MT: A simple prognostic index for patients with acute renal failure requiring dialysis. Ren Fail 1996; 18:585–592.

91. Lins R (personal communication).

92. Barton IK, Hilton PJ, Taub NA, et al: Acute renal failure treated by hemofiltration: factors affecting outcome. QJM 1993; 86:81–90.

93. Lange HW, Aeppli DM, Brown DC: Survival of patients with acute renal failure requiring dialysis after open heart surgery: early prognostic indicators. Am Heart J 1987; 113:1138–1143.

94. Hou SH, Bushinsky DA, Wish JB, et al: Hospital-acquired renal insufficiency: a prospective study. Am J Med 1983; 74:243–248.

95. Lohr JW, McFarlane MJ, Grantham JJ: A clinical index to predict survival in acute renal failure patients requiring dialysis. Am J Kidney Dis 1988; 11:254–259.

96. Schaefer JH, Jochimsen F, Keller F, et al: Outcome prediction of acute renal failure in medical intensive care. Intensive Care Med 1991; 17:19–24.

97. Gentric A, Cledes J: Immediate and long-term prognosis in acute renal failure in the elderly. Nephrol Dial Transplant 1991; 6:86–90.

98. Pascual J, Liaño F, and the Madrid Acute Renal Failure Study Group: Causes and prognosis of acute renal afilure in the very old. J Am Geriatr Soc 1998; 46:721–725.

99. Chertow GM, Lazarus JM, Paganini EP, et al: Predictors of mortality and the provision of dialysis in patients with acute tubular necrosis. J Am Soc Nephrol 1998; 9:692–698.

100. Knaus WA, Draper EA, Wagner DP, et al: APACHE II: a severity of disease classification system. Crit Care Med 1985; 13:818–829.

101. Knaus WA, Wagner DP, Draper EA, et al: The APACHE III prognostic system: risk prediction of hospital mortality for critically ill hospitalized adults. Chest 1991; 100:1619–1636.

102. Le Gall JR, Loirat P, Alperovitch A, et al: A simplified acute physiology score for ICU patients. Crit Care Med 1984; 12:975–977.

103. Le Gall JR, Lemeshow S, Saulnier F: A new Simplified Acute Physiology Score (SAPS II) based on a European/North American multicenter study. JAMA 1993; 270:2957–2963.

104. Lemeshow S, Teres D, Pastides H, et al: A method for predicting survival and mortality of ICU patients using objectively derived weights. Crit Care Med 1985; 13:519–525.

105. Lemeshow S, Teres D, Klar J, et al: Mortality probability models (MPM II) based on an international cohort of intensive care unit patients. JAMA 1993; 270:2478–2486.

106. Douma CE, Redekop WK, Van Der Meulen JHP, et al: Predicting mortality in intensive care patients with acute renal failure treated with dialysis. J Am Soc Nephrol 1997; 8:111–117.

107. Stott RB, Cameron JS, Ogg CS, et al: Why the persistently high mortality in acute renal failure? Lancet 1972; 1:75–78.

108. Woodrow G, Turney JH: Cause of death in acute renal failure. Nephrol Dial Transplant 1992; 7:230–234.

109. Weisberg LS, Allgren RL, Genter FC, et al: Cause of acute tubular necrosis affects its prognosis. Arch Intern Med 1997; 157:1833–1838.

110. Druml W: Prognosis of acute renal failure 1975–1995. Nephron 1996; 73:8–15.

111. van Bommel EFH, Bouvy ND, So KL, et al: High-risk surgical acute renal failure treated by continuous arteriovenous hemodiafiltration: metabolic control and outcome in sixty patients. Nephron 1995; 70:185–192.

112. Chertow GM, Lazarus JM, Christiansen CL, et al: Preoperative renal risk stratification. Circulation 1997; 95:878–884.

113. Cameron JS: Acute renal failure: the continuing challange. QJM 1986; 59:337–343.

114. Kraman S, Khan F, Patel S, et al: Renal failure in the respiratory intensive care unit. Crit Care Med 1979; 7:263–266.

115. Jalil R, Downey P, Jara A, et al: Insuficiencia renal aguda en adultos mayores: evaluación de factores pronósticos. Nefrología 1995; 15:343–348.

116. Sánchez JA, Martín J, Macias JF, et al: Shock séptico y fracaso renal agudo: análisis de los factores que intervienen en su evolución. Nefrología 1984; 4:197–203.

117. Abreo K, Moorthy V, Osborne M: Changing patterns and outcome of acute renal failure patients requiring dialysis. Arch Intern Med 1986; 146:1338–1341.

118. Beaman M, Turney JH, Rodger RSC, et al: Changing pattern of acute renal failure. QJM 1987; 62:15–23.

119. Rialp G, Roglan A, Betbesé AJ, et al: Prognostic indexes and mortality in critically ill patients with acute renal failure treated with different dialytic techniques. Ren Fail 1996; 18:667–675.

120. Chew SL, Lins RL, Daelemans R, et al: Outcome in acute renal failure. Nephrol Dial Transplant 1993; 8:101–107.

121. Yuasa S, Takahashi N, Shoji T, et al: A simple and early prognostic index for acute renal failure patients requiring renal replacement therapy. Artif Ogans 1998; 22:273–278.

122. Kleinknecht D, Landais P, Brivet F, et al: Prognosis and mortality in patients with multiple organ system failure. Ren Fail 1996; 18:347–353.

123. Mehta R, Farkas A, Pascual M, et al: Effect of delayed consultation on outcome from acute renal failure in the ICU. J Am Soc Nephrol 1995; 6:471–474.

124. Chertow GM, Sayegh MH, Allgren RL, et al: Is the administration of dopamine associated with adverse or favorable outcomes in acute renal failure? Am J Med 1996; 101:49–53.

125. Allgren RL, Marbury TC, Rhaman SN, et al: Anaritide in acute tubular necrosis. N Engl J Med 1997; 336:828–834.

126. Hirschberg R, Kopple J, Lipsett P, et al: Multicenter clinical trial of recombinant human insulin-like growth factor I in patients with acute renal failure. Kidney Int 1999; 55:2423–2432.

127. Himmelfarb J, Rubin NT, Chandran P, et al: A multicenter

comparison of dialysis membranes in the treatment of acute renal failure requiring dialysis. J Am Soc Nephrol 1998; 9:257–266.

128. Kjellstrand C: Acute Renal Failure in the 21st Century. In: Cantarovich F, Rangoonwala B, Verho M, eds: Progress in Acute Renal Failure 1998. Bridgewater, NJ: Hoechst Marion Roussel; 1998:329–340.

129. Levy EM, Viscoli CM, Horwitz RI: The effect of acute renal failure on mortality: a cohort analysis. JAMA 1996; 275:1489–1494.

130. Vincent JL, de MendonCa A, Cantraine F, et al: Use of the SOFA score to assess the incidence of organ dysfunction/failure in intensive care units: results of a multicenter, prospective study. Crit Care Med 1998; 26:1793–1800.

131. Liaño F: Severity of acute renal failure: the need of measurement. 1994; 9(suppl 4):229–238.

132. Randolph AG, Guyatt GH, Richardson WS: Prognosis in the intensive care unit: finding accurate and useful estimates for counseling patients. Crit Care Med 1998; 26:767–772.

133. Knaus WA, Zimmerman JE, Wagner DP, et al: APACHE—acute physiology and chronic health evaluation: a physiologically based classification system. Crit Care Med 1981; 9:591–597.

134. Castella X, Gilabert J, Torner F, et al: Mortality prediction models in intensive care: acute physiology and chronic health evaluation and mortality prediction model compared. Crit Care Med 1991; 19:191–197.

135. Beck DH, Taylor BL, Millar B, et al: Prediction of outcome from intensive care: a prospective cohort study comparing Acute Physiology and Chronic Health Evaluation II and III prognostic systems in a United Kingdom intensive care unit. Crit Care Med 1997; 25:9–15.

136. Moreau R, Soupison T, Vauquelin P, et al: Comparison of two simplified severity scores (SAPS and APACHE II) for patients with acute myocardial infarction. Crit Care Med 1989; 17:409–412.

137. Féry-Lemonner E, Landais P, Kleinknecht D, et al: Evaluation of severity scoring systems in ICUs—translation, conversion, and definition ambiguities as a source of inter-observer variability in APACHE II, SAPS, and OSF. Intensive Care Med 1995; 21:356–360.

138. Knaus WA, Draper EA, Wagner DP, et al: Prognosis in acute organ-system failure. Ann Surg 1985; 202:685–693.

139. Marshall JC, Cook DJ, Christou NV, et al: Multiple organ dysfunction score: a reliable descriptor of a complex clinical outcome. Crit Care Med 1995; 23:1638–1652.

140. Le Gall JR, Lemeshow S, Saulnier F, et al: The logistic organ dysfunction system: a new way to assess organ dysfunction in the intensive care unit. JAMA 1996; 276:802–810.

141. The SOFA (sepsis-related organ failure assessment) score to describe organ dysfunction/failure. Intensive Care Med 1996; 22:707–719.

142. Gainza FJ, Maynar J, Crral E, et al: Estudio prospectivo y multicéntrico del fracaso renal agudo con necesidad de tratamiento sustitutivo en pacientes críticos. Nefrología 1998; 18(suppl 3):25.

143. Paganini EP, Halstenberg WK, Goormastic M: Risk modeling in acute renal failure requiring dialysis: the introduction of a new model. Clin Nephrol 1996; 46:206–211.

144. Lombardi R, Zampedri L, Rodriguez I, et al: Prognosis in acute renal failure of septic origin: a multivariate analysis. Ren Fail 1998; 20:725–732.

145. Liaño F, García-Martin F, Gallego A, et al: Easy and early prognosis in acute tubular necrosis: a forward analysis of 228 cases. Nephron 1989; 51:307–313.

146. Halstenberg WK, Goormastic M, Paganini EP: Validity of four models for predicting outcome in critical ill acute renal failure patients. Clin Nephrol 1997; 47:81–86.

147. Radovic M, Ostric V, Djukanovic LI: Validity of prediction scores in acute renal failure due to polytrauma. Ren Fail 1996; 18:615–620.

148. Foni LG, Wright DA, Hilton PJ, et al: Prognostic stratification in acute renal failure. Arch Intern Med 1996; 156:1023–1027.

149. Liaño F, Solez K, Eliahou H, et al: Acute Renal Failure Scoring. In: Ronco C, Bellomo R, eds: Critical Care Nephrology. Dordrecht: Kluwer Academic Publisher; 1998:1535–1545.

150. Bellomo R, Mansfield D, Rumble S, et al: A comparison of conventional dialytic therapy and acute continuous hemodiafiltration in the management of acute renal failure in the critically ill. Ren Fail 1993; 15:595–602.

151. Schiffl H, Lang SM, Strasser T, et al: Biocompatible membranes in acute renal failure: prospective case-controlled study. Lancet 1994; 344:570–572.

152. Van Bommel E, Bouvy ND, So KL, et al: Acute dialytic support for the critically ill: intermittent hemodialysis versus continuous arteriovenous hemodiafiltration. Am J Nephrol 1995; 15:192–200.

153. Verde E, Ruiz F, Vozmediano MC, et al: Valor predictivo del APACHE II en el fracaso renal agudo de las unidades de cuidados intensivos. Nefrología 1996; 19:32.

154. Consentino F, Chaff C, Piedmonte M: The risk of dying with acute renal failure requiring dialysis in the intensive care unit: a multivariate analysis. J Am Soc Nephrol 1993; 4:314.

155. Cullen DJ, Chernow B: Predicting outcome in critically ill patients. Crit Care Med 1996; 22:1345–1348.

156. Braitman LE, Davidoff F: Predicting clinical status in individual patients. Ann Intern Med 1996; 125:406–412.

Index

Note: Page numbers followed by the letter f refer to figures; those followed by the letter t refer to tables.

Antibody–mediated vasculitis, direct, 280–285
Anticoagulation therapy, for atheroembolic disease, 257
Antidiuretic hormone, renal circulatory effects of, 14t
Antifungal agents, nephrotoxicity of, 355–356, 355t
Antiglomerular basement membrane glomerulonephritis, 280–282
  after renal transplantation, 332t
  clinical features of, 281
  pathogenesis of, 280–281
  treatment of, 281–282
Antihypertensive drugs, prerenal ARF and, 158, 159f
Antimetabolites, nephrotoxicity of, 367t, 370–371
Antimony, 416
Antimyeloperoxidase (anti-MPO) antibodies, 281
Antineoplastic agents
  ARF associated with, 365–373
  nephrotoxicity of, 365–373
    factors augmenting, 365–366
Antineutrophil cytoplasmic autoantibody (ANCA)–small vessel vasculitis, 276t, 280–285
Antinuclear antibodies, in lupus, 276–277, 277t
Antioxidant agents, for radiocontrast nephropathy, 379–380
Antithymocyte globulin (ATG)
  in cardiac transplantation, 337
  in renal transplantation
    for ischemic tubular necrosis, 325
    for rejection, 328, 329
Antitumor antibiotics, nephrotoxicity of, 367t, 371
Antiviral agents, nephrotoxicity of, 356–358, 357t
Anuria, renal artery embolism and, 258
APACHE II, 511, 513
APACHE III, 511, 512, 513, 514, 514f
Apical brush border, of tubular cells
  animal model of, 7–8
  injury to, 2, 2f, 101, 102f
  urinary markers of, 164
Apical microvillous alterations, 120, 121f
Apoptosis, 35–54
  antagonists of, 48–52
  biochemical pathways leading to, 31
  caspases and, 42–47, 43f, 44t
  causes of, 35–36
  cell biology of, 35–45
  cell injury and, 36
  cellular events associated with, 36–42, 37f
  condensation and fragmentation of nuclear chromatin in, 39
  deficiency of "survival factors" in, 35–36
  DNA damage and, 36
  DNA fragmentation and, 37–38, 38f
  end-labeling assays of, 38–39
  endonuclease activation and, 37–38, 38f
  Fas and related cell-surface death receptors in, 46–47
  heme oxygenase-1, 82–83
  in ARF in vivo, 52–53
    causes of, 53–54
    DNA damage and, 53
    ischemic and cytotoxic tubular cell injury and, 53
    receptor-mediated, 53–54
    survival factors and, 53
  in recovery from ARF, 443–445
  in renal proximal tubules, 101, 102f
  in transplant kidney, 9
  inducers of, 42–48, 50–52, 50t
  inhibition of, 54
    caspase inhibitors and, 54
  loss of nuclear envelope in, 39
  mediators of, 42–48
  mitochondrial changes in, 40–42

Apoptosis (Continued)
  mitochondrial dysfunction in, 31
  mitochondrial transmembrane potential loss in, 41–42
  molecular biology of, 42–53
  morphologic characteristics of, 30–31, 30t
  necrosis vs., 30–31, 30t
  nuclear changes in, 37–39, 38f
  of tubular cells, 3–5, 4f, 8
  phagocytic clearance of cells in, 42–54
  plasma membrane changes in, 39–40
  programmed cell death and, 35
  receptor-mediated, 35
  regulators of, 42–48
  survival pathways in, 48–50
  trigger of, 37, 37f
Apoptosis-inducing factor (AIF), 41
Apoptosis protease-activating factor 1 (Apaf-1), 41
Apoptosis signal-regulating kinase 1 (ASK-1), 52
Arachidonic acid
  in multiple organ system failure, 493t
  Na+,K+-ATPase and, 34
ARF. See Renal failure, acute (ARF).
Aristolochia fangchi, 386, 387f, 388
Aristolochia manshuriensis Kom (AMK), 386, 387f
Arp2/3 complex, 123, 124
Arsenic, nephrotoxicity of, 415
Arsine, nephrotoxicity of, 415
Arteriography, of renal artery embolism, 258, 259f
Aspirin, 410
ATF-2, 111
ATF-3, 111
Atheroembolic disease, 255–257
  clinical presentation of, 256
  differential diagnosis of, 257
  laboratory findings in, 256–257
  pathology of, 256, 256f
  predisposing factors for, 255–256
  treatment of, 257
Atherosclerotic ischemic renal disease, 261
Atractylis gummifera-L, 420
Atractyloside
  in apoptosis, 41
  nephrotoxicity from, 420
Atrial natriuretic peptide (ANP)
  for ARF, 432–433
  for radiocontrast nephropathy, 379
  renal circulatory effects of, 14t
Autoantibodies, in pauci-immune small vessel vasculitis, 283
Autoimmune hemolytic anemia, hemoglobinuria and, 216
5-Azacitidine, nephrotoxicity of, 367t, 371
Azathioprine
  for Goodpasture's disease, 281
  for lupus nephritis, 277
  for pauci-immune small vessel vasculitis, 283
  for renal disease, in pregnancy, 309
Azithromycin, nephrotoxicity of, 353
Azoles, nephrotoxicity of, 355t, 356
Azotemia, prerenal, from malignancies, 315–316

B

Bacitracin, nephrotoxicity of, 350t, 354
Bacteremia
  ARF from, 294–295
  rhabdomyolysis and, 222, 222t
Bacterial infections, ARF from, 292–296, 292t
Bacteriuria, in pregnancy, 305
BAPTA-AM, 138
Basal vascular tone, renal, 14–15
Bax subfamily, in apoptosis, 48, 50–52, 50t

Bcl-2 family, in apoptosis, 45t, 50–52, 50t, 444–445
Bcl-xL, in apoptosis, 50–51, 50t
Bee venom, 383t, 385, 419
Bence Jones protein
  acidosis and, 178
  myeloma and, 317
Benzene, hemoglobinuria from, 216
Beta-actin, 45, 45t, 148
Beta2-adrenergic agonists, for hyperkalemia, 176
Beta-adrenergic blockers, NSAID interaction with, 411
Beta-catenin, 45, 45t, 136f, 136t, 138–139, 139f
Beta2-glycoprotein 1, in apoptosis, 39
Beta1 integrin, tubular cell injury and, 7
Beta-lactams, nephrotoxicity of, 350t, 352, 352t
Beta2 microglobulin, urinary excretion of, 164, 164f
BH3 subfamily, in apoptosis, 50–52, 50t
BHRF1, in apoptosis, 50t
Bilirubin, heme oxygenase-1 and, 85
Biliverdin, 214
Biologic nephrotoxins, 367t, 371, 383–388, 383t
BiP, 146
Bismuth, 416
BK virus infection, in renal transplantation, 335
Black Creek Canal virus, 298
Black widow spider venom, 385
  rhabdomyolysis from, 224
Blackwater fever, hemoglobinuria from, 217
Bladder examination, in ARF diagnosis, 161
Bladder outlet obstruction
  from amphetamines, 398
  from malignancies, 312
Bleeding disorders
  dialysis for, 182
  in ARF, 181–183
  nondialytic treatment of, 182–183, 183t
Blood urea nitrogen (BUN), in ARF
  concentration of, 157–158, 158f, 346–347
  phases of, 425
  recovery from, 427, 510
BN 52021, 326
Bone marrow transplantation (BMT), 344–347
  ARF in, 344–347, 372
    detection of, 346–347
    epidemiology of, 344
    occurrence of, 344
    pathogenesis of, 344–346, 346t
    prevention of, 346
    treatment of, 347
  hemoglobinuria and, 217
  nephropathy from, 372–373
Bone morphogenic protein-7 (BMP-7), 104, 108
Brain-derived neutrophilic factor (BDNF), 110
BUN/creatine (SCr) ratio, in ARF, 157–158, 158f
Burn patients, 247–253
  ARF in, 249–250
    dialysis for, 252–253, 252t
    fluid therapy for, 251
    management of, 251–253
    nutritional support for, 251
    pathogenesis of, 250–251, 250f
    sepsis and, 251
    wound management in, 251
  circulating and local mediators in, 247–248
  complications of, 248
  electrical, 248
  electrolyte abnormalities and, 249
  glomerular filtration rate in, 248–249
  hematuria in, 249
  hemoglobinuria in, 217
  hemolytic-uremic syndrome in, 249
  hormonal changes in, 248
  immunologic response in, 248
  inhalation injury and, 248
  pathophysiology of, 247–249, 247f

Extracellular signal-regulated kinase (ERK) cascade *(Continued)*
in apoptosis, 49
Eye examination, in ARF diagnosis, 161
Ezrin, 124, 136t

F

F-actin, 120, 121f, 124–125, 126f
FADD-like ICE inhibitory protein (FLIP), 46
Famciclovir, nephrotoxicity of, 357–358, 357t
Fas, apoptosis and, 46, 47
Fas-associated death domain protein (FADD), 46, 47, 48
Fat emulsions, in nutritional support, 469, 477, 477f
Fatty acids, oxidation of, in ARF, 469
Fatty liver of pregnancy, acute, 306
Fibrinolytic therapy, for renal artery embolism, 259
  contraindications to, 261
Fibroblast growth factor(s), 104, 109
  in renal injury and repair, 105t, 107t, 109–110
  receptor of, 109–110
  types 1–17, 109
Fibronectin-EIIIA (FN-EIIIA), 108
FK506, in transplantation
  apoptosis and, 9–10
  inflammation and, 95
Flk1, 111
FLT1, 111
FLT4, 111
Fluid disorders, from nonsteroidal anti-inflammatory drugs, 410
Fluid restriction
  for hyponatremia, 173
  for volume overload, 170
Fluid therapy. *See* Volume replenishment.
Fluorescein, hemoglobinuria from, 216
Fluoroquinolones, nephrotoxicity of, 350t, 353
5-Fluorouracil, nephrotoxicity of, 367t, 370–371
Focal adhesion kinase (FAK), 45, 45t
Fodrin, 45t
Folic acid, CRRT and, 471
Follicle-stimulating hormone (FSH), levels of, in ARF, 184
Fomepizole, 417
Fong's disease, abdominal radiography of, 193
Foscarnet, nephrotoxicity of, 356–357, 357t
Four Corners virus, 298
Functional renal failure, 265. *See also* Hepatorenal syndrome (HRS).
Functional residual defects, from ARF, 427–428, 428f
Fungal infections, renal diseases from, 292
Furosemide
  adverse effects of, 170–171
  for ARF, 431
  for volume overload, 170–171, 171t

G

G protein(s)
  heterotrimeric, 134t
  tight junction regulation and, 138
G-actin, 120, 124, 125
GADD153, 150
GADD45α (β;γ), in apoptosis, 48
Gallium nitrate, nephrotoxicity of, 367t, 371
Gamma radiation, apoptosis and, 36
Gamma-catenin, 136t
Gamma-glutamyl transpeptidase (GGTP), tubular cell injury and, 2

Ganciclovir, nephrotoxicity of, 357–358, 357t
Gas2, 45t
Gastrointestinal bleeding, in ARF, 158, 159f, 169t
  management of, 182–183
Gastrointestinal tract, dysfunction of
  in multiple organ system failure, 491t, 493
  nutritional support for patients with ARF and, 473
Gated blood-pool scan, in ARF diagnosis, 165
Gelatin, nephropathy from, 394
Gelsolin, 45t
Gentamicin, nephrotoxicity of, 65–67, 65t
  anemia and, 181
  heme oxygenase-1 and, 83
  mononuclear cells in, 452t
  reactive nitrogen species and, 66–67
  reactive oxygen species and, 65–66, 66f
Glasgow Coma Scale, 493
Glial cell line–derived neurotrophic factor (GDNF), 104, 108
Glomerular basement membrane, lysis of, in ischemic injury, 20–21
Glomerular capillaries, 13, 14f
Glomerular capillary pressure, 16, 17f
Glomerular diseases, from malignancies, 318–319
Glomerular filtration, 13–14, 14f
Glomerular filtration rate (GFR)
  decline in, 13–14
    volume overload from, 169–170
  endothelin and, 232
  in burn patients, 248–249
  in hepatorenal syndrome, 268
  in mannitol nephropathy, 392–393
  in multiple organ system failure, 492
  in phases of ARF, 425–427
  in pyelonephritis in pregnancy, 305
  in radiocontrast nephropathy, 376, 377f
  in recovery from ARF, 427
  in sepsis, 295
  in tubular injury, 3, 119
  nonsteroidal anti-inflammatory drugs and, 406, 408, 410
  radionuclide measurement of, 200
  serum creatine (S_{Cr}) concentration and, 157
  vasoactive agent effect on, 14t
Glomeruli, in ARF, 6, 7f
Glomerulonephritis
  after renal transplantation, 332t
    de novo, 331
  antiglomerular basement membrane, 280–282
  from malaria, 298–299
  imaging of, 193, 193f
  in pregnancy, 308
  lupus, 276
  membranoproliferative, 318
  necrotizing, in pauci-immune small vessel vasculitis, 282–283
  postinfectious, 293
  prerenal ARF vs., 164
Glomerulosclerosis, focal segmental, recurring after renal transplantation, 331–332, 331f
Gloriosa superba, 419
Glucagon
  in ARF, 184
  in burn patients, 248
  renal circulatory effects of, 14t
    renal circulatory effects of, 14t
Gluconeogenesis, in patients with ARF, 468
Glucose
  for hyperkalemia, 176, 177t
  hyponatremia and, 173
  in parenteral nutrition, 476–477
  intolerance of, in ARF, 184
  metabolism of, CRRT and, 472
Glucose-6-phosphate dehydrogenase (G6PD)
  deficiency, hemoglobinuria and, 216, 217, 218

Glue sniffing, 401
Glutamic-oxaloacetic transaminase, in ARF, 162
Glutamine
  for burn patients, 251
  in parenteral nutrition, 478t, 479
Glutathione
  ischemia-reperfusion injury and, 62
  myoglobinuric ARF and, 68
Glutathione peroxidase deficiency
  ARF and, 471
  hemoglobinuria and, 217
Glutathione reductase deficiency, hemoglobinuria and, 217
Glycerol
  hypertonic, hemoglobinuria from, 216
  nephropathy from, 394
Glycerol model, of acute renal failure, 78, 79–80, 81
Glycogen synthetase kinase-3 (GSK-3), 138–139
Glycosuria, 220
Gold, 416
Gonadotropin–releasing hormone (GnRH), in ARF, 184
Goodpasture's disease, 280–282
  clinical features of, 281
  treatment of, 281–282
G-protein–coupled receptors (GPCR), in apoptosis, 49
Granzyme B, 44
Griseofulvin, nephrotoxicity of, 355t, 356
GroEL, 144
Growth factors
  in renal injury and repair, 101–112, 128, 439–440
    mitogen-activated protein kinase cascade and, 111–112, 112f
    role of specific factors in, 104–111, 105t, 106t, 107t, 440–441, 440t. *See also specific factors.*
  renal, 103–104
    development and, 103–104
    urinary excretion of, 164, 164f
Growth hormone, recombinant, for catabolism in patients with ARF, 468
Grp-78, 148, 151, 153
Grp-94, 146, 148, 153
GTPase-binding proteins, 126–127, 127f
Guanine nucleotide exchange factors (GEFs), 126, 127f
Guanmutong, 386
Guanosine nucleotide dissociation inhibitor, 126, 127f
Guanosine nucleotide exchange factors (GEFs), 126, 127f
Guanosine triphosphatases (GTPases), Rho, 135
  actin and, 126–128, 127f
  and junction regulation, 135, 137, 138
Guanosine triphosphate activating protein, 126, 127f

H

Haff disease, 223
Halogenated hydrocarbons, 416
Hantavirus infections, 297–298
Hantavirus pulmonary syndrome, 298
Haptoglobin, 214
  for burn patients, 252
Heart disease. *See* Cardiovascular disease.
Heart failure
  ARF and, 261
  congestive, in mannitol nephropathy, 393
  volume overload and, 169, 170f
Heart surgery, open, ARF after, 262
  prophylaxis for, 262

ISBN 0-7216-9174-9